DISCARD

GROVE CITY HIGH SCHOOL
LIBRARY, 4665 HOOVER ROAD,
GROVE CITY, OHIO 43123
614-801-3330

MW00589654

Salem Health

Community & Family Health Issues

An Encyclopedia of Trends,
Conditions & Treatments

Salem Health

Community & Family Health Issues

An Encyclopedia of Trends, Conditions & Treatments

Volume 3
N-W
Appendixes

Editors
Amber Bruggman, LCSW
Kimberly Ortiz-Hartman, PsyD, LMFT

SALEM PRESS

A Division of EBSCO Information Services, Inc.
Ipswich, Massachusetts

GREY HOUSE PUBLISHING

Salem $395.00 Sept. 2019

Copyright © 2017, by Salem Press, A Division of EBSCO Information Services, Inc., and Grey House Publishing, Inc.

All rights in this book are reserved. No part of this work may be used or reproduced in any manner whatsoever or transmitted in any form or by any means, electronic or mechanical, including photocopy, recording, or any information storage and retrieval system, without written permission from the copyright owner. For permissions requests, contact proprietarypublishing@ebsco.com.

∞ The paper used in these volumes conforms to the American National Standard for Permanence of Paper for Printed Library Materials, Z39.48–1992 (R2009).

Publisher's Cataloging-In-Publication Data
(Prepared by The Donohue Group, Inc.)

Names: Bruggman, Amber, editor. | Ortiz-Hartman, Kimberly, editor.
Title: Community & family health issues : an encyclopedia of trends, conditions & treatments / editors, Amber Bruggman, LCSW, Kimberly Ortiz-Hartman, PsyD LMFT.
Other Titles: Community and family health issues | Salem health | Salem health (Pasadena, Calif.)
Description: [First edition]. | Ipswich, Massachusetts : Salem Press, a division of EBSCO Information Services, Inc. ; [Amenia, New York] : Grey House Publishing, [2017] | Includes bibliographical references and index. | Contents: Volume 1. Abandoned Children-Divorce: Psychosocial Effects on Women -- Volume 2. Education, Social Work: Cultural Competence-Music Therapy and Stroke Rehabilitation -- Volume 3. Narcissistic Personality Disorder-Workplace Violence: Sexual Harassment.
Identifiers: ISBN 978-1-68217-337-4 (set) | ISBN 978-1-68217-339-8 (v.1) | ISBN 978-1-68217-340-4 (v.2) | ISBN 978-1-68217-640-5 (v.3)
Subjects: LCSH: Families--Health and hygiene--Encyclopedias. | Health--Encyclopedias. | Family medicine--Encyclopedias. | Public health--Encyclopedias. | Community health services--Encyclopedias.
Classification: LCC RA418.5.F3 C66 2017 | DDC 613--dc23

CONTENTS

N

NARCISSISTIC PERSONALITY DISORDER

MAJOR CATEGORIES: Behavioral & Mental Health, Medical & Health

DESCRIPTION

Narcissistic personality disorder (NPD) is one of 10 diagnosable personality disorders that appear in the *Diagnostic and Statistical Manual of Mental Disorders, 5th Edition* (*DSM-5*), all of which are retained from the fourth edition of the manual. NPD is grouped with antisocial personality disorder, borderline personality disorder, and histrionic personality disorder to form the cluster B personality disorders, which share the features of extreme affect, theatricality, and unpredictability. The general criteria for NPD are an exaggerated and unrealistic sense of superiority, a need for admiration, and an inability to understand the feelings of others, starting by early adulthood and present in different areas of functioning.

To diagnose NPD, at least five of the nine specific following criteria must be met: inflated and unjustified self-regard, with expectations that others will concur; an inordinate focus on having success, power, and unrealistic relationships; belief that one is superior and can only be understood by people or institutions with the same superior standing; a constant demand for attention and extreme praise; belief that one deserves special treatment above and beyond others, and that others should unquestioningly carry out any request; an exploitative view of relationships; failure to acknowledge or understand the feelings or needs of others; belief that others are envious, or being envious of others; and exhibiting arrogance in interpersonal interactions. The grandiosity and beliefs of a person with NPD may manifest as either fantasy or actual behavior. Furthermore, such fantasies and beliefs are different from the bizarre delusions associated with psychotic disorders in that the fantasies and beliefs are possible, in principle, no matter how embellished or distorted.

Although they are not included in the *DSM-5*, there are two subtypes of NPD recognized in the clinical setting: grandiose, or overt, and vulnerable, or covert. Individuals with the grandiose subtype of NPD tend more toward overt displays of self-importance, entitlement, fantasies of admiration, denial of weakness, and exploitative behavior, whereas those with the vulnerable subtype tend more toward hypersensitivity to insult; self-criticism; feelings of shame, helplessness, or inadequacy; and social withdrawal. It is theorized that the subtypes develop because of the different approaches of earlier caregiver(s): overly indulgent with extravagant praise versus cold with excessive expectations. Both approaches adversely affect attachment and development of healthy self-esteem..

It is important to note that even though the *DSM-5* retained the *DSM-IV* criteria for personality disorders, the *DSM-5* Section III (which includes potential models for future research) presents an alternative model in which personality disorders are characterized by impairments in personality functioning and pathological personality traits. The proposed diagnostic criteria for NPD in Section III of the *DSM-5* include significant impairments in personality functioning manifested in self functioning in four areas: identity, self-direction, empathy, and relationships. Furthermore, criteria for diagnosis of NPD in Section III of the *DSM-5* includes antagonism (i.e., active hostility) characterized by grandiosity (e.g., feeling above others, being condescending) and attention-seeking (e.g., trying an inordinate amount to get the attention of others). Researchers believe that the alternative model provided in Section III of the *DSM-5* represents a significant improvement in diagnostic criteria in comparison with the traditional model in Section II of the *DSM-5 and* that it is much more clinically useful (Ronningstam, 2014; Skodol et al., 2014).

The etiology of NPD is unresolved, with most literature attributing it to an interaction of genetically inherited traits and environmental influences, particularly the impact of early parenting on the ability to self-regulate emotions and other internal controls.

FACTS AND FIGURES

The *DSM-5* reports prevalence rates of NPD in community samples in the United States ranging from 0% to 6.2%, with 50% to 75% of individuals with NPD being male (American Psychiatric Association, 2013). Investigators performing analysis of the Wave 2 National Epidemiologic Survey on Alcohol and Related Conditions (Stinson et al., 2008) found rates of NPD among respondents with bipolar I disorder to be 31.1%; among those with panic disorder with agoraphobia, 23.9%; and among those with drug dependence, 34.9%. Other findings included greater rates of NPD among individuals who were separated, divorced, or widowed, and an inverse relationship between NPD and age, with the greatest decline after age 29 (Stinson et al., 2008). Unfortunately, there is a paucity of further NPD statistics.

RISK FACTORS

Risk factors include lack of parental empathy during early development or otherwise disrupted development of self-regulation skills. Some studies have found higher rates of NPD among children of individuals with NPD, but there is no conclusive evidence that genetic or environmental factors are the cause.

SIGNS AND SYMPTOMS

Signs and symptoms include grandiosity, fantasies of unlimited power and success, a need for admiration and to be associated with high-standing individuals or institutions, lack of empathy, exploitation of others, sense of entitlement, insecurity, feelings of being a fraud, excessive envy, and displays of arrogance. Individuals with NPD may appear to have fragile self-esteem, be hypersensitive to criticism, have high levels of achievement, have strong feelings of humiliation or shame, and possess a need to be the object of attention. They may appear manipulative, indifferent, inadequate, lonely, self-centered, and self-absorbed.

ASSESSMENT

Standard biopsychosocial-spiritual assessment, including risk for suicide. Individuals with NPD are more likely than others to present themselves in a favorable way and to omit or avoid unfavorable feelings or experiences.

Assessment for risk factors, including coexisting mental health conditions.

Observation of functioning and demeanor during interview.

Collateral information from family, friends, and coworkers is especially important because individuals with NPD frequently have limited insight into their own symptoms.

ASSESSMENTS AND SCREENING TOOLS

Care should be used with self-reporting screening tools due to the client's general lack of insight. Not all of the tools listed are specific to NPD but are used for general measurements of personality dysfunction.

Personality Inventory for DSM-5 (PID-5), a 220-item self-report designed to assess 25 personality traits.

Five-Factor Narcissism Inventory (FFNI), a 148-item self-report of 15 traits related to vulnerable and grandiose narcissism.

Pathological Narcissism Inventory (PNI), a 52-item self-report measuring traits related to vulnerable and grandiose narcissism.

Narcissistic Personality Inventory (NPI), a 40-item forced-choice self-report measure of grandiose narcissism.

TREATMENT

Researchers have found that NPD clients are at the highest risk of dropping out of psychotherapy compared to clients with other personality disorders (Ellison, Levy, Cain, Ansell, & Pincus, 2013).

Clinicians have to navigate the complexities of NPD, especially with clients who oscillate between grandiosity and vulnerability. The grandiosity may be evident as domineering and vindictive interpersonal behaviors, whereas the vulnerability may display as shame, agitation, and self-criticism (Pincus, Caine, & Wright, 2014).

Researchers indicate that progress can be made if barriers to treatment are avoided. The three most common barriers are strong and counterproductive feelings of countertransference; clinicians' belief (and covert communication of that belief to the individual being treated) in the myth of untreatability; and the provision of direct and specific advice on social functioning or personal problems, which usually produces dependence, noncompliance, or resentment. Establishing an appropriate therapeutic alliance with individuals with NPD may be particularly difficult. A first step in treatment of NPD is collaborative goal setting with regard to treatment; consistent attention to developing and maintaining therapeutic boundaries; and transparency in all interactions, including sharing diagnostic impressions with the client.

Clinicians can use an approach called transference-focused psychotherapy (TFP) with their clients with NPD. This therapy initially works on limit setting with the client to decrease destructive behaviors and then explores the client's mind and sense of identity. Clinicians using TFP usually meet with their client two times a week (Stern & Yeomans, n.d.).

Social workers should be aware of their own cultural values, beliefs, and biases and develop specialized knowledge about the histories, traditions, and values of their clients. Social workers should adopt treatment methodologies that reflect their knowledge of the cultural diversity of the communities in which they practice.

Problem	Goal	Intervention
Clinician has difficulty developing and maintaining a therapeutic alliance with client with NPD	Establish a long-term therapeutic alliance	Sharing diagnostic impressions and greater than usual inclusion of client in developing treatment goals, greater than usual attention to importance of tact, timing, and precise use of language. The clinician should be wary of unwittingly compromising boundaries and becoming a source of narcissistic supply for the client via overt, excessive tact
Client's heightened sensitivity to criticism is negatively affecting his or her ability to participate in treatment	Full engagement in treatment by client	Use of transference-focused psychotherapy (TFP) to accommodate client's hypersensitivity

LAWS AND REGULATIONS

Each jurisdiction (i.e., nation, state, or province) has its own standards, procedures, and laws for involuntary restraint and detention of persons who may be a danger to themselves or others. Individuals with NPD might be at risk for suicide. Local and professional reporting requirements for neglect and abuse should also be known and observed.

Each country has its own standards for cultural competency and diversity in social work practice. Social workers must be aware of the standards of practice set forth by their governing body (National Association of Social Workers, British Association of Social Workers, etc.) and practice accordingly.

SERVICES AND RESOURCES

- National Mental Health Consumers' Self-Help Clearinghouse, http://mhselfhelp.squarespace. com/clearinghouse-resources/category/personality-disorders

FOOD FOR THOUGHT

In contrast to most mental health disorders, some of the personality traits at the core of NPD are viewed as necessary for both intrapersonal and interpersonal functioning. Healthy development and maintenance of some degree of self-regard and belief in one's abilities and accomplishments, as well as validation and affirmation from external sources, are all needed for development of a robust personality.

RED FLAGS

Signs and symptoms of NPD are similar to those of other cluster B personality disorders and can be difficult to distinguish for diagnostic purposes. The myth that personality disorders are untreatable can be self-reinforcing when repeated among professionals involved in the treatment of NPD.

Clinicians report that clients with a comorbid diagnosis of NPD and borderline personality disorder can be the most challenging clients to treat because they tend to provoke or alienate the therapist in an effort to devalue the therapeutic relationship and treatment.

Physical illness and problems resulting from substance use can threaten the image of superiority held by persons with NPD; they may minimize these issues to preserve their sense of superiority.

NEXT STEPS

Review medication regimen and symptoms of adverse effects, if any, and make follow-up appointment with agency issuing prescription.

Instruct client to seek immediate attention for aggression and suicide ideation/attempts.

Provide education about the nature of NPD and the need for follow-up treatment if symptoms reappear.

Assess for stability of employment and housing.

Refer to appropriate treatment modality depending on severity and subtype of NPD.

Provide referrals for support and education of family members.

Written by Chris Bates, MA, MSW, and
Melissa Rosales Neff, MSW

Reviewed by Pedram Samghabadi

REFERENCES

American Psychiatric Association. (2013). *Diagnostic and statistical manual of mental disorders: DSM-5* (5th ed.). Washington, DC: American Psychiatric Publishing.

British Association of Social Workers. (2012, January). The code of ethics for social work: Statement of principles. Retrieved October 25, 2015, from http://cdn.basw.co.uk/upload/basw_112315-7.pdf

Diamond, D., Levy, K., Clarkin, J., Fischer-Kern, M., Cain, N., Doering, S., ... Buchheim, A. (2014). Attachment and mentalization in female patients with comorbid narcissistic and borderline personality disorder. *Personality Disorders, 5*(4), 428-433. doi:10.1037/per0000065

Dimaggio, G. (2012). Narcissistic personality disorder: Rethinking what we know. *Psychiatric Times, 29*(7), 17-25.

Ellison, W. D., Levy, K. N., Cain, N. M., Ansell, E. B., & Pincus, A. L. (2013). The impact of pathological narcissism on psychotherapy utilization, initial symptom severity, and early-treatment symptom change: A naturalistic investigation. *Journal of Personal Assessment, 95*(3), 291-300. doi:10.1080/0022 3891.2012.742904

International Federation of Social Workers. (2012, March 3). Statement of ethical principles. Retrieved October 25, 2015, from http://ifsw.org/policies/statement-of-ethical-principles/

Kealy, D., & Ogrodniczuk, J. S. (2012). Pathological narcissism: A front-line guide. *Practice: Social Work in Action, 24*(3), 161-174. doi:10.1080/09503153.2 012.679255

Levy, K. N. (2012). Subtypes, dimensions, levels, and mental states in narcissism and narcissistic personality disorder. *Journal of Clinical Psychology, 68*(8), 886-897. doi:10.1002/jclp.21893

Miller, J., McCain, J., Lynam, D., Few, L., Gentile, B., & MacKillop, J. (2014). A comparison of the criterion validity of popular measures of narcissism and narcissistic personality disorder via the use of expert ratings. *Psychological Assessment, 26*(3), 958-969. doi:10.1037/a0036613

Mizrahi, T., & Mayden, R. W. (2001). NASW standards for cultural competency in social work practice. Retrieved October 25, 2015, from http://www.socialworkers.org/practice/standards/NAS-WCulturalStandards.pdf

Pincus, A., Cain, N., & Wright, A. (2014). Narcissistic grandiosity and narcissistic vulnerability in psychotherapy. *Personality Disorders, 5*(4), 439-443.

Pincus, A. L., & Lukowitsky, M. R. (2010). Patho-logical narcissism and narcissistic person-ality disorder. *Annual Review of Clinical Psy-chology*, 6, 421-446. doi:10.1146/annurev.clinpsy.121208.131215

Ronningstam, E. (2010). Narcissistic personality dis-order: A current review. *Current Psychiatry Report*, 12(1), 68-75. doi:10.1007/s11920-009-0084-z

Ronningstam, E. (2014). Beyond the diagnostic traits: A collaborative exploratory diagnostic pro-cess for dimensions and underpinnings of narcis-sistic personality disorders. *Personality Disorders*, 5(4), 434-438. doi:10.1037/per0000034

Skodol, A., Bender, D., & Morey, L. (2014). Narcis-sistic personality disorder in DSM-5. *Personality Dis-orders*, 5(4), 422-427.

Stern, B., & Yeomans, F. (n.d.). Transference-focused psychotherapy (TFP). Retrieved October 25, 2015, from http://www.borderlinedisorders.com/trans-ference-focused-psychotherapy.php

Stinson, F. S., Dawson, D. A., Goldstein, R. B., Chou, S. P., Huang, B., Smith, S. M., ... Grant, B. F. (2008). Prevalence, correlates, disability, and comorbidity of DSM-IV narcissistic personality disorder: Results from the Wave 2 National Epidemiologic Survey on Alcohol and Related Conditions. *Journal of Clinical Psychiatry*, 69(7), 1033-1045.

NATIVE AMERICANS & POVERTY: PSYCHOSOCIAL ISSUES

MAJOR CATEGORIES: Behavioral & Mental Health, Cultural Competency, Homelessness

WHAT WE KNOW

Since 2015, poverty in the United States is defined by the government as a family of four living on an annual income of $24,250 or less. There are 5.2 mil-lion self-identified Native American individuals, sometimes addressed as Native Indians and Alaska Natives (NIAN), living in the United States; Native Americans make up 1.7 percent of the total U.S. population. Almost half belong to one of the 566 federally recognized tribes and live on reservations or tribal land. The number of NIAN households is 1.7 million. Of these, 39 percent are married-couple families, including those with children.

Native Americans have the highest poverty rate of all ethno-racial groups in the United States, at 27 per-cent; the poverty rate among blacks is 26 percent and among Latinos, 23 percent, and the overall U.S. rate is 14 percent.

Social science consistently demonstrates the ad-verse psychosocial and biophysical consequences of poverty on children, youth, and adults. Findings from neuroscience demonstrate that living in a low-income household also adversely affects brain de-velopment, indicating that poverty poses a threat to educational attainment and adult productivity. The impact of poverty can be severe largely because of the continual stress it places on the individual's psycho-biological system.

The presence or absence of financial and familial resources permeates an individual's ecosystem. Poverty can impair physical and mental health, lower cognitive achievement, and increase the risk of child maltreatment; in turn, each of these increases the risk of poverty. While it is important to note that not all adults living in poverty suffer mental health problems, have cognitive difficulties, or abuse their children, it is equally important to appreciate how the poverty cycle can entrap individuals, families, and communities.

In addition to the role of poverty in the develop-ment of psychosocial problems, members of Native American groups may have what is described as in-ternalized "intergenerational trauma" resulting from the historical exploitation and oppression of Native Americans in the United States.

Researchers utilizing the Historical Loss Scale and the Historical Loss Associated Symptoms Scale with Native American adults found that the majority of respondents thought about historical losses at least occasionally and that these thoughts caused psychosocial distress. Substance dependence, anx-iety disorders, and mood disorders were correlated with symptoms associated with historical loss.

Accounts of poverty in one study of Native American women underscore how it impedes their ability to parent. Providing food and housing can be challenging financially, especially for single mothers. Transportation can be a problem for individuals living in rural environments; lack of access to transportation has prevented mothers from visiting hospitalized infants.

Single Native American mothers highlight the absence of support from fathers.

Native American mothers express concern over the interruption of their education caused by raising children and how having children and lacking qualifications present barriers to employment in large part because they lack accessible, affordable, high-quality child care.

The Substance Abuse and Mental Health Administration (SAMHA) reports that in 2014, 8.8 percent of Native Americans ages 18 and up had co-occurring mental and substance use disorders in the past year compared to the national average of 3.3 percent. SAMHA also reported that the suicide rate among Native Americans ages 15 to 34 is 2.5 times higher than the national average.

Native American mothers have expressed that it is difficult to escape the "drug culture" in their communities. Both male and female adolescents report rates of alcohol use, cigarette use, marijuana use, and other nonprescription drug use that are higher than national averages. Similarly, they report rates of binge drinking and illicit drug use that are higher than national averages. This may be the result of viewing alcohol consumption as a family bonding activity.

Alcohol consumption is significantly associated with intimate partner violence (IPV); Native American women who drink alcohol, whether it is heavy or light drinking, are more likely to be victims of IPV than non-Hispanic-white women who drink).

Fetal alcohol spectrum disorders are a concern for all women of reproductive age who drink; binge drinking poses the greatest threat to the fetus.

Native American individuals experience what are described as "alarmingly high" rates of the following mental disorders: substance use disorder, posttraumatic stress disorder (PTSD), childhood conduct disorder, and suicidal behaviors. Results from a study from a mental health clinic indicate that the Native American youth being treated there have high rates of mood and adjustment disorders, alcohol and marijuana use, traumatic exposure, and PTSD.

The risk of schizophrenia has long been considered higher for Native Americans; however, a 2007 study showed comparable prevalence rates between Native Americans and the general U.S. population.

The rural and isolated location of many Native American communities creates a barrier to accessing mental health services. While most Indian Health Service (IHS) clinics and hospitals are located on reservations, the majority of Native Americans in the United States no longer reside on reservations and thus may experience difficulty accessing this care.

Researchers who have noted the disparities in health among the Native Americans in comparison to other U.S. populations state that these disparities may be the result of lack of access to primary care options. As stated above, the IHS clinics can be difficult to get to on reservations, so Native Americans are using emergency departments for their medical care instead of a primary care provider.

Gaming or casinos on reservations can make a positive impact on poverty. Researchers of a study found that for each slot machine added, the per capita income for Native Americans in the corresponding school district rose $541 and there was a corresponding 0.6 percent decrease in the percentage living in poverty. There was also a decrease in the probability that children would be overweight or obese.

Strengths and protective factors connected to Native American culture include a strong identification with culture, importance of family, connections to the past, traditional health practices or ceremonies, adaptability, and the wisdom of elders.

Social workers can use these factors help combat negative psychosocial impacts of poverty. Effective culturally based models of care emphasize therapeutic relationships that draw upon and respect cultural traditions.

WHAT CAN BE DONE

Become knowledgeable about the psychosocial issues that are experienced by Native Americans coping with poverty. Treatment methodologies should reflect the cultural values, beliefs, and biases of the individual in need of care and treatment.

Government policies that provide assistance with healthcare, food, education, and employment can provide a safety net for individuals who live in poverty and weaken its adverse consequences.

Learn about the challenges of poverty and advocate for policies that reduce the burden of poverty and end discrimination.

Multiple forms of discrimination experienced by ethnic, racial, and indigenous groups greatly increase the risk of poverty; efforts to eradicate all forms of discrimination must continue.

Learn about the challenges and barriers poverty imposes on Native American mothers.

Learn about successful culturally based interventions for Native American children, youth, and adults to improve service delivery for these groups and increase the potential for positive outcomes.

Written by Jan Wagstaff, MA, MSW

Reviewed by Lynn B. Cooper, D. Criminology and Jessica Therivel, LMSW-IPR

REFERENCES

Addressing the needs of vulnerable families during an economic crisis. (2008). *First Focus.* Retrieved November 29, 2014, from http://firstfocus. net/resources/report/addressing-needs-vulnerable-families-during-economic-crisis/

Adler, N. E., & Rehkopf, D. H. (2008). U.S. disparities in health: Descriptions, causes, and mechanisms. *Annual Review of Public Health, 29,*235-252. doi:10.1146/annurev.publhealth.29.020907.090852

American Psychiatric Association. (2014). Mental health disparities: American Indians and Alaska Natives. *APA Fact Sheet.* : American Psychiatric Association.

British Association of Social Workers. (2012). The code of ethics for social work: Statement of principles. Retrieved November 29, 2015, from http://cdn. basw.co.uk/upload/basw_112315-7.pdf

Croff, R. L., Rieckman, T. R., & Spence, J. D. (2013). Provider and state perspective on implementing cultural-based models of care for American Indian

and Alaska Native patients with substance use disorders. *Journal of Behavioral Health Services & Research,* 1-15. doi:10.1007/s11414-013-9322-6

Dickerson, D. L., & Johnson, C. L. (2012). Mental health and substance abuse characteristics among a clinical sample of urban American Indian/Alaska Native youths in a large California metropolitan area: A descriptive study. *Community Mental Health Journal, 48*(1), 56-62. doi:10.1007/s10597-010-9368-3

Docherty, S. L., Lowry, C., & Miles, M. S. (2007). Poverty as context for the parenting experience of low-income Lumbee Indian mothers with a medically fragile infant. *Neonatal Network, 26*(6), 361.

Duwe, E., Petterson, S., Gibbons, C., & Bazemore, A. (2014). Ecology of health care: The need to address low utilization in American Indians/Alaska Natives. *American Family Physician, 89*(3), 217-218.

Ehlers, C. L., Gizer, I. R., Gilder, D. A., Ellingson, J. M., & Yehuda, R. (2013). Measuring historical trauma in an American Indian community sample: Contributions of substance dependence, affective disorder, conduct disorder, and PTSD. *Drug Alcohol Depend, 133*(1), 180-187. doi:10.1016/j.drugalcdep.2013.05.011

Friese, B., Grube, J. W., Seringer, S., Paschall, M. I., & Moore, R. S. (2011). Drinking behavior and sources of alcohol: Differences between Native American and white youths. *Journal of Studies on Alcohol & Drugs, 72*(1), 53-60.

Gone, J. P., & Trimble, J. E. (2012). American Indian and Native mental health: Diverse perspectives on enduring disparities. *Annual Review of Clinical Psychology, 8,*131-160. doi:10.1146/annurev-clinpsy-032511-143127

International Federation of Social Workers. (2012, March 3). Statement of ethical principles. Retrieved November 29, 2015, from http://ifsw.org/policies/statement-of-ethical-principles

Jones-Smith, J. C., Dow, W. H., & Chichlowska, K. (2014). Association between casino opening or expansion and risk of childhood overweight and obesity. *JAMA,311*(9), 929-936. doi:10.1001/jama.2014.604

Lipina, S. J., & Posner, M. I. (2012). The impact of poverty on the development of brain networks. *Frontiers in Human Neuroscience, 6,*238. doi:10.3389/fnhum.2012.00238

Macartney, S., Bishaw, A., & Fontenot, K. (2013). Poverty rates for selected detailed race and Hispanic groups by state and place: 2007-2011. Retrieved November 29, 2014, from http://www.census.gov/prod/2013pubs/acsbr11-17.pdf

Matthews, K. A., & Gallo, L. C. (2011). Psychological perspectives on pathways linking socioeconomic status and physical health. *Annual Review of Psychology*, 62,501-530. doi:10.1146/annurev.psych.031809.130711

Montag, A., Clapp, J. D., Calac, D., Gorman, J., & Chambers, C. (2012). A review of evidence-based approaches for reduction of alcohol consumption in native women who are pregnant or of reproductive age. *The American Journal of Drug & Alcohol Abuse*, 38(5), 436-443. doi:10.3109/00952990.2012.694521

National Survey on Drug Use and Health. (2010). Substance use among American Indian or Alaska Native adolescents. Retrieved November 29, 2014, from http://www.samhsa.gov/data/2k11/WEB_SR_005/WEB_SR_005. htm

National Survey on Drug Use and Health. (2010). Substance use among American Indian or Alaska Native adults. Retrieved from http://www.samhsa.gov/data/2k10/182/AmericanIndianHTML.pdf

Robin, R. W., Gottesman, I. I., Albaugh, B., & Goldman, D. (2007). Schizophrenia and psychotic symptoms in families of two American Indian tribes. *BMC Psychiatry*, 7,30.

Substance Abuse and Mental Health Services Adminstration. (2015). Racial and ethnic minority populations. Retrieved November 29, 0205, from http://www.samhsa.gov/specific-populations/racial-ethnic-minority

Waller, M. W., Iritani, B. J., Christ, S. L., Kovach Clark, H., Moracco, K. E., Tucker Halpern, C., & Flewelling, R. L. (2012). Relationships among alcohol outlet density, alcohol use, and intimate partner violence victimization among young women in the United States. *Journal of Interpersonal Violence*, 27(10), 2062-2086. doi:10.1177/0886260511431435

U.S. Census Bureau. (2014). Facts for features: American Indian and Alaska native heritage month. Retrieved November 29, 0205, from http://www.census.gov/content/dam/Census/newsroom/facts-for-features/2014/cb14ff-26_aian_heritage_month.pdf

U.S. Department of Health and Human Services. (2015). 2015 poverty guidelines. Retrieved November 29, 2015, from http://aspe. hhs. gov/2015-poverty-guidelines

Wheeler, D. (2015). NASW standards and indicators for cultural competence in social work practice. Retrieved from http://www.socialworkers.org/practice/standards/PRA-BRO-253150-CC-Standards.pdf

Yoshikawa, H., Aber, J. L., & Beardslee, W. R. (2012). The effects of poverty on the mental, emotional, and behavioral health of children and youth: Implications for prevention. *American Psychologist*, 67(4), 272-284. doi:10.1037/a0028015

NEUROCOGNITIVE DISORDERS: DEMENTIA

MAJOR CATEGORIES: Behavioral & Mental Health; Medical & Health

DESCRIPTION

The *Diagnostic and Statistical Manual of Mental Disorders*, fifth edition (*DSM-5*), introduced a new conceptualization of the criteria for diagnosing dementia, as well as a new name: major and mild neurocognitive disorders. The primary difference between major and mild is the presence in major neurocognitive disorders of "substantial impairment" and interference with daily activities. Recognizing the pervasive use of the term *dementia* and that it is understood by patients and families, the *DSM-5* continues to use it in the etiological subtypes of neurocognitive disorder.

The dementia disorders as described in the *Diagnostic and Statistical Manual of Mental Disorders (DSM-IV-TR)* are characterized by a decline in cognitive abilities, including memory. This decline can be caused by a general medical condition, the persisting effects of a substance, or a combination of the two. Dementia usually is progressive, must be severe enough to interfere with social or occupational functioning, and usually is irreversible. As dementia progresses, individuals frequently develop symptoms of other mental health disorders, such as depression or psychosis, and behaviors such as aggression or wandering that may complicate treatment and care of the affected individual. The specific deficit in cognitive function usually is related to the area of the brain that is affected by the medical condition or substance, and may include the following:

Aphasia: language impairment including word-finding difficulty, word substitution, or mispronunciation. Language may eventually become incomprehensible.

Apraxia: impaired ability of motor function, such as loss of ability to operate familiar machines such as a dishwasher. May eventually lead to inability to dress or feed self.

Agnosia: failure to identify familiar objects or faces. May eventually lead to not recognizing self in a mirror. Also may cause lack of insight into degree of general impairment and unrealistic assessment of abilities.

Visuospatial dysfunction: loss of navigation skills and difficulty distinguishing an object from the background. May eventually lead to getting lost in familiar places.

Executive functioning decline: disturbance in planning, organizing, sequencing, and abstracting abilities. May lead to concrete thought patterns, inflexibility, impaired judgment, slowed thought processing, or impulsivity.

Diagnoses appearing in the *DSM-IV-TR* are differentiated based on etiology and include dementia of the Alzheimer's type, vascular dementia, dementia due to HIV disease, dementia due to head trauma, dementia due to Parkinson's disease, dementia due to Huntington's disease, dementia due to Pick's disease, dementia due to Creutzfeldt-Jakob disease, dementia due to other general medical condition, substance-induced persisting dementia, and dementia due to multiple etiologies.

A primary feature distinguishing dementia from delirium is memory impairment, which is always present in dementia in some form. Memory impairment may manifest as the inability to learn new information and skills or the inability to recall previously learned information and skills. Short-term memory usually is affected before long-term memory, and

procedural memory may be retained the longest. Impaired short-term memory may be the first outwardly visible sign of dementia and might include forgetting recent conversations or events, repetitive questions and storytelling, misplacing objects, forgetting appointments, or losing valuables. New information and skills cannot be learned, and there may be confusion or disorientation in new surroundings.

Dementia may be the result of any of a number of physiological diseases, disorders, conditions, or exposures, or a combination of them. The etiologies include the following:

- *Neurodegenerative*: Alzheimer's disease, dementia with Lewy bodies, frontotemporal dementia, Parkinson's disease, Huntington's disease;
- *Vascular*: infarction, Biswanger's disease, hemodynamic insufficiency;
- *Neurological disease*: multiple sclerosis, normal-pressure hydrocephalus, brain tumor;
- *Endocrine*: hypothyroidism, hypercalcemia, hypoglycemia;
- *Nutritional*: vitamin B12 deficiency, thiamine deficiency;
- *Infectious*: HIV, prion disease, neurosyphilis, cryptococcus;
- *Metabolic*: hepatic insufficiency, renal insufficiency, Wilson's disease, metachromatic leukodystrophy, neuroacanthosis;
- *Traumatic*: subdural hematoma, dementia pugilistica (boxing or other sports);
- *Exposure*: alcohol, heavy metals, irradiation, anticholinergic medications, carbon monoxide.

The progression of dementia includes slow, usually at first unnoticeable, onset with chronic course of gradual development over months or years, with the progressive deterioration spanning 3 to 10 years and eventually ending in death. Disruption in and loss of short-term memory is the first sign, with long-term memory failing slowly as the disorder progresses. Other areas of cognitive decline depend on the exact etiology of the dementia and vary as noted above. All dementias are progressive and may eventually lead to severe disruption of functioning. With the exception of dementia resulting from normal-pressure hydrocephalus and vitamin B12 deficiency, dementia is irreversible. Treatments vary depending on the etiology and progression of the dementia and may include medications, cognitive training or rehabilitation, various strategies to provide for comfort and safety, and eventually possible placement in a facility dedicated to the care of individuals with dementia. Palliative care should be considered for persons who are at the end of life.

FACTS AND FIGURES

It is estimated that 46.8 million people worldwide have dementia, with prevalence rates for most regions ranging from 5.6 percent to 7.6 percent of people 60 years and over (Alzheimer's Disease International, 2015). Typically, onset of dementia occurs after age 60, and prevalence doubles approximately every 5 years, until at age 85 and older approximately half the population is affected. Dementia occurs more often in women, which may be because of longer life expectancy (Aminoff & Kerchner, 2016). Alzheimer's disease is the leading cause of dementia in the United States, accounting for approximately two-thirds of dementia cases (Harper, Johnston, & Landefeld, 2016).

RISK FACTORS

Advanced age is the leading risk factor for most forms of dementia. Additional risk factors include any of the diseases or activities listed above, genetic predisposition or family history of dementia, lower educational status, sedentary lifestyle, and diabetes. Dementia occurs more often in women.

SIGNS AND SYMPTOMS

Signs and clinical presentation will vary depending on the exact cause of the dementia. In addition to the signs and symptoms of any of the diseases listed above, disruption of short-term memory usually is the first outward sign of dementia, with word-finding difficulty, visuospatial dysfunction, and executive function deterioration (e.g. distractibility, impulsivity, slowed processing speed, impaired judgment, decreased planning and organizational skills, mental inflexibility, concrete thought patterns) following. Individuals with signs or symptoms of repeated head trauma or abusive levels of substance consumption may also have signs or symptoms of dementia that are not apparent.

ASSESSMENT

Professionals working with people with dementia may perform some or all of the following assessments: Perform a standard biopsychosocial-spiritual history, including assessment for suicide and harm to self or others; observe functioning and demeanor during interview; and/or collect collateral information from family, friends, and coworkers. This is especially important because individuals frequently have limited insight into their memory loss and other declines in functioning.

Professionals may also use any or all of the following instruments to assess people with dementia: Clock drawing test, Folstein Mini-Mental Status Exam (MMSE), Reisberg Functional Assessment Staging (FAST), Cambridge Cognitive Examination (CAMCOG), Dementia Screening Questionnaire for Individuals with Intellectual Disabilities (DSQUID), and/or Alzheimer's Disease Assessment Scale (ADAS-Cog).

Professionals may also perform appropriate medical tests (e.g., blood tests, CT, MRI, PET, SPECT, lumbar puncture) to identify medical condition causing dementia and to specify which dementia disorder is present and appropriate tests for substances (including prescription medications) to identify substance use as possible cause of dementia.

TREATMENT

Person-centered care for people with dementia involves developing a holistic, strengths-based understanding of their strengths and needs and their social contexts. Treatment goals should be individually tailored but may include reducing or managing symptoms of dementia, treating comorbid mood disorders, managing behavioral issues, improving quality of life, and strengthening family and community supports.

Professionals may also review medication regimen and make follow-up appointment with agency issuing prescription, provide referrals for support and education for family members; discuss medical decision-making and power of attorney; review likely progression and next step(s) of treatment; establish a long-term care plan with person and family in anticipation of changes in needs; and review safety considerations, including driving.

Problem	Goal	Intervention
Disruption of memory and cognitive functioning, and/or secondary impacts such as depression or anxiety	Reduce and slow symptoms of dementia and address other symptoms such as depression or anxiety to make individual as comfortable as possible	Cognitive stimulation, training and/or rehab, pharmacological treatments for dementia symptoms. Cognitive behavioral therapy (CBT), psychodynamic therapy, counseling, psychoactive medication if indicated for symptoms of anxiety or depression. Follow up on medication adherence and effectiveness, including discussion of importance of adhering to prescription dosage and timing with family and caregivers. Continuously monitor medications as dementia progresses.
Social exclusion and marginalization as a result of disability	Strive to understand the emotions and behaviors of those with dementia within their own social circumstances and biographies and care for them as unique individuals	Learn about the background of each individual being cared for and design care and support appropriate to his or her unique needs and life story using person-centered values such as the importance of the perspective of the individual with dementia, the importance of relationships and interactions, and his or her individuality and unique life history and how that affects manifestation of dementia. Use effective communication strategies (e.g., ask simple, open-ended questions; attend to emotional cues and metaphors in expressions; allow time to gather thoughts and words). Look for support groups or an adult day care setting if appropriate that may reduce isolation.
Decline in ability to accomplish tasks of daily living and care for self and possible anxiety related to decline	Maximize independence and mobility; provide for physical, mental, and emotional well-being, comfort, and safety as well as reduction of anxiety if present	Wide variety of behavioral interventions as appropriate to individual and stage of dementia, such as physical exercise to maintain strength and mobility, strategies for communications, scheduling, nutritional concerns, toileting, wandering, and general safety. Also consideration of adult day care, in-home care, palliative/hospice care, or eventual placement in a care facility if needed.
Family and caregiver lack of information about dementia and how to treat it	Provide factual information and emotional support to family and caregivers	Educate family and caregivers about dementia, including the likely progression, home safety, and addressing behavioral problems. Provide references to peer-based support groups.

LAWS AND REGULATIONS

Each jurisdiction (i.e., nation, state, or province) has its own standards, procedures, and laws for involuntary restraint and detention of persons who may be a danger to themselves or others. Individuals with dementia may become aggressive or may lose the ability to care for themselves, and consideration may have to be given to involuntary care. Consideration should also be given to the legal ramifications of loss of executive functioning as it affects medical decision-making and to general power of attorney for life-changing decisions (e.g., wills, sale of assets, entering extended-care facilities). Individuals with dementia are at higher risk than their peers for abuse (including financial abuse) and neglect, and those involved in their care should be familiar with local reporting agencies and procedures. Locally applicable rules and regulations for suspension or removal of driver's licenses should also be considered.

SERVICES AND RESOURCES

Note: Enter "dementia" in the search box on each Web site mentioned below to access relevant information.

- Alzheimer's Disease and Dementia, http://www.alz.org/
- Brain & Behavior Research Foundation (formerly NARSAD), http://bbrfoundation.org/
- National Alliance on Mental Illness (NAMI), http://www.nami.org/
- U.S. National Institutes of Health (NIH), http://www.nih.gov/

FOOD FOR THOUGHT

The social model of disability focuses on secondary effects caused by societal factors that marginalize and exclude people with dementia and other disabling conditions. The importance of maintaining regard for the personhood and dignity of persons with dementia is emphasized.

RED FLAGS

Because of the gradual decline in the cognitive abilities needed to drive, it may become necessary to report the individual with a dementia disorder to appropriate authorities for removal of his or her driver's license or to remove his or her car or keys if the individual continues to drive after it is unsafe to do so.

The constantly (although frequently slowly) changing nature of dementia requires continual assessment and readiness to intervene as circumstances change.

Ethical considerations should be considered concerning decision-making, consent to treatments, and advance medical orders if present.

Psychoactive medications are associated with additional risks in older adults. Benzodiazepines have been associated with increased risk of falling, and antipsychotics have black box warnings associated with increased risk for death in the elderly.

Older adults admitted to acute care hospitals may have undiagnosed dementia. Investigators in a study in Ireland found that 25 percent of patients aged 70 years and older had dementia, but of these, only 35.6 percent had been previously diagnosed (Timmons et al., 2015).

Individuals with young-onset dementia (i.e., diagnosed before age 65) experience longer delays in diagnosis in part because professionals are not well-versed in the presentation of dementia in younger adults. Because they are generally stronger and more mobile than older clients with dementia and are in a different stage of life (e.g., employed, parenting dependent children), adults with young-onset dementia and their families also have difficulty locating services suited to their unique needs.

Written by Chris Bates, MA, MSW

Reviewed by Jessica Therivel, LMSW-IPR

REFERENCES

American Psychiatric Association. (2000). *Diagnostic and statistical manual of mental disorders* (4th ed., text revision ed.). Washington, DC: Author. American Psychiatric Association. (2013). *Diagnostic and statistical manual of mental disorders: DSM-5* (5th ed.). Arlington, VA: Author.

Aminoff, M. J., & Kerchner, G. A. (2016). Nervous system disorders. In S. J. McPhee & M. A. Papadakis (Eds.), *Current medical diagnosis and treatment* (55th ed., pp. 1002-1007). New York, NY: McGraw Hill Medical.

British Association of Social Workers. (2012, January). The code of ethics for social work: Statement of principles. Retrieved December 9, 2015, from http://cdn.basw.co.uk/upload/basw_112315-7.pdf

British Psychological Society. (2007). A NICE-SCIE guideline on supporting people with dementia and their carers in health and social care. Leicester, England: Author.

Cheung, K. S., Lau, B. H., Wong, P. W., Leung, A. Y., Lou, V. W., Chan, G. M., & Schulz, R. (2015). Multicomponent intervention on enhancing dementia caregiver well-being and reducing behavioral problems among Hong Kong Chinese: A translational study based on REACH II. *International Journal of Geriatric Psychiatry, 30*(5), 1-10. doi:10.1002/gps.4160

Council of Europe. (2003). Convention for protection of human rights and fundamental freedoms as amended by Protocol 11. Strasbourg, France: Author.

Farooq, U., & Siddiqui, N. H. (2015). Dementia. In F. J. Domino (Ed.), *The 5-minute clinical consult* (24th ed., p. 275). Philadelphia, PA: Wolters Kluwer Health.

Gareri, P., De Fazio, P., Manfredi, V. G., & De Sarro, G. (2014). Use and safety of antipsychotics in behavioral disorders in elderly people with dementia. *Journal of Clinical Psychopharmacology, 34*(1), 109-123. doi:10.1097/JCP.0b013e3182a6096e

Hayo, H. (2015). Diagnosis and support for younger people with dementia. *Nursing Standard, 29*(47), 36-40. doi:10.7748/ns.29.47.36.e9197

Heath, H., & Sturdy, D. (2009). Living well with dementia in a care home. Harrow, England: RCN Publishing. International Federation of Social Workers. (2012, March 3). Statement of ethical principles. Retrieved December 9, 2015, from http://ifsw.org/policies/statement-of-ethical-principles/

Harper, G. M., Johnston, C. B., & Landefeld, C. S. (2016). Geriatric disorders. In M. A. Papadakis & S. J. McPhee (Eds.), *Current medical diagnosis and treatment* (55th ed., pp. 55-60). New York, NY: McGraw Hill Medical.

Marder, K. (2012). Dementia and memory loss. In J. C. M. Brust (Ed.), *Current diagnosis and treatment neurology* (2nd ed., pp. 78-101). New York, NY: McGraw Hill Medical.

McEvoy, P., & Plant, R. (2014). Dementia care: Using empathic curiosity to establish the common ground that is necessary for meaningful communication. *Journal of Psychiatric and Mental Health Nursing, 21*(6), 477-482. doi:10.1111/jpm.12148

Ortega, V., Qazi, A., Spector, A.E., & Orrell, M. (2014). Psychological treatments for depression and anxiety in dementia and mild cognitive impairment and anxiety in dementia and mild cognitive impairment. *Cochrane Database of Systematic Reviews*, 1. Art. No.: CD009125. doi:10.1002/14651858. CD009125.pub2

Schnall, A. (2015). Public advocacy and community engagement: Interventions for individuals with young-onset dementia and their families. *The Psychiatric Clinics of North America, 38*(2), 353-362. doi:10.1016/j.psc.2015.01.006

Scottish Intercollegiate Guidelines Network. (2006). Management of patients with dementia: A national clinical guideline. Edinburgh, Scotland: Author.

Timmons, S., Manning, E., Barrett, A., Brady, N. M., Browne, V., O'Shea, E., ... Linehan, J. G. (2015). Dementia in older people admitted to hospital: A regional multi-hospital observational study of prevalence, associations and case recognition. *Age and Ageing, 44*(6), 993-999. doi:10.1093/ageing/afv131

Wheeler, D., ... McClain, A. (2015). NASW standards and indicators for cultural competence in social work practice. Retrieved December 9, 2015, from http://www.socialworkers.org/practice/standards/PRA-BRO-253150-CC-Standards.pdf

Wilson, J. A. (2011). Cognitive disorders. In N. J. Keltner, C. E. Bostrom, & T. M. McGuinness (Eds.), *Psychiatric nursing* (6th ed., pp. 322-342). St. Louis, MO: Elsevier Mosby.

Wilson, K., & Bachman, S. S. (2015). House calls: The impact of home-based care for older adults with Alzheimer's and dementia. *Social Work in Health Care, 54*(6), 547-558. doi:10.1080/00981389.2015.1045576

Alzheimer's Disease International. (2015). World Alzheimer report 2015: The global impact of dementia. Retrieved December 9, 2015, from http://www.alz.co.uk/research/WorldAlzheimerReport2015.pdf

O

OBESITY IN CHILDREN & ADOLESCENTS: HEALTHCARE COSTS

MAJOR CATEGORIES: Adolescents, Medical & Health

WHAT WE KNOW

Obesity is the most common health problem among children and adolescents in developed countries, and the numbers are on the rise, it is caused mostly by poor diet, caloric excess, and a lack of physical activity.

Childhood obesity is commonly defined as a body mass index (BMI [i.e., a measurement of body fat based on height and weight]) ≥ 95th percentile on the Centers for Disease Control and Prevention (CDC) BMI-for-age growth charts.

Obesity is due to an imbalance between how many calories are consumed by the child and how many calories are subsequently burned.

The prevalence of obesity in children and adolescents has increased dramatically worldwide during the last two decades.

The CDC reports that the prevalence of obesity among children (aged 6–11 years) and adolescents (aged 12–19 years) in United States in 1980 was estimated to be 7% and 5%, respectively; from 1980 to 2012, the prevalence of obesity increased to 18% for children and 21% for adolescents.

Results from the 2012 National Health and Nutrition Examination Survey (NHANES) indicated that 31.8% of youth were classified as overweight or obese, with 16.9% meeting criteria for being clinically obese.

Among infants and toddlers from birth to age 2 years, 8.1% were considered high weight for their length. Between boys and girls at this age there was a large difference in prevalence, with 5% of boys and 11.4% of girls meeting this high weight mark.

Among all youth, there was not a significant difference in prevalence based on sex, but there were racial and ethnic differences. 8.6% of non-Hispanic Asian youth were obese compared to 14.1% of non-Hispanic whites, 20.2% of non-Hispanic blacks, and 22.4% of Hispanics

- The prevalence of obesity in low-income, preschool children in the United States increased from 12.4% in 1998 to 14.6% in 2008.
- Public Health England reports that in 2013–2014, 9.5% of children aged 4–5 were obese and 19.1% of 10–11-year-olds were obese.
- In Canada, the prevalence rates of childhood obesity and overweight were 9.9% and 32.9%, respectively, in 2005.
- In Germany, 15.5% of children aged 5–7 years are overweight and 4.3% are obese

Genetic factors are thought to contribute to the rising rates of childhood obesity, but actually environmental factors play an even larger role. Primary contributing factors include poor parental diet; parental obesity; diet high in fat and convenience foods and low in nutrient-rich foods (e.g., whole grains, fruits and vegetables, lean protein); increased television watching and decreased physical activity; advertisement of less healthy foods, limited access to healthy foods that are affordable; increases in portion sizes in restaurants, vending machines, and grocery stores; and daily sleep duration of less than 9 hours.

Ethnic minority children and children of low socioeconomic households are more likely than White children or children of higher socioeconomic

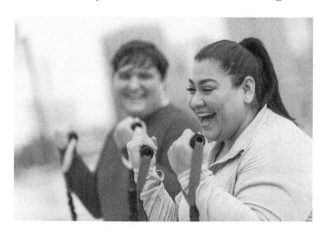

households to be overweight or obese, owing to the abundance of fast food restaurants in less affluent neighborhoods and the higher cost of nutrient-rich foods.

As a result of childhood and adolescent obesity there are increased healthcare costs such as increased hospitalization, outpatient/ emergency room visits and prescription drug use.

Other medical conditions associated with obesity include hypertension, mental disorders (e.g., depression, attention deficit disorder), metabolic disorders (e.g., hypothyroidism, hyperinsulinism, type 2 diabetes mellitus [DM2]), hyperlipidemia, sleep apnea, asthma, joint pain, Blount's disease (i.e., bowed legs), acanthosis nigricans (i.e., a skin disorder characterized by velvety brown markings within skin folds), and ventricular hypertrophy.

In 2014 investigators reviewed six U.S. studies to identify an estimate of lifetime medical costs for an obese child and concluded that the best estimate was $19,000. The investigators then took the lifetime medical cost estimate of $19,000 and multiplied that by the estimated number of children aged 10 years who are obese in the U.S. and determined a direct medical obesity cost of close to $14 billion for that age group.

An analysis of the Medical Expenditure Panel Survey (MEPS) found that parents or caregivers of overweight and obese children and adolescents aged 6–19 years spent $194 more on outpatient visits, $114 more on prescription drugs, and $12 more on emergency room visits than the parents or caregivers of their normal-weight or underweight peers.

There is a lack of evidence on optimal interventions for childhood obesity. One researched intervention includes family-based programs that modify diet, reduce sedentary behavior, and use behavioral techniques to boost motivation produce modest reductions in weight (1–3 kg/m decrease in BMI on average). However these interventions often are not cost-effective, are not effectively implemented, and they frequently fail to result in a reduction in obesity or related illness.

In contrast, researchers in another study found that the HOME Plus program (a community-based, family-focused intervention program that promotes families' preparing healthy food together and eating meals together) was extremely successful in reducing obesity and was cost-effective.

Interventions can be expensive if they are resource intensive. Results from one study indicated that a program called High Five for Kids, which is a primary care intervention, had a net cost of $196 per child, and the researchers recommended that further research be completed on the efficacy of the program to see if the cost is justified by its results.

Along with these programs, there have been countless different interventions and programs that have been researched and implemented into communities to work on this rising issue of childhood obesity. All of these programs include their own approaches to encouraging a healthier diet and increased physical activity.

WHAT CAN BE DONE

Learn about the multiple factors contributing to healthcare costs of obesity in children and adolescents so that you can assist yourself and other in making informed lifestyle modifications.

Explore obesity prevention strategies and treatments.

Seek emotional support and counseling that will be needed to reinforce major lifestyle modification and the relationship changes that come with this modification

Try to eat a diet high in fruits, vegetables, and lean protein and low in fat and convenience foods, and to get adequate sleep and routine physical exercise.

Explore your community to find out where to access affordable healthy food (e.g., community-supported agriculture [CSA], food co-op).

Explore the long-term costs they are facing versus the short-term increased expense in making healthier food choices..

Explore resources for financial assistance with meals, if needed (e.g., Supplemental Nutrition Assistance Program [SNAP], http://www.fns.usda.gov/snap/)

Written by Carita Caple, RN, BSN, MSHS

Reviewed by Jessica Therivel, LMSW-IPR

REFERENCES

Apfelbacher, C. J., Loerbroks, A., Cairns, J., Behrendt, H., Ring, J., & Krämer, U. (2008). Predictors of overweight and obesity in five to seven-year-old children in Germany: Results from cross-sectional studies. *BMC Public Health, 8*, 171. doi:10.1186/1471-2458-8-171

British Association of Social Workers. (2012, January). The code of ethics for social work: Statement of principles. Retrieved December 14, 2015, from http://cdn.basw.co.uk/upload/basw_112315-7.pdf

Centers for Disease Control and Prevention. (2009). Obesity prevalence among low-income, preschool-aged children-United States, 1998-2008. *MMWR Morbidity and Mortality Weekly Report, 58*(28), 769-773.

Centers for Disease Control and Prevention. (2014, July 11). About BMI for children and teens. Retrieved December 14, 2015, from http://www.cdc.gov/healthyweight/assessing/bmi/childrens_BMI/about_childrens_BMI.html

Centers for Disease Control and Prevention. (2015). Childhood obesity causes and consequences. Retrieved December 14, 2015, from http://www.cdc.gov/obesity/childhood/causes.html

Centers for Disease Control and Prevention. (2015). Childhood obesity facts. Retrieved December 14, 0205, from http://www.cdc.gov/healthyschools/obesity/facts.htm

Dunn, A. M. (2009). Nutrition. In C. E. Burns, A. M. Dunn, M. A. Brady, N. B. Starr, & C. G. Blosser (Eds.), *Pediatric primary care* (4th ed., pp. 220-224). St. Louis, MO: Saunders Elsevier.

Finkelstein, E. A., Graham, W. C., & Malhotra, R. (2014). Lifetime direct medical costs of childhood obesity. *Pediatrics, 133*(5), 854-862. doi:10.1542/peds.2014-0063

Flattum, C., Draxten, M., Horning, M., Fulkerson, J., Neumark-Sztainer, D., Garwick, A., ... Story, M. (2015). HOME Plus: Program design and implementation of a family-focused, community-based intervention to promote the frequency and healthfulness of family meals, reduce children's sedentary behavior, and prevent obesity. *International Journal of Behavioral Nutrition & Physical Activity, 12*(1), 1-9.

Gahagan, S. (2011). Overweight and obesity. In R. M. Kliegman, B. F. Stanton, J. W. I. I. I. Geme, N. F. Schor, & R. E. Behrman (Eds.), *Nelson textbook of pediatrics* (19th ed., pp. 179-188). Philadelphia, PA: Saunders Elsevier.

Gortmaker, S., Long, M., Resch, S., Ward, Z., Cradock, A., Barrett, J., & Wang, C. (2015). Cost-effectiveness of childhood obesity interventions: Evidence and methods for CHOICES. *American Journal of Preventative Medicine, 49*(1), 102-111. doi:10.1016/j.amepre.2015.03.032

Hughes, A. R., & Reilly, J. J. (2008). Disease management programs targeting obesity in children: Setting the scene for wellness in the future. *Disease Management and Health Outcomes, 16*(4), 255-266. doi:10.2165/00115677-200816040-00006

International Federation of Social Workers. (2012, March 3). Statement of ethical principles. Retrieved December 13, 2015, from http://ifsw.org/policies/statement-of-ethical-principles/

Jerrell, J. M., & Sakarcan, A. (2009). Primary health care access, continuity, and cost among pediatric patients with obesity hypertension. *Journal of the National Medical Association, 101*(3), 223-228.

Kwapiszewski, R. M., & Wallace, A. L. (2011). A pilot program to identify and reverse childhood obesity in a primary care clinic. *Clinical Pediatrics, 50*(7), 630-635. doi:10.1177/0009922811398389

Laurson, K. R., Eisenmann, J. C., Welk, G. J., Wickel, E. E., Gentile, D. A., & Walsh, D. A. (2008). Combined influence of physical activity and screen time recommendations on childhood overweight. *Journal of Pediatrics, 153*(2), 209-214. doi:10.1016/j.jpeds.2008.02.042

Newby, P. K. (2009). Plant foods and plant-based diets: Protective against childhood obesity? *American Journal of Clinical Nutrition, 89*(5), 1572s-1587s. doi:10.3945/ajcn.2009.26736G

Ogden, C. L., Carroll, M. D., Kit, B. K., & Flegal, K. M. (2014). Prevalence of childhood and adult obesity in the United States, 2011-2012. *JAMA, 311*(8), 806-814. doi:10.1001/jama.2014.732

Public Health England. (2015). Child obesity. Retrieved December 14, 2015, from http://www.noo.org.uk/NOO_about_obesity/child_obesity

Trasande, L., & Chatterjee, S. (2009). The impact of obesity on health service utilization and costs in childhood. *Obesity (Silver Spring, Md), 17*(9), 1749-1754. doi:10.1038/oby.2009.67

Veugelers, P. J., & Fitzgerald, A. L. (2005). Prevalence of and risk factors for childhood overweight and obesity. *CMAJ: Canadian Medical Association Journal, 173*(6), 607-613. doi:10.1503/cmaj.050445

Wake, M., Baur, L. A., Gerner, B., Gibbons, K., Gold, L., Gunn, J., & The, L. E. A. P. (2009). Outcomes and costs of primary care surveillance and intervention for overweight or obese children: The LEAP 2 randomised controlled trial. *BMJ (Clinical Research ed.)*, *339*, b3308. doi:10.1136/bmj.b3308

Wang, L. Y., Denniston, M., Lee, S., Galuska, D., & Lowry, R. (2010). Long-term health and economic impact of preventing and reducing overweight and obesity and adolescence. *Journal of Adolescent Health: Official Publication of the Society for Adolescent Medicine*, *46*(5), 467-473. doi:10.1016/j.jadohealth.2009.11.204

Wheeler, D. (2015). NASW Standards and Indicators for Cultural Competence in Social Work Practice.

Retrieved December 14, 2015, from http://www.socialworkers.org/practice/standards/PRA-BRO-253150-CC-Standards.pdf

Whittemore, B. J., Smaldone, A., & Steiner, R. D. (2013). Endocrine and metabolic disorders. In C. E. Burns, A. M. Dunn, M. A. Brady, N. B. Starr, C. G. Blosser, & D. L. Garzon (Eds.), *Pediatric Primary Care* (5th ed., pp. 547-548). Philadelphia, PA: Elsevier Saunders.

Wright, D. R., Taveras, E. M., Gillman, M. W., Horan, C. M., Hohman, K. H., Gortmaker, S. L., & Prosser, L. A. (2014). The cost of a primary care-based childhood obesity prevention intervention. *BMC Health Services Research*, *14*(1), 44. doi:10.1186/1472-6963-14-44

OPEN ADOPTION

MAJOR CATEGORIES: Adoption/Foster Care, Child & Family

WHAT WE KNOW

Adoption is the permanent, legal transfer of parental rights and responsibilities for a child from the child's birth parents (BPs) to adoptive parents (APs), with the goal of ensuring that children whose BPs are unwilling or unable to care for them have a legal family to nurture and support them. Adoption is also understood to be a lifelong process involving complex, dynamic relationships between children, their biological families, and their adoptive families, with these relationships taking place in the context of the children's and their biological and adoptive families' communities and cultures.

Adoptions may be independent and private, with the BPs voluntarily making plans for the adoption of their children, most often during infancy; or may occur through a public agency, consisting of a state or county social service department that makes plans for the adoption of children into foster care when their BPs cannot provide a safe home and the BPs' parental rights have been terminated; or may be an intercountry adoption, in which case children of BPs in one country are adopted by foster parents in another country.

During much of the twentieth century, adoption in many Western countries involved a high degree of confidentiality and secrecy, which was designed to protect the children and families whom it involved from the stigma associated with birth to unmarried women, or, because of infertility in the children's families, birth to surrogate mothers, and also to prevent BPs from intruding in children's adoptive families. Over the past several decades, however, the practice in adoption has increasingly shifted towards more openness, both in the sharing of information with children about their origins and BPs, and in the amount of contact between the BPs and APs of adopted children and the children themselves. This often involves ongoing relationships of an adopted child and APs with the child's BPs, and contrasts with closed adoption practices. These closed practices emphasize that the adoptive parents are replacement parents for a child, and in which, at the time of adoption, APs are given only nonidentifying information about a child's BPs (physical characteristics, educational level, religion, family medical/mental health history), and no contact occurs between BPs and APs. Barriers to open adoption include some professionals' and families' belief that closed adoption avoids confusion, dual loyalties, and competition between BPs and APs, and protects children.

Two further types of adoptions are mediated adoptions and fully disclosed adoptions. Mediated, or semiopen, adoptions are those in which a designated third party, often the agency that manages the adoption, facilitates the exchange of nonidentifying information, letters, photographs, and/or gifts between BPs and APs, who do not have direct contact with one another. Approximately 40 percent of adoptions in the United States are mediated adoptions. Fully disclosed, or "open" adoptions, in which the BPs and APs of a child meet and exchange identifying information at the beginning of its adoption and continue to communicate over time, constitute 55 percent of current adoptions in the United States. Almost half of these families involved in open adoptions have ongoing visits with one another.

Children in private domestic adoptions are those most likely (68 percent) to have contact with their BPs. Only 39 percent of children adopted through public agencies and 6 percent of children in intercountry adoptions have contact with their BPs.

OPENNESS IN ADOPTION

Openness in adoption can be conceptualized in terms of communication openness and structural openness. "Communication openness" refers to APs' practices in terms of telling children that they were adopted, facilitating adoption-related conversations with children, and responding to children's needs for information and for emotional processing of their adoption. "Structural openness" refers to the continuum of contact between a child's birth family and its adoptive family, and ranges from the exchange of letters and/or phone calls to in-person visits with one another of adopted children, their APs, and their BPs.

Adoption communication varies on a continuum from restricted (in which children's adoption status is revealed to them in a single conversation) to open and ongoing communication by APs with their adopted children about their adoption. One study found that preparing APs for adoption communication during the adoption process, the comfort of APs in speaking about their adopted child's origins, empathy for the child's BPs, and APs having more

open communication with one another as a couple were associated with more open and regular adoption communication. Although in the past it was common practice not to tell children that they were adopted until adulthood, if at all, the vast majority (97 percent) of currently adopted children aged 5 years and older have been told that they were adopted.

Children's understanding of adoption, and their need for adoption-related information, changes over the course of their development. Adopted children first begin to learn the "language of adoption" while they are preschoolers. Although they cannot yet comprehend the difference between their family and those of other children, introducing the concept of adoption when children are of preschool age lays the groundwork for open communication about it as they mature. Children first recognize the significance of biological relationships, and that being adopted also means the loss of a birth family, when they are of school age. They begin to wonder about how they came to be adopted and whether their BPs think of them or miss them. Adolescents can better grasp the implications of adoption than can younger children, and can potentially begin to understand their BPs' life decisions. They begin to integrate adoption and their connection to their birth families and adoptive families into their emerging identities. Adoption-related issues can continue to reemerge during the adulthood of adopted children, sometimes triggered by milestones such as getting married, having a baby, or the death of an AP.

Postadoption contact is more likely when an adopted child's BPs and APs can establish open communication, roles, and boundaries with one another before the adoption of the child. An agreement between the BPs and APs for postadoption contact, made at the time of adoption, and whether an implied agreement or a legal one, also increases the likelihood of contact after adoption. In the United States, 26 states and the District of Columbia have statutes allowing enforceable postadoption contact agreements. Although the provisions in such statutes are typically limited to BPs, courts in some states allow other significant members of a child's birth family to be included in having contact with the child.

Ongoing contact in adoption is associated with APs' having more positive feelings about birth mothers, helps APs feel less threatened by the BPs' ties to the adopted child, is linked with greater satisfaction by both APs and birth mothers with the adoption process, is linked with better postadoption adjustment by birth mothers, and assists the adopted child to integrate both families into the child's sense of itself and attain a more positive sense of its identity.

Contact between APs and BPs or openness in their communication has not shown any association with externalizing behaviors in the adopted children, such as negative behaviors directed at other persons or situations, and including attention-deficit/hyperactivity disorder (ADHD) or oppositional defiant disorder (ODD). Nor has such contact or openness in communication shown any association with adopted children's emotional or behavioral development. A longitudinal study of families who adopted infants and maintained open adoption arrangements throughout these infants' childhoods found that APs viewed the experience positively and felt that it was in their adopted children's best interests. The adoptees, as young adults, reported experiencing contact with their birth families as a normal part of their lives, and benefiting from it in a variety of ways. Nevertheless, although postadoption contact is positive in many situations, it is is not always feasible or in the best interests of the child, and its potential benefits and risks should be assessed individually for each child and family.

Visits between BPs and APs most often involve the birth mother of an adopted child, and adoptive mothers tend to be more involved than adoptive fathers in facilitating contact with BPs; contact between birth fathers and children is less common. Children adopted through intercountry adoption or foster care are less likely than those adopted privately to have postadoption contact with their BPs. During adolescence, youths who have not had contact with their BPs may seek it on their own or may respond to contact from older siblings or members of their birth families.

In adoptions of children by public agencies, psychosocial issues of the children's BPs, previous maltreatment of the children, and the children's preexisting relationships with their birth families sometimes raise concern that postadoption contact with the BPs could jeopardize the children's physical and/or psychological safety and their adjustment to adoption.

WHAT CAN BE DONE

The social worker involved in an adoption should be knowledgeable about adoption and openness in adoption so as to be able to accurately assess the personal characteristics and education needs of the APs, BPs, and children involved in it. The social worker can educate BPs and APs about the benefits and challenges of their ongoing communication and/or contact in adoption, help them in assessing their own situations and needs, and determine whether ongoing communication or contact between them would be in the adopted child's and in their own best interests. In addition to this, the social worker can help to set the ground rules for such communication and provide education, coaching, and support to assist APs to establish and/or maintain age-appropriate openness in communicating with their children about adoption and adoption-related issues. Any agreements for the contact of APs, BPs, and children after adoption should be sufficiently flexible as to allow these participants' needs to change over time, and should not create stress or anxiety for the participants.

Social workers involved in adoption should be aware of their own cultural values, beliefs, and biases; learn about the histories, traditions, and values of the APs and BPs with whom they work; and adopt treatment methodologies that reflect the cultural needs of these parents and the children involved in an adoption.

By Jennifer Teska, MSW

Reviewed by Laura McLuckey, MSW, LCSW

REFERENCES

Baden, A. L., Gibbons, J. L., Wilson, S. L., & McGinnis, H. (2013). International adoption: Counseling and the adoption triad. *Adoption Quarterly, 16*(3/4), 218-237. doi:10.1080/10926755.2013.794440

Barbosa-Ducharne, M. A., & Soares, J. (2016). Process of adoption communication openness in adoptive families: Adopters' perspective. *Psicologia: Reflexão e Crítica, 29*, 9. doi:10.1186/s41155-016-0024-x

British Association of Social Workers. (2012, January). The code of ethics for social work: Statement of principles. Retrieved May 7, 2016

Brodzinsky, D. M. (2011). Children's understanding of adoption: Developmental and clinical implications. *Professional Psychology: Research and Practice, 42*(2), 200-207. doi:10.1037/a0022415

Brodzinsky, D., & Smith, S. L. (2014). Post-placement adjustment and the needs of birthmothers who place an infant for adoption. *Adoption Quarterly, 17*, 165-184. doi:10.1080/10926755.2014.891551

Child Welfare Information Gateway. (2011). Post-adoption contact agreements between birth and adoptive families. Washington, DC: U.S. Department of Health and Human Services, Children's Bureau.

Farr, R. H., Flood, M. E., & Grotevant, H. D. (2016). The role of siblings in adoption outcomes and experiences from adolescence to emerging adulthood. *Journal of Family Psychology, 30*(3), 386-396. doi:10.1037/fam0000173

Farr, R. H., Grant-Marsney, H. A., & Grotevant, H. D. (2014). Adoptees' contact with birth parents in emerging adulthood: The role of adoption communication and attachment to adoptive parents. *Family Processes, 53*(4), 656-671. doi:10.1111/famp.12069

Ge, X., Natsuaki, M. N., Martin, D. M., Neiderhiser, J. M., Villareal, G., ... Reiss, D. (2008). Bridging the divide: Openness in adoption and post-adoption psychosocial adjustment among birth and adoptive parents. *Journal of Family Psychology, 22*(4), 529-540. doi:10.1037/a0012817

Grotevant, H. D., Rueter, M., Von Korff, L., & Gonzalez, C. (2011). Post-adoption contact, adoption communicative openness, and satisfaction with contact as predictors of externalizing behavior in adolescence and emerging adulthood. *Journal of Child Psychology and Psychiatry, 52*(5), 529-536. doi:10.1111/j.1469-7610.2010.02330.x

Grotevant, H. D., Wrobel, G. M., Von Korff, L., Skinner, B., Newell, J., Friese, S., & McRoy, R. G. (2008). Many faces of openness in adoption: Perspectives of adopted adolescents and their parents. *Adoption Quarterly, 10*(3-4), 79-101. doi:10.1080/10926750802163204

International Federation of Social Workers. (2012). Statement of ethical principles. Retrieved March 14, 2016, from http://ifsw.org/policies/statement-of-ethical-principles/

Juffer, F., Palacios, J., Le Mare, L., Sonuga-Barke, E. J. S., Tieman, W., ... Verhulst, F. C. (2011). Development of adopted children with histories of early adversity. *Monographs of the Society for Research in Child Development, 76*(4), 31-61. doi:10.1111/j.1540-5834.2011.00627.x

Logan, J. (2013). Contemporary adoptive kinship: A contribution to new kinship studies. *Child & Family Social Work, 18*(1), 35-45. doi:10.1111/cfs.12042

Mizrahi, T., & Davis, L. E. (Eds.). (2008). Adoption. In *Encyclopedia of Social Work* (20th ed., pp. 33-44). Washington, DC: NASW Press and Oxford University Press, Inc.

Neil, E. (2012). Making sense of adoption: Integration and differentiation from the perspective of adopted children in middle childhood. *Children and Youth Services Review, 34*(2), 409-416. doi:10.1016/j.childyouth.2011.11.011

Sales, S. (2015). Contested attachments: Rethinking adoptive kinship in the era of open adoption. *Child & Family Social Work, 20*(2), 149-158. doi:10.1111/cfs.12062

Siegel, D. H. (2013). Open adoption: Adoptive parents' reactions two decades later. *Social Work, 58*(1), 43-52. doi:10.1093/sw/sws053

Siegel, D. H., & Smith, S. L. (2012, March). Openness in adoption: From secrecy and stigma to knowledge and connections. *Evan B. Donaldson Adoption Institute.* NY: Evan B. Donaldson Adoption Institute. Retrieved March 7, 2016, from http://adoptioninstitute.org/old/publications/2012_03_OpennessInAdoption.pdf

Vandivere, S., Malm, K., & Radel, L. (2009). *Adoption USA: A chartbook based on the 2007 National Survey of Adoptive Parents.* Washington, D.C.: U.S. Department of Health and Human Services, Office of the Assistant Secretary for Planning and Evaluation.

Wright, L., Flynn, C. C., & Welch, W. (2006). Adolescent adoption and the birthfamily. *Journal of Public Child Welfare, 1*(1), 35-63. doi:10.1300/J479v01n01_03

ORPHANS: A GLOBAL PERSPECTIVE ON FOSTER CARE & ADOPTION

MAJOR CATEGORIES: Adoption/Foster Care

DESCRIPTION

Poverty, underdevelopment, natural disasters, epidemics, and war are conditions that produce a staggering number of orphans worldwide. The term orphan has been applied loosely throughout history, often to include children who are homeless, abandoned, or neglected. The United Nations Children's Education Fund (UNICEF) defines an orphan as a child who has lost one or both parents. Eighty percent of the world's orphans, amounting to more than 17.9 million children, live in sub-Saharan Africa (UNICEF, 2011). Most of these children are described as "true" or "double" orphans, having lost both parents to acquired immune deficiency syndrome (AIDS). A study in Zimbabwe found that in a sample of orphans, 40% had lost both parents through illnesses related to infection by human immunodeficiency virus (HIV), and that 17% had lost both parents through other causes (Mhaka-Mutepfa et al., 2014). It is well established that orphaned children experience more deficits in education, socialization, and nutrition than do non-orphaned children. Addressing the care of orphaned children requires an understanding of interconnected issues concerning local and kinship foster care and adoption; orphanage placements; and international adoption. In Nepal, a study reported in 2013 found that 70% of orphans living with HIV/AIDS were in kinship care settings, whereas 30% were in institutional care (Acharya et al., 2013). The Nepalese children who were in kinship care had more positive and optimistic outlooks on life and had more friends than those in institutional care (Acharya et al., 2013).

However, the large numbers of orphaned children in developing countries, especially in Africa, puts a strain on the traditional system of kinship care, in which children whose biological parents are deceased or unable to care for them are raised by relatives or close family friends. In many cases, family members who are not parents are too young or too old to adequately care for a child of relatives, and many cannot afford the care required for an additional child or children. For these and other reasons, many children taken in by relatives are treated differently from biological children; they often are subjected to discrimination and experience deprivation and exclusion.

Many become ill. Many children in kinship care have inadequate food, clothing, shelter, and education. Some children leave these situations to live on the streets, where they are vulnerable to other forms of abuse. Recruitment to armies and other types of forced labor, and recruitment into organized criminality, as well as exposure to sexual and physical abuse, prostitution, sexually transmitted diseases (STDs), and substance use, are common experiences among orphaned children in developing countries.

Children for whom kinship care is not an option may be raised in orphanages. However, large numbers of orphanages in developing countries lack adequate funding and have inadequate physical facilities and management. Although some orphanages provide consistent caregiving that is supportive and can help foster healthy attachment relationships, others are equipped only to meet the basic physical needs of children. Some researchers have found that orphanages can be detrimental to the psychosocial and physical development of children, especially children who have been traumatized by war. In contrast, other researchers have determined that children living in these institutions can have positive outcomes. Generalizations about institutional care should be avoided. Some community-based orphanages, even those described as existing in low-resource conditions (e.g., lacking clean water, lacking adequate physical facilities, lacking funding), try to mirror a familial environment and have the potential to meet children's developmental needs. It is important to note that a good-quality foster or adopting family environment is always optimal, and is described as the most significant factor in addressing childhood traumatization.

Although Africa in particular has many orphans and faces a crisis in the provision of orphan care, the countries of Africa do not generally support international adoption, and only a small number now permit it. Community-based solutions, such as kinship foster/adoption or familial-type orphanages, are considered preferable, but some scholars are encouraging international adoption in Africa as another option. Most orphaned children adopted by families in the United States from institutions in African countries arrive in the United States with attachment disorders or cognitive, social, or physical deficits from prolonged deprivation. The longer children have spent in poorly resourced orphanages, the more behavioral and other problems adopting parents encounter. Researchers studying Guatemalan orphans found that those who had been placed in Guatemalan foster care before adoption in the United States had better overall outcomes than those adopted from institutions (Miller et al., 2005). Research has shown that children with a range of difficulties at the time of their arrival for foster care can display remarkable gains when placed in stable families with adequate resources to address any medical or psychological needs (Judge, 2004).

Children in institutions that focus on strong caregiver-child interactions and attachments have shown improved social, emotional, mental, and physical development. In countries in which orphan and other homeless children cannot be deinstitutionalized, efforts to improve the existing institutions can improve child outcomes. These improvements may include lower caregiver-to-child ratios, improved physical facilities, and increased screening for any developmental issues (McCall, 2013). Some countries that rely heavily on kinship care for orphans are attempting to formulate official community-based orphan care programs that provide supplementary care and schooling for these children and funding for their caregivers (Maundeni & Malinga-Musamba, 2013).

The motivations of persons wishing to adopt a child from another country vary, but reasons commonly given are wanting to give a home to a disadvantaged child; general love for children; wanting to start a family; wanting to help with a refugee situation; or a desire to add to one's family.

FACTS AND FIGURES

In fiscal year 2013, there were 7,092 adoptions in the United States of children from other nations, a decrease from 8,668 in 2012 and from 22,734 in 2005 (U.S. Department of State, 2015). The five countries of origin of children adopted in the United States in 2013, in order from the most to the least number of children adopted, were China, Ethiopia, Russia, South Korea, and Ukraine (U.S. Department of State, 2015). Of the children involved in these adoptions, 7.6% were under 12 months of age, 37.8% were between 1 and 2 years old, 16% were between 3 and 4 years old, 28.6% were between 5 and 12 years

old, 9.3% were between 13 and 17 years old, and 0.6% were young adults 18 years old or older (U.S. Department of State, 2015).

RISK FACTORS

As noted earlier, diseases such as HIV/AIDS, and more recently Ebola, have created large numbers of orphans in some countries. Poverty and its resulting challenges can also increase the risk that a child will be orphaned. Children in kinship care or orphanages are vulnerable to developmental issues, human trafficking, or abuse. Also, because intercountry adoption is driven by demand, families in some countries may be coerced into allowing their children to be adopted rather than being informed of social services that may offer support and assistance that would allow the child to remain in the home. Besides this, prospective adopters are at risk of becoming engaged in fraudulent adoption practices, and may also experience emotional difficulties from the stresses related to foreign adoption. These stresses may include extended time frames for the completion of an international adoption, changes in various countries' policies on international adoptions while such adoptions are taking place, or countries shutting down all foreign adoptions even after a prospective family has been matched with a child.

SIGNS AND SYMPTOMS of Problems in Internationally Adopted Children

Families and other groups seeking to adopt orphaned children internationally can anticipate their experiencing signs and symptoms of developmental difficulties (e.g., developmental delays, attachment issues, health problems), particularly when a particular child has spent an extended period in an orphanage that lacked resources or that provided limited caregiving. The child may also have physical symptoms of borth defects, injury, and illness, such as a cleft lip and palate, stunted growth, heart disease, orthopedic issues, malnutrition, and infections.

APPLICABLE LAWS AND REGULATIONS

A child should not be considered legally available for adoption until the following three conditions are met: (1) the child meets the legal qualifications of eligibility for adoption of both the child's country of origin and the receiving country; (2) the adoption is determined to be in the best interest of the child; and

(3) a valid consent process has been completed with the child's biological family.

The United Nations Convention on the Rights of the Child is an international human rights treaty that recognizes that every child is entitled certain basic rights, including the child's best interests as the primary concern in decisions that affect the child, the right of a child to be raised by its own parent(s) or cultural group if possible, and the right to have a relationship with its parent(s) even if separated from them.

In international adoption, the laws of both the country in which the child lives and those of the country in which the adoptive parents live govern the process of adoption. In addition to these laws, countries may be party to the Hague Convention on Intercountry Adoption (HCIA) of 1993, which the United States ratified in 2008 and which acts as an international law, establishes procedural safeguards for intercountry adoption, and imposes additional requirements for adoption. A requirement of the Hague Convention is that prospective adopters be trained in the issues surrounding transracial adoption.

There are two processes for adopting internationally, depending on whether the country of origin is or is not a part to the Hague Convention. A fact sheet the legal requirements for international adoption set forth in the Hague Convention can be found at https://www.childwelfare.gov/pubs/factsheets/hague.pdf

ADOPTION PROCEDURE

Persons interested in international adoption typically proceed through the following steps:

Step 1: Become educated about international adoption.

Step 2: Have an understanding of the laws pertaining to adoption in the adoptive child's country of origin and their own country.

Step 3: Select an agency through which they can explore options for adoption. The social worker may be employed by this adoption agency or may be working with the persons interested in adoption in another capacity and be providing support for them as they pursue adoption.

Step 4: Complete a detailed home/family study conducted through a state adoption agency.

Step 5: Select a child for adoption.

Step 6: File the necessary legal documents for adoption.

A home/family study will be conducted during the foster or adoption application process for adoption or foster care. In addition to information gathering, this process includes the education and preparation of prospective parents, and can take from 2 to 10 months. The social worker assisting the persons seeking to adopt a child, or working with a foster-care setting for the child, should have access to any screening tools for abnormal behavior that have been used with the child.

Screenings of the child should be done for infectious diseases, hematologic issues, metabolic disorders, nutritional status, delayed development, and lead exposure, and a toxicology screening for drug and/or alcohol use may be done on the prospective adoptive parents or investigation for a medical history of drug and/or alcohol use made be done on the child's biological parents.

International adoption has been a controversial matter. Concerns have been raised globally about how children become available for adoption, the suitability of the adopting families for child care, and the regulation of the agencies or intermediaries involved in the adoption process. Persons who wish to adopt internationally but have concerns about the process for this can obtain relevant information about each step in the process at the Child Welfare Information Gateway, https://www.childwelfare.gov/pubPDFs/f_inter.pdf. This web site can help such persons in finding support and advice about foreign adoption; ensure that the persons interested in adoption has engaged a reputable adoption agency and is not being taken advantage of; and provide the client with emotional support and counseling for coping with the stresses and anxieties related to foreign adoptions.

Social workers participating in international adoptions should be aware of their own cultural values, beliefs, and biases, and develop specialized knowledge about the histories, traditions, and values of the children, families, and foster-care organizations with which they work. They should adopt treatment methods that reflect their knowledge of the cultural diversity of the communities in which they practice.

Social workers involved in international adoption need to recognize that in many countries where kinship care is utilized, such arrangements may not be subject to the legal requirements, reimbursements, or formal oversight that exist in more developed countries.

The existence of fraud and corruption in international adoption has important implications for social work: social workers involved in global adoption, including those who work with families involved in global adoption, need to be aware of the legal and ethical procedures pertaining to adoption in both the countries of origin and those of placement of the children for whom adoption is planned, and to speak up publicly if they encounter fraudulent or dangerous practices.

SERVICES AND RESOURCES
The following resources are available for information about international adoption:

- Center for Adoption Support and Education, http://adoptionsupport.org/
- About Social Workers, "Help Starts Here," http://www.helpstartshere.org/tag/adoption
- Bureau of Consular Affairs, U.S. Department of State, "Intercountry Adoption," http://adoption.state.gov
- UNICEF, http://www.unicefusa.org – search on adoption
- Holt International Children's Services, http://www.holtinternational.org/
- National Council for Adoption, http://www.adoptioncouncil.org/

Written by Jan Wagstaff, MA, MSW, and Jessica Therivel, LMSW-IPR

Reviewed by Lynn B. Cooper, D. Crim, and Laura McLuckey, MSW, LCSW

REFERENCES
Acharya, S. L., Pokhrel, B. R., Ayer, R., Belbase, P., Ghimire, M., & Gurung, O. (2013). *Journal of Nepal Health Research Council, 11*(23), 22-25.

Ahmad, A., & Mohamed, K. (1996). The socioemotional development of orphans in orphanages and traditional foster care in Iraqi Kurdistan. *Child Abuse & Neglect, 20*(12), 1161-1173.

Ahmad, A., Qahar, J., Siddiq, A., Majeed, A., Rasheed, J., Jabar, F., & von Knorring, A. L. (2005). A 2-year follow-up of orphans' competence, socioemotional problems and post-traumatic stress symptoms in traditional foster care and orphanages in Iraqi Kurdistan. *Child: Care, Health & Development, 32*(2), 203-215.

Boone, J. L., Hostetter, M. K., & Weitzman, C. C. (2003). The predictive accuracy of pre-adoption video review in adoptees from Russian and Eastern European orphanages. *Clinical Pediatrics, 42*(7), 585-590.

Breuning, M. (2013). What explains openness to intercountry adoption?. *Social Science Quarterly, 94*(1), 113-130. doi:10.1111/j.1540-6237.2012.00902.x

Feast, J., Grant, M., Rushton, A., & Simmonds, J. (2013). The British Chinese adoption study: Planning a study of lifecourse and outcomes. *European Journal of Social Work, 16*(3), 344-359. doi:10.1080/13691457.2012.660906

Freivalds, S. (2004). Wanting a daughter, needing a son: Abandonment, adoption and orphanage care in China [Review of the book by Johnson, K. A.]. *Adoption Quarterly, 7*(3), 93-95.

Judge, S. (2004). Adoptive families: The effects of early relational deprivation in children adopted from Eastern European orphanages. *Journal of Family Nursing, 10*(3), 338-356.

Lee, L. M., & Fleming, P. L. (2003). Estimated number of children left motherless by AIDS in the United States, 1978-1998. *Journal of Acquired Immune Deficiency Syndromes, 34*(2), 231-236.

Maundeni, T., & Malinga-Musamba, T. (2013). The role of informal caregivers in the well-being of orphans in Botswana: A literature review. *Child and Family Social Work, 18*(2), 107-116. doi:10.1111/j.1365-2206.2011.00820.x

McCall, R. B. (2013). Review: The consequences of early institutionalization: Can institutions be improved? Should they? *Child and Adolescent Mental Health, 18*(4), 193-201. doi:10.1111/camh.12025

Mhaka-Mutepfa, M., Cumming, R., & Mpofu, E. (2014). Grandparents fostering orphans: Influences of protective factors on their health and well-being. *Health Care for Women International, 35*(7-9), 1022-1039. doi:10.1080/07399332.2014.916294

Miller, L., Chan, W., Comfort, K., & Tirella, L. (2005). Health of children adopted from Guatemala: Comparison of orphanage and foster care. *Pediatrics, 115*(6), e710-e117.

Mizrahi, T., & Mayden, R. W. (2001). NASW Standards for Cultural Competence in Social Work Practice. Retrieved October 5, 2015, from http://www.socialworkers.org/practice/standards/NASWCulturalStandards.pdf

O'Sullivan, J., & McMahon, M. F. (2006). Who will care for me? The debate of orphanages versus foster care. *Policy, Politics & Nursing Practice, 7*(2), 142-148.

Roby, J.L., Rotabi, K., & Bunkers, K. M. (2013). Social justice and intercountry adoptions: The role of the U.S. social work community. *Social Work, 58*(4), 295-303. doi:10.1093/sw/swt033

Roby, J. L., & Shaw, S. A. (2006). The African orphan crisis and international adoption. *Social Work, 51*(3), 199-210.

Sanou, D., O'Brien, H., Ouedraogo, S., & Desrosiers, T. (2008). Caring for orphans and vulnerable children in a context of poverty and cultural transition: A case study of a group foster home programme in Burkina-Faso. *Journal of Children and Poverty, 14*(2), 139-155.

Tseng, W. S., Ebata, K., Miguchi, M., Egawa, M., & McLaughlin, D. G. (1990). Transethnic adoption and personality traits: A lesson from Japanese orphans returned from China to Japan. *American Journal of Psychiatry, 147*(3), 330-335.

Wallis, A., Dukay, V., & Mellins, C. (2010). Power and empowerment: Fostering effective collaboration in meeting the needs of orphans and vulnerable children. *Global Public Health, 5*(5), 509-522.

PAIN MANAGEMENT IN CHILDREN

MAJOR CATEGORIES: Child & Family, Medical & Health

WHAT WE KNOW

Acute pain and chronic pain can both occur in children, with chronic pain often creating serious health problems and pain-related disability (e. g., an interference with social and physical functioning such as school absence, missing sports or other activities) in those children affected by pain.

Acute pain results from a negative stimulus in the form of an attack from a mechanical source (e. g., pressure, swelling, growth of a tumor), a chemical source (e. g., toxic substance, buildup of lactic acid in the muscles), or a thermal source (e. g., extreme heat or cold).

Acute pain serves to act as a warning system against further injury or damage. Acute pain usually is caused by an injury, surgery, swelling, or an unknown source but typically dissipates after an anticipated period of time with healing.

Inadequate treatment of acute pain in children is common among healthcare professionals and may be due, at least in part, to difficulty assessing pain intensity in children, concern regarding administering opiate analgesia (e. g., morphine) to children, lack of training and experience, difficulty locating vascular access for an IV, and refusal by the child to take medication.

Inadequate pain management in children is associated with poor outcomes including delayed wound healing, inflammation, change in immune function, more intense pain response in subsequent painful experiences, and chronic pain.

Chronic pain can have more than one causal factor, does not usually involve nociceptive pain activation (i. e., pain from a physical cause such as a burn or broken leg), and does not serve as a protective or warning system. The intensity of chronic pain may not be in proportion to objective measurements or findings.

Chronic pain persists beyond the expected time of healing and lasts indefinitely, either as a constant pain or in an intermittent state. When treating chronic pain, the focus may need to change from trying to cure the pain to determining how to manage it.

Management of pain in children, especially children with chronic pain, must take into account that pain is a constantly changing combination of physical processes, psychological factors, social and cultural contexts, and the developmental trajectory of the child.

Biological and physical factors that need to be considered are the child's age, sex, genetic factors, and comorbid conditions.

Children grow and develop throughout the course of the pain, which makes pediatric chronic pain different from chronic pain in adults. The pain experienced by a child with type 1 diabetes, for instance, may differ in severity when he or she is 7 years old versus when he or she is 12.

Chronic pain is often more common as children approach puberty.

Anxiety, depression, and low self-esteem are psychological issues that often are present as a result of chronic pain.

Chronic pain can have a negative effect on socialization skills: children with chronic pain are more likely to have problems with victimization by other children, difficulty making friends, and self-isolation.

Children coping with chronic pain often have many school absences and trouble maintaining social contacts and appropriate social development as a result. School absence also affects parents, who may have to stay home with the child and miss work and socialization opportunities of their own.

The most common chronic illnesses that result in chronic pain in children are sickle cell disease, cancer, juvenile arthritis, and hemophilia.

Chronic pain in children often manifests as headaches, abdominal pain, back pain, or musculoskeletal pain.

Sickle cell disease is characterized by pain that is unpredictable, recurrent, persistent, and severe.

Accurate pain assessment in children is necessary because pain in children often is underreported, underdiagnosed, and not treated appropriately.

Drug absorption, distribution, and metabolism in children vary and are not always dependent on age and weight, so standard dosing protocols may not be appropriate. Accurate pain assessment is important.

Different pain-assessment scales are recommended for different age groups.

For children aged 2 months to 7 years, behavioral/physiological scales suitable for nonverbal children may be used, such as the FLACC (Face, Legs, Activity, Cry, Consolability) scale.

For children aged 4 years and older a graphic scale may be used, such as a color analog that moves from red to green to indicate level of pain.

Children aged 3 years and up can use a FACES scale, which is a simplified scoring tool using cartoon faces to indicate level of pain.

Children aged 7 years and up can understand and use a numerical rating scale, verbal or written, that asks them to rate their pain on a scale from 0 to 10.

Self-reports of pain in school-aged children can be accurate, but healthcare providers often do not assess pediatric clients by asking if they are in pain.

The authors of a study in an emergency department found that 40 percent of pediatric patients studied left the emergency department in moderate to severe pain. In the same study, children who felt they could communicate with the provider had higher patient satisfaction scores.

If children attempt to fake pain with facial expressions, parents and healthcare providers generally are able to detect the deception, but they sometimes miss suppressed pain when children try to hide pain.

Therapy is often multimodal in children with pain, with most children receiving pharmacology as part of their treatment plan. Many of the medications used in pediatric pain management may not have been approved for pediatric use or approved for the specific pain for which they are prescribed, especially when the pain is complex and chronic.

The most commonly prescribed medications for pain in children are acetaminophen and nonsteroidal anti-inflammatory drugs (NSAIDs) (e. g., ibuprofen), opioids (e. g., morphine, fentanyl, methadone), antidepressants, and anticonvulsants.

The main focus of any psychological intervention for pain control is to modify the child's subjective pain experience, maximize adaptive behaviors, and minimize negative behaviors. These interventions may include psychoeducation, cognitive behavioral therapy (CBT), guided imagery, and relaxation techniques.

Researchers utilizing a systematic review found that psychological interventions were beneficial in reducing pain intensity and disability, with 56 percent of the experimental subjects having reduced pain scores after treatment compared with only 22 percent of the control groups.

CBT is a common intervention in pain management for children.

A typical CBT intervention for pain will include relaxation training, cognitive therapy that works on identifying and changing negative thoughts, and behavior therapy that is directed toward the child (e. g., changing any maladaptive coping behaviors related to pain) but may also be directed toward the parent to work on the parent's negative thoughts and maladaptive behaviors (e. g., minimizing parental attention given to pain and helping the parent support the child in applying coping skills, improving parental coping skills, providing psychoeducation).

Acceptance and change therapy (ACT) is a CBT technique based on the concept that negative emotions, fear, negative memories, and pain symptoms will have a negative influence on behavior and can lead to avoidance and inflexibility. The client is taught to alter the associations he or she may have between pain and these negative thoughts and emotions in order to positively change behavior and improve functioning. By accepting the pain, the client can create positive coping strategies versus putting the pain into a negative construct.

Problem-solving skills training (PSST) uses modeling, behavior rehearsal, and performance feedback to teach problem-solving skills.

In a PSST program was developed for parents trying to manage chronic pain in children, the parents may learn how to identify automatic thoughts and feelings, generate positive self-statements, and generate approaches to positive problem-solving.

Researchers found that parents who underwent PSST had measurably improved problem-solving skills, decreased depressive symptoms, improved mood, and decreased catastrophic thinking.

Guided imagery is a cognitive-behavioral technique in which the social worker utilizes imaginary pictures, sounds, or sensations with the child to reduce or eliminate pain and/or the anxiety, fear, and tension that are connected to the pain.

The technique uses relaxation training, visualization, and positive suggestion.

Guided imagery has had success in children with sickle cell disease. Study authors found that children who used guided imagery had a significant increase in their sense of self-efficacy, had fewer pain episodes, and used less pain medication than children who did not use guided imagery.

Guided imagery is intended to teach the client how to shift focus from his or her pain and discomfort to more comfortable or enjoyable thoughts. Guided imagery should be avoided with clients who are actively psychotic, are unable to think abstractly, are unable to distinguish reality from fantasy, have hallucinations or delusions, or have moderate to advanced dementia or other cognitive issues that affect communication.

Common guided imagery techniques for pain include the following:

- Creating a mental image for the pain and then transforming that image into a more manageable or less frightening image;
- Imagining the pain disappearing;
- Imagining the pain as something that one has complete control over (e. g., if the pain is visualized as an electric current, the client can turn the electric switch off).

The coping skills and coping style of parents, and their self-efficacy regarding managing their child's pain, influence outcomes for children.

Catastrophic thinking by a parent of a child with pain can have adverse outcomes for both the parent and the child. Parents who engage in catastrophic thinking may have an increased risk for anxiety or depressive symptoms and their child may have increased pain intensity and decreased quality of life.

Catastrophic thinking may lead to avoiding activities that might increase pain. If a child continually avoids certain situations due to catastrophic thoughts related to pain, his or her disability can increase.

Parents trying to manage a child's pain at home after surgery often have concerns about administering pain medication and being able to manage the child's pain.

Even when children were reporting moderate pain, parents in one study were still only providing one half to two thirds of the amount of pain medication that was approved by the physician's orders. Parents were often giving the lowest dose and fewer doses per day even after receiving an education intervention.

WHAT CAN BE DONE

Learn about pain management in children to accurately assess the individuals' personal characteristics and health education needs.

Develop an awareness of your own cultural values, beliefs, and biases as well as the histories, traditions, and values of the individual in need of care. Look for treatment methodologies that reflect the cultural needs of clients.

Understand the differences between acute and chronic pain.

Ensure that pediatric clients are having pain accurately assessed.

Provide or refer clients to the appropriate specialists who can offer interventions to try to improve management of chronic pain.

Recognize that parents' negative thoughts can have a negative effect on a child's pain behaviors, so the parents may need to be targeted for interventions.

Educate parents returning home with children after surgery on proper pain management, including assessing for severity of pain, administering pain medication on a regular schedule, and ensuring that their child is adequately hydrated.

Familiarize yourself with the common pharmacological treatments for pain in children.

Written by Jessica Therivel, LMSW-IPR

Reviewed by Laura Gale, LCSW

REFERENCES

Altilio, T. (2011). In T. Mizrahi & L. E. Davis (Eds.), *Encyclopedia of social work: Vol.3, J-R* (1st ed., Vol.3, pp.335-337). Washington, D. C. : NASW Press.

Barrie, J., & Loughlin, D. (2014). Managing chronic pain in adults. *Nursing Standard, 29*(7), 50-58. doi:10.7748/ns.29.7.50. e9099

Boerner, K. E., Chambers, C. T., Craig, K. D., Riddell, R. R. P., & Parker, J. A. (2012). Caregiver accuracy in detecting deception in facial expressions of pain in children. *PAIN, 154*(4), 525-533. doi:10.1016/j. pain.2012.12.015

Brasher, C., Gafsous, B., Dugue, S., Thiollier, A., Kinderf, J., Nivoche, Y.,... Dahmani, S. (2914). Postoperative pain management in children and infants: An update. *Paediatric Drugs, 16*(2), 129-140. doi:10.1007/s40272-013-0062-0

British Association of Social Workers. (2012, January). The Code of Ethics for Social Work: Statement of Principles. Retrieved November 25, 2015, from http://cdn. basw.co.uk/upload/basw_112315-7.pdf

Burnett, J. (2012, October). Guided imagery as an adjunct to pharmacological pain control at end of life. Paper presented at North American Association of Christians in Social Work (NACSW) Convention, October, 2012, St. Louis, MO. Retrieved November 25, 2015, from http://www.nacsw.org/Publications/Proceedings2012/BurnettJGuidedImagery.pdf

Dobson, C. E., & Byrne, M. W. (2014). Original research: Using guided imagery to manage pain in young children with sickle cell disease. *AJN, 114*(4), 26-36. doi:10.1097/01. NAJ.0000445680.06812.6a

Eccleston, C., Palermo, T. M., Williams, A. C., Lewandowski Holley, A., Morley, S., Fisher, E., & Law, E. (2014). Psychological therapies for the management of chronic and recurrent pain in children and adolescents. *Cochrane Database of Systematic Reviews*, Issue 5. Art. No. : CD003968. doi:10.1002/14651858. CD003968. pub4

Dorkham, M. C., Chalkiadis, G. A., von Ungern Sternberg, B. S., & Davidson, A. J. (2014). Effective postoperative pain management of children after ambulatory surgery, with a focus on tonsillectomy: Barriers and possible solutions. *Paediatric Anesthesia, 24*(3), 239-248. doi:10.1111/pan.12327

Forgeron, P. A., & Stinson, J. (2014). Fundamentals of chronic pain in children and young people. Part 1. *Nursing Children and Young People, 26*(8), 29-34. doi:10.7748/ncyp.26.8.29. e498

Fortier, M. A., Wahi, A., Bruce, C., Maurer, E. L., & Stevenson, R. (2014). Pain management at home in children with cancer: A daily diary study. *Pediatric Blood & Cancer, 61*(6), 1029-1033. doi:10.1002/pbc.24907

Grégoire, M.-C., & Finley, G. A. (2013). Drugs for chronic pain in children: A commentary on clinical practice and the absence of cvidence. *Pain Research & Management, 18*(1), 47-50.

Hofmann, S. G., Sawyer, A. T., & Fang, A. (2010). The empirical status of the "New Wave" of cognitive behavioral therapy. *The Psychiatric Clinics of North America, 33*(3), 701-710. doi:10.1016/j. psc.2010.04.006

International Federation of Social Workers. (2012, March 3). Statement of Ethical Principles. Retrieved November 25, 2015, from http://ifsw.org/policies/statement-of-ethical-principles/

Johnson, P. N., Miller, J. L., & Hagemann, T. M. (2012). Sedation and analgesia in critically ill children. *AACN Advanced Critical Care, 23*(4), 415-434. doi:10.1097/NCI.0b013e31826b4dea

Kozlowski, L. J., Kost-Byerly, S., Colantuoni, E., Thompson, C. B., Vasquenza, K. J., Rothman, S. K.,... Yaster. (2014). Pain prevalence intensity, assessment and management in a hospitalized pediatric population. *Pain Management Nursing, 15*(1), 22-35. doi:10.1016/j. pmn.2012.04.003

Langer, S. L., Romano, J. M., Mancl, L., & Levy, R. L. (2014). Parental catastrophizing partially mediates the association between parent-reported child pain behavior and parental protective responses. *Pain Research and Treatment, 2014*, 751097. Advance online publication. doi:10.1155/2014/751097

Maxwell, L. G., Buckley, G. M., Kudchadkar, S. R., Ely, E., Stebbins, E. L., Dube, C.,... Yaster, M. (2014). Pain management following major intracranial surgery in pediatric patients: A prospective cohort study in three academic children's hospitals. *Paediatric Anaesthesia, 24*(11), 1132-1140. doi:10.1111/pan.12489

Murphy, A., Barrett, M. A., Cronin, J., McCoy, S., Larkin, P., Brenner, M.,... O'Sullivan, R. (2014). A qualitative study of the barriers to prehospital management of acute pain in children. *Emergency Medicine Journal, 31*(6), 493-498. doi:10.1136/emermed-2012-202166

National Association of Social Workers. (2005). How social workers help with pain management. Retrieved November 25, 2015, from http://www.helpstartshere.org/health-and-wellness/pain/

pain-how-social-workers-help-with-pain-management. html

Palermo, T. M., Law, E. F., Essner, B., Jessen-Fiddick, T., & Eccleston, C. (2014). Adaptation of problem-solving skills training (PSST) for parent caregivers of youth with chronic pain. *Clinical Practice in Pediatric Psychology, 2*(3), 212-223.

Stinson, J., & Naser, B. (2003). Pain management in children with sickle cell disease. *Paediatric Drugs, 5*(4), 229-241.

van der Veek, S. M. C., Derkx, B. H. F., Benninga, M. A., Boer, F., & de Haan, E. (2013). Cognitive behavior therapy for pediatric functional abdominal pain: A randomized controlled trial. *Pediatrics, 132*(5), e1163-e1172. doi:10.1542/peds.2013-0242

Vincent, C., Chiappetta, M., Beach, A., Kiolbasa, C., Latta, K., Maloney, R., & Van Roeyen, L. S. (2012). Parents' management of children's pain at home after surgery. *Journal for Specialists in Pediatric Nursing, 17*(2), 108-120. doi:10.11 11/j.1744-6155.2012.00326. x

Weingarten, L., Kircher, J., Drendel, A. L., Newton, A. S., & Ali, S. (2014). A survey of children's perspectives on pain management in the emergency department. *The Journal of Emergency Medicine, 47*(3), 268-276. doi:10.1016/j. jemermed.2014.01.038

Wheeler, D. (2015). NASW standards and indicators for cultural competence in social work practice. Retrieved November 25, 2015, from http://www. socialworkers.org/practice/standards/PRA-BRO-253150-CC-Standards.pdf

Yellon, R. F., Kenna, M. A., Cladis, F. P., Mcghee, W., & Davis, P. J. (2014). What is the best non-codeine postadenotonsillectomy pain management for children? *Laryngoscope, 124*(8), 1737-1738. doi:10.1002/lary.24599

PAIN MANAGEMENT: BIOFEEDBACK

MAJOR CATEGORIES: Medical & Health

WHAT WE KNOW

Biofeedback utilizes specific devices to monitor an individual's physical reaction to stress, which can cause pain or intensify pain symptoms. The device displays either auditory or visual information that reports the presence of stress to the client so the client can learn how to control and calm his or her physical reactions.

Pain and stress are closely linked: fear of pain causes stress and chronic pain amplifies the effect of stressors (e. g., emotional distress, physical

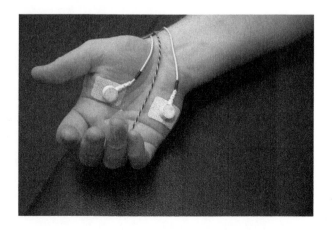

discomfort, anxiety). Biofeedback is a method to help clients understand this connection and gain awareness and control.

Biofeedback is meant to help clients identify, understand, and eventually control their physical, mental, and emotional responses to stress and pain. Biofeedback can also be effective in pediatric use for pain management. Investigators found that when children with frequent or severe headaches participated in two biofeedback sessions they experienced a greater than 50 percent reduction in headaches in a one-week period.

There are various modalities of biofeedback utilized for pain management, including electromyographic (EMG), electroencephalographic (EEG), temperature (i. e., thermal), electrodermal (i. e., galvanic), and heart rate variability (HRV).

In EMG muscle tension is measured by sensors or electrodes placed on the skin over particular muscle groups. The electrodes monitor the electrical activity that is causing the muscles to contract. EMG is most commonly used with back pain, neck pain, tension headaches, jaw pain, and fibromyalgia.

For example, if a client has identified shoulder muscles as being involved in his or her pain experience, a sensor placed on the shoulder muscle may relay a tone or beep when the muscle tenses or may show a visual cue on a monitor (e. g., a flower closing when the muscle tenses and opening when the muscle relaxes).

EEG biofeedback uses sensors placed on the scalp to monitor and measure the brain's electrical activity and provide visual or audio cues to the client to indicate stress reactions. For management of pain this form of biofeedback is most commonly used with headaches and pain related to traumatic brain injuries.

Thermal biofeedback employs sensors placed on the hands or feet to measure skin temperature. Individuals experiencing stress or pain often have lowered temperatures in their hands and feet because of decreased blood flow to the extremities. Clients who can learn to warm their hands or feet may experience a relaxation response. Thermal biofeedback is effective with many types of pain, but is used most often for migraines.

Galvanic skin response biofeedback uses sensors to measure the client's sweat gland activity and how much perspiration is on the skin. This device is used most often for excessive sweating and high blood pressure but may have pain applications as well.

HRV biofeedback uses a sensor on the finger or the earlobe using a photoplethysmographor sensors on the chest, lower torso, or wrists using an electrocardiograph to measure changes in the client's heart rate. HVR typically is used with abdominal pain but can be used for other sources of pain as well. The goal of HRV is to improve self-awareness and self-regulation of pain, increase low-frequency heart rhythms, and reduce stress.

The ideal heart rate has evenly spaced beats rather than dips and spikes, which are associated with stress reactions.

Clients with chronic pain who are most likely to benefit from biofeedback often have the following signs and symptoms:

- consistently high pain complaints;
- pain that worsens even with treatment;
- discontinued physical therapy because the therapy is too painful;
- exhibit signs or symptoms of substance use, especially misuse of prescription medicine;
- reduced activity levels;
- poor regulation of emotions;
- exaggerated or inconsistent pain behaviors;
- history of "shopping" for medications or prescribing physicians;
- history of abuse or trauma.

Integrating biofeedback with other rehabilitation therapies (e. g., physical therapy, occupational therapy) provides a comprehensive approach to pain management that can help reduce pain and improve quality of life.

To decide on the correct method of biofeedback to use, the social worker or therapist will complete a thorough evaluation to assess the client's symptoms, emotional regulation, cognitive functioning, past experiences with pain, and any trauma. Once a complete assessment is made, the correct modality can be utilized.

WHAT CAN BE DONE

Learn about biofeedback, including its risks and benefits, and share this information with others. Understand which pain disorders may be addressed effectively with biofeedback.

Develop an awareness of your own cultural values, beliefs, and biases as well as the histories, traditions, and values of the individual in need of care. Look for treatment methodologies that reflect the cultural needs of the individual.

Ask about a referral for a biofeedback pain or stress management program if appropriate.

Ask the individual about any pain.

By Jessica Therivel, LMSW-IPR

Reviewed by Laura Gale, LCSW

REFERENCES

Angoules, A. G., Balakatounis, K. C., Panagiotopoulou, K. A., Mavrogenis, A. F., Mitsiokapa, E. A., & Papagelopoulos, P. J. (2008). Effectiveness of electromyographic biofeedback in the treatment of musculoskeletal pain. *Orthopedics, 31*(10), e980-e984.

Benore, E., Banez, G. A., Sawchuk, T., & Bolek, J. (2014). Applied biofeedback in pediatric pain. *Biofeedback, 42*(3), 96-102. doi:10.5298/1081-5937-42.3.01

Blume, H. K., Brockman, L. N., & Breuner, C. C. (2012). Biofeedback therapy for pediatric headache: Factors associated with response. *Headache, 52*(9), 1377-1386. doi:10.1111/j.1526-466610.2012.02215. x

British Association of Social Workers. (2012). *The Code of Ethics for Social Work: Statement of principles.* Retrieved December 2, 2015, from http://cdn.basw.co.uk/upload/basw_112315-7.pdf

International Federation of Social Workers. (2012). Statement of ethical principles. Retrieved December 2, 2015, from http://ifsw.org/policies/statement-of-ethical-principles

Kent, P., Laird, R., & Haines, T. (2015). The effect of changing movement and posture using motion-sensor biofeedback, versus guidelines-based care, on the clinical outcomes of people with sub-acute or chronic low back pain-a multicenter, cluster-randomized, placebo-controlled, pilot trial. *BMC Musculoskeletal Disorders, 16*(1), 1-19. doi:10.1186/s12891-015-0591-5

Mayo Clinic. (2013). Biofeedback: Your brain vs. chronic pain. *Mayo Clinic Health Letter, 31*(11), 4-5.

Rabow, M. W., & Pantilat, S. Z. (2014). Palliative care & pain management. In M. A. Papadakis & S. J. McPhee (Eds.), *2014 Current medical diagnosis & treatment* (53rd ed., pp.71-82). New York: McGraw-Hill Medical.

Wheeler, D. (2015). NASW standards and indicators for cultural competence in social work practice. Retrieved December 2, 2015, from http://www.socialworkers.org/practice/standards/PRA-BRO-253150-CC-Standards.pdf

Whitney, A. (2014). Biofeedback: A way to regain some control over pain. *Journal of Family Practice, 63*(6), S12-S18.

Willmarth, E., Davis, F., & Fitzgerald, K. (2014). Biofeedback and integrative medicine in the pain clinic setting. *Biofeedback, 42*(3), 111-114. doi:10.5298/1081-5937-42.03.10

PAIN MANAGEMENT: COGNITIVE BEHAVIORAL THERAPY

MAJOR CATEGORIES: Behavioral & Mental Health, Medical & Health

WHAT WE KNOW

Cognitive behavioral therapy (CBT) is a set of techniques based on the premise that negative or maladaptive thoughts (i. e., cognitions) contribute to behaviors that increase stress, emotional distress, and/or pain responses.

CBT is considered to be an effective choice in the treatment of chronic or recurrent pain. In some situations (e. g., approaching a surgery, chemotherapy) it may be beneficial for individuals experiencing acute pain.

CBT treatment protocols have been developed to address a variety of disorders. Protocols for different types of pain may employ different therapeutic techniques. As a result, CBT refers to a family of intervention choices, not one treatment modality. There is not a single standard protocol of CBT for pain.

Pain is influenced by the cognitive, affective, and sensory experiences of the client. common elements in CBT therapies related to pain include relaxation training, behavioral goals, guidance in pacing (i. e., spending enough time and energy on an activity to get the most out of the activity without having pain), problem-solving skills training, and cognitive restructuring.

Pain is a subjective experience for the client. Pain may be chronic, acute, or acute pain that transitions into chronic pain. There are two types of pain, neuropathic and nociceptive; many clients with chronic pain experience a complex mix of both types. There is no laboratory test or diagnostic equipment that can definitively identify pain.

Neuropathic pain may originate in either the central nervous system (i. e., the brain, the spinal cord) or the peripheral nervous system (i. e., nerves outside the brain and spinal cord). Neuropathic pain often is caused by a disease or lesion involving the somatosensory system (e. g., bones, joints, skin, muscles, internal organs, cardiovascular system).

Nociceptive pain results when a physical cause stimulates the nociceptive pain receptors located in the area, which send a pain message through the sensory system to the brain (e. g., a burn, a twisted ankle, arthritis).

Chronic pain persists beyond the point at which healing would be expected and continues indefinitely; it may be constant or intermittent. Treatment of chronic pain may be management-oriented rather than cure-oriented. Chronic pain frequently results in negative emotional reactions such as depressive symptoms, including trouble sleeping, appetite disturbances, loss of interest or pleasure in activities or relationships, and isolation.

Depressive symptoms may also cause or intensify pain.

Clients with chronic pain often express positive reactions to CBT treatment for pain. In one study, 71 percent of participants receiving CBT treatment for pain stated that the CBT skills they learned were beneficial.

Cognitive components that were highlighted by participants were learning about the stress–pain connection (36 percent), automatic thoughts/catastrophic thoughts (21 percent), and examining beliefs (46 percent).

Behavioral components that were commented on most frequently by participants were relaxation techniques (75 percent), assertive communication (43 percent), expressive writing (36 percent), and coping self-statements (14 percent).

The main components of CBT for pain management are expanding the client's knowledge of pain, identifying and addressing any cognitions held by the client that limit his or her ability to engage in CBT activities, improving the client's coping and problem-solving skills while changing behaviors, and improving the client's social and physical activity levels.

Three cognitive variables consistently are found to have an adverse effect on pain: low pain self-efficacy beliefs, a high degree of catastrophizing, and a high fear of movement or re-injury with activity, which is also called "fear avoidance."

Pain disrupts the client's attention and affects the client's behavior on a frequent basis, causing disruption. Clients may be unable to complete tasks requiring attention (e. g., work assignments, memory tasks)in an acceptable manner or may be unable to complete tasks at all. This repeated interference negatively affects clients' sense of self and ability, resulting in feelings of weakness, worthlessness, and other negative thoughts.

Pain self-efficacy refers to the client's belief that he or she can accomplish various activities despite having pain. This can be measured with a tool such as the Pain Self-Efficacy Questionnaire (PSEQ).

Catastrophizing occurs when the client has a high frequency of escalating adverse thoughts while experiencing pain (e. g.,"I am never going to be pain-free");these thoughts are accompanied by feelings of helplessness.

Adverse thoughts can be measured with the catastrophizing scale on the Pain Response Self-Statements Scale (PRSS).

Clients may fear and avoid movement out of concern that activity will cause pain or re-injury.

The Tampa Scale for Kinesiophobia (TSK) may be used to measure this variable.

The Fear Avoidance Beliefs Questionnaire (FABQ) can also be utilized to measure these fears.

Fear and avoidance may exacerbate chronic pain: Inactivity and changes in posture that result from fears can lead to muscle atrophy and impaired postural control.

Studies have found success when CBT focuses on these three cognitive variables.

Researchers in Australia found that when CBT focusing on these variables was provided to a treatment group, there was significant improvement in measures of pain distress, overall disability, depression, fear-avoidance beliefs, catastrophizing, pain self-efficacy, and functional ability.

Researchers in Japan studying tension headaches found that those participants treated with CBT had a significant reduction in catastrophic thoughts and fear-avoidance behaviors. Participants who received CBT also felt more in control of their pain, which reduced feelings of helplessness and increased self-efficacy concerning pain.

Researchers in Sweden found great improvements in overall pain for individuals with chronic pain who participated in CBT. The individuals felt more control over their lives, experienced decreases in affective distress, and experienced improved social support.

Incorporating the concept of loss as it relates to chronic pain into CBT treatment is imperative.

Grief that accompanies chronic pain can be as severe as grief associated with a death.

To help clients adjust cognitions and behaviors to their situation of living with pain, the social worker needs to acknowledge and address their losses.

The most common losses that accompany chronic pain are loss of ability to engage in meaningful activities, loss of relation to others, and loss of self.

Clients with chronic pain often must give up work, social activities, physical activities, and hobbies as a result of their pain.

Chronic pain can affect relationships with spouses, partners, children, parents, and friends. Clients may feel that others question their pain and behavior and in turn they may stop communicating out of fear of seeming to complain. This often results in misunderstandings, conflicts, and a high degree of self-isolation.

Concentration and short-term memory may be affected by pain or medication taken to control pain, which may lead to feelings that one's overall mood or personality has been altered by pain. In addition, clients may feel they are not fulfilling their roles (e. g., parent, spouse, friend) as a result of limitations imposed by their pain.

A group CBT intervention can be appropriate for helping clients deal with the experiences of loss related to pain. A group environment can help clients to feel that they are in a space of trust, understanding, and safe disclosure among individuals who are experiencing the same issues. Researchers conducting a group intervention related to loss and pain management found that subjects reported feeling as if they had gained new perspectives and improved communication within the group setting, which participants felt would extend to improved communication outside the group setting.

Several subtypes of CBT may be used to address management of pain. These may have a different theoretical basis from traditional CBT but share the same techniques.

Acceptance and commitment therapy (ACT) is a CBT technique based on the concept that negative emotions (e. g., fear, negative memories, pain symptoms) negatively influence behavior, leading to avoidance and inflexibility. The client is taught to alter the associations he or she may have between pain and these negative thoughts and emotions in order to positively change behavior and improve functioning.

The goal of mindfulness-based cognitive therapy (MBCT) is to increase adaptive cognitive processes (e. g., acceptance) while decreasing negative cognitive processes (e. g., catastrophic thoughts) by incorporating daily meditation practices.

Clients are taught to be present-minded and to have nonjudgmental awareness. This is also referred to as teaching the client to "pay attention on purpose." Clients are discouraged from dwelling on the past or worrying about the future.

Meditation and yoga may be used to help reduce physical distress and improve the client's ability to understand his or her physical body and symptoms.

MBCT has been associated with successful relapse prevention.

Dialectical behavior therapy (DBT) utilizes the perspective that both acceptance and change are needed to regulate affect. This belief in opposing internal forces that are in a continual state of flux is called "the dialectical worldview." The client's ability to reconcile acceptance and change can create positive behavior change and improved affect.

Internet-delivered cognitive behavioral therapy (iCBT) involves the use of an Internet-connected computer to reach clients and engage them in a program to learn coping skills, relaxation techniques, and ways of challenging negative thoughts.

iCBT consists of structured online lessons that are either self-guided or clinician-guided.

Social workers need to be aware of clients' attitudes related to computers and any anxiety about using computers before recommending an iCBT therapy. iCBT can be appropriate even for clients who are using or misusing opioids to manage pain. Researchers in the United States found that even when subjects were using opioids, they were able to engage in an iCBT program and frequently had a decrease in misuse of opioids. These subjects also had improved self-efficacy, which was then associated with improved pain coping, pain thresholds, and tolerance for pain. iCBT may be appropriate when there are barriers in place that would otherwise prevent the client from engaging in a CBT group or individual therapy program.

In a randomized controlled trial in Australia, the treatment group that received iCBT had a greater than 30 percent improvement compared to the control group in disability, anxiety, depression, and pain, which was sustained at a 3-month follow-up point. The members of the control group were on a waiting list; during the time the treatment group received CBT, the control group did not receive pain management therapy.

Regardless of specific type, CBT programs incorporate common therapeutic techniques. These include the following:

Cognitive restructuring monitors the client's interpretation of his or her experience in order to help decrease feelings of emotional distress, helplessness, and hopelessness.

Modification of coping statements is a technique in which clients who are using defeatist self-statements are taught how to replace this negative self-talk with internal dialogues that increase feelings of calm and competence and positive coping skills.

Distraction techniques help the client refocus attention onto non-painful stimuli to distract him or her from the pain experience.

Self-monitoring through journals or diaries helps the client keep a personal history and externalize the thoughts, feelings, and behaviors that if internalized increase emotional distress.

Relaxation breathing with or without progressive muscle relaxation can alter the client's reaction to pain and stress in the behavioral, physical, and emotional realms. Family caregivers can be instructed on how to help clients with these techniques.

Guided imagery is a cognitive-behavioral technique in which the social worker encourages the use of imaginary pictures, sounds, or sensations to help the client reduce or eliminate pain and/or the anxiety, fear, or tension that are connected to the pain.

The technique uses relaxation training, visualization, and positive suggestion. Guided imagery is meant to teach the client how to shift focus from his or her pain and discomfort to more comfortable or enjoyable thoughts. Guided imagery should be avoided for clients who are actively psychotic, are unable to think abstractly, cannot distinguish reality from fantasy, are having hallucinations or delusions, have moderate to advanced dementia, or cannot communicate.

Common guided imagery techniques for pain include the following:

- creating a mental image for the pain and then transforming that image into a more manageable or less frightening image;
- imagining the pain disappearing;
- imagining the pain as something the client has complete control over (e. g., if the pain is an electric current, the client can turn the electric switch off).

There are barriers that contribute to the underutilization of CBT for pain management in spite of evidence supporting the effectiveness of CBT interventions. These include the following:

- financial (e. g., lack of insurance);
- environmental (e. g., trouble with transportation, no available providers);
- attitude-related (e. g., stigma associated with psychological assistance, belief that pain can be fixed only with medicine or surgery);
- healthcare system barriers (e. g., no referral system, providers unfamiliar with CBT).

WHAT CAN BE DONE

Learn about cognitive behavioral therapy for pain management to accurate assess an individual's personal characteristics and health and mental health education needs.

Develop an awareness of your own cultural values, beliefs, and biases as well as the histories, traditions, and values of the individual in need of care. Look for treatment methodologies that reflect the cultural needs of the individual.

Request referrals for the individuals to CBT pain management programs or groups when appropriate and available.

Assess the individual's pain regularly.

Work to eliminate any barriers to client access to CBT programs.

Assess the individual's self-efficacy for particular elements of the CBT program that may be challenging, such as comfort with computers for an iCBT program.

Assist client if needed in accessing an iCBT program.

Ask the individual for his or her preferences related to pain management to help determine appropriate interventions.

By Jessica Therivel, LMSW-IPR

Reviewed by Laura Gale, LCSW

REFERENCES

Akerblom, S., Perrin, S., Fischer, M. R., & McCracken, L. M. (2015). The mediating role of acceptance in multidisciplinary cognitive-behavioral therapy for chronic pain. *The Journal of Pain, 16*(7), 606-615. doi:10.1016/j. jpain.2015.03.007

Altilio, T. (2011). In M. T. & L. E. Davis (Eds.), *Encyclopedia of social work* (1st ed., pp.335-337). Washington, D. C. : NASW Press.

Altilio, T., Otis-Green, S., Hedlund, S., & Fineberg, I. C. (2012). Pain management and palliative care. In S. Gehlert & T. Browne (Eds.), *Handbook of health social work* (2nd ed., pp.590-626). Hoboken, NJ: John Wiley & Sons, Inc.

Barrie, J., & Loughlin, D. (2014). Managing chronic pain in adults. *Nursing Standard, 29*(7), 50-58. doi:10.7748/ns.29.7.50. e9099

Burnett, J. (2012, October). Guided imagery as an adjunct to pharmacological pain control at end of life. Paper presented at North American Association of Christians in Social Work (NACSW) Convention, St. Louis, MO. Retrieved from http:// www.nacsw.org/Publications/Proceedings2012/ BurnettJGuidedImagery.pdf

British Association of Social Workers. (2012). The code of ethics for social work: Statement of principles. Retrieved February 28, 2016, from http:// cdn. basw.co.uk/upload/basw_112315-7.pdf

Carter, J., Watson, A. C., & Sminkey, P. V. (2014). Pain management: Screening and assessment of pain as part of a comprehensive case management process. *Professional Case Management, 19*(3), 126-136. doi:10.1097/NCM.0000000000000029

Day, M. A., Thorn, B. E., & Kapoor, S. (2011). A qualitative analysis of a randomized controlled trial comparing a cognitive-behavioral treatment with education. *Journal of Pain, 12*(9), 941-952. doi:10.1016/j. jpain.2011.02.354

Day, M. A., Thorn, B. E., Ward, L. C., Rubin, N., Hickman, S. D., Scogin, F., & Kilgo, G. R. (2014). Mindfulness-based cognitive therapy for the treatment of headache pain: a pilot study. *The Clinical Journal of Pain, 30*(2), 152-161. doi:10.1097/ AJP.0b013e318287a1dc

Dear, B. F., Titov, N., Perry, K. N., Johnston, L., Wootton, B. M., Terides, M. D.,... Hudson, J. L. (2013). The Pain Course: A randomised controlled trial of a clinician-guided Internet delivered cognitive behaviour therapy program for managing chronic pain and emotional well-being. *Pain, 154*(6), 942-950. doi:10.1016/j. pain.2013.03.005

Ehde, D. M., Dillworth, T. M., & Turner, J. A. (2014). Cognitive-behavioral therapy for individuals with chronic pain: Efficacy, innovations, and directions for research. *American Psychologist, 69*(2), 153-166. doi:10.1037/a0035747

Harlaldseid, C., Dysvik, E., & Furnes, B. (2012). The experience of loss in patients suffering from chronic pain attending a pain management group based on cognitive-behavioral therapy. *Pain Management Nursing, 15*(1), 12-21. doi:v

Haraldseid, C., Dysvik, E., & Furnes, B. (2014). The experience of loss in patients suffering from chronic pain attending a pain management group based on cognitive-behavioral therapy. *Pain Management Nursing, 15*(1), 12-21. doi:10.1016/j. pmn.2012.04.004

Hofmann, S. G., Sawyer, A. T., & Fang, A. (2010). The empirical status of the "New Wave" of cognitive behavioral therapy. *Psychiatric Clinics of North America, 33*(3), 701-710. doi:10.1016/j. psc.2010.04.006

International Federation of Social Workers. (2012, March 3). Statement of Ethical Principles. Retrieved January 28, 2016, from http://ifsw.org/ policies/statement-of-ethical-principles/

Linden, M., Scherbe, S., & Cicholas, B. (2014). Randomized controlled trial on the effectiveness of cognitive behavior group therapy in chronic back pain patients. *Journal of Back and Musculoskeletal Rehabilitation, 27*(4), 563-80. doi:10.3233/ BMR-140518

Morley, S. (2011). Efficacy and effectiveness of cognitive behavior therapy for chronic pain: Progress and some challenges. *Pain, 152*(3 Suppl), S99-S106. doi:10.1016/j. pain.2010.10.042

Motoya, R., Oda, K., Ito, E., Ichikawa, M., Sato, T., Watanabe, T.,... Yabe, H. (2014). Effectiveness of cognitive behavioral therapy based on the pain sustainment/exacerbation model in patients with tension-type headache: A pilot study. *Fukushima Journal of Medical Science, 60*(2), 1-8.

National Association of Social Workers (NASW). (2005). How social workers help with pain management. Retrieved January 28, 2016, from http://www.helpstartshere.org/health-and-wellness/pain/pain-how-social-workers-help-with-pain-management. html

Nicholas, M. K., Asghari, A., Blyth, F. M., Wood, B. M., Murray, R., McCabe, R.,... Overton, S. (2013). Self-management intervention for chronic pain in older adults: A randomised controlled trial. *Pain, 154*(6), 824-835. doi:10.1016/j. pain.2013.02.009

Peilot, B., Andrell, P., Samuelsson, A., Mannheimer, C., Frodi, A., & Sundler, A. J. (2014). Time to gain trust and change–Experiences of attachment and mindfulness-based cognitive therapy among patients with chronic pain and psychiatric co-morbidity. *International Journal of Qualitative Studies on Health and Well-Being, 9.* doi:10.3402/qhw.v9.24420

Schneider, L. H., & Hadjistavropoulos, H. D. (2014). When in doubt, ask the audience: Potential users' perceptions of Internet-delivered cognitive behavioural therapy for chronic pain. *Pain Research & Management, 19*(4), 173-178.

Schneider, L. H., & Hadjistavropoulos, H. D. (2014). When in doubt, ask the audience: Potential users' perceptions of Internet-delivered cognitive behavioral therapy for chronic pain. *Pain Research and Management, 19*(4). doi:10.1016/j.pmn.2014.09.009

Wheeler, D. (2015). NASW Standards and Indicators for Cultural Competence in Social Work Practice. Retrieved January 28, 2016, from http://www.socialworkers.org/practice/standards/PRA-BRO-253150-CC-Standards.pdf

Wilson, M., Roll, J. M., Corbett, C., & Barbosa-Leiker, C. (2014). Empowering patients with persistent pain using an Internet-based self-management program. *Pain Management Nursing, 16*(4), 503-514.

PAIN MANAGEMENT: ROLE OF THE SOCIAL WORKER

MAJOR CATEGORIES: Health, Medical & Health

WHAT WE KNOW

Pain is a subjective experience for the client. Pain may be an acute reaction to an injury or it may become a chronic reaction. There are two types of pain, neuropathic and nociceptive; many clients with chronic pain experience a complex mix of both types. There are no laboratory or diagnostic tests that can definitively identify the presence of pain.

Pain acts as a signal to the body that there has been an injury that requires an action (e. g., healing, treatment). Neuropathic pain may originate in either the central nervous system (i. e. the brain, the spinal cord) or the peripheral nervous system (i. e., nerves outside the brain and spinal cord). Neuropathic pain often is caused by a disease or lesion involving the somatosensory system (e. g., bones, joints, skin, muscles, internal organs, cardiovascular system).

Nociceptive pain results when a physical cause stimulates the nociceptive pain receptors in the area, which send a pain message through the sensory system to the brain (e. g., a burn, a twisted ankle, arthritis).

Acute pain usually is caused by an injury, a surgery, swelling, or an unknown cause but typically dissipates after an anticipated period of time when the wound or injury has healed. Chronic pain persists beyond the point at which healing would be expected and continues indefinitely; it may be constant or intermittent.

Treatment of chronic pain may be management-oriented rather than cure-oriented. Chronic pain frequently results in negative emotional reactions including depressive symptoms, trouble sleeping, appetite disturbances, loss of interest or pleasure in activities or relationships, and isolation. Depressive symptoms can also cause or intensify pain.

Social work goals align closely with those of pain management: reducing suffering while enhancing quality of life. Social workers help clients manage pain in several ways.

Family caregivers of clients at end of life often are primarily responsible for managing the client's pain and frequently express uncertainty, anxiety, and trouble communicating with the client. Negative attitudes, fears, and beliefs regarding pain management can be addressed by the social worker.

A study of hospice social workers, who are closely involved in end-of-life care, reported that approximately 21 percent of their time was spent addressing issues related to pain management. 25.5 percent of the social workers reported that non-social-worker members of the interdisciplinary care team approached them at least once every 1–2 days to help a caregiver with concerns connected to pain management. Another 23.3 percent stated that this occurred at least once a week.

The most common barriers to effective pain management reported to social workers by caregivers were caregiver belief that pain cannot be controlled, desire to keep the client more awake and alert, and belief that the client would decline faster if given pain medicine. The social workers also found that caregivers often waited a long time before they would call hospice to report pain.

In the United States, chronic pain affects an estimated 100 million individuals. A 2011 report by the Institute of Medicine reported economic costs of chronic pain between $560 to $635 billion a year when loss of work was included.

Pain carries high social-emotional costs, which are linked to the following:
- Increased morbidity
- Higher rates of hospital admission
- Longer hospital stays
- Increased number of outpatient visits to healthcare providers
- Decreased ability to function

Pain often is underdiagnosed and undertreated. Reasons for this include biases related to gender, race, and age and physician fears related to opioid addiction. Use of a client-centered approach, in which the provider considers the goals and needs of the individual holistically rather than focusing on the immediate episode of pain, can improve pain management.

Age is a frequent source of bias in pain management: pain in older persons is more likely to go unrecognized and uncontrolled than pain in younger persons. Older clients may themselves feel that pain is expected with aging and may not acknowledge pain during an assessment or may describe the pain using mild language (e. g., aches, soreness). Older clients may fear becoming addicted to pain medications or have concerns about cost. Older adults are more likely to be experiencing cognitive impairments that interfere with their ability to describe their pain in an easily understandable way. Older clients may worry that they will be perceived as "bad" patients if they discuss pain.

Women are less likely to have reports of pain taken seriously by healthcare providers and are more likely to have their pain dismissed as being emotional or psychogenic in nature.

Minority clients historically have been less likely to receive adequate and appropriate pain management for both chronic and acute pain. If there are language barriers, the client may have trouble expressing his or her pain needs to staff and may have increased anxiety while trying to make those needs known.

Physicians may fail to prescribe opioids out of an exaggerated fear of overprescribing or encouraging dependence. This so-called opiophobia may cause some clients to continue to experience pain that could be alleviated with the correct use of opioids. Often clients do not receive the proper pain medications, receive an inadequate dose, or leave the emergency department or physician's office still in pain.

To help reduce physician anxiety related to prescribing opioids, the social worker may want to educate physicians on the use of an opioid agreement form. The first section of this form serves as an informed consent; the client acknowledges what the medication is being prescribed for and agrees to the following conditions in order to maintain the prescription:
- Discloses any other treatments he or she is participating in and agrees to taper or discontinue the opioid if other options are appropriate;
- Will take the medication only as prescribed;
- Will keep appointments;
- May receive opioid prescriptions from a single physician only;
- Will notify the pain clinic/physician if the client has an additional condition requiring a controlled narcotic or is hospitalized;
- Designates the single pharmacy that will be used;
- Agrees that early refills will not be honored and that if he or she loses medication or it is stolen, the medication will not be replaced;
- Will abstain from use of illegal or recreational drugs, including alcohol, and will submit to blood or urine testing if requested by doctor;
- Agrees to exact instructions regarding refills;
- Signs a release allowing the physician or staff members to discuss care with primary physician (if different) and any medical facilities providing care.

Pain is the most common reason for a visit to an emergency department, but emergency departments often present barriers to pain management. Social workers in the emergency department have an opportunity to advocate for clients and seek improved care. Barriers include failure by staff to acknowledge pain, to assess initial pain, to implement care according to the department's protocols or guidelines, to document pain, and to meet clients' expectations. All of the biases that affect pain management also take place in the emergency department and may require social work intervention.

The social worker in the emergency department setting should ensure that any assessment, whether completed by a social worker or a nurse, includes determining whether the client has had two or more visits to the emergency room within the last 6 months for pain and assessing whether the client is in fact drug-seeking or instead has poorly controlled pain. Not all drug-seeking behavior is intentional; it may result from a failure by the client to self-wean from pain medications after a physician has refused to refill prescriptions.

Red flags for potential misuse of opioids are prescription for minor reasons, prescriptions from multiple providers, and needing refills before the client should be out of medication, indicating the client is taking the medication more often or at higher amounts than prescribed.

Palliative care is an approach to care that frequently includes pain management. Barriers to effective pain management that social workers can identify and address in palliative care settings include the following:

- concerns about addiction that may be expressed by client, caregivers, or other professional members of the care team;
- tolerance of the pain medication, leaving the client undermedicated;
- stoicism about enduring pain by the client;
- fatalism about pain as a necessary part of life or aging;
- fears of side effects of pain medication such as drowsiness, confusion, constipation;
- perceived stigma regarding taking pain medications;
- fear of being a burden on caregivers and belief that reporting pain is being a burden;
- fear of overdosing on pain medications.

The social worker can also use screening tools along with a thorough biopsychosocial-spiritual assessment to determine client needs and effective interventions.

Two common screening tools are the Brief Pain Inventory, a 9-item inventory to assess pain, and the Patient Health Questionnaire (PHQ-9), which may be used to screen for depressive symptoms the client may be experiencing as a result of pain.

The social worker can also utilize the Physical Functional Ability Questionnaire (FAQ5) to assess whether chronic pain is limiting the client's ability to perform activities of daily living, instrumental activities of daily living, and lifting ability based on U.S. Department of Labor standards.

Interventions provided by social workers to help clients manage pain typically employ cognitive behavioral techniques meant to change negative behaviors and thoughts related to the pain and/or incorporate techniques such as supportive counseling, guided imagery, breathing exercises, and muscle relaxation.

Cognitive-behavioral techniques can be particularly effective during times of distress or feelings of lack of control by the client, which is common during procedures and testing.

Acceptance and commitment therapy (ACT) is based on the concept that negative emotions (e. g., fear, negative memories, pain symptoms) have a negative influence on behavior and can lead to avoidance and inflexibility. The client is taught to alter the associations he or she may have between pain and these negative thoughts and emotions in order to positively change behavior and improve functioning.

Cognitive restructuring monitors the client's interpretation of his or her experience in order to help decrease feelings of emotional distress, helplessness, and hopelessness.

Clients who are using defeatist self-statements can be taught how to replace negative self-talk with internal dialogues known as coping statements that will increase feelings of calm and competence and thereby enhance coping.

Distraction techniques help the client refocus his or her attention on non-painful stimuli to distract the client from his or her pain experience.

Self-monitoring though journals or diaries helps the client keep a personal history but also allows the client to externalize thoughts, feelings, and behaviors that may, if internalized, increase emotional distress.

Guided imagery is a cognitive-behavioral technique in which the social worker helps the client use imaginary pictures, sounds, or sensations to reduce or eliminate pain and/or the anxiety, fear, or tension that are connected to the pain.

The technique uses relaxation training, visualization, and positive suggestion.

Guided imagery teaches the client how to shift his or her focus away from his or her pain and discomfort to more comfortable or enjoyable thoughts.

Guided imagery should be avoided with clients who are actively psychotic, are unable to think abstractly, cannot distinguish reality from fantasy, are having hallucinations or delusions, have moderate to advanced dementia, or cannot communicate.

Common guided imagery techniques for pain include the following:

- creating a mental image for the pain and then transforming that image into a more manageable or less frightening image;
- imagining the pain disappearing; and
- imagining the pain as something the client has complete control over (e. g., if the pain is an electric current, the client can turn the electric switch off).

Relaxation breathing with or without progressive muscle relaxation can alter the client's reaction to pain and stress in the behavioral, physical, and emotional realms. Family caregivers can be instructed on how to help clients with these techniques.

Supportive counseling interventions work to clarify the relationship between pain and other psychosocial functioning, explore resources, validate the client's experience, and improve problem solving.

The social worker can develop a plan of care with the client to address the client's chronic pain. The plan of care should include the following areas of focus:

The client should list personal goals that may include improving functional ability and returning to work and/or specific personally enjoyable activities (e. g., hobbies, tasks, sports).

Sleep improvement may be achieved through having a specific sleep plan (e. g., no caffeine, no naps, relaxation techniques before bed, adherence to a target bedtime, no electronics in the bedroom) and listing any medications or homeopathic means that are being used to help with sleep.

The client should be aiming to increase physical activity. The care plan should address physical therapy, if appropriate, and stretching, aerobic exercise, and strengthening.

Stress management should be incorporated into the plan of care; this may take the form of formal interventions (e. g., counseling, support group, classes), daily practice of relaxation techniques, and/or medications for anxiety.

Decreasing pain should be addressed in the plan; between visits, the client should record times of his or her lowest and highest pain levels to assist with monitoring.

WHAT CAN BE DONE

Learn about the role of the social worker in pain management to accurately assess the client's unique characteristics and health/mental health education needs.

Treatment methodologies should reflect the cultural values, beliefs, and biases of the individual in need of care and treatment.

Understand the definitions of pain and the impact of pain on comorbidities.

Recognize the biases present in pain management and be prepared to advocate for those clients who are not receiving appropriate pain management as a result of bias.

Advocate for increased cultural sensitivity in areas of practice (e. g., hospitals, mental health agencies, nursing homes) to reduce disparities in pain management.

Include caregivers in any pain assessment and share any caregiver concerns related to pain with relevant healthcare team members.

Recognize the social worker's role in the emergency department to advocate for clients while also helping to assess for any substance abuse issues.

Social workers can educate clientson their strengths, areas of control, and areas of competence so they can feel more empowered in their pain management.

Social workers can teach clientsskills and strategies for coping with and managing pain, including relaxation techniques, guided imagery, and breathing techniques.

Utilize appropriate screening tools to assist in biopsychosocial-spiritual assessment.

Develop plans of care for clients that include needs related to pain management.

Refer clients to any appropriate pain management program or support group.

By Jessica Therivel, LMSW-IPR

Reviewed by Laura Gale, LCSW

REFERENCES

Altilio, T. (2011). Pain. In T. Mizrahi & L. E. Davis (Eds.), *Encyclopedia of social work* (1st ed., Vol.3, pp.335-337). Washington, D. C. : NASW Press.

Altilio, T., Otis-Green, S., Hedlund, S., & Fineberg, I. C. (2012). Pain management and palliative care. In S. Gehlert & T. Browne (Eds.), *Handbook of health social work* (2nd ed., pp.590-626). Hoboken, NJ: John Wiley & Sons, Inc.

Barrie, J., & Loughlin, D. (2014). Managing chronic pain in adults. *Nursing Standard, 29*(7), 50-58. doi:10.7748/ns.29.7.50. e9099

British Association of Social Workers. (2012, January). The code of ethics for social work: Statement of principles. Retrieved October 16, 2015, from http://cdn. basw.co.uk/upload/ basw_112315-7.pdf

Burnett, J. (2012, October). Guided imagery as an adjunct to pharmacological pain control at end of life. Paper presented at North American Association of Christians in Social Work (NACSW) Convention. St. Louis, MO. Retrieved October 16, 2015, from http://www.nacsw.org/Publications/Proceedings2012/BurnettJGuidedImagery.pdf

Cagle, J. G., & Altilio, T. (2011). The social work role in pain management and symptoms management. In T. Altilio & S. Otis-Green (Eds.), *Oxford textbook of palliative social work* (pp.271-286). New York, NY: Oxford University Press.

Carter, J., Watson, A. C., & Sminkey, P. V. (2014). Pain management: Screening and assessment of pain as part of a comprehensive case management process. *Professional Case Management, 19*(3), 126-136. doi:10.1097/ NCM.0000000000000029

Hanks-Bell, M., Halvey, K., & Paice, J. A. (2004). Pain assessment and management in aging. *The Online Journal of Issues in Nursing, 9*(3). Retrieved from http://www.nursingworld.org/MainMenuCategories/ANAMarketplace/ANAPeriodicals/OJIN/TableofContents/Volume92004/ No3Sept04/ArticlePreviousTopic/PainAssessmentandManagementinAging. aspx

Hooten, W. M., Timming, R., Belgrade, M., Gaul, J., Haake, B., Myers, C.,... Walker, N. (2013, November). Institute for Clinical Systems Improvement health care guideline: Assessment and management of chronic pain. Retrieved October 16, 2015, from https://www.icsi.org/_asset/bw798b/ ChronicPain.pdf

Relieving pain in America: A blueprint for transforming prevention, care, education, and research. (2011). *Institute of Medicine.* Washington, D. C. : The National Academies Press.

International Federation of Social Workers (IFSW). (2012). Statement of ethical principles. Retrieved October 16, 2015, from http://ifsw.org/ policies/statement-of-ethical-principles

Mizrahi, T., & Mayden, R. W. (2001). NASW Standards for Cultural Competency in Social Work Practice. Retrieved October 16, 2015, from http://www.socialworkers.org/practice/standards/NASWCulturalStandards.pdf

Motov, S. M., & Khan, A. N. (2009). Problems and barriers of pain management in the emergency department: Are we ever going to get better?. *Journal of Pain Research, 2,*5-11.

National Association of Social Workers (NASW). (2005). How social workers help with pain management. Retrieved October 16, 2015, from from http://www.helpstartshere.org/health-and-wellness/pain/pain-how-social-workers-help-with-pain-management. html

Oliver, D. P., Wittenberg-Lyles, E., Washington, K. T., & Sehrawat, S. (2009). Social work role in hospice pain management: A national survey. *Journal of Social Work in End-of-Life & Palliative Care, 5*(1-2), 61-74.

Otis-Green, S., Lucas, S., Spolum, M., Ferrell, B., & Grant, M. (2008). Promoting excellence in pain management and palliative care for social workers. *Journal of Social Work in End-of-Life & Palliative Care, 4*(2), 120-134.

PAIN MANAGEMENT: OLDER ADULTS

MAJOR CATEGORIES: Medical & Health

WHAT WE KNOW

Pain is a subjective experience for the older adult client that can start as an acute reaction to an injury or condition or become a chronic reaction to that injury or condition. Pain is categorized into two types, nociceptive and neuropathic, with many clients with chronic pain coping with a complex mix of both types. There are no laboratory tests or diagnostic equipment that can definitively identify pain.

Pain acts as a signal to the body that there has been an injury that requires an action (e. g., healing, removal from source of pain). Neuropathic pain may originate in the peripheral nerve system or come from another anatomical location but the nervous system is impacted and the pain is neurologically based. Neuropathic pain often comes from a disease or lesion impacting the somatosensory neurosystem.

Nociceptive pain results when a physical cause stimulates the nociceptive pain receptors located in the area, which send a pain message through the sensory system to the brain (e. g., a burn, a twisted ankle, arthritis).

Acute pain usually is caused by an injury, a surgery, swelling, or an unknown cause and will typically dissipate after an anticipated period of time with healing. Chronic pain is pain that persists beyond the point at which healing would be expected and lasts indefinitely; it may be constant or intermittent. When treating chronic pain, the focus may need to change from trying to cure the pain to determining how to manage it. Chronic pain frequently results in negative emotional reactions, including depressive symptoms, trouble sleeping, appetite disturbances, loss of interest or pleasure in activities or relationships, and isolation. Depressive symptoms can also cause pain or intensify pain the client is experiencing.

Chronic pain in older adults is associated with physical functional impairment, increased disability, slower rehabilitation from injuries, decreased quality of life, increased risk of falls, increased risk of mood changes and mood disorders, sleep and appetite disturbances, decreased socialization, greater healthcare utilization, higher healthcare costs, and increased risk of suicide. In a study, hospice social workers reported that approximately 21 percent of their time was spent on pain management. Investigators found that 25.5 percent of the social workers reported that non-social-work members of the interdisciplinary care team approached them at least one time a day or every other day to help a caregiver with concerns connected to pain management. Another 23.3 percent stated that this happened at least once a week.

Researchers conducting a longitudinal study found that the most commonly reported health conditions by adults age 50 and older were arthritis and back pain. One third of participants reported having pain that was troublesome and 23.6 percent reported pain so severe that typical activities such as work or household chores were difficult to complete. The group most likely to report this severe pain were frail, elderly women. In another study, researchers determined that 49 percent of older adult study participants with chronic pain were using one or more pain medications to try to manage pain. Of these individuals, 68.4 percent reported using at least one nonpharmacological solution for pain, with the most common being exercise, ointments, heat, and massage. For older adults with chronic pain, maintaining self-efficacy (i. e., belief in one's ability to accomplish a task) can be a protective factor against depressive symptoms, anxiety, activity avoidance, and perception of poor health.

In older adults with chronic pain, there is also an increased risk of depression as the number of comorbid conditions increases. In a recent study of adults aged 65 years and older without terminal illness or conditions resulting in functional decline (e. g., stroke, dementia), researchers found that 31.7 percent experienced moderate pain and 21 percent experienced mild pain. A high percentage of participants, 90 percent, had comorbidities, and depression scores were positively correlated with the number of comorbidities. The female participants had higher rates of depression and comorbidities than the male participants.

There are barriers that can make providing quality pain management to older adult clients difficult for the social worker. Pain, physical function, and cognitive function in older adults are linked. There is a direct relationship between pain and the older adult's physical functioning. Pain can also result in diminished cognitive functioning unrelated to any dementia, which then will also negatively affect physical functioning. When the individual is experiencing chronic pain, the focus and energy applied to coping with the pain can result in a decline in cognitive functioning. Attention and memory have both been identified as cognitive processes that can have a positive or negative effect on pain. Older adults with cognitive impairment in those areas may be at risk for more difficulties in managing pain.

Missed pain diagnoses and undertreatment of pain both are common in older adults. Researchers studying adult patients in an emergency department determined that older patients were less likely than younger patients to receive opioid pain medication for pain that was rated as moderate to severe; in turn, these older adults had a decreased reduction in pain. Another set of researchers studying older adults in an emergency department found that when these patients engaged in shared decision-making with the healthcare provider on managing their pain, they were more likely to be satisfied with the medication prescribed and to have a greater decrease in pain than clients who did not participate in the decision-making.

Older adults are more likely to underreport their pain. They may feel that pain is expected with aging and may not acknowledge pain during an assessment or may describe the pain with more mild language (e. g., aches, soreness) or have anxiety about becoming addicted to pain medications or concerns about cost.

Older clients are more likely to be experiencing cognitive impairments that interfere with their ability to express pain in an easily understandable way. They may worry that they will be perceived as "bad" patients if they discuss pain.

Cognitive impairment (e. g., dementia, delirium) in older adults can make obtaining an accurate verbal pain assessment difficult. These clients may need to be observed for pain behaviors, and if appropriate a proxy who knows the client may be utilized to help report on the client's pain.

Pain behaviors that are not speech-based may include agitation, confusion, withdrawal, grimacing, shouting, moaning, pacing, rocking, changes in interpersonal interactions (e. g., eating alone, easily agitated), changes in activity (e. g., not exercising),

protecting or favoring a body part, increased confusion, or new agitation.

Investigators studying nursing home residents found that only 17 percent of residents with dementia reported or exhibited signs of pain whereas 29 percent of residents without dementia did so.

Opioid pain medications, which are physician prescribed, as well as nonsteroidal anti-inflammatory drugs, which frequently are over the counter medications, both can have significant side effects (e. g., confusion, fatigue, constipation) in older adults.

Racial differences can be present in the reporting of pain by older adults. Investigators studying nursing homes found that, overall, 23 percent of residents reported or exhibited pain. Non-white residents were less likely to report or exhibit signs of pain when compared to white residents.

Nursing home residents are at risk for inadequate pain management. Researchers found that among nursing home residents who had pain, 44 percent did not have standing orders for pain control and also had not received any special services for pain management.

Untreated pain is a common problem for nursing home residents with cancer. Researchers found that more than 65 percent of nursing home residents with cancer who were surveyed had pain, with 13.5 percent reporting severe pain and 61.3 percent reporting moderate pain. More than 17 percent of residents with cancer reported daily pain. The researchers also found that older residents and residents with cognitive impairment were less likely to have daily pain documentation.

The social worker can develop a plan of care with the older adult client to address the client's chronic pain. The plan of care should include the following areas of focus:

Personal goals listed that include improving functional ability where improvement is feasible and a goal to return to specific personally enjoyable activities (e. g., hobbies, tasks, sports).

Sleep improvement to be achieved through having a specific sleep plan (e. g., no caffeine, no naps, relaxation techniques before bed, target bedtime, no electronics in the bedroom) and listing any medications or homeopathic means that are being used to help with sleep.

An increase in physical activity if appropriate. If the client is utilizing fear avoidance behaviors that are limiting physical activity, this may lead to more chronic pain. This aspect of the plan of care may include physical therapy if indicated, stretching, aerobic exercise, and strengthening.

Stress management needs to be incorporated into the plan of care, whether formal interventions (e. g., counseling, support group, classes), daily practice of relaxation techniques, and/or any medications for anxiety.

Decreasing pain, with the client tracking lowest and highest pain levels between visits to assist with tracking.

Social workers should be aware of the pain ladder approach to pain management to help advocate for clients and ensure that their pain needs related to medication are being met appropriately. The basis of the pain ladder approach to pain medication is that any pharmacological pain management regimen should start with the safest medications first and only escalate if the pain is not relieved.

After the plan of care is developed, the social worker can utilize an intervention that is appropriately tailored for working with an older adult. Frequently this will include cognitive behavioral therapy (CBT) with the addition of relaxation training and guided imagery, but it may also incorporate mobile health monitoring and other nonpharmacological interventions. CBT is a psychological technique based on the assumption that negative or maladaptive thoughts (i. e., cognitions) are linked to behaviors that increase stress, emotional distress, and/or pain responses as a result. Protocols for CBT are developed to address a variety of disorders, and even within treatment for pain different protocols for different types of pain may have different therapeutic techniques. As a result, CBT refers to a family of intervention choices, not a single treatment modality. There is not one standard protocol of CBT for pain. Common elements of CBT related to pain include relaxation training, behavioral goals, guidance in pacing, problem-solving skills training, and cognitive restructuring.

There are three common cognitive variables that are consistently found to have a negative effect on pain management. These variables cause interruption, interferences, and issues with identity. These are having low pain self-efficacy beliefs, a higher degree of catastrophizing, and a higher fear of movement or reinjury with activity, which is also called fear avoidance.

Mobile health technologies for pain management could be a successful source of support and assistance to older adults. Programs and applications are being developed that can track pain levels, monitor symptoms, monitor for falls, track side effects, give medication reminders, and provide client education and social support. 85 percent of older adults who were part of a focus group on mobile health demonstrated an interest in using these programs to help with pain management.

Nonpharmacological interventions can be used with older adults, who are vulnerable to medication side effects. These include exercise programs, acupuncture, and pain management support groups.

Social workers working with older adults need to incorporate the concept of loss into any intervention or plan of care in order to demonstrate to the client an understanding of these losses, to show compassion, and to help the client manage these losses in treatment. The common areas of loss for older adults are loss of the ability to engage in meaningful activities, loss of relation to others, and loss of self.

WHAT CAN BE DONE

Learn about pain management in older adults to accurately assess an individual's personal characteristics and health education needs.

Develop an awareness of your own cultural values, beliefs, and biases as well as the histories, traditions, and values of the individual in need of care. Look for treatment methodologies that reflect the cultural needs of your client.

Request referrals for your clients to CBT pain management programs or groups when appropriate or available.

Assess your client's pain regularly.

Ask your client for his or her preferences related to pain management to help determine appropriate interventions.

For the older adult client with cognitive impairment, educate family members and any caregivers on assessing the client's pain by observing pain behaviors.

Explore with client the relationships among the biological, psychological, cultural, spiritual, social, economic, and familial components of the client's pain experience to better understand his or her pain.

Work with the client to identify areas of strength, competency, and control in order to encourage self-efficacy and the belief that he or she has some control over his or her pain experience to reduce the likelihood of negative psychosocial symptoms.

Educate the client on relaxation strategies, breathing exercises, and guided imagery techniques to help with pain management.

Written by Jessica Therivel, LMSW-IPR

Reviewed by Laura Gale, LCSW

REFERENCES

Altilio, T. (2011). Pain. In T. Mizrahi & L. E. Davis (Eds.), *Encyclopedia of Social Work* (1st ed., Vol.3, J-R, pp.335-337). Washington, D. C.: NASW Press.

Altilio, T., Otis-Green, S., Hedlund, S., & Fineberg, I. C. (2012). Pain management and palliative care. In S. Gehlert & T. Browne (Eds.), *Handbook of health social work* (2nd ed., pp.590-626). Hoboken, NJ: John Wiley & Sons, Inc.

American Geriatrics Society Panel on the Pharmacological Management of Persistent Pain in Older Persons. (2009). Pharmacological management of persistent pain in older persons. *Journal of the American Geriatrics Society, AGS,57*(8), 1331-1346. doi:10.1111/j.1532-5415.2009.02376. x

Barrie, J., & Loughlin, D. (2014). Managing chronic pain in adults. *Nursing Standard, 29*(7), 50-58. doi:10.7748/ns.29.7.50. e9099

British Association of Social Workers. (2012, January). The Code of Ethics For Social Work: Statement of principles. Retrieved January 17, 2015, from http://cdn. basw.co.uk/upload/basw_112315-7.pdf

Carter, J., Watson, A. C., & Sminkey, P. V. (2014). Pain management: Screening and assessment of pain as part of a comprehensive case management process. *Professional Case Management, 19*(3), 126-136. doi:10.1097/NCM.0000000000000029

Diallo, B., & Kautz, D. D. (2014). Better pain management for elders in the intensive care unit. *Dimensions of Critical Care Nursing, 33*(6), 316-319. doi:10.1097/DCC.0000000000000074

Ehde, D. M., Dillworth, T. M., & Turner, J. A. (2014). Cognitive-behavioral therapy for individuals with chronic pain: Efficacy, innovations, and directions for research. *American Psychologist, 69*(2), 153-166. doi:10.1037/a0035747

Hanks-Bell, M., Halvey, K., & Paice, J. A. (2004). Pain assessment and management in aging. *The Online Journal of Issues in Nursing, 9*(3). Retrieved from http://www.nursingworld.org/MainMenuCategories/ANAMarketplace/ANAPeriodicals/OJIN/TableofContents/Volume92004/No3Sept04/ArticlePreviousTopic/PainAssessmentandManagementinAging. aspx

Haraldseid, C., Dysvik, E., & Furnes, B. (2014). The experience of loss in patients suffering from chronic pain attending a pain management group based on cognitive-behavioral therapy. *Pain Management Nursing: Official Journal of the American Society of Pain Management Nurses, 15*(1), 12-21. doi:10.1016/j. pmp.2012.04.004

Hermsen, L. A. H., Leone, S. S., Smalbrugge, M., Dekker, J., & van der Horst, H. E. (2014). Frequency, severity, and determinants of functional limitations in older adults with joint pain and comorbidity: results of a cross-sectional study. *Archives of Gerontology & Geriatrics, 59*(1), 98-106. doi:10.1016/j. archger.2014.02.006

Hofmann, S. G., Sawyer, A. T., & Fang, A. (2010). The empirical status of the "New Wave" of cognitive behavioral therapy. *Psychiatric Clinics of North America, 33*(3), 701-710. doi:10.1016/j. psc.2010.04.006

Hooten, W. M., Timming, R., Belgrade, M., Gaul, J., Haake, B., Myers, C.,... Walker, N. (2013, November). Institute for Clinical Systems Improvement health care guideline: assessment and management of chronic pain. Retrieved February 19, 2016, from https://www.icsi.org/_asset/bw798b/ChronicPain.pdf

Hugenschmidt, C. E., & Sink, K. M. (2015). No pain, functional gain: the importance of pain management in older adults with cognitive impairment. *Pain, 156*(8), 1377-1378.

Hwang, U., Richardson, L. D., Harris, B., & Morrison, R. S. (2010). The quality of emergency department pain care for older adult patients. *Journal of the American Geriatrics Society, 58*(11), 2122-2128. doi:10.1111/j.1532-5415.2010.03152. x

International Federation of Social Workers. (2012, March 3). *Statement of ethical principles.* Retrieved January 17, 2016, from http://ifsw.org/policies/statements-of-ethical-principles

Isaacs, C. G., Kistler, C., Hunold, K. M., Pereira, G. F., Buchbinder, M., Weaver, M. A.,... Platts-Mills, T. F. (2013). Shared decision-making in the selection of outpatient analgesics for older emergency department patients. *Journal of the American Geriatrics Society, 61*(5), 793-798. doi:10.1111/jgs.12207

Morley, S. (2011). Efficacy and effectiveness of cognitive behaviour therapy for chronic pain: progress and some challenges. *Pain, 152,* S99-S106. doi:10.1016/j. pain.2010.10.042

Morone, N. E., Abebe, K. Z., Morrow, L. A., & Weiner, D. K. (2014). Pain and decreased cognitive function negatively impact physical functioning in older adults with knee osteoarthritis. *Pain Medicine, 15*,9. doi:10.111/pme.12483

Morrissey, M. B., Viola, D., & Shi, Q. (2014). Relationship between pain and chronic illness among seriously ill older adults: expanding role for palliative social work. *Journal of Social Work in End-of-Life & Palliative Care, 10*(1), 8-33. doi:10.1080/15524256 .2013.877861

National Association of Social Workers (NASW). (2005). How social workers help with pain management. Retrieved January 17, 2016, from http://www.helpstartshere.org/health-and-wellness/pain/pain-how-social-workers-help-with-pain-management. html

Nicholas, M. K., Asghari, A., Blyth, F. M., Wood, B. M., Murray, R., McCabe, R.,... Overton, S. (2013). Self-management intervention for chronic pain in older adults: A randomised controlled trial. *Pain, 154*(6), 824-835. doi:10.1016/j. pain.2013.02.009

Oliver, D. P., Wittenberg-Lyles, E., Washington, K. T., & Sehrawat, S. (2009). Social work role in pain management with hospice caregivers: A national survey. *Journal of Social Work in End-of-Life & Palliative Care, 5*(1-2), 61-74.

Onubogu, U. D. (2014). Pain and depression in older adults with arthritis. *Orthopaedic Nursing, 33*(2), 102-108. doi:10.1097/NOR.0000000000000035

Parker, S. J., Jessel, S., Richardson, J. E., & Reid, M. C. (2013). Older adults are mobile too! Identifying the barriers and facilitators to older adults' use of mHealth for pain management. *BMC Geriatrics, 13*(43), 1-8. doi:10.1186/1471-2318-13-43

Pimental, C. B., Briesacher, B. A., Gurwitz, J. H., Rosen, A. B., Pimental, M. T., & Lapane, K. L. (2015). Pain management in nursing home residents with cancer. *Journal of the American Geriatrics Society, 63*(4), 633-641. doi:10.1111/jgs.13345

Sengupta, M., Bercovitz, A., & Harris-Kojetin, L. D. (2010). Prevalence and management of pain, by race and dementia among nursing home residents: United States, 2004. *NCHS Data Brief,* 1-8. Retrieved from

Stewart, C., Leveille, S. G., Shmerling, R. H., Samelson, E. J., Bean, J. F., & Schofield, P. (2012). Management of persistent pain in older adults: the MOBILIZE Boston study. *Journal of the American Geriatrics Society, 60*(11), 2081-2086. doi:10.1111/j.1532-5415.2012.04197. x

Wheeler, D. (2015). NASW Standards and Indicators for Cultural Competence in Social Work Practice. Retrieved January 17, 2016, from http://www.socialworkers.org/practice/standards/PRA-BRO-253150-CC-Standards.pdf

PALLIATIVE CARE FOR CHILDREN WITH CANCER

MAJOR CATEGORIES: Palliative & Hospice Care, Medical & Health

DESCRIPTION

Although rare in childhood, cancer is a leading cause of nonaccidental death in children. The most common cancers in children are leukemia and brain cancer. The causes of most childhood cancers are largely unknown; a diagnosis of Down syndrome, genetic abnormalities, and exposure to ionizing radiation explain a small number of cancer cases in children. Environmental causes of childhood cancer are suspected but difficult to confirm. Eighty percent of childhood cancers worldwide occur among children living in the developing world, where resources are scarce and many children with potentially treatable cancers die because therapies are unavailable.

Palliative care is both a philosophy of care and a system for delivering healthcare; it bridges the gap between cure-oriented medical treatments and symptom management. This approach to medical care involves an interdisciplinary palliative care team that includes physicians, nurses, clergy, social workers, hospice staff, the child, and the child's family. The goal of palliative care is to provide relief from painful and distressing physical, psychological, and emotional symptoms. It also offers a range of support services to families. Palliative care can span an extended period of time, encompassing the active treatment phase of the disease, periods of disease remissions, recurrences of the disease and symptoms, and the decline in health before death. Although not limited to end-of-life care, palliative care usually is provided for children with terminal illness.

Historically, palliative care has been provided by hospices, in which children with a life expectancy of 6 months or less abandon curative treatments. Hospice provides care of terminally ill children that focuses on pain and symptom management and the emotional and spiritual needs of the child. Yet there is growing recognition that palliative care should not be limited to the end of life but expanded to include caring for those with chronic illness and disease. Children with terminal cancer often experience considerable physical and psychosocial pain at the end of life. Palliative care services increasingly are offered to these children and their families, and studies suggest that palliative care should be introduced at the initial diagnosis of cancer. Prognostic uncertainty and hope for survival, however, can make the choice to pursue palliative care very difficult for families as long as palliative care is incorrectly perceived to be synonymous with end-of-life care.

Although there are some similarities, the palliative needs of children and adolescents are qualitatively different from those of adults. Children have unique developmental needs, their death is utterly untimely, and the family plays a more central role, especially because of the child's dependency. Children cannot legally consent to their own treatment. Treatment decisions tend to be made collectively with the family, although some parents have reported feeling excluded from the medical decision making process until the child is at the end of life. The parents may be distressed and have difficulty understanding the complex medical information about their child's diagnosis which can cause misunderstandings and confusion. Pain control and symptom management

in children is often inadequate and should take priority. Psychological and social risks and symptoms for the child with cancer and his or her family and friends include symptoms of anxiety, anger, and depression. Social workers should help facilitate the communication between the child and his or her family and between the family and healthcare professionals.

The grief for parents following the death of a child from cancer is much more intense than that resulting from the loss of a spouse/partner or parent; studies have shown that parents remain at risk for mental health problems for up to 5 years after the child's death. Although most siblings of sick and dying children are well adjusted, they have double the risk of developing mental health problems compared to children not living in such circumstances. Social workers should provide support and bereavement counseling and promote age-appropriate interventions for the siblings, friends, and family members. After a child dies, grief and bereavement services for siblings, parents, friends, schoolmates, and the extended community should continue.

FACTS AND FIGURES

The Centers for Disease Control and Prevention's (CDC) Cancer Statistics Working Group reported that in 2012 the rate of invasive cancer in the United States was 18 cases per 100,000 children younger than 19, with leukemia having the highest diagnosed rate at 4.4 cases per 100,000. The breakdown by race and ethnicity per 100,000 of each group's population was

- American Indian/Alaska Native, 11.4;
- Asian/Pacific Islander, 14.5;
- Black, 13.3;
- Hispanic, 17.2; and
- White, 18.8.

The World Health Organization (WHO) estimates that childhood cancer represents between 0.5 percent and 4.6 percent of all cancers worldwide, and that in high-income countries 80 percent of children diagnosed with cancer survive 5 or more years after diagnosis. The prognosis and life expectancy for children with cancer is much lower for children in low- and middle-income countries, but specific data are not available because of the lack of healthcare infrastructure.

RISK FACTORS

Different cancers have different risk factors. For adults, many cancers are linked to risk factors associated with lifestyle choices such as smoking, obesity, and not exercising. Because these risk factors take time to develop into cancer, however, they do not account for childhood cancer. A few environmental factors such as exposure to radiation might increase risk for childhood cancer, but most childhood cancers are thought not to have outside causes. Current research indicates that DNA mutation, either inherited or acquired after conception, is responsible for cancer in children.

SIGNS AND SYMPTOMS

The family can experience severe shock once a child receives a diagnosis of cancer, and there will likely be signs of anxiety, anger, and depression in family members. Parents of children diagnosed with cancer can experience strains and stresses within their parental roles and marriage. Following the death of a child, the parent and family responses to death vary widely, but symptoms of grief are often complicated by a range of additional mental health problems.

ASSESSMENT

The social worker should conduct a biological, psychological, social, and spiritual assessment of the child and family that includes information on any physical, mental, environmental, social, spiritual, financial, and medical factors that may affect the child or family. The assessment should include the whole family and the use of tools such as a genogram (map of family relationships) to assess family stability and communication styles.

ASSESSMENT AND SCREENING TOOLS

Standardized tools and assessments for screening or assessing children with cancer may be administered, such as the Distress Thermometer (DT), the Psychosocial Assessment Tool (PAT), and the SCREEM Family Resources Questionnaire, which measures family resources in six domains: social, cultural, religious, economic, educational, and medical.

TREATMENT

Communication by the medical team and social worker with families who have a child with cancer must be done with care and compassion. Cultural competence and knowledge of the family and child's healthcare beliefs is critical because it strongly influences the family and child's attitudes towards healthcare services and necessary advance care planning. Families indicate the need to hear comforting messages that validate that what they are experiencing is normal under the circumstances, and they need affirmation about the challenges they face. Pain and symptom management is often considered inadequate and must take priority in care decisions.

Social workers can assist families with completing their advance care directives (ACDs) and advance care planning (ACP), which require the consideration of a family's personal history. ACP is a process by which families can clarify their values and goals to guide possible future healthcare decisions that extend beyond medical decision making; social workers can assist the family and child in this planning process. Social workers can also help families think through ACDs that include curative medical treatment withdrawal.

INTERVENTION

If concerns are made known by the family or the social worker that the child may have signs and symptoms of cancer (fatigue, fever, unexplained bruising or pain, headaches), the social worker should assist in making a referral to the child's pediatrician or pediatric oncologist to determine whether the child has cancer. The medical team and social worker should use repetition and verification of understanding to ensure that any medical information or diagnosis discussed is understood by the family.

If cancer is diagnosed in childhood, the social worker should provide support and guidance to the family through the trauma of learning of the diagnosis and the expected prognosis. Relief from painful and distressing physical, psychological, emotional, and/or spiritual symptoms should be offered. The social worker assisting the family should collaborate with other healthcare professionals to deliver services that meet necessary palliative care goals. Roles of the social worker during this time may include translating medical information into understandable terms; advocating for adequate pain management; empowering the family and patient, providing counseling to the family and patient, and providing support; helping with developing ACPs and ACDs; and providing bereavement counseling to the family after the death of the child.

Parents may experience an anticipatory grief reaction to the child's diagnosis of cancer. Social workers should assist parents in coping with feelings of shock, fear, anger, confusion, and stress. The parents and family should be referred to peer support groups for coping with the child's cancer diagnosis. Medical professionals, palliative care team members, and the social worker should use repetition and verification of information with the family to ensure that the information regarding treatment and prognosis is understood.

The child may have feelings of loneliness, anxiety, anger, confusion, denial, depression, and fear regarding their diagnosis of cancer. The social worker should assist the child in processing and coping with any negative feelings about their cancer diagnosis. If needed, a referral to mental health services or support groups should be made. The social worker should help normalize the child's feelings about their diagnosis and provide necessary emotional support. The child's family and friends should be involved to increase the level of available support to the child.

APPLICABLE LAWS AND REGULATIONS

Children are not legally able to direct their own treatment. The age at which children can make their own treatment decisions varies by jurisdiction.

SERVICES AND RESOURCES

- National Cancer Institute, http://www.cancer.gov/types/childhood-cancers
- Cancer.Net, http://www.cancer.net
- U.S. Centers for Disease Control and Prevention (CDC), http://www.cdc.gov/cancer/
- World Health Organization (WHO), http://www.who.int/cancer/palliative/definition/en/
- National Association of Social Workers (NASW), http://www.socialworkers.org
- Bereaved Parents of the USA, http://www.bereavedparentsusa.org
- National Hospice and Palliative Care Organization, http://www.nhpco.org/learn-about-end-life-care
- The National Council for Palliative Care, http://www.ncpc.org.uk/

FOOD FOR THOUGHT

At the end of life, families typically prefer that all treatment take place at home. Many children die in critical-care settings, making the provision of peaceful, family-centered care at the time of the child's death a challenge.

Pediatric oncology social workers say they develop knowledge and skills on the job by listening to children and families.

Cultural competence extends to appreciating the contexts in which some immigrant families live. One study identified poverty and the absolute need to continue working as contributing to the parents' absence from children's bedside or from critical meetings, which should not be judged but understood with compassion by the treatment team. This challenge can also apply to nonimmigrant families struggling with poverty.

In attending to a family's psychological, practical, and spiritual needs, social workers need to consider how gender, race, and culture affect a family's value system, beliefs, and customs regarding illness and death.

Significant improvements are being made in palliative care for children dying from cancer in Germany, and there is a movement to develop similar standards in other European countries.

Parents often want to keep prognosis and treatment information from their child to protect him or her. However, parents should be encouraged to involve their child in the decision making process, as developmentally appropriate.

RED FLAGS

Children with cancer often experience considerable physical, psychological, and social pain at the end of life: Alleviating this pain should take priority in palliative care treatment plans. Parents of children dying of cancer report feeling excluded from the treatment decision making process until the child is at the end of life. There is a great need for retaining normalcy in families in which a child has cancer, yet achieving this can be profoundly difficult.

NEXT STEPS

The social worker should help educate the family regarding bereavement support and what to expect as the child's health declines. The social worker should encourage the family to address any feelings of grief and loss that arise with the decline and/or death of their child. The social worker should remain aware of where the family is in the grief process and make referrals to a mental health clinician if indicated (symptoms of depression, anxiety, posttraumatic stress disorder are reported).

Written by Jan Wagstaff, MA, MSW

Reviewed by Laura McLuckey, MSW, LCSW, and Chris Bates, MA, MSW

REFERENCES

American Cancer Society. (2015, January 1). Cancer in children: What are risk factors and causes of childhood cancer? Retrieved October 14, 2015, from http://www.cancer.org/cancer/cancerinchildren/detailedguide/cancer-in-children-risk-factors-and-causes

Black, D. (1998). Coping with loss: The dying child. *British Medical Journal, 316,* 7141. Retrieved October 14, 2015, from http://www.ncbi.nlm.nih.gov/pmc/articles/PMC1113075/

British Association of Social Workers. (2012, January). The code of ethics for social work: Statement of principles. Retrieved October 14, 2015, from http://cdn.basw.co.uk/upload/basw_112315-7.pdf

Contro, N., Davies, B., Larson, J., & Sourkes, B. (2010). Away from home: Experiences of Mexican American families in pediatric palliative care. *Journal of Social Work in End-of-Life and Palliative Care, 6*(3-4), 185-204. doi:10.1080/15524256.2010.529020

Csikai, E. L., & Black, K. (2009). Advance care planning in the delivery of adult protective services. *Journal of Social Service Research, 35*(4), 311-321. doi:10.1080/01488370903110811

Docherty, S. L., Brandon, D., Thaxton, C. A., & Barfield, R. C. (2015). Family-centered palliative care. In *Wong's nursing care of infants and children* (10th ed., pp. 791-801). St. Louis, MO: Elsevier Mosby.

Heitkemper, M. M. (2014). Palliative care at end of life. In S. L. Lewis, S. R. Dirksen, M. M. Heitkemper, L. Bucher, & M. M. Harding (Eds.), *Medical-surgical nursing: Assessment and management of clinical problems* (9th ed., pp. 140-153). St. Louis, MO: Mosby Elsevier.

Heyman, J. C., & Gutheil, I. A. (2010). Older Latinos' attitudes toward and comfort with end-of-life planning. *Health and Social Work, 35*(1), 17-26.

International Federation of Social Workers. (2012, March 3). Statement of ethical principles. Retrieved October 14, 2015, from http://ifsw.org/policies/statement-of-ethical-principles/

Jones, B. L. (2005). Pediatric palliative and end-of-life care: The role of social work in pediatric oncology. *Journal of Social Work in End-of-Life and Palliative Care, 1*(4), 35-61.

Jones, B. L. (2006). Companionship, control, and compassion: A social work perspective on the needs of children with cancer and their families at the end of life. *Journal of Palliative Medicine, 9*(3), 774-788. doi:10.1089/jpm.2006.9.774

Kazak, A. E., Brier, M., Alderfer, M. A., Reilly, A., Fooks-Parker, S.,... Barakat, L. P. (2013). Screening for psychosocial risk in pediatric cancer. *Pediatric Blood Cancer, 59*(5), 822-827. doi:10.1002/pbc.24166

McGrath, P. (2001). Findings on the impact of treatment for childhood acute lymphoblastic leukaemia on family relationships. *Child and Family Social Work, 6*(3), 229-237. doi:10.1046/j.1365-2206.2001.00200.x

Mizrahi, T., & Mayden, R. W. (2001). NASW standards for cultural competence in social work practice. Retrieved October 14, 2015, from http://www.socialworkers.org/practice/standards/NASWCulturalStandards.pdf

Pockett, R., Walker, E., & Dave, K. (2010). "Last orders": Dying in a hospital setting. *Australian Social Work, 63*(3), 250-265. doi:10.1080/0312407X.2010.497928

Riley, C. D. (2014). Cancer nursing. In N. S. M. (Ed.), *Lippincott manual of nursing practice* (10th ed., pp. 161-162). Philadelphia, PA: Wolters Kluwer Lippincott Williams & Wilkins.

Schmidt, P., Otto, M., Hechler, T., Metzing, S., Wolfe, J., & Zernikow, B. (2013). Did increased availability of pediatric palliative care lead to improved palliative care outcomes in children with cancer?. *Journal of Palliative Medicine, 16*(9), 1034-1039. doi:10.1089/jpm.2013.0014

Smith, P. (2009). The family caregivers journey in end of life care: Recognizing and identifying with the role of care. *International Journal on Disability and Human Development, 8*(1), 67-73. doi:10.1515/IJDHD.2009.8.1.67

Steliarova-Foucher, E., & Ullrich, A. (n.d.). International Childhood Cancer Day: 15

February 2015. Retrieved October 14, 2015, from http://www.who.int/cancer/media/news/Childhood_cancer_day/en/

U.S. Cancer Statistics Working Group. (2015). United States cancer statistics: 1999-2012 incidence and mortality. Retrieved October 14, 2015, from https://nccd.cdc.gov/uscs/childhoodcancerbyprimarysite.aspx

Van Beek, K., Woitha, K., Ahmed, N., Menten, J., Jaspers, B., Engels, Y.,... Hasselaar, J. (2013). Comparison of legislation, regulations and national health strategies for palliative care in seven European countries (results from the Europall Research Group): A descriptive study. *BMC Health Service Research, 13*, 275. Retrieved from http://www.ncbi.nlm.nih.gov/pmc/articles/PMC3720186/, doi:10.1186/1472-6963-13-275

Waldman, E., & Wolfe, J. (2013). Palliative care for children with cancer. *Clinical Oncology, 10*(2), 100-107.

Watts, J. H. (2013). Exploring the "social" of social work in palliative care: Working with diversity. *Illness, Crisis & Loss, 21*(4), 281-295. doi:10.2190/IL.21.4.b

Yeo, G. (2009). How will the U.S. healthcare system meet the challenge of the ethnogeriatric imperative? *Journal of the American Geriatrics Society, 57*(7), 1278-1285. doi:10.1111/j.1532-5415.2009.02319.x

PALLIATIVE CARE FOR OLDER ADULTS

MAJOR CATEGORIES: Palliative & Hospice Care, Medical & Health

DESCRIPTION

Palliative care is a worldwide movement comprising both a philosophy of care and a system for delivering healthcare. Palliative care bridges the gap between cure-oriented treatments and symptom management treatment. The goal of palliative care is to provide relief from painful and distressing physical symptoms with the integration of psychological, emotional, and spiritual/existential care. By definition, palliative care can span an extended period of time, encompassing the active treatment phase of disease, disease remissions, recurrences of disease, and the decline in health before death. Often these conditions and diseases are life-threatening or terminal and palliative care is strongly associated with end-of-life care.

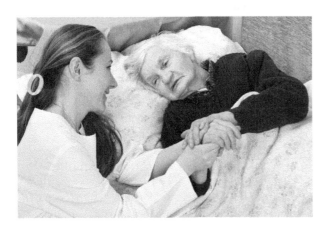

Increasingly, however, palliative care is not limited to those who are terminally ill but may be provided to all individuals in whom a serious illness or condition, including chronic pain, is diagnosed. Palliative care also includes services for families such as support with medical decision making and bereavement counseling after their loved one has died. This approach to care involves an interdisciplinary palliative care team that includes physicians, nurses, clergy, social workers, hospice staff, the patient, and the patient's family. The role of social workers in palliative care teams can be broad and may include advocating for the patient and family, providing counseling, and providing support to the patient and family as well as assisting patients in developing advance care plans (ACPs) and advance directives (ADs).

Older adults are persons over 65 years of age. The three leading causes of death in this age group are heart disease, cancer, and stroke. The number of older adults over 80 has significantly increased in recent decades, and these individuals often have multiple diseases, medical conditions, and increased frailty. Although surveys indicate that most persons have a strong preference to die at home, many older adults in their final years enter residential care facilities, long-term nursing homes, assisted living communities, or private community-based homes due to their medical needs and need for assistance with their care. The treatment for pain and symptom management for older adults living in these long-term care facilities are provided, along with the provided services and support for psychological, social, and spiritual needs, is inadequate, especially at the end of life. Increasingly, nursing homes are accessing palliative care for their residents by contracting with hospices for services. Individuals receive hospice care when they are not responsive to medical care or choose to stop curative treatments and death is anticipated within 6 months; hospices are considered the expert at providing palliative care.

The families of older adults often struggle with decisions about moving their relatives to residential care facilities such as nursing homes. They also encounter difficulties when attempting to make decisions about whether to limit or end curative treatment, especially when the benefits of treatment are uncertain. Within these conflicts, caregivers can become disconnected from the emotional needs of the older adult; ADs and ACPs can help ensure that patients' emotional needs are taken into account. ADs, sometimes called *living wills*, are legal documents in which patients specify what actions should be taken regarding their health should they become incapacitated and unable to make decisions regarding their medical care. ADs are intended to direct decision making for patients and support their autonomy, but in the event of an emergency they may prove inadequate.

The circumstances surrounding an end-of-life situation may necessitate the rewriting of an AD in collaboration with family and healthcare professionals. ACP is a broader process that extends beyond medical decision making: It focuses on establishing clear communication between the patient, family members, and healthcare professionals about the patient's healthcare wishes. Social workers can assist patients in clarifying their values and goals and help them identify principles that may guide care in the final years of life. It is worth noting that many dying people do not fear death, but above all value their autonomy, independence, and dignity and fear losing this.

FACTS AND FIGURES
Globally, the number of older adults will increase from 101 million in 2010 to 277 million by 2050. In the United States, approximately 16 percent of palliative care services are provided to patients over 85 years old, even though 39 percent of deaths occur in this age group. More than 25 percent of older adults

in the United States have not made any decisions regarding end-of-life care. In 2012–2013 nearly 50 percent of patients receiving palliative care in England died in their homes, compared to just over 20 percent in the rest of the United Kingdom.

RISK FACTORS
Older adults are at risk of experiencing unnecessary physical, psychological, emotional, and spiritual pain in their final years of life.

SIGNS AND SYMPTOMS
Some older adults near the end of life deteriorate erratically and suddenly, whereas others follow a predictable pattern of decline. Signs and symptoms vary depending on the diagnosis.

ASSESSMENT
Social workers can assist patients in writing ADs and ACPs, which require consideration of a patient's personal history. Therefore, a thorough biological, psychological, social, and spiritual assessment should be conducted with the patient and patient's family.

ASSESSMENT AND SCREENING TOOLS
Standardized assessment and screening tools may be used by social workers when assessing the need of the older adult patient. Possible assessment and screening tools that a social worker may use include the Palliative Care Outcome Scale (POS), the European Organization for Research and Treatment of Cancer Qualify of Life Questionnaire Core 15 Palliative (EORTC QLQ-C15-PAL), the Rest & Peace Scale (RPS), and the Patient Satisfaction Questionnaire-III (PSQ-III). The results of these scales and assessments will help direct the patient's advance directives and care plan.

TREATMENT
ACP is a process by which patients can clarify their values and goals to guide healthcare decisions that extend beyond medical decision making. Social workers can assist older patients with this planning process. They can also help patients think through ADs. Cultural competence is critical for social workers because culture strongly influences attitudes towards healthcare services and advance planning. It is important that the patient's cultural beliefs about healthcare and end-of-life decisions are taken into

account when discussing advanced care plans. Social workers should approach communication as a dialogue, communicate respectfully in various formats (verbally, in writing, and through demonstration), and avoid jargon when speaking with the patient and their family members. They should allow patients and family members to share their stories, thoughts, and feelings about the situation and be tactful when educating the family or patient if challenging cognitive distortions and beliefs are shared about the medical treatment. Contact information should be provided so patients can clarify information or ask questions when they need to. Social workers should educate patients about their rights, reminding them that they are in control during the decision making and advance care planning process.

INTERVENTION

Older adults may experience chronic physical and emotional pain in the final stages of life. Palliative care aims to help individuals maintain their autonomy and dignity by providing relief from painful and distressing physical, psychological, emotional, and spiritual symptoms at the end of life. Social workers work in collaboration with other healthcare professionals in delivering services to meet the patient's identified palliative care goals. Their role may include advocating for adequate pain management medication, providing counseling and support to the patient and family members, and helping patients write necessary ACPs and ADs.

APPLICABLE LAWS AND REGULATIONS

Nursing homes in the United States with 120 or more beds are required by law to employ a full-time social worker. In the United States, the Patient Self-Determination Act of 1990 requires that healthcare providers, including hospice and in-home care organizations, provide information about advance healthcare directives to adult patients upon their admission to the healthcare facility. In Germany, France, Poland, Spain, and the United Kingdom, the palliative healthcare policies vary between regions.

In 2013 the Palliative Care and Hospice Education Training Act was introduced in the House and Senate to improve palliative and hospice care.

In 2003 the National Association of Social Workers published "Standards of Social Work Practice in Palliative and End of Life Care (PELC)" to enhance

social workers' awareness and skills when dealing with patients and their families facing end-of-life issues. In 2010 the National Association of Social Workers published "Standards for Social Work Practice with Family Caregivers of Older Adults" to improve social work practice and standards in 12 domains (such as ethics and values, advocacy, collaboration). In 2015, the United States federal government proposed a policy to reimburse Medicare health providers for talking to beneficiaries about end-of-life care.

SERVICES AND RESOURCES

- Get Palliative Care, http://www.getpalliativecare.org
- International Association for Hospice & Palliative Care, http://www.hospicecare.com
- The Conversation Project, http://theconversationproject.org/
- National Hospice and Palliative Care Organization, http://www.nhpco.org/learn-about-end-life-care
- Palliative Care Matters, www.pallcare.info/
- American Geriatric Society's Health in Aging Foundation, www.healthinaging.org
- Aging with Dignity, www.agingwithdignity.org

FOOD FOR THOUGHT

Older adults are frequently devalued in society because individual worth is often measured by socioeconomic status and productivity and many older adults are unable to work. Only four countries (Germany, Japan, the Netherlands, and South Korea) have a dedicated insurance system for long-term care of older adults, but the fiscal sustainability of these services is threatened by declining birth rates and aging populations.

Many social workers and patients experience discomfort when discussing end-of-life issues. Terminally ill patients who are deeply connected to a religious community access hospice care less frequently and are less likely to pursue aggressive treatments than those who are terminally ill but not connected to a religious community. Integration of spiritual care and end-of-life discussions into a patient's treatment can reduce the use of aggressive treatments at the end of life. All older adult patients should be given the opportunity to express their wishes and preferences about end of life, so these conversations must take place as early as possible before patients lose the capacity to make decisions (for example, due to dementia).

RED FLAGS

In the United States, entering hospice care requires that a patient waive their other Medicare benefits such as paying for hospitalization and specialized nursing care related to terminal illness.

Homeless older adults in need of palliative care are an especially vulnerable group and encounter many barriers, such as funding needs, when seeking services.

NEXT STEPS

The social worker should encourage the patient and family to participate in activities they enjoy for as long as possible, to participate in religious or spiritual activities, if desired, and to avoid social isolation. The social worker should encourage older adult patients to prepare for possible end-of-life decision making needs while still living their lives fully through the completion of an AD and assignment of a healthcare proxy or representative. Patients and families should be encouraged to share their feelings about death and discuss any concerns they may have. Education regarding available bereavement support should be provided to the patient and family.

*Written by Jan Wagstaff, MA, MSW, and
Laura McLuckey, MSW, LCSW*

*Reviewed by Lynn B. Cooper, D Crim, and
Laura Gale, LCSW*

REFERENCES

Alzheimer's Disease International. (2013). World Alzheimer report 2013: Journey of caring: An analysis of long-term care for dementia. Retrieved December 14, 2015, from http://www.alz.co.uk/research/world-report-201

Balboni, T. A., Balboni, M., Enzinger, A. C., Gallivan, K., Paulk, M. E., Wright, A.,... Prigerson, H. G. (2013). Provision of spiritual support to patients with advanced cancer by religious communities and associations with medical care at the end of life. *JAMA Internal Medicine, 173*(12), 1109-1117. doi:10.1001/jamainternmed.2013.903

Bern-Klug, M., & Sabri, B. (2012). Nursing home social services directors and elder abuse staff training. *Journal of Gerontological Social Work, 55*(1), 5-20. doi:10.1080/01634372.2011.626016

British Association of Social Workers. (2012, January). The code of ethics for social work: Statement of principles. Retrieved December 14, 2015, from http://cdn.basw.co.uk/upload/basw_112315-7.pdf

Bye, R. A., Llewellyn, G. M., & Christi, K. E. (2009). Chapter 26: The end of life. In R. B. Bonder & V. Dal Bello-Haas (Eds.), *Functional performance in older adults* (3rd ed., pp. 633-652). Philadelphia, PA: F.A. Davis Company.

Cagle, J. G. (2009). Weathering the storm: Palliative care and elderly homeless persons. *Journal of Housing for the Elderly, 23*(1-2), 29-46. doi:10.1080/02763890802664588

Cagle, J. G., & Kovacs, P. J. (2009). Education: A complex and empowering social work intervention at the end of life. *Health & Social Work, 34*(1), 17-25. doi:10.1093/hsw/34.1.17

Centers for Medicare & Medicaid Services. (2015). Proposed policy, payment, and qualify provisions changes to the Medicare physician fee schedule for calendar year 2016. Retrieved December 14, 2015, from https://www.cms.gov/Newsroom/MediaReleaseDatabase/Fact-sheets/2015-Fact-sheets-items/2015-10-30-2.html

Congress.gov. (1990). H.R.4449 – Patient Self-Determination Act of 1990. Retrieved December 14, 2015, from https://www.congress.gov/bill/101st-congress/house-bill/4449

Correll Munn, J., & Adorno, G. (2008). By invitation only: Social work involvement at the end of life in long-term care. *Journal of Social Work in End-of-Life & Palliative Care, 4*(4), 333-357. doi:10.1080/15524250903081491

Csikai, E. L., & Black, K. (2009). Advance care planning in the delivery of adult protective services. *Journal of Social Service Research, 35*, 311-321. doi:10.1080/01488370903110811

Deodhar, J. K., & Muckaden, M. A. (2015). Continuing professional development for volunteers working in palliative care in a tertiary care cancer institute in India: A cross-sectional observation study of educational needs. *India Journal of Palliative Care, 21*(2), 158-163. doi:10.4103/0973-1075.156475

Doukas, N. (2014). Are methadone counselors properly equipped to meet the palliative care needs of older adults in methadone maintenance treatment?. *Implication for training. Journal of Social Work in End-of-Life & Palliative Care, 10*(2), 186-204. doi:10.1080/15524256.2014.906370

Gill, T. M., Gahbauer, E. A., Han, L., & Allore, H. G. (2010). Trajectories of disability in the last year of life. *New England Journal of Medicine, 362*(13), 1173-1180. doi:10.1056/NEJMoa0909087

Heyman, J. C., & Gutheil, I. A. (2010). Older Latinos' attitudes toward and comfort with end-of-life planning. *Health and Social Work, 35*(1), 17-26. doi:10.1093/hsw/35.1.17

Institute of Medicine. (2014). Dying in America: Improving qualify and honoring individual preferences near the end of life. Retrieved December 14, 2015, from https://iom.nation-alacademies.org/~/media/Files/Report percent-20Files/2014/EOL/Report percent20Brief.pdf

International Federation of Social Workers. (2012). Statement of ethical principles. Retrieved December 14, 2015, from http://ifsw.org/policies/statement-of-ethical-principles/

Kellehear, A. (2009). Dying old - and preferably alone? Agency, resistance and dissent at the end of life. *International Journal of Ageing and Later Life, 4*(1), 5-21.

Kelly, A., Conell-Price, J., Covinsky, K., Stijacic Cenzer, I., Chang, A., Boscardin, W. J., & Smith, A. K. (2010). Length of stay for older adults residing in nursing homes at the end of life. *Journal of the American Geriatrics Society, 58*(9), 1701-1706. doi:10.1111/j.1532-5415.2010.03005.x

Ko, F. C., & Morrison, R. S. (2014). Hip fracture: A trigger for palliative care in vulnerable older adults. *JAMA Internal Medicine, 174*(8), 1281-1282. doi:10.1001/jamainternmed.2014.999

Lepore, J. M., Miller, S. C., & Gozalo, P. (2010). Hospice use among urban black and white U.S. nursing home decedents in 2006. *The Gerontologist, 51*(2), 251-260. doi:10.1093/geront/gnq093

Lima, J. C., Miller, S. C., & Shield, R. (2009). Palliative and hospice care in assisted living: Reality or wishful thinking? *Journal of Housing for the Elderly, 23*, 47-65. doi:10.1080/02763890802664638

Lorenz, K. A., Rosenfeld, K., & Wenger, N. (2007). Quality indicators for palliative and end-of-life care in vulnerable elders. *Journal of the American Geriatrics Society, 55*(Suppl 2), 318-326. doi:10.1111/j.1532-5415.2007.01338.x

McCusker, M., Ceronsky, L., Crone, C., Epstein, H., Greene, B., Halvorson, J.,... Setterlund, L. (2013).

Palliative care for adults. Bloomington, MN: Institute for Clinical Systems Improvement. Retrieved December 14, 2015, from https://www.icsi.org/_asset/k056ab/PalliativeCare.pdf

McKnight's Staff. (2013). Palliative care legislation proposes $44 million in education and fellowship for nurses. Retrieved December 14, 2015, from http://www.mcknights.com/palliative-care-legislation-proposes-44-million-in-education-fellowships-for-nurses/article/285988/

National Association of Social Workers. (2015). NASW standards for social work practice in palliative and end of life care. Retrieved December 14, 2015, from https://www.socialworkers.org/practice/bereavement/standards/default.asp

National Association of Social Workers. (2010). NASW standards for social work practice with family caregivers of older adults. Retrieved from https://www.socialworkers.org/practice/standards/naswfamilycaregiverstandards.pdf

National survey of patient data for specialist palliative care services. (2014). *Public Health England.* Retrieved December 14, 2015, from http://www.endoflifecare-intelligence.org.uk/resources/publications/mds_report

Pal, L. M., & Manning, L. (2014). Palliative care for frail older people. *Clinical Medicine, 14*(3), 292-295. doi:10.7861/clinmedicine.14-3-292

Pockett, R., Walker, E., & Dave, K. (2010). "Last orders": Dying in a hospital setting. *Australian Social Work, 63*(3), 250-265. doi:10.1080/0312407X.2010.497928

Seymour, J., Payne, S., Chapman, A., & Holloway, M. (2007). Hospice or home? Expectations of end-of-life care among white and Chinese older people in the UK. *Sociology of Health & Illness, 29*(6), 872-890. doi:10.1002/9781444306606.ch5

Slort, W., Blankenstein, A. H., Schweitzer, B. P., Knol, D. L., von der Horst, H. E., Aaronson, N. K., & Deliens, L. (2014). Effectiveness of the palliative care "availability, current issues and anticipation" (ACA) communication training programme for general practitioners on patient outcomes: A controlled trial. *Palliative Medicine, 28*(8), 1036-1045. doi:10.1016/j.pec.2013.12.012

Sorensen, R., & Iedema, R. (2011). End-of-life care in an acute care hospital: Linking policy and practice. *Death Studies, 35*(6), 481-503. doi:10.1080/07481187.2011.553336

United States General Accounting Office. (1995). Patient Self-Determination Act: Providers offer information on advance directives but effectiveness uncertain. Retrieved December 14, 2015, from http://www.gpo.gov/fdsys/pkg/GAORE-PORTS-HEHS-95-135/pdf/GAOREPORTS-HEHS-95-135.pdf

Van Beek, K., Woitha, K., Ahmed, N., Menten, J., Jaspers, B., Engels, Y.,... Hasselaar, J. (2013). Comparison of legislation, regulations and national health strategies for palliative care in seven European countries (results from the Europall Research Group); A descriptive study. Retrieved from http://www.ncbi.nlm.nih.gov/pmc/articles/PMC3720186/

Waldrop, D., & Kirkendall, A. M. (2010). Rural-urban differences in end-of-life care: Implications for practice. *Social Work in Health Care, 49*(3), 263-289.

Wale, J. (2014). Exploring key topics in palliative care: Pain and palliative care for older people. *Clinical Medicine, 14*(4), 416-418. doi:10.7861/clinmedicine.14-4-416

Washington, K. T., Parker Oliver, D., Demiris, G., Wittenberg-Lyles, E., & Shaunfield, S. (2011). Family perspectives on the hospice experience in adult family homes. *Journal of Gerontological Social Work, 54*(2), 159-174. doi:10.1080/01634372.2010.536833

Wheeler, D. (2015). NASW standards and indicators for cultural competence in social work practice. Retrieved December 14, 2015, from http://www.socialworkers.org/practice/standards/PRA-BRO-253150-CC-Standards.pdf

World Wide Health Organization. (2012). Defusing the demographic "time-bomb" in Germany. *Bulletin of the World Wide Health Organization, 90*, 1. Retrieved December 14, 2015, from http://www.who.int/bulletin/volumes/90/1/12-020112/en/index.html

Yeo, G. (2009). How will the U.S. healthcare system meet the challenge of the ethnogeriatric imperative? *Journal of the American Geriatrics Society, 57*(7), 1278-1285. doi:10.1111/j.1532-5415.2009.02319.x

Palliative Care for the Neonate

Major Categories: Palliative & Hospice Care, Medical & Health

Description
Palliative care is a worldwide movement comprising both a philosophy and way of thinking about care and a system for delivering healthcare; it bridges the gap between cure-oriented treatment options and symptom management options. Palliative care aims to provide relief from painful and distressing physical, psychological, and emotional symptoms for the patient and family. It offers a range of support services to families, including bereavement counseling. Historically, palliative care has been provided to adults by hospices, in which patients who have 6 months or less to live abandon curative therapy and medical treatment in favor of pursuing only palliative care. However, there is growing recognition that palliative care should not be limited to the end of life, but expanded to include caring for those with chronic illness and disease, including children. A neonate is an infant who is less than 28 days old. Palliative care for both the infant and his or her family can begin at the limit of the infant's viability (less than a 50 percent chance of long-term survival), when lethal congenital anomalies have been diagnosed, or when the infant with a serious medical condition is not responding to medical treatment and therapy. For neonates, palliative care most often equates to end-of-life care, and palliative care service extends beyond the death of the child to encompass continued support for the family.

Any medical diagnosis and prognosis involving neonates can present parents with the need for critical, unanticipated decision making. The limited time that distressed parents may have to digest complex medical information may result in misunderstandings and confusion about the diagnosis and prognosis. Parents whose infants are born very prematurely often must immediately choose whether their baby should be resuscitated or receive palliative care. Many parents will face the traumatic decision of whether or not to discontinue therapeutic care for their neonate. They may also be faced with deciding whether to withdraw or withhold medically provided hydration or nutrition. Parents may have to consider the use of medications, such as opioids, that may relieve pain or discomfort but may also shorten their neonate's life. Most frequently, these decisions are made when there is no chance of survival or when the prognosis is extremely poor. Clear information on the child's condition and expected prognosis is vital for parents making these decisions. Other factors identified as assisting parents in the decision making process include the infant's visible deterioration, knowledge of the baby's likelihood of experiencing pain, and the parents being allowed to hold their sick baby. Holding and caring for the infant can also help parents through the grieving process, although some parents might find this too upsetting; parents should be encouraged to do what they feel is right for them.

Social workers can facilitate the critical communication between the family and the medical care team, which might include acting as an advocate for the family. They may also provide emotional support and bereavement counseling to the family. Collecting and storing material memories is important to some families and can help in the grieving process; social workers can help with this. Social workers can also help the family make funeral arrangements.

FACTS AND FIGURES
The World Health Organization (WHO) estimates that of children younger than age 5 who die, 40 percent are neonates, 75 percent of whom die during their first week of life. The WHO estimates that in 2014 there were 2,747,000 million neonate deaths worldwide: approximately 989,000 in Africa, 122,000 in the Americas, 454,000 in the Eastern Mediterranean, 71,000 in Europe, 926,000 in Southeast Asia, and 171,000 in the Western Pacific. The Centers for Disease Control and Prevention (CDC) recorded 15,893 neonate deaths during 2013 in the United States and 3,932,181 live births. The overall neonate mortality rate per 1,000 live births was 4.04; for American Indians or Alaska Natives it was 4.11, for Asian American or Pacific Islanders 2.99, for blacks 7.46, for Hispanics 3.55, and for whites 3.34.

A randomized controlled trial in which participants were asked to make choices regarding the hypothetical delivery of a 23-week gestation infant found that when participants were told that resuscitation was the hospital's default option, versus

comfort care (palliative care), 80 percent chose resuscitation. When told that comfort care was the hospital's default option, however, 39 percent chose resuscitation. Many neonatal intensive care units do not have written guidelines regarding the use of drugs for comfort care after intensive treatment is withdrawn. In a study of cases in which life-limiting conditions were diagnosed prenatally, 62 percent of the infants received comfort care, with a median age at death of 2 days, and 38 percent were resuscitated and received intensive care, with a median age at death of 2 days.

RISK FACTORS
Worldwide, the leading causes of neonatal death are preterm birth, infection, and asphyxia (lack of oxygen). Labor complications significantly increase the risk of neonatal death worldwide, and poverty is consistently associated with an increased risk of labor complications. In the United States, risk factors for neonatal death include premature birth; birth defects; complications during pregnancy, including preeclampsia (high blood pressure); complications involving the placenta, umbilical cord, and membranes; infections; and asphyxia.

The grief for parents following the death of a child at any age can be much more intense than that resulting from the loss of a spouse or parent. Studies have shown that grieving parents are at risk for mental health problems. Although most siblings of sick or dying children are well adjusted, they have double the risk of developing mental health problems.

SIGNS AND SYMPTOMS
Sick or dying neonates may experience a range of symptoms depending on the diagnosis. When a newborn's life is threatened, parents initially may express disbelief, experience symptoms of shock, denial, anger, and frustration; siblings can feel excluded and marginalized by their family and may experience symptoms of stress and guilt.

ASSESSMENT
The social worker should conduct a basic assessment of the family, including a genogram (graph of family dynamics and relationships) and an evaluation of current communication skills and styles. The assessment should include the psychological, social, biological,

and spiritual history and beliefs of the family. Taking the neonate and family history during the palliative care of a neonate may include providing support and helping the family process information and feelings about the situation.

ASSESSMENT AND SCREENING TOOLS

There are no diagnostic assessments or screening tools that may be used during the assessment process for palliative care with neonates.

TREATMENT

Cultural competence and education to the social worker is critical when working in palliative care because culture strongly influences attitudes towards healthcare services and providers. Parents indicate that they value emotional support that allows them to express their grief and that it is important for the social worker to call the neonate by his or her name. The responses of siblings need to be validated by the social worker as normal to the individual sibling and to the family as well. Studies have shown that siblings involved in their brother's or sister's death usually adjust better. Material memories can help families through their grieving process. Social workers can assist families in collecting and storing material memories, including footprints, locks of hair, and photographs. Families may need help in making funeral arrangements. Ongoing individual or group bereavement counseling for the family and siblings can help reduce mental health problems.

INTERVENTION

If a problematic diagnosis and/or prognosis for a neonate is determined by the medical team, the social worker should provide support and guidance to the parents through the trauma of the diagnosis and discussion of prognosis. Support should be provided for any painful and distressing physical, psychological, and emotional symptoms and/or spiritual pain the family may experience. The option of palliative care for the neonate should be discussed with the family. The social worker should collaborate with other healthcare professionals and the social worker's role may include translating medical information into understandable terms for the family, providing counseling and support to the family, advocating on the family's behalf to the medical team, helping the family compile material memories, and assisting the family in making funeral arrangements.

If a woman who is pregnant has received information that her infant will be born with a condition that will be incompatible with life, the social worker should assist the woman and her partner with advance care birth planning. The social worker should provide support and counseling grief experienced by the parent's while planning for the birth and possible immediate needs of the infant. The social worker should help the family explore and discuss the experience of the pregnancy and the impact the fetal diagnosis has had on the family. The social worker can foster and facilitate a therapeutic relationship with the family via provided support and assistance with shared decision making. Education should be provided to the family on the condition while also acknowledging uncertainties that are a reality in birth outcomes. The parents' goals and values should be recognized by the social worker and shared with the medical team.

APPLICABLE LAWS AND REGULATIONS

In the United States the Baby Doe Amendment to the Child Abuse Prevention and Treatment Act (CAPTA) of 1984 allows for withholding of federal funds if medical treatment (which could include anything from nutrition to complex surgery) is withheld from a newborn who is disabled or has medical condition(s) that threaten his or her life, regardless of the parents' wishes, unless at least one of three exceptions is met.

SERVICES AND RESOURCES

- March of Dimes, http://www.marchofdimes.org
- World Health Organization (WHO), http://www.who.int/en
- The Compassionate Friends, http://www.compassionatefriends.org
- Bereaved Parents of the USA, http://www.bereavedparentsusa.org
- National Association of Social Workers, http://socialworkers.org
- National Society of Genetic Counselors, http://www.nsgc.org

FOOD FOR THOUGHT

Engaging with the dying infant has been shown to assist some families in the grieving process; families should be encouraged to provide care for the infant when possible. Care of neonates with serious medical conditions typically consists of aggressive, curative interventions. As a result, when palliative care is enacted both the parents and staff may perceive this as a failure of treatment. Many neonatal deaths are related to congenital abnormalities.

Parents of a neonate who has died may need informed advice, including genetic counseling, before deciding whether to have more children. The ethical principle of double effect often is applied when providing palliative care to neonates. The principle of double effect occurs when an action is performed that has two possible outcomes. One outcome is good and one outcome is bad; the bad outcome, although foreseen, is not the intended outcome. A common example would be the provision of opioids for pain relief for the infant at end of life, even though those medications can inhibit breathing. In a survey, 96.7 percent of neonatologists reported the belief that palliative care should be a part of their training but almost 67 percent had received no formal training in palliative or end-of-life care.

RED FLAGS
Media accounts have helped to create a perception that all newborn problems can be fixed, which has been described as a "false sense of technological security." If an infant was delivered after 20 weeks' gestation, the mother will most likely be producing milk, which can be physically and emotionally painful if the neonate is not nursing; it will be necessary that the social worker assist with a referral to a lactation consultant.

The neonatal team can have difficulty making the transition to palliative care for the neonates in their care. A case study found that barriers to transitioning to palliative care felt by staff included fear that the neonate would experience respiratory depression if given opioids at end of life, conflict among staff, and feeling inadequately trained for end of life care. If the neonate has life-limiting congenital abnormalities and the family has decided to proceed with birth, the family should have a specific, individualized plan of care related to the birth and anticipated needs of the neonate.

NEXT STEPS
The social worker should continue providing support to the family with follow-up calls and visits to the family at home. The family should be encouraged to attend bereavement support groups, and individual counseling: these interventions are important

to avert adverse health outcomes due to associated symptoms of grief and loss.

The social worker should advocate for neonatal intensive care units to have clear guidelines regarding using drugs for comfort care after withdrawing intensive treatment. A trigger list of infant diagnoses and parental risk factors, which together will form criteria for a palliative care consult, should be developed and provided to the medical care team to encourage the use of palliative care.

Written by Jan Wagstaff, MA, MSW

Reviewed by Lynn B. Cooper, D Crim, and Jessica Therivel, LMSW-IPR

REFERENCES
Bhatia, J. (2006). Palliative care in the fetus and newborn. *Journal of Perinatology, 26*(Suppl. 1), S24-S26.

Black, D. (1998). The dying child. *BMJ (Clinical research ed.), 316*(7141), 1376-1378.

Boss, R. D., & Clarke-Pounder, J. P. (2012). Perinatal and neonatal palliative care: Targeting the underserved. *Progress in Palliative Care, 20*(6), 343-348. doi:10.1179/1743291X12Y.0000000039

British Association of Social Workers. (2012). The Code of Ethics for Social Work: Statement of principles. Retrieved October 5, 2015, from http://cdn.basw.co.uk/upload/basw_112315-7.pdf

Carter, B. S., & Jones, P. M. (2013). Evidence-based comfort care for neonates towards the end of life. *Seminars in Fetal & Neonatal Medicine, 18*(2), 88-92. doi:10.1016/j.siny.2012.10.012

Chaudhary, R., SIlwal, A., Gupta, A., & Kelsall, W. (2012). Drugs used for comfort care after withdrawal of intensive treatment in tertiary neonatal units in the U.K. *Archives of Disease in Childhood, Fetal, and Neonatal Edition, 97*(6), F487. doi:1136/fetalneonatal-2012-301883

Contro, N., Davies, B., Larson, J., & Sourkes, B. (2010). Away from home: Experiences of Mexican American families in pediatric palliative care. *Journal of Social Work in End-of-Life and Palliative Care, 6*(3-4), 185-204. doi:10.1080/15524256.2010.529020

Cortezzo, D. E., Sanders, M. R., Brownell, E., & Moss, K. (2013). Neonatologists' perspectives of palliative and end-of-life care in neonatal intensive care units. *Journal of Perinatology, 33*(9), 731-735. doi:10.1038/jp.2013.38

Craig, F., & Mancini, A. (2013). Can we truly offer a choice of place of death in neonatal palliative care?. *Seminars in Fetal & Neonatal Medicine, 18*(2), 93-98. doi:10.1016/j.siny.2012.10.008

Csikai, E. L., & Black, K. (2009). Advance care planning in the delivery of adult protective services. *Journal of Social Service Research, 35*(4), 311-321. doi:10.1080/01488370903110811

Docherty, S. L., Brandon, D., Thaxton, C. A., & Barfield, R. C. (2015). Family-centered palliative care. In *Wong's Nursing Care of Infants and Children* (10th ed., pp. 791-801). St. Louis, MO: Elsevier Mosby.

English, N. K., & Hessler, K. L. (2013). Prenatal birth planning for families of the imperiled newborn. *JOGNN: Journal of Obstetric, Gynecologic & Neonatal Nursing, 42*(3), 390-399. doi:10.1111/1552-6909.12031

Haward, M. F., Murphy, R. O., & Lorenz, J. M. (2012). Default options and neonatal resuscitation decisions. *Journal of Medical Ethics, 38*(12), 713-718. doi:10.1136/medethics-2011-100182

Heyman, J. C., & Gutheil, I. A. (2010). Older Latinos' attitudes toward and comfort with end-of-life planning. *Health and Social Work, 35*(1), 17-26.

Kliegman, R. M., Stanton, B. F., St Geme, J. W., III, Schor, N. F., & Behrman, R. E. (Eds.). (2011). *Nelson textbook of pediatrics* (19th ed.). Philadelphia, PA: Elsevier Saunders.

Larcher, V. (2013). Ethical considerations in neonatal end-of-life care. *Seminars in Fetal & Neonatal Medicine, 18*(2), 105-110. doi:10.1016/j.siny.2012.10.011

Lawn, J. E., Cousens, S., & Zupan, J. (2005). 4 million neonatal deaths: When? Where? Why?. *Lancet, 365*(9462), 891-900.

Martin, M. (2013). Missed opportunities: A case study of barriers to the delivery of palliative care on neonatal intensive care units. *International Journal of Palliative Nursing, 19*(5), 251-256.

Mathews, T. J., MacDorman, M. F., & Thoma, M. E. (2015). Infant mortality statistics from the 2013 period linked birth/infant death data set. *National Vital Statistics Reports, 64*(9), 1-30. Retrieved from http://www.cdc.gov/nchs/data/nvsr/nvsr64/nvsr64_09.pdf

McGraw, M., & Perlman, J. (2008). Reorientation of care in the NICU: A United States perspective. *Seminars in Fetal and Neonatal Medicine, 13*(5), 310:311.

Mizrahi, T., & Mayden, R. W. (2001). NASW standards for cultural competence in social work practice. Retrieved October 8, 2014, from http://www.socialworkers.org/practice/standards/NASWCulturalStandards.pdf

Parravicini, E., & Lorenz, J. M. (2014). Neonatal outcomes of fetuses diagnosed with life-limiting conditions when individualized comfort measures are proposed. *Journal of Perinatology, 34*(6), 483-487. doi:10.1038/jp.2014.40

Pockett, R., Walker, E., & Dave, K. (2010). "Last orders": Dying in a hospital setting. *Australian Social Work, 63*(3), 250-265. doi:10.1080/0312407X.2010.497928

Provoost, V., Cools, F., Mortier, F., Bilsen, J., Ramet, J., Vandenplas, Y., & Deliens, L. (2005). Medical end-of-life decisions in neonates and infants in Flanders. *Lancet, 365*(9467), 1315-1320.

Raman, V. T., & Weisleder, P. (2015). To rescind or not to rescind? Allow for a natural death (AND) orders during the perioperative period: A case-based commentary. *Clinical Pediatrics, 54*(7), 615-619. doi:10.1177/0009922814542483

Reid, S., Bredemeyer, S., den Berg, C., Cresp, T., Martin, T., Miara, N., & Wooderson, S. (2011). Palliative care in the neonatal nursery. *Neonatal, Paediatric and Child Health Nursing, 14*(2), 2-8.

Statement of ethical principles. (2012). *International Federation of Social Workers.* Retrieved October 5, 2015, from http://ifsw.org/policies/statement-of-ethical-principles

Vrakking, A. M., der Heide, A., Ontwuteaka-Philipsen, B. D., Keij-Deerenberg, I. M., der Maas, P. J., & der Wal, G. (2005). Medical end-of-life decision made for neonates and infants in the Netherlands, 1995-2001. *Lancet, 365*(9467), 1329-1331.

World Health Organization. (n.d.). Global health observatory data repository: Number of deaths (thousands) data. Retrieved October 5, 2015, from http://apps.who.int/gho/data/node.imr.CM130n?lang-en

World Health Organization. (2012, May). Newborns: Reducing mortality. Fact Sheet No. 333. Retrieved October 5, 2015, from http://www.who.int/mediacentre/factsheets/fs333/en

Yeo, G. (2009). How will the U.S. healthcare system meet the challenge of the ethnogeriatric imperative? *Journal of the American Geriatrics Society, 57*(7), 1278-1285. doi:10.1111/j.1532-5415.2009.02319.x

PALLIATIVE CARE: MANAGING CAREGIVER BURDEN

MAJOR CATEGORIES: Caregivers, Palliative & Hospice Care

WHAT WE KNOW

Palliative care (PC), or comfort care, is a specialized type of patient care that aims to promote comfort and maintain the highest quality of life of clients for as long as possible. By definition, PC can span an extended period of time, encompassing the active treatment phase of disease, disease remissions, recurrences of disease, and the decline in health before death. Although not limited to end-of-life care, PC usually is provided for patients with terminal illness.

This approach to care involves an interdisciplinary palliative care team (PCT), which includes physicians, nurses, clergy, social workers, hospice staff, the client, and the client's caregivers.

Caregivers are the persons who are responsible for the client's day-to-day care. PC is typically provided in the home setting by untrained caregivers, including spouses/partners, adult children, close friends, and relatives. These caregivers most often have no medical or nursing training yet assist the client in meeting his or her physical and psychological needs.

Historically, women have been the primary nonprofessional caregivers; according to a 2009 AARP study, however, the number of nonprofessional male caregivers has risen to nearly 40 percent of all caregivers.

The primary caregiver often lives with the ill person and receives some support from friends or members of the extended family.

Essential areas of PC, as recognized by caregivers, include the following:

- adequate pain management and symptom relief for the client;
- preserving client dignity;
- enabling the client to maintain a sense of control;
- helping the client prepare psychologically for death, when appropriate;
- strengthening relationships between the client and loved ones.

The client's illness and the intensity of his or her daily needs can have a negative impact on the caregivers' mental and physical health. Caregivers are in the unique position of giving care and support while requiring care and support from others themselves to help manage caregiver burden

Caregivers may need client health information and/or support for themselves at different times. As the client's disease progresses, a caregiver must cope with taking on new roles in his or her relationship with the client, trying to stay positive for the client, and/or acquiring new skills in caring for the client.

Caregiver challenges include lack of personal time, financial burdens related to the client's illness, isolation, and work schedule complications.

Caregiver burden may arise from having to use complex medical technology in caring for the client, having little or no respite from care, constraints on time, difficulty balancing the caregiver role with other work or family roles, social isolation, financial problems, and trouble accessing services.

Fatigue, both in clients receiving palliative care and in their caregivers, can increase the perceived caregiver burden. Researchers studying caregivers of cancer patients found that caregivers had fatigue scores that ranged from 23-26 on the Caregivers Strain Index, whereas scores of healthy control subjects averaged 19.9.

The caregiver's role often has a more negative impact on his or her mental health than it does on physical health. Emotional stressors can be triggered by fatigue, isolation, fear, and feeling overwhelmed or powerless. Depression and anxiety are commonly reported among caregivers, especially female caregivers. Depression and anxiety in the caregiver can lead to social isolation and lack of interest in previously pleasurable activities, as well as increased fear and restlessness.

Anxiety may be exacerbated by lack of information about available support services and ways of accessing these services as well as fear of a negative reaction from the healthcare team if such services are requested.

Caregivers should be provided with information about individual counseling and/or support groups and should be encouraged to maintain social contacts to cope with stress. Where appropriate, they should be given referrals for home nursing visits and information about telephone services (e.g., support hotlines) to help relieve caregiver burden.

Caregivers report the need to feel confident in the work they do and in the care the client is receiving. Trust in the healthcare team and belief that the team is there when needed can bring relief to caregivers and increase their sense of control and confidence in the care they provide to their loved one, which can lead to increased caregiver security.

Support from the PCT has been shown to decrease hospital admissions and facilitate the wishes of clients who want to die at home. Caregivers see communication among the client, family, and PCT as the key to providing optimal PC for the client.

Investigators have found that better communication is equated with higher caregiver satisfaction and better awareness of client wishes. Caregivers see improved communication as their greatest unmet need.

Scheduled family meetings between family caregivers, the client, and the PCT allow the client to express his or her wishes regarding PC. These meetings can serve as a forum for caregivers to ask questions and stay informed of treatment goals and illness progression. Family meetings may be a good time to discuss symptom control and plan for the future.

Interventions with caregivers designed to increase their sense of preparedness and competence can result in an overall improvement in their psychological well-being.

Caregivers' needs change as the client's illness progresses. Multiple factors can cause caregivers to feel that their needs are not being met. Caregivers may put the client's needs before their own, refrain from asking for what they need, feel that they should be able to do everything on their own, or have feelings of guilt that they are not doing enough for the client.

Seeing the needs of the ill person as primary, caregivers often fail to recognize their own needs. As the client's health declines, the PCT needs to anticipate the caregiver's changing needs and offer support.

Identifying secondary caretakers to provide respite and emotional support to primary caretakers can help reduce caregiver burden, yet secondary caretakers often are an underutilized resource.

Caregiver training has been shown to be helpful (e.g., using medical equipment, providing mouth care, managing medication, treating bedsores): the more skilled the caregiver and the greater his or her level of self-efficacy, the more effective he or she is in providing care to the loved one.

WHAT CAN BE DONE

Learn about the challenges of providing PC as seen by caregivers and clients; share this knowledge with your colleagues.

Develop an awareness of your own cultural values, beliefs, and biases and develop knowledge about the histories, traditions, and values of your clients. Adopt treatment methodologies that reflect the cultural needs of the client.

Learn and practice therapeutic communication skills with an emphasis on honesty, empathy, and patience. Use language the client and caregiver can easily understand. Be sure they are receiving the same information from each member of the PCT.

Be sure caregivers are familiar with members of the PCT and how to contact them. This will add to caregiver security and may allow the client to benefit from home care for a longer period of time.

Provide support to caregivers by recognizing their physical, emotional, and financial stresses and assessing their social supports.

As the client's disease progresses, assess the need for referrals to social service agencies, physical or occupational therapy, home nursing care, and healthcare assistants.

Encourage the caregiver to maintain or resume involvement in his or her own hobbies and activities, ask for help from others (e.g., friends, family), and take time for him- or herself, focusing on his or her physical, social, and spiritual well-being

Encourage the client and family to participate in activities they enjoy for as long as possible, to participate in religious or spiritual activities, and to avoid social isolation.

Encourage clients to prepare for end of life, while still living their life fully, through the use of an advance directive and assignment of a healthcare proxy. Encourage clients and families/caregivers to share their feelings about death.

Educate the caregiver regarding bereavement support and what to expect as the client's health declines.

Assist the caregiver in addressing feelings of grief and loss that arise with a loved one's decline and death. Be aware of where the caregiver is in the grief process and make referral to a mental health clinician if indicated (e.g., if client has symptoms of depression, anxiety, or posttraumatic stress disorder).

Encourage caregivers to obtain more information from the National Hospice and Palliative Care Organization at www.nhpco.org/i4a/pages/index.cfm?pageid=3254, Aging with Dignity at www.agingwithdignity.org/, the National Council for Palliative Care at http://www.ncpc.org.uk/, and World Health Organization at http://www.who.int/cancer/palliative/definition/en/.

Written by Laura McLuckey, MSW, LCSW

Reviewed by Lynn B. Cooper, D. Crim, and Jessica Therivel, LMSW-IPR

REFERENCES

National Alliance for Caregiving and AARP. (2009). Caregiving in the United States: Executive summary. Retrieved October 9, 2015, from http://assets.aarp.org/rgcenter/il/caregiving_09_es.pdf

Angelo, J. K., Egan, R., & Reid, K. (2013). Essential knowledge for family caregivers: A qualitative study. *International Journal of Palliative Nursing, 19*(8), 383-388. doi:10.12968/ijpn.2013.19.8.383

Brazil, K., Bainbridge, D., & Rodriguez, C. (2010). The stress process in palliative cancer care: A qualitative study on informal caregiving and its implication for the delivery of care. *American Journal of Hospice and Palliative Medicine, 27*(2), 111-116. doi:10.1177/1049909109350176

British Association of Social Workers. (2012, January). The code of ethics for social workers: Statement of principles. Retrieved October 9, 2015, from http://cdn.basw.co.uk/upload/basw_112315-7.pdf

Burns, C. M. (2013). Uncovering an invisible network of direct caregivers at the end of life: A population study. *Palliative Medicine, 27*(7), 608-615. doi:10.1177/0269216313483664

Family Caregiver Alliance. (2012). Selected caregiver statistics. Retrieved October 9, 2015, from http://caregiver.org/selected-caregiver-statistics

Funk, L. M., Allan, D. E., & Stajduhar, K. I. (2009). Palliative family caregivers' accounts of health care experiences: The importance of "security". *Palliative and Supportive Care, 7*(4), 435-447. doi:10.1017/S1478951509990447

Gough, K., & Hudson, P. (2009). Psychometric properties of the Hospital Anxiety and Depression Scale in family caregivers of palliative care patients. *Journal of Pain and Symptom Management, 37*(5), 797-806. doi:10.1016/j.jpainsymman.2008.04.012

Gueguen, J. A., Bylund, C. L., Brown, R. F., Levin, T. T., & Kissane, D. W. (2009). Conducting family meetings in palliative care: Themes, techniques, and preliminary evaluation of a communication skills module. *Palliative and Supportive Care, 7*(2), 171-179. doi:10.1017/S1478951509000224

Hasson, F., Spence, A., Waldron, M., Kernohan, G., McLaughlin, D., Watson, B., & Cochrane, B. (2009). Experiences and needs of bereaved carers during palliative and end-of-life care for people with chronic obstructive pulmonary disease. *Journal of Palliative Care, 25*(3), 157-163.

Heitkemper, M. M. (2014). Palliative care at end of life. In S. L. Lewis, S. R. Dirksen, M. M. Heitkemper, L. Bucher, & M. M. Harding (Eds.), *Medical-surgical nursing: Assessment and management of clinical problems* (9th ed., pp. 140-153). St. Louis, MO: Mosby Elsevier.

Henriksson, A., & Årestedt, K. (2013). Exploring factors and caregiver outcomes associated with feelings of preparedness for caregiving in family caregivers in palliative care: A correlational, cross-sectional study. *Palliative Medicine, 27*(7), 639-646. doi:10.1177/0269216313486954

Hudson, P., Trauer, T., Kelly, B., O'Connor, M., Thomas, K., Zordan, R., & Summers, M. (2013). Reducing the psychological distress of family caregivers of home based palliative care patients: Longer term effects from a randomized controlled trial. *Psycho-Oncology, 22*, 1987-1933. doi:10.1002/pon.3610

Hupcey, J. E., Fensternmacher, K., Kitko, L., & Penrod, J. (2010). Achieving medical stability: Wives' experiences with heart failure. *Clinical Nursing Research, 19*(3), 211-229. doi:10.1177/1054773810371119

International Federation of Social Workers. (2012, March 3). Statement of ethical principles. Retrieved October 9, 2015, from http://ifsw.org/policies/statement-of-ethical-principles/

Kayser, K., DeMarco, R. F., Stokes, C., DeSanto-Madeya, S., & Higgins, P. C. (2014). Delivering palliative care to patients and caregivers in inner-city communities: Challenges and opportunities. *Palliative & Supportive Care, 12*(5), 369-372. doi:10.1017/S1478951513000230

Wheeler, D. (2015). NASW standards and indicators for cultural competence in social work practice.

Retrieved December 2, 2015, from http://www.socialworkers.org/practice/standards/PRA-BRO-253150-CC-Standards.pdf

Mystakidou, K., Parpa, E., anagiotou, I., Tsilika, E., Galanos, A., & Gouliamos, A. (2013). Caregivers' anxiety and self-efficacy in palliative care. *European Journal of Cancer Care, 22*(2), 188-195. doi:10.1111/ecc.12012

Nelson, J. E., Puntillo, K. A., Pronovost, P. J., Walker, A. S., McAdam, J. L., Ilaoa, D.,... Penrod, J. (2010). In their own words: Patients and families define high-quality palliative care in the intensive care unit. *Critical Care Medicine, 38*(3), 808-818. doi:10.1097/CCM.0b013e3181c5887c

Oliver, M. A., Hillock, S., Moore, C., Goble, H., & Asbury, N. (2010). Comfort care packs: A little bit of hospice in hospital? *International Journal of Palliative Nursing, 16*(10), 511-515.

Peters, M. E., Goedendorp, M. M., Verhagen, S. A., Smilde, T. J., Bleijenberg, G., & van der Graaf, W. T. (2014). A prospective analysis of fatigue and experienced burden in informal caregivers of cancer patients during cancer treatment in the palliative phase. *Acta Oncologica, Early Online,* 1-7. doi:10.3109/0284186X.2014.953254

Rabow, M. W., & Pantilat, S. Z. (2015). Palliative care and pain management. In S. J. McPhee & M. A. Papadakis (Eds.), *Lange 2015 current medical diagnosis & treatment* (54th ed., pp. 71-92). New York, NY: McGraw-Hill Medical.

Reifsnyder, J. (2014). End-of-life care. In J. L. Hinkle & K. H. Cheever (Eds.), *Brunner & Suddarth's textbook of medical-surgical nursing* (13th ed., pp. 373-399). Philadelphia, PA: Wolters Kluwer Health/Lippincott Williams & Wilkins.

Riley, C. D. (2014). Cancer nursing. In S. M. Nettina (Ed.), *Lippincott manual of nursing practice* (10th ed., pp. 162-163). Philadelphia, PA: Wolters Kluwer Health/Lippincott Williams & Wilkins.

Sanderson, C., Lobb, E. A., Mowll, J., Butow, P. N., McGowan, N., & Price, M. A. (2013). Signs of post-traumatic stress disorder in caregivers following an expected death: A qualitative study. *Palliative Medicine2013, 27*(7), 625-631. doi:10.1177/0269216313483663

Smith, P. (2009). The family caregivers journey in end of life care: Recognising and identifying with the role of carer. *International Journal on Disability and Human Development, 8*(1), 67-73. doi:10.1515/IJDHD.2009.8.1.67

Stajduhar, K. I. (2013). Burdens of family caregiving at the end of life. *Clinical & Investigative Medicine, 36*(3), E121-E127.

Stajduhar, K. I., Funk, L., & Outcalt, L. (2013). Family caregiver learning- How family caregivers learn to provide care at the end of life: A qualitative secondary analysis of four datasets. *Palliative Medicine, 27*(7), 657-664. doi:10.1177/0269216313487765

PANCREATIC CANCER: RISK FACTORS

MAJOR CATEGORIES: Medical & Health

WHAT WE KNOW

The pancreas, located behind the stomach and in front of the spine, aids in digestion of food and regulation of glucose in the blood. Signs and symptoms of pancreatic cancer include jaundice, upper abdominal or back pain, nausea/vomiting, diarrhea, clay-colored stools, loss of appetite, weight loss, weakness, and fatigue.

Pancreatic cancer is one of the deadliest cancers worldwide, largely because of the inability to adequately screen for the disease and ineffective treatment methods. Individuals often are asymptomatic until their cancer is advanced, and the condition usually is fatal.

In the United Kingdom more than half of individuals with pancreatic cancer are at an advanced stage of the disease when it is diagnosed. Pancreatic cancer is the 5th most common cause of death and the 10th most common cancer in the United Kingdom.

The American Cancer Society estimated that pancreatic cancer would be diagnosed in approximately 53, 070 persons in the United States in 2016 and that 41, 780 persons would die of the disease. The incidence rate of pancreatic cancer in the United States has risen 1.2 percent a year since 2000, and the death rate has increased 0.4 percent yearly since 2000.

Pancreatic cancer has the highest mortality rate of all cancers; 94 percent of all persons with pancreatic cancer will die within 5 years of diagnosis, and 74 percent will die within the first year of diagnosis. Treatment strategies depend on the patient's status but may include radiation therapy (e.g., external beam), chemotherapy, nonchemotherapeutic targeted therapies, and/or surgery, together with palliative care.

Although the precise cause of pancreatic cancer is unknown, multiple risk factors have been directly and indirectly linked with its development. Most experts contend that its pathogenesis likely is multifactorial. The following are risk factors that have been most frequently associated with pancreatic cancer:

Age:

Older age has been identified as the most significant nonmodifiable risk factor. Pancreatic cancer affects primarily individuals over the age of 60, with a median age of 72 at diagnosis.

Sex:

Pancreatic cancer affects slightly more males than females.

Racial or ethnic background:

Pancreatic cancer is most common among black males in the United States and among males of Hawaiian, New Zealand Maori, Korean, Czech, and Latvian descent.

Social history:

Cigarette smoking is believed to be directly linked to development of pancreatic cancer and is considered the most important and most avoidable risk factor. Risk increases in direct proportion to the number of pack-years smoked (i.e., the quantity of cigarettes smoked and the duration of time spent smoking). Current smokers are about 2.5 times more likely to develop pancreatic cancer than nonsmokers.

The use of smokeless tobacco and exposure to environmental tobacco smoke may also increase risk. The results of clinical studies on the risk for pancreatic cancer resulting from alcohol intake have been mixed. Only heavy alcohol intake has been directly linked with pancreatic cancer, but even a moderate amount of alcohol use can increase risk for chronic pancreatitis, which increases the risk for pancreatic cancer

Mental health history:

Depression rates are high in clients with pancreatic cancer.

There may be a bi-directional link between pancreatic cancer and depression. A study of deaths due to pancreatic cancer in Sweden between 1991 and 2009 using the Swedish Multi-Generation Register and the death of a child as a measure of stress found that increased stress increased the risk for pancreatic cancer. The association was observed to be strongest in the first 5 years after the child's death and when the child's death was due to suicide.

Medical history:

Individuals who undergo partial gastrectomy (i.e., stomach removal) or cholecystectomy (i.e., gallbladder removal) have a 2- to 5-fold increased risk of developing pancreatic cancer within 20 years after surgery.

Individuals who have diabetes mellitus, and especially those who have had diabetes mellitus for at least 5 years, are more than twice as likely to develop pancreatic cancer as persons without diabetes mellitus.

Incretin based therapies for the management of type 2 diabetes mellitus may increase the risk of developing pancreatic cancer. Individuals who have had pancreatitis and/or chronic inflammation may also be at increased risk for pancreatic cancer.

Obesity:

Individuals who are overweight or obese (i.e., with body mass index [BMI] over 25 and 30, respectively) may be more likely to develop pancreatic cancer, and at a younger age, than individuals who are not obese. Risk was found to be higher for men than for women.

Dietary patterns:

Increased intake of fat and meat has been associated with increased risk, although the mechanism for this is not clear.

Soft-drink consumption may be associated with increased risk according to a 2010 clinical study conducted in Singapore; the study's authors postulated that individuals who consume soft drinks regularly may be increasing serum insulin levels to a degree that contributes to pancreatic cancer cell growth.

Genetics/family history:

Certain familial syndromes, including Peutz-Jeghers syndrome, Lynch syndrome, and familial atypical multiple mole melanoma (FAMMM) syndrome, predispose individuals to pancreatic cancer. Individuals with BRCA1 and BRCA2 mutation carriers are at increased risk for pancreatic cancer. As many as 10 percent of individuals with pancreatic cancer have a family history of pancreatic cancer. Risk is highest among first-degree relatives.

The risk for pancreatic cancer is increased in individuals with a family history of breast and ovarian cancer or nonpolyposis colorectal cancer

Researchers have found that blood type may be a risk factor for pancreatic cancer, with individuals with blood type A, B, or AB at increased risk of developing the disease compared to those with blood type O

WHAT CAN BE DONE

Learn more about risk factors for pancreatic cancer so that you can accurately assess your clients' personal characteristics and health education needs; share this knowledge with your colleagues.

Develop an awareness of your own cultural values, beliefs, and biases and develop knowledge about the histories, traditions, and values of your clients. Adopt treatment methodologies that reflect the cultural needs of clients.

Practice with awareness of and adherence to the NASW Code of Ethics core values of service, social justice, dignity and worth of the person, importance of human relationships, integrity, and competence. Become knowledgeable of the NASW ethical standards as they apply to pancreatic cancer, and practice accordingly.

Assess your clients' risk for pancreatic cancer. Collaborate with the treating clinician, registered dietician, and/or mental health clinician in providing strategies that may lower a client's individual risk (e.g., smoking cessation, a low-fat diet, weight loss, decreasing alcohol intake)

Encourage individuals who are identified as being at increased risk to discuss the need for increased surveillance with their treating clinician.

Screening by magnetic resonance cholangio-pancreatographic imaging (MRCP) or endoscopic ultrasound (EUS) in clients with a family history or genetic predisposition to pancreatic cancer can be useful for early diagnosis so that surgical resection can be performed, which may be curative.

Request a referral to a licensed mental health worker for clients who experience anxiety and/or depression as a result of their increased risk for pancreatic cancer or diagnosis of pancreatic cancer.

Assess for depression in any at-risk clients or clients in whom pancreatic cancer has been diagnosed

and encourage them to pursue the appropriate treatment, including pharmacotherapy, to improve their quality of life.

Obtain more information about pancreatic cancer from the American Cancer Society at http://www.cancer.org and Pancreatic Cancer UK at http://www.pancreaticcancer.org.uk/.

Written by Suzanne Pinto, MSW, and Carita Caple, RN, BSN, MSHS

Reviewed by Laura McLuckey, MSW, LCSW, and Chris Bates, MA, MSW

REFERENCES

American Association for Cancer Research. (2010). Soft drink consumption may increase risk of pancreatic cancer. *NEWS-Line for Nurse Practitioners, 16*(4), 7-8.

American Cancer Society. (2016). Cancer facts & figures 2016. Retrieved May 5, 2016, from http://www.cancer.org/acs/groups/content/@research/documents/document/acspc-047079.pdf

Beliveau, A. (2014). Incretin-based therapies and the risk of pancreatic cancer. *Canadian Adverse Reaction Newsletter, 24*(4), 1-2.

Ben, Q., Cai, Q., Li, Z., Yuan, Y., Ning, X., Deng, S., & Wang, K. (2011). The relationship between new-onset diabetes mellitus and pancreatic cancer risk: A case-control study. *European Journal of Cancer, 47*(2), 248-254. doi:10.1016/j.ejca.2010.07.010

Berry, L. (2013). Charity calls for much earlier diagnosis of pancreatic cancer. *Cancer Nursing Practice, 12*(8), 9.

British Association of Social Workers. (2012). *The code of ethics for social work: Statement of principles.* Retrieved May 5, 2016, from http://cdn.basw.co.uk/upload/basw_112315-7.pdf

Canto, M. I., Harinck, F., Hruban, R. H., Offerhaus, G. J., Poley, J. W., Kamel, I.,... Bruno, M. (2013). International cancer of the pancreas screening (CAPS) consortium summit on the management of patients with increased risk for familial pancreatic cancer. *Gut, 62*(3), 339-347. doi:10.1136/gutjnl-2012-303108

Chen, Y., Rubinson, D. A., Qian, Z. R., Chen, W., Kraft, P., Ying, B., & Wolpin, B. M. (2015). Survival among patients with pancreatic cancer and long-standing or recent-onset diabetes mellitus. *Journal* of *Clinical Oncology*, *33*(1), 29-35. doi:10.1200/JCO.2014.57.5688

Croghan, A., & Heitkemper, M. M. (2011). Liver, pancreas, and biliary tract problems. In S. L. Lewis, S. R. Dirksen, M. M. Heitkemper, L. Bucher, & I. M. Camera (Eds.), *Medical-surgical nursing: Assessment and management of clinical problems* (8th ed., pp. 1094-1095). St. Louis, MO: Mosby Elsevier.

Dragovich, T., Erickson, R. A., Larson, C. R., & Shabahang, M. (2014, October 8). Pancreatic cancer. *Medscape Reference*. Retrieved May 5, 2016, from http://emedicine.medscape.com/article/280605-overview

Dzeletovic, I., Harrison, E. M., Crowell, M. D., Pannala, R., Nguyen, C. C., Wu, Q., & Faigel, D. O. (2014). Pancreatitis before pancreatic cancer: Clinical features and influence on outcome. *Journal of Clinical Gastroenterology*, *48*(9), 801-805. doi:10.1097/MCG.0b013e3182a9f879

Feller, E. (2016). Pancreatic cancer. In F. J. Domino (Ed.), *The 5-minute clinical consult 2016* (24th ed., pp. 804-806). Philadelphia, PA: Wolters Kluwer Health/Lippincott Williams & Wilkins.

Helwick, C. (2010). The optimal Rx for pancreatic cancer: Stop it before it starts. *Oncology News International*, *19*(3), 7-9, 11.

Hirshberg Foundation for Pancreatic Cancer Research. (2016). Pancreatic cancer facts. Retrieved May 6, 2016, from http://www.pancreatic.org/site/c.htJYJ8MPIwE/b.5050503/k.40C9/Pancreatic_Cancer_Facts.htm

Huang, J., Valdimarsdottir, U., Fall, K., Ye, W., & Fang, F. (2014). Pancreatic cancer risk after loss of a child: A register-based study in Sweden during 1991-2009. *American Journal of Epidemiology*, *178*(4), 582-589. doi:10.1093/aje/kwt045

International Federation of Social Workers. (2012, March 3). Statement of ethical principles. Retrieved May 5, 2016, from http://ifsw.org/policies/statement-of-ethical-principles/

Kanji, Z. S., & Gallinger, S. (2013). Diagnosis and management of pancreatic cancer. *Canadian Medical Association Journal*, *185*(14), 1219-1226. doi:10.1503/cmaj.121368

Lai, H. C., Tsai, I. J., Chen, P. C., Muo, C. H., Chou, J. W., Pent, C. Y.,... Morisky, D. E. (2013). Gallstones, a cholecystectomy, chronic pancreatitis, and the risk of subsequent pancreatic cancer in diabetic patients: A population-based cohort study. *Journal*

of *Gastroenterology*, *48*(6), 721-727. doi:10.1007/s00535-012-0674-0

Li, D., Morris, J. S., Liu, J., Hassan, M. M., Day, R. S., Bondy, M. L., & Abbruzzese, J. L. (2009). Body mass index and risk, age of onset, and survival in patients with pancreatic cancer. *JAMA*, *301*(24), 2553-2562. doi:10.10011/jama.2009.886

Lin, J., Shu-Man, J., Yuan-Yuan, S., Yao-Xing, H., Yi-Jun, L., De-Rong, X., & Fa-Cao, Z. (2010). Investigation of the incidence of pancreatic cancer-related depression and its relationship with the quality of life of patients. *Digestion*, *82*(1), 4-9. doi:10.1159/000253864

Luca, A. L., Frado, L. E., Hwang, C., Kumar, S., Khanna, L. G., Levinson, E. J.,... Frucht, H. (2014). BRCA1 and BRCA2 germline mutations are frequently demonstrated in both high-risk pancreatic cancer screening and pancreatic cohorts. *Cancer*, *120*(13), 1960-1967. doi:10.1002/cncr.2866

Mayr, M., & Schmid, R. M. (2010). Pancreatic cancer and depression: Myth and truth. *BMC Cancer*, *10*(1), 569-575. doi:10.1186/1471-2407-10-569

National Association of Social Workers. (2008). Code of ethics. Retrieved May 12, 2016, from https://www.socialworkers.org/pubs/code/code.asp

National Association of Social Workers. (2015). NASW standards and indicators for cultural competence in social work practice. Retrieved March 29, 2016, from http://www.socialworkers.org/practice/standards/PRA-BRO-253150-CC-Standards.pdf

Risch, H. A., Lu, L, Want, J., Zhang, W., Ni, Q., Gao, Y., & Yu, H. (2013). ABO blood groups and risk of pancreatic cancer: A study in Shanghai and meta-analysis. *American Journal of Epidemiology*, *177*(12), 1326-1337. doi:10.1093/aje/kws458

Talamini, R., Polesel, J., Gallus, S., Dal Maso, L., Zucchetto, A., Negri, E., & La Vecchia, C. (2010). Tobacco smoking, alcohol consumption and pancreatic cancer risk: A case-control study in Italy. *European Journal of Cancer*, *46*(2), 370-376. doi:10.1016/j.ejca.2009.09.002

Wolfgang, C. L., Herman, J. M., Laheru, D. A., Klein, A. P., Erdek, M. A., Fishman, E. K., & Hruban, R. H. (2013). Recent progress in pancreatic cancer. *CA: A Cancer Journal for Clinicians*, *63*(5), 318-348. doi:10.3322/caac.21190

Zambirinis, C. P., Pushalkar, S., Saxena, D., & Miller, G. (2014). Pancreatic cancer, inflammation and microbiome. *Cancer Journal*, *20*(3), 195-202. doi:10.1097/PPO.0000000000000045

Zechner, D., Radecke, T., Amme, J., Burtin, A. C., Partecke, L. I., & Vollmar, B. (2015). Impact of diabetes type II and chronic inflammation on pancreatic cancer. *BMC Cancer*, *15*(1), 51-63. doi:10.1186/s12885-015-1047-x

PARANOID PERSONALITY DISORDER

MAJOR CATEGORIES: Behavioral & Mental Health

DESCRIPTION

Paranoid personality disorder (PPD) is one of 10 diagnosable personality disorders that appear in the *Diagnostic and Statistical Manual of Mental Disorders*, Fifth Edition (*DSM-5*), all of which are retained from the fourth edition (*DSM-IV*) of the manual. PPD is grouped with schizoid personality disorder and schizotypal personality disorder to form the cluster A personality disorders, which share the appearance of eccentricity and oddness. The *DSM-5* general criteria for all 10 personality disorders include significant variation in behavior and internal life experience from one's own cultural norms in at least two of the four areas of cognition, affectivity, interpersonal functioning, and impulse control, as well as a long-term and consistent history across a variety of life situations apparent since at least adolescence that has caused significant disturbances in functioning in important areas of life and which could be described as an abiding pattern, one that is not caused by another mental health disorder, including substance use disorder(s), impact of medications, or a medical condition.

The specific criterion for PPD is a deep and persistent distrust of others, including assuming that the intent to cause harm is present. To be diagnosed, at least four of seven specific criteria must be met. These include unfounded suspicions that others are out to exploit, harm, or deceive the individual; preoccupation with doubts related to the loyalty and trustworthiness of others; a reluctance to confide in others out of a fear of being used; interpretation of hidden threatening messages in benign comments or events; holding grudges that are persistent; perception of attacks on character that are not apparent to anyone else, with quick counterattack; and recurrent suspicions related to the fidelity of partner without justification. These criteria do not occur in association with a diagnosis of schizophrenia, bipolar or depressive disorders, or another psychotic disorder and are not caused by a medical condition. The absence of delusions and hallucinations distinguishes PPD from psychotic disorders, although short-lived delusions and hallucinations may occur. Delusions can be distinguished from paranoid thoughts by their complete lack of plausibility (believing the CIA has implanted a broadcasting device in one's head versus believing that a coworker is listening to one's private phone calls). Individuals with PPD may appear quick to make negative judgments, hostile, emotionally volatile or unemotional, cold in personal relationships, controlling, brittle, blaming, extremely independent, rigid in their thinking, uncompromising, quiet, aloof, quick to anger or rage, overly concerned about status and rank, and, above all, suspicious and extremely vigilant for perceived threats. Cultural considerations related to PPD include language/communication barriers and unfamiliarity with cultural norms that may be perceived as hostility. Persistent substance abuse may cause signs and symptoms similar to PPD and should be ruled out as a source of symptoms. There may be overlap with symptoms and diagnosis of other cluster A disorders.

Personality is generally agreed to refer to the internal organization and evolution of an individual's psychobiological and social inheritance and learning that enable him or her to live in, and adapt to, a constantly changing world. One model of personality is the five-factor model (FFM), which divides and measures personality using five traits: openness to experience, conscientiousness, extraversion, agreeableness, and neuroticism. Each trait is measured using a continuum for agreeableness, friendly/compassionate to cold/unkind). PPD can be viewed as a demonstration of the extreme cold/unkind end of the agreeableness trait, overwhelming all the other traits. To be considered disordered, the sum of these five traits must be dysfunctional on both an individual and a social level, and typically these traits are inflexible and outside the norms of the individual's culture. Furthermore, individuals with PPD usually lack awareness that there are problems in their personal or social functioning.

Controversy surrounds the personality disorders and is reflected by the inclusion in the *DSM-5* of a chapter titled "Alternative DSM-5 Model for Personality Disorders" in Section 3, "Emerging Measures and Models." The alternative model was introduced to address shortcomings in the current model, including that many individuals simultaneously meet the criteria for several personality disorders and that the general categories of "other specified" or "unspecified" are the most often diagnosed yet are uninformative about the individual. A larger question about the personality disorder diagnosis is its categorical nature (meaning either the criteria are met and there is a disorder/diagnosis, or the criteria are not met and there is no disorder/diagnosis) as opposed to the dimensional nature (meaning that personality traits occur along a continuum from not present at all to having overwhelming impact) of actual human behavior and lives. The *DSM-5* personality disorders remain categorical, yet the alternative model introduces the concept of dimensional assessment. Another issue of contention is the theory that personality disorders are actually a point on the continuum of a larger mental health disorder, usually at the less impactful end of a dimensional model. In the case of PPD, the debate centers on whether PPD and other disorders with a primary feature of delusion are on a continuum with schizophrenia or form their own spectrum of paranoid disorders.

The etiology of PPD is unresolved, with most literature attributing it to an interaction of genetically inherited traits and environmental influences, particularly maltreatment in childhood. Additionally, individuals with PPD rarely seek treatment unless there is another mental health disorder present or they are mandated to treatment by courts, both of which complicate assessment, treatment, and research into PPD. The viability of treatment for personality disorders is the subject of debate, with some literature claiming that individuals with personality disorders are unreceptive to treatment and some asserting that the problem with treatment lies with professionals who blame their countertransference and lack of success on the individuals with personality disorders. Individuals with PPD are much more likely to respond positively to treatment using individual rather than group modalities. Investigators recently reported success treating PPD using cognitive analytic therapy (CAT), a brief, structured intervention that incorporates cognitive strategies and transparency about the therapeutic process.

FACTS AND FIGURES

The nature of PPD makes it difficult to recruit individuals for studies, so facts and figures are difficult to verify. The *DSM-5* reports prevalence of between 2.3 and 4.4 percent and notes that PPD is more often diagnosed in men (p. 651). A review of admissions to a Danish psychiatric hospital between 1975 and 2000 for diagnosis of PPD on first admission found more males than females, equal division between urban and rural dwellers, and a distribution of education levels similar to that of the general population. Multiple studies have indicated racial differences in the diagnosis of PPD, with PPD diagnosed in more black individuals than in Caucasians. In some studies, the racial difference has been attributed in part to lower socioeconomic status. It is theorized that the victimization and cultural mistrust that is experienced by many blacks is assessed as meeting the paranoia criteria for PPD. Perceived discrimination can often be correlated with paranoid delusions. Furthermore, an increased belief in the supernatural among blacks may be behind the elevated levels of paranoia found in studies that compare rates of PPD among blacks and Caucasians. In one study that examined participants in a substance treatment program, researchers found that 24 percent of the black participants met the criteria for PPD, compared to 10 percent of the Caucasian participants.

RISK FACTORS

As with other aspects of PPD, identifying risk factors is complicated by the debate regarding the nature of the disorder and the difficulty of recruiting individuals for research. However, there is a generally agreed-upon higher risk for individuals with first-degree relatives in whom schizophrenia or other cluster A personality disorders have been diagnosed. Various environmental factors have been researched without conclusive findings, but some studies have found maltreatment or neglect during childhood to be possible markers for developing PPD. An additional childhood or adolescent trait that is considered a hallmark for development of PPD is an inability to experience pleasure (anhedonia). Traumatic brain injuries also can increase the risk for PPD. Substance abuse has been correlated with the development of PPD.

SIGNS AND SYMPTOMS

Signs and symptoms include broadly held distrust and suspiciousness, a formal and businesslike manner, poor eye contact, projection of blame for difficulties in life, extreme concern about the emotions and attitudes of others, difficulty in interpersonal relationships, social isolation, hypersensitivity, jealousy, rigidity, hypervigilance, antagonism, and aggression. Some signs and symptoms may appear contradictory.

ASSESSMENT

Professionals working with people with PPD may perform any or all of the following assessments: collecting standard biopsychosocial-spiritual history, including risk for suicide; observing functioning and demeanor during interview; collecting collateral information from family, friends, and coworkers—especially important because individuals frequently have limited insight into the inappropriateness of their beliefs and behavior.

Professionals may also use any or all of the following diagnostic or screening tools: Structured Clinical Interview for DSM-5 (Personality Disorders) (SCID-5-PD), Personality Diagnostic Questionnaire–Revised (PDQ-R), Minnesota Multiphasic Personality Inventory (MMPI), Millon Clinical Multiaxial Inventory (MCMI), Temperament and Character Inventory (TCI). Care should be used with self-reporting screening tools due to the person's general lack of insight.

Laboratory testing may include tests for the presence of alcohol or other substances at levels indicating abuse and examining any scans or past medical history that indicate a previous head trauma.

TREATMENT

Individuals with PPD rarely seek treatment, and if they do it is likely that another mental health disorder, most often depression or anxiety, has prompted them to consider services. Usually it is difficult to engage individuals with PPD in therapy because of the nature of the disorder: extreme distrust, suspicion of the motives of others, and belief that others are intent on causing harm. Lack of insight and concern about dysfunction further complicates engagement and progress in treatment, which may cause clinicians to lose interest in treatment. A commonly repeated myth holds that individuals with personality disorders are untreatable or that personality disorders are inflexible and cannot be treated. Research shows, however, that progress can be made if barriers to treatment are not erected. The three most common barriers are strong and counterproductive feelings of countertransference; the clinician's belief (and covert communication of this belief to the individual being treated) in the myth of untreatability; and the clinician's giving direct and specific advice on social functioning or personal problems, which usually produces dependence, noncompliance, or resentment. Establishing a therapeutic alliance with individuals with PPD is particularly difficult because of the profound distrust that is at the heart of PPD. Antianxiety or antipsychotic drugs may help manage anxiety and agitation. Some research suggests that medications may be helpful in decreasing paranoid ideation, yet distrust may forestall medication adherence. A first step in treatment of PPD is collaborative goal setting about treatment. Clinicians should immediately give constant attention to developing and maintaining a therapeutic alliance.

Professionals may also do any of the following to help in treatment. Review medication regimen and make follow-up appointment with the agency issuing the prescription, assess the stability of employment and living situation, refer to the appropriate treatment modality, assist the patient in locating support resources, and provide referrals for support and education for family members.

Problem	Goal	Intervention
Person with PPD is exhibiting signs of aggression and threatening behavior, causing severe disruption of social or occupational relationships, or presence of depression or anxiety.	Person will have a reduction in disruptive behavior and depression and anxiety symptoms.	Schedule appointment with mental health professional who can prescribe appropriate medications. Follow up with family and caregiver on medication adherence and effectiveness, including discussion of importance of adhering to prescription dosage and timing with family and caregivers while remaining sensitive to developing trust. Establish stability to allow for participation in other forms of treatment.
Person is having difficulty in establishing therapeutic alliance with social worker.	Establish a therapeutic alliance to allow for engagement in treatment interventions.	Use of patience, validation, and unconditional positive regard by the therapist. Care must be used not to let an overly warm or familiar manner be perceived as threatening: A more businesslike manner may be more effective in the beginning, and giving more control to the person may help him or her preserve a sense of autonomy.
Person is experiencing disrupted or inappropriate social or occupational interpersonal relationships	Establish or reestablish productive and functional social or occupational interpersonal relationships	Using individual rather than group methods, employ cognitive-behavioral methods, psychodynamic therapy, and skills training as appropriate.

APPLICABLE LAWS AND REGULATIONS

Each jurisdiction (nation, state, province) has its own standards, procedures, and laws for involuntary restraint and detention of persons who may be a danger to themselves or others. Individuals with PPD may be at risk for involvement with the criminal justice system due to aggressive behavior or their own initiation of legal action. Local and professional reporting requirements for neglect and abuse should also be known and observed.

Each country has its own standards for cultural competency and diversity in social work practice. Social workers must be aware of the standards of practice set forth by their governing body (National Association of Social Workers in the United States, British Association of Social Workers in the United Kingdom) and practice accordingly.

SERVICES AND RESOURCES

- National Alliance on Mental Illness (NAMI), http://www.nami.org/

- U.S. National Institutes of Health (NIH), http://www.nih.gov/
- U.S. National Institute of Mental Health (NIMH), http://www.nimh.nih.gov/index.shtml
- National Association of Social Workers (NASW), http://www.socialworkers.org/

FOOD FOR THOUGHT

The *DSM-5* states that the traits exhibited by individuals with PPD may be adaptive, meaning they may be beneficial to the individual in enabling functioning. In particular, the traits of PPD may be adaptive in threatening or hostile environments. Attention should be paid to the level of distress and/or the disruption in his or her social or occupational functioning before considering a diagnosis of PPD.

RED FLAGS

Individuals with PPD may engender strong positive or negative feelings in professionals that may lead to countertransference.

PPD may be difficult to diagnose because it is hard to distinguish from other cluster A personality disorders, from prodromal schizophrenia, and from delusional disorders.

The myth that personality disorders are untreatable can be self-reinforcing when repeated among professionals involved in treatment of PPD.

Written by Chris Bates, MA, MSW

Reviewed by Laura Gale, LCSW, and Jessica Therivel, LMSW-IPR

REFERENCES

American Psychiatric Association. (2013). Diagnostic and statistical manual of mental disorders. (5th ed.). Arlington, VA: American Psychiatric Publishing.

Bernstein, D. P., & Useda, J. D. (2007). Paranoid personality disorder. In W. O'Donohue, K. A. Fowler, & S. O. Lilienfeld (Eds.), *Personality disorders: Toward the DSM-V* (pp. 41-62). Thousand Oaks, CA: Sage Publications, Inc.

Birkeland, S. F. (2011). Paranoid personality disorder and sociodemography: A 25-year study of first admissions to a Danish general psychiatric hospital. *Nordic Psychology, 63*(3), 40-49. doi:10.1027/1901-2276/a000038

Bockian, N. R. (2006). Depression in paranoid personality disorder. In N. R. Bockian (Ed.), *Personality-guided therapy for depression* (pp. 41-62). Washington, DC: American Psychological Association.

British Association of Social Workers. (2012, January). The code of ethics for social workers: Statement of principles. Retrieved December 6, 2015, from http://cdn.basw.co.uk/upload/basw_112315-7.pdf

Cloninger, C. R., & Svrakic, D. R. (2009). Personality disorders. In B. J. Sadock, V. A. Sadock, & P. Ruiz (Eds.), *Kaplan & Sadock's comprehensive textbook of psychiatry* (9th ed., Vol. 2, pp. 2197-2240). Philadelphia, PA: Lippincott Williams & Wilkins.

Esterbery, M. L., Goulding, S. M., & Walker, E. F. (2010). Cluster A personality disorders: Schizotypal, schizoid, and paranoid personality disorders in childhood and adolescence. *Journal of Psychopathology & Behavioral Assessment, 32*(4), 515-528. doi:10.1007/s10862-010-9183-8

Horowitz, L. M. (2004). Obsessive-compulsive and paranoid personality disorder. In L. M. Horowitz (Ed.), *Interpersonal foundations of psychopathology* (pp. 131-146). Washington, DC: American Psychological Association.

Iacovino, J. M., Jackson, J. J., & Oltmanns, T. F. (2014). The relative impact of socioeconomic status and childhood trauma on Black-White differences in paranoid personality disorder symptoms. *Journal of Abnormal Psychology, 123*(1), 225-230. doi:10.1037/a0035258

International Federation of Social Workers. (2012, March 3). Statement of ethical principles. Retrieved December 6, 2015, from http://ifsw.org/policies/statement-of-ethical-principles

Janowsky, D. (2008). Personality disorders. In M. H. Ebert, P. T. Lossen, B. Nurcombe, & J. F. Leckman (Eds.), *Current diagnosis & treatment psychiatry* (2nd ed., pp. 513-519). New York, NY: McGraw Hill Medical.

Kellett, S., & Hardy, G. (2014). Treatment of paranoid personality disorder with cognitive analytic therapy: A mixed methods single case experimental design. *Clinical Psychology and Psychotherapy, 21*(5), 452-464. doi:10.1002/cpp.1845

Natsuaki, M. H., Diddhetti, D., & Rogosch, F. A. (2009). Examining the developmental history of child maltreatment, peer relations, and externalizing problems among adolescents with symptoms of paranoid personality disorder. *Development and Psychopathology, 21,* 1181-1193. doi:10.1017/S0954579409990101

Raza, G. T., DeMarce, J. M., Lash, S. J., & Parker, J. D. (2014). Paranoid personality disorder in the United States: The role of race, illicit drug use, and income. *Journal of Ethnicity in Substance Abuse, 13*(3), 247-257. doi:10.1080/15332640.2013.850463

Sadock, B.J., Sadock, V.A., & Ruiz, P. (2015). Personality disorders. In *Kaplan & Sadocks Synopsis of Psychiatry: Behavioral Sciences/Clinical Psychiatry* (11th ed., pp. 746-745). Philadelphia, PA: Wolters Kluwer Health/Lippincott Williams & Wilkins.

Triebwasser, J., Chemerinski, E., Roussos, P., & Siever, L. J. (2013). Paranoid personality disorder. *Journal of Personality Disorders, 27*(6), 795-805. doi:10.1521/pedi_2012_26_055

Wheeler, D.,... McClain, A. (2015). NASW standards and indicators for cultural competence in social work practice. Retrieved December 6, 2015, from http://www.socialworkers.org/practice/standards/PRA-BRO-253150-CC-Standards.pdf

PARENTAL BEREAVEMENT & GRIEF

MAJOR CATEGORIES: Child & Family, Behavioral & Mental Health

DESCRIPTION

Whether the death of a child is sudden or anticipated, whether it is a fetus that is lost or a child of any age, the grief response for parents typically is profound. The grief responses of parents have been described as a struggle to "accommodate a changed interpersonal reality"; this challenges the concept of grief as a linear process, experienced in specific stages and phases. Grief is primarily understood as a psychological condition affecting the mind, yet it is very often physical as well and has been described as a "whole body" experience. Losing a child undermines and defies what is considered the natural order of life. The grief experienced by parents is deeply personal and each response is unique. Grief's intensity can disrupt a parent's identity, bringing feelings of insecurity and vulnerability. It can adversely change and permanently impact both the individual and the family function.

Over half of the children who die each year in the United States die in hospital settings. Parents anticipate recovery in these clinical environments, so when a child dies it is often sudden and unexpected for them. Studies show that having an opportunity to say goodbye can be important to the adjustment and grieving process. The parents of children who die of violent causes are more likely to experience physical and mental health problems throughout their lives than parents whose loss results from disease or other natural causes. Grieving parents should be able to have their expression of grief facilitated, which may include rituals such as holding their child following her or his death.

Bereaved parents may demonstrate high levels of anger and hostility, as well as intense guilt about their perceived failure to protect their child. These responses can impair parents' interactions with surviving children: responding appropriately to the needs of siblings may be compromised, and grieving parents may be unable to provide a secure base for their surviving children. For grieving parents who return to work, it is often difficult to focus on their employment responsibilities when they are still working through strong feelings of guilt and mourning their child's loss. Furthermore, bereavement and grief can develop into complicated grief, which is grief that is prolonged, impacts daily functioning (going to work, school), impairs mental and physical health, and reduces the overall quality of a person's life. The *Diagnostic and Statistical Manual of Mental Disorders*, Fifth Edition (*DSM-5*), added proposed criteria for a possible diagnosable grief disorder, "persistent complex bereavement disorder," in the chapter titled Conditions for Further Study. The proposed disorder's criteria include at least 12 months of clinically significant disruption of functioning and six symptoms specific to reactive distress to the death or related social and identity disruption due to the death. Parents who develop complicated grief are at risk for suicide. More mothers (including female guardians) suffer complicated grief symptoms than fathers, which is thought to be related to the strength of the maternal attachment bond. Where there is limited partner closeness, or no partner, there is an increased risk of mental and physical health complications. Bereaved parents have higher rates of physical illnesses, including cancer and multiple sclerosis (MS), and increased mortality.

All members of families who lose children require ongoing emotional support services. The quality of the relationship between the parents can be critical to adjustment, especially once professional support has ceased, so social workers are advised to help couples strengthen their relationships. When grief becomes complicated, brief cognitive therapies have proven to be successful with helping parents adjust to their loss.

FACTS AND FIGURES

In the United States in 2011, there were approximately 6 neonatal and infant deaths per 1,000 live births. Over half of these deaths were attributed to one of five causes: congenital malformations, short gestation/low birthweight, sudden infant death syndrome, maternal complications, or unintentional injury. There are no data on the number of adults who die while their parents are still living.

Risk Factors

All parents who lose children are at risk of complicated grief symptoms. Women are at higher risk than men for complicated grief. Delayed or inhibited grief may also increase the risk for complicated grief. If parents decide to not have formalized or culturally appropriate rituals to mark the death of the child there may be an increased risk of complicated grief.

Signs and Symptoms

Physical symptoms of bereavement may include long-term sleep problems, fatigue, and anxiety. Psychological symptoms of bereavement may include cognitive deficits in concentration and memory processes. Parents grieving for a child lost to suicide or a traumatic event report posttraumatic stress responses such as flashbacks, intrusive memories, excessive rumination, and extreme guilt. Complicated grief symptoms are prolonged and include intense yearnings for the child, a sense of disbelief, anger, bitterness, and intrusive thoughts and preoccupations. Symptoms of complicated grief that persist for at least 6 months result in poor bereavement outcomes (divorce, neglect of other children) and are associated with mental health problems.

Assessment

The social worker should conduct a complete biological, psychological, social, and spiritual history of the parents, noting any mental health issues that may increase the risk of complicated grief and suicidal ideation.

Assessment and Screening Tools

Standardized assessments and screening tools may be helpful to further assess the individual's symptoms and needs. The *Diagnostic and Statistical Manual of Mental Disorders* (*DSM-5*) helps social workers differentiate between symptoms of a normal grief reaction and symptoms of a major depressive episode. The Complicated Grief Assessment has 10 questions that help diagnose complicated grief symptoms. The Perinatal Bereavement Grief Scale short version has 33 questions, helps distinguish bereavement from depression, and is available in English and Spanish. The Scale for Suicidal Ideation (SSI) measures the intensity, pervasiveness, and characteristics of suicidal ideation.

Treatment

Research shows that effectively helping those who are grieving involves "listening, responding with empathy and concern, and holding – with your presence, voice and eyes." Multiple sources of support, from family and friends as well as professional services, are important. When a child is terminally ill, access to counseling prior to the child's death is also critical. These support networks and services allow grieving parents to feel a sense of control over their grief and integrate it into their daily lives. A close marriage/partnership between the parents is an important coping resource in the short and long term following the death of a child, so interventions provided by social workers and other mental health professionals should enhance and/or facilitate this relationship. Some parents will benefit from engaging in specific activities such as attending clubs of interest or support groups, taking up hobbies, or getting regular exercise. Although the use of medications often is discouraged for managing symptoms of grief because of the risk of overuse and because they can inhibit the expression of grief, some parents may benefit from short-term medication use and should speak with their physician. Treatment therapies for complicated grief includes cognitive, short-term therapy that focuses on the individual revisiting his or her loss, reimagining his or her relationship with the dead child, and envisioning his or her future. Parents with complicated grief may need to be evaluated for suicide risk.

Family Bereavement Program (FBP) is designed to promote resilience in parents who have lost their children. FBP consists of 12 two-hour group sessions led by counselors or social workers, each of which involves the teaching of a particular skill (positive coping, good communication, problem solving), practicing the skill (role play), and assigning activities for practice at home. Evaluation of FBP has shown positive effects (better management of parent depression and grief, positive parent and surviving child relationship) at both 11-month and 6-year follow-ups.

For bereaved parents with a surviving child or children, a social worker can engage in therapeutic work with the parents to help them process and cope with their loss as well as maintain the ability to stay engaged, in tune with, and attached to their surviving children and reestablish a healthy family life. Part of this therapeutic approach will involve giving parents age-appropriate tools to help their children understand the loss of a sibling, learn about the grief that often accompanies that loss, and learn ways to maintain a bond with the deceased sibling (writing letters to sibling, drawing family pictures to include sibling).

An emerging intervention and resource for bereaved parents are peer supporters. Peer supporters are volunteers who have also lost a child who are trained in bereavement support. Peer supporters follow up with bereaved parents on the phone and through home visits, as well as invite them to bereavement support groups. Although more research is needed, initial feedback and evaluations indicate that bereaved parents appreciate and value peer supporters.

If a child dies in a hospital setting, bereavement photography may be an option offered prior to the death of the child. Investigators have found that families who decide to have a photographer take pictures of their child before the child dies or after the child dies appreciate the photos, which help them in their healing process. The photos can help make a horrible experience a treasured last moment. Photographers who perform bereavement photography tend to be extremely sensitive to the situation and create a therapeutic setting by taking photos in a documentary style versus a portrait style. Initial evaluations of bereavement photography suggest that it may contribute to the increased psychological wellness of a bereaved family.

INTERVENTION

A parent who has lost a child will experience symptoms of grief. Social workers should assist families in learning and maintaining healthy expressions of grief. A social worker may help the parents express and understand their grief. Support groups, individual therapy, couples counseling, and family therapy may be suggested. Bereaved parents should be encouraged to increase their social support network.

A parent who has lost a child may experience symptoms of complicated grief. The social worker may assist the parents adjust to the loss of their child and recover from complicated grief symptoms through support, counseling, and referrals to available resources. Counseling may include cognitive treatment that revisits the loss of the child with the

individual and has the individual reimagine an ongoing relationship with the child and reenvision a future life without the child. In addition, support groups, individual therapy, couples counseling, and family therapy should all be considered.

A parent who has lost a child may experience suicidal ideation. The goal of a social worker assisting the parent is to help eliminate the suicidal ideation and maintain safety. The social worker should assess the individual for suicide using a standardized screening tool such as SSI. It should be determined if the parent has a plan to accomplish his or her suicide. Parents who have suicidal ideation without a plan should see a mental health professional as soon as possible. If there is active suicidal ideation and a plan, the individual should be taken to an emergency room or mental health facility. If the individual refuses to go, the police can be called for involuntary detainment to ensure the individual's safety.

APPLICABLE LAWS AND REGULATIONS

Each jurisdiction (nation, state, or province) has its own standards, procedures, and laws for involuntary restraint and detention of persons who may be a danger to themselves or others. Because complicated grief may lead to suicide ideation it is important that the social worker, mental health professionals, and medical professionals working with bereaved parents are familiar with the local requirements for involuntary detention.

SERVICES AND RESOURCES

- Bereaved Parents of the USA, http://www.bereavedparentsusa.org
- The Compassionate Friends, http://www.compassionatefriends.org
- National Institute of Mental Health, http://www.nimh.nih.gov
- International Stillbirth Alliance, http://www.stillbirthalliance.org
- National Palliative Care Research Center, http://www.npcrc.org

FOOD FOR THOUGHT

There is no consensus on what exactly constitutes an unhealthy or complicated response when a parent loses a child. The accepted expression of bereavement differs across cultural and ethnic groups. Patterns of lifelong grieving and feelings of acute loss can serve to maintain the emotional connection between the parent and the dead child. Many bereaved parents welcome these emotions as a way to preserve the memory and value of their child.

Marital/relationship closeness can help some parents through their grieving process and with adjustment; however, many parents divorce following the death of a child. Bereaved parents have a greater risk for divorce than nonbereaved parents. Knowing this, social workers should offer to provide marriage and family counseling beyond the crisis stage following the child's death.

Unlike an orphan, a widower, or a widow, there is no name specific for a parent who has lost a child. Many parents who lose children to suicide will deny that their child took his or her own life. Motherhood itself can be a protective factor for bereaved mothers if they have other living children. Their other children can provide distraction from grief and can give them a sense of purpose and meaning in their day-to-day life.

RED FLAGS

Parents with symptoms of complicated grief are at higher risk for suicide. Support groups for grieving parents are more effective when the group is offered in the parents' first language.

NEXT STEPS

Families who lose children require ongoing emotional support services to assist them in adjustment to their bereavement.

Written by Jan Wagstaff, MA, MSW

Reviewed by Lynn B. Cooper, D Crim, and Melissa Rosales Neff, MSW

REFERENCES

Aho, A., Astedt-Kurki, P., & Paunonen, M. (2013). Peer supporters' experiences of bereavement follow-up intervention for grieving parents. Omega, 68(4), 347-366.

American Psychiatric Association. (2013). agnostic and statistical manual of mental disorders. Arlington, VA: American Psychiatric Publishing.

Arnold, J., & Gemma, P. B. (2008). The continuing process of parent grief. *Death Studies, 32*(7), 658-673.

Ayers, T., Wolchik, S., Sandler, I., Twohey, J., Weyer, J., Padgett-Jones, S.,... Kriege, G. (2013). The Family Bereavement Program: description of a theory-based prevention program for parentally bereaved children and adolescents. *Omega, 68*(4), 293-314.

Barrera, M., Agostino, N. M., Schneiderman, G., Tallet, S., Spencer, L., & Jovcevska, V. (2007). Patterns of parental bereavement following the loss of a child and related factors. *Omega, 55*(2), 145-167.

Blood, C., & Cacciatore, J. (2014). Parental grief and memento mori photography: Narrative, meaning, culture, and context. *Death Studies, 38*(4), 224-233. doi:10.1080/07481187.2013.788584

Bolton, J., Au, W., Walld, R., Chateau, D., Martens, P., Leslie, W.,... Sareen, J. (2014). Parental bereavement after the death of an offspring in a motor vehicle collision: A population-based study. *American Journal of Epidemiology, 179*(2), 177-285. doi:10.1093/aje/kwt247

Bugge, K., Darbyshire, P., Rokholt, E., Haugstvedt, K., Sulheim, T., & Solvi, H. (2014). Young children's grief: Parents' understanding and coping. *Death Studies, 38*(1), 36-43. doi:10.1080/07481187.2012.718037

Chidley, B., Khademi, M., Meany, K., & Doucett, M. (2014). Bereavement during motherhood: A mixed method pilot study exploring bereavement while parenting. *Bereavement Care, 33*(1), 19-27. doi:10.1080/02682621.2014.902614

Collings, C. (2008). That's not my child anymore! Parent grief after acquired brain injury (ABI): Incidence, nature, longevity. *British Journal of Social Work, 38*(8), 1499-1517.

Estes, E. B. (2002). Bereaved parents of the USA: Suicide. Retrieved October 9, 2014, from http://www.bereavedparentsusa.org/BP_Brochures.htm

Fortinash, K. M. (2012). Grief: in loss and death. In K. M. Fortinash, & P. A. Holoday (Eds.), *Psychiatric Mental Health Nursing* (5th ed., pp. 640-657). St. Louis, MO: Elsevier Mosby.

Gibson, J., Gallagher, M., & Jenkins, M. (2010). The experiences of parents readjusting to the workplace following the death of a child by suicide. *Death Studies, 34*(6), 500-528.

Gudmundsdottir, M. (2009). Embodied grief: Bereaved parents' narratives of their suffering body. *Omega, 59*(3), 253-269.

Kreicbergs, U. C., Lannen, P., Onelov, E., & Wolfe, J. (2007). Parental grief after losing a child to cancer: Impact of professional and social support on long-term outcomes. *Journal of Clinical Oncology, 25*(22), 3307-3312.

Lyngstad, T. H. (2013). Bereavement and divorce: Does the death of a child affect parents' marital stability?. *Family Science , 4*(1), 79-86. doi:10.1080/19424620.2013.821762

MacDorman, M. F., Hoyert, D. L., & Mathews, T. J. (2013). Recent declines in infant mortality in the United States, 2005-2011. U. S. Department of Health and Human Services, Centers for Disease Control and Prevention, NCHS Data Brief, 120, April 2013.

Michelson, K., Blehart, K., Hochberg, T., & James, K. (2013). Bereavement photography for children: Program development and health care professionals' response. *Death Studies, 37*(6), 513-528.

Michon, B., Balkou, S., Hivon, R., & Cyr, C. (2003). Death of a child: Parental perception of grief intensity - end-of-life and bereavement care. *Paediatric Child Health, 8*(6), 363-366.

Mizrahi, T., & Mayden, R. W. (2001). NASW standards for cultural competence in social work practice. Retrieved August 7, 2015, from http://www.socialworkers.org/practice/standards/NASWCulturalStandards.pdf

O'Leary, J. M. (2007). Pregnancy and infant loss: Supporting parents and their children. *Zero to Three, 27*(6), 42-49.

Sandler, I., Wolchik, S., Ayers, T., Tein, J., & Luecken, L. (2013). Family bereavement program (FBP) approach to promoting resilience following the death of a parent. *Family Science , 4*(1), 87-94. doi:10.1080/19424620.2013.821763

Song, J., Floyd, F. J., Seltzer, M. M., Greenberg, J. S., & Hong, J. (2010). Long-term effects of child death on parents' health-related quality of life: A dyadic analysis. *Family Relations, 59*(3), 269-282.

Statement of Ethical Principles. (2012, March 3). *International Federation of Social Workers.* Retrieved August 7, 2015, from http://ifsw.org/policies/statement-of-ethical-principles/

The Policy, Ethics, and Human Rights Committee, British Association of Social Workers. (2012, January). The Code of Ethics for Social Work: Statement of principles. Retrieved August 7, 2015, from http://cdn.basw.co.uk/upload/basw_112315-7.pdf

Tomita, T., & Kitamura, T. (2002). Clinical and research measures of grief: A reconsideration. *Comprehensive Psychiatry, 43*(2), 95-102.

Townsend, M. C. (2015). The bereaved individual. In M. C. Townsend (Ed.), *Psychiatric Mental Health Nursing: Concepts of Care in Evidence-Based Practice* (8th ed., pp. 830-850). Philadelphia: F.A.: Davis Company.

PARENTAL DEATH: CHILDHOOD & ADOLESCENCE—PSYCHOSOCIAL ISSUES

MAJOR CATEGORIES: Behavioral & Mental Health, Child & Family

DESCRIPTION

Children and adolescents who have experienced the death of a parent commonly express sadness, hopelessness, and despair, and periods of anger and agitation. The term childhood traumatic grief is generally used when grieving symptoms become so intense that they interfere with a child's grieving process and adjustment. When there are additional traumatic aspects to a parent's death, such as a death from suicide, war, AIDS, or a drug overdose, a child's or adolescent's emotional response may be described as complicated grief or childhood traumatic grief.

There is considerable variability in the emotional responses of children and adolescents to the death of a parent. The child or adolescent may seem to have a delayed response to the death or may alternate between appearing bereaved and appearing unaffected. The tasks of grief for the child or adolescent can include telling the death story; expressing and accepting the sadness, guilt, anger, and other feelings that may accompany death; reviewing the relationship with the deceased; exploring possibilities after loss; understanding processes and problems of grief; and being understood and accepted by others. Children and adolescents who experience the death of a parent may appear to the adults around them to have quickly overcome their loss or to not fully understand it.

Cultural standards of behavior can pressure a grieving child to get on with life as if it were normal, which may inhibit and/or worsen the process of grief. A parent' death may challenge a child's religious belief for other children faith can provide meaning or context for a parent's death. The child's relationship with his or her surviving parent or caregiver is critical to the child's adjustment and well-being. A depressed surviving parent may be unable to provide positive interactions, or the parenting may feel harsh to the child, both of which can have adverse effects. Some children will develop serious emotional problems. When trauma is involved in the death of a parent, the risk of anxiety and/or depression increases and behavior problems and disorders involving substance abuse may arise in adolescence. Post-traumatic stress disorder (PTSD) can be a persistent problem, and issues of physical health may also develop. Research has indicated that high levels of PTSD and childhood traumatic grief are common among children who have lost a parent, regardless of whether the death was sudden and/or violent or was expected.

Bereaved children can be helped to manage their belief systems and worldviews after losing a parent. Social workers can assist them in maintaining a bond with the deceased parent and ensuring that the child has opportunities to explore and experience his or her natural grieving process. A range of therapies can assist children with this. Facilitating positive relationships between the child and his or her surviving parent or caregiver, as well as with other adults and the child's peers, is very important. Helping the child establish relationships with children who have also experienced the death of a parent can be helpful. Children can benefit from physical exercise and participating in activities such as a team sport or bicycling to channel their emotions. In addition to addressing the emotions associated with the loss of a parent, bereaved children also need to experience the normal range of positive emotions in their daily lives to aid in the grieving process.

FACTS AND FIGURES

It is estimated that 153 million children worldwide have lost one or both parents. As of 2014, 13.3 million children had lost one or both parents to AIDS. Of

these children, 11 million lived in sub-Saharan Africa. In the United States, 3.4 percent of children and adolescents experience the death of a parent before age 18. In 2013, approximately 1.2 million children in the United States were receiving survivor's benefits from Social Security as a result of the death of a parent. About 1 in 5 children develop serious emotional symptoms a year or more after the death of a parent. In a poll of bereaved children and adolescents conducted in the United States in 2013, 33 percent reported that their current guardian or caregiver was having difficulty communicating with them about personal matters. In the same poll, 75 percent of the children and adolescents reported that the most pervasive emotion they felt during their grieving was sadness, followed by anger, being overwhelmed, and loneliness. Of the children and adolescents surveyed, 39 percent reported trouble sleeping and 45 percent reported having trouble concentrating at school. Adolescents who have experienced the loss of a parent are 3 times more likely to develop depression than those who have not.

RISK FACTORS

Children and adolescents who have lost a parent are at significant risk for depression, PTSD, symptoms of trauma, and other biologic, psychological, and social complications of such loss. The type of death of a parent may exacerbate grief in children, in that some deaths carry a stigma, such as those resulting from suicide, homicide, or AIDS. The type of a parent's death may also intensify grief if the death was the result of an accident, natural disaster, or terrorist attack, and/or if the child witnessed the death. The ability of the surviving parent and other adult caregivers to function both physically and emotionally will influence the child's adjustment. If the surviving parent/adult is in denial or ignores the loss of the deceased parent, the child may feel unable to openly grieve. The child's personality will also affect his or her adjustment to loss. A child who is anxious is likely to have a greater risk of experiencing complicated grief than is a child who is more pragmatic. Preexisting conditions and risk factors may also influence a child's ability to cope with a loss, including learning problems, social problems, or mental health concerns such as depression. Children's adjustment to the death of a parent may also be affected by family structure and functioning. Children in families in which communication is poor and conflict exists may have difficulty adjusting; they may feel guilt if their relationship with the deceased parent was characterized by turmoil. Families' coping with simultaneous stressors (e.g., financial problems, unstable living situations) creates a risk to the adjustment of the grieving child. The support systems available before, during, and after the loss can serve as protective factors for the grieving child or as risk factors if these systems are insufficient.

SIGNS AND SYMPTOMS

Psychological signs and symptoms of depression include feelings of depression (episodic or pervasive); hopelessness; isolation; denial; anger directed toward self, the deceased, or remaining caregivers; shame; guilt; fear; worthlessness; nervousness; irritability; loss of pleasure in activities; stress; feelings of stigma; reliving of traumatic events; hyperarousal; yearning to be with the deceased; numbness; curiosity about the circumstances of the death; anxious attachment to a surviving caregiver; distress about separation from the deceased parent; inability to focus; frustration; belief that one caused the death; preoccupation with the life of the person who died are among the effects on a child of the death of a parent or other close caregiver.

Behavioral effects of such a death include and increase or decrease in sleep, increase or decrease in appetite, inappropriate euphoria, aggression, agitation, loss of interest in activities, risk-taking behaviors, isolation, developmental delays or regression, nightmares, conduct disorder (e.g., breaking rules, lying, truancy).

Physical effects on a child of the death of a parent or close caregiver include somatic complaints (e.g., chronic muscle and back pain, headaches, fatigue, gastrointestinal problems), changes in weight, neglect of hygiene, and psychosomatic mirroring of health problems of the deceased person.

ASSESSMENT

A comprehensive biological, psychological, and social-spiritual assessment of the child who has experienced the death of a parent or other close caregiver should include information about any physical, mental, environmental, cultural, social, spiritual, and medical factors relating to the child and the child's family.

The assessment should include the child's answers to questions about any history of trauma and trauma-related symptoms, prior caregiving, attachment to the deceased parent/caretaker, family history, psychiatric symptoms or issues that might pose a risk to the child or to others (e.g., suicidality, self-harm, substance abuse, aggression, child-to-parent violence, fire setting, running away, harming animals, sexual perpetration). The assessment should include the child's stress-management and coping skills.

ASSESSMENTS AND SCREENING TOOLS

Screening for a child's well-being after the death of a parent or other close caregiver may be done with the following social-work, medical, and psychological tools: Clinician Administered PTSD Scale (CAPS), Beck Depression Inventory (BDI), Complicated Bereavement Risk Assessment (CBRA), Beck Anxiety Inventory (BAI), Childhood Traumatic Grief Symptom Scale (CTGSS), University of California–Los Angeles Post-Traumatic Stress Disorder Reaction Index, Extended Grief Inventory (EGI), Center for Epidemiological Studies Depression Scale (CES-D), Depression Anxiety Stress Scales (DASS), the Conflict Tactics Scale, Child Well-Being Scales, eco-map.

For adolescent clients, medical and other professionals treating the child may want to consider whether drug or alcohol testing is warranted.

TREATMENT

In narrative therapy, the child who has experienced the death of a parent or other close caregiver describes his or her experiences through writing (e.g., poetry, journals, letters), drawing, and drama. Children who establish an ongoing bond with their deceased parent have better outcomes. Using rituals, linking significant objects to the lost parent, looking at photographs of the lost parent, listening to music and/or recordings of the parent's voice, and engaging in activities such as tree planting to commemorate the parent's life can offer comfort, assist with adjustment, and help a child maintain a bond. Physical activity can be important in easing symptoms of grief and channeling emotions. The child's relationship its surviving parent is critical: Clinical attention should focus both on this and on the individual responses and psychological processes of the child.

Social workers can help the surviving parent to understand the significance of his or her role in the adjustment process of a child who has lost its other parent. Positive parenting, which is a combination of positive language and creating positive experiences, should be encouraged and supported. Relationships with other children can be helpful; it is especially important for bereaved children to meet with peers who are going through similar experiences. Youth camps are available for bereaved children through the Moyer Foundation. Although the ability to freely express anger and sadness is important to a child after the death of a parent, so too are opportunities for having fun and sharing humor and laughter.

The Family Bereavement Program (FBP) is designed to promote resilience in children who have lost a parent. The program consists of 12 two-hour group sessions led by two counselors or social workers. Each session involves teaching a skill (e.g., positive coping, communication skills, problem-solving skills), practicing that skill (e.g., through role playing), and assigning activities for practicing the skill at home. Evaluation of FBP has shown it to have positive effects at follow-up periods of both 11-months and 6-years after its application.

For children who show low levels of distress after the death of a parent, traditional interventions for managing bereavement may seem too intense or unnecessary. In such cases, a social worker may need to connect the child and his or her caregiver to an alternative form of intervention, such as a self-directed grief- support resource. An example of this type of resource is a video called Talk, Listen, Connect III: When Families Grieve, produced by Sesame Street. Using characters from the Sesame Street television show, the video provides education that encourages children with a psychological problem, and these children's caregivers, to communicate more with one another and develop a shared understanding of each other's experiences of grief. Both children and their caregivers report positive effects of viewing this video, including an enhanced ability to cope.

It is important to note that some children and adolescents will resolve bereavement without any professional support. A social worker, clinical psychologist, or other qualified healthcare professional can communicate with the caregiver of a bereaved child or adolescent to determine whether it needs any professional help. Bereavement is a natural process and should be normalized. Although individual and family therapy and other interventions are important for children who have experienced the death of a parent or other close caregiver, there is also a need for social workers to view bereavement and palliative care as a public health issue and work with their communities to provide education about these issues. Making bereavement education a public-health issue challenges the social stigma attached to talking about death. Educated teachers, religious leaders, and others such as family friends (persons a bereaved child knows and trusts) can help support grieving children on a longer-term and more sustained basis than can more limited or shorter-term treatments.

Educational information provided to bereaved children should be provided in a personally and culturally sensitive manner, in language that can be easily understood by the individual child and the child's family. If a client has a low literacy level, the use of pictograms (i.e., a symbol or picture representing a concept or idea) can be beneficial. It is important that any professional treatment provided to a bereaved child utilizes evidence-based practices, ensures the privacy and confidentiality of the child and its family, and is accurately recorded in the client's file.

INTERVENTION

When bereavement of a child or adolescent is anticipated, it is essential to promote their mental health. It is important that family members, friends, and professional counselors visit the child and family before the parent's death. Help should be provided toward any spiritual reconciliation. The child/adolescent who will be bereaved should be linked with other children/adolescents going through similar experiences. It is useful to suggest that the child or adolescent who will be bereaved attend support groups, which often are held at hospices and/or religious centers. The child/adolescent and family members who are to be affected should be educated about the psychological aspects of the bereavement process and the means for addressing them. The bereaved child or adolescent should be encouraged to maintain a bond with the deceased parent by visiting the parent's gravesite or keeping a journal (depending on child's age). The child or adolescent should be given space for the expression of grief that includes laughter as well as sadness, and should be linked with other children going through similar experiences. Opportunities should be provided for the affected child or adolescent to have physical exercise, and the surviving parent should be supported in his or her parenting

A child who has experienced the loss of a parent or other close caregiver is often angry, irritable, and/or aggressive, or may have decreased aggressive behaviors and a decrease in negative emotions. Individual therapy appropriate to the age and developmental level of the affected child or adolescent should be provided to help him or her to explore emotions, reduce anger, and develop coping strategies. Counseling should be given on alternatives to aggressive behaviors, and a referral should be provided for group grief therapy or a grief camp.

A child under age 12 who shows signs of developmental regression such as bedwetting, thumbsucking, or "baby talk" will still be able to express feelings and behave at a level appropriate to its stage of development.. Individual counseling with play, art, or music therapy elements can help the child in exploring emotions related to his or her loss. Professionally guided behavior modification can be used to reduce developmental regression and assist a bereaved child or adolescent in returning to an appropriate level of functioning. Family caregivers should be encouraged and supported in establishing routines and ways of helping the bereaved child or adolescent to feel more secure.

For adolescents engaging in risk-taking behaviors as components of the grieving process, efforts should be made to prevent or stop harmful behaviors such as cutting, substance/alcohol abuse, and promiscuity. The bereaved child or adolescent should be educated about feelings associated with grief to help normalize his or her feelings. This can be done with techniques such as psychotherapy, journaling, memorializing the deceased, peer support, relaxation, meditation, exercise, and other stress-reducing activities.

APPLICABLE LAWS AND REGULATIONS

In the United States, all social workers, mental-health clinicians, and healthcare professionals are bound by the "duty to warn," which requires that they inform the proper authorities if a person is found to be a danger to him- or herself or others. Professional persons working with bereaved children or adolescents

or their families should be aware of the regulations and procedures in their state's duty-to-warn law. In the United Kingdom, social services workers are not mandated by law to warn but are expected to act in the best interest of the child.

SERVICES AND RESOURCES

- Camps for grieving children are organized by the Moyer Foundation, http://www.moyerfoundation.org
- National Alliance for Grieving Children, https://childrengrieve.org/
- American Cancer Society, http://www.cancer.org
- Hello Grief, http://www.hellogrief.org/
- Childhood Bereavement Network, United Kingdom, http://www.childhoodbereavementnetwork.org.uk

FOOD FOR THOUGHT

Healthcare professionals working with bereaved children or adolescents and their families should attempt to assist them in avoiding and eliminating symptoms associated with grief, which may complicate the grieving process, and it is important to recognize that the risk for depression in adulthood is increased for persons who experience the death of a parent in childhood.

Helping children and adolescents to find meaning in life, as well as meaning in the life of a deceased parent or caregiver, can help them to move forward from traumatic grief to more normal grief (Dickens, 2014).

Children in the twenty-first century have much more exposure to a variety of ideas of death and afterlife through television, films, books, and the Internet than did children in the past. It is important to maintain an ongoing dialogue with children who have experienced the death of a parent because they may have questions about how their parent died, what happens after death, and other issues relating to death.

RED FLAGS

Symptoms of emotional trauma may be more common in bereaved children and adolescents than was once thought, regardless of the type of loss. Bereaved children, like other bereaved persons, can quickly come to feel that others do not wish to hear about their loss. Having the support of people who want to listen is an important part of the grieving process.

When children are not given age-appropriate information about the death of a loved one, they may make incorrect assumptions about the death, which increases their risk of experiencing complicated grief.

NEXT STEPS

It is important to determine whether a bereaved child or adolescent has unmet physical, medical, and psychological needs and to make referrals to the appropriate care providers as needed.

If possible, the bereaved child or adolescent should have regular contact, communication, and support throughout the initial grieving period. The a child or adolescent should be monitored for any complications for up to 1 year after a parent's death.

It is important to support the surviving parent with education about positive parenting and encouragement to be direct, honest, and open with the bereaved child or adolescent about the loss of the other parent.

The child or adolescent should be referred to one or more appropriate support group(s) as indicated.

Written by Jan Wagstaff, MA, MSW

REFERENCES

Ayers, T., Wolchik, S., Sandler, I., Twohey, J., Weyer, J., Padgett-Jones, S.,... Kriege, G. (2013). The Family Bereavement Program: Description of a theory-based prevention program for parentally bereaved children and adolescents. Omega: Journal of Death and Dying, 68(4), 293-314. doi:10.2190/OM.68.4.a

Berg, L., Rostila, M., & Hjern, A. (2014). Parental death during childhood and subsequent school performance. Pediatrics, 133(4), 682-689. doi:10.1542/peds.2013-2771

Brewer, J. D., & Sparkes, A. C. (2011). Young people living with parental bereavement: Insights from an ethnographic study of a UK childhood bereavement service. Social Science & Medicine, 72(2), 283-290. doi:10.1016/j.socscimed.2010.10.032

British Association of Social Workers. (2012). The code of ethics for social work: Statement of principles. Retrieved April 20, 2016, from http://cdn.basw.co.uk/upload/basw_112315-7.pdf

Cas, A. G., Frankenberg, E., Suriastini, W., & Thomas, D. (2014). The impact of parental death on child well-being: Evidence from the Indian Ocean tsunami. Demography, 51(2), 437-457. doi:10.1007/s13524-014-0279-8

Dickens, N. (2014). Prevalence of complicated grief and posttraumatic stress disorder in children and adolescents following sibling death. The Family Journal, 22(1), 119-126. doi:10.1177/1066480713505066

Edgar-Bailey, M., & Kress, V. E. (2010). Resolving child and adolescent traumatic grief: Creative techniques and interventions. Journal of Creativity in Mental Health, 5(2), 158-176. doi:10.1080/15401383.2010.485090

Fortinash, K. M. (2012). Grief: in loss and death. In K. M. Fortinash, & P. A. Holoday (Eds.), Psychiatric Mental Health Nursing (5th ed., pp. 640-657). St. Louis, MO: Elsevier Mosby.

Haine, R. A., Wolchik, S. A., Sandler, I. N., Millsap, R. E., & Ayers, T. S. (2006). Positive parenting as a protective resource for parentally bereaved children. Death Studies, 30(1), 1-28. doi:10.1080/07481180500348639

Hope, R. M., & Hodge, D. M. (2006). Factors affecting children's adjustment to the death of a parent: The social work professional's viewpoint. Child and Adolescent Social Work Journal, 23(1), 107-126. doi:10.1007/s10560-006-0045-x

Hung, N. C., & Rabin, L. A. (2009). Comprehending childhood bereavement by parental suicide: A critical review of research on outcomes, grief processes, and interventions. Death Studies, 33(9), 781-814. doi:10.1080/07481180903142357

International Federation of Social Workers. (2012, March 3). Statement of ethical principles. Retrieved April 20, 2016, from http://ifsw.org/policies/statement-of-ethical-principles/

Li, J., Vestergaard, M., Cnattingius, S., Gissler, M., Beck, B., Hammer Beck, B.,... Olsen, J. (2014). Mortality after parental death in childhood: A nationwide cohort study from three Nordic countries. PLoS Medicine, 11(7), e1001679. doi:10.1371/journal.pmed.1001679

Mannarino, A. P., & Cohen, J. A. (2011). Traumatic loss in children and adolescents. Journal of Child & Adolescent Trauma, 4(1), 22-33. doi:10.1080/19361521.2011.545048

McClatchey, I. S., Vonk, M. E., & Palardy, G. (2009). The prevalence of childhood traumatic grief - a comparison of violent/sudden and expected loss. Omega: Journal of Death and Dying, 59(4), 305-323. doi:10.2190/OM.59.4.b

Nader, K., & Salloum, A. (2011). Complicated grief reactions in children and adolescents. Journal of Child & Adolescent Trauma, 4(3), 233-257. doi:10.1080/19361521.2011.599358

National Alliance for Grieving Children. (2013). National poll of bereaved children & teenagers. Retrieved April 20, 2016, from http://www.childrengrieve.org/national-poll-bereaved-children-teenagers

National Association of Social Workers. (2003). Standards for the practice of social work with adolescents. Retrieved April 20, 2016, from https://www.socialworkers.org/practice/standards/Adolescents.asp

National Association of Social Workers. (2008). Code of ethics. Retrieved April 20, 2016, from https://www.socialworkers.org/pubs/code/code.asp

Ortiz, C., Cozza, S., Fullerton, C., & Ursano, R. (2013). Feasibility of a multimedia program for parentally bereaved children. Child & Youth Care Forum, 42(6), 489-506. doi:10.1007/s10566-013-9216-z

Paul, S. (2013). Public health approaches to palliative care: The role of the hospice social worker working with children experiencing bereavement. British Journal of Social Work, 43(2), 249-263. doi:10.1093/bjsw/bct017

Rostila, M., & Saarela, J. M. (2011). Time does not heal all wounds: Mortality following the death of a parent. Journal of Marriage and Family, 73(1), 236-249. doi:10.2307/29789570

Schoenfelder, E. N., Sandler, I. N., Wolchik, S., & MacKinnon, D. (2011). Quality of social relationships and the development of depression in parentally-bereaved youth. Journal of Youth and Adolescence, 40(1), 85-96. doi:10.1007/s10964-009-9503-z

Sherr, L., Croome, N., Clucas, C., & Brown, E. (2014). Differential effects of single and double parental death on child emotional functioning and daily life in South Africa. Child Welfare, 93(1), 149-172.

Smeltzer, S. C. (2014). End-of-life care. In J. L. Hinkle & K. H. Cheever (Eds.), Brunner & Suddarth's textbook of medical-surgical nursing (13th ed., Vol. 1, pp. 374-397). Philadelphia, PA: Wolters Kluwer Health/Lippincott Williams & Wilkins.

Social Security Administration. (2014). Fast facts & figures about Social Security, 2014. Retrieved April 20, 2016, from http://www.ssa.gov/policy/docs/chartbooks/fast_facts/2014/fast_facts14.pdf

SOS Children's Villages. (2014). Worldwide children's statistics. Retrieved April 20, 2016, from http://www.sos-usa.org/our-impact/childrens-statistics

Unicef. (2015). Protection, care and support for children affected by HIV and AIDS. Retrieved April 20, 2016, from http://www.data.unicef.org/hiv-aids/care-support.html

Way, P. (2013). A practitioner's view of children making spiritual meanings in bereavement. Journal of Social Work in End-of-Life & Palliative Care, 9(2/3), 144-157. doi:10.1080/15524256.2013.794032

Werner-Lin, A., & Biank, N. M. (2009). Along the cancer continuum: Integrating therapeutic support and bereavement groups for children and teens of terminally ill cancer patients. Journal of Family Social Work, 12(4), 359-370. doi:10.1080/10522150903321314

Wheeler, D. (2015). NASW Standards and Indicators for Cultural Competence in Social Work Practice. Retrieved from http://www.socialworkers.org/practice/standards/PRA-BRO-253150-CC-Standards.pdf

Wolchik, S. A., Coxe, A., Tein, J. Y., Sandler, I. N., & Ayers, T. S. (2008). Six-year longitudinal predictors of posttraumatic growth in parentally bereaved adolescents and young adults. Omega: Journal of Death and Dying, 58(2), 107-128.

Wolchik, S. A., Ma, Y., Tein, J., Sandler, I. N., & Ayers, T. S. (2008). Parentally bereaved children's grief: Self-system beliefs as mediators of the relations between grief and stressors and caregiver-child relationship quality. Death Studies, 32(7), 597-620. doi:10.1080/07481180802215551

Reviewer(s)

Melissa Rosales Neff, MSW, Cinahl Information Systems, Glendale, CA

Laura Gale, LCSW, Cinahl Information Systems, Glendale, CA

PARENTAL SUBSTANCE USE DISORDER: IMPACT ON FAMILIES

MAJOR CATEGORIES: Behavioral & Mental Health, Child & Family, Substance Abuse

WHAT WE KNOW

Parental substance use disorder is a significant problem that affects millions of children in the United States alone.

The *Diagnostic and Statistical Manual of Mental Disorders*, fifth edition (*DSM-5*) addresses substance use disorders and substance-induced disorders (intoxication, withdrawal, and other substance/medication-induced mental disorders). Thus it removes the distinction between abuse and dependence and instead divides each disorder into mild, moderate, and severe subtypes. Drug craving was added as a criterion for substance use disorder, whereas "recurrent legal problems" was removed. In the DSM-5, substance abuse is referred to as substance use disorder or substance dependence, whereas in the research literature it is still commonly referred to as substance abuse. The DSM-5 bases the diagnosis of a substance use disorder on criteria that reflect "a pathological pattern of behaviors related to use of the substance" (American Psychological Association, 2013, p.483), which may include impaired control over use; withdrawal from usual activities; interference with family, work, or social responsibilities; persistent use despite consequences; tolerance; and withdrawal.

It is estimated that, worldwide, 3.6 percent of persons ages 15–64 have a current alcohol use disorder (i. e., within the past 12 months). The African region has the lowest prevalence (1.1 percent), whereas higher prevalence rates are noted in the American region (encompassing North, South, and Central America and the Caribbean; 5.2 percent) and the Eastern European (10.9 percent) region.

Approximately 8.3 million children in the United States, or 11.9 percent of all U.S. children, live with at least one parent who abuses alcohol and/or drugs. When alcohol and illicit drugs are considered separately, 10 percent of children live with a parent who abuses alcohol and 3 percent with a parent who abuses an illicit drug.

According to data from England's National Drug Treatment Monitoring System, among adults in England starting drug treatment in 2010–2011, 21 percent lived with their own children, 20 percent were parents who did not live with their own children, and 13 percent were living with children other than their offspring (e. g., their partner's children or relatives).

Parental substance use disorder has substantial impacts on children and families. It often dominates family life, becoming the parent's primary focus and the organizing force in the household. The compulsion to obtain and use alcohol and/or drugs overrides considerations regarding children's safety and well-being; children's needs become peripheral to substance use. Preoccupied with securing and using substances, the parent may come and go unpredictably, leaving the children with relatives or other caregivers for extended periods. Parents may adopt practices that they believe shield their children from their use, such as locking themselves or their children in a separate room so they do not witness the parent's substance use, or they may bring drugs or drug-using friends into the home, use in front of their children, and/or leave paraphernalia in the children's reach.

Financial issues are one of the greatest stressors reported by families in which a family member abuses substances. A person with substance abuse issues may sell possessions, spend household funds, or steal or demand money to buy drugs or alcohol. This is a particular hardship for impoverished families, for whom housing and other necessities may be jeopardized.

Parental substance abuse is associated with inconsistent and unpredictable behaviors, changes in mood and personality, isolation, deceitfulness, irritability, and verbal and physical aggression. 70 percent of partners/spouses of persons who abuse substances report violence-related problems.

Parental substance use disorder is linked with an array of psychosocial issues. For mothers, the most common co-occurring problems include mental health issues, intimate partner violence, criminal activity, and a history of maltreatment as children. For fathers, the most common issues include criminal activities and mental health problems. Parental substance use disorder may also be associated with dangerous lifestyles.

Methamphetamine use is associated with particularly hazardous conditions for children because of dangers involved in the manufacture of the drug in home-based laboratories and the effects of the substance on the user (e. g., prolonged highs and periods of wakefulness that often lead to violence and paranoia, alternating with long periods of sleep).

Adult family members of individuals with substance use disorder report high rates of emotional, relational, and health problems. They report feeling anxious, worried, depressed, angry, guilty, and alone, and they may experience difficulty sleeping and eating or have other physical symptoms of distress. Potential effects of parental substance use disorder on children include feelings of fear, anxiety, and shame; isolation from support systems, diminished social competency, difficulties in peer relationships, disruptions in school attendance and/or behavior, and increased emotional/behavioral problems; insecure attachment; and parentification.

Parental substance use disorder also increases the risk of substance use disorder in youth as a result of modeling and normalization of substance use and possibly direct involvement in substance abuse with parents and other family members. Investigators conducting a study of adolescent girls in whom substance use disorder was diagnosed and who had a high rate of involvement with juvenile justice and/or child protective services described pervasive family drug use leading to normalization of drug use; traumatic events; exposure to street life (e. g., violence, drug traffic, gangs); and access to drugs and alcohol leading to early use at a mean age of 12 years.

Living with a non-substance-using parent or caregiver, absence of violence, social supports, and positive experiences outside of the home are considered to be protective factors that can reduce the adverse effects of parental substance abuse on children. Variables such as the gender of the affected parent may also moderate effects; for instance, children whose mothers abuse substances are more likely to feel a sense of rejection and shame, whereas children whose fathers abuse substances are at higher risk of exposure to violent or abusive behaviors.

Parental substance use disorder is also associated with an increased risk for child maltreatment, repeated instances of abuse and/or neglect, out-of-home care, extended stays in foster care, termination of parental rights, and adoption. It is a factor in a significant number of families involved with child welfare services, with estimates ranging from 25 percent to 80 percent of cases.

Parents preoccupied with substance use may fail to provide adequate care or supervision; may live in dangerous environments in which children may access drugs, drug paraphernalia, and other hazards; and may drive with children while under the influence. Of children in Finland whose mothers were treated in specialized clinics during pregnancy because of suspected or confirmed substance use, half had been placed in out-of-home care, 38 percent by age 2. Out-of-home care has been found to be more likely when both parents abuse substances and/or the child is an infant. Children in families in which parents abuse substances are at greater risk for repeat maltreatment, particularly in young children and in combination with parental mental health issues, conflict between parents, and social deprivation.

American family treatment drug courts, which are utilized for parents involved with child welfare services, provide intensive monitoring (e. g., frequent hearings and drug testing) and coordination among judicial, child welfare, and treatment providers. This model is gaining recognition as a result of positive effects on rates of treatment entry, time to entry, length of stay in treatment, successful completion among mothers involved with child welfare services, and family reunification.

Investigators reported the following findings from a study involving a cohort of 13,829 parents referred for expedited substance abuse assessment and/or treatment through the Child Protection Substance Abuse Initiative (CPSAI), a collaborative effort between child welfare and substance abuse organizations in New Jersey:

From the total cohort, 79 percent completed substance abuse assessments, of which 59 percent were referred to the appropriate level of treatment (e. g., outpatient, residential, halfway house). Of those referred, the enrollment rate was 40 percent;of those individuals who entered treatment, 55 percent either completed or were in the process of completing treatment. Of the 6,380 individuals determined eligible for treatment, 20 percent (1,282) successfully completed treatment.

Women were more likely than men to be assessed and to enroll in treatment; men were more likely than women to complete treatment.

Treatment completion was positively associated with being employed, having an open case in family court, and not having current involvement with the criminal justice system.

Although further research is needed, results of recent randomized controlled trials have given some indication that the impact of parental substance abuse on children can be moderated by interventions that improve parenting practices and strengthen parent–child relationships.

Providing parenting interventions concurrently with substance abuse treatment can have beneficial impacts in both areas. Issues that can be targeted include poor emotional regulation in parents with substance abuse issues, inadequate knowledge of child development and appropriate parenting, and less enjoyment of parenting. Interventions may need to be sequenced—for instance, focusing on strengthening the parent's capacity for emotional regulation prior to focusing on discipline techniques.

Parenting interventions may be predominately skill-based or attachment. Skill-based parenting interventions include parent–child interaction therapy (PCIT), triple P positive parenting program, Incredible Years, and Strengthening Families. These interventions often are based in cognitive behavioral theory and seek to change parenting behaviors. Attachment-based parenting interventions include attachment and biobehavioral catchup (ABC), Mothers and Toddlers Program (MTP), and Circle of Security. These interventions emphasize emotional bonds, including the parents' attachment and trauma history. Researchers reported that in a randomized controlled trial of brief strategic family therapy (BSFT), the BSFT intervention was associated with improved family functioning, lower alcohol use in parents, and decreased substance use in adolescents whose parents used drugs.

In a study examining the effects of an intensive, relationship-focused in-home treatment program for parents of young children, researchers reported that preliminary data showed that this approach, which combined individual therapy, substance abuse treatment and monitoring, support and guidance regarding parenting, and comprehensive case management, can be an effective means to stabilize families and prevent the need for out-of-home placement.

WHAT CAN BE DONE

Learn about the impact of parental substance abuse on families and children to accurately assess the client's personal characteristics and health education needs.

Treatment methodologies should reflect the cultural values, beliefs, and biases of the individual in need of care and treatment.

Treatment for parental substance abuse should be evidence based and integrative, addressing psychosocial issues as needed (e. g., mental health, vocational training, employment, housing, physical and dental healthcare, parenting).

Programs should also recognize and address barriers such as lack of transportation and child care, unmet basic needs, and stigma.

Once the parent is in active recovery, couples or family therapy or multifamily group treatment may be helpful to rebuild family relationships.

Continually assess risk of harm to self or others.

Peer support groups (e. g., Al-Anon, Alateen, Adult Children of Alcoholics, Nar-Anon) are especially helpful for children and families of individuals with substance abuse issues.

Recognize the impact of parental substance abuse on family members (e. g., child care or custodial responsibilities due to parent's incapacitation) and provide supportive services such as referrals for financial assistance and coaching regarding setting boundaries.

Substance abuse education and prevention are recommended for adolescents.

Refer to online resources for additional information, fact sheets, and other educational materials.

- Child Welfare Information Gateway, Substance Abuse Resources for Families, https://www.childwelfare.gov/topics/systemwide/substance/resources/.
- National Association for Children of Alcoholics (NACoA), http://www.nacoa.org/.
- National Center on Substance Abuse and Child Welfare, https://ncsacw. samhsa.gov/.
- National Institute on Drug Abuse, http://www.drugabuse.gov.

Written by Jennifer Teska, MSW

Reviewed by Melissa Rosales Neff, MSW

REFERENCES

American Psychiatric Association. (2013). Diagnostic and statistical manual of mental disorders: DSM-V. (5th ed.). Arlington, VA: Author.

Benishek, L. A., Kirby, K. C., & Dugosh, K. L. (2011). Prevalence and frequency of problems of concerned family members with a substance-using loved one. *The American Journal of Drug and Alcohol Abuse, 37*,82-88. doi:10.3109/00952990.2010.540276

British Association of Social Workers. (2012, January). *The code of ethics for social workers: Statement of principles.* Retrieved December 13, 2015, from http://cdn. basw.co.uk/upload/basw_112315-7. pdf

Calhoun, S., Conner, E., Miller, E., & Messina, N. (2015). Improving the outcomes of children affected by parental substance abuse: A review of randomized controlled trials. *Substance Abuse and Rehabilitation, 6*,15-24. doi:10.2147/SAR. S46439

Daley, D. C., & Ward, J. (2015). The impact of substance use disorders on parents, part II. *Counselor: The Magazine for Addiction Professionals, 16*(3), 27-30.

Forrester, D., & Harwin, J. (2008). Parental substance misuse and child welfare: Outcomes for children two years after referral. *British Journal of Social Work, 38*,1518-1535. doi:10.1093/bjsw/bcm051

Hanson, K. E., Saul, D. H., Vanderploeg, J. J., Painter, M., & Adnopoz, J. (2015). Family-based recovery: An innovative in-home substance abuse treatment model for families with young children. *Child Welfare, 94*(4), 161-183.

Hayward, R. A., Depanfilis, D., & Woodruff, K. (2010). Parental methamphetamine use and implications for child welfare intervention: A review of the literature. *Journal of Public Child Welfare, 4*,25-60. doi:10.1080/15548730903563095

Hedges, K. E. (2012). A family affair: contextual accounts from addicted youth growing up in substance using families. *Journal of Youth Studies, 15*(3), 257-272. doi:10.1080/13676261.2011.635194

Horigian, V. E., Feaster, D. J., Brincks, A., Robbins, M. S., Perez, M. A., & Szapocznik, J. (2015). The effects of Brief Strategic Family Therapy (BSFT) on parent substance use and the association between parent and adolescent substance use. *Addictive Behaviors, 42*,44-50. doi:10.1016/j. addbeh.2014.10.024

International Federation of Social Workers. (2012, March 3). Statement of Ethical Principles. Retrieved December 13, 2015, from http://ifsw.org/policies/statement-of-ethical-principles/

Laslett, A., Room, R., Dietze, P., & Ferris, J. (2012). Alcohol's involvement in recurrent child abuse and neglect cases. *Addiction, 107*,1786-1793. doi:10.1111/j.1360-0443.2012.03917. x

Melhuish, J. (2011). Crack cocaine use and parenting: An analysis of three parents' accounts of impact their crack cocaine use had on family life. *Practice: Social Work in Action, 23*(4), 201-213. doi:10.1080/09503153.2011.597203

National Treatment Agency for Substance Misuse. (2012). Parents with drug problems: How treatment helps families. London: NTA. Retrieved December 13, 2015, from http://www.nta. nhs. uk/uploads/families2012vfinali.pdf

Neger, E. N., & Prinz, R. J. (2015). Interventions to address parenting and parental substance abuse: Conceptual and methodological considerations. *Clinical Psychology Review, 39*,71-82. doi:10.1016/j. cpr.2015.04.004

Oliveros, A., & Kaufman, J. (2011). Addressing substance abuse treatment needs of parents involved with the child welfare system. *Child Welfare, 90*(1), 25-41.

Orford, J., Velleman, R., Copello, A., Templeton, L., & Ibanga, A. (2010). The experiences of affected family members: A summary of two decades of qualitative research. *Drugs: Education, Prevention, and Policy, 17*(S1), 44-62. doi:10.3109:09687637.2010.514192

Raitasalo, K., Holmila, M., & Makela, P. (2011). Drinking in the presence of underage children: Attitudes and behavior. *Addiction Research and Theory, 19*(5), 394-401. doi:10.3109/16066359.2011.560693

Renk, K., Boris, N. W., Kolomeyer, E., Lowell, A., Puff, J., Cunningham, A.,... McSwiggan, M. (2015). The state of evidence-based parenting interventions for parents who are substance-involved. *Pediatric Research,* 1-7. doi:10.1038/pr.2015.201

Sarkola, T., Kahila, H., Gissler, M., & Halmesmaki, E. (2007). Risk factors for out-of-home custody child care among families with alcohol and substance abuse problems. *Acta Paediatrica, 96*,1571-1576. doi:10.1111/j.1651.2227.2007.00474. x

Scaife, V. H. (2008). Maternal and paternal drug misuse and outcomes for children: Identifying risk and protective factors. *Children & Society*, 22,53-62. doi:10.1111/j.1099-0860.2007.00093. x

Substance Abuse and Mental Health Services Administration, Office of Applied Studies. (2009). The NSDUH report: Children living with substance-dependent or substance-abusing parents: 2002 to 2007. Rockville, MD: Author.

Templeton, L., Novak, C., & Wall, S. (2011). Young people's views on services to help them deal with parental substance misuse. *Drugs, Education, Prevention and Policy, 18*(3), 172-178. doi:10.3109/09 687637.2010.489081

Traube, D. E., He, A. S., Zhu, L., Scalise, C., & Richardson, T. (2015). Predictors of substance abuse assessment and treatment completion for parents involved with child welfare: One state's experience in matching across systems. *Child Welfare, 94*(5), 45-66.

Wheeler, D., & McClain, A. (2015). NASW standards and indicators for cultural competency in social work practice. Retrieved December 13, 2015, from http://www.socialworkers.org/practice/standards/PRA-BRO-253150-CC-Standards.pdf

Worcel, S. D., Furrer, C. J., Green, B. L., Burrus, S. W. M., & Finigan, M. W. (2008). Effects of family treatment drug courts on substance abuse and child welfare outcomes. *Child Abuse Review, 17*,427-443. doi:10.1002/car.1045

PARENTING TRANSGENDER CHILDREN & YOUTH

MAJOR CATEGORIES: Child & Family, Gender/Identify

DESCRIPTION

Transgender is an umbrella term used to describe individuals whose gender identity and behaviors fall outside gender norms and do not conform to these individuals' biological sex. Other terms used to describe such identify and behavior are *gender nonconformity* and *gender variance*. Transgender individuals are described as having either a male-to-female (MTF) identity or a female-to-male (FTM) identity.

Gender identity is thought to be determined by an interaction of biological, environmental, and sociological factors. The reasons for an individual's undergoing a transgender transformation are unknown; however, gender is increasingly understood as existing on a spectrum ranging from male to female and vice versa, rather than as a binary, purely

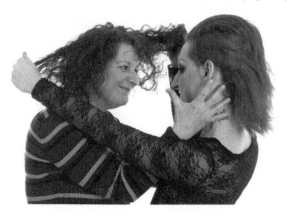

male or purely female characteristic, and there are gradations in one's internal experience of masculinity and femininity. Furthermore, the concepts of gender and sexual identity are often conflated, with gender combining gender identity, presentation, and role behavior, whereas sexual identity or orientation is based on the sex or gender of the persons to which an individual is attracted, and a transgender identity not implying a particular sexual orientation.

Gender diversity in children, adolescents, and adults is often misunderstood and pathologized. Social stigma is believed to be at the root of many of the problems experienced by transgender individuals. The fifth edition of the *Diagnostic and Statistical Manual of Mental Disorders* (*DSM-5*) contains the diagnosis of *gender dysphoria* in children, adolescents, and adults, defining this condition as a "marked incongruence between one's experienced/expressed gender and assigned gender, of at least 6 months' duration, as manifested by at least six of the following:

- A strong desire to be of the other gender or an insistence that one is a member of the other gender.
- In boys, a strong preference for cross-dressing or simulating female attire; in girls, a strong preference for wearing typically masculine clothing only and a strong resistance to the wearing of typically feminine clothing.

- A strong preference for cross-gender roles in make-believe play or fantasy play.
- A strong preference for the toys, games, and activities stereotypically used or engaged in by the other gender.
- A strong preference for playmates of the other gender.
- In boys, a strong rejection of typically masculine toys, games, and activities and a strong avoidance of rough-and-tumble play; in girls, a strong rejection of typically feminine toys, games, and activities.
- A strong dislike of one's sexual anatomy.
- A strong desire for the primary and/or secondary sex characteristics that match one's self-experienced gender.

The diagnosis named *gender dysphoria* in the *DSM-5* is a revision of what was named *gender identity disorder* in the fourth edition of the manual (*DSM-IV*). In the *DSM-5*, the word *disorder* has been removed, to emphasize that gender nonconformity is not itself a mental disorder. The *DSM-5* uses the term *gender dysphoria* because a specific diagnosis is required for the insurance coverage of any medical needs associated with a particular condition, including treatments associated with the transgender state (hormone therapy, gender reassignment surgery).

Moreover, the medical profession suggests that diagnosis of gender dysphoria can facilitate support, education, advocacy, and medical interventions such as hormone therapy for individuals with this condition. For children with a diagnosis of gender dysphoria, however, any medical interventions should be done with caution so as not to prevent the child's exploration of its sexual identity. Transgender children often feel a tension between their sex at birth and their preferred gender identity. As an example of this, a small proportion of infants may have been born with ambiguous genitalia, such as an unusually small penis or an unusually large clitoris, and underwent surgical alterations of their genitalia shortly after birth, and may subsequently struggle to reconcile their biological sex and their gender expression.

The social stigma attached to transgender individuals typically causes great distress. They may be subject to verbal attack and physical abuse from family members, peers, authority figures, and others. Puberty is an especially complex time for such individuals, with many experiencing the changes occurring in their bodies as traumatic.

The pressures and in some cases abuse experienced by transgender children and adolescents can lead to an array of biological, psychological, and social problems. Transgender individuals of dating age are more vulnerable to dating violence as well as higher levels of depression and suicidal ideation. They are at risk for lower grades in school and they commit a greater than average number of delinquent acts in their communities. Transgender adolescents and those in their twenties may run away from abusive home environments or be forced to leave home and become homeless. Their identities are often excessively sexualized, and because of this they are vulnerable to sexual abuse from predatory adults. The rejection by parents of a youngster of transgender identity may put the youngster at risk for substance abuse, depression, and suicidality, whereas their acceptance may be a protective factor that leads the youngster to higher self-esteem and better physical and mental health.

Although, as noted above, many parents of transgender children advocate for them, the family environments of these children are often unsupportive. Their fathers tend to be more critical of them than are their mothers, and many parents of transgender children discourage transgender behavior and send these children for sexual-orientation counseling. The parents may express fear for their children's future safety and happiness, and many attempt to balance the needs of their transgender children with limits, such as permitting transgender dressing only in certain environments. Parents raising a transgender child report having many of their core beliefs disrupted and their prejudices challenged. Some have reported secondary stigmatization as a result of negative social judgment by members of their extended families and their communities when they disclose that they have a transgender child. Many parents of transgender children struggle between supporting their children's self-expression and protecting them from the censorship and abuse that may result from their standing out as transgender individuals.

FACTS AND FIGURES

Limited data exist about the prevalence of transgenderism, but an estimated 2 to 5 percent of the world population is transgender (experiences some degree of nontypical gender identification). In the United

States, an estimated 0.3 percent of persons are transgender. A study of transgender youth found that 54 percent of their mothers and 63 percent of their fathers reacted negatively to their sons' or daughters' disclosure that they were transgender. The National Center for Transgender Equality Survey indicated that 78 percent of transgender or gender-nonconforming children in grades K–12 reported harassment, 53 percent reported physical assault, and 12 percent reported sexual assault.

RISK FACTORS

Parents, family, friends, teachers, and others frequently reject ambiguously gendered children. Transgender children and youth are stigmatized and have an increased risk of experiencing verbal and physical abuse. They may be condemned by religious authorities in their communities; they have an increased risk of having mental health problems, including depression, anxiety, self-abuse, substance abuse, and suicide; their identity is persistently oversexualized; they are extremely vulnerable to sexual abuse and sexually transmitted diseases (STDs); and they are at risk for academic difficulties and school dropout.

Transgender boys are more prone to anxiety and negative emotions and experience greater stress than do transgender girls. Puberty intensifies the distress felt by transgender youth; many describe this period as traumatic.

SIGNS AND SYMPTOMS

Data suggest that children learn about gender and gendered roles very early in their lives. Some children exhibit unconventional gender behaviors in the first year of life. Some children are born with ambiguous genitalia. Some children may undergo hormonal treatment and/or surgical intervention affecting these and other gender-related factors. There is controversy about the appropriateness of medical intervention for gender-related factors in young children because it can prevent a child from fully exploring his or her gender identity; however, follow-up studies of adolescents who have received medical treatment show that it can be effective in alleviating distress.

TREATMENT

The social worker assisting a transgender youth should conduct a standard biological, psychological,

social, and spiritual assessment of this youngster, including an assessment of his or her affect and risk for suicide, and of his or her family. The assessment should examine the youngster's developmental history, attainment of milestones, growth, physical abilities, communication, behavior, family and peer relationships, leisure activities, self-concept, life expectations, and social and environmental considerations. The assessment should also examine the parents' functioning; preconceived beliefs about transgender youth; understanding of and adjustment to their son's or daughter's gender identity, including possible guilt or grief and perceptions and hopes for the child; and awareness of the son's or daughter's needs. Beyond this, the assessment should examine the effect of the son's or daughter's transgender identity on his or her siblings, the parents' socioeconomic status, family or marital stress, social support, quality of life, and cultural factors.

There is a pressing need among parents of transgender youngsters for more information and assistance. Parents of such youngsters indicate that they need professional and peer support, along with parenting strategies and medical advice. A skilled social worker can counsel the family on treatment options for a transgender youngster, from hormone therapy to surgery; can ascertain the readiness of the youngster and family to make changes; can educate the family on issues they may face with their transgender youngster; and can provide tools for coping with factors that attend transgenderism, including strategies for managing the social stigma often associated with it. Of help with this is the Transgender Network (TNET) operated by Parents, Families, & Friends of Lesbians and Gays (PFLAG), which offers support and mentoring to transgender individuals and their families. In addition to this, social workers can advocate for and help create safe and respectful spaces in which transgender children and adolescents can explore and express their identities.

Social workers should be aware of their own cultural values, beliefs, and biases, and develop specialized knowledge about the psychosocial issues surrounding transgender youngsters and the histories, traditions, and values of the transgender youngsters with whom they work, and of these youngster's families. They should adopt treatment methods that reflect this knowledge.

APPLICABLE LAWS AND REGULATIONS

In 2011 the United Nations High Commission for Human Rights adopted Resolution 17/19, which explicitly supports the human rights of transgender individuals (as well as lesbian, gay, and bisexual individuals). The report presented to the High Commission in support of the resolution expressed grave concern about the global abuse and discrimination that confronts the lesbian, gay, transgender, and bisexual population.

In the United States, the scope of nondiscrimination laws and policies varies according to state and county jurisdiction. Some states have laws prohibiting discrimination on the basis of gender identity or expression, including discrimination in public employment. The Equal Employment Opportunity Commission in the United States (EEOC) enforces the prohibition against discrimination in employment, including transgender discrimination (also referred to as gender identity discrimination) that is contained in Title VII of the Civil Rights Act of 1964.

SERVICES AND RESOURCES

- Gender Spectrum, https://www.genderspectrum.org/
- Parents, Families, & Friends of Lesbians and Gays (PFLAG), http://community.pflag.org/transgender
- Lead with Love, http://leadwithlovefilm.com
- Gay Family Support, http://gayfamilysupport.com
- FTM International, http://www.ftmi.org
- Renaissance Transgender Association, http://www.ren.org
- Transgender Law Center, http://transgenderlawcenter.org
- Amplify Your Voice, http://www.amplifyyourvoice.org
- National Center for Transgender Equality, http://transequality.org
- National Coalition for Lesbian, Gay, Bisexual & Transgender Health, http://lgbthealth.webolutionary.com
- Lambda Legal, http://www.lambdalegal.org
- International Foundation for Gender Education, http://www.ifge.org
- Transgender Zone, http://www.transgenderzone.com/

Written by Jan Wagstaff, MA, MSW, and Melissa Rosales Neff, MSW

Reviewed by Laura McLuckey, MSW, LCSW

REFERENCES

American Psychiatric Association. (2013). *Diagnostic and statistical manual of mental disorders: DSM-5* (5th ed.). Arlington, VA: American Psychiatric Association.

Centers for Disease Control and Prevention. (2014). Lesbian, Gay, Bisexual and Transgender Health. Retrieved May 20, 2015, from http://www.cdc.gov/lgbthealth/about.htm

Craig-Oldsen, H., Craig, J. A., & Morton, T. (2006). Issues of shared parenting of LGBTQ children and youth in foster care: Preparing foster parents for new roles. *Child Welfare, LXXXV*(2), 267-280.

Dank, M., Lachman, P., Zweig, J., & Yahner, J. (2014). Dating violence experiences of lesbian, gay, bisexual, and transgender youth. *Journal of Youth and Adolescence, 43*(5), 846-857. doi:10.1007/s10964-013-9975-8

Dysart-Gale, D. (2010). Social justice and social determinants of health: Lesbian, gay, bisexual, transgendered, intersexed, and queer youth in Canada. *Journal of Child & Adolescent Psychiatric Nursing, 23*(1), 23-28.

Gates, G.J. (2011). How many people are lesbian, gay, bisexual and transgender? The William Institute. Retrieved August 21, 2015, from http://williamsinstitute.law.ucla.edu/research/census-lgbt-demographics-studies/how-many-people-are-lesbian-gay-bisexual-and-transgender/

Grant, J. M., Mottet, L. A., Tanis, J., Harrison, J., Herman, J. L., & Keisling, M. (2011). Injustice at every turn: A report of the National Transgender Discrimination Survey. Retrieved from http://endtransdiscrimination.org/PDFs/NTDS_Report.pdf

Grossman, A. H., Augelli, A. R., & Salter, N. P. (2006). Male-to-female transgender youth: Gender expression milestones, gender atypicality, victimization, and parents' responses. *Journal of GLBT Family Studies, 2*(1), 71-92.

Grossman, A. H., Augelli, A. R., Jarrett Howell, T., & Hubbard, S. (2005). Parents' reactions to transgender youths' gender nonconforming expression and identity. *Journal of Gay & Lesbian Social Services, 18*(1), 3-16.

Hill, D. B., & Menvielle, E. (2009). "You have to give them a place where they feel protected and safe and loved": The views of parents who have gender-variant children and adolescents. *Journal of LGBT Youth, 6*, 243-271.

Ignatavicius, S. (2013). Stress in female-identified transgender youth: A review of the literature on effects and interventions. *Journal of LGBT Youth, 10*(4), 267-286. doi:10.1080/19361653.2013.825196

International Federation of Social Workers. (2012). Statement of ethical principles. Retrieved September 4, 2015, from http://ifsw.org/policies/statement-of-ethical-principles/

Johnson, S., & Benson, K. (2014). "It's always the mother's fault" secondary stigmatization of mothering a transgender child. *Journal of GLBT Family Studies, 10*(1/2), 124-144. doi:10.1080/1550428X.2014.857236

Kenagy, G. P., & Hsieh, C. (2005). Gender differences in social service needs of transgender people. *Journal of Social Service Research, 31*(3), 1-21.

Kliegman, R. M., Stanton, B. F., Schor, N. F., St Geme, J. W., & Behrman, R. E. (2011). In *Nelson textbook of pediatrics* (19th ed., pp. 654-659). Philadelphia, PA: Elsevier Saunders.

Levine, D. A. (2013). Office-based care for lesbian, gay, bisexual, transgender, and questioning youth. *Pediatrics, 132*(1), e297-e313.

Levine, S. B., & Solomon, A. (2009). Meanings and political implications of "psychopathology" in a gender identity clinic: A report of 10 cases. *Journal of Sex & Marital Therapy, 35*, 40-57. doi:10.1080/00926230802525646

Meininger, E., & Remafedi, G. (2002). Gay, lesbian, bisexual, and transgender adolescents. In L. S. Neinstein (Ed.), *Adolescent health care: A practical guide* (5th ed., pp. 554-561). Philadelphia, PA: Lippincott Williams & Wilkins.

Mizrahi, T., & Mayden, R. W. (2001). NASW standards for cultural competence in social work practice. Retrieved May 20, 2015, from http://www.socialworkers.org/practice/standards/NASWCulturalStandards.pdf

Moch, H. (2013). In a historic move, Senate committee approves tran-inclusive ENDS. Retrieved August 21, 2015, from http://www.glaad.org/blog/historic-move-senate-committee-approves-trans-inclusive-enda

Newcomb, M. E., Heinz, A. J., Birkett, M., & Mustanski, B. (2014). A longitudinal examination of risk and protective factors for cigarette smoking among lesbian, gay, bisexual, and transgender youth. *Journal of Adolescent Health, 54*(5), 558-564. doi:10.1016/j.jadohealth.2013.10.208

Rands, K. E. (2009). Considering transgender people in education: A gender-complex approach. *Journal of Teacher Education, 60*(4), 419-431.

Riley, E. A., Sitharthan, G., Clemson, L., & Diamond, M. (2011). The needs of gender-variant children and their parents: A parent survey. *International Journal of Sexual Health, 23*(3), 181-195.

Riley, E., Clemson, L., Sitharthan, G., & Diamond, M. (2013). Surviving a gender-variant childhood: The views of transgender adults on the needs of gender-variant children and their parents. *Journal of Sex and Marital Therapy, 39*(3), 241-263. doi:10.1080/0092623X.2011.628439

Rosenthal, S. M. (2014). Approach to the patient: transgender youth: endocrine considerations. *The Journal of Clinical Endocrinology and Metabolism, 99*(12), 4379-4389. doi:10.1210/jc.2014-1919

Rosenthal, S.M. (2014). Approach to the patient: transgender youth: endocrine considerations. The Journal of Clinical Endocrinology and Metabolism, 99(12), 4379-4389. doi:10.1210/jc.2014-1919

Statement of ethical principles. (2012, March 3). *International Federation of Social Workers.* Retrieved May 20, 2015, from http://ifsw.org/policies/statement-of-ethical-principles/

The Policy, Ethics, and Human Rights Committee, British Association of Social Workers. (2012, October). The Code of Ethics for Social Work: Statement of principles. Retrieved May 20, 2015, from http://cdn.basw.co.uk/upload/basw_112315-7.pdf

TransCentralPA. (n.d.). Transgender issues: A fact sheet. Retrieved May 20, 2015, http://www.transcentralpa.org/_content/downloads/NGLTF_transfactsheet.pdf

Transgender issues: A fact sheet. (n.d.). *TransCentralPA.* Retrieved May 20, 2015, from http://www.transcentralpa.org/_content/downloads/NGLTF_transfactsheet.pdf

Transgender Law Center. (2004). Transgender health and the law: Identifying and fighting health care discrimination. Retrieved May 20, 2015, from http://www.thecentersd.org/pdf/health-advocacy/identifying-transgender.pdf

U.S. Equal Employment Opportunity Commission (EEOC). (n.d.). Facts about discrimination in federal government employment based on marital status, political affiliation, status as a parent, sexual orientation, or transgender (gender identity) status. Retrieved May 20, 2015, from http://www.eeoc.gov/federal/otherprotections.cfm

Veldorale-Griffin, A. (2014). Transgender parents and their adult children's experiences of disclosure and transition. Journal of GLBT Family Studies, 10(5), 475-501. doi:10.1080/1550 428X.2013.866063

PARKINSON DISEASE: PALLIATIVE CARE

MAJOR CATEGORIES: Palliative & Hospice Care

WHAT WE KNOW

Parkinson disease (PD) is a chronic, progressive, neurodegenerative disease caused by the lack of the neurotransmitter dopamine, which acts as a chemical messenger in the brain; it has no known cure. This deficit results in slow, reduced physical movement (bradykinesia), tremors, muscle stiffness, and postural and gait instability that affects all aspects of everyday living.

Parkinson disease is the second most common age-related neurodegenerative condition after Alzheimer disease, with prevalence of approximately 0.5 percent between ages 65 to 69 and 3 percent among persons 85 and older. It affects an estimated 1.5 million persons in the United States and 4 million people worldwide, with 1–2 percent of the world population over the age of 65 having the disease.

Symptoms can take 20 years or longer to develop and the trajectory of the disease varies from person to person.

Clinical features of Parkinson disease include the following:

- motor manifestations: tremors; bradykinesia (i. e., slowness of movement) and akinesia (i. e., loss of movement), which cause problems with dexterity and gait; weakness; rigidity; immobility
- nonmotor manifestations: constipation, urinary and sexual dysfunction
- cognitive manifestation: slowness in memory and thought
- psychiatric manifestations: depression, psychosis, hallucinations, dementia

Dementia is common in clients; up to 83 percent of clients develop dementia within 20 years of receiving a diagnosis. Aging increases the risk of dementia; there is likely some interplay between Parkinson disease and aging in the development of cognitive decline.

Palliative care, or comfort care, is a specialized type of client care that aims to promote comfort and dignity while maintaining the highest quality of life of clients for as long as possible. By definition, palliative care can span an extended period of time, encompassing the active treatment phase of disease, disease remissions, recurrences of disease, and the decline in health before death. Although not limited to end-of-life care, palliative care usually is provided for clients with terminal illness.

Palliative care is most commonly associated with advanced cancer, although it is critical in non-malignant conditions such as Parkinson disease.

Clients with Parkinson disease commonly do not receive palliative care or engage in discussions with their healthcare team regarding end-of-life choices, decisions, and treatment options. Researchers in the United Kingdom identified individuals who had died from Parkinson disease or related complications. They found that almost 50 percent died in the hospital. Of the 110 who died in the hospital, only three individuals had a recorded discussion with a physician about a preferred place of death. Only 15 were referred to palliative care.

Palliative care involves an interdisciplinary team that includes physicians, nurses, clergy, social workers, other healthcare personnel, the client, and the client's caregivers. Caregivers are the persons who are responsible for the client's day-to-day care. Palliative care often is provided in the home setting by untrained caregivers, including spouses/partners, adult children, relatives, and close friends.

Essential areas of palliative care, as recognized by caregivers, include managing the client's pain and relieving symptoms, preserving the client's dignity, enabling the client to maintain a sense of control, and helping the client prepare psychologically for death, when appropriate.

A widely used scale developed by Hoehn and Yahr categorizes persons with Parkinson disease into one of five stages.

Stage one. Clients typically have mild symptoms that may interfere with day-to-day tasks (e. g., tremors, poor posture, shaking). These symptoms usually are on one side of the body. Diagnosis can be difficult in the early stage; it is based on clinical presentation of symptoms and a thorough neurological examination to rule out other conditions.

Palliative care is important during the early stages of Parkinson disease to help provide a framework to guide treatment, provide clinical information, ensure effective symptom control, refer to community-based services, educate on progression of illness, provide emotional support, and refer to specific activities and services to optimize physical, emotional, psychological, and cognitive functioning. Palliative rehabilitation can increase clients' functioning, promote independence, and enable clients to adapt to disability.

Advance care planning is the cornerstone of palliative care. Advance care planning is a process of planning for future medical care before the client is unable to make decisions. It is a continual process, not a one-time event or the creation of a single document. Advance care planning helps reduce uncertainty by minimizing confusion and conflict over the client's medical care (e. g., the client's wishes regarding resuscitation, analgesia, artificial feeding) and preferred place of care and death.

Researchers have found that many healthcare professionals provide only limited information regarding disease progression (e. g., they may not indicate that Parkinson disease is incurable and will lead to global deterioration) for fear of causing feelings of hopelessness and distress that may delay advance care planning. However, it has been shown that discussing advance care planning with clients increases discussion about future care and is correlated with increased client satisfaction with the care they receive.

Pharmacological interventions are primarily for comfort or maintaining function rather than for curative purposes and are largely aimed at increasing dopamine levels during the early stage of the disease. Oral administration of the dopamine precursor levodopa is the most common therapy for Parkinson disease.

Stage two. Symptoms become more pronounced and often are bilateral, affecting both sides of the body. There is minimal disability and balance is still intact. Palliative care plays a key role in identifying changes in the client's level of functioning and titrating medication according to changing symptoms. Palliative care also helps to establish a baseline of the client's level of functioning and an opportunity to refer for additional services.

Stage three. Symptoms are moderately severe and balance is impaired, but the client can still function independently. There is a diminished benefit from anti-parkinson medications. Palliative care is important to support the client's physical and emotional needs and coordinate between primary and secondary care. Palliative care also helps to minimize distress and control pain, improving the quality of life of clients and their families facing the problems associated with PD.

Stage four. Symptoms are severe and include the inability to walk straight or even stand. The client is no longer able to live alone. The palliative care multidisciplinary team must be more active and the family should be fully engaged in discussions regarding the client's wishes.

Stage five. In the advanced stage of Parkinson disease the client has global deterioration, with severe physical and psychological symptoms. Clients use wheelchairs or are bedridden. During this final stage clients are at increased risk of acute life-threatening illnesses such as pneumonia, aspiration, and chest infection. Palliative measures to keep the client comfortable replace life-prolonging therapy.

Palliative care assists clients and their families to plan for future care and helps reduce the use of emergency medical resources at the end of life. Treatment focus shifts from maximizing function to minimizing suffering and maintaining the client's comfort and dignity. The palliative care team facilitates home-care services to assist with care and end of life (e. g., hospice, bereavement care).

Tools to screen for the symptoms of Parkinson disease and quality of life include the Parkinson's Disease Questionnaire (PDQ-39), Palliative Care Assessment (PACA), Unified Parkinson's Disease Rating Scale (UPDRS), and Palliative care Outcome Scale (POS-S).

DISCARD

WHAT CAN BE DONE

Learn about the challenges of providing palliative care to clients with Parkinson disease as seen by caregivers and clients; share this knowledge with your colleagues.

Treatment methodologies should reflect the cultural values, beliefs, and biases of the individual in need of care and treatment.

Practice with awareness of, and adherence to, the social work principles of respect for human rights and human dignity, social justice, and professional conduct as described in the International Federation of Social Workers (IFSW) Statement of Ethical Principles.

Be sure caregivers are familiar with members of the palliative care team and how to contact them. This will add to caregiver security and may allow the client to benefit from home care for a longer period of time.

Encourage clients to prepare for end of life while still living their lives fully through the use of advance care planning, an advance directive, and assignment of a healthcare proxy. Encourage clients and families to share their feelings about death.

Assist caregivers in addressing grief and loss feelings that arise with their loved one's decline. Be empathic and validate the caregivers' feelings.

Educate the caregiver regarding bereavement support.

Encourage caregivers to obtain more information from the one of the following:

- National Parkinson Foundation at http://www.parkinson.org/
- American Parkinson Disease Association at http://www.apdaparkinson.org
- Parkinson's UK at http://www.parkinsons.org. uk/
- National Hospice and Palliative Care Organization at http://www.nhpco.org/learn-about-end-life-care
- Get Palliative Care at http://www.getpalliativecare.org
- Aging with Dignity at www.agingwithdignity.org/

Encourage clients and caregivers to visit the National Hospice and Palliative Care Organization at http://www.caringinfo.org/ to create the appropriate advance directive for their state.

Written by Laura McLuckey, MSW, LCSW and Jessica Therivel, LMSW-IPR

Reviewed by Lynn B. Cooper, D. Criminology

REFERENCES

American Psychiatric Association. (2013). Diagnostic and statistical manual of mental disorders. (5th ed.). Washington, DC: American Psychiatric Publishing.

British Association of Social Workers. (2012). The code of ethics for social work: Statement of principles. Retrieved May 21, 2016, from http://cdn.basw.co.uk/upload/basw_112315-7.pdf

Bunting-Perry, L. K. (2006). Palliative care in Parkinson's disease: Implications for neuroscience nursing. *Journal of Neuroscience Nursing, 38*(2), 106-113.

Campbell, C. W., Jones, E. J., & Merrills, J. (2010). Palliative and end-of-life-care in advanced Parkinson's disease and multiple sclerosis. *Clinical Medicine, 10*(3), 290-292.

Feng, L. R., & Maguire-Zeiss, K. (2010). Gene therapy in Parkinson's disease: Rationale and current status. *CNS Drugs, 24*(3), 177-192.

Gueguen, J. A., Bylund, C. L., Brown, R. F., Levin, T. T., & Kissane, D. W. (2009). Conducting family meetings in palliative care: Themes, techniques, and preliminary evaluation of a communication skills module. *Palliative and Supportive Care, 7*(2), 171-179. doi:10.1017/S1478951509000224

Heitkemper, M. M. (2014). Palliative care at end of life. In S. L. Lewis, S. R. Dirksen, M. M. Heitkemper, L. Bucher, & M. M. Harding (Eds.), *Medical-surgical nursing: Assessment and management of clinical problems* (9th ed., pp.140-153). St. Louis, MO: Mosby Elsevier.

Hely, M. A., Reid, W. G., Adena, M. A., Halliday, G. M., & Morris, J. G. (2008). The Sydney multicenter study of Parkinson's disease: The inevitability of dementia at 20 years. *Movement Disorders, 23*(6), 837-844. doi:10.1002/mds.21956

Hoehn and Yahr Staging of Parkinson's Disease, Unified Parkinson Disease Rating Scale (UPDRS), and Schwab and England Activities of Daily Living. (2005). Retrieved May 21, 2016, from http://neurosurgery. mgh. harvard.edu/functional/pd-stages. htm

International Federation of Social Workers. (2012, March 3). Statement of ethical principles. Retrieved from http://ifsw.org/policies/statement-of-ethical-principles/

Kernohan, G., Waldron, M., & Hardyway, D. (2011). Palliative care in Parkinson's disease. *Nursing Times, 107*(24), 22-25.

McCoy, K., & Bass, P. F. (n. d.). Recognizing the stages of Parkinson's disease progression. Retrieved May 21, 2016, from http://www.everydayhealth.com/parkinsons-disease/parkinsons-disease-progression. aspx

McLaughlin, D., Hasson, F., Kernohan, W. G., Waldron, M., McLaughlin, M., Cochrane, B., & Chambers, H. (2010). Living and coping with Parkinson's disease: Perceptions of informal carers. *Palliative Medicine, 25*(2), 177-182.

National Association of Social Workers. (2015). Standards and Indicators for Cultural Competence in Social Work Practice. Retrieved May 21, 2016, from http://www.socialworkers.org/practice/standards/PRA-BRO-253150-CC-Standards.pdf

Niklasch, D. M., & Starkweather, A. (2014). Neurologic disorders. In S. M. Nettina (Ed.), *Lippincott manual of nursing practice* (10th ed., pp.521-524). Philadelphia, PA: Wolters Kluwer Health/Lippincott Williams & Wilkins.

Rabow, M. W., & Pantilat, S. Z. (2016). Palliative care and pain management. In M. A. Papadakis & S. J. McPhee (Eds.), *2016 Current Medical Diagnosis & Treatment* (55th ed., pp.71-93). New York, NY: McGraw Hill Education.

Richfield, E. W., Jones, J. J., & Alty, J. E. (2013). Palliative care for Parkinson's disease: A summary of the evidence and future directions. *Palliative Medicine, 27*(9), 805-810. doi:10.1177/0269216313495287

Riley, C. D. (2014). Cancer nursing. In S. M. Nettina (Ed.), *Lippincott manual of nursing practice* (10th ed., pp.161-162). Philadelphia, PA: Wolters Kluwer Health/Lippincott Williams & Wilkins.

Sadock, B., Sadock, V., & Ruiz, P. (2015). End of life issues. In *Kaplan & Sadock's comprehensive textbook of psychiatry* (11th ed., Vol.1, pp.1352-1371).

Philadelphia, PA: Wolters Kluwer Health/Lippincott Williams & Wilkins.

Saleem, T. Z., Higginson, I. J., Chaudhuri, K. R., Martin, A., Burman, R., & Leigh, P. N. (2013). Symptom prevalence, severity and palliative care needs assessment using the Palliative Outcome Scale: A cross-sectional study of patients with Parkinson's disease and related neurological conditions. *Palliative Medicine, 27*(8), 722-731. doi:10.1177/0269216312465783

Smith, P. (2009). The family caregiver's journey in end of life care: Recognizing and identifying with the role of care. *International Journal on Disability and Human Development, 8*(1), 67-73. doi:10.1515/IJDHD.2009.8.1.67

Waldron, M., Kernohan, G., Hasson, F., Foster, S., Cochrane, B., & Payne, C. (2011). Allied health professionals' views on palliative care for people with advanced Parkinson's disease. *International Journal of Therapy and Rehabilitation, 18*(1), 48-58.

Waldorn, M., Kernohan, W. G., Hasson, F., Foster, S., & Cochrane, B. (2013). What do social workers think about the palliative care needs of people with Parkinson's disease? *British Journal of Social Work, 43*(1), 81-98. doi:10.1093/bjsw/bcr157

Walker, R. W. (2013). Palliative care and end-of-life planning in Parkinson's disease. *Journal of Neural Transmission, 120*(4), 635-638. doi:10.1007/s00702-013-0967-3

Walker, R. W., Churm, D., Dewhurst, F., Samuel, M., Ramsell, A., Lawrie, C.,... Gray, W. K. (2014). Palliative care in people with idiopathic Parkinson's disease who die in hospital. *BMJ Supportive & Palliative Care, 4*(1), 64-67. doi:10.1136/bmjspcare-2012-000412

POSTADOPTION SERVICES

MAJOR CATEGORIES: Adoption/Foster Care, Child and Family

DESCRIPTION

Adoption is the permanent legal transfer of parental rights and responsibilities for a child from the child's birth parents (BPs) to adoptive parents (APs). Adoption is also understood to be a lifelong process involving complex, dynamic relationships between children, their birth families, and their adoptive families in the context of their community and culture. Postadoption services encompass an array of educational, material, and supportive services designed to assist children and families with mental health needs, adjustment, and other adoption-related issues that may arise during an adoptee's childhood.

Although most adoptions result in the successful integration of children into their adoptive families, most such families experience some normative adoption-related challenges, such as determining when and how to share their adopted child's birth/adoption story, incorporating the child's dual family relationships into their thinking, deciding whether to maintain contact with the child's birth family, and encouraging acceptance of the child. Adoptive parents may experience discordance between what they had expected of adoption and its reality; exclusion by their families and friends, who may not understand or support them; struggles to adjust to the demands of parenting; and changes in their lifestyle, household, and marital relationship. Some APs experience postadoption depression, which can lead them to negative parenting behaviors and affect the developing relationship between themselves and their adopted child. Adoptive parents may also experience stress-related physical symptoms or exacerbation of preexisting medical or mental health problems. Children who are adopted after infancy may have an array of challenges, including health issues, attachment problems, behavioral issues, and grief over loss of their birth families.

Establishing parent–child attachment between APs and adopted children, and integrating the adopted child into its immediate and extended adoptive families, can be challenging. This can be particularly true in the adoption of older children, who may have ambivalent feelings about adoption from having had negative experiences with previous caregivers, unresolved grief, and/or conflicting loyalties. Children with a history of deprivation, maltreatment, or multiple changes in their caregivers may resist entering into relationships from fear and a need for self-protection. Adoptive parents without sufficient training for parenthood may misinterpret their adopted children's behaviors and attempt to address difficulties by using discipline instead of recognizing the children's underlying needs and using a firm yet comforting response. This can result in a negative cycle of escalating behavior problems on the part of a child and harsh responses from the APs. Adopted children may begin to exhibit relationship problems and behavioral problems soon after being placed with their APs, and these problems often intensify during adolescence. Aggression, which an adopted child may have shown since early childhood, becomes more difficult to manage physically during adolescence,

and the child may have instances of being violent to its APs as well as towards siblings and pets.

Postadoption services are a vital support for families who adopt children with complex needs. The purpose of such services is that adoption "not only creates families but also enables them to be successful." Postadoption services may include information about and referral of BPs and APs to community resources, information about background and needs of the child being adopted, trainings/conferences, guidance about adoption issues, financial assistance, medical care, special education, mental health services for children and/or parents, respite, special events, support groups, mentoring, advocacy, assistance to APs in mediating contact with birth families, direct support to young people, case management, and/or crisis intervention. In the United States, most families adopting a child from foster care receive a financial subsidy and continued public health insurance for the child, based on a determination of "special needs," which consist of factors that the state defines as making it more difficult to place a child into adoption, such as the child's ethnic or racial background, age, disability, or placement of the child as part of a sibling group. Non-white families, kinship families (in which the adopted child is a biological relative), and those who adopt through private agencies are less likely than others to receive needed postadoption services.

Families adopting a child through private adoption services or through intercountry adoption (ICA) receive less support than those who adopt from public agencies. Thus, for instance, the child being adopted through private services or ICA usually does not qualify for healthcare coverage and must be enrolled in the APs' private health insurance, and in contrast to the situation in adoption from foster care, no adoption subsidies are available to the APs. Adoption agencies approved by the Council on Accreditation (COA) are required to provide or refer adopting families for postplacement developmental, educational, and mental health and therapeutic services; respite care; and re-placement if the adoptive child's placement is disrupted.

In some cases, APs are unwilling to engage in services to support or preserve their adoption. Parents who have had to address severe problems with their adopted child for an extended time often express feelings of guilt, inadequacy, and substantial anger with the child for not responding to their parenting, as well as expressing ambivalence about the child and regret about the adoption. Disruption occurs when a family decides against adopting a child who has been placed with them for adoption but before the adoption has been finalized. Postadoption placement, sometimes referred to as "displacement," occurs when a child who has been adopted leaves its adoptive home before reaching adulthood (for treatment of a mental health problem, by running away from home, or because of detention by legal authorities) but the APs maintain their legal rights as the child's parents. In such a case the child may subsequently return to its adoptive home after a period of treatment, or may remain in an alternative setting until reaching adulthood. Dissolution occurs when the legal relationship between a child and its APs is terminated by the APs voluntarily giving up or relinquishing their parental rights, or by court action. One study found that 17 percent of APs reported the dissolution of an adoption; dissolution was particularly linked with educational deficits and having an adopted child with substance abuse issues.

According to a study conducted in 2014, an estimated 9 percent to 15 percent of the more than 2 million children who were identified in the 2010 U.S. Census as adopted children experienced disruption before finalization of their adoptions. About 10 percent of adopted children return to foster care at some point following a finalized adoption, and dissolution occurs in from 1 percent to 10 percent of finalized adoptions). A significant number of children also leave their adoptive homes at some point other than through the intervention of child welfare authorities.

Despite such occurrences, adoption has been found to be a more stable permanent growth setting for children than either long-term foster care or guardianship. Because it forms a lifelong family, adoption supports a greater sense of long-term belonging and security in children. Although adopted children face varying degrees of challenge. depending on their age and the adversities they may have experienced before being adopted, most adopted children show improvements in development and functioning in their adoptive homes. Furthermore, although adopted children have a higher prevalence of disability than nonadopted children, adoptive families are more likely to have greater education and a higher

socioeconomic status than BPs, and are more likely to access services for their children. For families that face greater challenges, postadoption support and adoption-competent services can be instrumental in reducing the risk of displacement of an adopted child or the dissolution of an adoption.

FACTS AND FIGURES

Adopted children utilize mental health services at much higher rates than do nonadopted children. Among adopted children 5 years of age and older, 46 percent of children adopted from foster care use mental-health services, as do 35 percent of those adopted from ICA and 33 percent of those adopted in private, domestic adoptions, as compared with 10 percent of children in the general population. However, in a recent study, most APs (77 percent) reported that their children are well integrated into their families, and 80 percent felt that their children demonstrated improvement in social, emotional, and/or educational functioning. In another study, depression was found in about 25 percent of APs after adoption.

Adoptive families are increasingly likely to utilize postadoption services with the passage of time after adoption. In one study, the number of families reporting using postadoption services increased from 31 percent at 2 years after adoption to 81 percent at 8 years after adoption. Adoptive parents in a survey conducted in the United States rated support groups for parents, mental health services for children, and financial assistance as the most important postadoption services.

RISK FACTORS

Children who are adopted often have multiple risk factors for mental and physical disorders, including prenatal exposure to substance abuse by their BPs, low birthweight, trauma, and disrupted preadoption caregiving. Risk factors linked with serious difficulty or disruption in adoption include adoption at an older age; child maltreatment; severe externalizing behaviors, such as attention-deficit/hyperactivity disorder (ADHD); and strong attachment of a child to its birth mother. Adoptive parents who are inexperienced, have no prior relationship with the child they adopt, or have unrealistic expectations of adoption; those who have more defined preferences for an adoptive child (race, gender, background); have a tendency to attribute psychological or physical abnormalities to the child; have insufficient information about the child before adoption; and have insufficient preparation, training, and support; and couples who are not equally invested in the adoption; as well as the adoptive placement of a child by less experienced social workers, are all risk factors for troubled or failed adoption.

Risk factors for postadoption depression in APs are similar to those associated with postnatal depression (a parental history of depression or anxiety, idealization of parenthood, and history of difficulties in relationships; a lack of support systems; medical, developmental, and/or behavioral difficulties of an adopted child); multiple simultaneous adoptions; discrepancies between the expectations of APs and the realities of their bonding with their adoptive child; and the realities of the parenting experience.

SIGNS AND SYMPTOMS

Signs and symptoms of psychological problems in adopted children that are associated with difficulties in adoption include attachment issues, grief, depression, anxiety, anger/rage, physical and/or verbal aggression (including assaultive behavior towards the adoptive mother, siblings, and/or pets), severe tantrums, defiance, antisocial behavior, manipulation, lying, stealing, self-harm, hyperactivity, inattention, school difficulties, inappropriate sexual behaviors, soiling, sleep difficulties, night terrors, hoarding food, substance abuse, and running away. Children adopted through ICA often show signs of physical conditions such as cleft lip and palate, heart disease, orthopedic issues, malnutrition, and infections.

ASSESSMENT

Social workers involved in the process of adoption must be aware of the federal, state, and local legal and social standards for it, and should complete a comprehensive biological (medical), psychosocial, and spiritual assessment of the adopted child and adopting family with information on physical, mental, environmental, social, and financial factors relating to them. The social worker should ask about the child's history of trauma and trauma-related symptoms, attachment difficulties, the family history of its birth family and adoptive family, the care given to the child before adoption, circumstances that

led to its being placed for adoption, its adjustment to placement, any psychiatric symptoms or issues on the part of the child that might pose a risk to itself or others (suicidality, self-harm, substance abuse, aggression, fire setting, running away, harming animals, sexual perpetration, child-to-parent violence), any history of mental health treatment for the child, its involvement in other systems (school, corrections), and the family and community supports available to the child and its APs.

The adopting family should be asked about its household members, siblings and/or other children in the home; its awareness of and ability to meet the adopted child's basic needs; its parental functioning, efficacy and risk factors in its parenting, and risk factors (including unresolved issues that may affect its parenting capacity); any symptoms of depression in the family members; their perceptions and feelings about the adoptive child; their parenting practices regarding discipline, supervision, and nurturing; and supports available to the family and adopted child. A complete assessment of each family member is helpful for understanding the extent and nature of the effect that adoption has on the family and its effect on other areas of their lives. This is essential to ensure that an adopted child's individual needs are addressed and that APs have adequate training and support in their parental role. Ideally, the APs should be introduced to postadoption services before their adoption becomes final. It is important that in advance of adoption, the social worker review with the APs the adopted child's history, highlighting issues that are likely to emerge over time, and discuss the use of supports and services for the adoption.

Adopting parents may not disclose violent behavior on the part of an adopted child because of stigma and shame about it, but such violence is a leading cause of adoption disruption and should be routinely screened for when families seek postadoption services. Adopting parents who feel overwhelmed and unable to continue caring for an adopted child may resort to potentially dangerous alternatives such as independently "rehoming" it with a new family that has not had background checks or home studies and that may abuse or exploit the child.

Adoption-competent mental health services are important to ensuring that children, BPs, and APs involved in adoption receive adequate preparation and postadoption support. Families often report difficulties in finding providers of mental healthcare who are knowledgeable and experienced in matters relating to adoption. Competent therapy is critical to address psychological and emotional issues affecting an adopted child, such as trauma, attachment to parents and others, and identity formation. Intervention should occur as early as possible, and should include the APs.

TREATMENT

A range of promising evidence-based interventions may be helpful to an adopted child and the family that adopts it in solving adoption-related problems. Trauma-focused cognitive behavioral therapy (TF-CBT), the most recognized treatment for child trauma, is used with children ranging in age from 3 to 18 years who have posttraumatic stress disorder (PTSD) or other emotional problems related to trauma. This therapy integrates cognitive and behavioral interventions, such as the psychological education of patients about trauma and common reactions to it, parenting skills to manage children's emotional and behavioral reactions, individualized stress-management techniques and coping skills, and development by the patient of a trauma narrative to help organize feelings and thoughts related to traumatic experiences. Dialectical behavior therapy (DBT) is a modification of cognitive behavioral therapy (CBT) that may be used with adolescents. It uses a combination of group, family, and individual sessions focused on increasing skills in interpersonal relations, tolerance of distress, regulation of emotions, and mindfulness. Child–parent relationship therapy (CPRT) is a structured model that has been used successfully to address attachment and relationship problems in children of ages 3 to 10 years who have been adopted from foster care by training their adoptive parents to use interventions designed to increase these children's safety, acceptance of adoption, and connectedness to their APs and others.

Another treatment technique, parent–child interaction therapy (PCIT), is an intervention used with children aged 2 to 12 years who have serious behavior issues. During sessions of such therapy, the therapist, seated in an observation room and using a wireless earpiece, coaches the parents of an adopted child in practice interactions with the child. Initial sessions are child-directed and focused on enhancing the parent–child relationship, with later sessions being parent-directed and focused on behavior-management skills. Attachment and biobehavioral catch-up (ABC) is a home-based intervention designed for infants and toddlers from 0 to 2 years old who show signs of attachment difficulties related to maltreatment or disruptions in their care. Treatment in this technique focuses on assisting parents to interpret the child's signals in a way that elicits a nurturing response, and to provide a sensitive and responsive environment for the child. Trust-based relational intervention (TBRI) is an attachment-based program that incorporates principles of empowering an adopted child by addressing both its external and internal physical needs (sensory needs, nutrition, and hydration), connecting needs (attachment needs of the child; parent self-awareness, attunement to and playful engagement with the child), and correcting needs (behavioral needs such as boundaries, self-regulation) to increase the child's ability to feel safe and develop secure attachments.

Several further techniques for managing problems and assisting in adoption are also available. The Triple P Positive Parenting Program is a social-learning-based intervention that focuses on increasing parent knowledge of child development, enhancing positive behavior management and parenting skills, and reducing coercive or punitive parental behaviors. Incredible Years (IY) is a training program with child, parent, and teacher components. Children in the IY program are taught social interaction, emotional regulation, and problem solving skills in group settings in which practice is available with the children's peers and with therapists, while caregivers learn positive strategies and the use of calm, nurturing attention. Early intervention consists of an individualized package of developmental therapies and services provided to children from birth to age 3 years who have delays in cognitive, physical, communication, social-emotional, and/or adaptive skills, or a condition such as Down syndrome, cerebral palsy, or autism spectrum disorder (ASD). Theraplay integrates play, family therapy, and psychoeducation to provide children with reparative emotional experiences and to build their attachment to parents and others. A variation of this technique, known as whole-family Theraplay, has been used to also address family communication and adult relational skills. Video-feedback intervention to promote positive parenting (VIPP) uses a brief series of home-based video-feedback sessions to increase parents' sensitivity and responsiveness to an adopted child.

Adoptive parents may experience strain in their marriage from adoption-related issues (difficulty in maintaining a united front when dealing with challenging relationship dynamics or behaviors on the part of their adopted child, being ostracized from support systems when an adopted child's behaviors are severe). Marriage enrichment programs specifically for adoptive parents can help strengthen the parents' marriage and the overall stability of the family.

More intensive treatment, such as intensive adoption preservation services or residential treatment, may be needed for APs and adopted children, and medicinal or pharmacological treatment may be used to help stabilize and/or alleviate symptoms of thought disorders, mood disorders, and attention disorders and/or to regulate hyperarousal (sleep problems, anxiety) in an adopted child and in APs.

Social support, particularly from persons knowledgeable about adoption-related issues, is highly valued by APs, and referrals for peer mentoring and support groups are particularly beneficial. Support groups and/or mentoring have been found to be particularly helpful; counseling for postadoption depression, preexisting issues that may be contributing to parenting difficulties, and marital issues may also be indicated. The social worker should provide linkage to these and to other community services for adopted children and APs, such as referrals for medical, counseling, and educational services as appropriate. Adopting parents may also need assistance with childcare and respite from their duties, particularly if the child they adopt has significant behavioral problems or requires specialized care.

When possible, the social worker should maintain ongoing contact with adoptive families after finalization of their adoptions, through avenues such as newsletters, special events, and continuing education.

Social workers involved in adoption should be aware of their own cultural values, beliefs, and biases and develop specialized knowledge about the histories, traditions, and values of the individuals they serve. Social workers should adopt treatment methodologies that reflect their knowledge of the cultural diversity of the communities in which they practice.

To treat attachment issues, some social work and other practitioners have used coercive techniques such as "holding therapy," which involves confrontation and physical restraint of a child in order to break through its defenses and provide a "corrective experience"; these practitioners have also advocated the parental use of strict and sometimes harsh parenting practices to maintain control over a child. Such techniques are not supported by evidence, are considered harmful, and have led to several deaths.

SERVICES AND RESOURCES

- Center for Adoption Support and Education (C.A.S.E.), http://adoptionsupport.org
- Child Welfare Information Gateway, https://www.childwelfare.gov
- Council on Foster Care, Adoption, and Kinship Care, http://www2.aap.org/sections/adoption/index.html
- Hague Conference on Private International Law, Intercountry Adoption, https://www.hcch.net/en/instruments/conventions/specialised-sections/intercountry-adoption
- Medline Plus, http://www.nlm.nih.gov/medlineplus/adoption.html
- National Council for Adoption, http://www.adoptioncouncil.org/
- North American Council on Adoptable Children, www.nacac.org
- MedLinePlus, http://www.nlm.nih.gov/medlineplus/childmentalhealth.html
- Guidelines for the Alternative Care of Children, an international policy and practice guide that is focused on the well-being and protection of children who are at risk for being or who are deprived of parental care, https://www.unicef.org/protection/alternative_care_Guidelines-English.pdf

Written by Jennifer Teska, MSW

Reviewed by Laura McLuckey, MSW, LCSW

REFERENCES

Bergeron, J., & Pennington, R. (2013). Supporting children and families when adoption dissolution occurs. *Adoption Advocate, 62.* Retrieved February 24, 2016, from https://www.adoptioncouncil.org/publications/2013/08/adoption-advocate-no-62

British Association of Social Workers. (2012, January). The code of ethics for social work: Statement of principles. Retrieved October 11, 2015, from http://cdn.basw.co.uk/upload/basw_112315-7.pdf

Bryan, V., Flaherty, C., & Saunders, C. (2010). Supporting adoptive families: Participant perceptions of a statewide peer mentoring and support program. *Journal of Public Child Welfare, 4*(1), 91-112. doi:10.1080/15548730903563178

Carnes-Holt, K., & Bratton, S. C. (2014). The efficacy of child parent relationship therapy for adopted children with attachment disruptions. *Journal of Counseling & Development, 92*(3), 328-337. doi:10.1002/j.1556-6676.2014.00160.x

Child Welfare Information Gateway. (2012, June). Adoption disruption and dissolution. Washington, DC: U. S. Department of Health and Human Services, Children's Bureau. Retrieved February 24, 2016, from https://www.childwelfare.gov/pubPDFs/s_disrup.pdf

Child Welfare Information Gateway. (2012). Providing Postadoption Services. Washington, DC: U.S. Department of Health and Human Services, Children's Bureau.

Coakley, J., & Berrick, J. D. (2008). Research review: In a rush to permanency: Preventing adoption disruption. *Child and Family Social Work, 13*(1), 101-112. doi:10.1111/j.1365-2206.2006.00468.x

Egbert, S. C. (2015). Supporting and strengthening foster adoptive families: Utah's story of post-adoption service development, delivery, and ongoing evaluation. *Journal of Public Child Welfare, 9*(1), 88-113. doi:10.1080/15548732.2014.1001936

Festinger, T. (2014). extracurricular activities. In G. P. Mallon & P. M. Hess (Eds.), *Child welfare for the twenty-first century: A handbook of practices, policies, and programs* (pp. 452-468). New York, NY: Columbia University Press.

Festinger, T., & Maza, P. (2009). Displacement or post-adoption placement? A research note. *Journal of Public Child Welfare, 3*, 275-286. doi:10.1080/15548730903129889

Foli, K. J., South, S. C., Lim, E., & Hebdon, M. (2013). Depression in adoptive fathers: An exploratory mixed methods study. *Psychology of Men & Masculinity, 14*(4), 411-422. doi:10.1037/a0030482

Forbes, H., & Dziegielewski, S. F. (2003). Issues facing adoptive mothers of children with special needs. *Journal of Social Work, 3*(3), 301-320.

Faasse, K., Bobo, S. H., & Magnuson, A. (2014, December). The post-adoption life: Supporting adoptees, birth parents, and families after adoption. *Adoption Advocate, 78*, 1-12. Retrieved from http://www.adoptioncouncil.org/publications/2014/12/adoption-advocate-no-78

Gibbs, D., Barth, R. P., & Houts, R. (2005). Family characteristics and dynamics among families receiving postadoption services. *Families in Society: The Journal of Contemporary Social Services, 86*(4), 520-532.

Hartinger-Saunders, R. M., Trouteaud, A. R., & Johnson, J. M. (2015). The effects of postadoption service need and use on child and adoptive parent outcomes. *Journal of Social Service Research, 41*(1), 75-92. doi:10.1080/01488376.2014.953286

Hartinger-Saunders, R. M., Trouteaud, A. R., & Johnson, J. M. (2015). Underserved adoptive families: Disparities in postadoption access to information, resources, and services. *Journal of Family Strengths, 15*(1), Article 6. Retrieved from http://digitalcommons.library.tmc.edu/jfs/vol15/iss1/6

Hartinger-Saunders, R. M., Trouteaud, A. R., & Johnson, J. M. (2015). Post adoption service need and use as predictors of adoption dissolution: Findings from the 2012 National Adoptive Families Study. *Adoption Quarterly, 18*(4), 255-272. doi:10.1080/10926755.2014.895469

Harwood, R., Feng, X., & Yu, S. (2013). Preadoption adversities and postadoption mediators of mental health and school outcomes among international, foster, and private adoptees in the United States. *Journal of Family Psychology, 27*(3), 409-420. doi:10.1037/a0032908

Hegar, R. L., & Watson, L. D. (2013). Managing special needs and treatment approaches of intercountry adoptees and families. *Adoption Quarterly, 16*(3/4), 238-261. doi:10.1080/10926755.2013.79086

Hill, K., & Moore, F. (2015). The postadoption needs of adoptive parents of children with disabilities. *Journal of Family Social Work, 18*(3), 146-182. doi:10.1080/10522158.2015.1022846

Howe, D. (2006). Developmental attachment psychotherapy with fostered and adopted children. *Child and Adolescent Mental Health, 11*(3), 128-134. doi:10.1111/j.1475-3588.2006.00393.x

International Federation of Social Workers. (2012, March). Statement of ethical principles. Retrieved January 15, 2015, from http://ifsw.org/policies/statement-of-ethical-principles/

Ji, J., Barth, R. P., Brooks, D., & Kim, H. (2010). Beyond preadoptive risk: The impact of adoptive family environment on adopted youth's psychosocial adjustment. *American Journal of Orthopsychiatry, 80*(3), 432-442. doi:10.1111/j.1939-0025.2010.01046.x

Kreider, R. M., & Lofquist, D. A. (2014, April). Adopted children and stepchildren, 2010: Population characteristics. Washington, DC: U. S. Census Bureau. February 24, 2016,

Lieberman, A. F. (2003). The treatment of attachment disorder in infancy and early childhood: Reflections from clinical intervention with later-adopted foster care children. *Attachment & Human Development, 5*(3), 279-282. doi:10.1080/14616730310001596133

McKenzie, L. B., Purvis, K. B., & Cross, D. R. (2014). A trust-based home intervention for special-needs adopted children: A case study. *Journal of Aggression, Maltreatment & Trauma, 23*(6), 633-651. doi:10.1080/100926771.2014.920454

Mizrahi, T., & Davis, L. E. (Eds.). (2008). Adoption. In *Encyclopedia of Social Work* (20th ed., pp. 33-44). Washington, DC: NASW Press and Oxford University Press, Inc.

Mooradian, J. K., Hock, R. M., Jackson, R., & Timm, T. M. (2011). What couples who adopt children from child welfare want professionals to know about supporting their marriages. *Families in Society, 92*(4), 390-396. doi:10.1606/1044-3894.4155

Proctor, L. J., Van Dusen Randazzo, K., Litrownik, A. J., Newton, R. R., Davis, I. P., & Villodas, M. (2011). Factors associated with caregiver stability in permanent placements: A classification tree approach. *Child Abuse & Neglect, 35*(6), 425-436. doi:10.1016/j.chiabu.2011.02.002

Purvis, K. B., Cross, D. R., Dansereau, D. F., & Parris, S. R. (2013). Trust-based relational intervention (TBRI): A systemic approach to complex developmental trauma. *Child & Youth Services, 34*(4), 360-386. doi:10.1080/0145935X.2013.859906

Randall, J. (2009). Towards a better understanding of the needs of children currently adopted from care: An analysis of placements 2003-2005. *Adoption & Fostering, 33*(1), 44-55.

Randall, J. (2013). Failing to settle: A decade of disruptions in a voluntary adoption agency in placements made between 2001 and 2011. *Adoption & Fostering, 37*(2), 188-199. doi:10.1177/0308575913490493

Schwartz, A., Cody, P. A., Ayers-Lopez, S. J., McRoy, R. G., & Fong, R. (2014). Post-adoption support groups: Strategies for addressing marital issues.

Adoption Quarterly, 17(2), 85-111. doi:10.1080/109267555.2014.891544

Selwyn, J., Wijedasa, D., & Meakings, S. (2014, April). Beyond the adoption order: Challenges, interventions and adoption disruption. Research Brief. *Department for Education (UK)*. UK: Department for Education. Retrieved February 24, 2016, from https://www.gov.uk/government/uploads/system/uploads/attachment_data/file/302339/Final_Research_brief_-_3rd_April_2014.pdf

Smith, S. L. (2014, March). Keeping the promise: The case for adoption support and preservation. *Donaldson Adoption Institute*. Retrieved February 24, 2016, from http://adoptioninstitute.org/publications/keeping-the-promise-the-case-for-adoption-support-and-preservation/

Smith, S. L. (2014). Supporting and preserving adoptive families: Profiles of publicly funded post-adoption services. *Donaldson Adoption Institute*. Retrieved February 24, 2016, from http://adoptioninstitute.org/wordpress/wp-content/uploads/2014/04/Supporting-and-Preserving-Families.pdf

St-Andre, M., & Keren, M. (2011). Clinical challenges of adoption: Views from Montreal and Tel Aviv. *Infant Mental Health Journal, 32*(6), 694-706. doi:10.1002/imhj.20329

Vandivere, S., Malm, K., & Radel, L. (2009). Adoption USA: A Chartbook Based on the 2007 National Survey of Adoptive Parents. Washington, D.C.: The U.S. Department of Health and Human Services, Office of the Assistant Secretary for Planning and Evaluation.

Weir, K. N., Lee, S., Canosa, P., Rodrigues, N., McWilliams, M., & Parker, L. (2013). Whole family theraplay: Integrating family systems theory and theraplay to treat adoptive families. *Adoption Quarterly, 16*(3/4), 175-200. doi:10.1080/10926755.2013.844216

Wheeler, D. (2015). NASW standards and indicators for cultural competence in social work practice. Retrieved February 24, 2016, from http://www.socialworkers.org/practice/standards/PRA-BRO-253150-CC-Standards.pdf

Wind, L. H., Brooks, D., & Barth, R. P. (2007). Influences of risk history and adoption preparation on post-adoption services use in U.S. adoptions. *Family Relations, 56*(4), 378-389. doi:10.1111/j.1741-3729.2007.00467.x

POSTPARTUM DEPRESSION IN WOMEN SERVING IN THE MILITARY

MAJOR CATEGORIES: Behavioral & Mental Health

DESCRIPTION

Postpartum depression (PPD) is defined as clinical depression that has lasted for at least 2 weeks and has an onset within 4 weeks of giving birth. It can take up to a year to develop these depressive symptoms to still be diagnosed as PDD.

PPD is the most common complication of pregnancy and childbirth, with 10 percent of new mothers in the United States experiencing it.

There has been limited research on postpartum depression among women in the military, but some studies report that between 11 percent and 24 percent of new mothers in the military experience PDD.

Postpartum "baby blues" are experienced by up to 80 percent of new mothers; the symptoms are less severe than those of PPD and are transitory, not extending beyond 2 weeks postpartum.

Symptoms of PPD include sadness, tearfulness, decreased motivation, decreased interest in food and self-care, withdrawal from family, poor self-esteem regarding ability to parent, anxiety, mental confusion, feelings of shame and guilt, and/or loss of interest in the baby.

Approximately 15 percent of active-duty members of the military are females. The Navy and Marines have recently extended maternity leave from 6 weeks to 18 weeks. The Air Force and Army, however, still allow only 6 weeks of maternity leave. The Air Force recently changed its policy on postpartum deployment: whereas before women had a 6-month deferment after giving birth, they now have a 12-month deferment.

Researchers in a study of servicewomen who gave birth while on active-duty status found that 11 percent had met criteria for PPD. The highest prevalence (16.6 percent) was among women who had been deployed before childbirth and reported combat-related exposure and trauma symptoms.

It is unclear whether the increased risk for PPD among women who had been deployed in combat zones was attributable to combat exposure, experiencing childbirth, leaving another young child for deployment, or a combination of any of these factors.

Another study found that the prevalence of PPD among active-duty servicewomen was 9.9 percent.

The highest incidence was found in the Army, 12.0 percent, and the lowest in the Air Force, 7.3 percent.

Among servicewomen it was found that the youngest age group, 18- to 20-year-olds, was about 40 percent higher than that in the oldest age group, women over 40, to experience PPD.

It was also found that the risk of suicide was higher for servicewomen with PPD compared to those without PPD.

RISK FACTORS

There are several risk factors for postpartum depression, including the following:

- A prior history of depression or bipolar disorder diagnosis.
- A prior history of postpartum depression.
- Lack of social support, especially if missing from the father of the baby or the mother's partner (if the mother is a single parent or is unsupported in her relationship).
- Deployment can increase this lack of support from the father of the baby.
- A previous or current deployment.
- Personal, familial, and professional stressors common to military life, such as frequent moves, prolonged deployment in combat, and being away from extended family.
- A history of severe premenstrual syndrome.
- A family history of depression
- Lower socioeconomic status and/or financial stressors.
- An infant in poor health or one with a difficult temperament.
- Young age.

Women in the military may be hesitant to disclose mental health concerns for fear that this may have a negative effect on their military careers; because of this, symptoms of PPD in this population may go unidentified and untreated.

ASSESSMENT AND SCREENING TOOLS

There are screening tools available to both medical and mental health personnel to screen for postpartum depression or risk for postpartum depression if the woman is still pregnant. These are meant for screening only; they are not used to diagnose.

The Postpartum Depression Screening Scale (PDSS) is a 35-item self-reporting measure; higher scores indicate a higher degree of depressive symptoms present.

The Edinburgh Postnatal Depression Scale (EPDS) is a 10-item self-report measure in which items on the scale correspond to symptoms of clinical depression (suicidal ideation, anhedonia, sleep disturbances).

The Patient Health Questionnaire 2-item (PHQ-2) is another preferred screening tool of the U.S. Department of Veterans Affairs (VA).

The VA/Department of Defense recommends that women be screened for depression at both prenatal and postnatal appointments; use of the EPDS or PHQ-2 is preferred by the VA.

INTERVENTIONS

The interventions that typically are used for depression have been shown to be effective for PPD. These include mental health therapy including cognitive behavioral therapy (CBT), antidepressant medications, and medication combined with mental health therapy.

Support group therapy that incorporates mental health support and educational elements.

Other supports found to help reduce risk of PDD include social support services, recreational opportunities, financial assistance, and hospital-sponsored support programs.

The MIST (Maternal Infant Support Team) program at Camp Pendleton in San Diego hosts group meetings with case managers, social workers, medical officers, lactation consultants, pediatric nurses, professionals from military relief groups, community Women, Infants, and Children (WIC) staff, community program representatives, and community visiting nurses. The program also includes mental health counseling and a 10-week program, Moms in Transition, which offers education and support to active-duty women and civilian wives of military spouses who have recently given birth.

Written by Jessica Therivel, LMSW-IPR

Reviewed by Laura Gale, LCSW, and Chris Bates, MA, MSW

REFERENCES

The American Congress of Obstetrics and Gynecologists. (2015). Committee opinion: Screening for perinatal depression. Retrieved March 21, 2016, from http: //www.acog.org/Resources-And-Publications/Committee-Opinions/Committee-on-Obstetric-Practice/Screening-for-Perinatal-Depression

America's Navy. (2015). SECNAV announces new maternity leave policy. Retrieved March 21, 2016, from http: //www.navy.mil/submit/display.asp?story_id=87987

Appolonio, K. K., & Fingerhut, R. (2008). Postpartum depression in a military sample. *Military Medicine, 173*(11), 1085-1091.

Army Times. (2015). Army reviewing rules for maternity, paternity leave. Retrieved from http: //www.armytimes.com/story/military/careers/army/2015/08/07/army-reviewing-rules-maternity-paternity-leave/31285283/

Boland-Prom, K. W., & MacMullen, N. (2012). Expanding the postpartum depression construct using a social work paradigm. *Journal of Human Behavior in the Social Environment, 22*(6), 718-732. doi: 10.1080/10911359.2012.692563

British Association of Social Workers. (2012). The code of ethics for social work: Statement of principles. Retrieved March 21, 2016, from http: //cdn.basw.co.uk/upload/basw_112315-7.pdf

Centers for Disease Control and Prevention. (2016). Depression among women. Retrieved March 21, 2016, from http: //www.cdc.gov/reproductivehealth/depression/

Department of Veterans Affairs and Department of Defense. (2009). VA/DoD clinical practice guideline for management of major depressive disorder (MDD). Retrieved from http: //www.healthquality.va.gov/mdd/mdd_full09_c.pdf

Do, T., Hu, Z., Otto, J., & Rohrbeck, P. (2013). Depression and suicidality during the postpartum period after first time deliveries, active component service women and dependent spouses, U.S. Armed Forces, 2007-2012. *MSMR, 20*(9), 2-7.

Fagan, J., & Lee, Y. (2010). Perceptions and satisfaction with father involvement and adolescent mothers' postpartum depressive symptoms. *Journal of Youth and Adolescence, 39*(9), 1109-1121. doi: 10.1007/s10964-009-9444-6

International Federation of Social Workers. (2012). Statement of ethical principles. Retrieved March 21, 2016, from http: //ifsw.org/policies/statement-of-ethical-principles/

McDonagh, M. S., Matthews, A., Phillippi, C., Romm, J., Peterson, K., Thakurta, S., & Guise, J. M. (2014). Depression drug treatment outcomes in pregnancy and the postpartum period: A systematic review and meta-analysis. *Obstetrics & Gynecology, 124*(3), 526-534. doi: 10.1097/AOG.0000000000000410

National Institute of Mental Health. (2015). Postpartum depression facts. Retrieved from http: //www.nimh.nih.gov/health/publications/postpartum-depression-facts/index.shtml

Nguyen, S., Leardmann, C. A., Smith, B., Conlin, A. M., Slymen, D. J., Hooper, T. I.,... Smith, T. C. (2013). Is military deployment a risk factor for maternal depression?. *Journal of Women's Health, 22*(1), 9-18. doi: 10.1089/jwh.2012.3606

Pinheiro, R. T., Botella, L., Quevedo, L. D., Pinheiro, K. A. T., Jansen, K., Osorio, C. M., & da Silva, R. A. (2011). Maintenance of the effects of cognitive behavioral and relational constructivist psychotherapies in the treatment of women with postpartum depression: A randomized controlled trial. *Journal of Constructivist Psychology, 27*(1), 59-68.

Shivakumar, G., Anderson, E., & Suris, A. (2015). Managing posttraumatic stress disorder and major depression in women veterans during the perinatal period. *Journal of Women's Health, 24*(1), 18-22. doi: 10.1089/jwh.2013.4664

Spooner, S., Rastle, M., & Elmore, K. (2012). Maternal depression screening during prenatal and postpartum care at a Navy and Marine Corps military treatment facility. *Military Medicine, 177*(10), 1208-1211.

Wheeler, D. (2015). NASW standards and indicators for cultural competence in social work practice. Retrieved March 2, 2016, from http: //www.socialworkers.org/practice/standards/PRA-BRO-253150-CC-Standards.pdf

Yehia, D. B. M., Callister, L. C., & Hamdan-Mansour, A. (2013). Prevalence and predictors of postpartum depression among Arabic Muslim Jordanian women serving in the military. *Journal of Perinatal and Neonatal Nursing, 27*(1), 25-33. doi: 10.1097/JPN.0b013e31827ed6db

Postpartum Depression: An Overview

Major Categories: Behavioral & Mental Health

What We Know

Postpartum depression (PPD) is defined as clinical depression that has lasted for at least two weeks and has an onset within four weeks of giving birth. It is

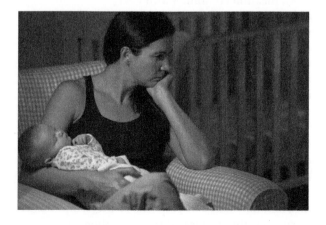

now understood that these depressive symptoms may take up to a year postpartum to begin.

PPD is the most common complication of pregnancy and childbirth, with approximately 12 percent of women experiencing it. "Postpartum blues" are experienced by up to 70 percent of new mothers; the symptoms are less severe than those of PPD and are shorter in duration, not extending beyond two weeks postpartum. PPD often is underidentified and undertreated: In as many as 50 percent of women experiencing PPD, symptoms are undetected by medical and mental health clinicians.

Women who have a history of depression outside of pregnancy have a 25 percent chance of developing PPD. Women who previously had PPD are at an increased risk of having it again with another pregnancy. PPD is five to ten times more likely to occur than gestational diabetes yet still is frequently missed.

Symptoms of PPD include sadness, tearfulness, decreased motivation, decreased interest in food and self-care, difficulty concentrating, poor maternal self-esteem, anxiety, mental confusion, feelings of shame and guilt, and loss of interest or ability to care for the baby. Decreased interest in the baby can have long-lasting consequences such as the baby struggling to form healthy attachments. Depressed mothers exhibit less affectionate behavior, are less responsive to cues from the infant, withdraw, and may even have hostile interactions with the infant. Women with PPD are at an increased risk of disrupted breastfeeding.

Suicide is the leading cause of death for women who are in the pregnancy and postpartum stages.

Although it has been suggested that there may be a connection between postpartum hormone changes and PPD, this has not yet been supported by research.

Risk factors for PPD include:

- A prior history of depression or bipolar disorder diagnosis
- A prior history of postpartum depression;women who had untreated PPD are 300 times more likely to experience PPD with future pregnancies
- A history of severe premenstrual syndrome
- A family history of depression

Problems with delivery and/or having a premature infant in the neonatal intensive care unit (NICU); the risk of PPD was found to increase as the length of the stay in the NICU went past 14 days, but then the risk leveled off and began to decrease after the baby was in the NICU for 31 days.

- Infant with poor health or difficult temperament
- Lower socioeconomic status and/or financial stressors
- History or current experience of intimate partner violence (IPV); IPV is a frequent cooccurrence with PPD even if there is not a causal relationship
- Poor-quality relationship between mother and intimate partner
- Expectations during pregnancy of a vaginal delivery and/or breastfeeding that did not occur
- Lack of social support, especially if missing from the father of the baby or a partner (single parent or unsupported in a couple)

Studies have found a higher rates of depression among lesbians than among heterosexual women, which leads to higher rates of PPD for both biological and nonbiological lesbian mothers.

- Being an adolescent mother

Exposure to a natural disaster such as the earthquake and tsunami in Japan in March 2011, which increased rates of PPD from a nationwide average of 13.9 percent to 21.3 percent.

There are screening tools available to both medical and mental health personnel to screen for postpartum depression or risk for postpartum depression if the patient is still pregnant. These are meant for screening only and are not able to conclude a PDD diagnosis.

The Postpartum Depression Screening Scale (PDSS) is a 35-item self-reporting measure, with higher scores indicating a higher degree of depressive symptoms present. The scale has seven symptom subscales: sleeping/eating disturbances, anxiety/insecurity, emotional lability, mental confusion, loss of self, guilt/shame, and suicidal thoughts.

The Edinburgh Postnatal Depression Scale (EPDS) is a 10-item self-reporting measure with items on the scale corresponding to symptoms for clinical depression (suicidal ideation, lack of pleasure, sleep disturbances).

There is an online version of the EPDS that can be utilized for online screening for PPD, which may helpful to combat the fear and stigma related to revealing PPD. This may also be helpful for women to understand what they are experiencing and whether they should seek mental health therapy or other supports.

Interventions typically used for depression have been shown to be effective for PPD include:

Cognitive behavior therapy (CBT);

- Medication combined with CBT;
- Interpersonal psychotherapy (IPT);
- Psychodynamic therapy;
- Educational interventions;
- Antidepressant medications;
- Postpartum support groups;
- Motherhood/breastfeeding circles.

Women with PPD often face barriers to receiving the needed diagnosis and treatment. Only 2 percent of women in one study sought mental health help for PPD in the first year postpartum.

Unfortunately some medical and mental health professionals may not respond to the symptoms reported by the patient, dismissing them as normal responses to new motherhood. This experience shuts down the mother from seeking the appropriate support she is needing. Regardless whether these struggles are normal, seeking support should always be offered and encouraged.

Other times women are offered medication from their medical provider without being encouraged to seek emotional support as well. It is incredibly important for new mothers to have a strong support network in order to manage this new life challenge. Medical professionals should always suggest additional supports and counseling when they are prescribing medication for PDD.

Some women may face cultural barriers to care. In some cultures, positive social support for new mothers, which serves as a protective factor, is the norm; in others, however, this type of support may not be present or there may be cultural biases against seeking help.

WHAT CAN BE DONE

Social workers should learn about postpartum depression so they can assess the needs of friends, family, and the patient for additional support. They should also develop an awareness of the patient's cultural values, beliefs, and biases and how they may be creating a barrier to seeking the support needed.

If the patient shows signs of suicidal, homicidal thinking or behavior, and/or abuse or neglect of the infant, the social worker should make sure to get help for the patient as soon as possible.

To reduce stress in the patient, the social worker should explore support systems; support may come from family, friends, spiritual/religious sources, support groups, or community mental health agencies.

The social worker should never ignore the signs or symptoms of postpartum depression. Becoming a new mother comes with many challenges, and she should be encouraged to seek out support early and often to help manage this transition in the healthiest way possible.

Written by Jessica Therivel, LMSW-IPR

Reviewed by Laura Gale, LCSW, and Chris Bates, MA, MSW

REFERENCES

Baker, L., Cross, S., Greaver, L., Wei, G., & Lewis, R. (2005). Prevalence of postpartum depression in a Native American population. *Maternal and Child Health Journal, 9*(1), 21-25.

Baker, L., & Oswalt, K. (2008). Screening for postpartum depression in a rural community. *Community Mental Health Journal, 44*(3), 171-180.

Banker, J. E., & LaCoursiere, D. Y. (2014). Postpartum depression: Risks, protective factors, and the couple's relationship. *Issues in Mental Health Nursing, 35*(7), 503-508. doi: 10.3109/01612840.2014.888603

Bina, R. (2008). The impact of cultural factors upon postpartum depression: A literature review. *Health Care for Women International, 29*(6), 568-592. doi: 10.1080/07399330802089149

Bledsoe, S. E., & Grote, N. K. (2006). Treating depression during pregnancy and the postpartum: A preliminary meta-analysis. *Research on Social Work Practice, 16*(2), 109-120. doi: 10.1177/1049731505282202

Boland-Prom, K. W., & MacMullen, N. (2012). Expanding the postpartum depression construct using a social work paradigm. *Journal of Human Behavior in the Social Environment, 22*(6), 718-732. doi: 10.1080/10911359.2012.692563

Borra, C., Iacovou, M., & Sevilla, A. (2015). New evidence on breastfeeding and postpartum depression: The importance of understanding women's intentions. *Maternal & Child Health Journal, 19*(4), 897-907.

British Association of Social Workers. (2012). *The Code of Ethics for Social Work: Statement of principles.* Retrieved December 2, 2015, from http: //cdn.basw.co.uk/upload/basw_112315-7.pdf

Drake, E., Howard, E., & Kinsey, E. (2014). Online screening and referral for postpartum depression: An exploratory study. *Community Mental Health Journal, 50*(3), 305-311. doi: 10.1007/s10597-012-9573-3

Fagan, J., & Lee, Y. (2010). Perceptions and satisfaction with father involvement and adolescent mothers' postpartum depressive symptoms. *Journal of Youth and Adolescence, 39*(9), 1109-1121. doi: 10.1007/s10964-009-9444-6

Houston, K. A., Kaimal, A. J., Nakagawa, S., Gregorick, S. E., Yee, L. M., & Kuppermann, M. (2015). Mode of delivery and postpartum depression: The role of patient preferences. *American Journal of Obstetrics & Gynecology, 212*(2), 229-231.

International Federation of Social Workers. (2012, March 3). Statement of ethical principles. Retrieved June 26, 2015, from http: //ifsw.org/ policies/statement-of-ethical-principles/

Maccio, E. M., & Pangburn, J. A. (2011). The case for investigating postpartum depression in lesbians and bisexual women. *Women's Health Issues: Official Publication of the Jacobs Institute of Women's Health, 21*(3), 187-190. doi: 10.1016/j.whi.2011.02.007

Mizrahi, T., & Mayden, R. W. (2001). *NASW Standards for Cultural Competency in Social Work Practice.* Retrieved June 26, 2015, from http: //www.socialworkers.org/ practice/standards/NASWCulturalStandards.pdf

Nishigori, H., Sugawara, J., Obara, T., Nishigori, T., Sato, K., Sugiyama, T.,... Yaegashi, N. (2014). Surveys of postpartum depression in Miyaga, Japan, after the great East Japan earthquake. *Archives of Women's Mental Health, 17*(6), 579-581.

Paris, R., Bolton, R. E., & Weinberg, M. K. (2009). Postpartum depression, suicidality, and mother-infant interactions. *Archives of Women's Mental Health, 12*(5), 309-321. doi: 10.1007/s00737-009-0105-2

Rhyne, E. P., & Borawski, A. (2014). Text messaging as an adjunct treatment for urban mothers with postpartum depression. *Journal of Pediatric Healthcare, 28*(6), e49.

Stuebe, A. M., Horton, B. J., Chetwynd, E., Watkins, S., Grewen, K., & Meltzer-Brody, S. (2014). Prevalence and risk factors for early, undesired weaning attributed to lactation dysfunction. *Journal of Women's Health, 23*(5), 404-412. doi: 10.1089/jwh.2013.4506

Thoppil, J., Riutcel, T. L., & Nalesnik, S. W. (2005). Early intervention for perinatal depression. *American Journal of Obstetrics & Gynecology, 192*(5), 1446-1448.

Trabold, N., Waldrop, D. P., Nochajski, T. H., & Cerulli, C. (2013). An exploratory analysis of intimate partner violence and postpartum depression in an impoverished urban population. *Social Work in Health Care, 52*(4), 332-350. doi: 10.1080/00981389.2012.751081

Vasa, R., Eldeirawi, K., Kuriakose, V. G., Nair, G. J., Newsom, C., & Bates, J. (2014). Postpartum depression in mothers of infants in neonatal intensive care unit: Risk factors and management strategies. *American Journal of Perinatology, 31*(5), 425-433. doi: 10.1055/s-0033-1352482

Wei, G., Greaver, L. B., Marson, S. M., Herndon, C. H., & Rogers, J. (2008). Postpartum depression: Racial differences and ethnic disparities in a tri-racial and bi-ethnic population. *Maternal and Child Health Journal, 12*(6), 699-707.

Wynter, K., Rowe, H., & Fisher, J. (2014). Interactions between perceptions of relationship quality and postnatal depressive symptoms in Australian, primiparous women and their partners. *Australian Journal of Primary Health, 20*(2), 174-181. doi: 10.1071/PY12066

Zittel-Palamara, K., Rockmaker, J. R., Schwabel, K. M., Weinstein, W. L., & Thompson, S. J. (2008). Desired assistance versus care received for postpartum depression: Access to care differences by race. *Archives of Women's Mental Health, 11*(2), 81-92. doi: 10.1007/s00737-008-0001-1

POSTPARTUM DEPRESSION: PSYCHOSOCIAL SUPPORT

MAJOR CATEGORIES: Behavioral & Mental Health

DESCRIPTION

Postpartum depression (PPD) is defined as clinical depression that has lasted for at least two weeks and has an onset within four weeks of giving birth. Symptoms of PPD include sadness, tearfulness, decreased motivation, decreased interest in food and self-care, difficulty concentrating, poor self-esteem regarding ability to parent, anxiety, mental confusion, feelings of shame and guilt, and/or loss of interest in the baby.

A significant risk factor for PPD is either thinking about or actually experiencing decreased levels of psychosocial support. Psychosocial support is looking at the impact of relational interactions on the mother's mental health. A new mother may be missing support in various areas of her life causing her to be at risk for PPD.

RISK FACTORS

The woman's family and friends may be absent, critical, or intrusive. The woman also may be experiencing emotional or physical abuse.

The practices of a woman's culture can serve as a protective factor or a risk factor depending on how that culture supports and assists new mothers.

The woman may be experiencing stress related to work (including the absence from work, the decision regarding whether to return to work, loss of career), money, and other potential losses.

Stress and how it relates to the parenting role has been consistently linked to PPD. This stress may be episodic stress or chronic stress. Episodic stressors are stressful life events, daily hassles, or catastrophic events. Chronic stress includes perceived stress, chronic strain, and parenting stress. Perceived stress is when a mother feels overwhelmed and unable to cope with her current situation. Chronic strain may come from low socioeconomic status, work demands, insufficient food, and the like.

Parenting stress can be measured and evaluated using three domains. These are parental distress, difficult child stress, and parent–child dysfunctional interaction (PCDI), Parental distress involves the mother's feelings of incompetence in parenting and the responsibilities that go along with parenting. Difficult child stress is related to the mother's perception of how challenging the child is. PCDI measures how the mother feels about her interactions with the child. This stressor can be affected by partner support, and if the mother is working outside the home, reduced interaction occurs naturally.

In 2014, the Centers for Disease Control and Prevention (CDC) published information from 2009 reporting that in the United States, 11.9 percent of women between the ages of 18 and 44 who gave birth experienced symptoms of depression.

Women with PPD may feel tearful, anxious, hopeless, and inadequate at caring for the baby; may have difficulty sleeping and experience loss of appetite; may experience inability to experience pleasure and memory problems; and may develop suicidal thinking.

Parenthood, whether through childbirth or adoption, can be a time of crisis for new parents due to drastic change in someone's identity. It causes transitions in roles, relationships, and patterns of interpersonal functioning. Emotions are more difficult to regulate. Social expectations that new mothers will experience joyful bonding with their infants may serve to minimize the stress and discomfort that may also be present.

Because it is assumed that adoption is a desired, positive experience, adoptive parents can feel as though they are unable to seek help or express negative emotions even though they may encounter the same issues of loss of identity, independence, career, and so on that biological parents experience.

SUPPORT

Instrumental support includes actual physical assistance such as meals preparation, laundry, or house cleaning.

Informational support consists of advice or suggestions.

Emotional support produces expressions of love, caring, and compassionate support.

Relationship quality between parents, rather than marital status, provides the protective social support.

Single mothers did not show a higher rates of PPD when relationship quality was taken out of the equation.

Another aspect that can reduce the risk of developing PDD includes validating or supportive statements (called appraisal support) such as "I trust your judgment" or "You are doing a good job."

Today, new mothers can find these kinds of supports through online education, social media, message boards, forums, and support groups.

Adolescent mothers are at a higher risk for PPD because they often lack these supports.

Often women need less actual support than believed; however, they seem to benefit from awareness that the support exists if needed.

Parental self-efficacy refers to the beliefs held by a parent about his or her abilities, powers, and capabilities to complete the needed tasks to care for a child. High self-efficacy in a new mother has shown to reduce the risk of PDD.

Psychosocial support (referrals to education, support groups, and assistance with home/childcare) offered by the social worker will only be useful if the woman feels this support meets needs that she has identified and if it is acknowledged that she may be experiencing PPD.

Often women may not seek treatment for PPD until symptoms are severe or family and/or friends ask them to get help.

Women may be ashamed to recognize a need for help and may not know how or where to find help.

Women may intellectually understand PPD but not recognize the symptoms in themselves.

Commonly, new mothers will minimize their symptoms and may deny the severity of their depression.

Partner and/or family support can be the most beneficial even when support is coming from other sources.

Cultural considerations may affect whether women seek treatment, and PPD is more likely to go undetected and untreated in minority groups.

Social hierarchy and cultural disadvantages can increase risk for PPD.

Women in minority groups may feel shame related to PPD, perceive stigma, or be coping with cultural beliefs that minimize depression by seeing mental health issues as a sign of weakness or with a cultural bias against disclosing any negative feelings to family or friends. This is a common experience, as minority groups overall seek less mental health treatment. For example, some black mothers reported a community belief that "strong" mothers do not "catch" PPD.

Research showed that the most beneficial interventions used to reduce risk of PDD were interpersonal psychotherapy, home visits conducted by a postpartum nurse or midwife, postpartum peer-based phone support, and flexible postpartum care by midwives.

ASSESSMENT

There are screening tools that measure social supports for women. The Maternal Support Scale is an index of emotional, informational, childcare, financial, respite, household, and other supports that may or may not be available from the baby's father, mother's parents, in-laws, and extended family. The Postpartum Social Support Questionnaire (PSSQ) is a 50-item questionnaire that measures emotional and instrumental social support from spouse/partner, parents, in-laws, other family members, and friends.

The stress and coping model for PPD theorizes that it is the psychosocial stressors listed above that are a main risk factor for PPD. The model proposes that positive actual supports or perceived supports will help the woman to have improved self-confidence, general satisfaction, and positive self-evaluation.

TREATMENT

Any counseling interventions for PPD will be more likely to have positive outcomes if they work to build up the new mother's ability to cope with stress and enhance her support system through advocacy and finding resources.

Organizations exist that provide community-based psychosocial support for women experiencing PPD by linking them with volunteers who have survived PPD and with healthcare workers/clinicians who are specialists in the treatment of PPD.

Support groups such as Postpartum Education and Support and Postpartum Support International were created to help women with PPD and their families. Support is provided through outreach, education, and local referrals for treatment, services, and volunteer contacts. These groups project a common message of validation that the woman is are not alone, reassurance that it is not her fault, and hope that she will be able to overcome PDD.

It is important for women experiencing PDD to reach out for support. They should do their own research to find the resources and supports for PDD in their community.

SERVICES AND RESOURCES

- Postpartum Education and Support, http: // pesnc.org
- Postpartum Support International, http: //www. postpartum.net

REFERENCES

Abrams, L. S., & Curran, L. (2007). Not just a middle-class affliction: Crafting a social work research agenda on postpartum depression. *Health & Social Work*, *32*(4), 289-296.

Akincigil, A., Munch, S., & Niemczyk, K. C. (2010). Predictors of maternal depression in the first year postpartum: Marital status and mediating role of relationship quality. *Social Work in Health Care*, *49*(3), 227-244. doi: 10.1080/00981380903213055

Baker, L., Cross, S., Greaver, L., Wei, G., & Lewis, R. (2005). Prevalence of postpartum depression in a Native American population. *Maternal and Child Health Journal*, *9*(1), 21-25.

Banker, J. E., & LaCoursiere, D. Y. (2014). Postpartum depression: Risks, protective factors, and the couple's relationship. *Issues in Mental Health Nursing, 35*(7), 503-508. doi: 10.3109/01612840.2014.888603

Bertram, L. (2009). Helping women make the emotional transition to motherhood–first of two articles. *Independent Nurse, 18*, 42-43.

Bina, R. (2008). The impact of cultural factors upon postpartum depression: A literature review. *Health Care for Women International, 29*(6), 568-592. doi: 10.1080/07399330802089149

Boland-Prom, K. W., & MacMullen, N. (2012). Expanding the postpartum depression construct using a social work paradigm. *Journal of Human Behavior in the Social Environment, 22*(6), 718-732. doi: 10.1080/10911359.2012.692563

British Association of Social Workers. (2012, January). *The Code of Ethics for Social Work: Statement of principles.* Retrieved September 16, 2015, from http: //cdn.basw.co.uk/upload/basw_112315-7. pdf

Brown, J. D., Harris, S. K., Woods, E. R., Buman, M. P., & Cox, J. E. (2012). Longitudinal study of depressive symptoms and social support in adolescent mothers. *Maternal and Child Health Journal, 16*(4), 894-901. doi: 10.1007/s10995-011-0814-9

Centers for Disease Control and Prevention (CDC). (2014, April 25). Surveillance summaries - Core state preconception health indicators: Pregnancy Risk Assessment Monitoring System and Behavioral Risk Factor Surveillance System, 2009. *MMWR, 63*(ss03), 1-62.

Dagher, R. K., McGovern, P. M., Alexander, B. H., Dowd, B. E., Ukestad, L. K., & McCaffrey, D. J. (2009). The psychosocial work environment and maternal postpartum depression. *International Journal of Behavioral Medicine, 16*(4), 339-346. doi: 10.1007/s12529-008-9014-4

Dennis, C. L., & Dowswell, T. (2014). Psychosocial and psychological interventions for preventing postpartum depression. *Cochrane Database of Systematic Reviews, 2.* Art. No.: CD001134.

Evans, M., Donelle, L., & Hume-Loveland, L. (2012). Social support and online postpartum depression discussion groups: A content analysis. *Patient Education and Counseling, 87*(3), 405-410. doi: 10.1016/j.pec.2011.09.011

Gair, S. (1999). Distress and depression in new motherhood: Research with adoptive mothers highlights important contributing factors. *Child and Family Social Work, 4*(1), 55-66.

Gruen, D. S. (1990). Postpartum depression: A debilitating yet often unassessed problem. *Health & Social Work, 15*(4), 261-270.

Haga, S. M., Ulleberg, P., Slinning, K., Kraft, P., Steen, T. B., & Staff, A. (2012). A longitudinal study of postpartum depressive symptoms: Multilevel growth curve analyses of emotion regulation strategies, breastfeeding self-efficacy, and social support. *Archives of Women's Mental Health, 15*(3), 175-184. doi: 10.1007/s00737-012-0274-2

Honikman, J. I. (2006). The role of Postpartum Support International in helping perinatal families. *Journal of Obstetric, Gynecologic, and Neonatal Nursing, 35*(5), 659-661. doi: 10.1111/j.1552-6909.2006.00088.x

International Federation of Social Workers. (2012, March 3). Statement of ethical principles. Retrieved September 16, 2015, from http: //ifsw. org/policies/statement-of-ethical-principles/

Leahy-Warren, P., McCarthy, G., & Corcoran, P. (2012). First-time mothers: Social support, maternal parental self-efficacy, and postnatal depression. *Journal of Clinical Nursing, 21*(3-4), 388-397. doi: 10.1111/j.1365-2702.2011.03701.x

McCarthy, M., & McMahon, C. (2008). Acceptance and experience of treatment for postnatal depression in a community mental health setting. *Health Care for Women International, 29*(6), 618-637. doi: 10.1080/07399330802089172

McManus, B. M., & Poehlmann, J. (2012). Maternal depression and perceived social support as predictors of cognitive function trajectories during the first 3 years of life for preterm infants in Wisconsin. *Child: Care, Health & Development, 38*(3), 425-434. doi: 10.1111/j.1365-2214.2011.01253.x

Mizrahi, T., & Mayden, R. W. (2001). NASW standards for cultural competency in social work practice. Retrieved September 16, 2015, from http: // www.socialworkers.org/practice/standards/NAS-WCulturalStandards.pdf

Paris, R., Bolton, R. E., & Weinberg, M. K. (2009). Postpartum depression, suicidality, and mother-infant interactions. *Archives of Women's Mental Health, 12*(5), 309-321. doi: 10.1007/s00737-009-0105-2

Sheng, X., Le, H., & Perry, D. (2010). Perceived satisfaction with social support and depressive symptoms in perinatal Latinas. *Journal of Transcultural Nursing, 21*(1), 35-44. doi: 10.1177/1043659609348619

Sampson, M., Duron, J. F., Torres, M. I. M., & Davidson, M. R. (2014). A disease you just caught: Low-income African American mothers' cultural beliefs about postpartum depression. *Women's Healthcare*. Retrieved September 16, 2015, from http: //npwomenshealthcare.com/wp-content/ uploads/2014/10/PostPart_N14.pd

Thomason, E., Volling, B. L., Flynn, H. A., McDonough, S. C., Marcus, S. M., Lopez, J. F., & Vazquez, D. (2014). Parenting stress and depressive symptoms in postpartum mothers: Bidirectional or unidirectional effects?. *Infant Behav Dev, 37*(3), 406-415.

Yim, I. S., Stapleton, L. R. T., Guardino, C. M., Hahn-Holbrook, J., & Schetter, C. D. (2015). Biological and psychosocial predictors of postpartum depression: Systematic review and call for integration. *Annual Review of Clinical Psychology, 11*, 99-137.

POSTPARTUM PSYCHOSIS

MAJOR CATEGORIES: Behavioral & Mental Health

DESCRIPTION

Psychosis refers to specific symptoms such as hallucinations, delusions, grossly disorganized thought, abnormal motor behaviors, , and looks at their severity, and their duration. (For more information on psychosis, see *T709378*.) Experiencing these symptoms does not automatically lead to a psychotic diagnosis. Currently postpartum psychosis (PPP) is not a distinct diagnosis in the *DSM-5*. The classifications "with peripartum onset" or "with postpartum onset" can be applied to a variety of mood disorders as an impacting element. Despite its absence from the *DSM-5* there is consensus on which elements of psychosis combine in the syndrome called PPP. There is also consensus that PPP is the most extreme manifestation of postpartum psychological occurrences, which range from so-called baby blues through postpartum depression to PPP.

Briefly, baby blues are transient disturbances or problems of adjustment that usually appear within the first few days after giving birth and that do not significantly impair function. Between 50 percent and 70 percent of postpartum women experience baby blues, which may include tearfulness, headaches, low self-esteem, emotional lability, fatigue, and ambivalent feelings toward the new infant. Postpartum depression includes the same symptoms as major depressive disorder; it impacts functioning and affects 10 percent to 20 percent of women who have recently given birth, usually within 12 weeks of delivery with an onset up to a year postpartum. Since the mother's functioning is impacted by mood disturbances such as depressed mood loss of interest in normal activities, and possibly intrusive thoughts about harming the newborn or guilt about not being a good mother it is extremely important to seek professional assessment and treatment as soon as possible. In more severe cases where the mothers level of functioning is significantly impacted and the health and development of the newborn may be compromised it may be necessary to have involvement of agencies such as Child Protective Services (CPS).

Due to the severity of the symptoms, PPP is a medical emergency that requires immediate intervention. Early intervention is necessary to address the increased risk of suicide and harm to the baby and to decrease the impact of the current episode. Onset is sudden and rapid, usually from 2 days to 4 weeks after delivery, and most often starts with mania (hyperactivity or elevated mood) or other mood symptoms and progresses rapidly to symptoms that may include delusions (frequently centered on the new baby), mood lability, hallucinations, bizarre behavior, mania, severe depression, confusion, and obsessions (frequently centered on the new baby). Although PPP frequently occurs in women with a history of mental health diagnoses, the symptoms of PPP appear suddenly. PPP has a profound negative impact on functioning, although if mania is present the mother's vastly increased activity level may mask the impairment. It was found that 73 percent of women who developed PPP recalled symptoms appearing within 3 days of giving birth and that the most common symptoms were feeling excited, elated, or "high" (52 percent); not needing sleep or not being able to sleep (48 percent); feeling active or energetic (37 percent); and being very talkative (31 percent). Symptoms of

PPP may appear similar to those of a primary psychotic disorder (e.g., schizophrenia) or a mood disorder (e.g., bipolar disorder). Aside from the obvious factor of recently having given birth, other factors associated with the onset of PPP are a history of mental health disorder(s), including previous PPP, family history of psychotic illness, recent stressful events beyond the immediate impact of giving birth, absence of a family or social support system, delivering one's first child, emergency caesarean section or otherwise complicated birth, and perinatal death.

Numerous causes for postpartum psychological distress have been investigated, including increased levels of emotional stress caused by pregnancy and the responsibilities of child rearing, sudden endorphin decrease with labor, abrupt hormone level changes after delivery, low serum levels of free tryptophan (which is an essential amino acid associated with the development of major depression), thyroid gland dysfunction, a prior mental health diagnosis, a family history of mental health disorder(s), occurrence of unexpected adverse life events, lack of social or family support, genetic factors, and maternal age ≥ 35 years. One approach (Spinelli, 2009) views PPP as the manifestation of a lifetime vulnerability to mood disorders that is precipitated by childbirth. The outcome varies with speed of diagnosis and treatment. Most women recover within 12 weeks, but up to 15 percent continue to experience depressive symptoms for more than 24 weeks. Approximately 40 percent have the same symptoms again after a subsequent pregnancy. Treatment may include voluntary or involuntary hospitalization, medications, and psychoeducational therapy for the affected individual and the family.

FACTS AND FIGURES

Heron (2008) and Spinelli (2009) report that PPP occurs in 1–2 mothers per 1, 000 deliveries. Spinelli reports that approximately 4 percent of women with PPP commit infanticide. Sadock (2015) reports that 50 to 60 percent of PPP episodes occur after the birth of a first child, that 50 percent of cases involve women with a family history of mood disorders, and that 50 percent of cases involve deliveries that had complications of a non-psychiatric nature.

RISK FACTORS

Risk factors include a personal or family history of a mental health disorder(s), particularly a mood or psychotic disorder; a prior episode of PPP; recent stressful events; lack of social or family support; first delivery; emergency caesarean section or other delivery complications, including perinatal death; and lack of sleep.

SIGNS AND SYMPTOMS

Signs and clinical presentation include recent childbirth, sudden and rapid onset of symptoms, hallucinations, delusions (frequently centered on the infant), withdrawal and disconnection, disorganized thinking and behavior, mood lability, obsessions (frequently involving birth or the new infant), and sleep deprivation. Mania (hyperactive or elevated mood) frequently is present and may be mistaken for better than average adjustment to the presence of a new baby.

ASSESSMENT

Shame about not being able to care for a newborn infant may prevent or delay seeking treatment. A brief assessment for postpartum depression and PPP should be conducted at every contact with women who have recently delivered a baby. If the brief assessment indicates there is a need, an in-depth assessment using relevant diagnostic and assessment tools should be conducted.

When assessing for PPP consider the following:

- Complete a standard bio-psycho-social-spiritual history;
- Thoroughly assess personal and family mental health history, including prior mental health diagnoses and medication;
- Assess for suicidal thinking or thoughts of harming the baby and otherwise harming self or others; and
- Assess family support and care system for the newborn.

ASSESSMENTS AND SCREENING TOOLS

- Postpartum Bonding Questionnaire (PBQ)
- Edinburgh Postnatal Depression Scale (EPDS)
- Postpartum Depression Screening Scale (PDSS)
- Mood Disorder Questionnaire (MDQ)

TREATMENT

Treatment of PPP should start with preventive measures throughout the pregnancy, including assessment of prior PPP or other mental health disorders, family history of mental health disorders, education about possible postpartum mood lability ranging from baby blues to PPP, involvement of family and support network with the pregnancy, and brief assessments of mood at every visit.

When PPP does occur treatment should first include considerations of the safety, health, and well-being of the newborn. Appropriate referrals should be made immediately for assessment and intervention if needed to care for the newborn. Child Protective Services or analogous agencies may need to be involved. There may be times when the best interests of the mother and those of the child are in conflict.

It is important to be aware of cultural values, beliefs, and biases when working with different people. Treatment should include knowledge about the histories, traditions, and values of the people with whom you are working.

APPLICABLE LAWS AND REGULATIONS

Each jurisdiction (e.g., nation, state, province) has its own standards, procedures, and laws for involuntary restraint and detention of persons who may be a danger to themselves or others. The lack of a formal *DSM-5* diagnosis for PPP may complicate legal and detention issues. It is important to understand protocols in your jurisdiction to best help support mothers struggling with PPP.

As mandated reporters all medical and mental health professionals must report any suspicion of neglect or abuse of a child to Child Protective Services or local agency.

Since 1922 the laws of England have recognized the biological and psychiatric circumstances that may surround infanticide, and probation and psychiatric treatment are mandated when appropriate. Twenty-nine other countries have made similar adjustments to their laws; however, the U.S. judicial system continues to punish rather than treat mothers with postpartum mental disorders who kill their children.

Each country has its own standards for cultural competency and diversity in social work practice. Social workers must be aware of the standards of practice set forth by their governing body (e.g., National Association of Social Workers in the United States, British Association of Social Workers in England), and practice accordingly.

SERVICES AND RESOURCES

- Brain & Behavior Research Foundation (formerly NARSAD), http://bbrfoundation.org/

- National Alliance on Mental Illness (NAMI), http://www.nami.org/
- U.S. National Institutes of Health (NIH), http://www.nih.gov/
- U.S. National Institute of Mental Health (NIMH), http://www.nimh.nih.gov/index.shtml
- National Association of Social Workers (NASW), http://www.socialworkers.org/
- Royal College of Psychiatrists (RCP), http://rcpsych.ac.uk

FOOD FOR THOUGHT

The case of Andrea Yates, the Texas woman who drowned her five children in June 2001, encapsulates many issues surrounding PPP and infanticide, including the failure of family, society, and failure of the mental health and legal communities to intervene appropriately. Yates had been pregnant or breastfeeding for 7 years, cared for her bedridden father, home-schooled her older children, taught evening Bible study, baked cookies, designed crafts, made costumes—in short, she was a "super mom." However, she also had a history of psychiatric illness, with the first reported psychotic episode after the birth of her first child, two suicide attempts that were attributed to efforts to resist satanic voices commanding her to kill her fourth child soon after birth, numerous other hospitalizations and disrupted medication regimens, plus an immediate family history of bipolar disorder and major depressive disorder. At her first trial the jury acknowledged the tragedy of the situation and their own conflicted feelings by returning a guilty verdict after 3 and one half hours of deliberations and by taking only 35 minutes to deny the prosecutor's request for the death penalty. The incident was treated as a legal question rather than a mental health issue when Yates was sentenced to life in prison rather than to intensive treatment. A second trial overturned the first verdict on a technicality and she is now in a state mental hospital. This case highlights the fact that PPP is an extremely serious mental health crisis where immediate intervention is necessary.

RED FLAGS

Assess for suicidal, infanticidal, or homicidal ideation.

Monitor changing medication regimens, or non-adherence to regimen, particularly if breastfeeding.

Evaluate mother-child attachment, as it may be adversely impacted by PPP.

Social workers are mandated reporters for abuse and neglect of children and must report any suspicions that abuse or neglect is happening to CPS or the appropriate local agency.

Written by Chris Bates, MA, MSW

Reviewed by Lynn B. Cooper, D. Crim, and Melissa Rosales Neff, MSW

REFERENCES

American Psychiatric Association. (2013). Diagnostic and Statistical Manual of Mental Disorders. Fifth edition. DSM-5. In (5th ed., pp. 45-47). Washington, DC: American Psychiatric Publishing.

Doucet, S., Dennis, C. L., Letourneau, N., & Blackmore, E. R. (2009). Differentiation and clinical implications of postpartum depression and postpartum psychosis. *Journal of Obstetric, Gynecologic & Neonatal Nursing, 38*(13), 269-279.

Hall, S. D., & Bean, R. A. (2008). Family therapy and childhood-onset schizophrenia: Pursuing clinical and bio/psycho/social competence. *Contemporary Family Therapy, 30*(2), 61-74.

Heron, J., McGuinness, M., Blackmore, E. R., Craddock, N., & Jones, I. (2008). Early postpartum symptoms in puerperal psychosis. *BJOG: An International Journal of Obstetrics & Gynaecology, 115*(3), 348-353.

Jones, D. W. (2004). Families and serious mental illness: Working with loss and ambivalence. *British Journal of Social Work, 34*(7), 961-979.

Mizrahi, T., & Mayden, R. W. (2001). NASW standards for cultural competency in social work practice. Retrieved from http://socialworkers.org/practice/standards/NASWCulturalStandards.pdf

Monzon, C., di Scalea, T. L., & Pearlstein, T. (2014). Postpartum psychosis: Updates and clinical issues. *Psychiatric Times, 31*(1), 1-6.

Noorlander, Y., Bergink, V., & den Berg, M. P. (2008). Perceived and observed mother-child interaction at time of hospitalization and release in postpartum depression and psychosis. *Archives of Women's Mental Health, 11*(1), 49-56.

Posmontier, B. (2010). The role of midwives in facilitating recovery in postpartum psychosis. *Journal of Midwifery and Women's Health, 55*(5), 430-437.

Sadock, R. J., Sadock, V. A., & Ruiz, P. (2015). Kaplan & Sadock's synopsis of psychiatry: behavioral sciences/clinical psychiatry. In (pp. 831-840). Philadephia, PA: Wolters Kluwer.

Sit, D., Rothschild, A. J., & Wisner, K. L. (2006). A review of postpartum psychosis. *Journal of Women's Health, 15*(4), 352-368.

Spinelli, M. G. (2004). Maternal infanticide associated with mental illness: Prevention and the promise of saved lives. *American Journal of Psychiatry, 161*(9), 1548-1557.

Spinelli, M. G. (2009). Postpartum psychosis: Detection of risk and management. *American Journal of Psychiatry, 166*(4), 405-408.

Statement of ethical principles. (n.d.). *International Federation of Social Workers.* Retrieved from http://ifsw.org/policies/statement-of-ethical-principles/

The Policy, Ethics, and Human Rights Committee, British Association of Social Workers. (2012, January). The Code of Ethics for Social Work: Statements of principles. Retrieved March 24, 2014, from http://cdn.basw.co.uk/upload/basw_112315-7.pdf

Walther, V. N. (1997). Postpartum depression: A review for perinatal social workers. *Social Work in Health Care, 24*(3/4), 99-111.

POSTTRAUMATIC STRESS DISORDER IN ADULTS

MAJOR CATEGORIES: Behavioral & Mental Health

DESCRIPTION

In the past, posttraumatic stress disorder (PTSD) was classified as an anxiety disorder that affected military personnel and war veterans. Today, the fifth edition of the *Diagnostic and Statistical Manual of Mental Disorders* (*DSM-5*) identifies PTSD as a trauma and stress-related disorder that can develop in anyone who has been exposed to a traumatic or stressful event. PTSD may develop after an individual witnesses or otherwise experiences an event involving death, the threat of death, serious physical injury, or a threat to the individual's physical safety, and continues to experience such a traumatic event in the form of thoughts, flashbacks, dreams, delusions, or phobias.

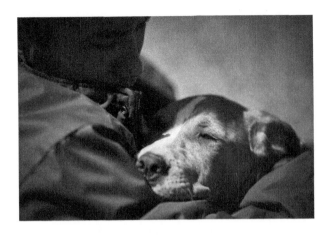

The *DSM-5* names the following eight criteria as being required for a diagnosis of PTSD:

Criterion A: Stressor: Experiencing, witnessing, or being confronted with a traumatic or life-threatening event.

Criterion B: Intrusion symptoms: Persistent reexperiencing of the event that triggered PTSD in the form of thoughts, flashbacks, nightmares, illusions, or hallucinations.

Criterion C: Avoidance: Avoidance of stimuli associated with the traumatic event that triggered PTSD (avoidance of thoughts, avoidance of people or places, detachment, inability to recall details of the events).

Criterion D: Negative alterations in cognition and moods: Worsening of thoughts and moods (persistent negative beliefs, feelings of alienation, constricted affect, diminished interest in activities) following the onset of PTSD.

Criterion E: Arousal: Alterations in arousal and reactivity (irritability, aggressive ehavior, hypervigilance, intense anxiety, difficulty concentrating) following the onset of PTSD.

Criterion F: Duration: Persistence of symptoms for more than 1 month.

Criterion G: Functional significance: Significant distress or functional impairment.

Criterion H: Exclusion: Exclusion of medication, substance abuse, or illness as a cause of psychological disturbance.

FACTS AND FIGURES

PTSD is one of the most common of all psychiatric disorders, and is diagnosed in twice as many women as men (lifetime prevalence 10 to 14 percent for women and 5 to 6 percent for men), with 50 percent of cases in women related to sexual assault. In the United States the estimated lifetime prevalence of PTSD ranges from 7.8 to 12.3 percent. Approximately 30 percent of men and women who have spent time in a war zone experience symptoms that meet the criteria for PTSD. Among U. S. military personnel who served in the Afghanistan and Iraq wars, 15 percent developed PTSD.

Remission rates for PTSD vary. Results from a recent meta-analysis showed that almost half of the subjects with PTSD experienced a remission after a mean of 3 years. Remission rates in studies of these rates within 5 months after the traumatic event that triggered PTSD were higher, averaging 51.7 percent, whereas rates in studies that examined remission after 5 months averaged 36.9 percent, indicating that PTSD at this stage is more likely to be chronic. A lower prevalence of PTSD found among older adults may be due in part to confounding factors, such as the greater likelihood that older adults will report psychological symptoms as somatic complaints, and older adults' reluctance to disclose trauma. The assessment of older adults for PTSD can also be more difficult if they have any concurrent cognitive or sensory problems.

RISK FACTORS

In terms of the risk of an individual's developing PTSD, persons at greater-than-average risk of witnessing or experiencing a traumatic event include undereducated males, persons with extroverted personalities, and those with a personal history of conduct problems or of psychiatric illness. The risk factors for development of PTSD after a traumatic experience include female gender, neuroticism, a lower level of social support, a lower intelligence quotient (IQ), preexisting psychiatric illness, a traumatic brain injury, and a family history of mood, anxiety, or substance abuse disorders. Individuals who are victims of violence (terror attacks, childhood abuse, sexual assault) and military veterans are at a high risk for PTSD. Men who have sex with men who have been victims of childhood sexual abuse are also at high risk for PTSD. Persons who experience severe trauma in the first decade of life may have a greater risk of developing PTSD after experiencing a traumatic event during adulthood. Persons with extended exposure to a traumatic event, those exposed to more than one traumatic event, or those who experience extreme violence are at greater than average risk of developing chronic PTSD.

Individuals with PTSD are at increased risk for other psychiatric disorders, including panic disorders, obsessive-compulsive disorder, social phobias, specific phobias, major depressive disorder, and suicidal and homicidal behaviors. Because PTSD increases the risk of suicidal thinking, persons with the disorder should be continually assessed for the risk of suicide.

SIGNS AND SYMPTOMS

Posttraumatic stress disorder is typically characterized by the combination of a number of psychological, behavioral, physical, and social effects. Its psychological effects include negative thoughts and perceptions; hallucinations, delusions, nightmares, flashbacks, suicidal ideation, and exaggerated reactions to stimuli; symptoms of depression and anxiety; memory loss, especially regarding details of the traumatic event that triggered PTSD; trouble in concentrating; poor impulse control; and feelings of guilt or fear.

Behavioral effects of PTSD include issues with substance use; perpetration of intimate partner violence (IPV); sexual dysfunction; marital discord; the detachment from reality known as dissociation, demonstrated by attempts to avoid places, persons, thoughts, conversations, or activities associated with the causative traumatic event of PTSD; agitation; intense anger; and feelings of numbness.

Physical manifestations of PTSD can include dishevelment, poor personal hygiene; somatic complaints, including gastrointestinal disturbances, muscle aches, and headaches.

Social effects of PTSD include withdrawal; self-isolation; limited friendships; poor social support; reduced emotional intimacy; trouble in performing daily tasks (cleaning, grooming, cooking); and an impaired ability to work and reintegrate into society.

TREATMENT

The social worker assisting an individual with PTSD should ask about the individual's history and response to the traumatic event responsible for the disorder; note the individual's overall presentation,

level of functioning, and any physical findings that may relate to the individual's PTSD; assess the individual's psychiatric history and ask about any history of substance abuse, childhood abuse, and exposure to violence; and conduct a biological, psychological, social, and spiritual assessment to include information on physical, mental, environmental, social, financial, and medical factors that may relate to the individual's condition. The social worker should also assess the individual's stress management skills and coping mechanisms, and obtain permission to interview the individual's family members for relevant information.

Persons with PTSD will often benefit from supportive psychotherapy and instruction in stress reduction techniques. The sooner treatment is initiated, the better the prognosis. The successful treatment of PTSD is best achieved through early intervention with cognitive behavioral therapy (CBT) with a focus on trauma, which is the most effective and widely used treatment for PTSD and helps the patient identify irrational beliefs and replace them with more adaptive thought processes. This method has evolved to include education on stress response, breathing training, and prolonged mental recounting of the event that caused PTSD in order to decrease the emotional response to it and other stress stimuli. CBT is currently considered the standard of care for PTSD by the U.S. Department of Defense (DOD). Other treatment techniques for PTSD are group therapy, eye movement desensitization and reprocessing (EMDR), a version of CBT that involves the use of imagery and rapid eye movement to desensitize an individual with PTSD through prolonged exposure to stimuli, and strengths-focused approaches.

Persons with PTSD should be referred for a psychiatric evaluation to determine whether they may benefit from pharmacologic therapy with beta blocker drugs (propranolol); selective serotonin reuptake inhibitors (SSRIs, such as sertraline, fluoxetine), which can help ease panic attacks, sleep disruption, and severe symptoms of hyperarousal; antianxiety agents (benzodiazepines); or antipsychotic drugs (risperidone). Pharmacologic therapy may be needed to address sleep disruption, nighttime hyperarousal, and nightmares that are associated with PTSD. Social workers should be aware of their own cultural values, beliefs, and biases and develop specialized knowledge about the histories, traditions, and values of their patients. Social workers should adopt treatment methodologies that reflect their knowledge of the cultural diversity of the communities in which they practice.

Factors associated with a good prognosis in PTSD include early initiation of treatment, ongoing social support, avoidance of reexposure to trauma, and the absence of other psychiatric disorders and substance abuse.

Social workers assisting persons with PTSD should practice with awareness of and adherence to the social work principles of respect for human rights and human dignity, cultural competency, social justice, and professional conduct.

SERVICES AND RESOURCES

- U.S. Department of Veterans Affairs National Center for PTSD, http://www.ptsd.va.gov
- National Institute of Mental Health, http://www.nimh.nih.gov
- National Alliance on Mental Illness, http://www.nami.org

Written by Nikole Seals, MSW, ACSW

Reviewed by Laura Gale, LCSW, and Jessica Therivel, LMSW-IPR

REFERENCES

American Psychiatric Association. (2013). Panic Disorder. In *Diagnostic and statistical manual of mental disorders: DSM-5* (5th ed., pp. 481-589). Washington, DC: American Psychiatric Publishing. http://cdn.basw.co.uk/upload/basw_112315-7.pdf

Choi, G. (2011). Secondary traumatic stress of service providers who practice with survivors of family or sexual violence: A national survey of social workers. *Smith College Studies in Social Work, 81*(1), 101-119. doi: 10.1080/00377317.2011.543044

Compton, K., & May, A. C. (2016). Posttraumatic stress disorder. In F. F. Ferri (Ed.), *2016 Ferri's clinical advisor: 5 books in 1* (pp. 993-994). Philadelphia, PA: Elsevier.

Craig, C. D., & Sprang, G. (2010). Factors associated with the use of evidence-based practices to treat psychological trauma by psychotherapists with trauma treatment expertise. *Journal of Evidence-Based Social Work, 7*(5), 488-509. doi: 10.1080/15433714.2010.528327

Dinnen, S., Simiola, V., & Cook, J. M. (2015). Posttraumatic stress disorder in older adults: A systematic review of the psychotherapy treatment literature. *Aging and Mental Health, 19*(2), 144-150. doi: 10.1080/13607863.2014.920299

Gill, I. J., Mullin, S., & Simpson, J. (2014). Psychosocial and psychological factors associated with post-traumatic stress disorder following traumatic brain injury in adult civilian populations: A systematic review. *Brain Injury, 28*(1), 1-14. doi: 10.3109/02699052.2013.851416

International Federation of Social Workers. (2012, March 3). Statement of ethical principles. Retrieved April 19, 2016, from http://ifsw.org/policies/statement-of-ethical-principles/

Morina, N., Wicherts, J. M., Lobbrecht, J., & Priebe, S. (2014). Remission from post-traumatic stress disorder in adults: A systematic review and meta-analysis of long term outcome studies. *Clinical Psychology Review, 34*(3), 249-255. doi: 10.1016/j.cpr.2014.03.002

National Association of Social Workers. (2008). Code of ethics. Retrieved April 4, 2016, from https://www.socialworkers.org/pubs/code/code.asp

National Association of Social Workers. (2015). NASW standards and indicators for cultural competence in social work practice. Retrieved March 2, 2016, from http://www.socialworkers.org/practice/standards/PRA-BRO-253150-CC-Standards.pdf

Olthuis, J., Watt, M., Bailey, K., Hayden, J., Stewart, S., Olthuis, J.,... Stewart, S. (2015). Therapist-supported Internet cognitive behavioral therapy for anxiety disorders in adults. *Cochrane Database of Systematic Reviews,* (Issue 2), CD011565.

Sadock, B. J., Sadock, V. A., & Ruiz, P. (2015). Trauma and stressor related disorders. In B. J. Sadock, V. A. Sadock, & P. Ruiz (Eds.), *Kaplan & Sadock's comprehensive textbook of psychiatry* (11th ed., pp. 437-446). Philadelphia, PA: Wolters Kluwer Health/Lippincott Williams & Wilkins.

POSTTRAUMATIC STRESS DISORDER IN CHILDREN

MAJOR CATEGORIES: Behavioral & Mental Health

DESCRIPTION

Posttraumatic stress disorder (PTSD) is a trauma- and stressor-related disorder that can develop in anyone who has experienced a stressful or traumatic event. The etiology of PTSD includes direct exposure to a traumatic event. The biological basis for the disorder includes complex activity in the brain that results in memories of the causative traumatic event(s) that are deeply engraved in the part of the brain responsible for memory. PTSD is increasingly being viewed as a disorder of the brain's limbic system and as being brought on by changes in this system that result from the traumatic event that triggers the disorder.

According to the fifth edition of the D*iagnostic and Statistical Manual of Mental Disorders* (*DSM-5*), published by the American Psychiatric Association, an individual must experience at least one symptom in each of the following eight criteria for a diagnosis of PTSD.

Criterion A: Stressor: Experiencing, witnessing, or being confronted with a traumatic or life-threatening event.

Criterion B: Intrusion symptoms: Persistent reexperiencing of the event that triggered PTSD in the form of thoughts, flashbacks, nightmares, illusions, or hallucinations.

Criterion C: Avoidance: Avoidance of stimuli associated with the traumatic event that triggered PTSD (avoidance of thoughts, avoidance of people or places, detachment, inability to recall details of the events).

Criterion D: Negative alterations in cognition and moods: Worsening of thoughts and moods (persistent negative beliefs, feelings of alienation, constricted affect, diminished interest in activities) following the onset of PTSD.

Criterion E: Arousal: Alterations in arousal and reactivity (irritability, aggressive ehavior, hypervigilance, intense anxiety, difficulty concentrating) following the onset of PTSD.

Criterion F: Duration: Persistence of symptoms for more than 1 month.

Criterion G: Functional significance: Significant distress or functional impairment.

Criterion H: Exclusion: Exclusion of medication, substance abuse, or illness as a cause of psychological disturbance.

These criteria are used to diagnose symptoms in adults, adolescents, and children older than 6 years. Although the assessment of adolescents is similar to that of adults, diagnosing PTSD in children under the age of 6 can be challenging because they may not have the ability to verbalize their feelings or describe symptoms. The *DSM-5* includes a specific age-related subtype of PTSD that takes into account the developmental differences in the expression and description of symptoms of PTSD for children under the age of 6. In the absence of verbal statements by children in this age group, social workers can use behavioral indicators to determine the presence and chronicity of symptoms of PTSD (extreme temper tantrums, reenactment in play of the traumatic event responsible for PTSD, and performance or behavioral problems in school).

The set of tools for the diagnosis of PTSD in children (administered questionnaires, observation, family interviews) differs from that for adults. For children as for adults, reexperiencing the traumatic event that triggered PTSD may induce nightmares, intrusive memories and thoughts, frightening dreams that do not reference the event, recurrent recollections, and reenactment in play, during which themes of the trauma are expressed. Avoidant behaviors in children may appear in the form of isolation, amnesia, emotional numbing, diminished interest in activities, developmental regression, restricted affect, and avoidance of stimuli associated with the causative traumatic event. Hyperarousal may manifest as poor concentration, sleep problems (night terrors, night waking), agitation, extreme startle responses, and hypervigilance, as further discussed in the section below on Signs and Symptoms.

FACTS AND FIGURES

The lifetime prevalence of PTSD in persons in the United States is 8 to 9 percent. It was reported that 60.4 percent of individuals are exposed to a traumatic event during childhood or adolescence. Results of a meta-analysis of data relating to PTSD indicated that approximately 1 in 6 children and adolescents exposed to trauma developed the disorder.

RISK FACTORS

Children who experience a traumatic event such as an automobile accident, personal injury, a medical diagnosis of a serious disorder, a natural disaster (fire, flood, hurricane, earthquake), war or terrorism, sexual abuse, physical abuse, domestic violence (as a witness or victim of injury during an episode), or severe maltreatment are at risk for PTSD. Victims of sexual abuse are the most likely to develop PTSD. Children previously exposed to trauma, those with a history of psychopathology or externalizing behaviors (difficult temperament, antisocial characteristics, hyperactivity), and those who have parents with a history of anxiety disorders are at a greater than average risk for having PTSD. Girls are more likely than boys to develop PTSD. Research has identified the four most significant factors in the development of PTSD as (1) the severity of the trauma that caused the disorder, (2) the parental reaction to the causative traumatic event (parent becomes overprotective or fearful), (3) the type of the causative traumatic event, and (4) whether the victim was involved in the causative traumatic event or was a witness to it. Caregiver behavior can influence the risk of PTSD developing in a child, with a greater likelihood of its occurrence in children whose caregivers have a history of mental health problems, who engage in domestic violence or other criminal behaviors, or who exhibit psychological aggression or abusive behaviors.

SIGNS AND SYMPTOMS

Psychological effects of PTSD in children can include reexperience of the trauma that induced PTSD through nightmares, flashbacks, or irrational fears; depression, anxiety, and feelings of guilt; memory, especially regarding details of the causative traumatic event; and somatic complaints

Behavioral effects of PTSD in children under the age of 5 years may include the expression of fear in the form of crying, whimpering, screaming, immobility, frightened facial expressions, fear of separation from a parent, or regressive behavior (thumb-sucking, bedwetting), or disorganized or agitated behavior. Children aged 5 years and older may exhibit extreme withdrawal, disruptive behavior, regressive behaviors

(fear of the dark, fear of being alone), eating difficulties, sexual acting out, substance abuse, self-injurious behaviors, or suicidal ideation. Children with PTSD may experience poor concentration and impulse control; young children may have tantrums or be noncompliant with behavioral standards.

Physical manifestations of PTSD in children may include signs of self-injurious behaviors such as cuts (cutting), missing patches of hair (hair pulling), or open/infected wounds (picking at skin or burning); changes in general appearance (dishevelment, poor personal hygiene); somatic complaints, including gastrointestinal disturbances, aches and pains, headaches; and sleep disturbances.

Social effects of PTSD in children may include the refusal to attend school or difficulties with schoolwork, and fear of strangers. Social effects in adolescents may include running away from home, delinquent behavior; withdrawal from family and peers; and the expression of changes in significant aspects of life (changes in goals, dreams, and aspirations).

ASSESSMENT

Social workers assisting children with PTSD should ensure that they are safe in the care of their parents or other caregivers; interview children with PTSD and their family members to obtain a history of these children's specific responses to traumatic event(s); note the overall demeanor and level of functioning of each child; and conduct a biological, psychological, social, and spiritual study that includes information about physical, mental, environmental, social, financial, spiritual, and medical factors affecting the child.

The social worker should educate the child's family members about the risk factors and signs of PTSD so as to equip them to provide support and seek help if and as it is needed; educate them about resources in their community that can assist and support them; encourage them to adhere to a plan of care for the child; and provide them with hotline information and emergency contacts to use during times of crisis.

Assessing a child for a history of abuse by a parent(s) is critical during treatment, as the most important goal of treatment is to maintain the safety of the child; any concerns should be reported to the relevant child protective services agency. The social worker should also assess the child's parents' ability to cope; its interfamilial relationships; whether any member of the family has a history of PTSD or other mental health problems, or a history of substance abuse; and the safety of the child's home and neighborhood environment. Because specific symptoms and displays of distress vary from among cultures, it is also important to be aware that PTSD may manifest differently in children of different cultures.

In working with children who may have PTSD, the social worker should use the alternative diagnostic tools for young children to determine whether the criteria for diagnosis of the disorder are met.

TREATMENT

The treatment of children with PTSD is based on a multidimensional approach. Research has established that for children, family therapy is an effective intervention, in addition to individual, group, and school-based therapy, as well as pharmacotherapy if it is needed. It is essential that if at all possible, parents and family members be involved in the treatment of PTSD in a child, to foster an environment of support, understanding, and reassurance for the child; family involvement has been found to be a strong predictor of successful treatment of the disorder.

Cognitive behavioral therapy (CBT), as either individual or group therapy, and with a focus on trauma, can be used with children who have PTSD to reduce hyperarousal and gradually reduce discomfort associated with stimuli that trigger symptoms of the disorder. The most common and effective form of CBT is individual therapy with a focus on trauma, which helps to reduce the fear associated with the traumatic event responsible for PTSD, to reorganize thoughts, and to improve adaptive behaviors. The focus should be on helping the child transition from having the mindset of a victim to one of a survivor. Research indicates that trauma-focused CBT (TF-CBT) is effective with 8- to 17-year-olds in reducing symptoms of PTSD, anxiety, and depression through a program of 12 sessions. Researchers are investigating whether TF-CBT would be effective with 3- to 8-year-olds with PTSD. Preliminary studies look promising, but more research is needed.

Narrative therapy (having an affected child write narratives or keep a journal of thoughts, emotions, and experiences associated with PTSD) or play therapy (drawing, playing with puppets) may be particularly useful with children who have PTSD.

Eye movement desensitization and reprocessing therapy can also be effective in easing symptoms PTSD in children. This method involves the use of imagery, and of rapid eye movement on the part of someone who has PTSD, to desensitize them to various stimuli through prolonged exposure to these stimuli.

Children who have severe or persistent symptoms of PRSD should be referred for a psychiatric assessment to determine whether they might benefit from pharmacologic therapy, such as with a beta blocker drug, antidepressant, or mood stabilizer, which may help with severe symptoms of anxiety, hyperarousal, and avoidance, and with any coexisting disorders such as depression. With regard to the pharmacologic treatment of PTSD in children, the U.S. Food and Drug Administration (FDA) issued an advisory in 2003 about a potential risk of suicide in patients under the age of 18 being treated with antidepressant drugs for major depression. A larger study by the Group Health Cooperative in 2013 found that the risk of suicide in this population increased with the use of antidepressants.

Social workers should be aware of their own cultural values, beliefs, and biases and develop specialized knowledge about the histories, traditions, and values of the children with whom they are working. Social workers should adopt treatment methodologies that reflect their knowledge of the cultural diversity of the communities in which they practice.

APPLICABLE LAWS AND REGULATIONS

State and local jurisdictions have requirements for reporting the abuse and neglect of children, and these should be known and observed.

SERVICES AND RESOURCES

- National Center for PTSD, http://www.ptsd. va.gov/professional/treatment/children/ptsd_ in_children_and_adolescents_overview_for_pro- fessionals.asp
- National Institute of Mental Health, http://www. nimh.nih.gov/health/topics/post-traumatic- stress-disorder-ptsd/index.shtml

Written by Nikole Seals, MSW, ACSW

Reviewed by Lynn B. Cooper, D Crim, and Chris Bates, MA, MSW

REFERENCES

Alisic, E., Zalta, A., Van Wesel, F., Floryt, L., Hafstad, S., Hassanpour, G., & Smid, G. (2014). Rates of post-traumatic stress disorder in trauma-exposed children and adolescents: Meta-analysis. *British Journal of Psychiatry, 204*(5), 335-340. doi: 10.1192/bjp.bp.113.131227

American Psychiatric Association. (2013). Panic Disorder. In *Diagnostic and statistical manual of mental disorders: DSM-5* (5th ed., pp. 481-589). Washington, DC: American Psychiatric Publishing. http://cdn.basw.co.uk/upload/basw_112315-7.pdf

Compton, K., & May, A. C. (2016). Posttraumatic stress disorder. In F. F. Ferri (Ed.), *2016 Ferri's clinical advisor: 5 books in 1* (pp. 993-994). Philadelphia, PA: Elsevier.

Dalgleish, T., Goodall, B., Chadwick, I., Werner-Seidler, A., McKinnon, A., Morant, N.,... Meiser-Stedman, R. (2015). Trauma-focused cognitive behaviour therapy versus treatment as usual for post-traumatic stress disorder (PTSD) in young children aged 3 to 8 years: Study protocol for a randomized controlled trial. *Trials, 16*(1), 116. doi: 10.1186/s13063-015-0632-2

Group Health Cooperative. (2013). Adult and adolescent depression: Screening, diagnosis, and treatment guideline. Retrieved March 11, 2016, from https://www.ghc.org/all-sites/guidelines/depression.pdf

International Federation of Social Workers. (2012, March 3). Statement of ethical principles. Retrieved March 11, 2016, from http://ifsw.org/policies/statement-of-ethical-principles/

Lubit, R. H. (2010). Posttraumatic stress disorder in children. *Medscape Reference*. Retrieved March 11, 2016, from http://emedicine.medscape.com/article/918844-overview

Rosenberg, D. R., Vandana, P., & Chiriboga, J. A. (2011). Anxiety disorders. In R. M. Kliegman, B. F. Stanton, N. F. Schor, J. W. St. Geme, III, & R. E. Behrman (Eds.), *Nelson textbook of pediatrics* (19th ed., pp. 77-82). Philadelphia, PA: Elsevier Saunders.

Sadock, B. J., Sadock, V. A., & Ruiz, P. (Eds.). (2015). Posttraumatic stress disorder of infancy, childhood, and adolescence. In *Kaplan & Sadock's Synopsis of Psychiatry* (11th ed., pp. 1221-1226). Philadelphia, PA: Wolters Kluwer Health/Lippincott Williams & Wilkins.

Sadock, B. J., Sadock, V. A., & Ruiz, P. (2015). Trauma and stressor related disorders. In B. J. Sadock, V. A. Sadock, & P. Ruiz (Eds.), *Kaplan & Sadock's comprehensive textbook of psychiatry* (11th ed., pp. 437-446). Philadelphia, PA: Wolters Kluwer Health/Lippincott Williams & Wilkins.

Scheeringa, M. S. (2013). PTSD for children 6 years and younger. U.S. Department of Veterans Affairs. Retrieved March 11, 2016, from http://www.ptsd.va.gov/professional/PTSD-overview/ptsd_children_6_and_younger.asp

Scheeringa, M., Weems, C., Cohen, J., Amaya-Jackson, L., & Guthrie, D. (2011). Trauma-focused cognitive-behavioral therapy for posttraumatic stress disorder in three through six year-old children: A randomized clinic trial. *Journal of Child Psychology and Psychiatry, 52*(8), 853-860. doi: 10.1111/j.1469-7610.2010.02354.x

Smith, P., Yule, W., Perrin, S., Tranah, T., Dalgleish, T., & Clark, D. (2007). Cognitive-behavioral therapy for PTSD in children and adolescents: A preliminary randomized controlled trial. *Journal of the American Academy Child Adolescent Psychiatry, 46*(8), 1051-1061. doi: 10.1097/CHI.0b013e318067e288

Stafford, B. (2011). Child & Adolescent Psychiatric disorders & psychosocial aspects of pediatrics. In W. W. Hay, M. J. Levin, J. M. Sondheimer, & R. R. Deterding (Eds.), *Current diagnosis & treatment pediatrics* (pp. 197-198). New York, NY: McGraw-Hill Medical.

Wheeler, D. (2015). NASW standards and indicators for cultural competence in social work practice. Retrieved March 2, 2016, from http://www.socialworkers.org/practice/standards/PRA-BRO-253150-CC-Standards.pdf

POSTTRAUMATIC STRESS DISORDER IN MILITARY PERSONNEL & VETERANS

MAJOR CATEGORIES: Military & Veterans, Behavioral & Mental Health

DESCRIPTION

Posttraumatic stress disorder (PTSD) was first identified during World War I and was initially referred to as *shell shock*. The American Psychiatric Association officially recognized PTSD as a type of anxiety disorder in 1980, introducing a conceptual change in which symptoms of PTSD were considered to result from trauma rather than being viewed as an internal weakness or inability to cope. After 1980, an individual's cognitive and emotional processes were seen as the factors that determined whether that individual was able to recover from trauma or would develop symptoms of PTSD. Although traumatic events can take many forms (natural disasters, severe injury, abuse, brushes with death), some events, such as rape, torture, and combat-related stress, are more likely than others to be experienced as traumatic.

Since its recognition as a distinct psychiatric disorder, PTSD has been reclassified as a disorder related to trauma and stress, and is the most common psychiatric disorder experienced by military personnel. Symptoms of PTSD may wax and wane over time, which can affect the way in which PTSD manifests itself in those who have it. Symptoms of PTSD may not be present immediately after the trauma that causes it, but may develop later and worsen with the passage of time. Symptoms of PTSD may also appear and disappear in response to various triggering factors. According to the fifth ddition of the *Diagnostic and Statistical Manual of Mental Disorders* (*DSM-5*), published by the American Psychiatric Association, the following criteria are used in making a diagnosis of PTSD:

Criterion A: Stressor: Experiencing, witnessing, or being confronted with a traumatic or life-threatening event.

Criterion B: Intrusion symptoms: Persistent reexperiencing of the event that triggered PTSD in the form of thoughts, flashbacks, nightmares, illusions, or hallucinations.

Criterion C: Avoidance: Avoidance of stimuli associated with the traumatic event that   triggered PTSD (avoidance of thoughts, avoidance of people or places, detachment, inability to recall details of the events).

Criterion D: Negative alterations in cognition and moods: Worsening of thoughts and moods (persistent negative beliefs, feelings of alienation, constricted affect, diminished interest in activities) following the onset of PTSD.

Criterion E: Arousal: Alterations in arousal and reactivity (irritability, aggressive ehavior, hypervigilance, intense anxiety, difficulty concentrating) following the onset of PTSD.

Criterion F: Duration: Persistence of symptoms for more than 1 month.

Criterion G: Functional significance: Significant distress or functional impairment.

Criterion H: Exclusion: Exclusion of medication, substance abuse, or illness as a cause of psychological disturbance.

Men and women who serve in the military are at the highest risk for developing PTSD because they are more likely to be exposed to trauma and to experience more severe trauma than nonmilitary persons. Sources of trauma for military personnel include combat trauma, sexual trauma (sexual harassment, sexual assault), witnessing or participating in death and injury, and living in extreme conditions (exposure to heat or cold, radiation, infectious disease, or unsanitary conditions).

Additionally, times of transition within the military setting (beginning a deployment, returning from deployment, exiting active duty) may cause stress, which in turn may trigger PTSD. Individuals in these transition periods may need to be encouraged to undergo transition coaching, which is available to veterans and active-duty service members through the U.S. Veterans Administration (VA) system.

The effective treatment of PTSD in military personnel involves helping them to recognize the fear-related memories of the event that triggered their PTSD, incorporate new meanings for those memories, and develop stress management skills and mechanisms for coping with these memories. Standard methods of treatment for PTSD include cognitive behavioral therapy (CBT), cognitive processing therapy (CPT), group therapy, and eye-movement desensitization and reprocessing (EMDR). This last method involves the use of imagery and rapid eye movement to desensitize the individual with PTSD through prolonged exposure to stimuli. Medications can be used to stabilize and manage severe symptoms of PTSD. Persons with PTSD should be assessed to determine whether they may benefit from pharmacologic therapy: beta blocker drugs, antidepressants, and mood stabilizers can help ease panic attacks, sleep disruption, and severe symptoms of hyperarousal caused by PTSD.

FACTS AND FIGURES

The lifetime prevalence rate of PTSD among Americans who have not served in the military is 7.8 percent. From 2004 to 2012, the percentage of active-duty military personnel in whom PTSD was diagnosed rose from 1 percent to 5 percent. In 2012, 13.5 percent of members of the Army, 10 percent of members of the Marine Corps, 4 percent of members of the Navy, and 4 percent of members of the Air Force had PTSD at some point during the year. In that same year, approximately half a million armed forces veterans sought treatment for PTSD through the Veterans Health Administration (VHA). The increase in diagnoses of PTSD in United States military personnel is attributed to an increase in the number and duration of military deployments, the difficulty in modern military conflicts of distinguishing enemy combatants from civilians, and an increased likelihood of surviving combat wounds and injuries.

With combat, sexual assault is one of the two most commonly reported traumas among military personnel and veterans. In 2014, 4.3 percent of women on active military duty in the United States armed forces reported experiencing unwanted sexual contact; in the same period, the percentage of men on active duty reporting unwanted sexual contact was 0.9 percent. In 2012 the VA spent $3 billion and the Department of Defense (DOD) spent $294 million on the treatment of PTSD in military personnel.

RISK FACTORS

Factors that may increase the risk of a member or veteran of the United States armed forces developing chronic PTSD include exposure to trauma as a result of combat, personal injury, involvement in atrocities, and a perceived threat to life. Military personnel of non-white race, lower socioeconomic status, lower intelligence, or younger age, and those with a history of familial discord, behavioral problems in childhood, or psychopathology predating a traumatic experience are also at increased risk for PTSD. Active-duty personnel and veterans who have experienced a traumatic event are more likely to develop PTSD if they have a low level of social support, negative homecoming experiences, and poor coping skills. Military personnel who were victims of violence (terror attacks, childhood abuse, sexual assault, criminal acts) before a traumatic event are also at increased risk for PTSD.

SIGNS AND SYMPTOMS

Posttraumatic stress disorder is typically characterized by having combinations of a number of psychological, behavioral, physical, and social effects. Its psychological effects include negative thoughts and perceptions; hallucinations, delusions, nightmares, flashbacks, suicidal ideation, and exaggerated reactions to stimuli; symptoms of depression and anxiety; memory loss, especially regarding details of the traumatic event that triggered PTSD; trouble in concentrating; poor impulse control; and feelings of guilt or fear.

Behavioral effects of PTSD include issues with substance use; perpetration of intimate partner violence (IPV); sexual dysfunction; marital discord; the detachment from reality known as dissociation, demonstrated by attempts to avoid places, persons, thoughts, conversations, or activities associated with the causative traumatic event of PTSD; agitation; intense anger; and feelings of numbness.

Physical manifestations of PTSD can include dishevelment, poor personal hygiene; somatic complaints, including gastrointestinal disturbances, muscle aches, and headaches.

Social effects of PTSD include withdrawal; self-isolation; limited friendships; poor social support; reduced emotional intimacy; trouble in performing daily tasks (cleaning, grooming, cooking); and an impaired ability to work and reintegrate into society.

TREATMENT

It is important for social workers assisting military personnel and veterans to understand the language and structure of the military as well as service members' commitment to mission, honor, and sacrifice. Stigma is reported by both active-duty personnel and veterans as a major barrier to seeking treatment for problems in mental health such as PTSD. The fear of such stigma is based on the belief that seeking help or acknowledging the existence of a mental health condition will have a negative effect on such individuals' military evaluation, possible promotion in rank, or service record, or otherwise undermine the individual's military career.

For individuals experiencing symptoms that are common in PTSD, the social worker should conduct a complete biological, psychological, social, and spiritual assessment. This should include an assessment of the individual's personal, family, and spiritual beliefs; family history, family structure, and roles; military deployments; and the effect of reentry into the family and community after these deployments, as well as past exposure to violence, childhood trauma, substance use, and support systems. The social worker should also assess the individual's stress management skills and coping mechanisms, as well as the family and/or other support systems available to the individual, and should ask for permission to interview members of the individual's family and/or collateral sources. The social worker should also provide hotline information and emergency contacts to persons with PTSD for use during times of crisis.

Besides these considerations, veterans with PTSD often have a concurrent substance use disorder, especially with alcohol, and concurrent PTSD and alcohol misuse are associated with a significant increase in violence and aggression in veterans. Additionally, a high number of veterans with PTSD use cannabis or derivative products to control PTSD symptoms. Because of the high rate of substance use among persons with PTSD, it may be appropriate for military personnel and veterans to undergo drug testing as part of their treatment for PTSD.

When working with military personnel on active duty, social workers should be aware of military regulations regarding confidentiality and recognize that they may be a barrier to an individual's disclosure of traumatic events. Social workers are required to explain the limits on the confidentiality of the information that a member or veteran of the armed forces can disclose to a social worker or other therapist, and such persons must sign a "limits to confidentiality" document before treatment is begun. Before 1999, there was no patient–therapist confidentiality protection in the military setting. However, a presidential executive order issued in 1999, known as Military Rule of Evidence 513, established a privilege for members of the military to disclose confidential information to therapists, although it does not protect military members' rights as strongly as federal laws protect the legal rights of civilians in therapy.

The treatment of PTSD is based on the active discussion and exploration of the traumatic experience that caused it with the individual who has the condition. For persons who meet the criteria for acute or chronic PTSD, including hyperarousal in response to stimuli and symptoms of mood disorder, treatment typically involves trauma-focused interventions such as cognitive behavioral therapy (CBT), which has evolved to include education on stress response, breathing training, and the mental recounting of traumatic events in order to decrease the emotional response to them. The U.S. DOD currently considers CBT to be the standard of care for PTSD. Another treatment technique for PTSD is eye movement desensitization and reprocessing (EMDR), in which the patient is instructed to imagine a painful traumatic memory and experience the negative feelings associated with it, such as guilt or shame, while focusing visually on the therapist's rapidly moving forefinger. This technique has produced significant clinical improvements with only a few sessions of treatment, and may be better tolerated than other treatments by individuals who are resistant to recounting traumatic events. Stress-reduction techniques (relaxation, meditation, and exercise techniques) can also provide immediate reduction of symptoms in persons with PTSD.

An additional promising intervention for veterans with PTSD is mindfulness-based stress reduction (MBSR). This intervention involves 9 weekly sessions that include seated and walking meditations, yoga, body scans, and discussions of pain, stress, and mindfulness. Results indicate that MBSR produces significant reductions in symptoms of PTSD such as depression, anxiety, and suicidal ideation. Persons with PTDSD should be referred for a psychiatric evaluation to determine whether they may benefit from pharmacologic treatment with beta blocker medications (propranolol); specific serotonin reuptake inhibitors (SSIs) such as sertraline, fluoxetine; antianxiety agents (benzodiazepines); or antipsychotic drugs (risperidone).

Because it is typical for veterans to attend one or two sessions of treatment for PTSD and not return, social workers and clinicians must take the steps needed to ensure such persons' regular attendance and active engagement in the treatment process.

To assist persons with PTSD in coping with future stressors and trauma, they can be taught stress management skills and a relapse prevention plan. The social worker can link the individual with PTSD to resources and support groups as part of a relapse prevention plan. The social worker can also educate the family members of military personnel and veterans about the risk factors and signs of PTSD so that they are equipped to lend support and seek help for these if it is needed.

SERVICES AND RESOURCES

- U.S. Department of Veterans Affairs National Center for PTSD, http://www.ptsd.va.gov
- National Institute of Mental Health, http://www.nimh.nih.gov/health/topics/post-traumatic-stress-disorder-ptsd/index.shtml

Written by Nikole Seals, MSW, ACSW, and Jessica Therivel, LMSW-IPR

Reviewed by Lynn B. Cooper, D Crim, and Laura Gale, LCSW

REFERENCES

American Psychiatric Association. (2013). Panic Disorder. In *Diagnostic and statistical manual of mental disorders: DSM-5* (5th ed., pp. 481-589). Washington, DC: American Psychiatric Publishing.

Beder, J. (2011). Preface to special issue: Social work with the military: Current practice challenges and approaches to care. *Social Work in Health Care, 50*(1), 1-3. doi: 10.1080/00981389.2010.517011

Betthauser, K., Pilz, J., & Vollmer, L. (2015). Use and effects of cannabinoids in military veterans with posttraumatic stress disorder. *American Journal of Health-System Pharmacy, 72*(15), 1279-1284. doi: 10.2146/ajhp140523

Bramson, R., Brown, M. L., & Shurtz, S. (2015). Posttraumatic stress disorder. In F. J. Domino, R. A. Baldor, J. Golding, & J. A. Grimes (Eds.), *The 5-minute clinical consult 2016* (24th ed., pp. 892-893). Philadelphia, PA: Wolters Kluwer Health/ Lippincott Williams & Wilkins.

British Association of Social Workers. (2012). The code of ethics for social work: Statement of principles. Retrieved April 13, 2016, from http://cdn. basw.co.uk/upload/basw_112315-7.pdf

Chaumba, J., & Bride, B. E. (2010). Trauma experiences and posttraumatic stress disorder among women in the United States military. *Social Work in Mental Health, 8*(3), 280-303. doi: 10.1080/15332980903328557

Compton, K., & May, A. C. (2016). Posttraumatic stress disorder. In F. F. Ferri (Ed.), *2016 Ferri's clinical advisor: 5 Books in 1* (pp. 993-994). Philadelphia, PA: Elsevier Mosby.

Defraia, G. S., Lamb, G. O., Resnick, S. E., & McClure, T. D. (2014). Continuity of mental health care across military transitions. *Social Work in Mental Health, 12*(5/6), 523-543. doi: 10.1080/15332985.2013.870103

Department of Defense. (2015). Department of Defense annual report on sexual assault in the military: Fiscal year 2014. Retrieved April 13, 2016, from http://sapr.mil/public/docs/reports/ FY14_Annual/FY14_DoD_SAPRO_Annual_Report_on_Sexual_Assault.pdf

Elbogen, E., Johnson, S., Wagner, R., Sullivan, C., Taft, C., & Beckham, J. (2014). Violent behavior and posttraumatic stress disorder in US Iraq and Afghanistan veterans. *British Journal of Psychiatry, 204*(5), 368-375.

Friedman, M. J. (2013). PTSD history and overview. *U.S. Department of Veterans Affairs*. Retrieved April 13, 2016, from http://www.ptsd.va.gov/professional/PTSD-overview/ptsd-overview.asp

Fuehrlein, B., Ralevski, E., O'Brien, E., Serrita, J., Arias, A., & Petrakis, E. (2014). Characteristics and drinking patterns of veterans with alcohol dependence with and without post-traumatic stress disorder. *Addictive Behaviors, 39*(2), 374-378. doi: 10.1016/j.addbeh.2013.08.026

Halim, R., & Halim, H. (2015). Risk among combat veterans with post-traumatic stress disorder: The impact of psychosocial factors on the escalation of suicidal risk. *Archives of Neuropsychiatry, 52*(3), 263-266. doi: 10.5152/npa.2015.7592

Institute of Medicine. (2014). Treatment for post-traumatic stress disorder in military and veteran populations: Final assessment, executive summary. Retrieved from http://www.iom.edu/~/media/Files/Report percent20Files/2014/PTSD-II/PTSD-II-RB.pdf

International Federation of Social Workers. (2012). Statement of ethical principles. Retrieved April 13, 2016, from http://ifsw.org/policies/statement-of-ethical-principles/

National Association of Social Workers. (n.d.). Psychotherapist-patient privilege in the military. Retrieved April 13, 2016, from http://www.socialworkers.org/ldf/legal_issue/200507.asp?back=yes

National Association of Social Workers. (2008). Code of ethics. Retrieved April 13, 2016, from http://socialworkers.org/pubs/code/code.asp

National Association of Social Workers. (2012). NASW standards for social work practice with service members, veterans, and their families. Retrieved April 13, 2016, from http://www.social-workers.org/practice/military/documents/MilitaryStandards2012.pdf

National Association of Social Workers. (2015). Standards and indicators for cultural competence in social work practice. Retrieved April 13, 2016, from http://www.socialworkers.org/practice/standards/PRA-BRO-253150-CC-Standards.pdf

O'Malley, P. (2015). In veterans with PTSD, mindfulness-based group therapy reduced symptom severity. *ACP Journal Club, 163*(12), JC9. doi: 10.7326/ACPJC-2015-163-12-009

Polusny, M., Erbes, C., Thuras, P., Moran, A., Lamberty, G., Collins, R.,... Lim, K. (2015). Mindfulness-based stress reduction for posttraumatic stress disorder among veterans: A randomized clinical trial. *JAMA: Journal of the American Medical Association, 314*(5), 456-465. doi: 10.1001/jama.2015.8361

Sadock, B. J., Sadock, V. A., & Ruiz, P. (Eds.). (2015). Trauma and stressor related disorders. In *Kaplan & Sadock's comprehensive textbook of psychiatry* (11th ed., pp. 437-446). Philadelphia, PA: Wolters Kluwer Health/Lippincott Williams & Wilkins.

Solomon, Z., Bensimon, M., Greene, T., Horesh, D., & Ein-Dor, T. (2015). Loneliness trajectories: The role of posttraumatic symptoms and social support. *Journal of Loss and Trauma, 20*(1), 1-21. doi: 10.1080/15325024.2013.815055

Steenkamp, M., Litz, B., Hoge, C., & Marmar, C. (2015). Psychotherapy for military-related PTSD: A review of randomized clinical trials. *JAMA, 314*(5), 489-500. doi: 10.1001/jama.2015.8370

Walker, S. (2010). Assessing the mental health consequences of military combat in Iraq and Afghanistan: A literature review. *Journal of Psychiatric and Mental Health Nursing, 17*(9), 790-796. doi: 10.1111/j.1365-2850.2010.01603.x

Yarvis, J. S. (2011). A civilian social worker's guide to the treatment of war-induced PTSD. *Social Work in Health Care, 50*(1), 51-72. doi: 10.1080/00981389.2010.518856

POSTTRAUMATIC STRESS DISORDER: FEMALE MILITARY SERVICE PERSONNEL

MAJOR CATEGORIES: Military & Veterans

DESCRIPTION

Posttraumatic stress disorder (PTSD), as defined by the *Diagnostic and Statistical Manual of Mental Disorders,* Fifth Edition (*DSM-5*), can occur when an individual has experienced or witnessed a traumatic event, learned of a traumatic event happening to a close family member or friend, or experiences repeated or extreme exposure to the details of the event. The event needs to involve actual or threatened death or serious injury or involve a perceived threat to the physical safety of the affected individual or others.

Women now make up close to 15 percent of active-duty forces in the U.S. military. Female servicemembers and veterans who have experienced combat often encounter physically and psychologically traumatic situations and as a result are at risk for developing PTSD. In addition to combat-related trauma, female military personnel are at significant risk for military sexual trauma (MST). MST is a term that is defined by the U.S. Department of Veterans Affairs (VA) as "sexual harassment that is threatening in character or physical assault of a sexual nature that occurred while the victim was in the military, regardless of geographic location of the trauma, gender of the victim, or the relationship to the perpetrator." MST encompasses both the harassment/assault as well as the trauma associated with the assault. Exacerbating such experiences is the fact that a female in the military cannot always easily transfer to another duty station or quit, so she may be subject to repeated interactions or casual contact with the perpetrator.

Female military service personnel and veterans have a higher rate of premilitary stressors and traumatic life experiences than nonmilitary women. Females in the military have very high rates of nonmilitary service–related trauma, including sexual assault, childhood abuse, adult abuse, and intimate partner violence (IPV). Researchers have found that many women join the military to escape violent or traumatic home situations. This nonmilitary service–related trauma can lead to an increased risk for PTSD. In addition, because females are underrepresented in the military, the unit cohesion that is present as a social support for male soldiers may be absent.

FACTS AND FIGURES

Demand by veterans for treatment for PTSD has greatly increased in the last 10 years. Veterans Affairs records indicate that 155,704 veterans were treated for PTSD in 1998; by 2008 this number had grown to 438,248. Prevalence estimates of PTSD in veterans of current foreign wars range from 12 to 24 percent. Individuals with PTSD frequently also abuse alcohol and other substances: it is estimated that 35 to 50 percent of those in whom a substance use disorder has

been diagnosed also have a diagnosis of PTSD. These individuals also often have more severe drug use and worse outcomes than patients without PTSD. Many more veterans receive a diagnosis of PTSD than receive treatment: VA and Department of Defense (DOD) data show that only about half of veterans in whom the disorder is diagnosed receive treatment. Female veterans also contend with a lower diagnosis rate than male veterans. Results from a study indicate that 59 percent of males received a diagnosis whereas 62.7 percent met the criteria for diagnosis of PTSD; female veterans had a 19.8 percent diagnosis rate whereas 40.1 percent met the criteria.

Studies have reported conflicting findings with respect to differences in risk for PTSD between males and females. A systematic review identified seven studies that found servicewomen postdeployment at a higher risk for PTSD than servicemen, four studies with servicewomen at a decreased risk, and seven studies in which no gender difference was determined. A study of veterans found that female veterans were more likely to have internalizing symptoms related to concentration and distress from reminders of the traumatic events. Male veterans were more likely to have externalizing symptoms including nightmares, hypervigilance, and emotional numbing. Researchers in a study found that women veterans who had been exposed to combat reported higher levels of PTSD, depression, and alcohol misuse than women veterans who had not been exposed to combat.

RISK FACTORS

Factors that may increase the risk for PTSD in female military personnel and veterans include combat experience; long deployments; multiple deployments; having been wounded; having witnessed death; service on graves registration duty; being tortured or captured by the enemy; exposure to stress that is unpredictable and uncontrollable; poor social support; poor family support; MST; previous lifetime traumas history of physical or sexual abuse in childhood or adulthood); mild traumatic brain injury (TBI); and alcohol dependence and/or substance use. Meta-analysis has shown that lack of social support may be the primary risk factor for developing PTSD. The symptoms of PTSD have a negative effect on relationships, which serves to reduce the social support that is needed to combat the PTSD. Female servicemembers who have been sexually assaulted in the military have a 9 times greater chance of developing PTSD. Being a member of a particular racial or ethnic group has not been determined to increase one's vulnerability to developing PTSD; although rates of PTSD differ across racial and ethnic groups, it is not clear whether these differences stem from greater exposure to traumatic stress, from sociodemographic factors, or from true ethnic vulnerability. This finding was supported in a study of female veterans that found more similarities than differences with respect to rates of PTSD between Caucasian, Hispanic, and African American subjects.

SIGNS AND SYMPTOMS

Psychological symptoms include anxiety, depression, anger, emotional detachment, numbing, hallucinations, dissociative episodes, and restricted range of affect.

Behavioral problems include sleep disturbances (trouble falling asleep, trouble staying asleep, nightmares), alcohol or substance use, excessive smoking, not exercising, aggression, overeating, decreased appetite and dietary intake, avoidance behaviors, physical abuse of partner or children, diminished interest in activities that were normally of interest, and increased risk taking behaviors.

Sexual symptoms include decreased interest in sexual activity or increased interest in sexual activity.

Physical problems involve increased risk of diabetes, obesity, and heart disease; exaggerated startle reflex; trouble concentrating; elevated heart rate; elevated blood pressure; and elevated risk for premature mortality possibly due to medical conditions connected to poor health behaviors (smoking, drinking, obesity) but also from chronic stress.

Social problems may include marital or relationship distress, difficulty parenting, and isolation and withdrawal from family and friends.

ASSESSMENT

Professionals who are helping those with PTSD may perform any or all of the following assessments:

perform a complete bio-psycho-social-spiritual history to explore all potential symptoms or manifestations of PTSD, assess risk factors for PTSD, and/or assess and explore social and family functioning and measure available supports.

Professionals may also use screening tools such as Combat Exposure Scale (CES) (determines exposure to combative situations and enemy contact from light to heavy, which can provide information regarding risk for PTSD), PTSD Checklist—Military (PCL-M), Clinician-Administered PTSD Scale (CAPS), Beck Depression Inventory (BDI), Dissociative Experiences Scale (DES), Impact of Event Scale (IES), Traumatic Life Event Questionnaire (TLEQ), The State-Trait Anger Expression Inventory-2 (STAXI-2), The PTSD Symptom Scale Interview (PSS-1), The Mississippi Scale for Combat-Related PTSD, and/or The Inventory of Psychosocial Functioning (IPF) (specific to active-duty military personnel and veterans).

Professionals may also perform laboratory testing for alcohol and illegal drug use or an MRI or CT scan to determine if a TBI is a comorbidity that may be indicated depending on symptom clusters.

TREATMENT

Accurate assessment of PTSD is important to correctly guide treatment. Having an accurate assessment will improve treatment planning and also help with determination of disability. Treatment for PTSD will most likely involve counseling and/or medication. The most common therapeutic intervention for the treatment of PTSD is one of the variations of cognitive behavioral therapy (CBT), specifically cognitive processing therapy (CPT), prolonged exposure therapy (PE), or imagery rehearsal (IR), which can be provided to individuals or groups. In group-based work, participants work towards a common goal, which is an experience familiar to them from military culture. Some clinicians who specialize in trauma work and have the appropriate training may also use an intervention called eye movement desensitization and reprocessing (EMDR). All of the therapeutic interventions are goal-oriented, active, engaging, and skill-based. The most commonly prescribed medications for treatment are the selective serotonin reuptake inhibitors (SSRIs).

CPT can work for people who are feeling stuck in memories or recurrent thoughts related to the trauma. CPT focuses on learning about symptoms, becoming aware of thoughts and feelings, learning skills to challenge these thoughts and feelings (cognitive restructuring), and understanding how trauma typically affects one's beliefs.

PE therapy helps to address the avoidance symptoms and behaviors that the person may be utilizing. Repeating exposure to the thoughts, situations, and emotions that the person has been avoiding can help them learn that these reminders do not have to be avoided. PE has four main parts: (1) education on symptoms and how treatment can provide symptom relief, (2) breathing retraining to assist with relaxation and decrease distress, (3) real-world rehearsals (in vivo exposure) in a safe environment to reduce emotional distress in avoidance situations, and (4) imaginal exposure (talking through the trauma) to regain control over emotions and cognitions.

In IR, the person takes an image or nightmare related to the trauma and actively works on changing the image or nightmare so it is less upsetting and then mentally rehearses the changed image or nightmare. Elements of psychoeducation and muscle relaxation are included as well.

EMDR has the person focus on hand movements or tapping motions while she relays information about the traumatic memories. The rapid eye movements have been found to help the brain process the memories. Over time, the person will change her reaction to the memories and learn relaxation strategies. EMDR has four main parts: (1) identifying a specific targeted memory, belief, or image related to the trauma, (2) desensitizing and reprocessing, which is the process of the eye movements, (3) learning how to replace negative images with positive images and thoughts, and (4) learning how to complete a body scan: she will look for areas of tension or unusual sensations to identify any additional areas that need to be addressed.

Yoga has emerged as a potential treatment for symptoms of hyperarousal (anger, sleep problems). In a study in which participants attended yoga sessions researchers found a significant decrease in hyperarousal symptoms. Results from a similar study of veterans with PTSD who had participated in yoga and meditation sessions for 8 to 12 weeks indicated statistically significant reduction of stress, anxiety, and depression as well as improvements in quality of sleep, social functioning, and spiritual well-being.

Many veterans with PTSD do not receive the treatment they need because of barriers such as stigma related to going to a mental health treatment facility, time constraints, and lack of transportation. To reduce barriers for veterans with PTSD, the VA is implementing a telephone-based collaborative care model, which utilizes care teams consisting of nurse care managers, pharmacists, psychologists, and psychiatrists who provide care by phone or videoconference. The nurses manage care, the pharmacists review medication histories, the psychologists deliver CPT via interactive video, and the psychiatrists supervise the team and provide consultations. Initial results from studies of this new model indicate that it is effective in reducing PTSD symptoms and in providing care for veterans who would not otherwise have sought treatment.

Professionals who work with female military service personnel or veterans need to understand the unique features of military culture for female veterans in order to appropriately refer for any follow-up care. They may also need to educate the person and families about PTSD, including the need for good self-care to reduce symptoms and negative side effects, refer to specialized PTSD programs and clinicians as appropriate, encourage person to join a PTSD support group (preferably a military-supported group), encourage evaluation by physician and/or psychiatrist to address physical symptoms (sleep disturbances, shortness of breath, tension), advocate as needed with the VA or Social Security Administration for benefits or services, and safeguard confidentiality and privacy and maintain awareness of what impact releasing records can have on the woman's military service record and military career.

Problem	Goal	Intervention
Person is exhibiting signs and symptoms of PTSD.	Person will have relief from PTSD symptoms and return to baseline functioning.	Review assessments and tools to learn where symptoms are clustering and in what areas the person is experiencing the most distress. Evaluate for drug or alcohol use that may be exacerbating symptoms. Evaluate available supports and enlist as appropriate. Begin therapeutic intervention (CPT, PE, EMDR) or refer to outside mental health resource. Refer for group support if appropriate and if the person is receptive.
Person is experiencing high levels of anger and increased potential to be violent.	Decrease anger and violent impulses. Improve safety for person and family and social supports.	Screen for IPV risk or perpetration. Address any physical aggression and what the triggers are. Work on behavioral interventions and breathing exercises to help reduce anger and violent impulses. Show how repeated stress due to violence will destabilize the family. Establish a safety plan.
Person has disclosed that she experienced sexual trauma in the military and is now exhibiting signs and symptoms of PTSD.	Person will have a reduction in symptoms and feel empowered and more in control of her personal safety.	Utilize CBT to work on symptom reduction. Access a self-defense or personal safety empowerment intervention that will reduce feelings of fear and help her feel she is in control of her personal safety and will not suffer a sexual trauma again.
Person's family is experiencing negative symptoms such as stress, family discord, anxiety, and depression as a result of the patient's PTSD.	Reduce negative symptoms and improve family coping and family support.	Address numbing and avoidance behaviors that create the most conflict with relationships and family functioning. Encourage the woman to be more expressive and regain emotional intimacy with her partner and/or family. Reduce self-isolation from family members and friends by breaking cycle of avoidance and withdrawal. If the woman has been away for a long period, educate on the age-appropriate needs of and discipline for her children. Encourage positive parent-child interactions.

APPLICABLE LAWS AND REGULATIONS

PTSD has been used in the criminal justice system as an insanity defense and stress from exposure to combat has been allowed in consideration for sentencing.

The U.S. Supreme Court has officially recognized the need for defendants' military service including mental health issues to be taken under consideration in capital cases.

Since 2008, many states have established veterans' treatment courts to serve criminal defendants who are veterans and have mental health and/or substance use issues. These dockets usually involve a combination of biweekly court appearances, random drug/alcohol testing, and mandatory treatment/counseling sessions. State legislation is required to establish these courts; many state legislators have specifically named PTSD as the rationale for the veterans-only docket and treatment model.

The VA and the DOD have set forth clinical practice guidelines for psychosocial rehabilitation of veterans (job training, social skills training, self-care, education, employment, psychoeducation, peer counseling, and intensive case management). These include the following:

- The safety of the veteran is paramount.
- The veteran should have a discharge plan that includes a plan for safe, stable housing.
- The veteran should have an option of work or another productive activity.
- The veteran and family should be educated about his or her disorders and provided with resources, including referral to support groups.
- The veteran should be assigned a case manager if needed.
- The veteran should receive job skills training.
- The veteran must be assigned to a primary care team in either a medical or mental health setting.
- The veteran must have access to psychiatrists, psychologists, social workers, and/or nurses as needed.

Professionals need to be aware of military regulations regarding confidentiality when providing mental health services to active-duty personnel and recognize that these limits may be a barrier to disclosure of traumatic events. Before President Clinton's executive order in1999, there was no patient-therapist confidentiality protection in the military setting. Military Rules of Evidence, Rule 513 (MRE 513), does not protect rights as strongly as federal laws for civilians do, however. If the professional is court-ordered to reveal information, he or she may ask the judge to include a protective order to admit only portions of the records, not the records in their entirety, and to seal the record of the hearing in order to safeguard privacy. Under MRE 513, there are several exceptions to confidentiality: Deceased patient; evidence of spousal abuse or child abuse; mandatory reporting under federal, state, or military law; danger to any person, including the patient; fraud committed by the patient; a constitutional requirement (the accused's right to due process may be weighed against the accuser's right to privacy); or the need to ensure the safety and security of military personnel, military dependents, military property, classified information, or the accomplishment of a military mission. This military mission inclusion is considered a grey area: it gives the military great leeway in requesting records.

SERVICES AND RESOURCES

The VA maintains the National Center for PTSD, which is a vast source of information for patients and professionals, http://www.ptsd.va.gov

The VA also has a veterans' crisis hotline: 1-800-273-8255. This hotline connects veterans in crisis or their loved ones with a qualified responder through the Department of Veteran Affairs.

The VA has PTSD-specific treatment programs that include outpatient programs and intensive programs that may be inpatient or residential. PTSD specialists are available at VA medical centers.

Every VA medical center also has on staff a women veterans program manager to serve as an advocate and referral source.

Female-specific programs and treatments include women's stress disorder treatment teams; outpatient mental health programs with a primary focus on PTSD and other issues related to experienced trauma; specialized inpatient and residential programs for female veterans who require more intensive support; and women's comprehensive health centers, which are female-specific VA health centers located in some VAs that often provide outpatient mental health services.

The National Alliance on Mental Illness (NAMI) has a veterans resource center with resources on PTSD, treatments, programs, news and media reports, and online discussion forums, http://www.nami.org/template.cfm?section=ptsd

FOOD FOR THOUGHT

In 2009, a jury in Oregon found a defendant who had killed an unarmed man guilty but legally insane due to PTSD. The defendant was being treated for service-connected PTSD; he faced a 25-year prison sentence but instead was committed to a psychiatric hospital.

Some police departments are training their crisis response teams in management of suspects who have PTSD (hostage situations in which the hostage-taker is a veteran with PTSD).

Veterans with PTSD and mild traumatic brain injuries (TBI) have an increased risk for suicide only if the PTSD symptoms are severe. Having a mild TBI and mild PTSD symptoms does not increase risk for suicide.

Accidental motor vehicle death rates may be higher among veterans because of an increase in high-risk behaviors (not using seatbelts, driving while intoxicated).

A new area of research is using personal safety training or self-defense training to empower female veterans who have been traumatized sexually and who have PTSD. This is in effect a behavior therapy technique that shows promise but needs further testing and evaluation.

Women serving in Iraq or Afghanistan are more likely to be unmarried and poorer than their male counterparts. The combination of less social support and increased financial stress can increase the risk of PTSD.

Seeking Safety is a CBT-based group intervention for women with PTSD and a co-occurring substance use disorder that has had successful outcomes.

Partners and family members living with veterans with PTSD can experience emotional strain, intimacy problems (for partners), and low satisfaction with life. It is important to include partners and family members in PTSD treatment if they are willing and able to address the social support relationships.

RED FLAGS

Suicide is the third leading cause of death among members of the military currently serving in combat zones, with suicide rates among active-duty personnel at record highs.

In one study, veterans with PTSD were found to have a higher incidence of IPV perpetration than veterans who do not have PTSD. Fifty-three percent of the veterans in the study identified at least one physically aggressive act they had perpetrated in the previous 4 months. Sixty percent of veterans who had current or recent partners reported mild-to-moderate IPV perpetration some time in the past 6 months.

If a person is in crisis (suicidal ideation, ongoing trauma), the crisis problems need to be resolved before beginning any type of CBT treatment.

Written by Jessica Therivel, LMSW-IPR, and Melissa Rosales Neff, MSW

Reviewed by Lynn B. Cooper, D Crim, and Laura Gale, LCSW

REFERENCES

American Psychiatric Association. (2013). Diagnostic and statistical manual of mental disorders. (5th ed.). Arlington, VA: American Psychiatric Publishing.

Barnes, S. M., Walter, K. H., & Chard, K. M. (2012). Does a history of mild traumatic brain injury increase suicide risk in veterans with PTSD? *Rehabilitation Psychology, 57*(1), 18-26. doi:10.1037/a0027007

Boden, M. T., Kimerling, R., Jacobs-Lentz, J., Bowman, D., Weaver, C., Carney, D.,... Trafton, J. A. (2012). Seeking safety treatment for male veterans with a substance use disorder and post-traumatic stress disorder symptomatology. *Addiction, 107*(3), 578-576. doi:10.1111/j.1360-0443.2011.03658.x

Buckley, T. C., Holohan, D., Greif, J. L., Bedard, M., & Suvak, M. (2004). Twenty-four hour ambulatory assessment of heart rate and blood pressure in chronic PTSD and non-PTSD veterans. *Journal of Traumatic Stress, 17*(2), 163-171.

Castro, F., Hayes, J. P., & Keane, T. M. (2011). Issues in assessment of PTSD in military personnel. In B. A. Moore & W. E. Penk (Eds.), *Treating PTSD in military personnel: A clinical handbook* (pp. 23-41). New York, NY: The Guilford Press.

C'de Baca, J., Castillo, D., & Qualls, C. (2012). Ethnic differences in symptoms among female veterans diagnosed with PTSD. *Journal of Traumatic Stress, 25*(3), 353-357. doi:10.1002/jts.21709

Clark, S., McGuire, J., & Blue-Howells, J. (2010). Development of veterans treatment courts: Local and legislative initiatives. *Drug Court Review, 7*(1), 171-208.

Crum-Cianflone, N. F., & Jacobson, I. (2014). Gender differences of postdeployment post-traumatic stress disorder among service members and veterans of the Iraq and Afghanistan conflicts. *Epidemiologic Reviews, 36*(1), 5-18. doi:10.1093/epirev/mxt005

David, D., Woodward, C., Esquenazi, J., & Mellman, T. A. (2004). Comparison of comorbid physical illnesses among veterans with PTSD and veterans with alcohol dependence. *Psychiatric Services, 55*(1), 82-85.

David, W. S., Simpson, T. L., & Cotton, A. J. (2006). Taking charge: A pilot curriculum of self-defense and personal safety training for female veterans with PTSD because of military sexual trauma. *Journal of Interpersonal Violence, 21*(4), 555-565.

Department of Defense. (2015). Active duty military personnel by service by rank/grade. Retrieved June 22, 2015, from https://www.dmdc.osd.mil/appj/dwp/dwp_reports.jsp

Department of Veterans Affairs (VA) Veterans Health Initiative. (2004, January). Military sexual trauma: independent study course. Retrieved June 22, 2015, from http://www.publichealth.va.gov/docs/vhi/military_sexual_trauma.pdf

Dobie, D. J., Kivlahan, D. R., Maynard, C., Bush, K. R., McFall, M., Epler, A. J., & Bradley, K. A. (2002). Screening for post-traumatic stress disorder in female Veterans Affairs patients: Validation of the PTSD checklist. *General Hospital Psychiatry, 24*(6), 367-374.

Drescher, K. D., Rosen, C. S., Burling, T. A., & Foy, D. W. (2003). Causes of death among male veterans who received residential treatment for PTSD. *Journal of Traumatic Stress, 16*(6), 535-543.

Elhai, J. D., Frueh, B. C., Gold, P. B., Hamner, M. B., & Gold, S. N. (2003). Posttraumatic stress, depression and dissociation as predictors of MMPI-2 Scale 8 scores in combat veterans with PTSD. *Journal of Trauma and Dissociation, 4*(1), 51-64.

Fiore, R., Nelson, R., & Tosti, E. (2014). The use of yoga, meditation, mantram, and mindfulness to enhance coping in veterans with PTSD. *Therapeutic Recreation Journal, 48*(4), 337-340.

Fontana, A., Rosenheck, R., & Desai, R. (2010). Female veterans of Iraq and Afghanistan seeking care from VA specialized PTSD programs comparison with male veterans and female war zone veterans of previous eras. *Journal of Women's Health, 19*(4), 751-757. doi:10.1089/jwh.2009.1389

Fortney, J., Pyne, J., Kimbrell, T., Hudson, T., Robinson, D., Schneider, R.,... Schnurr, P. (2015). Telemedicine-based collaborative care for post-traumatic stress disorder: a randomized clinical trial. *JAMA Psychiatry, 72*(1), 58-67. doi:10.1001/jamapsychiatry.2014.1575

Garcia, H. A., Finley, E. P., Lorber, W., & Jakupcak, M. (2011). A preliminary study of the association between traditional masculine behavior norms and PTSD symptoms in Iraq and Afghanistan veterans. *Psychology of Men and Masculinity, 12*(1), 55-63. doi:10.1037/a0020577

Gavloski, T., & Lyons, J. A. (2004). Psychological sequelae of combat violence: A review of the impact of PTSD on the veteran's family and possible interventions. *Aggression and Violent Behavior, 9*(5), 477-501.

Gerlock, A. A., Grimesey, J. L., Pisciotta, A. K., & Harel, O. (2011). Documentation of screening for perpetration of intimate partner violence in male veterans with PTSD. *American Journal of Nursing, 111*(11), 26-34. doi:10.1097/01.NAJ.0000407296.10524.d7

Harb, G. C., Cook, J. M., Gehrman, P. R., Gamble, G. M., & Ross, R. J. (2009). Post-traumatic stress disorder nightmares and sleep disturbance in Iraq war veterans: A feasible and promising treatment combination. *Post-traumatic stress disorder nightmares and sleep disturbance in Iraq war veterans: A feasible and promising treatment combination, 18*(5), 516-531.

Haskell, S. G., Gordon, K. S., Mattocks, K., Duggal, M., Erdos, J., Justice, A., & Brandt, C. A. (2010). Gender differences in rates of depression, PTSD, pain, obesity, and military sexual trauma among Connecticut war veterans of Iraq and Afghanistan. *Journal of Women's Health, 19*(2), 267-271. doi:10.1089/jwh.2008.1262

Hassija, C., Jakupcak, M., Maguen, S., & Shipherd, J. (2012). The influence of combat and interpersonal trauma on PTSD, depression, and alcohol misuse in U.S. Gulf War and OEF/OIF women veterans. *Journal of Traumatic Stress, 25*(2), 216-219. doi:10.1002/jts.21686

Hoerster, K., Jakupcak, M., Stephenson, K., Fickel, J., Simons, C., Hedeen, A.,... Felker, B. (2015). A pilot trial of telephone-based collaborative care management for PTSD among Iraq/Afghanistan war veterans. *Telemedicine Journal and E-Health, 21*(1), 42-47. doi:10.1089/tmj.2013.0337 I

nstitute of Medicine of the National Academies. (2012). Treatment for posttraumatic stress disorder in military and veteran populations:

Initial assessment. *Report Brief*, 1-3. International Federation of Social Workers. (2012, March 3). *Statement of ethical principles*. Retrieved June 22, 2015, from http://ifsw.org/policies/statement-of-ethical-principles

Katzman, M., Bleau, P., Blier, P., Chocca, P., & Van Ameringen, M. (2014). Canadian clinical practice guidelines for the management of anxiety, post-traumatic stress and obsessive-compulsive disorders. *BMS Psychiatry, 14*(Suppl 1).

Kelly, U. A., Skelton, K., Patel, M., & Bradley, B. (2011). More than military sexual trauma: Interpersonal violence, PTSD, and mental health in women veterans. *Research in Nursing & Health, 34*(6), 457-467. doi:10.1002/nur.20453

Keltner, N. L., & McGuinness, J. P. (2011). War-related psychiatric disorders in soldiers. N. L. Keltner, C. E. Bostrom, & T. M. McGuinness (Eds.), *Psychiatric nursing* (6th ed.). St. Louis, MO: Elsevier Mosby.

King, M. W., Street, A. E., Gradus, J. L., Vogt, D. S., & Resnick, P. A. (2013). Gender differences in posttraumatic stress symptoms among OEF/OIF veterans: An item response survey analysis. *Journal of Traumatic Stress, 26*(2), 175-183. doi:10.1002/jts.21802

Kirby, A. C., Hertzberg, B. P., Collie, C. F., Yeatss, B., Dennis, M. F., McDonald, S. D.,... Beckham, J. C. (2008). Smoking in help-seeking veterans with PTSD returning from Afghanistan and Iraq. *Addictive Behaviors, 33*(11), 1448-1453. doi:10.1016/j.addbeh.2008.05.007

Kuhn, E., Drescher, K., Ruzek, J., & Rosen, C. (2010). Aggressive and unsafe driving in male veterans receiving residential treatment for PTSD. *Journal of Traumatic Stress, 23*(3), 399-402. doi:10.1002/jts.20536

Laffaye, C., Cavella, S., Drescher, K., & Rosen, C. (2008). Relationships among PTSD symptoms, social support, and support source in veterans with chronic PTSD. *Journal of Traumatic Stress, 21*(4), 394-401. doi:10.1002/jts.20348

Lewis-Fernandez, R., Turse, N., Neria, Y., & Dohrenwend, B. P. (2008). Elevated rates of current PTSD among Hispanic veterans in the NVVRS: True prevalence of methodological artifact? *Journal of Traumatic Stress, 21*(2), 123-132. doi:10.1002/jts.20329

MacDonell, G., Thorsteinsson, E., Bhullar, N., & Donald, W. (2014). Psychological functioning of partners of Australian combat veterans: Contribution of veterans' PTSD symptoms and partners' caregiving distress. *Australian Psychologist, 49*(5), 305-312. doi:10.1111/ap.12069

McDevitt-Murphy, M. E. (2011). Significant other enhanced cognitive-behavioral therapy for PTSD and alcohol misuse in OEF/OIF veterans. *Professional Psychology, Research and Practice, 42*(1), 40-46.

Middleton, K., & Craig, C. D. (2012). A systematic literature review of PTSD among female veterans from 1990 to 2010. *Social Work in Mental Health, 10*(3), 233-352. doi:10.1080/15332985.2011.639929

Mizrahi, T., & Mayden, R. W. (2001). *NASW standards for cultural competence in social work practice.* Retrieved June 22, 2015, from http://www.socialworkers.org/practice/standards/NASWCultural-Standards.pdf

National Association of Social Workers. (n.d.). Psychotherapist-patient privilege in the military. In NASW. Retrieved June 22, 2015, from http://www.socialworkers.org/ldf/legal_issue/200507.asp?back=yes

National Center for PTSD, United States Department of Veterans Affairs. (2011, February). Understanding PTSD treatment. Retrieved from http://www.ptsd.va.gov/public/understanding_TX/booklet.pdf

Penk, W. E., Little, D., & Ainspan, N. (2011). Psychosocial rehabilitation. In B. A. Moore & W. E. Penk (Eds.), *Treating PTSD in military personnel: A clinical handbook* (pp. 173-194). New York, NY: The Guilford Press.

The Policy, Ethics, and Human Rights Committee, British Association of Social Workers. (2012, January). The Code of Ethics for Social Work: Statement of principles. Retrieved June 22, 2015, from http://cdn.basw.co.uk/upload/basw_112315-7.pdf

Ready, D. J., Sylvers, P., Worley, V., Butt, J., Mascaro, N., & Bradley, B. (2012). The impact of group-based exposure therapy on the PTSD and depression of 30 combat veterans. *Psychological Trauma: Theory, Research, Practice, & Policy, 4*(1), 84-93.

Staples, J. K., Hamilton, M. F., & Uddo, M. (2013). A yoga program for the symptoms of post-traumatic stress disorder in veterans. *Military Medicine, 178*(8), 854-860. doi:10.7205/MILMED-D-12-00536

Suris, A., Lind, L., Kashner, T. M., Borman, P. D., & Petty, F. (2004). Sexual assault in women veterans:

An examination of PTSD risk, health care utilization, and cost of care. *Psychosomatic Medicine, 66*(5).

Sutherland, R. J., Mott, J. M., Lanier, S. H., Williams, W., Ready, D. J.,... Teng, E. J. (2012). A pilot study of a 12-week model of group-based exposure therapy for veterans with PTSD. *Journal of Traumatic Stress, 25*(2), 150-156. doi:10.1002/jts.21679

Teten, A. L., Miller, L. A., Sanford, M. S., Petersen, N. J., Bailey, S. D., Collins, R. L.,... Kent, T. A. (2010). Characterizing aggression and its association to anger and hostility among male veterans with post-traumatic stress disorder. *Military Medicine, 175*(6), 405-410.

Warner, C., Warner, C., Appenzeller, G., & Hoge, C. (2013). Identifying and managing posttraumatic stress disorder. *American Family Physician, 88*(12), 827-834. Yambo, T., & Johnson, M. (2014). An integrative review of the mental health of partners of veterans with combat-related post-traumatic stress disorder. *Journal of the American Psychiatric Nurses Association, 20*(1), 31-41. doi:10.1177/1078390313516998

POVERTY IN THE UNITED STATES: PSYCHOSOCIAL EFFECTS ON ADULTS

MAJOR CATEGORIES: Behavioral & Mental Health

WHAT WE KNOW

The 2014 U.S. Census reported that 46.7 million persons in the United States are living in poverty and 13.5 percent of adults ages 18–64 were living in poverty in 2012.

The federal poverty level (FPL) for 2015is an annual household income of $15,930 for a family of two and $24,250 for a family of four. Poverty limits an individual's ability to meet basic human needs including food, adequate shelter, and healthcare, including mental health treatment. Impoverished adults often live in impoverished or rural communities, which tend to have fewer resources to alleviate the effects of poverty (e. g., charitable organizations, educational institutions, low-income housing, food banks, subsidized childcare). A 2011 study found that of impoverished adults living in urban areas 9.1 percent had completed less than a high school education compared with 16.5 percent of those living in rural areas.

Impoverished adults often have untreated physical and mental health conditions due to lack of financial resources, limited insurance, and the inability to access resources that promote a healthy lifestyle (e. g., preventive healthcare). Public health agencies and low-income health insurance plans are less likely than private insurers to provide oral healthcare. Poor dental health can lead to gum disease, tooth loss, heart disease, and lung infection and can further complicate diabetes.

Poverty has a strong relationship with mental illness (e. g., anxiety, depression). Impoverished adults have limited means to pay for mental health treatment and often live in impoverished or rural communities with inadequate mental health services (e. g., therapists, psychiatrists, public mental health clinics).

Obesity is more prevalent among poor adults than non-poor adults. Impoverished adults are less likely to be able to afford tools that promote weight management (e. g., fitness centers, healthy foods). A 2013 study indicated that having limited financial resources did not lead to a reduction in tobacco use. The subjects in the study would often choose tobacco products over food in times of limited financial resources. Tobacco use can cause heart disease, cancer, and lung disease.

The social conditions of poverty (e. g., financial strain, inability to meet basic needs, violent communities) can lead to psychological distress, including stress, anxiety, post-traumatic stress disorder (PTSD), and depression. High levels of stress and anxiety increase risk for depression. High levels of anxiety, stress, and depression together with minimal financial resources for mental healthcare can lead to substance abuse.

Impoverished adults are more likely to live in unsafe communities and experience high levels of danger, exposure to violence, and crime, which increases risk for developing PTSD. Persons living in poor communities are more likely to be victimized by repeated episodes of sexual assault than those living in communities whose residents have greater financial resources.

Adults with physical and mental disabilities make up one of the largest groups of impoverished persons in the United States. Disabled people often are unable to work. Federal benefit programs including Supplemental Security Income (SSI) and Social Security Disability Insurance (SSDI) do not provide enough financial assistance to bring an individual above the FPL.

Impoverished adults are more likely to be dissatisfied with their lives, marriages, and jobs than non-poor adults. This dissatisfaction is related to the inability to afford higher education, which leads to fewer work opportunities, greater familial financial dependence, and poor psychological health.

Young adults in poverty are more likely to be unable to experience an extended period of emerging adulthood (i. e., the period of development between the ages of 18 and 25). Impoverished families are unable to financially support young adults through college and emerging adulthood; instead, impoverished young adults must enter the workforce and take on adult responsibilities earlier than peers with greater financial resources. An extended period of emerging adulthood is beneficial to human development by allowing the young adult to explore career options and relationships without the pressure to make lifetime commitments. Increasing numbers of impoverished young black men are spending their emerging adulthood in prison, which limits future educational, occupational, and social opportunities.

The disadvantages of poverty (e. g., health problems, limited education, mental illness) make it difficult for an individual to exit poverty; children raised in poverty often become impoverished adults. Impoverished parents are more likely to raise children in single-parent households, to be unable financially to meet children's needs (e. g., food, clothing, shelter, education), and to live in unsafe communities. Impoverished parents are likely to experience high levels of stress, leading to less patience in parenting and greater use of physical punishment and violence against children.

WHAT CAN BE DONE

Learn about the psychosocial effects of poverty to accurately assess the client's personal characteristics, mental health needs, and immediate needs for food, clothing, shelter, and healthcare.

Become knowledgeable about the resources available in your community, including food banks, vocational assistance, mental health services, and emergency housing.

Poverty has a strong relationship with mental and physical health problems. Social workers should accurately assess clients to provide them with appropriate interventions and referrals for services to meet their mental and physical health needs.

Assist your clients to identify and capitalize on their strengths to help cope with challenges incurred as a result of poverty, including difficulty parenting, stress, unstable housing, and unemployment.

Treatment methodologies should reflect the cultural values, beliefs, and biases of the individual in need of care and treatment.

Written by Emma Tiffany-Malm, MSW

Reviewed by Jessica Therivel, LMSW-IPR. and
Melissa Rosales Neff, MSW

REFERENCES

Bennett, K. J., Probst, J. C., & Pumkam, C. (2011). Obesity among working age adults: The role of county-level persistent poverty in rural disparities. *Health & Place, 17*(5), 1174-1181.

Berzin, S. C., & De Marco, A. C. (2010). Understanding the impact of poverty on critical events in emerging adulthood. *Youth & Society, 42*(2), 278-300. doi:10.1177/0044118X09351909

Comfort, M. (2012)."It was basically college to us": Poverty, prison, and emerging adulthood. *Journal of Poverty, 16*(3), 308-322.

Duncan, G. J., Kalil, A., & Ziol-Guest, K. M. (2010). Early-childhood poverty and adult attainment, behavior, and health. *Child Development, 81*(1), 306-325. doi:10.1111/j.1467-8624.2009.01396. x

Edwards, J. B., Gomes, M., & Major, M. A. (2013). The charged economic environment: Its role in parental psychological distress and development of children, adolescents, and young adults. *Journal of Human Behavior in the Social Environment, 23*(2), 256-266. doi:10.1080/10911359.2013.747350

Ferdous, T., Cederholm, T., Kabir, Z. N., Hamadani, J. D., & Wahlin, A. (2010). Nutritional status and cognitive function in community-living rural

Bangladeshi older adults: Data from the Poverty and Health in Ageing Project. *Journal of the American Geriatrics Society, 58*(5), 919-924. doi:10.11 11/j.1532-5415.2010.02801. x

Frigerio, A., Costantino, E., Ceppi, E., & Barone, L. (2013). Adult attachment interviews of women from low-risk, poverty, and maltreatment risk samples: comparisons between hostile/helpless and traditional AAI coding systems. *Attachment & Human Development, 15*(4), 424-442. doi:10.1080/1 4616734.2013.797266

Hernandez, D. C., & Pressler, E. (2014). Accumulation of childhood poverty on young adult overweight or obese status: Race/ethnicity and gender disparities. *Journal of Epidemiology and Community Health, 68*(5), 478-484. doi:10.1136/ jech-2013-203062

International Federation of Social Workers. (2012, March 3). Statement of ethical principles. Retrieved January 27, 2015, from http://ifsw.org/ policies/statement-of-ethical-principles/

Kendig, S. M., Mattingly, M. J., & Bianchi, S. M. (2014). Childhood poverty and the transition to adulthood. *Family Relations, 63*(2), 271-286. doi:10.1111/fare.12061

Kim, J., Richardson, V., Park, B., & Park, M. (2013). A multilevel perspective on gender differences in the relationship between poverty status and depression among older adults in the United States. *Journal of Women & Aging, 25*(3), 207-226. doi:10.1 080/08952841.2013.795751

Klest, B. (2012). Childhood trauma, poverty, and adult victimization. *Psychological Trauma: Theory, Research, Practice, and Policy, 4*(3), 245-251. doi:10.1037/a0024468

Li, N., Pang, L., Chen, G., Song, X., Zhang, J., & Zheng, X. (2011). Risk factors for depression in older adults in Beijing. *Canadian Journal of Psychiatry, 56*(8), 466-473.

Lipman, E. L., Georgiades, K., & Boyle, M. H. (2011). Young adult outcomes of children born to teen mothers: Effects of being born during their teen or later years. *Journal of the American Academy of Child & Adolescent Psychiatry, 50*(3), 232-241. doi:10.1016/j.jaac.2010.12.007

Mallon, A. J., & Stevens, G. V. G. (2012). Children's well-being, adult poverty, and jobs-of-last-resort. *Journal of Children and Poverty, 18*(1), 55-80. doi:10. 1080/10796126.2012.657047

Manrique-Espinoza, B., Salinas-Rodriguez, A., Mojarro-Iniguez, M. G., Tellez-Rojo, M. M., Perez-Nunez, R., & Ventura-Alfaro, C. E. (2010). Tooth loss and dental healthcare coverage in older rural Mexican adults living in poverty. *Journal of the American Geriatrics Society, 58*(4), 804-805. doi:10.11 11/j.1532-5415.2010.02785. x

Wheeler, D. (2015). *NASW Standards and Indicators for Cultural Competence in Social Work Practice.* Retrieved February 23, 2016, from http://www. socialworkers.org/practice/standards/PRA-BRO-253150-CC-Standards.pdf

Najman, J. M., Hayatbakhsh, M. R., Clavarino, A., Bor, W., O'Callaghan, M. J., & Williams, G. M. (2010). Family poverty over the early life course and recurrent adolescent and young adult anxiety and depression: A longitudinal study. *American Journal of Public Health, 100*(9), 1719-1723. doi:10.2105/ AJPH.2009.180943

Palomar-Lever, J., & Victorio-Estrada, A. (2011). Personality and social psychology: Factors that influence emotional disturbance in adults living in extreme poverty. *Scandinavian Journal of Psychology, 53*(2), 158-164. doi:10.11 11/j.1467-9450.2011.00921. x

Peterson, L. E., & Litaker, D. G. (2010). County-level poverty is equally associated with unmet health care needs in rural and urban settings. *The Journal of Rural Health, 26*(4), 373-382. doi:10.11 11/j.1748-0361.2010.00309. x

Singh, P. N., Washburn, D., Yel, D., Kheam, T., & Job, J. S. (2013). Poverty does not limit tobacco consumption in Cambodia: Quantitative estimate of tobacco use under conditions of no income and adult malnutrition. *Asia-Pacific Journal of Public Health, 25*(5S), 75S-83S. doi:10.1177/1010539513486919

Soffer, M., McDonald, K. E., & Blanck, P. (2010). Poverty among adults with disabilities: Barriers to promoting asset accumulation in individual development accounts. *American Journal of Community Psychology, 46*(3-4), 376-385. doi:10.1007/ s10464-010-9355-4

Stransky, M. L., & Mattingly, M. J. (2011). Poverty and mental health during the transition to adulthood. Paper presented at the annual meeting of the American Sociological Association, Las Vegas, NV, August 2011.

Torres, J. M., & Wong, R. (2013). Childhood poverty and depressive symptoms for older adults in Mexico: A life-course analysis. *Journal of Cross-Cultural Gerontology, 28*(3), 317-337. doi:10.1007/s10823-013-9198-1

Number in poverty and poverty rate: 1959 to 2014. (n. d.). *United States Census Bureau.* Retrieved October 23, 2015, from https://www.census.gov/hhes/www/poverty/data/incpovhlth/2014/figure4.pdf

British Association of Social Workers. (2012, January). The code of ethics for social work: Statement of principles. Retrieved March 15, 2016, from http://cdn. basw.co.uk/upload/basw_112315-7.pdf

(2015). 2015 HHS Poverty Guidelines. *U.S. Department of Health and Human Services.* Retrieved November 16, 2015, from http://aspe. hhs.gov/2015-poverty-guidelines

Wells, N. M., Evans, G. W., Beavis, A., & Ong, A. D. (2010). Early childhood poverty, cumulative risk exposure, and body mass index trajectories through young adulthood. *American Journal of Public Health, 100*(12), 2507-2512. doi:10.2105/AJPH.2009.184291

United States Census Bureau. (n. d.). Income and poverty in the United States: 2014. Retrieved November 16, 2015, from https://www.census.gov/content/dam/Census/library/publications/2015/demo/p60-252.pdf

POVERTY IN THE UNITED STATES: PSYCHOSOCIAL ISSUES FOR CHILDREN

MAJOR CATEGORIES: Behavioral & Mental Health; Community

WHAT WE KNOW

The federal poverty level (FPL) for 2013 was an annual household income of $15,730 for a family of two and $23,550 for a family of four. In 2013 19.9 percent of children in the United States were living in poverty. Black children had a poverty rate of 36.9 percent in 2013; Hispanic children, 30.4 percent; and non-Hispanic white children, 10.7 percent. The poverty rate for children living in single-mother households in 2013 was 45.8 percent; in married-couple households, 9.5 percent.

Children in poverty are more likely to experience impoverished neighborhoods, family conflict, food insecurity, low-quality education, and financial stress than children not living in poverty are. Impoverished neighborhoods have higher crime rates, limited public resources (e. g., libraries, schools, parks), lower-quality schools, and more convenience stores than groceries, limiting access to nutritious foods. They are exposed more often than other children to high levels of family conflict and instability at home, including parental stress, absence of adult supervision, teen mothers, intimate partner violence (IPV), single parents, forceful discipline, and physical punishment.

Impoverished families have little disposable income, which limits access to resources, including education, childcare, housing, food, healthcare, and mental health services. Children living in poverty often are expected to take on adult roles (e. g., paying household bills, caring for younger siblings) earlier than peers not living in poverty.

The social conditions of poverty (e. g., impoverished neighborhoods, low-quality education, family conflict, limited healthcare, poor nutrition) adversely affect childhood health, which can lead to significant health problems and conditions in adulthood, including weakened immune systems, obesity, heart disease, poor dental health, and diabetes.

Children who live in poverty have limited access to preventive healthcare as a result of the absence of health services in poor neighborhoods, limited financial resources, and inadequate health insurance coverage.

As a result of poor nutrition, obesity is prevalent among children who live in poverty. Childhood obesity can lead to chronic health conditions in adulthood (e. g., diabetes, heart disease).

Female children in poverty are more likely than male children to experience prolonged obesity from childhood through young adulthood.

Children in impoverished neighborhoods are less likely to have safe outdoor recreation areas and have less adult supervision as a result of parents working long hours. Risk for obesity decreases in neighborhoods in which children have access to play outdoors and among children who receive adult supervision.

Many children living in poverty are unable to afford or access dental care (e. g., because they do not have dental insurance or they have difficulty finding a dentist who will accept Medicaid). Dental health is negatively affected by improper diet and the inability to afford nutritious food. Unmet dental needs can lead to increased vulnerability to tooth loss, infection, and heart disease.

The social conditions of poverty, including impoverished neighborhoods, family conflict, poor nutrition, and limited healthcare, negatively affect the mental health of impoverished children.

Children living in poverty have more behavioral problems in school, lower cognitive functioning, and lower language and math comprehension than non-poor children do, which leads to lifetime disadvantages in education and work. These challenges arise from limited access to mental health services, exposure to violence at home or in the community, inadequate nutrition, parental absence due to long work hours, and low academic achievement of parents.

Black children living in poverty are more likely to be exposed to harsh discipline and physical punishment from parents than are white children living in poverty. Harsh discipline and physical punishment increase the risk of developing behavioral problems.

Poor communities often have underfunded and overcrowded schools that are unable to address the behavioral problems and individual educational needs of students.

Living in impoverished neighborhoods, exposure to violence, poor nutrition, and family conflict increase the risk that a child will develop mental health problems, including depression, anxiety, posttraumatic stress disorder (PTSD), attention deficit hyperactivity disorder (ADHD), and conduct disorder.

Children in poverty often experience chronic stress from unsafe neighborhoods, limited financial resources, and family conflict. Poor nutrition (e. g., high-sugar foods, caffeinated beverages) can further impair a child's ability to cope with stress, control impulses, and focus. Stress negatively affects a child's ability to concentrate and control impulses, which can lead to behavioral problems, conduct disorder, and ADHD.

Children living in poverty are more likely to be exposed to violence from parents and neighborhoods, leading to an increased risk of developing PTSD, exhibiting antisocial behavior, and engaging in delinquent or high risk activity (e. g., substance use, unprotected sex, absence from school).

The mental health problems of children who live in poverty often go untreated due to carers' inability to afford or access mental health services (e. g., no insurance, no services in the community). Untreated mental and behavioral health problems can lead to mental illness, substance abuse, and a propensity to commit crime.

The disadvantages of childhood poverty (e. g., mental health problems, cognitive impairments, low educational achievement, limited preventive healthcare) make it difficult to leave poverty; many impoverished children become impoverished adults. Limited access to preventive healthcare and mental health services impairs the physical and psychological development of children living in poverty. Physical and mental health problems negatively affect the ability to maintain stable employment as adults.

Children raised in poverty are less likely to graduate from high school and to attend college because of cognitive impairments, low academic achievement, and inability to afford higher education, leading to difficulty finding employment and poor job satisfaction.

Children living in poverty acquire adult responsibilities in the home (e. g., paying bills, caring for younger siblings) earlier than peers not living in poverty. This impairs their ability to attend school and explore career options, leading to unstable employment as adults.

WHAT CAN BE DONE

Learn about the psychosocial issues to which children in poverty are vulnerable (e. g., mental health problems, nutritional deficiencies, violent neighborhoods, family conflict) to accurately asses and treat the individual's health and mental health needs.

Share your knowledge about the psychosocial issues of childhood poverty with your colleagues.

Learn about community resources in your area, including mental health services, emergency shelters, food banks, subsidized childcare, educational programs, and public healthcare, so you can refer clients to appropriate resources.

Become knowledgeable about programs and services available through public health or community behavioral health agencies that offer early intervention strategies for low-income children and parents. Early intervention is the best tool for preventing lifetime consequences from childhood behavioral, health, and mental health problems.

Learn evidence-based interventions to improve outcomes of treatment. For example, a family-centered approach has been demonstrated to be more successful than a victim-perpetrator approach when working with impoverished families in the child welfare system.

Advocate for policies, legislation, and programs that can provide necessary services for impoverished children (e. g., free school lunches, vaccine education, mental health services in schools).

Treatment methodologies should reflect the cultural values, beliefs, and biases of the individual in need of care and treatment.

Written by Emma Tiffany-Malm, MSW

Reviewed by Laura Gale, LCSW, and
Chris Bates, MA, MSW

REFERENCES

Anthony, E. L., King, B., & Austin, M. J. (2011). Reducing child poverty by promoting child well-being: Identifying best practices in a time of great need. *Children and Youth Services Review, 33*(10), 1999-2009. doi:10.1016/j. childyouth.2011.05.029

Briceno, A. C. L., de Feyter, J. J., & Winsler, A. (2013). The school readiness of children born to low-income, adolescent Latinas in Miami. *American Journal of Orthopsychiatry, 83*(2, pt.3), 430-442. doi:10.1111/ajop.12021

Burchinal, M., McCartney, K., Steinberg, L., Crosnoe, R., Friedman, S. L., McLoyd, V., & Pianta, R. (2011). Examining the Black-White achievement gap among low-income children using the NICHD study of early child care and youth development. *Child Development, 82*(5), 1404-1420. doi:10.11 11/j.1467-8624.2011.01620. x

De Fonseca, M. A. (2012). The effects of poverty on children's development and oral health. *Pediatric Dentistry, 34*(1), 32-38.

Department of Health and Human Services. (2014). *Information on poverty and income statistics: A summary of 2014 current population survey data. ASPE Issue Brief.* Retrieved October 6, 2015, from http:// aspe. hhs.gov/report/information-poverty-and-income-statistics-summary-2014-current-population-survey-data

Dowd, J. B., Palermo, T. M., & Aiello, A. E. (2012). Family poverty is associated with cytomegalovirus antibody titers in U.S. children. *Health Psychology, 31*(1), 5-10. doi:10.1037/a0025337

Duncan, G. J., Kalil, A., & Ziol-Guest, K. M. (2010). Early-childhood poverty and adult attainment, behavior, and health. *Child Development, 81*(1), 306-325. doi:10.1111/j.1467-8624.2009.01396. x

Effects of poverty, hunger and homelessness on children and youth. (n. d.). *American Psychological Association.* Retrieved October 6, 2014, from https://www.apa.org/pi/families/poverty. aspx

American Psychological Association. (n. d.). Ethnic and racial minorities & socioeconomic status. Retrieved October 6, 2015, from http://www.apa.org/pi/ses/resources/publications/factsheet-erm. aspx

Fox, R. A., Mattek, R. J., & Gresl, B. L. (2013). Evaluation of a university-community partnership to provide home-based, mental health services for children from families living in poverty. *Community Mental Health Journal, 49*(5), 599-610. doi:10.1007/s10597-012-9545-7

Hernandez, D. C., & Pressler, E. (2014). Accumulation of childhood poverty on young adult overweight or obese status: race/ethnicity and gender disparities. *Journal of Epidemiology and Community Health, 68*(5), 478-484. doi:10.1136/jech-2013-203062

Holzer, H. J., Schanzenbach, D. W., Duncan, G. J., & Ludwig, J. (2008). The economic costs of childhood poverty in the United States. *Journal of Children and Poverty, 14*(1), 41-61. doi:1080/10796120701871280

Hotez, P. J. (2013). Pediatric tropical diseases and the world's children living in extreme poverty. *Journal of Applied Research on Children, 4*(2), 1-12.

International Federation of Social Workers. (2012, March). Statement of ethical principles. Retrieved January 15, 2015, from http://ifsw.org/policies/statement-of-ethical-principles/

Jarrett, R. L., Bahar, O. S., & Taylor, M. A. (2011)."Holler, run, be loud:" Strategies for promoting child physical activity in a low-income, African American neighborhood. *Journal of Family Psychology, 25*(6), 825-836. doi:10.1037/a0026195

Kaminski, J. W., Perou, R., Visser, S. N., Scott, K. G., Beckwith, L., Howard, J.,... Danielson, M. L. (2013). Behavioral and socioemotional outcomes through age 5 years of the legacy for children public health approach to improving developmental outcomes among children born into poverty. *American Journal of Public Health, 103*(6), 1058-1066. doi:10.2105/AJPH.2012.300996

Kendig, S. M., Mattingly, M. J., & Bianchi, S. M. (2014). Childhood poverty and the transition to adulthood. *Family Relations, 63*(2), 271-286. doi:10.1111/fare.12061

Leiner, M., Puertas, H., Caratachea, R., Avila, C., Atluru, A., Briones, D., & de Vargas, C. (2012). Children's mental and collective violence: a binational study on the United States-Mexico border. *Revista Panamericana De Salud Pública (Pan American Journal of Public Health), 31*(5), 411-416.

Loman, L. A., & Siegel, G. L. (2012). Effects of anti-poverty services under the differential response approach to child welfare. *Children and Youth Services Review, 34*(9), 1659-1666. doi:10.1016/j.childyouth.2012.04.023

Luby, J., Belden, A., Botteron, K., Marrus, N., Harms, M. P., Babb, C.,... Barch, D. (2013). The effects of poverty on childhood brain development: The mediating effects of caregiving and stressful life events. *JAMA Pediatrics, 167*(12), 1135-1142. doi:10.1001/jamapediatrics.2013.3139

Wheeler, D. (2015). *NASW standards for cultural competency in social work practice.* Retrieved March 3, 2015, from http://www.socialworkers.org/practice/standards/PRA-BRO-253150-CC-Standards.pdf

Purtell, K. M., & McLoyd, V. C. (2013). Parents' participation in a work-based anti-poverty program can enhance their children's future orientation: Understanding pathways of influence. *Journal of Youth and Adolescence, 42*(6), 777-791. doi:10.1007/s10964-012-9802-7

Rossen, L. M. (2014). Neighbourhood economic deprivation explains racial/ethnic disparities in overweight and obesity among children and adolescents in the USA. *Journal of Epidemiology & Community Health, 68*(2), 123-129. doi:10.1136/jech-2012-202245

British Association of Social Workers. (2012, January). The code of ethics for social work: Statement of principles. Retrieved October 11, 2015, from http://cdn. basw.co.uk/upload/basw_112315-7.pdf

United States Department of Helath and Human Services. (n. d.). *2013 HHS poverty guidelines.* Retrieved October 6, 2015, from http://www.aspe.hhs.gov/poverty/13poverty. cfm

Vernon-Feagans, L. (2013). VI. Discussion and implications for children living in rural poverty. *Monographs of the Society for Research in Child Development, 78*,5. doi:10.1111/mono.12052

Wadsworth, M. E., Raviv, T., Reinhard, C., Wolff, B., Santiago, C. D., & Einhorn, L. (2008). An indirect effects model of the association between poverty and child functioning: The role of children's poverty-related stress. *Journal of Loss and Trauma, 13*(2-3), 156-185.

Waldman, H. B., Cannella, D., & Perlman, S. P. (2012). Dentistry and childhood poverty in the United States. *The Journal of Clinical Pediatric Dentistry, 37*(1), 113-116.

PREGNANCY IN ADOLESCENCE: PREVENTION—BEYOND ABSTINENCE

MAJOR CATEGORIES: Adolescents

WHAT WE KNOW
In the United States, unplanned pregnancies account for almost half of all pregnancies and nearly a quarter of births. Most adolescents are not ready to take on the responsibilities of parenthood, and most who become pregnant are not actively choosing to become parents. In 2014, the adolescent birth rate was 24 births for every 1,000 adolescent girls, which is about a 9 percent decline from 2013 and a 61 percent decline since a peak in 1991. Declines in

adolescent birth rates ranging from 9 percent to 11 percent were reported for every racial and ethnic group.

A significant proportion of adolescents have intercourse. Males are more likely to be sexually experienced than females. Sexual activity increases with age.

Visits to primary healthcare providers are opportunities for those providers to address pregnancy prevention with adolescent girls. Investigators in Minnesota found that in a population of pregnant adolescents, these adolescents had a mean of 4.1 visits to a primary care provider in the 12 months before they became pregnant.

Adolescents who become mothers are at an increased risk for negative economic and social repercussions. These include the following:

- decreased likelihood of receiving a high school diploma or equivalent;
- decreased likelihood of going to and completing college;
- increased likelihood of living in poverty.

There are increased physical and social/environmental risks for children whose mothers were adolescents at the time of their birth versus children born to women who delayed having children until adulthood. These include increased risks for:

- premature birth;
- low birth weight;
- mental retardation;
- living in poverty;
- having absentee fathers;
- poor school performance;
- receiving welfare benefits;
- receiving substandard healthcare;
- receiving inadequate parenting; and
- being victims of abuse and neglect.

The choices adolescents make regarding contraception are based on available contraceptive options but also on attitudes, values, and beliefs that arise from their cultural, social, and economic circumstances.

Teen birth rates are higher in areas with a high degree of cultural cohesion and low literacy rates. Gender roles in communities of American Indians can increase risk of adolescent pregnancy because of the social pressure to be a young mother. Prevention programs in these communities should include redefining gender roles and norms by empowering adolescent girls to seek out contraception options.

Barriers to contraceptive use include the following:

- insufficient knowledge about contraceptives and the correct way to use them
- limited access to health services including transportation
- the high costs of care
- lack of health insurance
- concerns about confidentiality

Adolescents have named their parents as having the most influence over what decisions the adolescents make regarding sexual activity; therefore parental involvement is crucial. Peer influence also affects adolescents' decisions. Adolescents overestimate how sexually active their peers are while underestimating the negative consequences of sexual activity.

Parental involvement can have a strong positive influence on lowering teen birth rates, but there is less evidence that including parental involvement as a formalized part of a teen pregnancy prevention program has a positive effect. Programs that have allowed parental involvement and are abstinence-only have been found to be less effective than more comprehensive sexual education programs. Parental notification requirements related to consent for contraception can present a barrier for adolescents in accessing health services and deter them from pursuing care.

Most U.S. states have laws regarding the authority of minors to consent to contraceptive services. The District of Columbia and 26 other states allow minors over the age of 12 to consent to contraceptives. Twenty states allow consent for minors in certain categories (e. g., minors who are pregnant, married, or already a parent). Four states have no case law on contraception and minors.

The confidentiality of a minor's medical records related to contraceptive use is managed by the Health Insurance Portability and Accountability

Act (HIPAA). Normally a parent has access to a minor child's medical records except in the follow circumstances:

when the minor is the one who consents to the care and the consent of the parent is not required by that state or through other laws

when the minor receives the care at the direction of a court or court-appointed representative

when the parent has agreed that the minor and the provider can have a confidential relationship

Adolescent pregnancy prevention programs should focus on helping adolescents with their ability to receive and process information in order to make informed decisions about engaging in sexual activity. The Obama administration has focused on evidence-based programs and moved away from the strict abstinence-only programs that were prevalent from 1996 to 2009.

The Office of Adolescent Health (OAH), which is part of the Department of Health and Human Services, provides a list of the 28 evidence-based models it has found to be effective and thus appropriate for communities, school systems, and organizations to employ. Several are abstinence-only models, but many aim to increase use of contraceptives among adolescents.

Successful programs provide the following information:

Information about the benefits of abstinence

Information about condoms and other contraceptives

Information about early detection and prevention of sexually transmitted diseases (STDs)

Information on how to resist peer pressure

Information on how to improve communication with partners (e. g., how to say no, how to inform partner of boundaries).

An effective adolescent pregnancy prevention program will:

- convince adolescents not to have sex or, if they are having sex, persuade them to use contraception regularly and correctly;
- be of a sufficient length (i. e., longer than a few weeks);
- have leaders who are trained and believe in the program and its mission statement;

- be personalized to the participants by reflecting the culture, age, and sexual experience of the participants;
- address peer pressure and related issues; and
- enhance participants' communication skills.

WHAT CAN BE DONE
Learn about the prevention of adolescent pregnancy beyond abstinence so you can adequately advise and assist adolescents.

Develop community or school-based programs that will educate adolescents about abstinence but also provide strategies to reduce the risks involved with sexual activity.

For maximum success, programs should include the following:
- parental involvement to help foster self-esteem, improve the adolescents' interpersonal skills, and help with planning for the future through discussion and participation in the pregnancy prevention program;
- a peer component, with peers leading sections of the education and modeling appropriate choices;
- an empowerment aspect that helps the adolescents feel in control of their decisionmaking.

Look for any underlying social causes that may be leading to higher adolescent pregnancy rates.

Ensure that minor clients are aware of confidentiality and consent issues.

Lobby for adolescent pregnancy prevention programs in areas experiencing increases in teen birth rates and STDs.

Provide referrals to community health services.

Provide access to community supports.

Educate and encourage primary care providers to look for opportunities for pregnancy prevention during healthcare visits.

Treatment methodologies should reflect the cultural values, beliefs, and biases of the individual in need of care and treatment.

Written by Tricia Peneku, MS, PPS, and Jessica Therivel, LMSW-IPR

Reviewed by Chris Bates, MA, MSW, and Laura Gale, LCSW

REFERENCES

British Association of Social Workers. (2012, January). The code of ethics for social work: Statement of principles. Retrieved October 30, 2015, from http://cdn. basw.co.uk/upload/basw_112315-7.pdf

Furstenberg, F. (2007). *Destinies of the disadvantaged.* New York, NY: Russell Sage.

Manlove, J., Terry-Humen, E., Minicieli, L., & Moore, K. (2008). Kids having kids: Economic costs and social consequences of teen pregnancy. In S. Hoffman & R. Maynard (Eds.), *Kids having kids: Economic costs and social consequences of teen pregnancy* (2nd ed., pp.161-196). Washington, DC: Urban Institute Press.

Mizrahi, T., & Mayden, R. W. (2001). NASW standards for cultural competence in social work practice. Retrieved October 30, 2015, from http://www.socialworkers.org/practice/standards/NASWCulturalStandards.pdf

Sisson, G. (2012). Finding a way to offer something more: Reframing teen pregnancy prevention. *Sexuality Research and Social Policy, 9*(1), 57-69. doi:10.1007/s13178-011-0050-5

Solomon-Fears, C. (2013). Teenage pregnancy prevention: Statistics and programs. *Congressional Research Service (CRS) Report for Congress.* Retrieved from https://www.fas.org/sgp/crs/misc/RS20301.pdf

The National Campaign to Prevent Teen and Unplanned Pregnancy. (2001). *Halfway there: A prescription for continued progress in preventing teen pregnancy.* Washington, DC: The National Campaign to Prevent Teen Pregnancy. Retrieved October 30, 2015, from http://hivhealthclearinghouse. unesco.org/library/documents/halfway-there-prescription-continued-progress-preventing-teen-pregnancy

Statement of ethical principles. (2012, March 3). *International Federation of Social Workers.* Retrieved October 30, 2015, from http://ifsw.org/policies/statement-of-ethical-principles

Collins, L. R., Felderhoff, B. J., Kim, Y. K., Mengo, C., & Pillai, V. K. (2014). State-wise variation in teenage birth rates in the United States: Role of teenage birth prevention policies. *International Journal of Child and Adolescent Health, 7*(3), 239-248.

Guttmacher Institute. (2015, June 1). An overview of minors' consent law. Retrieved June 23, 2015, from http://www.guttmacher.org/statecenter/spibs/spib_OMCL.pdf

Hanson, J. D., McMahon, T. R., Griese, E. R., & Kenyon, D. B. (2014). Understanding gender roles in teen pregnancy prevention among American Indian youth. *American Journal of Health and Behavior, 38*(6), 807-815. doi:10.5993/AJHB.38.6.2

Kharbanda, E. O., Stuck, L., Molitor, B., & Nordin, J. D. (2014). Missed opportunities for pregnancy prevention among insured adolescents. *JAMA Pediatrics, 168*(12), e142809. doi:10.1001/jamapediatrics.2014.2809

Martin, J. A., Hamilton, B. E., Osterman, M. J. K., Curtin, S. C., & Matthews, T. J. (2015, January 15). Births: Final data for 2013. *National Vital Statistics Report, 64*(1). Retrieved from http://www.cdc.gov/nchs/data/nvsr/nvsr64/nvsr64_01.pdf

Silk, J., & Romero, D. (2014). The role of parents and families in teen pregnancy prevention: An analysis of programs and policies. *Journal of Family Issues, 35*(10), 1339-1362. doi:10.1177/0192513X13481330

National Campaign to Prevent Teen and Unplanned Pregnancy. (n. d.). National and state data. Retrieved October 30, 2015, from http://thenationalcampaign.org/data/landing

U.S. Department of Health and Human Services. (2006, March 14). Does the HIPAA Privacy Rule allow parents the right to see their children's medical records? Retrieved October 30, 2015, from http://www.hhs.gov/ocr/privacy/hipaa/faq/right_to_access_medical_records/227.html

PREGNANCY IN ADOLESCENCE: PREVENTION—EMERGENCY CONTRACEPTION

MAJOR CATEGORIES: Adolescence, Medical & Health

DESCRIPTION

Adolescent pregnancy and birth rates in the United States have decreased steadily since the early 1990s. Yet teen pregnancy remains an important medical, social, and public health issue; teenage pregnancy rates are much higher in the United States than in other industrialized countries, with approximately 900,000 adolescent females becoming pregnant each year. Failure to use contraceptives, or using them improperly or inconsistently, is the primary cause of teenage pregnancy. Emergency contraception decreases the risk of pregnancy following unprotected intercourse or contraceptive failure.

There are two methods of emergency contraception available, hormonal (emergency contraceptive pills [ECPs] that contain the progestin levonorgestrel, such as Plan B) and nonhormonal (such as the copper T intrauterine device, or IUD [ParaGard]). ECPs work by preventing or delaying ovulation and causing changes in the cervical mucus that make it more difficult for sperm to reach the ova. Side effects are rare but include nausea, vomiting, and spotting. There are no contraindications to providing ECPs other than an allergy to levonorgestrel, undiagnosed vaginal bleeding, or known pregnancy (because levonorgestrel can inhibit implantation by altering the endometrium). ECPs must be taken within 72 hours of contraception failure. Each packet of Plan B or Plan B One-Step contains a tablet of levonorgestrel, which when taken can reduce the risk for pregnancy by almost 95 percent. The sooner the pill is taken, the more effective the method. Plan B or Plan B One-Step may work in one of the following ways: preventing or delaying ovulation, interfering with fertilization of an egg, or preventing implantation of a fertilized egg in the uterus by altering the uterine lining. Plan B or Plan B One-Step is not the same as RU-486, which is an abortion pill. ECPs do not cause a miscarriage or abortion. They do not stop development of a fetus once the fertilized egg implants in the uterus and will not work if already pregnant when taken. Researchers have found that providing ECPs to adolescents in advance of sexual activity increases the likelihood of use without decreasing the use of other contraceptive methods or increasing the likelihood of sexual activity. Adolescents are twice as likely to use ECPs if they already have them in their possession; education alone is not enough to increase ECP use. Some clinicians believe that all female victims of sexual assault should be offered ECPs.

ParaGard, which many women use for regular birth control, may also be used for emergency contraception and is the most effective method for this purpose. It prevents 99 percent of pregnancies by creating an environment that is toxic to sperm. ParaGard is as effective as sterilization in preventing pregnancy. The most common side effects are heavier and more painful menses. IUDs are underused in adolescents because of fears that they may increase the risk of pelvic inflammatory disease (PID). Investigators have found that the risk of infection is related to the insertion procedure and not the device itself. Screening for and treating existing infections prior to insertion can reduce the risk of PID.

FACTS AND FIGURES

In the United States, the teen birth rate in 2013 was 273,105 births among girls ages 15 to 19, a 10-percent decrease from 2012 and a 57-percent decrease from its peak in 1991.

When adolescents use contraceptives, they often use them incorrectly (missed pills, condom breakage), resulting in method failure. One third of female adolescents taking oral contraceptives miss at least one pill a month, and many report missing three pills a month. Errors (missed pills) increase the failure rate from 0.3 percent to 8 percent; some studies estimate a failure rate as high as 25 percent in adolescents. The risk of pregnancy is greatest if pills are missed at the beginning or end of the nonplacebo portion of the pill cycle.

A survey showed that 84 percent of adolescents were not aware that pregnancy could be prevented after intercourse. Once they received information about emergency contraception, 87 percent of sexually active adolescents stated that they would consider using emergency contraception.

Investigators in a global study on contraception use in lower- and middle-income countries found a wide range of rates of contraceptive use, from 21 percent to 64 percent, in unmarried adolescents ages 15 to 19. They also reported that of the 16 million adolescents ages 15 to 19 worldwide who give birth each year, 95 percent are from lower- and middle-income countries.

RISK FACTORS

Risk factors for adolescent sexual activity and/or pregnancy include physical and sexual abuse, poverty, lack of parental supervision and/or support, early puberty, lack of knowledge, psychological factors, and lack of access to contraceptives.

Adolescents who live in families with little parental support, little restriction of risky behaviors, and poorly defined goals are more likely to become sexually active and are more likely to become adolescent parents.

Early physical maturation has widened the gap between reproductive capacity and cognitive and emotional maturation, increasing the risk of unintended pregnancy among adolescents.

Adolescents may believe that they cannot get pregnant in their first sexual encounter or that they are too young to become pregnant. Adolescents may lack information about available contraceptive methods and where to obtain contraceptives.

Psychological factors may also lead to risk factors. Adolescents may fear side effects of contraceptives, real or assumed, or be embarrassed to obtain contraceptives. They may be unable or unwilling to discuss contraceptive use with their partners, or their partners may refuse to use available methods.

Clinicians may not address sexuality and contraceptive use with adolescent patients, may be unwilling to prescribe contraceptives, or may be overtly judgmental about sexual activity among teens.

SIGNS AND SYMPTOMS

Adolescents who need emergency contraception may experience psychological symptoms such as anxiety, embarrassment, tearfulness, and/or guilt.

SOCIAL WORK ASSESSMENT

Professionals working with teens who may need emergency contraception should take a complete history through a bio-psycho-social-spiritual assessment with particular attention to the risk factors mentioned above.

Standardized urine tests may have been administered by a clinician to screen for pregnancy.

TREATMENT

A complete bio-psychsosocial-spiritual assessment is helpful to understand the extent and nature of risk factors. This is essential for careful diagnosis, appropriate case management, and successful treatment. Providers should use standardized screening tools, assessment instruments, and interview protocols that have been established for adolescents. It is important to consider the clinical risks versus benefits of contraceptives, as well as the adolescent's ability to use them consistently and correctly, motivation, cost, involvement of partner and/or parents, access, and confidentiality, and to explore possible barriers to access (health insurance, transportation, cost, emotional/psychological concerns) and provide referrals to reduce potential obstacles. Providers should be aware of whether school nurses in their area are able to administer emergency contraception and whether there are local pharmacies that provide free emergency contraception.

Professionals may also provide sex/contraception education, provide referrals to medical services, ensure appropriate education regarding risks of sexual activity and how to protect herself from unwanted pregnancy and sexually transmitted diseases (STDs), and ensure that the adolescent is aware of how to access emergency contraception.

Problem	Goal	Intervention
Adolescent is sexually active.	Reduce risk for unwanted pregnancy and need for emergency contraception.	Conduct a complete bio-psycho-social-spiritual history related to pregnancy risk factors. Determine need for contraceptives. Refer for medical evaluation/treatment.
Adolescent is demonstrating that she is at risk for unwanted pregnancy due to misinformation.	Ensure that adolescent has the correct information regarding pregnancy, STDs, and sexual intercourse.	Access the appropriate information and educational materials. Provide if appropriate.
Adolescent lacks parental supervision and support.	Increase parental involvement, supervision, and support.	With permission, involve parent(s) in discussion. Educate parent(s) on reality of adolescent's sexual activity and need for increased supervision and support.
Adolescent reports sexual or physical maltreatment.	Ensure that adolescent is in a safe environment and has resolution she desires regarding reporting the maltreatment.	Use active listening to encourage adolescent to share her story. Assess whether she wishes to pursue further action. Educate her on the professional's role as a mandated reporter since she is a minor and follow appropriate protocol regarding reporting of maltreatment. Assess current situation and ensure safety.
Adolescent lacks consistent access to contraception.	Adolescent will have access to contraception.	Determine why she cannot access contraception. Assist her in navigating barriers to access and obtaining needed contraception.
Adolescent is expressing emotional anxiety and concerns about using emergency contraception.	Reduce anxiety.	Provide education on emergency contraception. Assess source of anxiety (worry about side effects, religious beliefs about conception). Depending on source of anxiety, use therapeutic techniques to reduce anxiety.

APPLICABLE LAWS AND REGULATIONS

The age of consent (the age the law states that one is considered legally competent to agree to sex) varies from state to state, but typically is 16 to 18 years of age.

Each country has its own standards for cultural competency and diversity in social work practice. Social workers must be aware of the standards of practice set forth by their governing body (National Association of Social Workers, British Association of Social Workers) and practice accordingly.

Each state or nation may have its own regulations regarding mandated reporting of maltreatment of minors by social workers working with those minors. Each social worker needs to be aware of the laws and regulations in his or her region of practice.

SERVICES AND RESOURCES

- National Campaign to Prevent Teen and Unplanned Pregnancy, http://thenationalcampaign.org
- Planned Parenthood, www.plannedparenthood.org

FOOD FOR THOUGHT

Adolescents in the United States and Europe have comparable rates of sexual activity, but adolescents in Europe generally use contraceptives more often and use more effective methods than adolescents in the United States, resulting in lower pregnancy rates.

The American Academy of Pediatrics is in favor of prescribing emergency contraception to adolescents in advance of any immediate need to increase the likelihood that adolescents will use it.

Food and Drug Administration (FDA) approval for emergency contraception is now for all women of child-bearing potential without age limitations.

RED FLAGS

Physical and sexual abuse are potential issues with any adolescent and can be a risk factor for early sexual activity. The social worker should complete a thorough history to determine whether either type of abuse is a part of the adolescent's history.

Written by Tricia Peneku, MS, PPS, and Jessica Therivel, LMSW-IPR

Reviewed by Lynn B. Cooper, D Crim

REFERENCES

American Academy of Pediatrics. (2014). Contraception for adolescents. *Pediatrics, 134*(4), e.1244-e1256. doi:10.1542/peds.2014-2299

American Academy of Pediatrics, Committee on Adolescence. (2012). Emergency contraception. Retrieved August 18, 2015, from http://pediatrics.aappublications.org/content/130/6/1174

Chandra-Mouli, V., McCarraher, D. R., Phillips, S. J., Williamson, N..E., & Hainsworth, G. (2014). Contraception for adolescents in low and middle income countries: Needs, barriers, and access. *Reproductive Health, 11*(1), 1. doi:10.1186/742-4755-11-1

Dixon, V. (2014). Special considerations when providing contraception advice and information to young people. *British Journal of School Nursing, 9*(4), 170-175.

Duffy, K., Wimberly, Y., & Brooks, C. (2009). Adolescent contraceptive care for the practicing pediatrician. *Adolescent Medicine, 20*(1), 168-187.

Federal Drug Administration (FDA). (2013, June 20). FDA approves Plan B One-Step emergency contraceptive for use without a prescription for all women of child-bearing potential. Retrieved from http://www.fda.gov/NewsEvents/Newsroom/PressAnnouncements/ucm358082.htm

Gupta, N., Corrado, S., & Goldstein, M. (2008). Hormonal contraception for the adolescent. *Pediatrics in Review, 29*(11), 386-396. doi:10.1542/pir.29-11-386

Haynes, K. A. (2007). An update on emergency contraception use in adolescents. *Journal of Pediatric Nursing, 22*(3), 186-195. doi:10.1016/j.pedn.2006.08.004

Hoffman, S. D. (2008). Kids having Kids: Economic costs and social consequences of teen pregnancy. Washington, DC: The Urban Institute Press.

International Federation of Social Workers. (2012). Statement of Ethical Principles. Retrieved January 21, 2015, from http://ifsw.org/policies/statement-of-ethical-principles/

Kann, L., Kinchen, S., Shanklin, S. L., Flint, K. H., Hawkins, J., Harris, W. A.,... Zaza, S. (2014). Youth risk behavior surveillance—United States, 2013. *Morbidity and Mortality Weekly Report, 63*(4), 1-168.

Mizrahi, T., & Mayden, R. W. (2001). NASW standards for cultural competence in social work practice. Retrieved from http://www.socialworkers.org/practice/standards/NASWCulturalStandards.pdf

Sanfilippo, J. S., & Lara-Torre, E. (2009). Adolescent gynecology. *Obstetrics and Gynecology, 113*(4), 935-947. doi:10.1097/AOG.0b013e31819b6303

Santelli, J., Sandfort, T., & Orr, M. (2008). Transnational comparisons of adolescent contraceptive use: What can we learn from these comparisons?. *Archives of Pediatrics & Adolescent Medicine, 162*(1), 92-94. doi:10.1001/archpediatrics.2007.28

Waller, L., & Bryson, W. (2007). Can emergency contraception help to reduce teen pregnancy?. *Journal of the American Academy of Physician Assistants, 20*(6), 42-46.

Whitaker, A. K., & Gilliam, M. (2008). Contraceptive care for adolescents. *Clinical Obstetrics and Gynecology, 51*(2), 268-280. doi:10.1097/GRF.0b013e31816d713e

(2015). National birth rates for teens, aged 15-19. *National Campaign to Prevent Teen and Unplanned Pregnancy.* Retrieved from http://thenationalcampaign.org/data/landing

The code of ethics for social work: Statement of principles. (2012). *British Association of Social Workers.* Retrieved August 18, 2015, from http://cdn.basw.co.uk/upload/basw_112315-7.pdf

PREGNANCY IN ADOLESCENCE: PREVENTION—FEMALE USE OF CONTRACEPTION

MAJOR CATEGORIES: Adolescents

DESCRIPTION

Adolescent pregnancy and birth rates in the United States have decreased steadily since the early 1990s. Yet teen pregnancy remains an important medical, social, and public health issue; teenage pregnancy rates are much higher in the United States than in other industrialized countries. In 2010, there were 614,000 pregnancies among 15- to 19-year olds in the United States, a pregnancy rate of approximately 6 percent. Failure to use contraceptives during sexual activity, or using them improperly or inconsistently, is the primary cause of teenage pregnancy. Methods of contraception not requiring a prescription that may be used by female adolescents include withdrawal, the sponge, spermicides, and female condoms. Withdrawal is up to 74 percent effective in preventing pregnancy but is not effective in preventing sexually transmitted diseases (STDs), including HIV/AIDS. Male condoms used by the female adolescent's partner are effective in preventing pregnancy, are the only method that offers protection against most STDs, and are inexpensive and easy to obtain. Proper use of condoms is required for them to be effective, however; in addition, they may decrease sensation, and cooperation by the male partner is required for the use of a condom. Methods of contraception that require a prescription are oral contraceptive pills, hormone-releasing transdermal patches, hormone-releasing vaginal rings, hormonal injections, hormone-releasing implants, cervical caps, diaphragms, and intrauterine devices (IUDs).

FACTS AND FIGURES

In the United States, there were 273,105 births in 2013 among girls ages 15 to 19, a decrease of 10 percent from 2012 and 57 percent from 1991, the year in which the highest number of births to adolescents was recorded.

Investigators for a global study on contraceptive use in low- and middle-income countries found a wide range of rates of use among 15- to 19-year-olds, from 21 percent to 64 percent. They also reported that 16 million 15- to 19-year-olds give birth each year, 95 percent of whom are from low- and middle-income countries.

More than half of all female adolescents using contraception choose oral contraceptive pills (OCPs), which are 99 percent effective in preventing pregnancy.

Approximately 62 percent of adolescent females continue to use the transdermal patch at 3 months, with 87 percent reporting perfect compliance.

The vaginal ring (NuvaRing) is a form of combined hormonal contraception; it is placed in the vagina, where it slowly releases hormones. The ring has many of the same side effects as OCPs, but it may also cause discomfort and increased vaginal discharge; in addition, adolescent females may be concerned that the ring may be felt by their partner or may not want to have to insert their fingers into the vagina to insert/remove the ring.

Injectable progestin (depot medroxyprogesterone [DMPA], trade name Depo-Provera) is the third most common method of contraception used by adolescents, after OCPs and condoms. DMPA may be a desirable option for female adolescents because it can be used without partner knowledge, does not require daily dosing, and does not require any action at the time of intercourse. Roughly 75 percent of adolescents using DMPA discontinue use within the first year, with the most common reasons for discontinuation being irregular bleeding and weight gain.

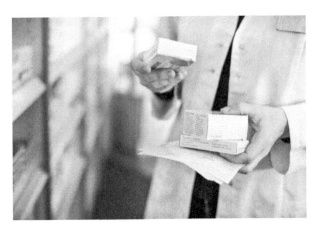

Menses usually becomes lighter and may stop altogether. Other common side effects are acne, headaches, breast tenderness, and mood changes; DMPA may worsen depression and should be used cautiously in patients with a history of depression. DMPA has also been associated with a decrease in bone mineral density.

The etonogestrel implant (Implanon) is a small rod that is implanted under the skin and slowly releases etonogestrel, a progestin, offering 3 years of highly effective contraception. Implanon may be desirable to female adolescents because it can be used without partner knowledge, does not require daily dosing, and does not require any action at the time of intercourse. As with progestin injections, irregular bleeding is the most common reason for discontinuation; weight gain is another.

IUDs are nearly 100 percent effective in preventing pregnancy for the life of the device (5-10 years), and their effects are completely reversible with removal. They can be used without partner knowledge, do not require daily dosing, and do not require any action at the time of intercourse, making them an excellent choice for use by many adolescents. There are two types of IUD, the copper T IUD (ParaGard) and the levonorgestrel-releasing IUD (Mirena). IUDs can be used in adolescents, including those who have not been pregnant before, and according to some experts are underprescribed for adolescents.

Prescription barrier methods (diaphragms and cervical caps) rarely are used by adolescent females because they must be stored properly, require action at the time of intercourse, and may be felt by partners.

RISK FACTORS

Risk factors for adolescent sexual activity and/or pregnancy include physical and sexual abuse, poverty, lack of parental supervision and/or support, early puberty, lack of knowledge, psychological factors, and lack of access to contraceptives.

Adolescents who live in families with little parental support, little restriction of risky behaviors, and poorly defined goals are more likely to become sexually active and are more likely to become adolescent parents.

Early physical maturation has widened the gap between reproductive capacity and cognitive and emotional maturation, increasing the risk of unintended pregnancy among adolescents.

Adolescents may believe that they cannot get pregnant in their first sexual encounter or that they are too young to become pregnant. Adolescents may lack information about available contraceptive methods and where to obtain contraceptives.

Psychological factors may also lead to risk factors. Adolescents may fear side effects of contraceptives, real or assumed, or be embarrassed to obtain contraceptives. They may be unable or unwilling to discuss contraceptive use with their partners, or their partners may refuse to use available methods.

Clinicians may not address sexuality and contraceptive use with adolescent patients, may be unwilling to prescribe contraceptives, or may be overtly judgmental about sexual activity among teens.

SIGNS AND SYMPTOMS

Adolescents who need contraception may have psychological symptoms including anxiety, depression, embarrassment, and feelings of guilt.

Adolescents who use contraceptives may have the behavioral symptoms that include mood and appetite changes or physical symptoms that include weight gain, lighter/heavier menses, skin irritation/acne, increased vaginal discharge, and headaches.

ASSESSMENT

Professionals who work with adolescents may evaluate for pregnancy risk factors and obtain adolescent history through a bio-psycho-social-spiritual assessment, with particular attention to the risk factors mentioned above. If family members are present, professionals may attempt to obtain information from them as well.

Standardized urine tests can be administered to screen for pregnancy.

TREATMENT

A complete bio-psycho-social-spiritual assessment is helpful to understand the extent and nature of risk factors. This is essential for careful diagnosis, appropriate case management, and successful treatment. Providers should use standardized screening tools, assessment instruments, and interview protocols that have been established for adolescents. It is important to consider the clinical risks versus the benefits of contraceptives, as well as the adolescent's ability to use them consistently and correctly, motivation, cost, involvement of partner and/or parents, access, and confidentiality, as well as to explore possible barriers to treatment (health insurance, transportation, emotional/psychological concerns) and provide referrals to reduce potential obstacles. Professionals should advocate for and assist in creating adolescent-friendly health services. Part of being adolescent-friendly is making sure that services are easily accessible, as accessibility can be a major obstacle for adolescents.

Professionals may also provide sex and contraception education, provide referrals to medical services, ensure appropriate education regarding risks of sexual activity and how to protect herself from unwanted pregnancy and sexually transmitted diseases, and ensure adolescent knows how to access contraception.

Problem	Goal	Intervention
Adolescent is sexually active and has disclosed that she is not utilizing any type of contraception.	Reduce risk for unplanned pregnancy.	Conduct a complete bio-psycho-social-spiritual history related to pregnancy risk factors. Determine need for contraceptives. Refer for medical evaluation/treatment.
Adolescent is demonstrating that she has incorrect information regarding basic sexuality and is at risk for unplanned pregnancy.	Ensure that she has accurate information regarding sexuality, sexual intercourse, pregnancy, and STDs.	Access the appropriate information and educational materials. Provide if appropriate. Educate on strategies to improve adherence to any contraceptive treatment plan (reminders about returning for hormone injections, text reminders to take birth control pills).
Adolescent lacks parental supervision and support.	Increase parental involvement with increased supervision and support.	With permission, involve parent(s) in discussion. Educate parent(s) on reality of adolescent's sexual activity and need for increased supervision and support.
Adolescent reports sexual or physical maltreatment.	Ensure that adolescent is in a safe environment and has resolution she desires regarding reporting the maltreatment.	Use active listening to encourage adolescent to share her story. Assess whether she wishes to pursue further action. Educate her on the professional's role as a mandated reporter since she is a minor and follow appropriate protocol regarding reporting of maltreatment. Assess current situation and ensure safety.
Adolescent has lack of consistent access to contraception.	Adolescent will have access to contraception.	Determine why she cannot access contraception. Assist her in navigating barriers to access and obtaining needed contraception.
Adolescent is expressing emotional anxiety and concerns about using contraception.	Reduce anxiety.	Provide education on contraception. Assess source of anxiety (worry about side effects, religious beliefs about conception). Depending on source of anxiety, use therapeutic techniques to reduce anxiety.

APPLICABLE LAWS AND REGULATIONS

The age of consent (the age at which one legally is considered competent to agree to sex) varies from state to state, but typically is 16 to 18 years of age.

Most states in the United States have laws regarding consent for contraception. The District of Columbia and 26 states allow minors over the age of 12 to consent to contraceptives. Twenty states allow consent for minors in certain categories (minors who are pregnant, who are married, who already are parents). Four states have no case law on access to contraception for minors.

Confidentiality of medical information between healthcare professionals and adolescents is addressed in the Health Insurance Portability and Accountability Act (HIPAA). Under HIPAA, a parent generally is allowed access to the medical records of his or her minor child except in instances in which the minor is afforded protection by state law; therefore, professionals need to be aware of state laws regarding confidentiality.

SERVICES AND RESOURCES

- National Campaign to Prevent Teen and Unplanned Pregnancy, www.thenationalcampaign.org
- Planned Parenthood, www.plannedparenthood.org.

FOOD FOR THOUGHT

Adolescents in the United States and Europe have comparable rates of sexual activity, but adolescents in Europe generally use contraceptives more often and use more effective methods than adolescents in the United States, resulting in lower pregnancy rates.

RED FLAGS

Physical and sexual maltreatment are a potential issue with any adolescent and can be a risk factor for early sexual activity. The social worker should complete a thorough history to determine if either type of abuse is a part of the adolescent's history.

Written by Tricia Peneku, MS, PPS, and Jessica Therivel, LMSW-IPR

Reviewed by Lynn B. Cooper, D Crim

REFERENCES

American Academy of Pediatrics. (2014). Contraception for adolescents. *Pediatrics, 134*(4), e.1244-e1256. doi:10.1542/peds.2014-2299

British Association of Social Workers. (2012). The code of ethics for social work: Statement of principles. Retrieved from http://cdn.basw.co.uk/upload/basw_112315-7.pdf

Chandra-Mouli, V., McCarraher, D. R., Phillips, S. J., Williamson, N..E., & Hainsworth, G. (2014). Contraception for adolescents in low and middle income countries: Needs, barriers, and access. *Reproductive Health, 11*(1), 1. doi:10.1186/742-4755-11-1

Cox, J. E. (2008). Teenage pregnancy. In L. S. Neinstein, C. M. Gordon, D. R. Katzman, D. S. Rosen, & E. R. Woods (Eds.), *Adolescent Health Care: A practical guide* (5th ed., pp. 1056-1066). Philadelphia, PA: Lippincott, Williams, & Wilkins.

Dixon, V. (2014). Special considerations when providing contraception advice and information to young people. *British Journal of School Nursing, 9*(4), 170-175.

Duffy, K., Wimberly, Y., & Brooks, C. (2009). Adolescent contraceptive care for the practicing pediatrician. *Adolescent Medicine, 20*(1), 168-187.

Gabzdyl, E. M. (2010). Contraceptive care of adolescents: Overview, tips, strategies, and implications for school nurses. *Journal of School Nursing, 26*(4), 267-277. doi:10.1177/1059840510374459

Gupta, N., Corrado, S., & Goldstein, M. (2008). Hormonal contraception for the adolescent. *Pediatrics in Review, 29*(11), 386-396. doi:10.1542/pir.29-11-386

International Federation of Social Workers. (2012). Statement of Ethical Principles. Retrieved January 21, 2015, from http://ifsw.org/policies/statement-of-ethical-principles/

Kost, K., & Henshaw, S. (2014, May). U.S. teenage pregnancies, births, and abortions, 2010: National and state trends by age, race, and ethnicity. Retrieved April 13, 2015, from http://www.guttmacher.org/pubs/USTPtrends10.pdf

Mizrahi, T., & Mayden, R. W. (2001). NASW standards for cultural competency in social work practice. Retrieved from http://www.socialworkers.org/practice/standards/NASWCulturalStandards.pdf

Santelli, J., Sandfort, T., & Orr, M. (2008). Transnational comparisons of adolescent contraceptive use: What can we learn from these comparisons?. *Archives of Pediatrics & Adolescent Medicine, 162*(1), 92-94. doi:10.1001/archpediatrics.2007.28

State policies in brief: An overview of minors' consent law. (2015). *Guttmacher Institute.* Retrieved February 4, 2015, from http://www.guttmacher.org/statecenter/spibs/spib_OMCL.pdf

National Campaign to Prevent Teen and Unplanned Pregnancy. (2015). National and state data. Retrieved February 4, 2015, from http://thenationalcampaign.org/data/landing

PREGNANCY IN ADOLESCENCE: PREVENTION—MALE USE OF CONTRACEPTION

MAJOR CATEGORIES: Adolescents

DESCRIPTION

Adolescent pregnancy and birth rates in the United States have decreased steadily since the early 1990s. Yet adolescent pregnancy remains an important medical, social, and public health issue; teenage pregnancy rates are much higher in the United States than in other industrialized countries. In 2010, the most recent year for which data are available, there were 625,000 pregnancies in females age 20 or younger, approximately 6 percent of this age group. Among sexually active adolescents, failure to use contraceptives, or using them improperly or inconsistently, is the primary cause of adolescent pregnancy. To prevent pregnancy, males have a limited number of options: abstinence, condoms, outercourse (sexual stimulation without penetration by the penis), vasectomy, and withdrawal. The most commonly used contraceptive for adolescent males is the condom. The use of condoms is an effective way to include the adolescent male in the responsibility of pregnancy prevention. Condoms are also easily accessible and inexpensive compared to many other contraceptive means. Adolescent clients need to recognize that relying on condoms as the only method of protection means that the client must commit to using a condom for every sex act or risk pregnancy. Often condom use will decrease over time in an ongoing adolescent relationship.

FACTS AND FIGURES

Adolescents in the United States have relatively high levels of sexual activity. Researchers for the 2013 Youth Risk Behavior Surveillance System survey found that 46.8 percent of all ninth- through twelfth-graders had ever been sexually active, with the highest rate found among black male adolescents, at 68.4 percent, followed by Hispanic male adolescents at 51.7 percent and white male adolescents at 42.2 percent.

The same investigators found that condom use among high school students had increased: In 1991, a condom was used in the last sexual experience of 46.2 percent of students and in 2013 in 59.1 percent of students. Adolescent males were more likely to report condom use

(65.8 percent) than adolescent females (53.1 percent). Black adolescent males had the highest rate of condom use, at 73.0 percent, followed by Hispanic male adolescents at 66.5 percent, and white male adolescents at 61.8 percent.

Condoms can be very effective in preventing pregnancy, offer protection against sexually transmitted diseases (STDs), are inexpensive, and are easy to obtain. However, consistent use of any contraceptive method, including condoms, is challenging for most adolescents. Proper use of condoms is required for them to be effective.

Condoms may break or leak during use; misapplication of the condom or failure to grasp hold of the condom prior to withdrawal further increases the risk for breakage or leaking. As a result, for adolescents, an estimated rate for condom failure is 18 percent.

Condoms may interfere with sexual pleasure. Because some adolescents use condoms to protect against STD and HIV/AIDS infection and not to provide birth control, they discontinue using them once they feel comfortable and safe with a partner.

RISK FACTORS

Males are slightly more likely to be sexually experienced than females, and sexual activity increases with high school grade. Black adolescents have the highest rate of early sexual activity, followed by Latino and white adolescents.

A majority of fathers in a study of adolescent parents had wanted their partner to become pregnant or were ambivalent about a pregnancy outcome. Significantly, the pregnancy intentions (desire to become a parent) of the mother and father often differed, and often they were unaware of each other's intentions. Fathers who wanted their partner to become pregnant or who were ambivalent reported less use of contraception.

There are psychosocial, socioeconomic, and cultural barriers to effective use of contraceptives by adolescents. Adolescents may be uncomfortable discussing contraceptive use with their parents, sexual partner(s), or medical professionals. Male adolescents may feel that contraception is the responsibility of their female partner. It is a socially and culturally supported belief that contraception is a female's responsibility. Adolescents and their partners may fear that confidentiality will be breached by healthcare providers if they request contraceptives or reproductive counseling.

Cultural and ethnic factors appear to play a role in contraceptive use: Fewer Hispanic adolescents use contraceptives than do adolescents of other ethnic or racial backgrounds, whereas African American adolescents are the most likely to use contraceptives.

Adolescents may be too emotionally or cognitively immature to realize the repercussions of having sex without the use of contraceptives. Early puberty increases the risk for being sexually active at an emotionally or cognitively immature age; emotionally or cognitively immature adolescents have lower rates of contraceptive use and higher rates of unintended pregnancy.

Use of alcohol or drugs increases risky sexual behavior, including having sex without the use of condoms.

Adolescents may be inadequately and incorrectly educated about contraceptive use, and those interested in using contraceptives may not have access to them. Research indicates that giving adolescents freer access to condoms is not associated with increased sexual activity but does increase condom use among sexually active adolescents.

Healthcare providers may not initiate discussions of sexuality with their adolescent patients and may be reluctant to dispense condoms without the knowledge of their parents.

SIGNS AND SYMPTOMS
Adolescents who need to discuss sexual activity or contraception may have psychological signs and symptoms such as anxiety, emotional/cognitive immaturity, and embarrassment.

ASSESSMENT
Professionals working with adolescents who may have need of contraceptives may evaluate for risk factors; obtain history through a bio-psycho-social-spiritual assessment, and obtain information from family members if possible.

Professionals may also find laboratory tests related to STDs of use in conversations about contraception use by males.

TREATMENT
A complete bio-psycho-social-spiritual assessment is helpful to understand the extent and nature of risk factors. This is essential for careful diagnosis, appropriate case management, and successful treatment. Providers should use standardized screening tools, assessment instruments, and interview protocols that have been established for the male population served. It is important to consider clinical risks versus benefits of contraceptives as well as the adolescent's ability to use them consistently and correctly, motivation, involvement of partner and/or parents, access, and confidentiality. Possible barriers to access should be explored (health insurance, transportation, cost, emotional/psychological concerns) and referrals provided to reduce potential obstacles.

Professionals may also provide education on sexuality and contraception, provide referrals to medical services, and ensure that the adolescent knows how to access contraception and is aware of any condom availability programs.

Problem	Goal	Intervention
Male adolescent is sexually active.	Determine need for contraceptives.	Assess level of education on contraception/sexual health. Educate on available contraception choices.
Male adolescent feels anxious and is embarrassed to discuss contraception.	Adolescent will feel comfortable discussing contraception options and will practice safe sex.	Educate on confidentiality and provide reassurances to address his anxiety and embarrassment. Stress the importance of the subject matter to protect him and his partner from unintended consequences. Educate on available contraception choices. Assess current level of education on contraception and correct any misconceptions.

APPLICABLE LAWS AND REGULATIONS

The age of consent—the age at which the law states that an individual is considered legally competent to agree to sex—varies from state to state.

Most states in the United States have laws regarding consent for contraception. The District of Columbia and 26 states allow minors over the age of 12 to consent to contraceptives. Twenty states allow consent for minors in certain categories (minors who are pregnant, who are married, who already are parents). Four states have no case law on access to contraception by minors.

Confidentiality of medical information between healthcare professionals and adolescents is addressed in the Health Insurance Portability and Accountability Act (HIPAA). Under HIPAA, a parent generally is allowed access to the medical records of his or her minor child except in instances in which the minor is afforded protection by state law.

SERVICES AND RESOURCES

- National Campaign to Prevent Teen and Unplanned Pregnancy, http://thenationalcampaign.org/.
- Planned Parenthood, http://www.plannedparenthood.org/.

FOOD FOR THOUGHT

Without contraception, there is a 90 percent chance of pregnancy within a year for sexually active teens.

Abstinence is 100 percent effective in preventing pregnancy. However, most adolescents either refuse to or are unable to abstain from sexual intercourse.

Pediatricians and other clinicians with hospitalized adolescents may want to consider discussing issues of sexual health and contraception with those adolescents while they are inpatients. Researchers found that 44 percent of hospitalized male adolescents expressed an interest in wanting to learn more about contraception and/or abstinence while they were hospitalized.

Adolescents will often utilize the Internet to look for sexual health information. Clinicians need to be aware that in this subject area, adolescents may be receiving misinformation. There are websites created by crisis pregnancy centers to offer abortion alternatives while targeting adolescents through content

and free screenings for sexually transmitted infections and pregnancy. Investigators found that of 254 crisis pregnancy center websites, 33.5 percent gave information on male condoms, whereas 63.5 percent discouraged the use of condoms. Most promoted abstinence and offered negative or misleading information on the use of condoms to prevent sexually transmitted infections, in contradiction to commonly accepted public health knowledge.

The American Academy of Pediatrics recommends abstinence as the most effective method to prevent sexually transmitted infections and pregnancy but states that pediatricians and other clinicians should support and encourage adolescents to utilize condoms consistently and correctly for prevention.

RED FLAGS

If the adolescent has experienced physical or sexual abuse in the past, this may affect his perceptions regarding relationships and sexuality.

Written by Tricia Peneku, MS, PPS

Reviewed by Lynn B. Cooper, D Crim, and Chris Bates, MA, MSW

REFERENCES

American Academy of Pediatrics. (2013, November). Condom use by adolescents. *American Academy of Pediatrics*. Retrieved November 4, 2015, from http://pediatrics.aappublications.org/content/107/6/1463

Bryant-Comstock, K., Bryant, A. G., Narasimhan, S., & Levi, E. E. (2015). Information about sexual health on crisis pregnancy center websites: Accurate for adolescents? *Journal of Pediatric Adolescent Gynecology*. Advance online publication. doi:10.1016/j.jpag.2015.05.008

Centers for Disease Control and Prevention (CDC). (2015, April 22). Unintended pregnancy prevention: Contraception. Retrieved December 6, 2015, from http://www.cdc.gov/reproductivehealth/unintendedpregnancy/contraception.htm

Cox, J. E. (2008). Teenage pregnancy. In L. S. Neinstein, C. M. Gordon, D. R. Katzman, D. S. Rosen, & E. R. Woods (Eds.), *Adolescent Health Care: A practical guide* (5th ed., pp. 1056-1066). Philadelphia, PA: Lippincott, Williams, & Wilkins.

Gabzdyl, E. M. (2010). Contraceptive care of adolescents: Overview, tips, strategies, and implications for school nurses. *Journal of School Nursing, 26*(4), 267-277. doi:10.1177/1059840510374459

Guss, C. E., WUnsch, C. A., McCulloh, R., Donaldson, A., & Alverson, B. K. (2015). Using the hospital as a venue for reproductive health interventions: A survey of hospitalized adolescents. *Hospital Pediatrics, 5*(2), 67-73. doi:10.1542/hpeds.2014-0043

Guttmacher Institute. (2015). State policies in brief: An overview of minors' consent law. Retrieved December 6, 2015, from http://www.guttmacher.org/statecenter/spibs/spib_OMCL.pdf

International Federation of Social Workers. (2012, March 3). *Statement of ethical principles.* Retrieved November 5, 2015, from http://ifsw.org/policies/statement-of-ethical-principles

Kost, K., & Henshaw, S. (2014, May). U.S. teenage pregnancies, births, and abortions, 2010: National and state trends by age, race, and ethnicity. Retrieved December 6, 2015, from http://www.guttmacher.org/pubs/USTPtrends10.pdf

Lewin, A., Mitchell, S. J., Hodgkinson, S., Gilmore, J., & Beers, L. S. (2014). Pregnancy intentions among expectant adolescent couples. *Journal of Pediatric and Adolescent Gynecology, 27*(3), 172-176. doi:10.1016/j.jpag.2013.09.012

Martinez, G., Copen, C. E., & Abma, J. C. (2011). Teenagers in the United States: Sexual activity, contraceptive use, and child bearing, 2006-2010 National Survey of Family Growth. *Vital Health Statistics, 23*(31), 1-44.

Santelli, J. S., Morrow, B., Anderson, J. E., & Lindberg, L. D. (2006). Contraceptive use and the pregnancy risk among U.S. high school students, 1991-2003. *Perspectives on Sexual and Reproductive Health, 38*(2), 106-111. doi:10.1111/j.1931-2393.2006.tb00067.x

Wheeler, D. (2015). NASW standards and indicators for cultural competence in social work practice. Retrieved December 6, 2015, from http://www.socialworkers.org/practice/standards/PRA-BRO-253150-CC-Standards.pdf

The Policy, Ethics, and Human Rights Committee, British Association of Social Workers. (2012, January). The Code of Ethics for Social Work: Statement of Principles. Retrieved November 19, 2014, from http://cdn.basw.co.uk/upload/basw_112315-7.pdf

Centers for Disease Control and Prevention (CDC). (2014, June 13). Youth Risk Behavior Surveillance – United States, 2013. *Morbidity and Mortality Weekly Report, 63*(SS04), 24-26.

(2014). Contraception for adolescents. *Pediatrics, 134*(4), e1244. doi:10.1542/peds.2014-2299

U.S. Department of Health and Human Services. (n.d.). Health information privacy: Personal representatives and minors. Retrieved December 6, 2015, from http://www.hhs.gov/ocr/privacy/hipaa/faq/personal_representatives_and_minors/

PREGNANCY IN ADOLESCENCE: PREVENTION—NONHORMONAL CONTRACEPTION

MAJOR CATEGORIES: Adolescents

DESCRIPTION

Although adolescent pregnancy and birth rates in the United States have decreased steadily since the early 1990s, adolescent pregnancy continues to be an important medical, social, and public health issue; approximately 900,000 adolescent females become pregnant each year in the United States, where teenage pregnancy rates remain much higher than in other advanced industrialized countries.

Failure to use contraceptives, or using them improperly or inconsistently, is the primary cause of teenage pregnancy. Adolescents may prefer nonhormonal methods of contraception for a range of reasons: concern about the adverse effects of hormonal contraception (weight gain, mood changes, acne), a preference for a nonprescription method, a lack of information or misinformation about hormonal contraception, lack of access to a doctor to obtain a prescription, or lack of health insurance or the ability to pay for a prescription. Nonhormonal contraception may be practiced using a variety of forms and methods, both prescription and nonprescription. Abstinence, withdrawal, the rhythm method, the sponge, spermicides, and condoms are nonprescription methods. Prescription barrier methods such as the diaphragm rarely are used by adolescents because they must be stored, require action at the time of intercourse, and may be felt by partners. Sterilization (vasectomy, tubal ligation) is a permanent method of contraception that rarely is indicated for use in adolescents.

FACTS AND FIGURES

Nonprescription methods other than condoms have failure rates approaching 30 percent among adolescents because adolescents rarely use them consistently or correctly.

In the United States, the teen birth rate in 2013 was 273,105 births among girls ages 15 to 19, a 10 percent decrease from 2012 and a 57 percent decrease from its peak in 1991.

In 2011, 95.9 percent of sexually experienced girls between 15 and 19 years old had a partner use a condom and 1.5 percent used the female condom.

RISK FACTORS

Risk factors for adolescent sexual activity and/or pregnancy include physical and sexual abuse, poverty, lack of parental supervision and/or support, early puberty, lack of knowledge, psychological factors, and lack of access to contraceptives.

Adolescents who live in families with little parental support, little restriction of risky behaviors, and poorly defined goals are more likely to become sexually active and are more likely to become adolescent parents.

Early physical maturation has widened the gap between reproductive capacity and cognitive and emotional maturation, increasing the risk of unintended pregnancy among adolescents.

Adolescents may believe that they cannot get pregnant in their first sexual encounter or that they are too young to become pregnant. Adolescents may lack information about available contraceptive methods and where to obtain contraceptives.

Psychological factors may also lead to risk factors. Adolescents may fear side effects of contraceptives, real or assumed, or be embarrassed to obtain contraceptives. They may be unable or unwilling to discuss contraceptive use with their partners, or their partners may refuse to use available methods.

Clinicians may not address sexuality and contraceptive use with adolescent patients, may be unwilling to prescribe contraceptives, or may be overtly judgmental about sexual activity among teens.

SIGNS AND SYMPTOMS

Psychological symptoms include anxiety and/or embarrassment for adolescents who are not comfortable asking for or discussing contraception.

ASSESSMENT

Professionals may obtain client bio-psycho-social-spiritual history with particular attention to the risk factors mentioned above. They may also administer a standardized urine test to screen for pregnancy.

TREATMENT

A complete bio-psycho-social-spiritual assessment is helpful to understand the extent and nature of risk factors. This is essential for careful diagnosis, appropriate case management, and successful treatment. Providers should use standardized screening tools, assessment instruments, and interview protocols that have been established for adolescents. It is important to consider clinical risks versus benefits of contraceptives, as well as the adolescent's ability to use them consistently and correctly, motivation, cost, involvement of partner and/or parents, access, and confidentiality, as well as to explore possible barriers to treatment (health insurance, transportation, cost, emotional/psychological concerns) and provide referrals to reduce potential obstacles. Professionals should advocate for and assist in creating adolescent-friendly health services. To be adolescent-friendly, services should be accessible, acceptable, appropriate, and effective. Adolescent-friendly services need to be in an environment that is acceptable for this age group (not a clinic that is picketed by antiabortion protesters).

Professionals may also provide sex/contraception education, ensure adolescent has appropriate education regarding risks of sexual activity and how to protect from unwanted pregnancy and sexually transmitted diseases (STDs), ensure adolescent is aware of nonhormonal contraception options, and provide referrals to medical services

Problem	Goal	Intervention
Adolescent is sexually active.	Reduce risk for unplanned pregnancy.	Conduct a complete bio-psycho-social-spiritual history related to pregnancy risk factors. Determine need for contraceptives. Refer for medical evaluation/treatment.
Adolescent is demonstrating that he or she is at risk for unplanned pregnancy due to misinformation.	Ensure that adolescent has the correct information regarding pregnancy, STDs, and sexual intercourse.	Access the appropriate information and educational materials. Provide if appropriate.
Adolescent lacks parental supervision and support.	Increase parental involvement, supervision, and support.	With permission, involve parent(s) in discussion. Educate parent(s) on reality of adolescent's sexual activity and need for increased supervision and support.
Adolescent reports sexual or physical maltreatment.	Ensure that adolescent is in a safe environment.	Use active listening to encourage adolescent to share his or her story. Assess whether he or she wishes to pursue further action. Educate adolescent on the professional's role as a mandated reporter since he or she is a minor and follow appropriate protocol regarding reporting of maltreatment. Assess current situation and ensure safety.
Adolescent lacks consistent access to contraception.	Adolescent will have access to contraception.	Determine why adolescent cannot access contraception. Assist adolescent in navigating barriers to access and obtaining needed contraception.
Adolescent is expressing emotional anxiety and concerns about using contraception.	Reduce anxiety.	Provide education on contraception. Assess source of anxiety (worry about side effects, religious beliefs about conception). Depending on source of anxiety, use therapeutic techniques to reduce anxiety.

APPLICABLE LAWS AND REGULATIONS

The age of consent (the age the law states that one is considered legally competent to agree to sex) varies from state to state, but typically is 16 to 18 years of age.

Most U.S. states have laws regarding the authority of minors to consent to contraceptive services. The District of Columbia and 26 other states allow minors over the age of 12 to consent to contraceptives.

Twenty states allow consent for minors in certain categories (minors who are pregnant, married, already a parent). Four states have no case law on contraception and minors.

Confidentiality of communication between healthcare professionals and adolescents and of adolescents' medical information is addressed in the Health Insurance Portability and Accountability Act (HIPAA). In most cases, under HIPAA a parent is

1417

allowed access to a minor's medical records except in instances in which the minor is afforded privacy protection by state law, such as laws that give minors the right to consent to contraceptives.

SERVICES AND RESOURCES
- National Campaign to Prevent Teen and Unplanned Pregnancy, www.thenationalcampaign.org.
- Planned Parenthood, www.plannedparenthood.org.

FOOD FOR THOUGHT
Adolescents in the United States and Europe have comparable rates of sexual activity, but adolescents in Europe generally use contraceptives more often and use more effective methods than adolescents in the United States, resulting in lower pregnancy rates.

Male condom use is the most common means of contraception utilized by adolescents. This may be due to condoms being low cost, easily accessible, and available without a prescription.

RED FLAGS
Physical and sexual abuse are potential issues with any adolescent client and can be a risk factor for early sexual activity.

Written by Tricia Peneku, MS, PPS

Reviewed by Lynn B. Cooper, D Crim, and Jessica Therivel, LMSW-IPR

REFERENCES
American Academy of Pediatrics. (2014). Contraception for adolescents. *Pediatrics, 134*(4), e.1244-e1256. doi:10.1542/peds.2014-2299

British Association of Social Workers. (2012). The code of ethics for social work: Statement of principles. Retrieved August 18, 2015, from http://cdn.basw.co.uk/upload/basw_112315-7.pdf

Centers for Disease Control and Prevention (CDC). (2011, October). Teenagers in the United States: Sexual activity, contraceptive use, and childbearing, 2006-2010 National Survey of Family Growth. Retrieved February 4, 2015, from http://www.cdc.gov/nchs/data/series/sr_23/sr23_031.pdf

Chandra-Mouli, V., McCarraher, D. R., Phillips, S. J., Williamson, N..E., & Hainsworth, G. (2014). Contraception for adolescents in low and middle income countries: Needs, barriers, and access. *Reproductive Health, 11*(1), 1. doi:10.1186/742-4755-11-1

Dixon, V. (2014). Special considerations when providing contraception advice and information to young people. *British Journal of School Nursing, 9*(4), 170-175.

Duffy, K., Wimberly, Y., & Brooks, C. (2009). Adolescent contraceptive care for the practicing pediatrician. *Adolescent Medicine, 20*(1), 168-187.

Fuller, J. M. (2007). Adolescents and contraception: The nurse's role as counselor. *Nursing for Women's Health, 11*(6), 546-556.

Guttmacher Institute. (2014). Facts on American teens' sexual and reproductive health. Retrieved February 4, 2015, from http://www.guttmacher.org/pubs/FB-ATSRH.html

International Federation of Social Workers. (2012). Statement of ethical principles. Retrieved August 18, 2015, from http://ifsw.org/policies/statement-of-ethical-principles/

Mizrahi, T., & Mayden, R. W. (2001). NASW standards for cultural competence in social work practice. Retrieved August 18, 2015, from http://www.socialworkers.org/practice/standards/NASWCulturalStandards.pdf

Santelli, J., Sandfort, T., & Orr, M. (2008). Transnational comparisons of adolescent contraceptive use: What can we learn from these comparisons?. *Archives of Pediatrics & Adolescent Medicine, 162*(1), 92-94. doi:10.1001/archpediatrics.2007.28

State policies in brief: An overview of minors' consent law. (2015). *Guttmacher Institute*. Retrieved August 18, 2015, from http://www.guttmacher.org/statecenter/spibs/spib_OMCL.pdf

National Campaign to Prevent Teen and Unplanned Pregnancy. (2015). National and state data. Retrieved August 18, 2015, from http://thenationalcampaign.org/data/landing

PREGNANCY IN ADOLESCENCE: PREVENTION—PROGESTIN-ONLY CONTRACEPTION

MAJOR CATEGORIES: Adolescence

DESCRIPTION

Adolescent pregnancy and birth rates in the United States have decreased steadily since the early 1990s. Yet adolescent pregnancy remains an important medical, social, and public health issue; teenage pregnancy rates remain much higher in the United States than in other industrialized countries. Failure to use contraceptives, or using them improperly or inconsistently, is the primary cause of teenage pregnancy.

Progestin-only hormonal methods of female contraception come in many forms, including daily and emergency pills, injections, implants, and intrauterine devices (IUDs), all of which require a prescription. Progestin-only contraception commonly is selected for the wide range of delivery methods or because of contraindication to oral contraceptive pills (OCPs) that contain estrogen (breastfeeding, migraines). Progestin-only pills (POPs) are less effective than pills that combine estrogen and a progestin (combined OCPs). POPs require strict, consistent use; missing one dose by 3 or more hours increases the risk for pregnancy. Because of this, POPs are not an optimal method of contraception for adolescents. POPs do not have placebo pills, and irregular bleeding is a common side effect.

Progestin-only injection (depot medroxyprogesterone [DMPA], such as Depo-Provera) is the third most common method of contraception used by adolescents, after OCPs and condoms. The hormone is injected every 10 to 15 weeks and prevents pregnancy by suppressing ovulation, thinning the endometrial lining, and altering cervical mucus to prevent sperm penetration. Menses usually is lighter and can cease altogether. Other common side effects are acne, headaches, breast tenderness, and mood changes. DMPA can worsen depression and should be used cautiously in adolescents with a history of depression. DMPA has been associated with decreased bone mineral density related to suppressed ovarian estrogen production. Because more than 50 percent of a woman's bone mass is accumulated during adolescence, there are concerns that bone loss during adolescence may increase the risk of fracture later in life. Hormonal implants (Implanon) are small, subcutaneously implanted rods that slowly release etonogestrel, a progestin that offers 3 years of highly effective contraception. Implanon has a 99-percent efficacy rate. Insertion of the etonogestrel rod requires a small incision; insertion and removal take 1 to 2 minutes. Like DMPA, hormonal implants can be used without a partner's knowledge and do not require storage or action at the time of intercourse. Additionally, implants do not require frequent visits to a clinician. Irregular bleeding is the most common reason for discontinuation. Weight gain, acne, breast tenderness, and headaches also are side effects.

The levonorgestrel-releasing IUD Mirena provides 5 years of contraception. Mirena thickens cervical mucus, thins the endometrial lining, and in some cases suppresses ovulation. Levonorgestrel has the same benefits as other forms of progestin-only contraception and can cause irregular bleeding. It is as effective as sterilization in preventing pregnancy and the effects are completely reversible with removal, making it an excellent choice for many adolescents. Adolescents have a slightly higher risk of expelling an IUD than older women because the adolescent uterus often is smaller, particularly in adolescents who have never had children. It is thought that IUDs are underprescribed to adolescents out of concern that devices may increase the risk for pelvic inflammatory disease. Recent research shows that the risk of infection is related to the insertion procedure and not to the devices themselves. No increase in the incidence of sexually transmitted diseases (STDs) or infertility has been reported with this method.

FACTS AND FIGURES

The factors that must be evaluated when considering a method of contraception for adolescents include the risks versus the benefits, the ability to use the contraceptive agent or device consistently and correctly, the motivation, the cost, the involvement of the partner and/or parents, access to the agent or device, and confidentiality (visibility of the method to others, storage requirements).

In 2014 in the United States, there were approximately 24 births for every 1,000 adolescent females ages 15 to 19, a total of 249,067 births to teen girls.

In 2013, the Centers for Disease Control and Prevention (CDC) reported the following results from the Youth Risk Behavior Surveillance System.

- 46.8 percent of ninth- to twelfth-graders had engaged in sexual intercourse. This number has decreased fairly steadily since 1991, when it was 54.1 percent of ninth- to twelfth-graders.
- 13.7 percent of those who had intercourse used no protection at all; 1.6 percent either used or their partner used an IUD; 4.7 percent used or their partner used a DMPA injection, a transdermal patch, or a birth control ring (NuvaRing).

The failure rate of POPs is as high as 10 percent within the first year, as compared to 0.3 percent for OCPs.

With typical use, the failure rate of DMPA in adolescents is 3 percent. DMPA might also be preferred by female adolescents because it can be used without partner knowledge and does not require storage or action at the time of intercourse. Approximately 75 percent of adolescents using DMPA discontinue use within the first year, most commonly for irregular bleeding and belief that the DMPA is responsible for weight gain.

Over time, IUD is one of the most cost-effective forms of contraception.

Emergency contraceptive pills (ECPs, such as Plan B, Plan B One-Step) must be taken within 72 hours of contraception failure. Each packet of Plan B or Plan B One-Step contains a tablet of levonorgestrel, which when taken can reduce the risk for pregnancy by almost 95 percent. The sooner the pill is taken, the more effective the method. Researchers are noting that ECPs may not be as effective for women over 164 pounds or obese women, but more research is needed to confirm this. Plan B or Plan B One-Step may work in one of the following ways: It may prevent or delay ovulation, it may interfere with fertilization of an egg, and/or it may prevent implantation of a fertilized egg in the uterus by altering its lining. Plan B or Plan B One-Step is not the same as RU-486, which is an abortion pill. It does not cause a miscarriage or abortion. It does not stop development of a fetus once the fertilized egg implants in the uterus, and it will not work if already pregnant when taken.

RISK FACTORS

Risk factors for adolescent pregnancy include the following:

High rates of frequency of sexual activity: Results from studies indicate that one third of high school students had engaged in sexual activity within the last 3 months, which suggests that a significant proportion of teens are having intercourse. Males are slightly more likely to be sexually experienced than females, and sexual activity increases with high school grade. African American teens have the highest rate of early sexual activity, followed by Latino and white teens.

Physical and sexual abuse: Abusive relationships are common features in the lives of adolescent mothers. Sexual victimization may increase risk of pregnancy.

Economic concerns: Adolescents who live in poverty face many obstacles that may increase their risk of pregnancy. In 2010, 48 percent of mothers ages 15 to 19 lived below the poverty line.

Cultural values: Adolescents who live in families with little parental support, little restriction of risky behaviors, and poorly defined goals are more likely to become sexually active and are more likely to become adolescent parents. Other cultural factors include peer pressure, early dating, and lack of religious affiliation. Some religions oppose any sex education that includes contraception or discusses any method of pregnancy prevention other than abstinence. A cycle of adolescent pregnancy can occur.

Psychological factors: Although psychological factors, such as depression, may have an influence on an adolescent's decision to engage in sexual activity, the role of psychological and behavioral antecedents is unclear. The Youth Risk Behavior Surveillance System survey indicated that 22.4 percent of adolescents used alcohol or drugs when having sex.

Early puberty: Early physical maturation has widened the gap between reproductive capacity and cognitive and emotional maturation and has increased the risk of unintended pregnancy in this age group.

Developmental issues: Many developmental characteristics of adolescents, particularly younger adolescents, interfere with decision making regarding sexual activity and the successful use of contraceptives.

Many factors influence adolescents' decisions regarding sexual activity and contraception and often act as barriers to contraceptive use:

Inaccurate and misleading information: Many adolescents have misinformation regarding conception and reproduction, including the belief that they cannot get pregnant in their first sexual encounter, that they are too young to become pregnant, or that parental consent is required for emergency contraception.

Accessibility: Many adolescents lack information about available contraceptive methods, do not know their legal rights to healthcare, do not know where to obtain contraceptives, and have concerns regarding cost and confidentiality. Health services that provide contraceptives also may not be readily available.

Contraceptive acceptability: Adolescents may have fear of specific methods and perceived side effects, concern regarding whether contraceptives might affect future fertility, embarrassment over the acquisition or use of the method, and concern that the method may interfere with pleasure.

Partner issues: Adolescents may be unable to discuss contraceptive use with their partners, or their partners may refuse to use available methods.

Intended pregnancy: Adolescents may desire to have a baby to solidify a relationship, have someone to love and take care of, change their status in the family or establish independence, escape an abusive family by creating their own family, or establish their fertility.

Provider problems: Providers may not address sexuality and contraceptive use with adolescent clients, they may be unwilling to prescribe contraceptives, or they may be overtly judgmental about sexual activity among teens.

SIGNS AND SYMPTOMS

Signs and symptoms that may be present with adolescents when discussing sexual activity or if a pregnancy is present include psychological signs including anxiety, depression, or embarrassment; behavioral signs including mood changes; physical symptoms including weight gain, skin irritation/acne, or headaches.

ASSESSMENT

A complete bio-psycho-social-spiritual assessment is helpful for understanding the extent and nature of risk factors. This is essential for careful diagnosis, appropriate case management, and successful treatment. Professionals should evaluate for risk factors and obtain as much information as possible from family members. Professionals may wish to use standardized urine tests to screen for pregnancy.

TREATMENT

Providers should use standardized screening tools, assessment instruments, and interview protocols that have been established for the adolescent population served. It is important to weigh clinical risks and benefits of contraceptives, as well as the adolescent's ability to use them consistently and correctly, motivation, cost, involvement of partner and/or parents, access, and confidentiality. It is also important to explore possible barriers to access (health insurance, transportation, cost, emotional/psychological concerns) and provide referrals to reduce potential obstacles.

Professionals may also ensure that adolescents have accurate information to make informed decisions by providing sex/contraception education, educate adolescents on their rights regarding consent to contraception according to the laws of the state or nation in which they live, and provide referrals to medical services.

Problem	Goal	Intervention
Adolescent is sexually active.	Determine need for contraceptives.	Conduct a complete bio-psycho-social-spiritual history related to pregnancy risk factors. Refer for medical evaluation/treatment.
Adolescent is demonstrating that he or she has incorrect information regarding basic sexuality and sex education.	Ensure that the adolescent has the correct information regarding pregnancy, STDs, and sexual intercourse.	Access the appropriate information and educational materials. Provide if appropriate.

APPLICABLE LAWS AND REGULATIONS

The age of consent—the age at which the law states that one is considered legally competent to agree to sex—varies from state to state.

In the United States, the age at which adolescents are legally allowed to consent to contraceptives varies among states. Twenty-six states and the District of Columbia allow all adolescents age 12 and older to consent to contraceptives. Twenty states allow only certain categories of minors to consent (typically those who are married, pregnant, or already parents). Four states have no statutes or case law concerning age of consent for contraceptives.

SERVICES AND RESOURCES

- National Campaign to Prevent Teen and Unplanned Pregnancy, http://thenationalcampaign.org/.
- Planned Parenthood, https://www.plannedparenthood.org/.

FOOD FOR THOUGHT

Without contraception, there is a 90 percent chance of pregnancy within a year for sexually active teens.

Abstinence is 100 percent effective in preventing pregnancy. However, most adolescents either refuse to or are unable to abstain from sexual intercourse.

Some adolescents may stop DMPA injections under the misconception that DMPA is responsible for weight gain. A recent review shows that DMPA does not cause weight gain and should not be a reason for refusal or nonadherence.

RED FLAGS

Physical and/or sexual abuse is a potential issue with any adolescent and can be a risk factor for early sexual activity. The social worker should complete a thorough history to try to determine whether either type of abuse is a part of the adolescent's history

Adolescents who are misinformed or lacking accurate knowledge about contraception have an increased risk for pregnancy.

Written by Jessica Therivel, LMSW-IPR

Reviewed by Lynn B. Cooper, D Crim,
Laura Gale, LCSW, and
Melissa Rosales Neff, MSW

REFERENCES

British Association of Social Workers. (2012, January). The code of ethics for social work: Statement of principles. Retrieved December 21, 2015, from http://cdn.basw.co.uk/upload/basw_112315-7.pdf

Centers for Disease Control and Prevention. (2014). Youth risk behavior surveillance, 2013. Retrieved December 21, 2015, from http://www.cdc.gov/mmwr/pdf/ss/ss6304.pdf

Duffy, K., Wimberly, Y., & Brooks, C. (2009). Adolescent contraceptive care for the practicing pediatrician. *Adolescent Medicine, 20*(1), 168-187.

Gupta, N., Corrado, S., & Goldstein, M. (2008). Hormonal contraception for the adolescent. *Pediatrics in Review, 29*(11), 386-396. doi:10.1542/pir.29-11-386

Guttmacher Institute. (2015, December). State policies in brief: an overview of minors' consent law. Retrieved November 21, 2014, from http://www.guttmacher.org/statecenter/spibs/spib_OMCL.pdf

International Federation of Social Workers. (2012, March 3). Statement of ethical principles. Retrieved December 21, 2015, from http://ifsw.org/policies/statement-of-ethical-principles/

Kann, L., Kinchen, S., Shanklin, S. L., Flint, K. H., Hawkins, J., Harris, W. A.,... Zaza, S. (2014). Youth risk behavior surveillance—United States, 2013. *Morbidity and Mortality Weekly Report, 63*(4), 1-168. Martinez, G., Copen, C. E., & Abma, J. C. (2011). Teenagers in the United States: Sexual activity, contraceptive use, and child bearing, 2006-2010 National Survey of Family Growth. *Vital Health Statistics, 23*(31), 1-44.

National Campaign to Prevent Teen and Unplanned Pregnancy. (2012). Why it matters: Teen childbearing, education, and economic well-being. Retrieved December 21, 2015, from http://thenationalcampaign.org/sites/default/files/resource-primary-download/childbearing-education-economicwellbeing.pdf

National Campaign to Prevent Teen and Unplanned Pregnancy. (2015). National and state data. Retrieved December 21, 2015, from http://thenationalcampaign.org/data/landing

National Institute for Health and Care Excellence (NICE). (2014). Contraceptive services with a focus on young people up to the age of 25. *NICE Public Health Guidance, 51,* 1-70. Sanfilippo, J. S., &

Lara-Torre, E. (2009). Adolescent gynecology. *Obstetrics & Gynecology, 113*(4), 935-947. doi:10.1097/AOG.0b013e31819b6303

Waller, L., & Bryson, W. (2007). Can emergency contraception help to reduce teen pregnancy? *Journal of the American Association of Physician Assistants, 20*(6), 42-46. doi:10.1097/01720610-200706000-00009

Wheeler, D. (2015). NASW standards and indicators for cultural competence in social work practice. Retrieved December 21, 2015, from http://www.socialworkers.org/practice/standards/PRA-BRO-253150-CC-Standards.pdf

Whitaker, A. K., & Gilliam, M. (2008). Contraceptive care for adolescents. *Clinical Obstetrics & Gynecology, 51*(2), 268-280. doi:10.1097/GRF.0b013e31816d713e

Yancey, J. R., & Raleigh, M. (2014). Progestin-only contraceptives: Effects on weight. *American Family Physician, 89*(9), 715-716.

Young, T., Turner, J., Denny, G., & Young, M. (2004). Examining external and internal poverty as antecedents of teen pregnancy. *American Journal of Health Behavior, 28*(4), 361-373. doi:10.5993/AJHB.28.4.8

PREGNANCY IN ADOLESCENCE: ABORTION TRENDS—GLOBAL PERSPECTIVE

MAJOR CATEGORIES: Adolescents

WHAT WE KNOW

Global abortion rates have been declining over recent decades but they remain high. An estimated 85 million women aged 15–44 have unintended pregnancies each year, of which 12.3 million are in more developed countries and 72.6 million are in less developed countries. Approximately half of all unintended pregnancies end in abortion (54 percent in more developed countries and 49 percent in less developed countries). Approximately 16 million births each year are to adolescent girls (aged 15–19). Although the average global birth rate for adolescent girls is 49 per 1,000 girls, birth rates vary considerably from country to country, with sub-Saharan Africa having the highest rate (299 per 1,000 girls).

Due to social stigma and political and religious censuring of abortion, underreporting of abortion is considered frequent.

Researchers in a study of global adolescent pregnancy and abortion rates found that the availability of accurate data regarding abortion among adolescents varies, depending in part on how liberal or restrictive the country's abortion laws are. Among countries that have liberal abortion laws and complete statistics (i. e., at least 90 percent of abortions are counted), the United States has the highest rate of adolescent pregnancy (57 pregnancies per 1,000 girls) and an abortion rate of 15 per 1,000 girls.

The Netherlands, Singapore, and Slovenia have the lowest rate of adolescent pregnancy (14 pregnancies per 1,000 girls). England, Wales, and Sweden have the highest rate of adolescent abortion (20 per 1,000 girls), and Switzerland has the lowest (5 per 1,000 girls).

In countries with restrictive abortion rates, official statistics are not available. Estimates based on studies for five countries (Burkina Faso, Ethiopia, Kenya, Malawi, and Mexico) found that these countries had higher adolescent pregnancy rates (ranging from 121 pregnancies per 1,000 girls in Ethiopia to 187 pregnancies per 1,000 girls in Burkina Faso). Abortion rates ranged from 11 per 1,000 girls in Ethiopia to 44 per 1,000 girls in Mexico.

Forty-eight percent of abortions worldwide are unsafe and have a high mortality and morbidity risk.

An important factor that contributes to high adolescent pregnancy rates is limited access to and knowledge about contraception. Adolescents are often uninformed about and unreliable users of contraception. In some countries religious and cultural beliefs—for instance that premarital sex is viewed as culturally deviant—prevent adolescents from using contraception. Premarital sex is viewed as culturally deviant in many countries. Condoms for adolescents are viewed as taboo in many parts of Africa.

Sexual assault is another significant factor. Adolescent girls report higher rates of forced sex than older women. Coerced sex contributes to the number of unwanted pregnancies and abortions each year.

Abortion rates decline when women and adolescents have access to contraception. Contraception use can reduce poverty and hunger and avert 32 percent of all maternal deaths and 10 percent of childhood deaths.

Consequences of adolescent pregnancy can be social, economic, and medical. Adolescent pregnancy often is associated with disruption of education, social disadvantages, and perpetuation of poverty. Rates of low birth weight, prematurity, and infant mortality are higher among babies born to adolescent mothers. Pregnancy under the age of 15 is associated with suboptimal growth for the mothers themselves because the fetus and mother are competing for nutrients at a time when the mother's body is still growing.

The World Health Organization (WHO) defines unsafe abortion as "a procedure for terminating an unintended pregnancy, carried out either by persons lacking the necessary skills or in an environment that does not conform to minimal medical standards, or both." WHO reported in 2012 that worldwide 22 million unsafe abortions take place annually. This number increased from 20 million in 2003 to 22 million in 2008and has remained unchanged since 2008. Approximately 47,000 pregnancy-related deaths occur annually worldwide as a result of complications of unsafe abortions. Additionally, five million women are reported to become disabled annually as a result of complications of unsafe abortions.

Treating complications that result from unsafe abortions strain healthcare systems in developing countries.

Rates of unsafe abortion are highest in countries that have the most restrictive abortion laws. Globally, during the 21st century, there has been a trend to liberalize laws surrounding abortion. Most countries have laws that permit abortion under prescribed circumstances. However, these laws vary greatly from country to country and are influenced by cultural and religious beliefs and perspectives. A "global gag" prevents organizations supported with funding from the United States government, regardless of amount, from advising or assisting women with reproductive healthcare if the organizations offer information on pregnancy termination.

Ninety-eight percent of all unsafe abortions are in developing countries. In developing countries, 2.5 million adolescents have unsafe abortions each year. Twenty-five percent of unsafe abortions among adolescents occur in Africa, 15 percent in Latin America and the Caribbean, and 10 percent in Asia.

Research demonstrates that women who have an abortion have subsequent abortions at a higher frequency than the overall population.

Women and adolescent girls seeking second abortions are judged harshly.

The use of medical abortion (i. e., use of medications to induce abortion) in place of surgical abortion is increasing. Medical abortion is easy to administer and is as safe taking place at home as in a clinic.

In industrialized countries, there is ongoing debate about the prevalence of post-abortion psychological problems. Recent research indicates that adolescent girls are not at increased risk for mental health problems following safe abortion.

The strongest predictors of any psychological problems among adolescents are low self-esteem and depression prior to having an abortion.

WHAT CAN BE DONE

Learn about the factors that contribute to pregnancy and abortion in adolescents so we can accurately assess our clients' personal characteristics and health education needs.

Develop an awareness of personal cultural values, beliefs, and biases as well as the histories, traditions, and values of the individual. Look for treatment methodologies that reflect the cultural needs of the client.

Become knowledgeable about reproductive health and ensure a nonjudgmental approach.

A strengths-based approach is recommended with pregnant teenage girls who have chosen an abortion resolution.

Clients having abortions report they need quality, safe, and affordable abortion care that provides empathy and privacy.

Remember that timely information is critical when considering pregnancy resolutions with teenagers.

Attend to the adolescent's psychosocial needs by completing a biopsychosocialspiritual assessment; screen for depression.

Clients who are pregnant as a result of rape may need more extensive therapy to address possible guilt, shame, or trauma from the sexual assault in addition to the abortion.

Empower girls to protect themselves from unwanted sex and unwanted pregnancy.

When seeing clients with unwanted pregnancies, clinicians need to be alert to any coercion to either have an abortion or prohibit an abortion and to possible intimate partner violence.

Work with families to help their pregnant teenager decide how to handle the pregnancy.

Family planning counseling is important following abortion.

Become knowledgeable about the consequences of unwanted and unplanned pregnancies, and help reduce them by advocating for and supporting comprehensive family-planning services.

Written by Melissa Rosales Neff, MSW, and Jennifer Teska, MSW

Reviewed by Lynn B. Cooper, D. Crim, and Laura McLuckey, MSW, LCSW

REFERENCES

Baba, S., Goto, A., & Reich, M. (2014). Recent pregnancy trends among early adolescent girls in Japan. *Journal of Obstetrics & Gynaecology Research, 40*(1), 125-132. doi:10.1111/jog.12138

Bearinger, L. H., Sieving, R. E., Ferguson, J., & Sharma, V. (2007). Global perspectives on the sexual and reproductive health of adolescents: Patterns, prevention, and potential. *Lancet, 369*(9568), 1220-1231. doi:10.1016/S0140-6736(07)60367-5

Blyth, E. (2008). Inequalities in reproductive health: What is the challenge for social work and how can it respond? *Journal of Social Work, 8*(3), 213-232. doi:10.1177/1468017308091037

British Association of Social Workers. (2012, January). *The code of ethics for social work: Statement of principles.* Retrieved October 19, 2015, from http://cdn.basw.co.uk/upload/basw_112315-7.pdf

Cleland, J., Bernstein, S., Ezeh, A., Faundes, A., Glasier, A., & Innis, J. (2006). Family planning: The unfinished agenda. *Lancet, 368*(9549), 1810-1827. doi:10.1016/S0140-6736(06)69480-4

Dahlbäck, E., Maimbolwa, M., Kasonka, L., Bergström, S., & Ransjö-Arvidson, A.-B. (2007). Unsafe induced abortions among adolescent girls in Lusaka. *Health Care for Women International, 28*(7), 654-676. doi:10.1080/07399330701462223

Ely, G. E., & Dulmus, C. N. (2008). A psychosocial profile of adolescent pregnancy termination patients. *Social Work in Health Care, 46*(3), 69-83.

Glasier, A., Gülmezoglu, A. M., Schmid, G. P., Moreno, C. G., & Van Look, P. (2006). Sexual and reproductive health: A matter of life and death. *Lancet, 368*(9547), 1595-1607. doi:10.1016/S0140-6736(06)69478-6

Grimes, D. A., Benson, J., Singh, S., Romero, M., Ganatra, B., Okonofua, F. E., & Shah, I. H. (2006). Unsafe abortion: The preventable pandemic. *The Lancet, 368*(9550), 1908-1919. doi:10.1016/S0140-6736(06)69481-6

Grimes, D. A., & Raymond, E. G. (2011). Medical abortion for adolescents: Seems to be as effective and safe as in older women. *BMJ, 342*(7804), 935-936. doi:10.1136/bmj.d2185

Hung, S. L. (2010). Access to safe and legal abortion for teenage women from deprived backgrounds in Hong Kong. *Reproductive Health Matters, 18*(36), 102-110. doi:10.1016/S0968-8080(10)36527-X

International Federation of Social Workers. (2012, March 3). *Statement of ethical principles.* Retrieved October 19, 2015, from http://ifsw.org/policies/statement-of-ethical-principles/

McCarraher, D. R., Chen-Mok, M., Oronoz, A. S., Brito-Anderson, S., Grey, T., Tucker, H., & Bailey, P. E. (2010). Meeting the needs of adolescent post-abortion care patients in the Dominican Republic. *Journal of Biosocial Science, 42*(4), 493-509. doi:10.1017/S0021932010000015

Michaud, P., Berg-Kelly, K., Macfarlane, A., Renteria, S., Wyss, D., & Benaroyo, L. (2009). Addressing ethical dilemmas in the clinical care of adolescents: An international view. *Adolescent Medicine: State of the Art Reviews, 20*(3), 949-960.

National Association of Social Workers. (2001). *NASW standards for cultural competence in social work practice.* Retrieved October 18, 2015, from http://www.socialworkers.org/practice/standards/NASWCulturalStandards.pdf

Ngo, T. D., Park, M. H., Shakur, H., & Free, C. (2011). comparative effectiveness, safety and acceptability of medical abortion at home and in a clinic: A systematic review. *The Bulletin of the World Health Organization, 89*(5), 360-370.

Okereke, C. I. (2010). Assessing the prevalence and determinants of adolescents' unintended pregnancy and induced abortion in Owerri, Nigeria. *Journal of Biosocial Science, 42*(5), 619-632. doi:10.1017/S0021932010000179

Pazol, K., Creanga, A. A., Burley, K. D., Hayes, B., & Jamieson, D. J. (2013). Abortion surveillance—United States, 2010. *Morbidity and Mortality Weekly Report (MMWR), 62*(8), 1-44.

Renner, R.-M., de Guzman, A., & Brahmi, D. (2014). Abortion care for adolescent and young women. *International Journal of Gynaecology and Obstetrics: The Official Organ of the International Federation of Gynaecology and Obstetrics, 126*(1), 1-7. doi:10.1016/j. ijgo.2013.07.034

Rowlands, S. (2007). More than one abortion. *Journal of Family Planning & Reproductive Health Care, 33*(3), 155-158.

Sastre, M. T., Peccarisi, C., Legrain, E., Mullet, E., & Sorum, P. (2007). Acceptability in France of induced abortion for adolescents. *American Journal of Bioethic, 7*(8), 26-32. doi:10.1080/15265160701462368

Sedgh, G., Finer, L. B., Bankole, A., Eilers, M. A., & Singh, S. (2015). Adolescent pregnancy, birth, and abortion rates across countries: Levels and recent trends. *The Journal of Adolescent Health, 56*(2), 223-230. doi:10.1016/j. jadohealth.2014.09.007

Sedgh, G., Henshaw, S., Singh, S., Åhman, E., & Shah, I. H. (2007). Induced abortion: Estimated rates and trends worldwide. *Lancet, 370*(9595), 1338-1345. doi:10.1016/S0140-6736(07)61575-X

Sedgh, G., Singh, S., & Hussain, R. (2014). Intended and unintended pregnancies worldwide in 2012 and recent trends. *Studies in Family Planning, 45*(3), 301-314. doi:10.1111/j.1728-4465.2014.00393. x

Warren, J. T., Harvey, S. M., & Henderson, J. T. (2010). Do depression and low self-esteem follow abortion among adolescents? Evidence from a national study. *Perspectives on Sexual and Reproductive Health, 42*(4), 230-235. doi:10.1363/4223010

Weitz, T. A., & Cockrill, K. (2010). Abortion clinic patients' opinions about obtaining abortions from general women's health care providers. *Patient Education and Counseling, 81*(3), 409-414. doi:10.1016/j. pec.2010.09.003

World Health Organization (WHO). (n. d.). Maternal, newborn, child and adolescent health: Adolescent pregnancy. Retrieved October 19, 2015, from http://www.who. int/maternal_child_adolescent/topics/maternal/adolescent_pregnancy/en/

World Health Organization (WHO). (2006). *Frequently asked clinical questions about medical abortion.* Retrieved October 19, 2015, from http://www.gynmed. at/sites/default/files/faq-medical-abortion.pdf

World Health Organization (WHO). (2014). Adolescent pregnancy (Fact sheet N°364). Retrieved October 19, 2015, from http://www.who. int/mediacentre/factsheets/fs364/en/

World Health Organization, Department of Reproductive Health and Research. (2012). *Safe abortion: Technical and policy guidance for health systems (2nd ed.).* Retrieved October 19, 2015, from http://www.who. int/reproductivehealth/publications/unsafe_abortion/9789241548434/en/

Zakus, G., & Wilday, S. (1987). Adolescent abortion option. *Social Work in Health Care, 12*(4), 77-91. doi:10.1300/J010v12n04_06

PREGNANCY IN ADOLESCENCE: RISK FACTORS

MAJOR CATEGORIES: Adolescents, Medical & Health, Gender/Identity, Homelessness

WHAT WE KNOW

The rate of adolescents ages 15–19 giving birth in the United States was 24.2 births per 1,000 adolescents in 2014, a decrease of 9 percent from 2013. Although birth rates have declined by 61 percent since 1991, adolescent pregnancy rates in the United States are still much higher than those in other developed countries. The birth rate is highest for adolescents ages 18–19 with 43.8 births per 1,000 adolescents. The birth rate for teens ages 15–17 is 10.9 births per 1,000 adolescents. The birth rate for girls ages 14 years or younger is significantly lower than that of older teens with 0.3 births per 1,000 girls.

Birth rates for adolescents ages 15–19 vary considerably among states, ranging in 2014 from 10.6 births per 1,000 adolescents in Massachusetts to 39.5 births per 1,000 adolescent females in Arkansas.

Birth rates for adolescents ages 15–19 were highest for Hispanic teens (38 births per 1,000 Hispanic teens) and black teens (34.9 births per 1,000 black teens), compared with 17.3 births per 1,000 for white teens.

Among adolescents ages 15–19 enrolled in the military healthcare system as dependents, the birth rate is lower than the national rate (15.8 births per 1,000 adolescents). Among females enlisted in the military, almost one third of first births are to females under 21 years of age. Sexual activity combined with not using contraceptives or using them improperly or inconsistently is the major cause of pregnancy among adolescents. Most first-time pregnancies in adolescence occur within 6 months of first sexual intercourse, and most pregnancies in adolescence are unplanned.

At least 80 percent of adolescents who are 15 years or older when they first initiate sexual activity start using contraceptives during the same month, compared with a little over half of those who first have sex at 12–14 years of age or younger. In the 2013 National Youth Risk Behavior survey, almost 47 percent of students in grades 9–12 reported having had sexual intercourse. Among the 34 percent of students who reported being currently sexually active, 13.7 percent reported not using any form of contraceptive during their last sexual intercourse.

Ecological systems theory can be used to conceptualize the multiple, interacting risk factors associated with adolescent pregnancy. Based upon the ecological systems theory, the risk factors for adolescent pregnancy can be characterized as individual, partner-related, family-related, and social/environmental. Individual risk factors for pregnancy in adolescence in the United States include non-white race, early menarche (i.e., age at first menstruation), early sexual debut (i.e., younger age at first intercourse), higher number of sexual partners, absent or ineffective use of contraception, positive or ambivalent perception of pregnancy, history of pregnancy, history of sexual or physical abuse, history of neglect, mental health problems, lower intelligence or learning disability, lower educational attainment, poor school performance, being in foster care, risky sexual behavior, lack of knowledge regarding contraception and consequences of risky sexual behavior, substance use, and delinquency.

Researchers in a large study found that adolescent girls involved with the juvenile justice system were more than 3 times more likely to give birth as teens than their peers who had not been involved with the juvenile justice system. Prior pregnancy is a significant risk factor in adolescent females. Just under 20 percent of births to teen mothers are to teens who have given birth at least once previously, and nearly 70 percent of these repeat births occur within 18 months, increasing the risk for preterm birth.

Partner characteristics also contribute to the risk for pregnancy in adolescence. The likelihood that a female adolescent will become pregnant increases if she perceives that the relationship with her partner is not casual, if she has little decision-making power in the relationship, or if her male partner has any of the following characteristics: is older than she is; has a history of being sexually abused; is involved in gang activity; or is incarcerated (pregnancy usually occurs after the partner is released).

The greatest risk factor for adolescent pregnancy is pregnancy intention. If the male partner intends to impregnate his female partner or she perceives that he desires her to become pregnant, the likelihood of pregnancy increases. In a United States study, 6 percent of males ages 15–19 reported ever being involved in a pregnancy. Researchers found that the prevalence of pregnancy involvement increased significantly among males with specific clusters of risk factors. The highest pregnancy-involvement prevalence (87 percent) was found in a cluster of adolescent males who at some point sought HIV testing, who reported having more than 4 lifetime sexual partners and 2 sexual partners in the past year, who expected to feel less pleasure with condom use, and whose highest educational attainment was below 11th grade.

Although research regarding the impact of sexual abuse on fatherhood is limited, male partners who have been sexually abused may perceive fathering a child as a way of restoring their masculinity. Having a male partner who is a member of a gang increases the risk for pregnancy in adolescent females. Membership of an adolescent female in a gang, however, does not appear to affect pregnancy risk.

Familial/parental characteristics that contribute to the risk for pregnancy in adolescence include maternal history of adolescent pregnancy, emotional abuse from a mother, exposure to family violence, having single or divorced parents, having an incarcerated household member, poor family communication, having a greater number of siblings, having an older sibling who is sexually active, pregnant, or parenting, lack of parental supervision, disengagement from family, poor parent–child relationship, and harsh or inconsistent discipline by parents. A maternal history of adolescent pregnancy increases the risk for adolescent pregnancy by 66 percent. Youth in foster care are at increased risk for pregnancy.

Social/environmental risk factors for teen pregnancy include peer pressure, association with peers who engage in sexual activity or use drugs or alcohol, lack of access to confidential contraceptive services, fewer economic resources or fewer enrichment opportunities (e.g., afterschool programs), and a cultural background that supports adolescent pregnancy.

Academic achievement, school attendance, and involvement in school and/or plans for higher education result in a reduced rate of adolescent pregnancy. Students participating in school programs that foster attachment to school or dropout reduction programs have lower rates of adolescent pregnancy even when the program does not directly address sexuality. In areas where parental notification is required for contraceptive services, teens delay seeking contraceptive services.

Homeless or runaway teens become pregnant at a rate 4 times higher than that of teens who are not homeless or runaways. This risk increases with the amount of time the adolescent has been homeless. Homeless and runaway teens may trade sex for food or money. The expense and feasibility of using contraception may be prohibitive for homeless/runaway teens. Many homeless/runaway adolescents also have other risk factors for pregnancy, including being a member of an ethnic minority group, dropping out of school, a history of early sexual debut, substance use, or family dysfunction/abuse (particularly emotional abuse by the teen's mother).

Adolescent females from disadvantaged backgrounds with few professional opportunities may choose early motherhood as an alternative to a finding a career. Culture also affects adolescent females' perception of early motherhood. Latino cultures often promote motherhood as the ideal female role.

WHAT CAN BE DONE

Social workers can learn about the risk factors for adolescent pregnancy, as well as pregnancy prevention, treatment (e.g., prenatal care, pregnancy termination), and health outcomes in order to accurately assess clients' personal, medical and mental health needs. Social workers should complete an assessment of the adolescent's risk factors for pregnancy, including assessing for violence, statutory rape, substance abuse, and mental health issues, which is critical to providing appropriate client care. Assessments should include information about the adolescents' and families' attitudes toward pregnancy and parenthood, including exploring family, cultural, and religious influences. Prevention efforts should address individual, peer, and family risk factors for adolescent pregnancy and should be introduced during pre-teen years. Longer programs (over 6 months–1 year) are more effective at supporting the retention of knowledge and targeted behaviors.

Education may be provided to adolescent clients, both male and female, about methods of pregnancy prevention. The social worker should promote self-efficacy and teach strategies for dealing with peer pressure, risky situations, and refusing sex. Pregnancy prevention programs may be enhanced by incorporating education about gender roles and additional risk factors such as substance use. Adolescent clients should be encouraged to maintain school involvement, academic achievement, and regular school attendance.

Social workers can educate parents about the importance of remaining connected with their adolescents and providing support and supervision. Family-based programs may be utilized to strengthen parent–child relationships and communication styles. Motivational interviewing may be a helpful technique that social workers can use to engage adolescents in discussions of health-related behaviors such as substance abuse, risky sexual behaviors, and pregnancy prevention.

Social workers must follow facility protocols regarding confidentiality rules, parental notification/consent needs, rules on the dispensing of birth control, and mandated reporting laws if an adolescent is a victim of statutory rape or abuse. Social workers may provide referrals for adolescent-focused prenatal care, academic programs that focus on helping pregnant teens complete high school, parenting classes, support groups, childcare, transportation, legal assistance for abuse victims, and substance abuse treatment, if appropriate.

More information can be obtained from the following resources:

- Advocates for Youth, http://www.advocatesforyouth.org
- GuttmacherInstitute, https://www.guttmacher.org/
- Healthy Teen Network, http://www.healthyteen-network.org/
- Office of Adolescent Health, Reproductive Health, http://www.hhs.gov/ash/oah/adolescent-health-topics/reproductive-health
- Planned Parenthood Federation of America, http://www.plannedparenthood.org
- The National Campaign to Prevent Teen and Unplanned Pregnancy, http://www.thenationalcampaign.org

*Written by Gilberto Cabrera, MD, and
Jennifer Teska, MSW*

*Reviewed by Jessica Therivel, LMSW-IPR, and
Laura McLuckey, MSW, LCSW*

REFERENCES

Aparicio, E., Pecukonis, E. V., & Zhou, K. (2014). Sociocultural factors of teenage pregnancy in Latino communities: Preparing social workers for culturally responsive practice. *Health & Social Work, 39*(4), 238-243. doi:10.1093/hsw/hlu032

Barrett, D., Katsiyannis, A., Zhang, D., & Kingree, J. (2015). Predictors of teen childbearing among delinquent and non-delinquent females. *Journal of Child & Family Studies, 24*(4), 970-978. doi:10.1007/s10826-014-9907-6

British Association of Social Workers. (2012, January). The code of ethics for social work: Statement of principles. Retrieved April 11, 2016, from http://cdn.basw.co.uk/upload/basw_112315-7.pdf

Burr, J. E., Roberts, T. A., & Bucci, J. R. (2013). Dependent adolescent pregnancy rates and risk factors for pregnancy in the military health care system. *Military Medicine, 178*(4), 412-415. doi:10.7205/MILMED-D-12-00461

Connery, H. S., Albright, B. B., & Rodolico, J. M. (2014). Adolescent substance use and unplanned pregnancy: strategies for risk reduction. *Obstetrics & Gynecology Clinics of North America, 41*(2), 191-203. doi:10.1016/j.ogc.2014.02.011

Finley, C. (2013). Integrating evidence-based teen pregnancy prevention in child welfare: Outcomes and impact for youth and systems. *Policy & Practice, 71*(6), 16-19.

Finner, L. B., & Philbin, J. M. (2013). Sexual initiation, contraceptive use, and pregnancy among young adolescents. *Pediatrics, 131*(5), 886-891. doi:10.1542/peds.2012-3495

Francisco, M. A., Hicks, K., Powell, J., Styles, K., Tabor, J. L., & Hulton, L. J. (2008). The effect of childhood sexual abuse on adolescent pregnancy: An integrative research review. *Journal for Specialists in Pediatric Nursing, 13*(4), 237-248. doi:10.1111/j.1744-6155.2008.00160.x

Glassman, J. R., Franks, H. M., Baumler, E. R., & Coyle, K. K. (2014). Mediation analysis of an adolescent HIV/STI/pregnancy prevention intervention. *Sex Education, 14*(5), 497-509. doi:10.1080/14681811.2014.914025

Hamilton, B. E., Martin, J. A., Osterman, M. J. K., Curtin, S. C., & Mathews, T. J. (2015). Births: Final data for 2014. *National Vital Statistics Reports, 64 (2)*. Retrieved April 11, 2016, from http://www.cdc.gov/nchs/data/nvsr/nvsr64/nvsr64_12.pdf

Helfrich, C. M., & McWey, L. M. (2014). Substance use and delinquency: High-risk behaviors as predictors of teen pregnancy among adolescents involved with the child welfare system. *Journal of Family Issues, 35*(10), 1322-1338. doi:10.1177/0192513X13478917

Hoskins, D., & Simons, L. (2015). Predicting the risk of pregnancy among African American youth: Testing a social contextual model. *Journal of Child & Family Studies, 24*(4), 1163-1174. doi:10.1007/s10826-014-9925-4

International Federation of Social Workers. (2012). Statement of ethical principles. Retrieved May 17, 2015, from http://ifsw.org/policies/statement-of-ethical-principles/

Kann, L., Kinchen, S., Shanklin, S. L., Flint, K. H., Hawkins, J., Harris, W. A.,... Zaza, S. (2014). Youth Risk Behavior Surveillance – United States, 2013. *Morbidity and Mortality Weekly Report (MMWR)*. Retrieved May 23, 2015, from http://www.cdc.gov/mmwr/pdf/ss/ss6304.pdf?utm_source=rss&utm_medium=rss&utm_campaign=youth-risk-behavior-surveillance-united-states-2013-pdf

Killebrew, A. E., Smith, M. L., Nevels, R. M., & Weiss, N. H. (2014). African-American adolescent females in the southeastern United States: Associations among risk factors for teen pregnancy. *Journal of Child & Adolescent Substance Abuse, 23*(2), 65-77. doi:10.1080/1067828X.2012.748591

King, B., Putnam-Hornstein, E., Cederbaum, J. A., & Needell, B. (2014). A cross-sectional examination of birth rates among adolescent girls in foster care. *Children and Youth Services Review, 36,* 179-196. doi:10.1016/j.childyouth.2013.11.007

Kirby, D. (2002). The impact of schools and school programs upon adolescent sexual behavior. *Journal of Sex Research, 39*(1), 27-33. doi:10.1080/00224490209552116

Klein, D. A., & Adelman, W. P. (2008). Adolescent pregnancy in the U. S. military: What We Know and what we need to know. *Military Medicine, 173*(7), 658-665. doi:10.7205/milmed.173.7.658

Lau, M., Lin, H., & Flores, G. (2015). Clusters of factors identify a high prevalence of pregnancy involvement among US adolescent males. *Maternal & Child Health Journal, 19*(8), 1713-1723. doi:10.1007/s10995-015-1685-2

Lee, Y. M., Cintron, A, & Kocher, S. (2014). Factors related to risky sexual behaviors and effective STI/HIV and pregnancy intervention programs for African American adolescents. *Public Health Nursing, 31*(5), 414-427. doi:10.1111/phn.12128

Leonard, S. M., & Suellentrop, K. (2013). Integrating pregnancy prevention in child welfare: Supporting youth in care to prevent teen pregnancy. *Policy & Practice, 71*(4), 24-31.

Madigan, S., Wade, M., Tarabulsy, G. M., & Shouldice, M. (2014). Association between abuse history and adolescent pregnancy: A meta-analysis. *Journal of Adolescent Health, 55*(2), 151-159. doi:10.1016/j.jadohealth.2014.05.002

Meade, C. S., Kershaw, T. S., & Ickovics, J. R. (2008). The intergenerational cycle of teenage motherhood: An ecological approach. *Health Psychology, 27*(4), 419-429. doi:10.1037/0278-6133.27.4.419

Minnis, A. M., Moore, J. G., Doherty, I. A., Rodas, C., Auerswald, C., Shiboski, S., & Pandian, N. S. (2008). Gang exposure and pregnancy incidence among female adolescents in San Francisco: Evidence for the need to integrate reproductive health with violence prevention efforts. *American Journal of Epidemiology, 167*(9), 1102-1109. doi:10.1093/aje/kwn011

Murphy-Erby, Y., Stauss, K., & Estupinian, E. F. (2013). Participant-informed model for preventing teen pregnancy in a rural Latino community. *Journal of Family Social Work, 16*(1), 70-85. doi:10.1080/1052 2158.2012.749187

National Association of Social Workers. (2003). NASW standards for the practice of social work with adolescents. Retrieved April 11, 2016, from http://socialworkers.org/practice/standards/Adolescents.asp

National Association of Social Workers. (2015). Standards and indicators for cultural competence in social work practice. Retrieved April 11, 2016, from http://www.socialworkers.org/practice/standards/PRA-BRO-253150-CC-Standards.pdf

Nerlander, L., Callaghan, W., Smith, R., & Barfield, W. (2015). Short interpregnancy interval associated with preterm birth in U.S. adolescents. *Maternal & Child Health Journal, 19*(4), 850-858. doi:10.1007/s10995-014-1583-z

Noll, J. G., & Shenk, C. E. (2013). Teen birth rates in sexually abused and neglected females. *Pediatrics, 131*(4), e1181-e1187. doi:10.1542/peds.2012-3072

Noll, J. G., Shenk, C. E., & Putnam, K. T. (2009). Childhood sexual abuse and adolescent pregnancy: A meta-analytic update. *Journal of Pediatric Psychology, 34*(4), 366-378. doi:10.1093/jpepsy/jsn098

Secor-Turner, M., McMorris, B., Sieving, R., & Bearinger, L. H. (2013). Life experiences of instability and sexual risk behaviors among high-risk adolescent females. *Perspectives on Sexual & Reproductive Health, 45*(2), 101-107. doi:10.1363/4510113

Sedgh, G., Finer, L. B., Bankole, A., Eilers, M. A., & Singh, S. (2015). Adolescent pregnancy, birth, and abortion rates across countries: Levels and recent trends. *Journal of Adolescent Health, 56*(2), 223-230. doi:10.1016/j.jadohealth.2014.09.007

Thompson, S. J., Bender, K. A., Lewis, C. M., & Watkins, R. (2008). Runaway and pregnant: Risk factors associated with pregnancy in a national sample of runaway/homeless female adolescents. *Journal of Adolescent Health, 43*(2), 125-132. doi:10.1016/j.jadohealth.2007.12.015

Whalen, M. L., & Loper, A. B. (2014). Teenage pregnancy in adolescents with an incarcerated household member. *Western Journal of Nursing Research, 36*(3), 346-361. doi:10.1177/0193945913496873

PRENATAL CARE, HEALTHCARE COSTS IN THE UNITED STATES

MAJOR CATEGORIES: Medical & Health

WHAT WE KNOW

Prenatal care (PNC) is an important part of maintaining a healthy pregnancy. The typical schedule for PNC in the United States includes visiting a medical professional (such as an OBGYN or Midwife) about once each month during the first 6 months of pregnancy, every 2 weeks during the 7th and 8th months of pregnancy, and weekly in the last month of pregnancy, for a total of about 14 visits. PNC should begin as soon as a woman suspects she is pregnant.

In 2013, an analysis was conducted of PNC costs in the United States. Investigators found that in 2010, average total charges for a vaginal birth were $29,800 for Medicaid and $32,093 for commercial insurance. For cesarean births, charges were $50,373 for Medicaid and $51,125 for commercial insurance.

PNC includes a medical history, establishing a due date to assist in monitoring fetal growth, a physical exam, a pelvic exam, diagnostic tests (e.g., blood type and Rh factor; rubella titer; screenings for syphilis and hepatitis B; urinalysis), discussion of lifestyle issues (e.g., nutrition, prenatal vitamins, exercise), and fetal ultrasound.

Costs for diagnostic tests during pregnancy typically were about $1,000 in 2004; costs may increase if the pregnancy is high-risk (requiring more tests) or if a woman chooses to undergo additional, optional tests (e.g., genetic testing).

Costs vary by site of care. In 2007, for instance, Kaiser Permanente, a self-insured provider, reported that PNC and hospital delivery cost on average about $10,000 per pregnancy in 2004.

The costs incurred during the inpatient stay related to birth account for the majority of the total cost related to pregnancy.

In 2014, researchers in California found that charges for delivery varied widely depending on hospital. In studying uncomplicated births in 2011, the researchers found that for a vaginal delivery, charges ranged from $3,296 to $37,227; for a cesarean delivery, they ranged from $8,312 to $70,908. Market-level (i.e., location) and institution-level differences (i.e., different hospitals charging different amounts for same services) accounted for only about 35 percent of the variation between hospitals, leaving approximately two thirds of the variation unexplained.

From 2004 to 2010 the average amount paid by commercial insurance plans for maternal care increased substantially: payments for cesarean births increased 41 percent and those for vaginal birth increased 49 percent. Out-of-pocket costs for mothers increased almost 4-fold in this same time period.

In 2007, about 75 percent of pregnancy-related prescription drug expenses were for prenatal vitamins and other nutritional supplements.

When complications develop during pregnancy, they are responsible for a significant increase in healthcare costs. Complications during pregnancy often are associated with high-risk pregnancy, which can increase the length of hospital stay and costs associated with care.

Pre-pregnancy factors that may make a pregnancy high-risk include younger or older maternal age, being overweight or underweight, having complications in previous pregnancies (e.g., pregnancy-induced hypertension, preterm labor), and certain medical conditions, such as high blood pressure, diabetes, and HIV infection.

Conditions occurring during pregnancy that make a pregnancy high-risk include preeclampsia and eclampsia, gestational diabetes, HIV infection/AIDS, multiple births, and preterm labor.

In the last 30 years, the percentage of women over age 40 having twins or higher multiples has increased 200 percent.

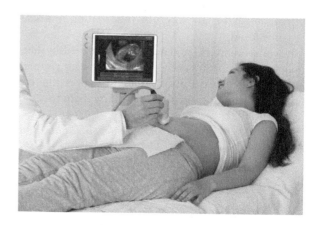

The Affordable Care Act (ACA) identified PNC as an essential health benefit, but prior to the act, in 2011, 62 percent of individuals and families who purchased their own health insurance did not have maternity coverage.

Because all plans purchased through the health insurance exchanges created by the ACA cover pregnancy and childbirth, it was anticipated that in 2014, 8.7 million Americans would be able to obtain maternity coverage.

Prenatal healthcare programs may be able to reduce costs overall.

Home visits by clinicians during a high-risk pregnancy may reduce overall pregnancy-related healthcare costs.

Prenatal care provided in a group setting (e.g., the Centering Pregnancy model) improves birth outcomes and is cost-effective.

Centering Pregnancy brings together pregnant women with similar due dates for a series of clinician-facilitated educational discussions and health evaluation activities that provide a social setting in which the women can receive care and build a support network.

WHAT CAN BE DONE

Learn about PNC healthcare costs so you can accurately assess personal characteristics and health education needs; share this knowledge with friends and family.

Maintain good health and become educated regarding the details of positive lifestyle changes before and during pregnancy, including:

- seeing a medical professional to evaluate preconception health;
- beginning PNC early and maintaining consistent PNC;
- maintaining a healthy weight;
- how to initiate and maintain a regular exercise program that is approved by the treating medical professional;
- the components of good nutrition and a healthy diet;
- taking at least 400 micrograms of folic acid supplementation every day prior to and during pregnancy;
- avoiding smoking, alcohol, and illicit drug use.

Written by Amy E. Beddoe, RN, PhD, and Jessica Therivel, LMSW-IPR

Reviewed by Jessica Therivel, LMSW-IPR, and Melissa Rosales Neff, MSW

REFERENCES

Agency for Healthcare Research and Quality, AHRQ Health Care Innovations Exchange. (2013, November 6). Telephone-based case management and periodic home visits reduce neonatal intensive care unit utilization and overall costs for high-risk pregnant women and their babies. Retrieved March 29, 2016, from https://innovations.ahrq.gov/profiles/telephone-based-case-management-and-periodic-home-visits-reduce-neonatal-intensive-care

Agency for Healthcare Research and Quality, AHRQ Health Care Innovations Exchange. (2015). Group visits focused on prenatal care and parenting improve birth outcomes and provider efficiency. Retrieved March 29, 2016, from https://innovations.ahrq.gov/profiles/group-visits-focused-prenatal-care-and-parenting-improve-birth-outcomes-and-provider

Akkerman, D., Cleland, L., Croft, G., Eskuchen, K., Heim, C., Levine, A.,... Westby, E. (2012). Health care guideline. Routine prenatal care. Retrieved March 29, 2016, from http://www.icsi.org/_asset/13n9y4/Prenatal.pdf

Anastas, J. W., & Clark, E. J. (2013). NASW standards for social work case management. Retrieved April 5, 2016, from http://www.socialworkers.org/practice/naswstandards/CaseManagementStandards2013.pdf

Briery, C. M., & Morrison, J. (2013, May). Overview of High-Risk Pregnancy. Retrieved March 29, 2016, from http://www.merckmanuals.com/home/womens_health_issues/pregnancy_at_high-risk/definition_of_high-risk_pregnancy.html

British Association of Social Workers. (2012, January). The code of ethics for social work: Statement of principles. Retrieved March 29, 2016, from http://cdn.basw.co.uk/upload/basw_112315-7.pdf

Eunice Kennedy Shriver National Institute of Child Health and Human Development, National Institutes of Health. (2013). High-risk pregnancy. Retrieved March 29, 2016, from http://www.nichd.nih.gov/health/topics/high-risk/Pages/default.aspx

Hsia, R. Y., Antwi, Y. A., & Weber, E. (2014). Analysis of variation in charges and prices paid for vaginal and caesarean section births: A cross-sectional study. *BMJ Open, 4*(1), e004017. doi:10.1136/bmjopen-2013-004017

International Federation of Social Workers. (2012, March 3). *Statement of ethical principles.* Retrieved March 29, 2016, from http://ifsw.org/policies/statement-of-ethical-principles/

Machlin, S. R., & Rohde, F. (2007). Research findings no. 27: Health care expenditures for uncomplicated pregnancies. Agency for Healthcare Research and Quality. Retrieved March 29, 2016, from http://www.meps.ahrq.gov/mepsweb/data_files/publications/rf27/rf27.pdf

Martin, J. A., Hamilton, B. E., & Osterman, M. J. K. (2012). Three decades of twin births in the United States, 1980-2009. *NCHS Data Brief, No. 80,* 1-8.

National Association of Social Workers. (2015). *Standards for cultural competence in social work practice.* Retrieved March 26, 2016, from http://www.socialworkers.org/practice/standards/PRA-BRO-253150-CC-Standards.pdf

Pollitz, K., Kofman, M., Salganicoff, A., & Ranji, U. (2007). Maternity care and consumer-driven health plans: Executive summary. *The Henry J. Kaiser Family Foundation.* Retrieved March 29, 2016, from http://kff.org/health-costs/report/maternity-care-and-consumer-driven-health-plans/

Truven Health Analytics. (2013, January). The cost of having a baby in the United States: Executive summary. Retrieved March 29, 2016, from http://transform.childbirthconnection.org/wp-content/uploads/2013/01/Cost-of-Having-a-Baby-Executive-Summary.pdf

U.S. Department of Health and Human Services. (2011). Essential health benefits: Individual market coverage. *ASPE Issue Brief.* Retrieved March 29, 2016, from http://aspe.hhs.gov/health/reports/2011/individualmarket/ib.shtml

PROBATION OFFICERS

MAJOR CATEGORIES: Incarceration/Probation

WHAT WE KNOW

The global practice of probation began over 150 years ago. John Augustus, a boot maker in Boston, came upon a man who was being charged by a judge as a drunkard and took pity on him. Augustus asked the judge to release the man to his care. The judge agreed, making Augustus the first American probation officer. From then on, respected citizens could act as "trusted bondsmen" to supervise offenders, provide moral guidance, and assist them in finding lodging and employment. The probation movement grew as more citizens volunteered to oversee offenders. In Europe, volunteer organizations were founded to provide supervision for individuals in lieu of prison time in the nineteenth century.

By the mid-twentieth century, probation had become formalized and was overseen by professional counselors. However, many probation officers had high caseloads and were underfunded. In the 1960s and 1970s, there was a movement toward shifting resources away from institutions such as prison and to community alternatives such as probation.

The Bureau of Justice Statistics (BJS) defines probation as "a court-appointed period of correctional supervision in the community, generally as an alternative to incarceration." Probation sometimes takes the form of incarceration followed by supervision in the community.

Parole is different from probation. Parole is "a period of conditional supervised release in the community following prison. It includes parolees released through discretionary or mandatory supervised release from prison, those released through other types of post-custody conditional supervision (serving a sentence in the community instead of prison) and those sentenced to a term of supervised release."

In 2013, 4,751,400 individuals in the United States (1 in 50) were under community supervision, which includes probation and parole. Of those, 82 percent were on probation. In 2012, there were approximately 90,300 probation officers and corrections specialists in the United States.

With nearly 5 million individuals on probation, caseloads for some probation officers are as high as 150–200 persons. Probation officers work with both youths (juvenile probation) and adults to help offenders obey the law (to prevent further crimes), rehabilitating offenders, and keeping society in general safe. The specific responsibilities of the probation officer vary depending on local laws, the perceived risk of the probationer, and the severity of the offense.

During the initial assessment, the probation officer reviews the offender's case file to estimate the offender's risk of recidivism based on the pre-sentence investigation report. The probation officer decides the type of supervision the offender will receive using risk assessment tools with the information from the report.

The probation officer uses standardized risk-assessment tools to determine the likelihood of recidivism. Both "static" information and "dynamic" information may be used in assessing the offender's risk of reoffending. The static information is information about the individual such as sex, age at first conviction, number of previous prison sentences, and type of offense. The dynamic risk factors considered are education, training, and employability; residence; relationships; lifestyle; drug and alcohol misuse; and emotional well-being. The levels of monitoring vary depending on each case.

Probation officers can work on a regular basis with offenders by seeing them weekly and developing a case-management plan to help them establish employment and find housing. If needed, probation officers may also make referrals to mental health services. Some cases may require a probation officer to make unscheduled visits to an offender's home or workplace and monitor him or her using a GPS system through an ankle bracelet. Some cases (for lower-level offenses) do not even require that the probation office check in with the offender.

Probation officers have a variety of educational backgrounds. In the United Kingdom, a diploma of probation studies is offered specifically for individuals who want to become probation officers. Probation officers in South Africa have social work backgrounds and have the skill set to provide rehabilitative services to individuals (as opposed to making referrals to local services for counseling, employment help, etc.). In the United States, probation officers typically have a bachelor's degree in criminal justice. They also receive training in investigation guidelines, report writing, substance abuse and mental health treatment, firearms, and safety.

There is often an overlap between social work and criminal justice, but there still are not many master's-level programs in the United States for social work that include this content. Researchers found that only 18 percent of Master's in Social Work (MSW) programs in the United States offer a dual-degree program combining an MSW with either a law or a criminal justice degree. 43 percent offered at least one criminal justice course as part of their MSW offerings.

Of a sample of 257 students in the United Kingdom working toward their diploma in probation studies in the UK, 70 percent were female, 73.8 percent were white, and 91.1 percent were heterosexual. The individuals in the study reported that they wanted to be probation officers because they wanted to help people, exercise their abilities to solve problems, exercise control and authority, wear a uniform, and be personally fulfilled.

Research has described the psychosocial effects of work on probation officers. Individuals working in justice occupations experience stress and burnout (emotional exhaustion). In a 2013 study, investigators found that burnout, role conflict (when incompatible demands are placed on an employee), and work stress are predictors of depressive symptoms among probation officers. Depressive symptoms can affect work performance and cause absenteeism.

WHAT CAN BE DONE

Treatment methodologies should reflect the cultural values, beliefs, and biases of the individual in need of care and treatment.

Learn about probation officers and their work to accurately assess the client's needs as related to probation.

Partner with probation officers when working in various contexts with juveniles (e. g., child welfare, group homes, schools) and with adults (e. g., in courts, providing psychological assessments for offenders).

Advocate for organizational changes that can alleviate stress and burnout among probation officers.

Advocate for more inclusion of criminal justice offerings in social work programs and field placements for master's in social work candidates within the criminal justice system (e. g., in prisons, in probation services) to increase their knowledge of the criminal justice system, skills in assessing risk of recidivism, and ability to write court reports.

If in a therapeutic setting, provide probation officers with strategies to deal with work-related stress and burnout (e. g., relaxation techniques, establishment of boundaries between work and personal life).

Written by Melissa Rosales Neff, MSW

Reviewed by Laura Gale, LCSW

REFERENCES

Bureau of Justice Statistics. (2015). Probation and parole in the United States, 2013. Retrieved October 31, 2015, from http://www.bjs.gov/content/pub/pdf/ppus13.pdf

Gayman, M. D., & Bradley, M. S. (2013).organizational climate, work stress and depressive symptoms among probation and parole officers. *Criminal Justice Studies, 26*(3), 326-346. doi:10.1080/1478601X.2012.742436

Gxubane, T. (2008). Agents of restorative justice? Probation officers in the child justice system. *SA Crime Quarterly, 25*(11-16).

Hek, R. (2012). Is it possible to develop and sustain non-traditional placements? An evaluation of the development of practice learning opportunities in partnership with the police and probation services in the West Midlands. *Social Work Education, 31*(4), 512-529. doi:10.1080/02615479.2011.570328

International Federation of Social Workers. (2012, March 3). Statement of ethical principles. Retrieved October 31, 2015, from http://ifsw.org/policies/statement-of-ethical-principles/

Knight, C. (2007). Why choose probation?. *British Journal of Community Justice, 5*(2), 55-69.

Lambert, E. G., Hogan, N. L., Cheeseman, D. K., Jiang, S., & Khondaker, M. (2012). Is the job burning me out? An exploratory test of the job characteristics model on the emotional burnout of prison staff. *The Prison Journal, 92*(1), 3-23. doi:10.1177/0032885511428794

Lancaster, E., & Lumb, J. (2006). The assessment of risk in the National Probation Service in England and Wales. *Journal of Social Work, 6*(3), 275-291. doi:10.1177/1468017306071176

Louden, J. E., & Skeem, J. L. (2013). How do probation officers assess and manage recidivism and violence risk for probationers with mental disorder? An experimental investigation. *Law and Human Behavior, 37*(1), 22-34. doi:10.1037/h0093991

Mizrahi, T., & Mayden, R. W. (2001). NASW standards for cultural competence in social work practice. Retrieved October 31, 2015, from http://www.socialworkers.org/practice/standards/NASWCulturalStandards.pdf

Peters, C. M. (2011). Social work and juvenile probation: Historical tensions and contemporary convergences. *Social Work, 56*(4), 355-365. doi:10.1093/sw/56.4.355

Perrault, R. T., Paiva-Salisbury, M., & Vincent, G. M. (2012). Probation officers' perceptions of youths' risk of reoffending and use of risk assessment in case management. *Behavioral Sciences & The Law, 30*(4), 487-505. doi:10.1002/bsl.2015

Phelps, M. (2011). Mass incarceration and (mass) probation: The two faces of punitiveness or differing strategies control? Conference paper presented at the American Sociological Association, Las Vegas, NV.

Svensson, K. (2004). An integrated organization for institutionalised caring power: Prison and probation in Sweden. *British Journal of Community Justice, 3*(1), 57-68.

British Association of Social Workers. (2012, January). The code of ethics for social work: Statement of principles. Retrieved October 31, 2015, from http://cdn. basw.co.uk/upload/basw_112315-7.pdf

Probation and pretrial officers and officer assistants. (n. d.). *United States Courts*. Retrieved October 31, 2015, from http://www.uscourts.gov/services-forms/probation-and-pretrial-services/probation-and-pretrial-officers-and-officer

Occupational outlook handbook: Probation officers and correctional treatment specialists. (2014). *Bureau of Labor Statistics*. Retrieved October 31, 2015, from http://www.bls.gov/ooh/community-and-social-service/probation-officers-and-correctional-treatment-specialists. htm

Epperson, M. W., Roberts, L. E., Ivanoff, A., Tripodi, S. J., & Gilmer, C. N. (2013). To what extent is criminal justice content specifically addressed in MSW programs in the United States? Retrieved October 31, 2015, from http://diginole. lib. fsu.edu/cgi/viewcontent. cgi?article=1007&context=csw_faculty_publications

PROBATION: EFFECTIVENESS

MAJOR CATEGORIES: Incarceration/Probation

WHAT WE KNOW

The United States Bureau of Justice Statistics defines probation as "a court-appointed period of correctional supervision in the community, generally as an alternative to incarceration." More rarely, probation follows a period of incarceration. At the end of 2013, 4,751,400 individuals (approximately 1 in 51 adult Americans) were under supervision in the community, which includes probation and parole (i..e., community supervision following a prison term). Of these persons, 82 percent were on probation. There are approximately 100,000 probation and parole officers in the United States. Caseloads for some probation officers can be as high as 150–200 persons.

The purposes of probation are to help probationers obey the law (to prevent further crimes), to rehabilitate them (i. e., reintegrate them into society), and to protect public safety. Probation sentences vary depending on local laws, the perceived risk posed by the probationer, and the severity of the offense.

The probation officer is responsible for assessing the risk that the probationer will commit new crimes by using standardized risk-assessment tools as well as "static" and "dynamic" information to assess the probationer's risk of reoffending. Static information consists of basic facts about the individual such as sex, age at first conviction, number of previous prison sentences, and type of offense(s). Dynamic information includes potential strengths and risk factors such as education level; vocational experience and employability; residence; relationships; lifestyle; drug and alcohol misuse; and emotional well-being.

Some cases do not require that the probation officer have contact with the offender. These are referred to as "banked" probation caseloads, in which there is little or no supervision. This type of probation limits the time spent and resources used by a probation officers working with a probationer, allowing officers only to make referrals for the probationer to local services. Banked caseloads represent the majority of probationers in the United States.

More involved cases may require the probation officer to make unscheduled visits to probationers' home or workplace and/or monitor them electronically (e. g., through GPS). These are considered specialized intensive cases (cases involving sexual or drug offenses) and have a "caseworker" model. Probation officers can develop case-management plans to help probationers establish employment and find housing; they may also provide individual counseling. Given the increased resource utilization required by this model, few cases are handled in this fashion.

In a study, researchers found that probation officers were incorporating evidence-based correctional strategies in their work with probationers with mental health issues. These strategies included spending time discussing mental health needs (versus strategies that focused on deterring the probationer from committing new crimes), teaching problem-solving skills, and affirming the probationers' efforts to rehabilitate such as attending counseling and group therapy and achieving therapeutic goals.

Numerous studies have examined the effectiveness of probation. Probation is considered cost-effective because probation services cost approximately $10 per day per person versus $100 or more per day per person for incarceration. Juvenile out-of-home placements can cost up to $250 per child per day.

Mental-health-specific caseloads in which probation officers help probationers receive treatment and connect to appropriate resources (e. g., motivational interviewing, cognitive behavioral interventions, alcohol and drug treatment, sexual offending counseling) are more likely to facilitate long-term behavior change than incarceration alone. A review of outcomes for probationers assigned to specialized mental health caseload (SMHC) probation officers in New Jersey in 2010 found that they had significantly fewer arrests, fewer days spent in jail, and improved mental health outcomes (e. g., improved work performance, reduced impact of emotional instability on day-to-day functioning) during the first 6 months of assignment to SMHC than probationers assigned to a probation agent who did not specialize in mental health cases.

In a 2010 study of 47 juveniles on probation for violent crimes, significant decreases in violent behavior and violence toward others were self-reported by those who completed 16 sessions of an intervention that used an ecological approach to violence, examining violence in all parts of the juveniles' lives. A study of 2,504 juveniles who committed a violent first-time offense in Los Angeles County between 2003 and 2005 and were assigned to in-home probation, probation camp, or group-home probation determined that those sentenced to in-home probation had the lowest rate of re-arrest (13 percent); those placed in probation camp had twice this rate, at 26 percent, and the rate for those in group homes was 17 percent.

Parental involvement in juvenile probation can reduce recidivism and reduce violations of probation. Parent involvement may take the form of communication with the probation officer by phone or in person to talk about their child's progress. Also, parents can report to the probation officer when their child is breaking probation rules.

The mental health and resiliency of probation officers themselves is a key aspect of the effectiveness of probation for probationers. Having an excessive caseload has a negative impact on probation officers and compromises their ability to provide timely and effective services for probationers. Working in the corrections system can lead to stress and burnout (i. e., emotional exhaustion) for probation officers. A study in 2013 found that burnout, role conflict (i. e., when incompatible demands are placed on an employee), and work stress are predictors of depressive symptoms among probation officers. Depressive symptoms can affect one's work performance and cause absenteeism in the workplace.

WHAT CAN BE DONE
Treatment methodologies should reflect the cultural values, beliefs, and biases of the individual in need of care and treatment.

Become knowledgeable about the effectiveness of probation to accurately assess a client's personal characteristics and needs concerning mental health, substance abuse, and reentry into the community.

Share information about probation with your colleagues.

Partner with probation officers when working with juveniles in various contexts such as child welfare, group homes, and schools, and when working with

adults in the court system such as by providing psychological assessments for offenders.

Advocate for organizational changes that can alleviate work stress and burnout in probation officers such as lower caseloads.

Advocate for more field placements within the criminal justice system (e. g., in prisons, in probation services) for master of social work candidates to increase their knowledge of the criminal justice system, build skills in assessing clients in the system for risk of recidivism, and learn to write court reports (i. e., objective reports on the progress of clients in the criminal justice system for judges and attorneys).

Written by Melissa Rosales Neff, MSW

REFERENCES
Herberman, E. J., & Bonczar, T. P. (2015). Probation and parole in the United States, 2013. Bulletin, U.S. Department of Justice, Bureau of Justice Statistic, NCJ 248029. Retrieved November 6, 2015, from http://www.bjs.gov/content/pub/pdf/ppus13.pdf

Why is probation effective and efficient? *Carver County [Minnesota].* Retrieved December 7, 2015, from http://www.co. carver. mn. us/county_government/courts/court_services/success_factors. asp

Gayman, M. D., & Bradley, M. S. (2013).organizational climate, work stress and depressive symptoms among probation and parole officers. *Criminal Justice Studies, 26*(3), 326-346. doi:10.1080/1478601X.2012.742436

Hek, R. (2012). Is it possible to develop and sustain non-traditional placements? An evaluation of the development of practice learning opportunities in partnership with the police and probation services in the West Midlands. *Social Work Education, 31*(4), 512-529. doi:10.1080/02615479.2011.570328

International Federation of Social Workers. (2012, March 3). Statement of ethical principles. Retrieved December 7, 2015, from http://ifsw.org/policies/statement-of-ethical-principles/

Khoury-Kassabri, M., Sharvet, R., Braver, E., & Livneh, C. (2010). An evaluation of a group treatment program with youth referred to the juvenile probation service because of violent crime.

Research on Social Work Practice, 20(4), 403-409. doi:10.1177/1049731509338935

Lambert, E. G., Hogan, N. L., Cheeseman, D. K., Jiang, S., & Khondaker, M. (2012). Is the job burning me out? An exploratory test of the job characteristics model on the emotional burnout of prison staff. *The Prison Journal, 92*(1), 3-23. doi:10.1177/0032885511428794

Lancaster, E., & Lumb, J. (2006). The assessment of risk in the National Probation Service in England and Wales. *Journal of Social Work, 6*(3), 275-291. doi:10.1177/1468017306071176

Louden, E., Skeem, J., Camp, J., Vidal, S., & Peterson, J. (2012). Supervision practices in specialty mental health probation: What happens in officer-probationer meetings?. *Law and Human Behavior, 36*(2), 109-119. doi:10.1037/h0093961

Wheeler, D. (2015). NASW standards and indicators for cultural competence in social work practice. Retrieved December 7, 2015, from http://www.socialworkers.org/practice/standards/PRA-BRO-253150-CC-Standards.pdf

Peters, C. M. (2011). Social work and juvenile probation: Historical tensions and contemporary convergences. *Social Work, 56*(4), 355-365. doi:10.1093/sw/56.4.355

Perrault, R. T., Paiva-Salisbury, M., & Vincent, G. M. (2012). Probation officers' perceptions of youths' risk of reoffending and use of risk assessment in case management. *Behavioral Sciences & The Law, 30*(4), 487-505. doi:10.1002/bsl.2015

Phelps, M. (2011). Mass incarceration and (mass) probation: The two faces of punitiveness or differing strategies of social control? Conference paper presented at the American Sociological Association, Las Vegas, NV. August 29, 2011,

Schwalbe, C. S., & Maschi, T. (2010). Patterns of contact and cooperation between juvenile probation officers and parents of youthful offenders. *Journal of Offender Rehabilitation, 49*(6), 398-416. doi:10.1080/10509674.2010.499055

British Association of Social Workers. (2012, January). The code of ethics for social work: Statement of principles. Retrieved December 7, 2015, from http://cdn.basw.co.uk/upload/basw_112315-7.pdf

United States Courts. (n. d.). Probation and pretrial officers and officer assistants. Retrieved December 7, 2015, from http://www.uscourts.gov/Federal-Courts/ProbationPretrialServices/Officers. aspx

Ryan, J. P., Abrams, L. S., & Huang, H. (2014). First-time violent juvenile offenders: Probation, placement, and recidivism. *Social Work Research, 38*(1), 7-18. doi:10.1093/swr/svu004

Wolff, N., Epperson, M., Shi, J., & Huenig, J. (2014). Mental health specialized probation caseloads: Are they effective? *International Journal of Law and Psychiatry, 37*(464-472). doi:10.1016/j.ijlp.2014.02.019

PROBLEMATIC INTERNET USE

MAJOR CATEGORIES: Behavioral & Mental Health

DESCRIPTION

The Internet has grown rapidly, from approximately 400 million users worldwide in 2000 to 3.2 billion in 2015. During this time there has also been a tremendous expansion in the types of online activities available to users and in the types of devices with which users can access the Internet. As the Internet has come to play an increasingly prominent role in daily life, some individuals report levels of Internet use that are high enough to have a negative impact on other areas of their lives. Problematic Internet use (PIU) is an emerging field of research and clinical practice.

A growing body of literature uses the term *Internet addiction* to describe individuals whose Internet use is characterized by preoccupation with online activities, decreased control over use to the extent that responsibilities and basic drives are neglected, and continued use despite experiencing distress and/or other negative consequences. Various theoretical models for Internet addiction have been proposed, with some researchers including additional criteria such as craving, tolerance, withdrawal, and use as a means of managing negative moods. However, at this time, there is insufficient data to support the inclusion of PIU in the fifth edition of the *Diagnostic and Statistical Manual of Mental*

Disorders (DSM-5), with the exception of one subset of PIU, Internet gaming disorder, which is included in the *DSM-5* as a condition that warrants more research before being classified as a formal disorder.

In the absence of established diagnostic criteria, a number of self-reporting tests and scales have been developed to identify and measure the prevalence of PIU. Although the characteristics of PIU are similar to those of other behavior- and substance-related addiction disorders, there are as yet no standard definition, criteria, or procedures for assessment. Some researchers have proposed that problematic use may not be focused on the Internet itself, but rather on specific activities delivered through the Internet, such as gaming, social media, email and texting, and/or sexual activities such as online pornography or cybersex. Respondents in one study indicated that they would greatly reduce their Internet use or not use the Internet at all if their preferred activity was no longer available. PIU is predominantly understood as being similar to obsessive-compulsive and impulse control disorders. Some scholars argue that PIU is a symptom of an existing disorder such as anxiety, depression, or attention-deficit/hyperactivity disorder (ADHD). For some individuals, Internet use may serve as a maladaptive coping strategy for dealing with boredom, loneliness, low self-esteem, stressors, or general dissatisfaction with life. On a global level, prevalence rates of PIU are higher in countries in which people have lower levels of self-reported life satisfaction. PIU is linked with a number of negative consequences, including sleep deprivation, mental distress, diminished performance at school and work, withdrawal from other activities, relationship problems, and social isolation. No evidence-based treatment for PIU is currently identified, in part due to insufficient research. Studies have indicated that individual and family therapy, multifamily group therapy, cognitive behavioral therapy (CBT), and psychosocial support can be effective in reducing PIU. Harm reduction techniques encourage individuals to select alternative activities, set time limits for use, and take regular breaks.

FACTS AND FIGURES

The percentage of households accessing the Internet ranges from 6.7 percent in the least developed countries to 81.3 percent in developed countries.

Investigators report that 74.4 percent of U.S. households reported Internet use in 2013. Internet use in the United States was more likely among younger households, Asians, whites, those living in metropolitan areas, and those with a bachelor's degree or higher.

A 2006 study in the United States found that 68.9 percent of adults reported regular Internet use. Of these, 5.9 percent felt their relationships suffered as a result of their use; 8.7 percent attempted to conceal nonessential use; 3.7 percent felt preoccupied by the Internet when offline; 13.7 percent found it very hard to stay away from the Internet; 8.2 percent used the Internet to escape problems or relieve a negative mood; 12.3 percent had tried to cut back (and 93.8 percent of the users who had tried to cut back had been successful); and 12.4 percent often stayed online longer than intended.

Because there is not a standardized definition of PIU, prevalence rates are largely based on individual self-report on various screening tools and they vary widely depending on the instrument and cutoff scores used. Researchers conducting a meta-analysis of several studies worldwide that used the Young Diagnostic Questionnaire or Internet Addiction Test (IAT) to assess PIU estimated the global prevalence rate of PIU to be 6 percent. Researchers in a study of U.S. college students who identified themselves as intensive Internet users found that the students first accessed the Internet at an average age of 9 years, and initially perceived their use as problematic at an average age of 16 years. Overuse of the Internet may have negative effects on an individual's response inhibition and impulse control.

Researchers in a study of Chinese adolescents described 7.5 percent of the adolescents as problematic Internet users and noted that these users were found to have lower levels of well-being. Researchers in a study of Polish adolescents found that 1.8 percent of the adolescents studied met the criteria for Internet addiction specified by the IAT and 33.2 percent were considered at risk for PIU. Of the Polish study participants, over half played violent games and over 40 percent used pornography sites. Among adolescents in general, PIU has been linked with higher rates of both victimization and perpetration of cyberbullying and online sexual solicitation.

RISK FACTORS

Men and women who suffer from depression, anxiety, and/or who have low self-esteem are at risk for PIU. Higher rates of PIU have been found for both adolescent and adult males compared to PIU rates of females, although this may be mediated by specific types of online use, in particular online gaming and sexual activities. Parental depression, family conflict, and less parental mediation of Internet use; poor academic performance; ADHD; and online game play have been linked with a higher risk of PIU in adolescents.

SIGNS AND SYMPTOMS

Signs and symptoms of PIU include a preoccupation with the Internet, use of the Internet as a means of coping with mood states or stress, a need to spend increasingly long periods online, neglect of one's basic needs and responsibilities, persistent and/or unsuccessful attempts to reduce use, tension, irritability or depression when reducing Internet use, time-management problems, withdrawal from relationships and activities, problems at work or in relationships with family and/or friends stemming from one's Internet use, deception regarding time spent online and types of activities pursued, and excessive fatigue.

ASSESSMENT

A biological, psychological, social, and spiritual assessment will assist in understanding the nature of the PIU within the individual's ecosystem (home and social system) and help direct necessary interventions. Information about the individual's patterns of Internet use, time spent on the Internet, and possible negative consequences of Internet use should be discussed by the social worker with the individual and family. Availability of social supports, friendships, and so forth should be identified. The assessment should also include a screening for signs and symptoms of depression and anxiety.

ASSESSMENT AND SCREENING TOOLS

Standardized assessments and screening tools may be utilized to further gather information regarding the individual's PIU. The Internet Addiction Test (IAT) is a screening tool that has 20 items that measure mild, moderate, and severe levels of addiction. The Internet Addiction Diagnostic Questionnaire (IADQ) is an assessment tool that consists of eight

criteria for PIU. The Compulsive Internet Use Scale (CIUS) has 14 items evaluated on a Likert scale. The Internet Addiction Scale (IAS) is a 20-item questionnaire in which each item is rated on a five-point scale; higher scores correspond with a higher degree of Internet addiction. The Chen Internet Addiction Scale (CIAS) is a 26-item self-report questionnaire.

INTERVENTION

Individuals who experience signs and symptoms of PIU may need support in discussing and identifying the problematic Internet activities. The social worker should explore individuals' motivation to change their Internet use prior to determine what intervention is necessary. Any underlying issues driving the excessive use should be explored. The social worker should help the individual identify situations or cognitions that trigger the PIU and plan alternative strategies and activities to avoid the PIU. Appropriate time limits for Internet use should be established. The use of time limits or increase in alternative activities may decrease the individual's PIU and increase the individual's self-esteem. A thorough assessment for depression, anxiety, and any other suspected disorders should also be completed. Referrals for mental health services may be made, if necessary.

APPLICABLE LAWS AND REGULATIONS

Employees with PIU whose employment has been terminated for Internet abuse at work have sued for wrongful termination under the Americans with Disabilities Act.

SERVICES AND RESOURCES

- The Center for Internet Addiction, http://www.netaddiction.com
- The Network for Internet Investigation and Research Australia has information and resources available for professionals and the public, http://www.niira.org.au
- Global Addiction is an organization that provides resources and information about all forms of addiction; he Internet Addiction Test is available at http://www.globaladdiction.org/scales.php
- Restart offers treatment for PIU; the Compulsive Internet Use Scale is also available at http://www.netaddictionrecovery.com/the-problem/Internet-addiction/compulsive-Internet-use-scale-cius.html

FOOD FOR THOUGHT

User-generated content, such as social media, wikis, and blogging, is an increasingly common feature of the Internet, which was not a part of earlier Internet use and is a new area of focus for studies of PIU. The American Psychiatric Association considers the research insufficient to conclusively diagnose PIU as an addiction; it recommends more research on the subject. There is evidence that use of computers enhances visual-spatial skill and increases brain function in older adults. Findings from various imaging studies have linked PIU with changes in brain structure and activity.

RED FLAGS

Heavy use of the Internet is not necessarily PIU. Family members may rationalize and discount an adolescent's Internet use as a phase. Abstinence from the Internet is especially difficult in a computerized society. The *DSM-5* discusses only Internet gaming disorder as a condition warranting more research, but many researchers feel that cybersex, social media, online shopping, and information search should be included as areas of risk for PIU. There have been multiple studies that have linked PIU with co-occurring psychiatric conditions, including alcohol use issues, ADHD, depression, and anxiety.

NEXT STEPS

Individuals may need ongoing support and referral to counseling for issues with relationships, work, or their social life due to PIU.

*Written by Jessica Therivel, LMSW-IPR, and
Jennifer Teska, MSW*

Reviewed by Laura Gale, LCSW

REFERENCES

Aboujaoude, E., Koran, L. M., Gamel, N., Large, M. D., & Serpe, R. T. (2006). Potential markers for problematic internet use: A telephone survey of 2,513 adults. *CNS Spectrums, 11*(10), 750-755.

Al-Gamal, E., Alzayyat, A., & Ahmad, M. M. (2015). Prevalence of Internet addiction and its association with psychological distress and coping strategies among university students in Jordan. *Perspectives in Psychiatric Care*. doi:10.1111/ppc.12102

American Psychiatric Association. (2013). Diagnostic and Statistical Manual of Mental Disorders (DSM-5). Arlington, CA: Author. Retrieved from http://www.w3.org

Brand, M., Young, K. S., & Laier, C. (2014). Prefrontal control and internet addiction: A theoretical model and review of neuropsychological and neuroimaging findings. *Frontiers in Human Neuroscience, 8*, 375. doi:10.3389/fnhum.2014.00375

British Association of Social Workers. (2012). The code of ethics for social work: Statement of principles. Retrieved April 25, 2015, from http://cdn.basw.co.uk/upload/basw_112315-7.pdf

Chang, F. C., Chiu, C. H., Miao, N. F., Chen, P. H., Lee, C. M., Chiang, J. T., & Pan, Y. C. (2015). The relationship between parental mediation and Internet addiction among adolescents, and the association with cyberbullying and depression. *Comprehensive Psychiatry, 57*, 21-28. doi:10.1016/j.comppsych.2014.11.013

Chen, Y. L., Chen, S. H., & Gau, S. S. (2015). ADHD and autistic traits, family function, parenting style, and social adjustment for Internet addiction among children and adolescents in Taiwan: A longitudinal study. *Research in Developmental Disabilities, 39*, 20-31. doi:10.1016/j.ridd.2014.12.025

Cheng, C., & Li, A. Y. (2014). Internet addiction prevalence and quality of (real) life: A meta-analysis of 31 nations across seven world regions. *Cyberpsychology, Behavior, and Social Networking, 17*(12), 755-760. doi:10.1089/cyber.2014.0317

Chou, W. J., Liu, T. L., Yang, P., Yen, C. F., & Hu, H. F. (2015). Multi-dimensional correlates of Internet addiction symptoms in adolescents with attention-deficit/hyperactivity disorder. *Psychiatry Research, 225*(1-2), 122-128. doi:10.1016/j.psychres.2014.11.003

File, T., & Camille, R. (2014). Computer and Internet Use in the United States: 2013. American Community Survey Reports, ACS-28. Washington, DC: U.S. Census Bureau. Retrieved July 17, 2015, from http://www.census.gov/content/dam/Census/library/publications/2014/acs/acs-28.pdf

Gilbert, R. L., Murphy, N. A., & McNally, T. (2011). Addiction to the 3-dimensional Internet: Estimated prevalence and relationship to real world addictions. *Addiction Research & Theory, 19*(4), 380-390.

Greenfield, P. M. (2009). Technology and informal education: What is taught, what is learned. *Science, 323,* 69-71.

Griffiths, M. (2003). Internet abuse in the workplace: Issues and concerns for employers and employment counselors. *Journal of Employment Counseling, 40,* 87-96.

Ho, R. C., Zhang, M. W., Tsang, T. Y., Toh, A. H., Pan, F., Lu, Y.,... Mak, K. K. (2014). The association between internet addiction and psychiatric co-morbidity: a meta-analysis. *BMC Psychiatry, 14,* 183. doi:10.1186/1471-244X-14-183

International Federation of Social Workers. (2012, March 3). *Statement of ethical principles.* Retrieved April 25, 2015, from http://ifsw.org/policies/statement-of-ethical-principles/

Kalaitzaki, A. E., & Birtchnell, J. (2014). The impact of early parenting bonding on young adults' Internet addiction, through the mediation effects of negative relating to others and sadness. *Addictive Behaviors, 39*(3), 733-736. doi:10.1016/j.addbeh.2013.12.002

Khazaal, Y., Chatton, A., Atwi, K., Zulino, D., Khan, R., & Billieux, J. (2011). Arabic validation of the Compulsive Internet Use Scale (CIUS). *Substance Abuse Treatment, Prevention, & Policy, 6*(32), 1-6.

Ko, C., Liu, G., Hsiao, S., Yen, J., Yang, M., Lin, W.,... Chen, C. (2009). Brain activities associated with gaming urge of online gaming addiction. *Journal of Psychiatric Research, 43*(7), 739-747.

Kuss, D. J., Griffiths, M. D., Karila, L., & Billieux, J. (2014). Internet addiction: A systematic review of epidemiological research for the last decade. *Current Pharmaceutical Design, 20*(25), 4026-4052.

Lam, L. T. (2015). Parental mental health and Internet addiction in adolescents. *Addictive Behaviors, 20,* 20-23. doi:10.1016/j.addbeh.2014.10.033

Li, B., Friston, K. J., Liu, J., Liu, Y., Zhang, G., Cao, F.,... Hu, D. (2014). Impaired frontal-basal ganglia connectivity in adolescents with internet addiction. *Scientific Reports, 4,* 5027. doi:10.1038/srep05027

Li, W., O'Brien, J. E., Snyder, S. M., & Howard, M. O. (2015). Characteristics of Internet addiction/pathological Internet use in U.S. university students: A qualitative-method investigation. *PLoS ONE, 10*(2), e0117372. doi:10.1371/journal.pone.0117372

Liu, Q. X., Fang, X. Y., Yan, N., Zhou, Z. K., Yuan, X. J., Lan, J., & Liu, C. Y. (2015). Multi-family group

therapy for adolescent Internet addiction: Exploring the underlying mechanisms. *Addictive Behaviors, 42,* 1-8. doi:110.1016/j.addbeh.2014.10.021

Mitchell, K. J., & Wells, M. (2007). Problematic Internet experiences: Primary or secondary presenting problems in person seeking mental health care?. *Social Science & Medicine, 65*(6), 1136-1141.

National Association of Social Workers. (2001). NASW standards for cultural competence in social work practice. Retrieved April 25, 2015, from http://www.socialworkers.org/practice/standards/NASWCulturalStandards.pdf

Morahan-Martin, J. (2005). Internet abuse: Addiction? Disorder? Symptom? Alternative explanations?. *Social Science Computer Review, 23*(1), 39-48.

Muller, K. W., Glaesmer, H., Brahler, E., Woelfling, K., & Beutel, M. E. (2014). Prevalence of internet addiction in the general population: Results from a German population-based survey. *Behaviour & Information Technology, 33*(7), 757-766. doi:10.1080/0144929X.2013.810778

Nichols, L. A., & Nicki, R. (2004). Development of a psychometrically sound internet addiction scale: A preliminary step. *Psychology of Addictive Behaviors, 18*(4), 381-384.

Pawowska, B., Zygo, M., Potembska, E., Kapka-Skrzypczak, L., Dreher, P., & Kdzierski, Z. (2015). Prevalence of Internet addiction and risk of developing addiction as exemplified by a group of Polish adolescents from urban and rural areas. *Annals of Agriculture and Environmental Medicine, 22*(1), 129-136. doi:10.5604/12321966.1141382

Petry, N. M. (2010). Commentary on Van Rooij et al. (2011): 'Gaming addiction' - a psychiatric disorder or not?. *Addiction, 106*(1), 213-214.

Pontes, H. M., Szabo, A., & Griffiths, M. D. (2015). The impact of Internet-based specific activities on the perceptions of Internet addiction, quality of life, and excessive usage: A cross-sectional study. *Addictive Behaviors Reports, 1,* 19-25. doi:10.1016/j.abrep.2015.03.002

Rumpf, H. J., Vermulst, A. A., Bischof, A., Kastirke, N., Gurtler, D., Bischof, G.,... Meyer, C. (2014). Occurrence of internet addiction in a general population sample: A latent class analysis. *European Addiction Research, 20*(4), 159-166. doi:10.1159/000354321

Senol-Durak, E., & Durak, M. (2011). The mediator roles in life satisfaction and self-esteem between the affective components of psychological well-being and the cognitive symptoms of problematic internet use. *Social Indicators Research, 103*(1), 23-32.

Sun, Y., Ying, H., Seetohul, R. M., Xuemei, W., Ya, Z., Qian, L.,... Ye, S. (2012). Brain fMRI study of crave induced by cue pictures in online game addicts (male adolescents). *Behavioral Brain Research, 233*(2), 563-576.

Sung, M., Shin, Y. M., & Cho, S. M. (2014). Factor structure of the Internet Addiction Scale and its associations with psychiatric symptoms for Korean adolescents. *Community Mental Health Journal, 50*(5), 612-618. doi:10.1007/s10597-013-9689-0

Tao, R., Huang, X., Wang, J., Zhang, H., Zhang, Y., & Li, M. (2010). Proposed diagnostic criteria for internet addiction. *Addiction, 105*(3), 556-564. doi:10.1111/j.1360-0443.2009.02828.x

Van Rooij, A. J., & Prause, N. (2014). A critical review of "Internet addiction" criteria with suggestions for the future. *Journal of Behavioral Addictions, 3*(4), 203-213. doi:10.1556/JBA.3.2014.4.1

Wang, C. W., Chan, C. L., Mak, K. K., Ho, S. Y., Wong, P. W., & Ho, R. T. (2014). Prevalence and correlates of video and internet gaming addiction among Hong Kong adolescents: A pilot study. *The Scientific World Journal, 2014*, 874648. doi:10.1155/2014/874648

Wang, L., Luo, J., Bai, Y., Kong, J., Gao, W., & Xinying, S. (2013). Internet addiction of adolescents in China: Prevalence, predictors, and association with well-being. *Addiction Research and Theory, 21*(1), 62-69. doi:10.3109/16066359.2012.690053

Weinstein, A., Dorani, D., Elhadif, R., Bukovza, Y., & Yarmulnik, A. (2015). Internet addiction is associated with social anxiety in young adults. *Annals of Clinical Psychiatry, 27*(1), 4-9.

Weinstein, A., & Lejoyeux, M. (2010). Internet addiction or excessive internet use. *The American Journal of Drug & Alcohol Abuse, 36*(5), 277-283.

Wieland, D. M. (2014). Internet addiction: opportunities for assessment and treatment by psychiatric mental health nurses. *Journal of Psychosocial Nursing and Mental Health Services, 52*(7), 3-5. doi:10.3928/02793695-20140530-01

Wolfling, K., Beutel, M. E., Dreier, M., & Muller, K. W. (2014). Treatment outcomes in patients with Internet addiction: A clinical pilot study on the effects of a cognitive-behavioral therapy program. *BioMed Research International*, ID 425924. doi:http://dx.doi.org/10.1155/2014/425924

Yilmaz, S., Herguner, S., Bilgic, A., & Isik, U. (2015). Internet addiction is related to attention deficit but not hyperactivity in a sample of high school students. *ational Journal of Psychiatry in Clinical Practice, 19*(1), 18-23. doi:10.3109/13651501.2014.979834

Young, K. (2004). Internet addiction: A new clinical phenomenon and its consequences. *American Behavioral Scientist, 48*(4), 402-415.

Zhu, Y., Zhang, H., & Tian, M. (2015). Molecular and functional imaging of Internet addiction. *BioMed Research International, 2015*, 378675. doi:10.1155/2015/378675

ICT Facts and Figures: The World in 2015. Geneva: ITU. (2015). *International Telecommunications Union.* Retrieved July 17, 2015, from http://www.itu.int/en/ITU-D/Statistics/Pages/facts/default.aspx

PROBLEMATIC INTERNET USE IN ADOLESCENTS

MAJOR CATEGORIES: Adolescents, Behavioral & Mental Health

DESCRIPTION

Problematic Internet use (PIU) occurs when Internet use adversely affects an individual's life. PIU is use that is risky, impulsive, or excessive and is leading to negative consequences in various areas of daily functioning, such as work, school, or relationships. It presently is understood as an impulse control disorder. Brain research indicates similarities between PIU and addiction to substances, such as cocaine. The American Psychiatric Association has not included PIU in the *Diagnostic and Statistical Manual of Mental Disorders,* fifth edition (*DSM-5*), because of insufficient research. However, the *DSM-5* has included proposed criteria for Internet gaming disorder in section III of the manual as a condition to be considered for future research.

PIU may include excessive online gaming, preoccupation with online sexual content, and/or

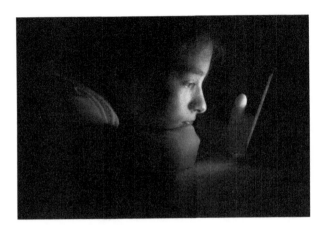

excessive email and text messaging. Problematic Internet use tends to occur in adolescents who are lonely and/or shy. It may be a cause of family and individual dysfunction, an effect of family or individual dysfunction, or both.

Marketers heavily target adolescents for gaming. Many online games allow adolescents to construct their own identities in virtual worlds that can be more fulfilling and exciting than real life. Many shy or lonely adolescents find that the anonymity of online relationships eases their social anxiety; they may find that the ability to control the timing of responses during online interactions makes this means of communicating easier than face-to-face interactions.

Adolescents who are lacking social support in real life may turn to the Internet for acceptance, social support, and interactions in a virtual arena. Many adolescents who turn to the Internet for this support may not be presenting their true or authentic self online either because they use avatars (i.e., an icon or figure that represents an individual in the online world) or present misinformation due to poor self-esteem.

Adolescents report that Internet communities created by gaming, chat rooms, or social media also can feel more supportive than family environments. It is important to understand that adolescents are drawn to these communities because they satisfy their need for social interaction in the short term. However, it is important for adolescents to develop meaningful relationships and social skills with peers outside of the virtual setting. Adolescents with problematic Internet use can fail to acquire these skills.

As contemporary life becomes increasingly enmeshed with technology, the number of hours that constitutes problematic Internet use is difficult to establish. Researchers have found that 20 hours or more a week is problematic; however, the central question for clinicians working with adolescents is whether the Internet use is impairing the adolescent's ability to function. Adolescents with problematic or excessive use can lose their sense of time or neglect basic drives such as eating and sleep. They can suffer fatigue and insomnia from overuse. They may have eye and back strain and develop carpal tunnel syndrome. They may withdraw and feel anger, tension, or depression when the Internet is inaccessible and may increase their amount of use over time. They may begin to argue and lie, their relationships may break down, and their academic performance may decline.

Violent video games can lead to desensitization and aggressive behavior. Adolescents can become socially isolated except when online. Researchers have found that PIU in adolescents can lead to risky behaviors, problematic alcohol use, poor school performance, aggression, attention-deficit/hyperactivity disorder, and self-injurious behavior. In a 2014 study in Taiwan researchers found that Taiwanese adolescents with PIU were more likely to have suicidal ideations and attempt suicide. PIU is associated with symptoms of depression, low self-esteem, and poor family support, which are all factors that increase suicide risk.

Because there is little research on PIU, evidence-based treatment has not been developed. However, researchers have indicated that abstinence programs, individual counseling, and cognitive behavioral therapy can be effective in reducing problematic use. It is important that parents and clinicians understand the alliances adolescents have made online. Therapy that helps families behave in different ways and address the unmet needs that adolescents are seeking to fulfill online has been successful in reducing PIU. Harm reduction techniques recommend that families promote alternative activities to internet use, increase supervision of the adolescent, set time limits on Internet use and enforce regular breaks, and encourage switching to games that are not played online.

FACTS AND FIGURES

The prevalence of PIU in adolescents varies among countries. Researchers in the Netherlands found a prevalence rate of 11 percent. In Turkey, the rate was found to be 9.3 percent in high school girls and 20.4 percent in high school boys.

Researchers have also found an association between duration of Internet use and drug use. Adolescents who use the Internet more than 20 hours per week were found to be twice as likely to use cannabis as adolescents who used the Internet less than this weekly. In 2014 PIU was found in 5.2 percent of adolescents in the United Kingdom, similar to the rate in Spain of 5 percent.

RISK FACTORS

The primary risk factor of problematic internet use in adolescents is the ease of accessibility of the Internet. When that access is combined with low levels of parental monitoring of Internet use and/or high levels of conflict in the family, PIU is more likely to occur. Adolescents with substance abusing parents or parents who engage in intimate partner violence are at risk for problematic internet use. Those adolescents with low self-esteem and who are shy and/or lonely are at risk. Those who have low emotional stability are at increased risk of PIU. Adolescents with avoidant or anxious attachment styles towards others can increase the risk for PIU.

SIGNS AND SYMPTOMS

Signs and symptoms of problematic internet use include a preoccupation with the Internet, a need to spend increasingly long periods online, repeated attempts to reduce use, experiencing withdrawal symptoms when reducing Internet use, time-management problems, environmental stressors (concerning family, school, and friends), deception regarding the amount of time spent online, and changes in the adolescent's mood.

ASSESSMENT

A biological, psychological, social, and spiritual assessment of the adolescent and family will assist in understanding the context of the internet addiction within the individual's ecosystem (personal and social life) and help direct necessary interventions.

ASSESSMENTS AND SCREENING TOOLS

Standardized assessment and screening tools may be utilized to further determine the needs of the adolescent. The Internet Addiction Test (IAT) is

an assessment that has 20 items that measure mild, moderate, and severe levels of addiction. The Compulsive Internet Use Scale (CIUS) has 14 items that are evaluated on a Likert scale. The Problematic Internet Use Scale (PIUS) is a 33-item self-report scale. The Generalized Problematic Internet Use Scale (GPIUS) is a 29-item scale evaluated on a Likert scale that examines to what degree the client experiences thoughts, behaviors, and outcomes that are connected to Internet use. There are no laboratory tests to determine problematic internet use in adolescents.

INTERVENTION

Parents or caregivers may express concern over the increasing internet use by an adolescent. Parents, caregivers, and adolescents should be educated on the potential problems with internet overuse. Support and assistance in helping the family and adolescent select alternative activities, such as increased outdoor activities with friends and family, and increased parental supervision through the use of set time limits or placing computers in family spaces may help decrease the adolescent's problematic internet use.

Additional interventions may include recommending regular breaks (every 20 minutes) or proposing switching to games that are not played online. The adolescent may be empowered to change their habits through mastering a sport, a musical instrument, or a challenging board game. Increased communication within the family and increased self-confidence in the adolescent may be achieved through individual and family therapy. The family and adolescent should be supported through therapy to assist in developing new ways in which the adolescent and family interact and behave. The adolescent may need to be referred for specific therapy such as CBT, if necessary.

APPLICABLE LAWS AND REGULATIONS

Adolescents receiving and sending sexual images over the Internet have been prosecuted for disorderly conduct, illegal use of a minor in nudity-oriented material, sexual abuse of children, criminal use of a communications facility, and open lewdness.

SERVICES AND RESOURCES

- The Center for Internet Addiction has information and resources for professionals, http://www.netaddiction.com

- The Children's Digital Media Center, Los Angeles, http://www.cdmc.ucla.edu/Welcome.html
- The Network for Internet Investigation and Research Australia has information and resources available for professionals and the public, http://www.niira.org.au
- Livestrong offers suggestions for individuals with problematic Internet use, http://www.livestrong.com/article/10360-overcome-internet-addiction
- Global Addiction Association is an organization that provides resources and information about all forms of addiction. The Internet Addiction Test is available here, http://www.globaladdiction.org/scales.php
- Restart offers treatment for problematic Internet use; the Compulsive Internet Use Scale (CIUS) is also available here, http://www.netaddiction-recovery.com/the-problem/internet-addiction/compulsive-internet-use-scale-cius.html

FOOD FOR THOUGHT

PIU may co-occur with the diagnosis of obsessive-compulsive disorder and attention-deficit/hyperactivity disorder. Loneliness as a result of isolation from their families and peers and boredom-proneness among adolescents are significantly correlated with rates of PIU. The American Psychiatric Association considers the research of PIU insufficient to conclusively diagnose PIU as an addiction and recommends more studies be completed.

Adolescents are active participants in creating the online cultures they participate in. There is evidence that adolescents' use of computers is enhancing their visual-spatial skills. Physical activity may reduce risk for PIU because physical activity has positive effects on sleep quality and stress. Adolescents who are sleeping better and feel less stress are less likely to have PIU.

RED FLAGS

Family members may rationalize and discount an adolescent's Internet use as a "phase". Adolescents with PIU frequently have a strong alliance with one parent, which can affect family dynamics and treatment of PIU. A major negative consequence of PIU in adolescents is sleep deprivation. Among adolescents with PIU, 26 percent to 60 percent report poor sleep quality; rates vary by country and cultural context.

NEXT STEPS

Families may need ongoing support and resources for further help should the problem reemerge.

Written by Jan Wagstaff, MA, MSW, and Melissa Rosales Neff, MSW

Reviewed by Lynn B. Cooper, D. Crim, and Laura Gale, LCSW

REFERENCES

An, J., Sun, Y., Wan, Y., Chen, J., Wang, X., & Tao, F. (2014). Associations between problematic Internet use and adolescents' physical and psychological symptoms: Possible role of sleep quality. *Journal of Addiction Medicine, 8*(4), 282-287. doi:10.1097/ADM.0000000000000026

British Association of Social Workers. (2012). *The code of ethics for social work: Statement of principles.* Retrieved March 26, 2016, from http://cdn.basw.co.uk/upload/basw_112315-7.pdf

Cao, F., & Su, L. (2006). Internet addiction among Chinese adolescents: Prevalence and psychological features. *Child: Care, Health & Development, 33*(3), 275-281.

Chong, W. H., Chye, S., Huan, V. S., & Ang, R. P. (2014). Generalized problematic Internet use and regulation of social emotional competence: The mediating role of maladaptive cognitions arising from academic expectation stress on adolescents. *Computers in Human Behavior, 38,* 151-158. doi:10.1016/j.chb.2014.05.023

der Aa, N., Overbeek, G., Engels, R. C., Scholte, R. H., Meerkerk, G. J., & den Eijnden, R. J. (2009). Daily and compulsive Internet use and well-being in adolescence: A diathesis-stress model based on big five personality traits. *Journal of Youth and Adolescence, 38*(6), 765-776.

Deryakulu, D., & Ursavas, O. F. (2014). Genetic and environmental influences on problematic Internet use: A twin study. *Computers in Human Behavior, 39,* 331-338. doi:10.1016/j.chb.2014.07.038

Ding, W. N., Sun, J. H., Sun, Y. W., Chen, X., Zhou, Y., Zhuang, Z. G.,... Du, Y. S. (2014). Trait impulsivity and impaired prefrontal impulse inhibition function in adolescents with Internet gaming addiction revealed by a Go/No-Go fMRI study. *Behavioral and Brain Functions, 10*(1), 20-29. doi:10.1186/1744-9081-10-20

Gilbert, R. L., Murphy, N. A., & McNally, T. (2011). Addiction to the 3-dimensional Internet: Estimated prevalence and relationship to real world addictions. *Addiction Research & Theory, 19*(4), 380-390. doi:10.3109/16066359.2010.530714

Gong, J., Chen, X., Zeng, J., Li, F., Zhou, D., & Wang, Z. (2009). Adolescent addictive internet use and drug abuse in Wuhan, China. *Addiction Research & Theory, 17*(3), 291-305.

Greenfield, P. M. (2004). Developmental considerations for determining appropriate Internet use guidelines for children and adolescents. *Applied Developmental Psychology, 25*(6), 751-762.

Greenfield, P. M. (2009). Technology and informal education: What is taught, what is learned. *Science, 323*(5910), 69-71. doi:10.1126/science.1167190

International Federation of Social Workers. (2012, March 3). *Statement of ethical principles.* Retrieved March 26, 2016, from http://ifsw.org/policies/statement-of-ethical-principles/

Jelenchick, L. A., Hawk, S. T., & Moreno, M. A. (2016). Problematic internet use and social networking site use among Dutch adolescents. *International Journal of Adolescent Medicine and Health, 28*(1), 119-121. doi:10.1515/ijamh-2014-0068

Johansson, A., & Götestam, K. G. (2004). Internet addiction: Characteristics of questionnaire and prevalence in Norwegian youth (12-18 years). *Scandinavian Journal of Psychology, 45*(3), 223-229.

Kaltiala-Heino, R., Lintonen, T., & Rimpelä, A. (2004). Internet addiction? Potentially problematic use of the Internet in a population of 12-18 year-old adolescents. *Addiction Research & Theory, 12*(1), 89-96.

Khazaal, Y., Chatton, A., Atwi, K., Zulino, D., Khan, R., & Billieux, J. (2011). Arabic validation of the Compulsive Internet Use Scale (CIUS). *Substance Abuse Treatment, Prevention, & Policy, 6*(32), 1-6.

Ko, C., Liu, G., Hsiao, S., Yen, J., Yang, M., Lin, W., & Chen, C. (2009). Brain activities associated with gaming urge of online gaming addiction. *Journal of Psychiatric Research, 43*(7), 739-747. doi:10.1016/j.jpsychires.2008.09.012

Kuss, D. J., Antonius, J., Shorter, G. W., Griffiths, M. D., & van de Mheen, D. (2013). Internet addiction in adolescents: prevalence and risk factors. *Computers in Human Behavior, 29*(5), 1987-1996. doi:10.1016/j.chb.2013.04.002

Li, M., Chen, J., Li, N., & Li, X. (2014). A twin study of problematic internet use: Its heritability and genetic association with effortful control. *Twin Research & Human Genetics, 17*(4), 279-287. doi:10.1017/thg.2014.32

Lin, C., Lin, S., & Wu, C. (2009). The effects of parental monitoring and leisure boredom on adolescents' Internet addiction. *Adolescence, 44*(176), 993-1004.

Lin, I. H., Ko, C. H., Chang, Y. P., Liu, T. L., Wang, P. W., Lin, H. C.,... Yen, C. F. (2014). The association between suicidality and Internet addiction and activities in Taiwanese adolescents. *Comprehensive Psychiatry, 55*(3), 504-509. doi:10.1016/j.comppsych.2013.11.012

Lopez-Fernandez, O., Honrubia-Serrano, M. L., Gibson, W., & Griffiths, M. D. (2014). Problematic Internet use in British adolescents: An exploration of the addictive symptomatology. *Computers in Human Behavior, 35*, 224-233.

Mitchell, K. J., & Wells, M. (2007). Problematic Internet experiences: Primary or secondary presenting problems in person seeking mental health care? *Social Science & Medicine, 65*(6), 1136-1141. doi:10.1016/j.socscimed.2007.05.015

National Association of Social Workers (NASW). (2015). NASW standards for cultural competency in social work practice. Retrieved March 26, 2016, from http://www.socialworkers.org/practice/standards/PRA-BRO-253150-CC-Standards.pdf

Nichols, L. A., & Nicki, R. (2004). Development of a psychometrically sound internet addiction scale: A preliminary step. *Psychology of Addictive Behaviors, 18*(4), 381-384. doi:10.1037/0893-164X.18.4.381

Park, S. (2014). Associations of physical activity with sleep satisfaction, perceived stress and problematic Internet use in Korean adolescents. *BMC Public Health, 14*(1), 1143. doi:10.1186/1471-2458-14-1143

Park, S., Kang, M., & Kim, E. (2014). Social relationship on problematic Internet use (PIU) among adolescents in South Korea: A moderated mediation model of self-esteem and self-control. *Computers in Human Behavior, 38*, 349-357.

Park, S. K., Kim, J. Y., & Cho, C. B. (2009). Prevalence of internet addiction and correlations with family factors among South Korean adolescents. *Family Therapy, 36*(3), 163-177.

Petry, N. M. (2011). "Gaming addiction"–A psychiatric disorder or not? *Addiction, 106*(1), 213-214.

Schimmenti, A., Passanisi, A., Gervasi, A. M., Manzella, S., & Fama, F. I. (2014). Insecure attachment attitudes in the onset of problematic Internet use among late adolescents. *Child Psychiatry & Human Development, 45*(5), 588-595. doi:10.1007/s10578-013-0428-0

Secades-Villa, R., Calafat, A., Fernandez-Hermida, J. R., Juan, M., Duch, M., Skarstrand, E.,... Talic, S. (2014). Duration of Internet use and adverse psychosocial effects among European adolescents. *Adicciones, 26*(3), 247-253.

Senol-Durak, E., & Durak, M. (2011). The mediator roles of life satisfaction and self-esteem between the affective components of psychological well-being and the cognitive symptoms of problematic internet use. *Social Indicators Research, 103*(1), 23-32. doi:10.1007/s11205-010-9694-4

Shek, D. L., Tang, V. M., & Lo, C. Y. (2009). Evaluation of an internet addiction treatment program for Chinese adolescents in Hong Kong. *Adolescence, 44*(174), 359-373.

Sun, Y., Ying, H., Seetohul, R. M., Xuemei, W., Ya, Z., Qian, L., & Ye, S. (2012). Brain fMRI study of crave induced by cue pictures in online game addicts (male adolescents). *Behavioral Brain Research, 233*(2), 563-576. doi:10.1016/j.bbr.2012.05.005

Tao, R., Huang, X., Wang, J., Zhang, H., Zhang, Y., & Li, M. (2010). Proposed diagnostic criteria for internet addiction. *Addiction, 105*(3), 556-564. doi:10.1111/j.1360-0443.2009.02828.x

Tayyar, S., Oner, S., Kurt, A., Yapici, G., Yazici, A., Bugdayci, R., & Sis, M. (2014). Prevalence and risk factors of Internet addiction in high school students. *European Journal of Public Health, 24*(1), 15-20. doi:10.1093/eurpub/ckt051

van Rooij, A. J., Schoenmakers, T. M., Vermulst, A. A., den Eijnden, R. J., & de Mheen, D. (2010). Online video game addiction: Identification of addicted adolescent gamers. *Addiction, 106*(1), 205-212.

Wan, C., & Chiou, W. (2007). The motivations of adolescents who are addicted to online games: A cognitive perspective. *Adolescence, 42*(165), 179-197.

Weinstein, A., & Lejoyeux, M. (2010). Internet addiction or excessive Internet use. *The American Journal of Drug & Alcohol Abuse, 36*(5), 277-283. doi:10.3109/00952990.2010.491880

Yang, S. C., & Tung, C. (2007). Comparison of Internet addicts and non-addicts in Taiwanese high schools. *Computers in Human Behavior, 23*(1), 79-96.

Young, K. (2004). Internet addiction: A new clinical phenomenon and its consequences. *American Behavioral Scientist, 48*(4), 402-415. doi:10.1177/0002764204270278

Young, K. (2009). Understanding online gaming addiction and treatment issues for adolescents. *The American Journal of Family Therapy, 37*, 355-372.

Zhong, X., Zu, S., Sha, S., Tao, R., Zhao, C., Yang, F., & Sha, P. (2011). The effect of a family-based intervention model on internet-addicted Chinese adolescents. *Social Behavior & Personality, 39*(8), 1021-1034.

PROSTATE CANCER: RISK FACTORS & PREVENTION

MAJOR CATEGORIES: Medical & Health

WHAT WE KNOW

The prostate gland produces fluid that increases the viability of sperm cells. Typically about the size of a walnut, the prostate is located below the bladder and in front of the rectum. In the United States prostate cancer is the second most commonly diagnosed cancer in men over the age of 50 (after skin cancer) and is the second leading cause of death from cancer in males.

Prostate cancer is complex and the onset of symptoms is greatly influenced by genetic and hormonal factors.

There are significant racial and ethnic disparities in prostate cancer incidence, mortality, and risk factors. In the United States, a disproportionate number of black males develop prostate cancer and die from prostate cancer than compared with white males. Black males experience barriers to health-promoting behavior and resources that may prevent the early detection of prostate cancer, some barriers which may apply to all men, include the reluctance to undergo regular prostate screenings, the lack of willingness to make lifestyle and nutritional modifications, discomfort in discussing health problems with healthcare clinicians, lack of information/education about the prostate cancer disease process, and fear that prostate cancer and its treatment are painful or greatly interfere with sexual function. In a study in Mississippi, researchers found that about 40 percent of the predominantly black study population could not identify the body organs, symptoms, and screening exams that were related to prostate cancer.

In addition to ethnicity and race, nonmodifiable factors that increase the risk of developing prostate cancer include age and family history. Age is an important nonmodifiable risk factor since prostate cancer has the steepest age-incidence curve of any cancer with the risk of prostate cancer increasing with older age. Having a family history of prostate cancer, especially in a first-degree relative such as a parent or sibling, increases an individual's risk for developing prostate cancer. Men who are a carrier of the BRCA1/2 gene mutation have an increased risk for prostate cancer. Individuals who are mutation carriers of the BRCA2 gene have both an increased risk of prostate cancer and risk for a more aggressive occurrence of the cancer.

Modifiable factors that increase the risk of developing prostate cancer include cigarette smoking; occupational exposure (e.g., to chemicals and/or substances such as pesticides and other agricultural products, cadmium, paint, rubber products, polyaromatic hydrocarbons from coal, liquid fuel combustion products, metallic dust, and certain types of lubricating oil and grease); history of frequent urinary tract infections; obesity, which increases risk of aggressive prostate cancer; diet, specifically high consumption of meat (e.g., red and processed meat), consumption of dairy products, calcium, animal fat, and trans fat, and low consumption of vegetables and fruits; high consumption of red meat, processed meat, and consumption of meat cooked at high temperatures which has been associated with increased risk of advanced and metastatic prostate cancer.

A study of 2, 720 Vietnam-era veterans found that exposure to Agent Orange (an herbicide used by the American military to kill vegetation in Vietnam) was associated with a 52 percent increase in risk of prostate cancer and a 75 percent increase in risk of high-grade prostate cancer (an aggressive form of prostate cancer with a Gleason score of greater than 8; Gleason score is a system of scoring cancer tissue in which the numbers 2-10 are assigned to describe normal to abnormal cells seen under a microscope).

Investigators reported that men who were involved in rescue and/or recovery efforts at the World Trade Center site of the September 11, 2001, terrorist attacks in the United States were 43 percent more likely to develop prostate cancer than men who were not involved. Researchers who tracked 21, 660 male physicians in the United States for 28 years found that study participants who drank more than 2.5 servings of dairy products per day had a 12 percent increased risk of developing prostate cancer. Consumption of skim and low-fat milk was positively associated with risk of low-grade prostate cancer, early-stage prostate cancer, and identification of prostate cancer during screening. The intake of whole milk was positively associated with death from prostate cancer.

According to the American Cancer Society, reduction of prostate cancer risk may be achieved by daily consumption of at least 2.5 cups of a variety of fruits and vegetables, engaging in regular physical activity, maintaining a healthy weight, and possibly limiting calcium intake.

Researchers who have conducted population-based and cohort studies of the effects of animal products, calcium, green tea, folic acid, lycopene, and fish consumption have not produced sufficiently robust results to warrant phase III clinical trials(i.e., in which new treatment is compared with a standard treatment in a large group of people). Although strategies to prevent prostate cancer have largely involved making behavioral changes, including dietary management, increased physical activity, and smoking cessation, the use of certain supplements and medications has been proposed for preventing prostate cancer.

Although the use of many supplements and dietary regimens has been evaluated, there is inadequate evidence to recommend them for prevention of prostate cancer. Results of several epidemiologic studies show that the use of nonsteroidal anti-inflammatory drugs (NSAIDs) reduced prostate cancer risk. Researchers in a 2012 study of nearly 30, 000 men concluded that daily aspirin use was associated with reduced prostate cancer risk and daily use of ibuprofen was not associated with reduced risk. Prostate cancer may be detected early using one of two methods: a digital rectal exam (DRE) or a prostate-specific antigen (PSA) blood test. Methods of testing that differentiate low-risk prostate cancers from more aggressive types of the cancer would improve disease management in men with prostate cancer.

WHAT CAN BE DONE

Social workers can learn about prostate cancer including the risk factors, symptoms, screening methods, and treatment options available to accurately assess clients' personal, medical, and mental health needs regarding prostate cancer treatment. Social workers may provide education to clients about the benefits of prostate cancer screening and the importance of early detection and prompt treatment. Education may also be provided regarding their personal risk for prostate cancer and the benefits of reducing their risk through smoking cessation and dietary changes, such as decreasing consumption of saturated fats and increasing consumption of fruits and vegetables.

Social workers may assist clients in accessing weight-loss programs and/or smoking cessation therapies through location of services and referrals. Social workers may help clients locate healthier food options and programs available in their community. Social workers may collaborate with the treating facility or agency's continuing education department to provide education on prostate cancer for clinicians of all specialties and to establish culturally sensitive prostate cancer screening programs targeting high-risk ethnic groups.

Written by Carita Caple, RN, BSN, MSHS, and Tanja Schub, BS

Reviewed by Jessica Therivel, LMSW-IPR, and Melissa Rosales Neff, MSW

REFERENCES

American Cancer Society. (2014). Prostate cancer prevention and early detection. Retrieved October 27, 2015, from http://www.cancer.org/acs/groups/cid/documents/webcontent/003182-pdf.pdf

Ansbaugh, N., Shannon, J., Mori, M., Farris, P. E., & Garzotto, M. (2013). Agent Orange as a risk factor for high-grade prostate cancer. *Cancer, 119*(13), 2399-2404. doi:10.1002/cncr.27941

Azzouni, F., & Mohler, J. (2012). Role of 5 alpha reductase inhibitors in prostate cancer prevention and treatment. *Urology, 79*(6), 1197-1205.

British Association of Social Workers. (2012). The code of ethics for social work: Statement of principles. Retrieved December 8, 2015, from http://cdn.basw.co.uk/upload/basw_112315-7.pdf

Carpenter, W. R., Godley, P. A., Clark, J. A., Talcott, J. A., Finnegan, T., Mishel, M., & Mohler, J. L. (2009). Racial differences in trust and regular source of patient care and the implications for prostate cancer screening use. *Cancer, 115*(21), 5048-5059. doi:10.1002/cncr.24539

Cuzick, J., Thorat, M. A., Andriole, G., Brawley, O. W., Brown, P. H., Culig, Z.,... Wolk, A. (2014). Prevention and early detection of prostate cancer. *The Lancet. Oncology, 15*(11), e484-e492. doi:10.1016/S1470-2045(14)70211-6

Ekundayo, O. T., & Tataw, D. B. (2013). Barriers to prostate cancer prevention and community recommended health education strategies in an urban African American community in Jackson, Mississippi. *Social Work in Public Health, 28*(5), 520-538. doi:10.1080/10911359.2013.763707

Henriquez-Hernandez, L., Valenciano, A., Foro-Arnalot, P., Alvarez-Cubero, M., Cozar, J., Suarez-Novo, J.,... Lara, P. C. (2014). Single nucleotide polymorphisms in DNA repair genes as risk factors associated to prostate cancer progression. *BMC Medical Genetics, 15*(1), 143. doi:10.1186/s12881-014-0143-0

Huncharek, M., Haddock, K. S., Reid, R., & Kupelnick, B. (2010). Smoking as a risk factor for prostate cancer: A meta-analysis of 24 prospective cohort studies. *American Journal of Public Health, 100*(4), 693-701. doi:10.2105/AJPH.2008.150508

International Federation of Social Workers. (2012, March 3). Statement of Ethical Principles.

Retrieved October 27, 2015, from http://ifsw.org/policies/statement-of-ethical-principles/

Jiang, L., Yang, K. -H., Tian, J. -H., Guan, Q. -L., Yao, N., Cao, N.,... Yang, S. -H. (2010). Efficacy of antioxidant vitamins and selenium supplement in prostate cancer prevention: A meta-analysis of randomized controlled trials. *Nutrition and Cancer, 62*(6), 719-727. doi:10.1080/01635581.2010.494335

John, E. M., Stern, M. C., Sinha, R., & Koo, J. (2011). Meat consumption, cooking practices, meat mutagens, and risk of prostate cancer. *Nutrition and Cancer, 63*(4), 525-537. doi:10.1080/01635581.2011.539311

Kushi, L. H., Doyle, C., McCullough, M., Rock, C. L., Denmark-Wahnefried, W., Bandera, E. V., & Gansler, T. (2012). American Cancer Society guidelines on nutrition and physical activity for cancer prevention: Reducing the risk of cancer with healthy food choices and physical activity. *CA: A Cancer Journal for Clinicians, 62*(1), 30-67. doi:10.3322/caac.20140

Li, J., Cone, J. E., Kahn, A. R., Brackbill, R. M., Farfel, M. R., Greene, C. M.,... Stellman, S. D. (2012). Association between World Trade Center exposure and excess cancer risk. *JAMA: Journal of the American Medical Association, 308*(23), 2479-2488. doi:10.1001/jama.2012.110980

Odedina, F. T., Scrivens, J. J., Jr, Larose-Pierre, M., Emanuel, F., Adams, A. D., Dagne, G. A., & Odedina, O. (2011). Modifiable prostate cancer risk reduction and early detection behaviors in black men. *American Journal of Health Behavior, 35*(4), 470-484. doi:10.5993/AJHB.35.4.9

Shebl, F. M., Sakoda, L. C., Black, A., Koshiol, J., Andriole, G. L., Grubb, R., & Hsing, A. W. (2012). Aspirin but not ibuprofen use is associated with reduced risk of prostate cancer: A PLCO study. *British Journal of Cancer, 107*(1), 207-214. doi:10.1038/bjc.2012.227

Song, Y., Chavarro, J. E., Cao, Y., Qiu, W., Mucci, L., Sesso, H. D.,... Ma, J. (2013). Whole milk intake is associated with prostate cancer-specific mortality among U.S. male physicians. *Journal of Nutrition, 143*(2), 189-196. doi:10.3945/jn.112.168484

Szymanski, K. M., Wheeler, D. C., & Mucci, L. A. (2010). Fish consumption and prostate cancer risk: A review and meta-analysis. *American Journal of Clinical Nutrition, 92*(5), 1223-1233. doi:10.3945/ajcn.2010.29530

U.S. Preventive Services Task Force. (2012, May). Understanding task force recommendations: Screening for prostate cancer: consumer guide. Retrieved October 27, 2015, from http://www.uspreventiveservicestaskforce.org/Page/Document/UpdateSummaryFinal/prostate-cancer-screening

Violette, P. D., & Saad, F. (2012). Chemoprevention of prostate cancer: Myths and realities. *Journal of the American Board of Family Medicine, 25*(1), 111-119. doi:10.3122/jabfm.2012.01.110117

Walker, R., Louis, A., Horsburgh, S., Bristow, R. G., & Trachtenberg, J. (2014). Prostate cancer screening characteristics in men with BRCA1/2 mutations attending a high-risk prevention clinic. *Canadian Urological Association Journal, 8*(11-12), E783-E788. doi:10.5489/cuaj.1970

Wheeler, D. (2015). NASW Standards and Indicators for Cultural Competence in Social Work Practice. Retrieved December 8, 2015, from http://www.socialworkers.org/practice/standards/PRA-BRO-253150-CC-Standards.pdf

Xu, X., Dailey, A. B., Talbott, E. O., Ilacqua, V. A., Kearney, G., & Asal, N. R. (2010). Associations of serum concentrations of organochlorine pesticides with breast cancer and prostate cancer in U.S. adults. *Environmental Health Perspectives, 118*(1), 60-66. doi:10.1289/ehp.0900919

PROSTITUTION

MAJOR CATEGORIES: Behavioral & Mental Health

DESCRIPTION

Prostitution is the delivery of sexual services to an individual who is not a spouse, partner, or friend in exchange for money, housing, food, or drugs. The individuals who engage in prostitution usually are women or girls; men or boys can prostitute themselves as well. Prostitution is illegal in 49 U.S. states; in some counties in Nevada prostitution is legal if provided in a licensed brothel. Prostitution may be off-street, in which services are provided by an escort or call-girl service with prearrangement of time and place or provided in a brothel setting. Prostitution also commonly is provided at the street level, meaning the prostitute is found by the customer on the street and not in a prearranged meeting. The street-level prostitute and client might then go to a motel, apartment, car. Globally, some countries have legalized prostitution by adult prostitutes or decriminalized elements of prostitution by legalizing the sale but not the purchase of sexual services.

Social, economic, and cultural factors create marked differences in the societal perception of prostitution. One view sees prostitution as a crime involving high degrees of violence, discrimination, and human rights violations. The opposite viewpoint regards prostitution as an acceptable occupational choice. Juvenile prostitution is understood and responded to very differently from adult prostitution. Because juveniles are not of legal age to consent to sex, the assumption is made that any engagement in prostitution by a juvenile is coerced. Juveniles should thus be considered victims of prostitution, not criminal offenders, although this is not always how they are treated. Juvenile prostitution is a significant problem both in the United States and internationally.

Professionals come into contact with those who are currently prostituting themselves or have in the past in a variety of practice areas, including in the areas of criminal justice, substance use, mental health, trauma, and child welfare. Such settings can be courts, hospitals, public health clinics, substance abuse treatment programs, homeless shelters, domestic and sexual violence centers, child protective services, and counseling centers/private practice. Professionals need to recognize this population as being very vulnerable and disenfranchised. Even though technically both the client and the adult prostitute are guilty of breaking the law, the customers of prostitutes are much less likely to be arrested than the prostitute. Many individuals engaged in street prostitution have very poor physical

health; it is estimated that HIV rates among prostitutes are high, with hepatitis B and C, gonorrhea, herpes, syphilis, and human papillomavirus (HPV) also common. Prostitutes are also at risk for violence, substance abuse, exploitation, and coercion, as well as isolation from social support.

To address the individual and economic costs of prostitution, some communities are instituting diversion programs for arrested prostitutes to try to stop the cycle of arrest, jail, and release.

FACTS AND FIGURES

An accurate estimate of prostitution is hard to obtain because most data derive only from those prostitutes who are arrested and do not include the prostitutes who are not arrested. Professionals can encounter prostitutes in practice knowingly or unknowingly depending on the population with which they work. Prostitution will often result in risky behavior choices due to risk of violence and substance use. Street prostitution is a violent experience for those who provide it. In the United States, rates of physical and sexual abuse of prostitutes range from 60 to 93.5 percent. British researchers found that 92 percent of prostitutes expressed having experienced violence in their lifetime; 72 percent had experienced abuse as children. A Portland, Oregon, program that assists prostitutes to leave prostitution found a history of childhood sexual abuse in 85 percent of the program participants. Many studies also have found links between prostitution and high rates of posttraumatic stress disorder (PTSD) symptoms. Prostitutes who report abuse or assaults to authorities are not always given the proper attention; the criminal justice system sometimes is reluctant to investigate or prosecute claims of violent victimization made by prostitutes. In the United States almost 3 percent of female homicide victims are women working as prostitutes; women involved in prostitution have a risk of death 12 times greater than that of similarly aged women.

There is also a strong association between substance use and prostitution. There is disagreement in the research community over whether drug use precedes prostitution or prostitution leads to substance abuse. At one health clinic, 86 percent of women engaged in prostitution were using illegal drugs compared to 23 percent of the total female clinic population. In a study of current and former prostitutes in the United Kingdom, researchers found that 83 percent were either currently addicted or had been addicted to drugs or alcohol when they were working as prostitutes. Researchers interviewing providers of drug and alcohol services in the United Kingdom found that approximately 25 percent of service users were women who were exchanging sex for money and/or drugs. The researchers also found that only 34.7 percent of providers offered information on prostitution and only 23.9 percent had harm reduction programs on prostitution. In contrast, 87.5 percent of programs designed for helping individuals exit prostitution had counseling and information on substance use, and 93.7 percent had harm reduction programs.

RISK FACTORS

Incidents of child abuse and family dysfunction in childhood have been reported in the background history of many of the individuals involved in prostitution.

School truancy can be a risk factor for juvenile prostitution.

Young people who run away from home can turn to prostitution as "survival sex," in which they exchange sex for resources.

In the United States, blacks have the highest rate of juvenile entry into prostitution.

Individuals who entered prostitution as juveniles are also at a higher risk of suicide.

Many prostitutes abuse substances; individuals might prostitute themselves to pay for their drug habits and they might use substances as a means of coping with prostituting themselves.

SIGNS AND SYMPTOMS

There are no obvious physical or emotional signs and symptoms that will indicate that a person is or has been a prostitute. A professional needs to complete a thorough bio-psycho-social-spiritual assessment while providing a nonjudgmental setting for the person to feel comfortable to disclose.

ASSESSMENT

A professional should perform a comprehensive bio-psycho-social-spiritual assessment that includes the person's past prostitution history, relevant family history, family relationships, substance use history, any childhood abuse, and other traumatic events.

A detailed interview and history with a self-reporting questionnaire should be the primary screening tool to help determine whether a person has been involved in prostitution, which can have a major impact on need for services. Other screening tools can identify whether a person has risk factors that can lead to prostitution. These screening tools may include the Child Trauma Questionnaire—Short Form (assesses childhood physical and sexual abuse using a Likert scale), the Davidson Trauma Scale or the Trauma Symptom Checklist (assesses the frequency and severity of PTSD symptoms), and the Impact of Event Scale—Revised (determines the impact of traumatic events on the client's life experiences). If indicated by history, the Addiction Severity Index can be used to evaluate the behaviors and problems associated with substance use.

Depending on the setting, a blood alcohol screening or drug test may either be required or medically ordered, and testing for sexually transmitted diseases (STDs) may be appropriate, including HIV and hepatitis.

TREATMENT

The Eaves study in the United Kingdom resulted in a five-stage model for exiting prostitution that professionals may utilize. This model is not linear or rigid but can serve as a guideline. The stages are readiness/engagement, treatment/support, transition/stabilization, reconstruction/rebuilding, and new roles/identities. Women who are involved in prostitution and are seeking counseling support may also benefit from a person-centered approach with elements of psychodynamic work and attachment theory.

Problem	Goal	Intervention
Person is actively prostituting self, putting self at risk.	Successfully exiting prostitution if the person wants to exit and receiving necessary formal support services to avoid re-entry. Enhanced safety and self-care through harm-reduction strategies for the person who wants to continue to be a sex worker.	Prioritize and address active problems that are linked to prostitution (substance abuse, depression, PTSD). Design treatment plan to address active problems and minimize risk of reentry into prostitution. Provide individual and/or group therapy to address underlying issues. Establish safety plan if there is risk of violence from a pimp who has threatened person working as street prostitute.
Person is prostituting self to support substance addiction.	Person will be drug and alcohol free and will not need to prostitute self to support addiction.	Detoxification if medically necessary. Assist in accessing appropriate drug treatment program to address addiction and provide the means to be sober or pursue a harm-reduction model of recovery if appropriate. Provide supportive environment for sobriety. Assist in finding appropriate housing/social support to maintain sobriety or harm reduction. Counsel and support to improve low self-esteem and reduce negative emotions that are being experienced.

APPLICABLE LAWS AND REGULATIONS

Prostitution is illegal in 49 U.S. states.

Some U.S. cities and counties have formal diversion programs in which arrested prostitutes are directed to specific programs to treat underlying issues (drug use) rather than being sentenced to jail or prison.

Human trafficking laws may help minors engaged in prostitution in the United States. As of 2014, six states (Illinois, Mississippi, Nebraska, North Carolina, Tennessee, and Vermont) have laws that provide immunity from prosecution for all minors who engage in prostitution, under the assumption that because minors cannot give consent, they are victims of human trafficking. Under so-called safe harbor laws, 19 states allow the minor who is under 18 and arrested for prostitution to enter an affirmative defense that his or her prostitution was due to trafficking. Connecticut's safe harbor law applies only to minors who are age 15 or younger.

SERVICES AND RESOURCES

Many individuals who are prostitutes may qualify for benefits or programs to address physical or mental health needs, but because of stigma or fear of arrest they will not or cannot access the services. Many need help with housing, employment, medical care, drug treatment, and mental health services, but low self-esteem, depression, resistance by providers to helping them, and the structure of the criminal justice system can all be barriers to access. The stigmatization of prostitutes often is internalized by the individual, who then feels he or she is not worthy of being helped.

Sex Industry Survivors Anonymous is a peer-support group for men or women who are either trying to escape prostitution or need support and recovery after leaving prostitution, http://www.sexindustry-survivors.com/

Arizona, California, Washington, D.C., Hawaii, Illinois, Maryland, Minnesota, Missouri, Nebraska, Nevada, New York, Ohio, Oregon, Washington, and

Wisconsin have programs and resources for individuals trying to leave prostitution.

Food for Thought

In a study, researchers found that in the United States, trafficked U.S. women who were engaging in prostitution received less empathy from study subjects than foreign trafficked women. There was a tendency by study subjects to believe that women should have known better and a tendency to blame those who participate in prostitution.

Research indicates that secure housing is a major need that must be met for individuals to be able to leave prostitution.

The illegal status of prostitution compounded by strong moral judgments make prostitutes a difficult population to study.

A formal support process improves the success rate of programs designed to assist individuals in exiting prostitution. In the absence of formal programs, many prostitutes try to exit while utilizing substance abuse treatment or domestic violence shelters but have less success.

Participants in Ohio's CATCH (Changing Actions to Change Habits) court program, for women who have been arrested multiple times for solicitation, have lower rates of rearrest for prostitution. Women who meet the program criteria are able to enter a two-year treatment program that addresses the physical, mental health, social, and community consequences of prostitution.

Engaging in prostitution leaves individuals vulnerable to loss of social services, removal of children and termination of parental rights, and expulsion from family or church social support. The stigma attached to prostitution makes it difficult for individuals to return to legitimate employment.

Red Flags

Providers working with this population need to be alert to signs of secondary or vicarious traumatization. While counseling with or working with this population, hearing about the traumas experienced can result in traumatic stress for the provider.

Written by Jessica Therivel, LMSW-IPR

Reviewed by Lynn B. Cooper, D Crim, and Laura Gale, LCSW

References

Begun, A. L., & Hammond, G. C. (2012). CATCH court: A novel approach to "treatment as alternative to incarceration" for women engaged in prostitution and substance abuse. *Journal of Social Work Practice in the Addictions, 12*(3), 328-331. doi:10.1080/1533256X.2012.703920

British Association of Social Workers. (2012). *The Code of Ethics for Social Work: Statement of Principles.* Retrieved January 27, 2016, from http://cdn.basw.co.uk/upload/basw_112315-7.pdf

Clarke, R. J., Clarke, E. A., Roe-Sepowitz, D., & Fey, R. (2012). Age at entry into prostitution: Relationship to drug use, race, suicide, education level, childhood abuse, and family experiences. *Journal of Human Behavior in the Social Environment, 22*(3), 270-289. doi:10.1080/10911359.2012.655583

Heilemann, T., & Santhiveeran, J. (2011). How do female adolescents cope and survive the hardships of prostitution? A content analysis of existing literature. *Journal of Ethnic & Cultural Diversity in Social Work, 20*(1), 57-76. doi:10.1080/15313204.2011.545945

Holly, J., & Lousley, G. (2014). The challenge of change – improving services for women involved in prostitution and substance use. *Advances in Dual Diagnosis, 7*(2), 80-89. doi:10.1108/ADD-02-2014-0005

International Federation of Social Workers. (2012). *Statement of ethical principles.* Retrieved January 27, 2016, from http://ifsw.org/policies/statement-of-ethical-principles/

Jackson, C. (2014). An upward spiral: Exiting prostitution. *Therapy Today, 25*(5), 10-13.

Jung, Y. E., Song, J. M., Chong, J., Seo, H. J., & Chae, J. H. (2008). Symptoms of post-traumatic stress disorder and mental health in women who escaped prostitution and helping activists in shelters. *Yonsei Medical Journal, 49*(3), 372-382. doi:10.3349/ymj.2008.49.3.372

Kurtz, S. P., Surratt, H. L., Kiley, M. C., & Inciardi, J. A. (2005). Barriers to health and social services for street-based sex workers. *Journal of Health Care for the Poor and Underserved, 16*(2), 345-361. doi:10.1353/hpu.2005.0038

Levin, L., & Peled, E. (2011). The Attitudes toward Prostitutes and Prostitution Scale: A new tool for measuring public attitudes toward prostitutes and prostitution. *Research on Social Work Practice, 21*(5), 582-593. doi:10.1177/1049731511406451

Love, R. (2015). Street level prostitution: A systematic literature review. *Issues in Mental Health Nursing, 36*(8), 568-576. doi:10.3109/01612840.2015.1020462

Mizrahi, T., & Davis, L. E. (2008). Prostitution. In *Encyclopedia of social work* (20th ed., Vol. 3). Washington, DC: NASW Press. National Association of Social Workers. (2012). Prostituted people, commercial sex workers, and social work practice policy statement. *Social Work Speaks, National Association of Social Workers Policy Statements 2012-2014* (9th ed.). Washington, DC: NASW Press.

National Conference of State Legislatures. (2014, May 9). Human trafficking overview. Retrieved January 27, 2016, from http://www.ncsl.org/research/civil-and-criminal-justice/human-trafficking-overview.aspx

Prostitution Research and Education. (n.d.). Services for survivors. Retrieved February 19, 2016, from http://prostitutionresearch.com/resources/services-for-survivors/

Roe-Sepowitz, D., Hickle, K. E., & Cimino, A. (2012). The impact of abuse history and trauma symptoms on successful completion of a prostitution-exiting program. *Journal of Human Behavior in the Social Environment, 22*(1), 65-77. doi:10.1080/10911359.2011.598830

Roe-Sepowitz, D., Hickle, K. E., Loubert, M. P., & Egan, T. (2011). Adult prostitution recidivism: Risk factors and impact of a diversion program. *Journal of Offender Rehabilitation, 50*(5), 272-285. doi:10.1080/10509674.2011.574205

Sallmann, J. (2010). "Going hand-in-hand": Connections between women's prostitution and substance use. *Journal of Social Work Practice in the Addictions, 10*(2), 115-138. doi:10.1080/1533256100373015

Sallmann, J. (2010). Living with stigma: Women's experiences of prostitution and substance use. *Journal of Women and Social Work, 25*(2), 146-159. doi:10.1177/0886109910364362

Silver, K. E., Karakurt, G., & Boysen, S. (2015). Predicting prosocial behavior toward sex-trafficked persons: the roles of empathy, belief in a just world, and attitudes toward prostitution. *Journal of Aggression, Maltreatment, & Trauma, 24*(8), 932-954. doi:10.1080/10926771.2015.1070231

Wheeler, D. (2015). NASW standards and indicators for cultural competency in social work practice. Retrieved January 27, 2016, from http://www.socialworkers.org/practice/standards/PRA-BRO-253150-CC-Standards.pdf

Wiechelt, S. A., & Shdaimah, C. S. (2011). Trauma and substance abuse among women in prostitution: Implications for a specialized diversion program. *Journal of Forensic Social Work, 1*(2), 159-184. doi:10.1080/1936928X.2011.598843

PSYCHOSIS: OVERVIEW

MAJOR CATEGORIES: Behavioral & Mental Health

DESCRIPTION

The severe mental disorder known as a psychosis, in which an individual's thinking and emotions are so impaired as to prevent the individual from having contact with external reality, is not a single disorder, but is instead a collection of symptoms that vary with the specific nature of the disorder. The duration and severity of these symptoms play prominent roles in defining a particular psychotic disorder and in its diagnosis and treatment.

A psychosis may include the following elements, individually or in combination.

Delusions: Irrational or false beliefs that are maintained despite clear and consistent evidence that they are not true; frequently these beliefs are paranoid, persecutory, religious, grandiose, or somatic.

Hallucinations: Sensory perceptions that are experienced in the absence of external and objective stimulation; they are frequently auditory, but may also be visual, tactile, olfactory, or gustatory.

Disorganized thought or speech: Thought or speech marked by a looseness of associations, incoherence, lack of logic, neologisms, echolalia, incoherence, flights of ideas, blocking (a sudden and unanticipated emptying of all thoughts from the mind), circumstantiality (the insertion of irrelevant or unimportant remarks into a conversation), pressured speech, phonemic paraphasia (the substitution of a word with a nonword that has similar phonic components), and other verbal abnormalities.

Grossly disorganized behavior: Behavior marked by inappropriate dress, frequent crying, poor hygiene, and other abnormalities.

Catatonic behavior: An extreme loss of motor movement, or constant hyperactive motor movement, including stereotyped, repetitive movements and holding rigid poses.

Negative symptoms: Behavioral, verbal, and other features that represent an absence or lack of normal activity (lack of normal emphasis in speech; decreased speech, or alogia; avolition, or a decreased self-starting of activities; anhedonia, or a decreased ability to experience pleasure; and asociality, or lack of interest in interacting with other people).

Loss of ego boundaries: The inability to differentiate between internal and external experiences.Gross impairment of reality testing: The inability to accurately distinguish between what is real and what is not real.

The diagnosis of a psychotic disorder is directly related to its origin and cause. Psychoses may result from the interaction of biological and psychosocial factors or purely social factors, or from organic medical conditions. Research is currently examining a range of possible causes for various psychoses, including genetic abnormalities, substance use (particularly marijuana), and human migration as a social factor that influences susceptibility to psychotic disorders. The prognosis and treatment of a psychosis depend on its eventual diagnosis.

The accurate assessment of a psychosis requires its grading on the three scales of its symptoms, severity, and duration. The mere presence of psychotic features of an individual's behavior does not mean that the individual has a specific psychotic disorder among the disorders described in the fifth edition of the *Diagnostic and Statistical Manual of Mental Disorders* (*DSM-5*). The particular psychotic symptoms exhibited in a psychotic disorder, as well as their prominence, severity, and duration, determine the type of the psychosis as given in the *DSM-5*. For example, the psychoses known as schizophrenia, schizophreniform disorder, schizoaffective

disorder, and brief psychotic disorder are characterized by delusions, prominent hallucinations, disorganized speech, negative symptoms, and/or disorganized or catatonic behavior. In a psychotic disorder caused by a general medical condition, and in a substance-induced psychotic disorder, psychosis refers to delusions or hallucinations unaccompanied by insight, defined as the ability to objectively understand the reality of a situation. In the case of delusional disorder and shared psychotic disorder, psychosis is synonymous with delusions. In addition, neurocognitive disorders (major or mild neurocognitive disorder due to Alzheimer's disease), bipolar disorder, and major depressive disorder may all include symptoms that appear similar to the psychotic symptoms listed above.

The condition known as attenuated psychosis syndrome (APS), distinguished by a mild onset of symptoms such as delusions, hallucinations, and disorganized speech, occurring at least once a week for a month, was added to the *DSM-5* as a condition requiring further study. Researchers have noted that early intervention for the treatment of APS can decrease the likelihood of its progressing to cause more severe psychotic symptoms.

Accurate assessment and diagnosis, and subsequently treatment, of the first episode of a psychosis are vital because each subsequent episode carries an increased risk of the development of persistent psychotic symptoms. Furthermore, recurrent episodes of a psychosis are associated with a loss of brain tissue that may reduce the effectiveness of medications for treating the psychosis. Multiple episodes of a psychosis also interfere with the educational, vocational, and social development of the individual in whom it occurs, with an adverse effect on the long-term outcomes of the affected individual.

FACTS AND FIGURES

A study reported in 2010 found that up to 40 percent of the initial diagnoses of psychotic disorders are changed within 3 months after their first episodes. A diagnosis of schizophrenia is made after a first episode of psychosis in from 50 percent to 70 percent of those who experience it; a diagnosis of schizoaffective disorder is made in approximately 20 percent of individuals experiencing a first psychotic episode; a diagnosis of bipolar disorder in 6 percent; and a diagnosis of one of a wide variety of other disorders in approximately 10 percent. One year after early intervention for the treatment of a first episode of psychosis, at least 66 percent of those it affects are in remission and 25 percent are experiencing residual symptoms. Five years after early intervention for a first episode of psychosis, approximately 15 percent of affected individuals are symptom free, 15 percent continue to be regularly institutionalized, and from 30 to 40 percent live in the community while continuing to experience psychotic symptoms.

RISK FACTORS

Biological sources of psychosis include genetics; abnormalities in the biochemistry of the neurotransmitter substances that convey signals between nerve cells; abnormalities in the structure of the brain; premature birth and various factors in prenatal development; traumatic brain injury or other organic factors; and the effects of various medications or their erroneous dosing. Daily use of marijuana, and of the substances known as cannabinoids derived from marijuana, can induce a psychosis, and psychotic symptoms and syndromes occur in as many as 40 percent of users of methamphetamine). Environmental factors that may result in a psychosis include low socioeconomic status, family dysfunction, physical or emotional abuse/neglect, exposure to trauma, and stress. The stigma associated with the diagnosis of a psychotic disorder may exacerbate its symptoms.

SIGNS AND SYMPTOMS

The signs and symptoms of psychotic disorders vary according to their specific nature, but may include social withdrawal or socially inappropriate behavior; a decrease in personal hygiene and self-care; inappropriate and often flattened or diminished affect; rapid changes in affect; hallucinations; auditory and other delusions; disrupted thought processes and speech; and confusion.

TREATMENT

The social worker assisting an individual in whom a diagnosis of a psychotic disorder has been made should conduct a standard biological, psychological, social, and spiritual assessment of the individual, including an assessment of his or her risk for suicide and inflicting harm on him- or herself and others. This should include observation of the individual's behavior and demeanor, with particular attention

to the duration and changes in the severity of symptoms, and the collection of information on any prior episodes of mental disturbance in the affected individual. The individual undergoing assessment should be questioned about any medications or substances that he or she may be using, and should be referred for medical tests done to eliminate a medical condition as the cause of the individual's psychotic disorder. The assessment should also include the collection of collateral information from the individual's family, friends, and coworkers.

The initial treatment of a psychotic disorder often includes the use of medication to relieve its symptoms. Further, specific treatments for a psychotic disorder depend on its diagnosis and may include individual or group psychotherapy, training of the affected individual in social skills, and family-oriented therapy. Severe symptoms of a psychosis that endanger the physical welfare or life of the individual or others require voluntary or involuntary hospitalization of the affected individual. Hallucinations, delusions, or erratic or self-destructive behavior require antipsychotic medication, which should be prescribed by a mental health professional. This should be followed by monitoring of the treated individual for adherence to the medication regimen and the observation and notation of changes in his or her behavior.

In the case of families confronted with or distressed by a first episode of psychosis in a family member, both the family itself and the affected member should be provided with an environment that is safe for the expression of his or her feelings. Assistance should involve facilitating dialogue among family members and education of the family about the affected individual's psychosis or specific diagnosis, and referral of the family to appropriate assistive organizations if and as needed.

Recovery from a psychotic illness is conceptualized as a process rather than a point at which treatment ends. Themes that guide recovery include hope, rebuilding of the affected individual's self, and rebuilding of his or her life towards the goal of an acceptable quality of life. A study of persons ranging from 16 to 25 years of age who had psychotic disorders found that they were not only interested in treatment to address the symptoms of their disorders but also to help them build personal skills across a wide range of psychosocial areas (communication skills, decision making skills, conflict management skills) and in various practical areas (writing a resume, finding housing, getting a driver's license).

Social workers assisting individuals with psychotic disorders and their families should be aware of their own cultural values, beliefs, and biases, and develop specialized knowledge about the histories, traditions, and values of these individuals and their families. They should adopt treatment methods that reflect knowledge of the cultural diversity of these people and their communities.

APPLICABLE LAWS AND REGULATIONS
Both the United States Government and individual states have own standards, procedures, and laws for the involuntary restraint and detention of persons who may be a danger to themselves or others. Because many persons experiencing a first episode of psychosis are at high risk for attempted suicide, it is important to be familiar with local and state requirements for involuntary detention. Local and professional reporting requirements for neglect and abuse should also be known and observed.

SERVICES AND RESOURCES
- Brain & Behavior Research Foundation (formerly NARSAD), https://bbrfoundation.org/
- National Alliance on Mental Illness (NAMI), http://www.nami.org/
- U.S. National Institutes of Health (NIH), https://www.nih.gov/
- U.S. National Institute of Mental Health (NIMH), http://www.nimh.nih.gov/index.shtml
- National Association of Social Workers (NASW), http://www.socialworkers.org/

Written by Chris Bates, MA, MSW

Reviewed by Lynn B. Cooper, D Crim

REFERENCES
Alvarez-Jimenez, M., Parker, A. G., Hetrick, S. E., McGorry, P. D., & Gleeson, J. F. (2011). Preventing the second episode: A systematic review and meta-analysis of psychosocial and pharmacological trials in first-episode psychosis. *Schizophrenia Bulletin, 37*(3), 619-630.
American Psychiatric Association. (2013). Diagnostic and Statistical Manual of Mental Disorders. In (5th ed., p. 41). Washington, DC: American Psychiatric Publishing.
Archie, S. (2010). Early detection, assessment, and optimal treatment of a first episode of psychosis. *JCOM, 17*(7), 323-334.
Berthelot, N., Paccalet, T., Gilbert, E., Moreau, I., Merette, C., Gingras, N.,... Maziade, M. (2015). Childhood abuse and neglect may induce deficits in cognitive precursors of psychosis in high-risk children. *Journal of Psychiatry & Neuroscience, 40*(5), 336-343.
British Association of Social Workers. (2012, January). The Code of Ethics for Social Work: Statement of principles. Retrieved March 23, 2016, from http://cdn.basw.co.uk/upload/basw_112315-7.pdf
DiForti, M., Sallis, H., Allegri, F., Trotta, A., Ferraro, L., Stilo, S., & Khondoker, M. (2014). Daily use, especially high-potency cannabis, drives the earlier onset of psychosis in cannabis users. *Schizophrenia Bulletin, 40*(6), 1509-1517. doi:10.1093/schbul/sbt181
Glasner-Edwards, S., & Mooney, L. (2014). Methamphetamine psychosis: epidemiology and management. *CNS Drugs, 28*(12), 1115-1126. doi:10.1007/s40263-014-0209-8
(2011). Psychosis. In R. J. Hoffman, V. J. Wang, & R. J. Scarfone (Eds.), *Fleisher and Ludwig's 5-minute pediatric emergency medicine consult* (1st ed., pp. 782-783). Philadelphia, PA: Wolters Kluwer Health/Lippincott Williams & Wilkins.
International Federation of Social Workers. (2012). Statement of ethical principles. Retrieved March 23, 2016, from http://ifsw.org/policies/statement-of-ethical-principles/
Law, H., & Morrison, A. P. (2014). Recovery in psychosis: A Delphi study with experts by experience. *Schizophrenia Bulletin, 40*(6), 1347-1355. doi:10.1093/schbul/sbu047
Mitchison, D., Jakes, S., Kelly, S., & Rhodes, J. (2015). Are young people hospitalized with psychosis interested in psychological therapy? *Clinical Psychology & Psychotherapy, 22*(1), 22-31. doi:10.1002/cpp.1864
National Association of Social Workers. (2015). Standards and Indicators for Cultural Competence in Social Work Practice. Retrieved March 23, 2016, from http://www.socialworkers.org/practice/standards/PRA-BRO-253150-CC-Standards.pdf
Sadock, R. J., Sadock, V. A., & Ruiz, P. (2015). Schizophrenia spectrum and other psychotic disorders

(Chapter 7). In *Kaplan & Sadock's synopsis of psychiatry: behavioral sciences/clinical psychiatry* (pp. 300-346). Philadephia, PA: Wolters Kluwer.

(2015). Schizophrenia spectrum and other psychotic disorders. In B. J. Sadock, V. A. Sadock, & P. Ruiz (Eds.), *Kaplan & Sadocks's comprehensive textbook of psychiatry* (11th ed., pp. 1594-1605). Philadelphia, PA: Wolters Kluwer Health/Lippincott Williams & Wilkins.

Schultze-Lutter, F., Michel, C., Ruhrmann, S., & Schimmelmann, B. (2014). Prevalence and clinical significance of DSM-5 Attenuated Psychosis Syndrome in adolescents and young adults in the general population: The Bern Epidemiological At-Risk (BEAR) Study. *Schizophrenia Bulletin, 40*(6), 1499-1508. doi:10.1093/schbul/sbt171

Stain, H., Bronnick, K., Hegelstad, W., Ioa, T., Johannessen, J., Langeveld, J.,... Larsen, T. (2014). Impact of interpersonal trauma on the social functioning of adults with first-episode psychosis. *Schizophrenia Bulletin, 40*(6), 1491-1498. doi:10.1093/schbul/sbt166

PULMONARY DISEASE: CHRONIC OBSTRUCTIVE IN OLDER ADULTS

MAJOR CATEGORIES: Medical & Health

WHAT WE KNOW

Chronic obstructive pulmonary disease (COPD) is a debilitating and life-threatening disease state that is defined by the Global Initiative for Chronic Obstructive Lung Disease as being "characterized by persistent airflow limitation that is usually progressive and associated with enhanced chronic inflammatory response in the airways and the lung to noxious particles or gases." Clients with COPD experience troublesome symptoms such as coughing, breathlessness, chronic sputum production, anxiety/panic, depression, and sleep disturbances. Prevalence and severity of COPD increase with age.

COPD often is associated with several comorbid conditions including malnutrition, obesity, cardiovascular disease, skeletal muscle dysfunction, and sleep apnea. Older adults may also have cognitive impairment, osteoporosis, lack of caregiver involvement, or problems with medication adherence, or be institutionalized. COPD is most commonly diagnosed for individuals in their 50s and 60s, though usually symptoms had been present for on average 10 years.

COPD in older adults often is complicated by other age-related conditions. As one ages, airflow limitations increase, resulting in decreased pulmonary lung function, narrowing of the airways in the lungs, and hypoxia (i. e., lack of sufficient oxygen). These limitations place older adults at greater risk for complications including respiratory infections, pulmonary hypertension, pneumothorax (i. e., collapsed lung), acute and chronic respiratory failure, arrhythmia (i. e., abnormal heartbeat), and nocturnal hypoxia.

Studies suggest that COPD and cognitive impairment may be interrelated: The more severe the COPD, the more one is at risk for cognitive decline. In 2015, researchers studying older adults with COPD found that for 56.6 percent of participants who died, respiratory-specific disease was the cause; 20.5 percent died from cardiovascular causes, 15.7 percent from cancer, and 7.2 percent from other causes. As the disease progresses, clients typically experience decreasing functional capacity and increasing social isolation. The burden of coping with symptoms coupled with functional limitations often reduces clients' quality of life.

By 2020 COPD is projected to rank as the third leading cause of chronic morbidity and mortality worldwide. In the United States, it affects 14.2 percent of adults age 65 and older. In Europe it accounts for nearly half of the €102 billion spent annually on lung disease. Over 12 million adults in the United States have COPD, which is the fourth leading cause of death in the nation. It is the fifth leading cause of mortality in Australia and costs approximately A$8.8 billion in health-related expenses annually.

Risk factors for COPD include smoking tobacco, exposure to secondhand smoke, occupational exposure to carcinogens (e. g., firefighters), exposure to air pollution, aging (i. e., being over age 50), childhood respiratory infections, and antiprotease deficiency (i. e., protease enzymes end up becoming overactive, causing lung issues).

Smoking tobacco is the single leading risk factor for COPD because it irritates the lungs and increases inflammation in the respiratory system. Clients who quit smoking slow the progression of the disease. The sooner a smoker quits, the more lung function is preserved. Even in older adults it is important to emphasize the benefits of smoking cessation to reduce mortality and improve health.

Although advances have been made in the management of COPD and its physical symptoms, the psychosocial burden of the disease is largely unrecognized and untreated.

COPD often leads to a gradual and progressive decline in lung function, which results in increased dyspnea (i. e., shortness of breath) and reduced ability to perform daily activities. This decline in functioning alters the client's relationships, social roles, and self-perception, resulting in the need for continual psychological adjustment. Impaired ability to participate in physical and social activities often leads to a sedentary lifestyle, which increases dyspnea and fatigue. This in turn leads to social isolation, an inability to participate in many activities of daily living (ADL), and reduced QOL.

Poor coping skills can result in increased stress and anxiety, panic, loss of control and independence, anger, loss of intimacy, irritability, alteration in relationships, lifestyle changes, and a sense of worthlessness. A feeling of control or sense of mastery over the disease helps one to cope with chronic symptoms.

There are challenges specific to advanced age that can negatively affect older adults with COPD. Older adults with COPD frequently have balance impairments, so clients may need to have their balance and fall risks assessed by appropriate providers. They are at an increased risk for hospitalizations. When researchers examined hospitalization data, they found that there were 40.2 hospitalizations per 1,000 adults with COPD from ages 55 to 64 years old, but this increased to 131 per 1,000 for adults ages 65 and older. Medications can be expensive, with high out-of-pocket costs for older adults, who may be on a fixed income. Investigators found that when older adults with COPD had out-of-pocket pharmacy costs that went above $20, there were higher rates of nonadherence.

Cognitive impairment can be a major concern as a co-occurring condition with COPD. These cognitive impairments can result in overuse or underuse of medications related to COPD and increase the likelihood of negative side effects or exacerbations.

Depression and anxiety are common among older adult clients with COPD. Prevalence rates of depression and anxiety are higher among older adult clients with COPD than among older adult clients with other chronic diseases. Effective treatment of anxiety and depression in clients with COPD may include a combination of individual and group therapy, cognitive behavioral therapy (CBT), support groups, pharmacological interventions, psychoeducation, relaxation techniques, and pulmonary rehabilitation. Effective treatment results in improved QOL.

As with all clients who have a chronic medical condition, it is important with clients with COPD, especially older adults, to address advance directives (AD), establishment of a healthcare proxy, palliative care (PC), and end-of-life decisions. ADs provide specific instructions on care and treatment and provide instructions to help guide the client's appointed representative to serve as a proxy in making healthcare decisions.

Palliative care, which aims to promote comfort and maintain the highest quality of life for clients, encompasses psychological care, which enables clients to express thoughts, feelings, and fears regarding their diagnosis and end-of-life decisions. It can include but is not limited to hospice care. Essential areas include adequate pain management and symptom relief, preservation of clients' dignity, enabling clients to maintain a sense of control, hospice care, and helping clients prepare psychologically for death, when appropriate.

Family meetings may allow clients to express their wishes regarding palliative care. These meetings can serve as a forum for clients and family members to ask questions and stay informed about treatment goals and illness progression and may be a good time to discuss symptom control and plan for the future.

Addressing concerns proactively at an appropriate time can help clients plan for end-of-life care. Allowing clients the opportunity to discuss specific issues—for example, where they would like to die—can help alleviate anxieties and give them a sense of control.

WHAT CAN BE DONE

Become knowledgeable about COPD in older adults to better understand the various health and mental health education needs there may be.

Treatment methodologies should reflect the cultural values, beliefs, and biases of the individual in need of care and treatment.

As with other diseases that increase the risk of mental health issues, be aware of risk of suicide.

Learn communication skills that encourage honesty, empathy, cultural sensitivity, and patience. Use language that the individual and his or her family or caregivers can understand.

Emphasize the importance of keeping medical appointments to allow continued monitoring of the condition and to support the individual's quality of life.

Assess clients for financial difficulties that may affect adherence and provide support resources.

Provide emotional support by taking sufficient time to assess the needs of individual by listening actively and answering questions and encouraging the individual and family members to discuss their fears, concerns, and questions regarding COPD and future disease-related implications.

As a client's disease progresses, assess the need for referrals to social service agencies, physical or occupational therapy, home nursing care, healthcare assistance, palliative care, and hospice.

Encourage clients and family members to participate in activities they enjoy for as long as possible, to participate in religious and spiritual activities if desired, and to avoid social isolation.

Encourage the person with COPD to prepare for end of life, while still living their lives fully, through the use of an AD and assignment of a healthcare proxy.

Provide educational information to help clients and their family members learn about how to improve quality of life.

Provide written education material on COPD, including:

- COPD-Support: http://www.copd-support.com/.
- COPD International: http://www.copd-international.com/index. htm.

If appropriate, provide written education material about smoking cessation and websites for information and support, including:

- Smoke Free: http://smokefree.gov.

- About.com smoking cessation: http://quitsmoking. about.com/.
- Educate the caregiver/family regarding bereavement support and provide referrals, including:
- Palliative Care Matters: www.pallcare. info.
- Aging with Dignity: www.agingwithdignity.org.
- The Conversation Project: www.theconversation-project.org.

Written by Laura McLuckey, MSW, LCSW

Reviewed by Pedram Samghabadi, and Jessica Therivel, LMSW-IPR

REFERENCES

Aboussouan, L. S., & Messinger-Rapport, B. (2014). COPD in the elderly: Diagnostic and management challenges. *Geriatric Times, Spring 2014,*6-9. Retrieved from http://my. clevelandclinic.org/ccf/media/files/Geriatrics/Geriatric-Times/geriatric-times-spring-2014.pdf

Black, K. (2007). Advance care planning throughout the end-of-life: Focusing the lens for social work practice. *Journal of Social Work in End-of-Life & Palliative Care, 3*(2), 39-57. doi:10.1300/J457v03n02_04

Bostock-Cox, B. (2011). COPD series 3. Optimising quality of life using inhaler therapy. *Practice Nursing, 22*(4), 205-209. doi:http://dx. doi.org/10.12968/pnur.2011.22.4.205

British Association of Social Workers. (2012). The code of ethics for social work. Retrieved October 30, 2015, from http://cdn. basw.co.uk/upload/basw_112315-7.pdf

Brooks, J. A. (2014). Management of patients with chronic pulmonary disease. In J. L. Hinkle & K. H. Cheever (Eds.), *Brunner and Suddarth's textbook of medical-surgical nursing* (13th ed., pp.618-637). Philadelphia, PA: Wolters Kluwer Health/Lippincott Williams & Wilkins.

Caress, A., Luker, K., & Chalmers, K. (2010). Promoting the health of people with chronic obstructive pulmonary disease: Patients' and carers' views. *Journal of Clinical Nursing, 19*(3-4,564-573). doi:10.1111/j.1365-2702.2009.02982. x

Castaldi, P. J., Rogers, W. H., Safran, D. G., & Wilson, I. B. (2010). Inhaler costs and medication nonadherence among seniors with chronic pulmonary disease. *Chest, 138*(3), 614-620. doi:10.1378/chest.09-3031

Chang, S. S., Chen, S., McAvay, G. J., & Tinetti, M. E. (2012). Effect of coexisting chronic pulmonary disease and cognitive impairment on health outcomes in older adults. *The American Geriatrics Society, 60*(10), 1839-1894. doi:10.1111/j.1532-5415.2012.04171. x

Chen, C. Z., Ou, C. Y., Yu, C. H., Yang, S. C., Chang, H. Y., & Hslue, T. R. (2015).comparison of global initiative for chronic obstructive pulmonary disease 2013 classification and body mass index, airflow obstruction, dyspnea, and exacerbations index in predicting mortality and exacerbations in elderly adults with chronic obstructive pulmonary disease. *Journal of the American Geriatrics Society, 63*(2), 244-250. doi:10.1111/jgs.13258

Chestnutt, M. S., & Prendergast, T. J. (2015). Pulmonary disorders: chronic obstructive pulmonary disease. In M. A. Papadakis, S. J. McPhee, & M. W. Rabow (Eds.), *Lange 2015 current medical diagnosis and treatment* (54th ed., pp.256-262). New York, NY: McGraw-Hill Education.

Cox, K. (2011). Smoking cessation buddies in COPD. *Nursing Times, 107*(44), 22-23.

Cropp, A. J. (2014). Chronic obstructive pulmonary disease and emphysema. In F. J. Domino, R. A. Baldor, J. Golding, & J. A. Grimes (Eds.), *The 5-minute clinical consult 2015* (23rd ed., pp.240-241). Philadelphia, PA: Wolters Kluwer Health/Lippincott Williams & Wilkins.

Ford, E. S., Croft, J. B., Mannino, D. M., Wheaton, A. G., Zhang, X., & Giles, W. H. (2013). COPD surveillance – 1999-2011. *Chest, 144*(1), 284-305. doi:10.1378/chest.13-0809

DynaMed. (2014, October 8). COPD. Ipswich, MA: EBSCO Publishing. Retrieved October 20, 2014, from http://search. ebscohost.com/login. aspx?direct=true&db=dme&AN=115557

Global Initiative for Chronic Obstructive Lung Disease (GOLD). (2015). Global strategy for the diagnosis, management, and prevention of chronic obstructive pulmonary disease. Retrieved October 30, 2015, from http://www.goldcopd.org/uploads/users/files/GOLD_Report_2015_Apr2.pdf

Gooneratne, N., Patel, N. P., & Corcoran, A. (2010). Chronic obstructive pulmonary disease diagnosis and management in older adults. *The American Geriatrics Society, 58*(6), 1153-1162. doi:10.1111/j.1532-5415.2010.02875. x

Gupta, B., & Kant, S. (2009). Health related quality of life (Hrqol) in COPD. *Internet Journal of Pulmonary Medicine, 11*(1), 1-9.

Halbert, R. J., Natoli, J. L., Gano, A., Badamgarav, E., Buist, A. S., & Mannino, D. M. (2006). Global burden of COPD: Systematic review and meta-analysis. *Eur Respir J,28*(3), 523-532. doi:10.1183/09031936.06.00124605

Jacome, C., Cruz, J., Gabriel, R., Figueiredo, D., & Marques, A. (2014). Functional balance in older adults with chronic obstructive pulmonary disease. *Journal of Aging & Physical Activity, 22*(3), 357-363. doi:10.1123/japa.2012-0319

Jehn, M., Schnidler, C., Meyer, A., Tamm, M., Schmidt-Trucksass, A., & Stolz, D. (2012). Daily walking intensity as a predictor of quality of life in patients with chronic obstructive pulmonary diseas. *Medicine & Science in Sports & Exercise, 44*(7), 1212-1218. doi:10.1249/MSS.0b013e318249d8d8

Kelly, C., & Lynes, D. (2008). Psychological effects of chronic lung disease. *Nursing Times, 104*(47), 82-85.

Luker, K. A., Chalmers, I., Caress, A. L., & Salmon, M. P. (2007). Smoking cessation interventions in chronic obstructive pulmonary disease and the role of the family: A systematic literature review. *Journal of Advanced Nursing, 59*(6), 559-568. doi:10.1111/j.1365-2648.2007.04379. x

McHugh, G., Chalmers, K., & Luker, K. A. (2007). Caring for patients with COPD and their families in the community. *British Journal of Community Nursing, 12*(5), 219-222. doi:10.12968/bjcn.2007.12.5.23356

Miravitlles, M., Naberan, K., Cantoni, J., & Azpeitia, A. (2011). Socioeconomic status and health-related quality of life with chronic obstructive pulmonary disease. *Respiration, 82*(5), 402-408. doi:10.1159/000328766

Mizrahi, T., & Mayden, R. W. (2001). NASW standards for cultural competence in social work practice. Retrieved October 30, 2015, from http://www.socialworkers.org/practice/standards/NASWCulturalStandards.pdf

Nelson, J. E., Puntillo, K. A., Pronovost, P. J., Walker, A. S., McAdam, J. L., Ilaoa, D.,... Penrod, J. (2010). In their own words: Patients and families define high-quality palliative care in the intensive care unit. *Critical Care Medicine, 38*(3), 808-818. doi:10.1097/CCM.0b013e3181c5887c

Probst, V. S., Kovelis, D., Hernandes, N. A., Camillo, C. A., Cavalheri, V., & Pitta, F. (2011). Effects of exercise training programs on physical activity and daily life in patients with COPD. *Respiratory Care, 56*(11), 1799-1807. doi:10.4187/respcare.01110

Rabow, M. W., & Pantilat, S. Z. (2015). Palliative care and pain management. In S. J. McPhee & M. A. Papadakis (Eds.), *Lange 2015 current medical diagnosis & treatment* (54th ed., pp.71-92). New York, NY: McGraw-Hill Medical.

Ringbaek, T., Brondum, E., Martinez, G., Thogersen, J., & Lange, P. (2010). Long-term effects of 1-year maintenance training on physical functioning and health status in patients with COPD: A randomized control study. *Journal of Cardiopulmonary Rehabilitation & Prevention, 30*(1), 47-52. doi:10.1097/HCR.0b013e3181c9c985

Saini, B. (2013). COPD: A hidden epidemic. *Pharmacy News*, 29-32.

Sin, D. D., McAlister, F. A., Man, S. F., & Anthonisen, N. R. (2003). Contemporary management of chronic obstructive pulmonary disease: Scientific view. *JAMA, 290*(17), 2301-2312. doi:10.1001/jama.290.17.2301

Van Schayck, C. P., Kaper, J., Wagena, E. J., Wouters, E. F. M., & Severens, J. L. (2009). The cost-effectiveness of antidepressants for smoking cessation in chronic obstructive pulmonary disease (COPD) patients. *Addiction, 104*(12), 2110-2117. doi:10.1111/j.1360-0443.2009.02723. x.

Yawn, B. P., Giardino, N. D., & Criner, G. J. (2007). Don't overlook the impact of these comorbidities COPD and mood disorders, part 1: Anxiety and depression. *The Journal of Respiratory Diseases, 28*(3), 94-103.

Zhang, M. W., Ho, R. C. M., Cheung, M. W., Fu, E., & Mak, A. (2011). Prevalence of depression symptoms in patients with chronic obstructive pulmonary disease: A systematic review, meta-analysis and meta-regression. *General Hospital Psychiatry, 33*(3), 217-223. doi:10.1016/j.genhosppsych.2011.03.009

Statement of ethical principles. (2012, March 3). *International Federation of Social Workers*. Retrieved October 30, 2015, from http://ifsw.org/policies/statement-of-ethical-principles/

PULMONARY DISEASE: CHRONIC OBSTRUCTIVE—ANXIETY & DEPRESSION

MAJOR CATEGORIES: Behavioral & Mental Health, Medical & Health

WHAT WE KNOW

Chronic obstructive pulmonary disease (COPD) is a debilitating and potentially life-threatening disease state that is defined by the Global Initiative for Chronic Obstructive Lung Disease as being "characterized by persistent airflow limitation that is usually progressive and associated with enhanced chronic inflammatory response in the airways and the lung to noxious particles or gases."

Clients with COPD experience troublesome symptoms such as coughing, breathlessness, chronic sputum production, anxiety/panic, depression, and sleep disturbances. It often is associated with several comorbid conditions that include malnutrition, obesity, cardiovascular disease, skeletal muscle dysfunction, hypertension, osteoporosis, and sleep apnea.

By 2020 COPD is projected to rank as the third leading cause of mortality worldwide and in 2040 as the fourth leading cause of mortality. In Europe COPD contributes to nearly half of the €102 billion spent annually on lung disease. Over 12 million adults in the United States have COPD, which is the fourth leading cause of death in the nation. In the United Kingdom, there are currently approximately 835,000 people who have a current diagnosis of COPD. COPD is the fifth leading cause of mortality in Australia, costing approximately A$8.8 billion in health-related expenses annually.

Smoking tobacco is the single greatest risk factor for COPD because it irritates the lungs of clients with COPD, increasing inflammation in the respiratory system. Those who quit smoking slow the progression of the disease. The sooner a smoker quits, the more lung function is preserved.

Anxiety and depression are common among clients with COPD. Prevalence rates of anxiety and depression are higher among clients with COPD than among those with other chronic diseases. Anxiety may be manifested as excessive worry or rumination, irritability, feelings of dread, avoidance behaviors including social isolation, diminished concentration, fear of losing control, fatigue, sleep disturbance, dry mouth, and panic. Among clients with mild-to-moderate or stable COPD, the prevalence of anxiety is 10 percent–19 percent. Among clients with severe COPD, the prevalence of anxiety is 50 percent–75 percent.

Depression may be manifested as loss of interest in daily activities; feeling sad or hopeless; excessive feelings of guilt or worthlessness; changes in sleep or appetite; difficulty concentrating, thinking, or making decisions; unintentional weight changes; psychomotor retardation or agitation; fatigue; and recurrent thoughts of death, suicidal ideation including plans, or actual suicide attempts. Among clients with mild-to-moderate or stable COPD, the prevalence of depression is 10 percent–42 percent. Among clients with severe COPD, the prevalence of depression is 37 percent–71 percent.

Risk factors for depression and anxiety in clients with COPD include hypoxia (reduction of oxygen supply to tissue), hypercapnia (excess carbon dioxide in the blood), dyspnea (difficult or labored breathing), use of supplemental oxygen, certain medications, physical disability, poor social support, poor coping skills, cognitive impairment, and being under age 60 when COPD is diagnosed. Clients who smoke are at increased risk for anxiety and depression. Female clients with COPD have a higher rate of both anxiety and depression.

Some screening tools for depression and anxiety have been validated to use with COPD clients. These include the Geriatric Depression Scale (GDS) and the 15-item short form (GDS-15), the Hospital Anxiety and Depression Scales (HADS), the Geriatric Anxiety Inventory (GAI), the Anxiety Inventory for Respiratory Disease (AIR), and the Brief Assessment Schedule Depression Cards (BASDEC).

Clinicians should use any screening tool with caution because of the possibility of a high rate of false positives as a result of the overlap between symptoms of depression and anxiety and those of COPD.

Research suggests a cycle of deleterious effects of COPD on physical, social, and psychological well-being that includes symptoms of depression and anxiety. Dyspnea leads to impaired mobility and social isolation. Clients with COPD whose anxiety causes hyperventilation (i. e., breathing more than the body needs) may experience worsened shortness of breath. This may include lung hyperinflation, in which more effort is required to breathe and less air can be drawn into the lungs.

Clients with COPD experience a number of losses as they progress through the disease: loss of independence, loss of activities, and loss of relationships as a result of isolation. Social isolation may result in depression, further impaired mobility, and dyspnea. Acute exacerbation of COPD is known to result in depression. Anxiety and depression result in increased social isolation, more frequent hospitalization, longer length of hospital stays, more frequent physician visits, and premature mortality. Depression and anxiety lower clients' quality of life and lead to decreased adherence to treatment plans.

Researchers studied both a low–treatment adherence group of COPD patients and a high–treatment adherence group. They found that the low–treatment adherence group had higher depression scores, lower vitality scores, and more dyspnea than the high–treatment adherence group did. Also, 41.4 percent of the low–treatment adherence group were still smoking, whereas only 12.1 percent of the high–treatment adherence group continued to smoke.

Depression and anxiety often coexist in clients with COPD and can exacerbate the adverse effects of the disease. Anxiety, depression, and smoking result in an increased risk of death. Researchers found that participants with COPD who smoked and had symptoms of depression had a 3.8-fold increased risk of death. Study participants who smoked and had anxiety symptoms had a 4.3-fold increased risk of death.

Effective treatment of anxiety and depression in clients with COPD results in improved QOL. Treatment may include a combination of individual and group therapy, cognitive behavioral therapy (CBT), Internet-based CBT, support groups, pharmacological interventions, psychoeducation, and pulmonary rehabilitation.

CBT for anxiety in those with COPD may include techniques that teach distraction, breathing control, and relaxation. The cognitive portion includes education on the flight-or-fight response and the influence of adrenaline to help clients recognize and respond to the physical symptoms of anxiety (e. g., shaking, feeling out of breath, hot flashes, palpitations). CBT for depression related to COPD focuses on reducing negative or maladaptive thoughts, increasing activity levels, reducing isolation, increasing engagement, and problem-solving.

Problem-solving therapy (PST) is a specific CBT intervention that has resulted in decreased depression in clients with COPD. This technique has the client work on enhancing and improving problem-solving skills for major life events and day-to-day needs. The social worker can help clients in changing their approaches to problems and navigating the challenges that come up in their daily life experience.

Pharmacotherapy is often used with clients who have COPD and depression, but its efficacy is questionable in part because of a lack of studies.

There have been no randomized controlled trials conducted within a primary care setting with an acceptable sample size or long enough follow-up. The studies that have been conducted on selective serotonin reuptake inhibitors (SSRIs) have had weak methodology including small sample sizes, heterogeneous samples, and variability in the screening tools used to diagnose and monitor the subjects' depressive symptoms. Only one study on tricyclic antidepressants showed significant improvements in depression, anxiety, and quality of life.

There are also issues with lack of adherence to pharmacotherapy treatment plans, which may be the result of the impairment of cognitive function that can be present in COPD clients, the lack of motivation and energy to be compliant, and the complexity of overall COPD treatment.

Controlled breathing programs, in which physiotherapists teach clients pursed-lip breathing and active expiration (i. e., contraction of abdominal muscles with diaphragm displacement) along with relaxation exercises, can result in reduced anxiety and depression.

Pulmonary rehabilitation can improve dyspnea, improve clients' exercise tolerance, and reduce clients' overall disability, which in turn can improve symptoms of anxiety and depression.

The effectiveness of pulmonary rehabilitation can be more limited if a client is experiencing depression or anxiety that will interfere with making health behavior changes. Screening clients for depression and anxiety prior to their entering a pulmonary rehabilitation program can improve outcomes.

WHAT CAN BE DONE
Learn about COPD and anxiety and depression to better understand the various health and mental health education needs there may be.

Treatment methodologies should reflect the cultural values, beliefs, and biases of the individual in need of care and treatment.

Recognize the signs and symptoms of clinical depression and anxiety.

Emphasize the importance of keeping medical appointments to allow continued monitoring of clients' condition and provide support for clients' anxiety and/or depression.

Provide emotional support by taking sufficient time to listen actively, answer questions, and encourage clients to discuss their fears, concerns, and questions regarding COPD and future disease-related implications.

Seek out mental health interventions for clients' needs.

Provide written educational material on COPD and anxiety and depression and direct clients to sources of COPD information and support, including:
- COPD Support: http://www.copd-support.com/.
- American Lung Association: http://www.lung.org/lung-disease/copd/getting-and-giving-support/social-support. html.

Provide written education material about smoking cessation and direct clients to sources of information and support, including:
- Smoke Free: http://smokefree.gov.
- About.com smoking cessation: http://quitsmoking. about.com/.
- Centers for Disease Control and Prevention: http://www.cdc.gov/tobacco/.

For clients who smoke but do not plan to quit, provide them with contact information for smoking cessation programs should they choose to quit.

Written by Nikole Seals, MSW, ACSW, and Sharon Richman, MSPT

Reviewed by Jessica Therivel, LMSW-IPR

REFERENCES

British Association of Social Workers. (2012, January). The Code of Ethics for Social Work: Statement of principles. Retrieved January 15, 2016, from http://cdn. basw.co.uk/upload/basw_112315-7.pdf

Brooks, J. A. (2014). Management of patients with chronic pulmonary disease. In J. L. Hinkle & K. H. Cheever (Eds.), *Brunner and Suddarth's textbook of medical-surgical nursing* (13th ed., pp.618-637). Philadelphia, PA: Wolters Kluwer Health/Lippincott Williams & Wilkins.

Caress, A., Luker, K., & Chalmers, K. (2010). Promoting the health of people with chronic obstructive pulmonary disease: patients' and carers' views. *Journal of Clinical Nursing, 19*(3-4), 564-573. doi:10.1111/j.1365-2702.2009.02982. x

Cox, K. (2011). Smoking cessation buddies in COPD. *Nursing Times, 107*(44), 22-23.

Global Initiative for Chronic Obstructive Lung Disease (GOLD). (2015). Global strategy for the diagnosis, management, and prevention of chronic obstructive pulmonary disease. Retrieved July 29, 2015, from http://www.gold-copd.org/uploads/users/files/GOLD_Report_2015_Apr2.pdf

Heslop, K. (2014). Non-pharmacological treatment of anxiety and depression in COPD. *Nurse Prescribing, 12*(1), 43-47. doi:10.12968/npre.2014.12.1.43

Lou, P., Chen, P., Zhang, P., Yu, J., Wang, Y., Chen, N.,... Zhao, J. (2014). Effects of smoking, depression, and anxiety on mortality in COPD patients: A prospective study. *Respiratory Care, 59*(1), 54-61. doi:10.4187/respcare.02487

Luker, K. A., Chalmers, I., Caress, A. L., & Salmon, M. P. (2007). Smoking cessation interventions in chronic obstructive pulmonary disease and the role of the family: A systematic literature review.

Journal of Advanced Nursing, 59(6), 559-568. doi:10.1111/j.1365-2648.2007.04379. x

Maurer, J., Rebbapragada, V., Borson, S., Goldstein, R., Kunik, M. E., Yohannes, A. M., & Hanania, N. A. (2008). Anxiety and depression in COPD: Current understanding, unanswered questions, and research needs. *Chest, 134*(Suppl.4), 43S-56S. doi:10.1378/chest.08-0342

McHugh, G., Chalmers, K., & Luker, K. A. (2007). Caring for patients with COPD and their families in the community. *British Journal of Community Nursing, 12*(5), 219-222. doi:10.12968/bjcn.2007.12.5.23356

McHugh, G., Chalmers, K., & Luker, K. A. (2007). Caring for patients with COPD and their families in the community. *British Journal of Community Nursing, 12*(5), 219-222. doi:10.12968/bjcn.2007.12.5.23356

Mizrahi, T., & Mayden, R. W. (2001). NASW standards for cultural competence in social work practice. Retrieved October 20, 2014, from http://www.socialworkers.org/practice/standards/NASWCulturalStandards.pdf

Sin, D. D., McAlister, F. A., Man, S. F., & Anthonisen, N. R. (2003). Contemporary management of chronic obstructive pulmonary disease: Clinical applications. *JAMA, 290*(17), 2301-2312. doi:10.1001/jama.290.17.2313

Saini, B. (2013). COPD: A hidden epidemic. *Pharmacy News,* 29-32. Retrieved from

Valenza, M. C., Valenza-Pena, G., Torres-Sanchez, I., Gonzalez-Jimenez, E., Conde-Valero, A., & Valenzaq-Demet, G. (2014). Effectiveness of controlled breathing techniques on anxiety and depression in hospitalized patients with COPD: A randomized clinical trial. *Respiratory Care, 59*(2), 209-215. doi:10.4187/respcare.02565

Van Schayck, C. P., Kaper, J., Wagena, E. J., Wouters, E. F. M., & Severens, J. L. (2009). The cost-effectiveness of antidepressants for smoking cessation in chronic obstructive pulmonary disease (COPD) patients. *Addiction, 104*(12), 2110-2117. doi:10.1002/14651858. CD001007. pub2

Yawn, B. P., Giardino, N. D., & Criner, G. J. (2007). Don't overlook the impact of these comorbidities COPD and mood disorders, part 1: Anxiety and depression. *The Journal of Respiratory Diseases, 28*(3), 94-103.

Zhang, M. W., Ho, R. C. M., Cheung, M. W., Fu, E., & Mak, A. (2011). Prevalence of depressive symptoms in patients with chronic obstructive pulmonary disease: a systematic review, meta-analysis and meta-regression. *General Hospital Psychiatry, 33*(3), 217-223. doi:10.1016/j. genhosppsych.2011.03.009

Statement of ethical principles. (2012, March 3). *International Federation of Social Workers.* Retrieved October 20, 2014, from http://ifsw.org/policies/statement-of-ethical-principles/

Avari, J. N., & Alexopoulos, G. S. (2015). Models of care for late-life depression of the medically ill: Examples from chronic obstructive pulmonary disease and stroke. *erican Journal of Geriatric Psychiatry, 23*(5), 477-487.

Fan, V. S., & Meek, P. M. (2014). Anxiety, depression, and cognitive impairment in patients with chronic respiratory disease. *Clinical Chest Medicine, 35,*399-409.

Heslop, K. (2014). Non-pharmacological treatment of anxiety and depression in COPD. *Nurse Prescribing, 12*(1), 43-47. doi:10.12968/npre.2014.12.1.43

Lou, P., Chen, P., Zhang, P., Yu, J., Wang, Y., Chen, N.,... Zhao, J. (2014). Effects of smoking, depression, and anxiety on mortality in COPD patients: A prospective study. *Respiratory Care, 59*(1), 54-61. doi:10.4187/respcare.02487

Pumar, M. I., Gray, C. R., Walsh, J. R., Yang, I. A., Rolls, T. A., & Ward, D. L. (2014). Anxiety and depression: Important psychological comorbidities of COPD. *Journal of Thoracic Disease, 6*(11), 1615-1631. doi:10.3978/j. issn.2072-1439.2014.09.28

Turan, O., Yemez, B., & Itil, O. (2013). The effects of anxiety and depression symptoms on treatment adherence in COPD patients. *Primary Healthcare Research and Development, 15*(3), 244-251.

Vestbo, J., Hurd, S., Augusti, A., Jones, P. W., Vogelmeier, C., Anzueto, A.,... Rodriguez-Roisin, R. (2013). Global strategy for the diagnosis, management, and prevention of chronic obstructive pulmonary disease: GOLD executive summary. *American Journal of Respiratory Critical Care Medicine, 187*(4), 347-365.

Yohannes, A., & Alexopoulos, G. (2014). Pharmacological treatment of depression in older patients with chronic obstructive pulmonary disease: Impact on the course of disease and health outcomes. *Drugs & Aging, 31*(7), 483-492. doi:10.1007/s40266-014-0186-0

PULMONARY DISEASE: CHRONIC OBSTRUCTIVE—FATIGUE

MAJOR CATEGORIES: Behavioral & Mental Health, Medical & Health

WHAT WE KNOW

Chronic obstructive pulmonary disease (COPD) is a debilitating and potentially life-threatening disease state that is defined by the Global Initiative for Chronic Obstructive Lung Disease as being "characterized by persistent airflow limitation that is usually progressive and associated with enhanced chronic inflammatory response in the airways and the lung to noxious particles or gases." Clients with COPD experience troublesome symptoms such as coughing, breathlessness, chronic sputum production, anxiety/panic, depression, fatigue, and sleep disturbances.

COPD often is associated with several comorbid conditions including malnutrition, obesity, cardiovascular disease, skeletal muscle dysfunction, and sleep apnea. By 2020 COPD is projected to rank as the third leading cause of mortality worldwide and by 2040 as the fourth leading cause of mortality. In Europe COPD contributes to nearly half of the €102 billion spent annually on lung disease. Over 12 million adults in the United States have COPD, making it the fourth leading cause of death in the United States. COPD is the fifth leading cause of mortality in Australia and costs approximately A$8.8 billion in health-related expenses annually.

Risk factors for COPD include smoking tobacco, exposure to secondhand smoke, occupational exposure (e. g., firefighters), exposure to air pollution, aging (i. e., being over age 50), childhood respiratory infections, and anti-protease deficiency.

Smoking tobacco is the single leading risk factor for COPD. Smoking irritates the lungs of persons with COPD, increasing inflammation in the respiratory system. Clients who quit smoking slow the progression of the disease. The sooner a smoker quits, the more lung function is preserved.

Potential complications of COPD include respiratory infections, pulmonary hypertension, pneumothorax (i. e., collapsed lung), acute and chronic respiratory failure, arrhythmia, and nocturnal hypoxia.

Fatigue is a prominent symptom of COPD. Even though it is a common symptom of COPD, there is not a universally utilized definition of fatigue. This is in part because fatigue is a subjective feeling;studies may use this term to represent states varying from general tiredness and lack of energy to complete exhaustion. A general explanation of fatigue characterizes it as a vague, unpleasant feeling that is always present. It results in a diminished capacity for physical or mental work, generalized tiredness, a desire to rest or sleep, and lack of motivation and interest in one's surroundings. These symptoms do not resolve with rest or food. This fatigue is different from normal fatigue, which is attributable to an identified exertion, is rapid in onset and brief in duration, and can be relieved with restorative sleep.

Fatigue is associated with dyspnea (i. e., shortness of breath), exercise intolerance, poor quality of life , and depression. Because the symptoms of fatigue overlap with those of dyspnea, it can be difficult to distinguish the two sets of symptoms in treatment and research. Many clients with COPD believe that fatigue is a natural consequence of the disease and, being resigned to this, will not express or disclose their fatigue to healthcare professionals.

Researchers for a COPD study found that many study participants who had COPD disclosed that they had not received any explanation or education on fatigue from their healthcare providers. COPD can progress to the point that the work of breathing is energy-depleting for the client. Muscle fatigue contributes to exercise intolerance. Reduced activity leads to loss of muscle mass and deconditioning, which further reduces capacity for physical activity.

Research suggests that men and women are equally likely to experience fatigue (frequency, duration, and severity) as a result of COPD. Some clients may experience fatigue related to exercise intolerance as a combination of muscle fatigue and respiratory fatigue.

Fatigue is an important indicator of health-related quality of life, which includes the person's perceived physical health, mental health, and functional status. In 2014, researchers found that, compared to healthy test subjects, test subjects with COPD had lower energy levels, decreased physical abilities, and greater social isolation, all of which contribute to a decreased HRQOL.

Many individuals with COPD report that they have never received an explanation of fatigue from physicians or that they have attended pulmonary rehabilitation programs that focus on physical activity but provide no education on fatigue.

Clients with fatigue often report feeling hopeless about the fatigue and that the fatigue is controlling their lives.

Pulmonary rehabilitation (PR) is a program of education and exercise for clients with COPD that addresses lifestyle modification, including how to perform activities with less dyspnea. PR can reduce fatigue and deconditioning, decrease the number of hospitalizations, decrease mortality, and improve HRQOL and the ability to perform activities of daily living (ADL). In a study that evaluated change in five dimensions of fatigue—general fatigue, physical fatigue, change in reduced activity, change in reduced motivation, and change in mental fatigue—pulmonary rehabilitation was found to result in improvements in the fatigue scores of most study participants, although improvements were not distributed equally across all five dimensions. Researchers in a 2014 study found that study participants who attended pulmonary rehabilitation programs learned about physical activity but not fatigue.

COPD often leads to a gradual and progressive decline in lung function, which results in increased dyspnea and reduced ability to perform ADLs. This decline in functioning affects the client's relationships, social roles, and self-perception, resulting in the need for continual psychological adjustment.

Inability to participate in physical and social activities often leads to a sedentary lifestyle that exacerbates dyspnea and fatigue. This in turn may lead to social isolation and inability to participate in many ADLs.

Understanding clients' perception of their disease burden is necessary in determining their coping abilities. Poor coping skills can result in increased stress and anxiety, panic, loss of control and independence, anger, loss of intimacy, irritability, alteration in relationships, lifestyle changes, and a sense of worthlessness. A feeling of control or a sense of mastery over the disease is an important aspect of coping with chronic symptoms. Helping clients learn how to plan, prioritize, and be flexible with day-to-day activities can help them feel they are gaining control over the fatigue.

Depression and anxiety are common among clients with COPD and often affect sleep, which can contribute to fatigue. Prevalence rates of depression and anxiety are higher among persons with COPD than among those with other chronic diseases. Depression and anxiety can be difficult to diagnose; fewer than one third of COPD clients with depression or anxiety receive treatment.

Effective treatment of anxiety and depression in clients with COPD may include a combination of individual and group therapy, cognitive behavioral therapy (CBT), support groups, pharmacological interventions, psychoeducation, relaxation techniques, and pulmonary rehabilitation. Effective treatment results in improved QOL.

Palliative care that aims to promote comfort and maintain the highest quality of life for clients is essential to the management of their symptoms. This includes psychological care that enables them to express thoughts, feelings, and fears.

Family meetings may allow clients to express their wishes regarding palliative care. These meetings can serve as a forum for clients and family members to ask questions and stay informed about treatment goals and illness progression. Family meetings may be a good time to discuss symptom control and plan for the future.

End-of-life care is an important component of palliative care that addresses concerns proactively at an appropriate time. Providing clients the opportunity to discuss specific issues—for example, where they would like to die—can help alleviate their anxieties and give them a sense of control.

WHAT CAN BE DONE

Learn about COPD and fatigue to better understand the various health and mental health education needs there may be.

Treatment methodologies should reflect the cultural values, beliefs, and biases of the individual in need of care and treatment.

Ensure that clients with COPD are receiving education on fatigue from healthcare providers.

Assess fatigue in clients with COPD.

A client history should include questions about alcohol and tobacco use, unintentional weight loss, activity restrictions, alterations in fatigue levels, sleep patterns, and current medication.

Emphasize the importance of keeping medical appointments to allow continued monitoring of the client's condition and the provision of support for the client's fatigue.

Provide emotional support in the following ways:
- taking sufficient time to assess needs by listening actively and answering questions
- encouraging them to discuss fears, concerns, and questions regarding having COPD

Provide written education material on COPD, including from the following:
- COPD-Support, http://www.copd-support.com/.
- COPD International, http://www.copd-international.com/index. htm.

If appropriate, provide written education material about smoking cessation, including websites that offer information and support, including the following:
- Smoke Free, http://smokefree.gov.
- About.com smoking cessation, http://quitsmoking. about.com/.
- Request a referral to PR for clients with symptoms of fatigue and dyspnea.

Written by Laura McLuckey, MSW, LCSW

Reviewed by Jessica Therivel, LMSW-IPR

REFERENCES

Bachasson, D., Wuyam, B., Pepin, J. L., Tamisier, R., Levy, P., & Verges, S. (2013). Quadriceps and respiratory muscle fatigue following high-intensity cycling in COPD patients. *Plos One, 8*(12), e83432. doi:10.1371/journal. pone.0083432

Boardman, M. B. (2008). Chronic obstructive pulmonary disease. In T. M. Buttaro, J. Trybulski, P. P. Bailey, & J. Sandberg-Cook (Eds.), *A collaborative practice* (3rd ed., pp. 433-443). St. Louis, MO: Mosby Elsevier.

British Association of Social Workers. (2012). The code of ethics for social work: Statement of principles. Retrieved March 10, 2015, from http://cdn.basw.co.uk/upload/basw_112315-7.pdf

Brooks, J. A. (2014). Management of patients with chronic pulmonary disease. In J. L. Hinkle & K. H. Cheever (Eds.), *Brunner and Suddarth's textbook of medical-surgical nursing* (13th ed., pp.618-637). Philadelphia, PA: Wolters Kluwer Health/Lippincott Williams & Wilkins.

Calik-Kutukcu, E., Savci, C., Salam, M., Vardar-Yagli, N., Inal-Ince, D., Arikan, H.,... Coplu, R. (2014). A comparison of muscle strength and endurance, exercise capacity, fatigue perception, and quality of life in patients with chronic obstructive pulmonary disease and healthy subjects: A cross-sectional study. *BMC Pulmonary Medicine, 14*(6). doi:10.1186/1471-2466-14-6

Caress, A., Luker, K., & Chalmers, K. (2010). Promoting the health of people with chronic obstructive pulmonary disease: patients' and carers' views. *Journal of Clinical Nursing, 19*(3-4), 564-573. doi:10.1111/j.1365-2702.2009.02982. x

Casaburi, R. (2006). Impacting patient-centered outcomes in COPD: Deconditioning. *European Respiratory Review, 15*(99), 42-46. doi:10.1183/09059180.00009904

Centers for Disease Control. (2011, March 17). HRQOL concepts. Retrieved October 30, 2015, from http://www.cdc.gov/hrqol/concept. htm

Cox, K. (2011). Smoking cessation buddies in COPD. *Nursing Times, 107*(44), 22-23.

Cropp, A. J. (2014). Chronic obstructive pulmonary disease and emphysema. In F. J. Domino, R. A. Baldor, J. Golding, & J. A. Grimes (Eds.), *The 5-minute clinical consult 2015* (23rd ed., pp.240-241). Philadelphia, PA: Wolters Kluwer Health/Lippincott Williams & Wilkins.

Global Initiative for Chronic Obstructive Lung Disease (GOLD). (2015). Global strategy for the diagnosis, management, and prevention of chronic obstructive pulmonary disease. Retrieved October 30, 2015, from http://www.goldcopd.org/uploads/users/files/GOLD_Report_2015_Apr2.pdf

Kelly, C., & Lynes, D. (2008). Psychological effects of chronic lung disease. *Nursing Times, 104*(47), 82-85.

Lewko, A., Bidgood, P. L., Jewell, A., & Garrod, R. (2014). Evaluation of multidimensional COPD-related subjective fatigue following a pulmonary rehabilitation programme. *Respiratory Medicine, 108*(1), 95-102. doi:10.1016/j. rmed.2013.09.003

Luker, K. A., Chalmers, I., Caress, A. L., & Salmon, M. P. (2007). Smoking cessation interventions in chronic obstructive pulmonary disease and the role of the family: A systematic literature review. *Journal of Advanced Nursing, 59*(6), 559-568. doi:10.1111/j.1365-2648.2007.04379. x

McHugh, G., Chalmers, K., & Lukers, K. A. (2007). Caring for patients with COPD and their families in the community. *British Journal of Community Nursing, 12*(5), 219-222. doi:10.12968/bjcn.2007.12.5.23356

Mizrahi, T., & Mayden, R. W. (2001). NASW standards for cultural competence in social work practice. Retrieved October 30, 2015, from http://www.socialworkers.org/practice/standards/NASWCulturalStandards.pdf

Saini, B. (2013). COPD: A hidden epidemic. *Pharmacy News,* 29-32.

Sin, D. D., McAlister, F. A., Man, S. F., & Anthonisen, N. R. (2003). Contemporary management of chronic obstructive pulmonary disease: Clinical applications. *JAMA,290*(17), 2301-2312. doi:10.1001/jama.290.17.2313

Stridsman, C., Lindberg, A., & Skar, L. (2014). Fatigue in chronic obstructive pulmonary disease: A qualitative study of people's experiences. *Scandinavian Journal of Caring Sciences, 28*(1), 130-138. doi:10.1111/scs.12033

Theander, K., & Unosson, M. (2011). No gender differences in fatigue and functional limitations due to fatigue among patients with COPD. *Journal of Clinical Nursing, 20*(9/10), 1303-1310. doi:10.1111/j.1365-2702.2010.03625. x

Trendall, J. (2001). Assessing fatigue in patients with COPD. *Professional Nurse, 16*(7), 1217-1220.

VanSchayck, C. P., Kaper, J., Wagena, E. J., Wouters, E. F. M., & Severens, J. L. (2009). The cost-effectiveness of antidepressants for smoking cessation in chronic obstructive pulmonary disease (COPD) patients. *Addiction, 104*(12), 2110-2117. doi:10.1002/14651858. CD001007. pub2

Yawn, B. P., Giardino, N. D., & Criner, G. J. (2007). Don't overlook the impact of these comorbidities COPD and mood disorders, part 1: Anxiety and depression. *The Journal of Respiratory Diseases, 28*(3), 94-103.

Zhang, M. W., Ho, R. C. M., Cheung, M. W., Fu, E., & Mak, A. (2011). Prevalence of depression symptoms in patients with chronic obstructive pulmonary disease: A systematic review, meta-analysis and meta-regression. *General Hospital Psychiatry, 33*(3), 217-223. doi:10.1016/j.genhosppsych.2011.03.009

International Federation of Social Workers. (2012, March 3). Statement of ethical principles. Retrieved October 30, 2015, from http://ifsw.org/policies/statement-of-ethical-principles/

Stridsman, C., Lindberg, A., & Skar, L. (2014). Fatigue in chronic obstructive pulmonary disease:

A qualitative study of people's experiences. *Scandinavian Journal of Caring Sciences, 28*(1), 130-138. doi:10.1111/scs.12033

Vestbo, J., Hurd, S., Augusti, A., Jones, P. W., Vogelmeier, C., Anzueto, A.,... Rodriguez-Roisin, R. (2013). Global strategy for the diagnosis, management, and prevention of chronic obstructive pulmonary disease: GOLD executive summary. *American Journal of Respiratory Critical Care Medicine, 187*(4), 347-365. doi:10.1164/rccm.201204-0596PP

PULMONARY DISEASE: CHRONIC OBSTRUCTIVE—QUALITY OF LIFE

MAJOR CATEGORIES: Behavioral & Mental Health, Medical & Health

WHAT WE KNOW

Chronic obstructive pulmonary disease (COPD) is a debilitating and potentially life-threatening disease that is defined by the Global Initiative for Chronic Obstructive Lung Disease as "characterized by persistent airflow limitation that is usually progressive and associated with an enhanced chronic inflammatory response in the airways and the lung to noxious particles or gases." Troublesome symptoms include coughing, breathlessness, and chronic sputum production. Anxiety/panic, depression, fatigue, loss of appetite, and weight loss are also common.

COPD often is associated with several comorbid conditions including cardiovascular disease, lung cancer, skeletal muscle dysfunction, osteoporosis, metabolic disorder, and chronic psychiatric conditions. Diagnosis is made by a physician utilizing a medical history (e. g., symptoms, history of exposure to risk factors, family history of COPD), physical exam, and spirometric testing.

Potential complications of COPD include respiratory infections, pulmonary hypertension, pneumothorax (i. e., collapsed lung), acute and chronic respiratory failure, arrhythmia, and nocturnal hypoxia.

COPD is one of the leading causes of chronic morbidity and mortality worldwide. In Europe COPD accounts for nearly half of the €102 billion spent annually on lung disease. Over 12 million adults in the United States have COPD, which is the fourth leading cause of death in the United States. COPD is the fifth leading cause of death in Australia and costs approximately A $8.8 billion in health-related expenses annually.

Risk factors for COPD include smoking tobacco, exposure to secondhand smoke, occupational exposure (e. g., firefighters), exposure to air pollution, aging (i. e., being over age 50), childhood respiratory infections, and antiprotease deficiency.

Smoking tobacco is the single leading risk factor for COPD. It irritates the lungs of persons with COPD, increasing inflammation in the respiratory system. Smoking cessation is the most important measure in preventing COPD and/or slowing its progression.

COPD is classified based on post-bronchodilator spirometric assessment of airflow limitation: GOLD 1 (mild), GOLD 2 (moderate), GOLD 3 (severe), and GOLD 4 (very severe). These classifications do not predict health-related quality of life. Combined COPD assessment incorporates both severity of symptoms and risk of exacerbations, placing clients in one of four groups: less severe symptoms and lower risk of exacerbations (group A), more severe symptoms and lower risk of exacerbations (group B), less severe symptoms and higher risk of exacerbations (group C), or more severe symptoms and higher risk of exacerbations (group D).

As COPD progresses, clients typically experience decreasing functional capacity and increasing social isolation. The burden of coping with symptoms coupled with functional limitations reduces the client's quality of life, including social engagement/isolation, independence/dependence, satisfaction/dissatisfaction, effective coping/ineffective coping, and self-efficacy/helplessness. Factors affecting QOL include physical signs and symptoms, physical and social activity, and psychological and spiritual status.

Characteristics associated with reduced quality of life include older age, female sex, decreased lung function, poor health status, low level of exercise capacity, comorbid diabetes mellitus, lower education level, lower socioeconomic status, and experiencing exacerbation of COPD symptoms.

In a French study of gender differences among persons with COPD, investigators reported that, compared with men, women were younger, were more likely to live alone, had lower tobacco use but were more likely to be current smokers, had higher rates of past anxiety and depression, had less impairment of lung function, and reported lower QOL. Men were more likely than women to have cardiovascular comorbidities, sleep apnea, and alcoholism.

Researchers in Finland found that individuals with COPD were more likely than matched controls to have comorbid disorders such as mental health problems, alcohol abuse, diabetes, and cardiovascular disease. These comorbid conditions were found to be significant contributors to QOL.

Low quality of life was linked with higher rates of mortality. Depression and anxiety, which commonly co-occur with COPD, are associated with lower QOL in clients with COPD. Individuals commonly report decreased quality of life resulting from worry, sadness, nervousness, irritability, and difficulty concentrating. Pain and anemia have also been associated with lower QOL. Avoiding a continual focus on COPD symptoms and not viewing oneself as being disabled are associated with a higher QOL. Self-efficacy has been associated with better functional capacity and higher QOL.

Although there is no universal method of measuring health status/QOL in clients with COPD, questionnaires are most commonly used. The St. George's Respiratory Questionnaire (SGRQ) is a comprehensive, 50-item questionnaire; shorter comprehensive questionnaires include the COPD Assessment Test (CAT) and COPD Control Questionnaire (CCQ). Using QOL assessment questionnaires, clients rate how their disease affects their everyday lives. Assessment domains include levels of fatigue, sleep disturbance, pain, social isolation, physical incapacitation, and dyspnea (i. e., shortness of breath).

Treatment of COPD may include pharmacologic treatment (e. g., bronchodilators, corticosteroids), continuous oxygen therapy for clients with hypoxia, surgery (e. g., removal of enlarged airspaces called bullae that may compress lungs, or lung volume reduction in some clients with advanced disease), pulmonary rehabilitation, preventive care strategies to reduce risk of acute exacerbations, and prompt medical attention for acute exacerbations.

Pulmonary rehabilitation (PR) includes various components associated with improved QOL, reduced COPD symptoms, and increased independence with activities of daily living. A PR program will include education regarding COPD and self-management of the disease (e. g., nutrition, daily breathing exercises, regular physical activity, how to perform activities with less dyspnea), smoking cessation, and advance directives.

Exercise training will also be included. Low-intensity exercise training has been shown to improve QOL for persons with COPD(15). Use of a pedometer and web-based exercise program has been linked with increased activity and improved QOL compared to a wait-listed control group. An intervention period of longer than 3 months may be needed in order for an exercise-based intervention to support maintenance of regular physical activity.

After clients complete an initial program of pulmonary rehabilitation, its positive effects on QOL decrease over time; a maintenance program in which supervised rehabilitation therapy is conducted at least once a month is recommended.

WHAT CAN BE DONE

Learn about COPD and quality of life to better understand the various health and mental health education needs there may be.

Assess quality of life in clients with COPD.

Taking a client's history should include asking about alcohol and tobacco use, unintentional weight loss, activity restrictions, alterations in fatigue levels, sleep patterns, and current medical conditions and medication.

Emphasize the importance of keeping medical appointments to enable continued monitoring of the client's condition and support for his or her QOL.

Provide emotional support in the following ways:
- take sufficient time to assess his or her needs by listening actively and answering questions
- encourage the client to discuss his or her fears, concerns, and questions regarding having COPD

Provide written education material on COPD, including:
- American Lung Association, http://www.lung.org/lung-health-and-diseases/lung-disease-lookup/copd/.
- COPD Foundation, http://www.copdfoundation.org/.
- COPD Support, Inc., http://www.copd-support.com/.

If appropriate, provide written education material, in suitable language and comprehension level, about smoking cessation and refer to websites for information and support, including:
- Smoke free, http://smokefree.gov.
- About.com smoking cessation, http://quitsmoking.about.com/.

Request a referral to PR to help improve QOL in clients with COPD. PR focuses on increasing activity tolerance; reducing symptoms of dyspnea, fatigue, and depression; and increasing their sense of control. Encourage clients to maintain the activity level they achieve in PR to retain its benefits.

Seek out educational information to help clients and their family members learn how to improve QOL.

Written by Laura McLuckey, MSW, LCSW and Jennifer Teska, MSW

Reviewed by Lynn B. Cooper, D. Crim

REFERENCES

Bentsen, S. B., Miaskowski, C., & Rostøen, T. (2014). Demographic and clinical characteristics associated with quality of life in patients with chronic obstructive pulmonary disease. *Quality of Life Research, 23*(3), 991-998. doi:10.1007/s1136-013-0515-5

Bostock-Cox, B. (2011). COPD series 3. Optimising quality of life using inhaler therapy. *Practice Nursing, 22*(4), 205-209. doi:http://dx.doi.org/10.12968/pnur.2011.22.4.205

Brooks, J. A. (2014). Management of patients with chronic pulmonary disease. In J. L. Hinkle & K. H. Cheever (Eds.), *Brunner and Suddarth's textbook of medical-surgical nursing* (13th ed., pp.618-637). Philadelphia, PA: Wolters Kluwer Health/Lippincott Williams & Wilkins.

British Association of Social Workers. (2012). The code of ethics for social Work: statement of principles. Retrieved from http://cdn. basw.co.uk/upload/basw_112315-7.pdf

Caress, A., Luker, K., & Chalmers, K. (2010). Promoting the health of people with chronic obstructive pulmonary disease: patients' and carers' views. *Journal of Clinical Nursing, 19*(3-4), 564-573. doi:10.1111/j.1365-2702.2009.02982. x

Cox, K. (2011). Smoking cessation buddies in COPD. *Nursing Times, 107*(44), 22-23.

Cropp, A., & Vehnovich, B. (2015). Chronic obstructive pulmonary disease and emphysema. In F. J. Domino, R. A. Baldor, J. Golding, & M. B. Stephens (Eds.), *The 5-minute clinical consult standard 2016* (24th ed., pp.206-207). Philadelphia, PA: Wolters Kluwer Health.

Ferrari, M., Manea, L., Anton, K., Buzzone, P., Menghello, M., Zamboni, F.,... Testi, R. (2015). Anemia and hemoglobin serum levels are associated with exercise capacity and quality of life in chronic obstructive pulmonary disease. *BMC Pulmonary Medicine, 15*,58. doi:10.1186/s12890-015-0050-y

Global Initiative for Chronic Obstructive Lung Disease (GOLD). (2015). Global strategy for the diagnosis, management, and prevention of chronic obstructive pulmonary disease. Retrieved December 29, 2015, from http://www.goldcopd.org/uploads/users/files/GOLD_Report_2015.pdf

Gupta, B., & Kant, S. (2009). Health related quality of life (Hrqol) in COPD. *Internet Journal of Pulmonary Medicine, 11*(1), 1-9.

International Federation of Social Workers. (2012). Statement of Ethical Principles. Retrieved December 29, 2015, from http://ifsw.org/policies/statement-of-ethical-principles

Jackson, B. E., Coultas, D. B., Ashmore, J., Russo, R., Peoples, J., Uhm, M., & Bae, S. (2014). Domain-specific self-efficacy is associated with measures of functional capacity and quality of life among patients with moderate to severe chronic obstructive pulmonary disease. *Annals of the American Thoracic Society, 11*(3), 310-315. doi:10.1513/AnnalsATS.201308-273BC

Jehn, M., Schindler, C., Meyer, A., Tamm, M., Schmidt-Trucksäss, A., & Stolz, D. (2012). Daily walking intensity as a predictor of quality of life in patients with chronic obstructive pulmonary disease. *Medicine & Science in Sports & Exercise, 44*(7), 1212-1218. doi:10.1249/MSS.0b013e318249d8d8

Koskela, J., Kilpeläinen, M., Kupiainen, H., Mazur, W., Sintonen, H., Boezen, M., & Laitinen, T. (2014). Co-morbidities are the key nominators of the health related quality of life in mild and moderate COPD. *BMC Pulmonary Medicine, 14*,102. doi:10.1186/1471-2466-14-102

Luker, K. A., Chalmers, I., Caress, A. L., & Salmon, M. P. (2007). Smoking cessation interventions in chronic obstructive pulmonary disease and the role of the family: A systematic literature review. *Journal of Advanced Nursing, 59*(6), 559-568. doi:10 .1111/j.1365-2648.2007.04379. x

McHugh, G., Chalmers, K., & Lukers, K. A. (2007). Caring for patients with COPD and their families in the community. *British Journal of Community Nursing, 12*(5), 219-222. doi:10.12968/ bjcn.2007.12.5.23356

Mehta, J. R., Ratnani, I. J., Dave, J. D., Panchal, B. N., Patel, A. K., & Vala, A. U. (2014). Association of psychiatric co-morbidities and quality of life with severity of chronic obstructive pulmonary disease. *East Asian Archives of Psychiatry, 24*(4), 148-155.

Miravitieles, M., Naberan, K., Cantoni, J., & Azpeitia, A. (2011). Socioeconomic status and health-related quality of life with chronic obstructive pulmonary disease. *Respiration, 82*(5), 402-408. doi:10.1159/000328766

Mouser, A. L. (2014). Health-related quality of life in patience with moderate to severe chronic obstructive pulmonary disease: A concept analysis. *International Journal of Nursing Knowledge, 25*(2), 73-79. doi:10.1111/2047-3095.12014

Moy, M., Collins, R. J., Martinez, C. H., Kadri, R., Roman, P., Holleman, R. G., & Richardson, C. R. (2015). An internet-mediated pedometer-based program improves health-related quality-of-life domains and daily step counts in COPD. *Chest, 148*(1), 128-137. doi:10.1378/chest.14-1466

Probst, V. S., Kovelis, D., Hernandes, N. A., Camillo, C. A., Cavalheri, V., & Pitta, F. (2011). Effects of exercise training programs on physical activity and daily life in patients with COPD. *Respiratory Care, 56*(11), 1799-1807. doi:10.4187/respcare.01110

Raherison, C., Tillie-Leblond, I., Prudhomme, A., Taillé Biron, E., Nocent-Ejnaini, C., & Ostinelli, J. (2014). Clinical characteristics and quality of life in women with COPD: An observational study. *BMC Women's Health, 14*,31. doi:10.1186/1472-6874-14-31

Ringbaek, T., Brondum, E., Martinez, G., Thogersen, J., & Lange, P. (2010). Long-term effects of 1-year maintenance training on physical functioning and health status in patients with COPD: A randomized controlled study. *Journal of Cardiopulmonary Rehabilitation & Prevention, 30*(1), 47-52. doi:10.1097/ HCR.0b013e3181c9c985

Saini, B. (2013). COPD: A hidden epidemic. *Pharmacy News*, 29-32.

Sin, D. D., McAlister, F. A., Man, S. F., & Anthonisen, N. R. (2003). Contemporary management of chronic obstructive pulmonary disease: Clinical applications. *JAMA,290*(17), 2301-2312. doi:10.1001/jama.290.17.2313

Steele, B. G., Belza, B., Cain, K., Coppersmith, J., Howards, J., Lakshminarayan, S., & Haselkorn, J. (2010). The impact of chronic obstructive pulmonary disease exacerbation on pulmonary rehabilitation and functional outcomes. *Journal of Cardiopulmonary Rehabilitation & Prevention, 30*(1), 53-60. doi:10.1097/HCR.0b013e3181c85845

Van Schayck, C. P., Kaper, J., Wagena, E. J., Wouters, E. F. M., & Severens, J. L. (2009). The cost-effectiveness of antidepressants for smoking cessation in chronic obstructive pulmonary disease (COPD) patients. *Addiction, 104*(12), 2110-2117. doi:10.1002/14651858. CD001007. pub2

Wheeler, D., & McClain, A. (2015). NASW standards for cultural competence in social work practice. Retrieved December 29, 2015, from http://www. socialworkers.org/practice/standards/PRA-BRO-253150-CC-Standards.pdf

PULMONARY DISEASE: CHRONIC OBSTRUCTIVE—SMOKING CESSATION

MAJOR CATEGORIES: Behavioral & Mental Health, Medical & Health

WHAT WE KNOW

Chronic obstructive pulmonary disease (COPD) is a debilitating and potentially life-threatening disease state that is defined by the Global Initiative for Chronic Obstructive Lung Disease as being "characterized by persistent airflow limitation that is usually progressive and associated with enhanced chronic inflammatory response in the airways and the lung to noxious particles or gases." Clients with COPD experience troublesome symptoms such as coughing, breathlessness, chronic sputum production, anxiety/panic, depression, and sleep disturbances.

COPD often is associated with several comorbid conditions including malnutrition, obesity, cardiovascular disease, skeletal muscle dysfunction, sleep apnea, depression, and anxiety. By 2020 COPD is projected to rank as the third leading cause of mortality worldwide and in 2040 as the fourth leading cause of mortality. In Europe COPD accounts for nearly half of the €102 billion spent annually on lung disease. Over 12 million adults in the United States have COPD, which is the fourth leading cause of death in the United States. COPD is the fifth leading cause of mortality in Australia and costs approximately A$8.8 billion in health-related expenses annually. In the United Kingdom, approximately 835,000 people have a current diagnosis of COPD.

Smoking tobacco is the single leading risk factor for COPD. Smoking irritates the lungs of persons with COPD, increasing inflammation in the respiratory system. Clients who quit smoking slow the progression of the disease. Smoking cessation is the single most important intervention for COPD and the cornerstone of management of chronic COPD.

Smoking cessation is the term used for the process of quitting smoking. The most common forms of quitting smoking are stopping completely and abruptly, gradual reduction of nicotine use, nicotine replacement therapy (NRT), nicotine patches, and pharmacological interventions (e. g., bronchodilators, inhaled corticosteroids, antidepressants). It is difficult to compare the different pharmacological interventions because the same medications and protocols are not universally utilized.

Researchers conducted a meta-analysis on smoking cessation with COPD clients and determined an average quit rate of 13.19 percent; the most commonly used individual technique was to boost the motivation and self-efficacy of the client. Interventions within a clinical setting and with group elements had the most success. Out of 17 interventions, four behavior change techniques had the most success. These include the following:

- facilitation of action planning and developing treatment plan;
- prompting self-recording;
- advising on methods of weight control; and
- advising on/facilitate use of social support.

Two techniques had a negative effect on COPD smokers trying to quit: assessing nicotine dependence and boosting motivation/self-efficacy. Clients sometimes felt that assessments of nicotine dependence stressed the addiction aspect and reduced the clients' self-efficacy. Too many attempts to boost motivation and self-efficacy could result in over motivation; more success was found when techniques included changing motivation into actual action.

Researchers conducting another systematic review found that in smoking cessation programs combining psychosocial interventions with pharmacotherapy, on average 35.5 percent of the members of the experimental groups successfully quit smoking and maintained cessation for 12 months, compared to 10 percent of those in the control groups.

A greater likelihood of success with smoking cessation was shown when interventions had an increased intensity via increased length, and an increased number of sessions of counseling as well as multiple sessions of interventions a week. Individual counseling, hypnosis, group therapy, and participation in support groups such as Smokers Anonymous that emphasize behavior change may be helpful for clients.

Cognitive behavioral therapy (CBT) is an effective therapy to help smokers quit. CBT examines the cognitions and thoughts that underlie the behavior the client is attempting to change. Research indicates that CBT combined with other quitting strategies (e. g., pharmacotherapy) helps clients maintain abstinence from smoking. CBT is also effective for people who exhibit depression or anxiety and/or who abuse substances (e. g., alcohol, marijuana, heroin, prescription medications).

Behavior modification programs can help clients stop smoking by breaking the stimulus–response cycle that triggers the urge to smoke. To improve cessation rates, social workers need to have a clear understanding of the influences on clients' ability to quit in order to improve motivation. Researchers in Sweden found the following common reasons given for not quitting:

- Clients reported that it is very difficult to break a lifetime or long-term habit.
- Clients felt as though they had no control over quitting.
- Clients wanted help and support but felt patronized.

Social workers need to be aware that quitting smoking can increase respiratory symptoms initially: As the lungs recover, changes in the cells that line the bronchi can trigger symptoms. Although this may result in increased hospitalizations, smoking cessation ultimately results in positive long-term effects.

Smoking cessation can be very difficult. Often it requires many attempts on the part of the client and considerable support from family, friends, and healthcare professionals. Because the family likely plays an important role in clients' health and health behaviors, utilizing a family systems approach is helpful. The smoker, nonsmoker, attempter, or planner (SNAP) model can help social workers determine which state of change a smoker self-classifies as and proceed accordingly. For this model:

- Smoker – currently smoking without any plans to quit
- Nonsmoker – not currently smoking
- Attempter – in the process of trying to quit
- Planner – smoking, but planning to quit

United States Public Health Clinical Practice guidelines recommend that mental health clinicians use an evidence-based smoking cessation protocol known as the five As. Social workers should ask these questions in a person-centered manner to really explore the clients' feelings and beliefs:

Ask clients at every office visit if they smoke.

Advise all smokers to quit using language that is clear, strong, and personalized, including strong warnings about the health effects of smoking and exposure to secondhand smoke, especially for children.

Assess clients' willingness to quit and provide motivation to do so

Assist clients in their attempts to quit by determining a quit date, helping them identify triggers, providing encouragement, and providing counseling and pharmacotherapy as appropriate.

Arrange follow-up with clients.

WHAT CAN BE DONE

Learn about COPD and smoking cessation to better understand the various health and mental health education needs there may be.

Develop an awareness of your own cultural values, beliefs, and biases as well as the histories, traditions, and values of the individual in need of care. Look for treatment methodologies that reflect the cultural needs of the individual.

Assess the smoking history of clients with COPD (e. g., number of years clients have smoked, how much they smokes, smoking cessation attempts).

Utilize the SNAP model to assess clients' state of change.

Assist clients in identifying triggers (e. g., stress, drinking alcohol) for their smoking behavior and look for ways to minimize, avoid, and/or respond to those triggers.

Social workers can educate clients on what to expect during and after smoking cessation.

Emphasize the importance of keeping medical appointments to allow continued monitoring of clients' condition and support clients' efforts to quit smoking.

Evaluate clients' motivation to quit smoking.

If a client is not motivated, explore the reasons for the lack of motivation.

Introduce the concept of the lethality of tobacco, using data from health literature.

Identify toxins found in cigarettes (e. g., arsenic, tar, benzene).

Emphasize the role of eating healthfully and exercising if weight gain is a concern related to smoking cessation.

Provide emotional support in the following ways:

- recognizing and acknowledging that quitting smoking is difficult and may require multiple attempts ; and
- taking sufficient time to assess clients' needs by listening actively and answering questions.

Provide written education material about smoking cessation and websites for information and support, including:

- Smoke Free, http://smokefree.gov.
- About.com smoking cessation, http://quitsmoking. about.com/.
- Centers for Disease Control and Prevention, Smoking and Tobacco Use, http://www.cdc.gov/tobacco.

For clients who smoke but do not plan to quit, provide them with contact information for smoking cessation programs should they choose to quit.

Written by Laura McLuckey, MSW, LCSW

Reviewed by Jessica Therivel, LMSW-IPR, and Lynn B. Cooper, D. Crim

REFERENCES

Abu Hassan, H., Abd Aziz, N., Hassan, Y., & Hassan, F. (2014). Does the duration of smoking cessation have an impact on hospital admission and health-related quality of life amongst COPD patients?. *International Journal of Chronic Obstructive Pulmonary Disease, 9*,493-499. doi:10.2147/COPD. S56637

Attar-Zadeh, D. (2014). Smoking cessation and COPD: A case study. *Practice Nursing, 25*(6), 284-289. doi:http://dx. doi.org/10.12968/pnur.2014.25.6.284

Bartlett, Y. K., Sheeran, P., & Hawley, M. S. (2014). Effective behavior change techniques in smoking cessation interventions for people with chronic obstructive pulmonary disease: A meta-analysis. *British Journal of Health Psychology, 19*(1), 181-203. doi:10.1111/bjhp.12071

British Association of Social Workers. (2012, January). The code of ethics for social work: Statement of principles. Retrieved October 30, 2015, from http://cdn.basw.co.uk/upload/basw_112315-7.pdf

Brooks, J. A. (2014). Management of patients with chronic pulmonary disease. In J. L. Hinkle & K. H. Cheever (Eds.), *Brunner and Suddarth's textbook of medical-surgical nursing* (13th ed., pp.618-637). Philadelphia, PA: Wolters Kluwer Health/Lippincott Williams & Wilkins.

Caress, A., Luker, K., & Chalmers, K. (2010). Promoting the health of people with chronic obstructive pulmonary disease: Patients' and carers' views. *Journal of Clinical Nursing, 19*(3-4), 564-573. doi:10.1111/j.1365-2702.2009.02982. x

Centers for Disease Control and Prevention. (2015, May 21). Quitting smoking. Retrieved October 30, 2015, from http://www.cdc.gov/tobacco/data_statistics/fact_sheets/cessation/quitting/index. htm

Cox, K. (2011). Smoking cessation buddies in COPD. *Nursing Times, 107*(44), 22-23.

Eklund, B. M., Nilsson, S., Hedman, L., & Lindberg, I. (2012). Why do smokers diagnosed with COPD not quit smoking? –A qualitative study. *Tobacco Induced Diseases, 10*,17. doi:10.1186/1617-9625-10-17

Global Initiative for Chronic Obstructive Lung Disease (GOLD). (2015). Global strategy for the diagnosis, management, and prevention of chronic obstructive pulmonary disease. Retrieved October 30, 2015, from http://www.goldcopd.org/uploads/users/files/GOLD_Report_2015_Apr2.pdf

Heslop, K. (2014). Non-pharmacological treatment of anxiety and depression in COPD. *Nurse Prescribing, 12*(1), 43-47. doi:10.12968/npre.2014.12.1.43

Luker, K. A., Chalmers, I., Caress, A. L., & Salmon, M. P. (2007). Smoking cessation interventions in chronic obstructive pulmonary disease and the role of the family: A systematic literature review. *Journal of Advanced Nursing, 59*(6), 559-568. doi:10.1111/j.1365-2648.2007.04379. x

McHugh, G., Chalmers, K., & Lukers, K. A. (2007). Caring for patients with COPD and their families in the community. *British Journal of Community Nursing, 12*(5), 219-222. doi:10.12968/bjcn.2007.12.5.23356

Mizrahi, T., & Mayden, R. W. (2001). NASW standards for cultural competence in social work practice. Retrieved October 30, 2015, from http://www.socialworkers.org/practice/standards/NASWCulturalStandards.pdf

Pires-Yfanttouda, R., Absalom, G., & Clemens, F. (2013). Smoking cessation interventions for COPD: A review of the literature, *58*(1), 1955-1962. doi:10.4187/respcare.01923

Saini, B. (2013). COPD: A hidden epidemic. *Pharmacy News*, 29-32.

Sin, D. D., McAlister, F. A., Man, S. F., & Anthonisen, N. R. (2003). Contemporary management of chronic obstructive pulmonary disease: Clinical applications. *JAMA,290*(17), 2301-2312. doi:10.1001/jama.290.17.2313

Stead, L. F., & Lancaster, T. (2005). Group behavior therapy programmes for smoking cessation. *Cochrane Database of Systematic Reviews.* Art. No. : CD001007. doi:10.1002/14651858. CD001007. pub2

Steinberg, M. B., Greenhaus, S., Schmelzer, A. C., Bover, M. T., Foulds, J., Hoover, D. R., & Carson, J. L. (2009). Triple-combination pharmacotherapy for medically ill smokers: A randomized trial. *Annals of Internal Medicine, 150*(7), 447-454.

U.S. Department of Health and Human Services. (2008). Helping smokers quit: A guide for clinicians. Retrieved August 14, 2015, from http://www.ahrq.gov/professionals/clinicians-providers/guidelines-recommendations/tobacco/clinicians/references/clinhlpsmkqt/index. html

Van Schayck, C. P., Kaper, J., Wagena, E. J., Wouters, E. F. M., & Severens, J. L. (2009). The cost-effectiveness of antidepressants for smoking cessation in chronic obstructive pulmonary disease (COPD) patients. *Addiction, 104*(12), 2110-2117. doi:10.1002/14651858. CD001007. pub2

Vestbo, J., Hurd, S., Augusti, A., Jones, P. W., Vogelmeier, C., Anzueto, A.,... Rodriguez-Roisin, R. (2013). Global strategy for the diagnosis, management, and prevention of chronic obstructive pulmonary disease: GOLD executive summary. *American Journal of Respiratory Critical Care Medicine, 187*(4), 347-365. doi:10.1164/rccm.201204-0596PP

Virtual Medical Centre. (2015, June 22). Cognitive-behavioural therapy (CBT) for quitting smoking. Retrieved October 30, 2015, from http://www.virtualmedicalcentre.com/treatment/cognitive-behavioural-therapy-cbt-for-quitting-smoking/178

Statement of ethical principles. (2012, March 3). *International Federation of Social Workers.* Retrieved October 30, 2015, from http://ifsw.org/policies/statement-of-ethical-principles/

RABIES: RISK IN ORGAN TRANSPLANTATION

MAJOR CATEGORIES: Medical & Health

WHAT WE KNOW

Rabies is an acute, progressive, and fatal *encephalitis* (inflammation of the brain tissue) caused by a virus that spreads primarily by animal saliva from a bite. Other, less common modes of transmission include inhalation of the aerosolized (fine spray) virus in caves and laboratories, organ transplantation, and mucous membranes' coming into contact with infected saliva.

Rabies transmission from an infected donor is a rare but fatal consequence of organ transplantation. Rabies has been documented in eight corneal (front section of the eye) transplant recipients in five countries (Thailand, India, Iran, the United States, and France). The corneal donor in the United States exhibited signs of neurological dysfunction, which is associated with rabies.

In 2004, the first U.S. case of rabies resulting from solid organ transplantation was reported. The organ donor experienced nausea and difficulty swallowing and in the emergency department showed signs and symptoms of altered mental status, fever, elevated systolic blood pressure, and, finally, seizures and coma. Diagnosis of a *subarachnoid hemorrhage* (i.e., bleeding into the compartment surrounding the brain) was made, ultimately leading to death. It was later reported that the donor had been bitten by a bat.

Four deaths resulting from *encephalitis* (sudden inflammation of the brain) were reported in transplant recipients of the liver, kidneys, and iliac artery from this donor. The recipients developed symptoms and signs of encephalitis (i.e., altered mental status, seizures, fever), with rapid deterioration, respiratory failure, and death.

Diagnostic images (i.e., MRI) demonstrated diffuse changes in temporal lobes, basal ganglia, and hippocampal structures in the brain. Rabies was confirmed based on examination of body tissues under a microscope.

In 2005, three recipients in Germany died after receiving organs from a donor infected with rabies.

The organ donor, a 26-year-old female, sought care because of fever, headache, and behavioral changes, and received a diagnosis of toxic psychosis. She suffered a cardiac arrest and was pronounced brain dead. It was later reported that she had been bitten by a dog during a visit to a country where rabies is commonly found.

Six patients were recipients of organs from this donor (i.e., liver, pancreas, lung, kidneys, and corneas). Three patients died after rapid clinical deterioration, and three survived. Two cornea recipients were not infected after their grafts were removed. One donor recipient had been vaccinated against rabies and survived the liver transplantation.

In the past 50 years there has been only one reported death from raccoon-type rabies virus in the United States. In 2013, the U.S. Centers for Disease Control and Prevention (CDC) confirmed that a man in Maryland died after receiving an organ from a donor infected with a raccoon-type rabies virus. Tissue samples from the donor and from the recipient who died were tested, and they confirmed that rabies had been contracted through organ transplantation.

Although the rabies disease can take 1 to 3 months to develop symptoms, the organ transplant occurred more than a year before the recipient was symptomatic and died. Cases of long rabies incubation are rare but have been reported.

The spread of rabies from transplantation brings into question the mode of rabies transmission from solid organs. No cases have been reported through blood transfusions, so a *hematological* (transferred through blood) route is doubtful. Some researchers have proposed transmission from neural tissue contained in the transplanted organs.

The study of the rabies disease has changed considerably over the past 20 years, especially in the United States, as a result of changes in the animal vectors and strain of the virus.

In the past, classic rabies was transmitted primarily through infected saliva by bites of rabid dogs. Most cases in the United States and in South America now result from bat bites, which produce small, needle-like punctures that are relatively painless and unnoticeable, which can make diagnosis difficult. In addition, bat bites carry strains of the virus that have been found to infect neural and non-neural cells.

In the United States all potential donors are screened and tested for potential risk to the recipient.

Organizations that find organs for donation are responsible for evaluating potential donors. In addition to a patient's health history as recalled by family and contacts, organ eligibility is determined through physical examination and blood testing for syphilis and for selected viral pathogens such as HIV and hepatitis B and C.

Rabies testing of the organ is not performed as a standard procedure in determining organ eligibility in the United States.

Definitive laboratory diagnosis of rabies cannot be determined from brain tissue until the death of the donor; testing the organ donor after death can result in delays in transplantation.

Despite the increasing numbers of organs transplanted in the United States, the CDC assesses the risk of rabies transmission by organ transplantation to be extremely low because only 1 to 3 cases of rabies are reported in the United States each year, and the CDC considers the benefits of organ donation to outweigh the risk of infectious disease transmission from screened donors.

WHAT CAN BE DONE

Become knowledgeable about rabies, including signs and symptoms, animal vectors, transmission, treatment, and prevention.

Be aware of the medical conditions in the organ donor's history, recent travel to countries where rabies is endemic and, particularly, if the organ donor experienced any signs and symptoms of rabies such as pain and/or numbness; prickly, stinging, or burning feeling at or near a wound, bite, or scratch; and fever, cough, sore throat, malaise, nausea, vomiting, and/or anorexia progressing to neurologic forms of furious or paralytic rabies.

Signs of furious rabies include confusion, delirium, hallucinations, seizures, hyperactivity, tachycardia (i.e., fast or irregular heart rate), hyperthermia,

hypertension, hydrophobia (i.e., fear of water), and aerophobia (i.e., fear of a draft of air or fresh air) progressing to coma. Hydrophobia is exhibited by gagging or choking upon seeing or drinking water, and aerophobia manifests as choking or gagging when air is blown on the patient's face.

Signs of paralytic rabies include paralysis that affects the extremities and possibly the respiratory muscles, eventually progressing to coma.

Be aware that in the United States federal officials are considering adding rabies to the list of viral pathogens screened for before an organ is transplanted.

Be aware that it is recommended that tissues or organs from a client with a neurologic disease with a viral or immune pathology should not be used for transplantation.

If transplant recipient is symptomatic with rabies, provide support and grief counseling to family.

Educate yourself about rabies, including prevention and treatment.

Be aware that the CDC recommends post-exposure treatment following a needle stick injury involving a client with rabies. The CDC does not consider exposure to feces, blood, urine, or other bodily fluids a risk in rabies transmission.

If indicated, notify appropriate personnel according to hospital policies and procedures for mandatory reporting.

For more information on rabies, go to the CDC website at www.cdc.gov/rabies/ and the Global Alliance for Rabies Control at https://rabiesalliance.org/

Written by Renee Matteucci, MPH, and
Gilberto Cabrera, MD

Reviewed by Jessica Therivel, LMSW-IPR, and
Laura McLuckey, MSW, LCSW

REFERENCES

British Association of Social Workers. (2012). The code of ethics for social work: Statement of principles. Retrieved March 12, 2016, from http://cdn.basw.co.uk/upload/basw_112315-7.pdf

Bronnert, J., Wilde, H., Tepsumethanon, V., Lumlertdacha, B., & Hemachudha, T. (2007). Organ transplantations and rabies transmission. *Journal of Travel Medicine, 14*(3), 177-180. doi:10.1111/j.1708-8305.2006.00095.x

Centers for Disease Control and Prevention (CDC). (2013). Questions and answers ??? human rabies due to organ transplantation, 2013. Retrieved March 12, 2016, from http://www.cdc.gov/rabies/resources/news/2013-03-15.html

Dietzschold, B., & Koprowski, H. (2004). Rabies transmission from organ transplants in the USA. *Lancet*, *364*(9435), 648-649. doi:10.1016/S0140-6736(04)16912-2

Global Alliance for Rabies Control. (2013). Organ transplants and rabies: What are the risks?. Retrieved March 12, 2016, from http://rabiesalliance.org/media/news/organ-transplants-and-rabies-what-are-the-risks

Houff, S. A., Burton, R. C., Wilson, R. W., Henson, T. E., London, W. T., Baer, G. M., & Sever, J. L. (1979). Human-to-human transmission of rabies virus by corneal transplant. *New England Journal of Medicine*, *300*(11), 603-604. doi:10.1056/NEJM197903153001105

International Federation of Social Workers. (2012, March 3). Statement of ethical principles. Retrieved from http://ifsw.org/policies/statement-of-ethical-principles/

Jackson, A. C. (2004). Screening of organ and tissue donors for rabies. *Lancet*, *364*(9451), 2094-2095. doi:10.1016/S0140-6736(04)17545-4

Kotton, C. N. (2007). Zoonoses in solid-organ and hematopoietic stem cell transplant recipients. *Clinical Infectious Diseases*, *44*(6), 857-866. doi:10.1086/511859

Manning, S. E., Rupprecht, C. E., Fishbein, D., Hanlon, C. A., Lumlertdacha, B., Guerra, M., & Hull, H. F. (2008). Human rabies prevention - United States, 2008: Recommendations of the Advisory Committee on Immunization Practices.

Recommendations and Reports: Morbidity and Mortality Weekly Report, 57. Retrieved from http://www.cdc.gov/mmwr/pdf/rr/rr57e507.pdf

Mattner, F., Henke-Gendo, C., Martens, A., Drosten, C., Schulz, T. F., Heim, A., & Strueber, M. (2007). Risk of rabies infection and adverse effects of postexposure prophylaxis in healthcare workers and other patient contacts exposed to a rabies virus-infected lung transplant recipient. *Infection Control and Hospital Epidemiology*, *28*(5), 513-518. doi:10.1086/513614

National Center for Emerging and Zoonotic Infectious Diseases (NCEZID). (2011). Update on investigation of rabies infections in an organ donor and transplant recipients. Retrieved March 12, 2016, from http://www.cdc.gov/rabies/resources/news/2004-07-02.html

Srinivasan, A., Burton, E. C., Kuehnert, M. J., Rupprecht, C., Sutker, W. L., Ksiazek, T. G., & Zaki, S. R. (2005). Transmission of rabies virus from an organ donor to four transplant recipients. *New England Journal of Medicine*, *352*(11), 1103-1111. doi:10.1056/NEJMoa043018

Vora, N. M., Basavaraju, S. V., Feldman, K. A., Paddock, C. D., Orciari, L., Gitterman, S., ... Griese, S. (2013). Raccoon rabies virus variant transmission through solid organ transplantation. *Journal of the American Medical Association*, *310*(4), 398-407. doi:10.1001/jama.2013.7986

Wheeler, D. (2015). NAWS standards and indicators for cultural competence in social work practice. Retrieved March 12, 2016, from http://www.socialworkers.org/practice/standards/PRA-BRO-253150-CC-Standards.pdf

REFUGEE CHILDREN: FOSTER CARE & ADOPTION

MAJOR CATEGORIES: Child & Family, Adoption/Foster Care

DESCRIPTION

The United States Immigration and Nationality Act defines a refugee as "a person who is outside his/her country of nationality or habitual residence and has a well-founded fear of persecution because of his/her race, religion, nationality, membership in a particular social group or political opinion; and is unable or unwilling to avail himself/herself of the protection of that country, or to return there, for fear of persecution" (United States Citizenship and Immigration Services, Immigration and Nationality Act (INA), Section 101(a)(42)(A)).

Under international law, countries have an obligation to protect the human rights of all refugees entering

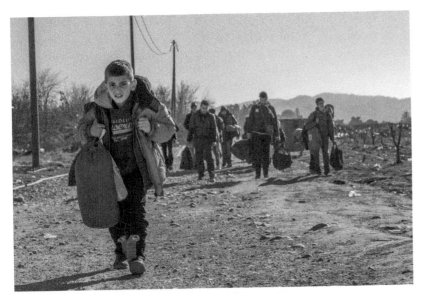

them. Armed conflicts and natural disasters force millions of children from their homes and native countries every year, most of whom are taken in by developing nations. Many such refugee children are orphaned and others are abandoned by their parents. Existing international conventions and guidelines for ethical adoption practice do not recommend that refugee children be adopted at the height of an emergency (Donaldson Adoption Institute, 2005). The United Nations Children's Fund (UNICEF) recommends that these children be given foster care, preferably with relatives or members of the child's own community, and this approach has been shown to result in the best overall outcomes for children displaced from their homes.

A small percentage of refugee children, sometimes unaccompanied, arrive in Western countries seeking asylum. Although there is growing recognition of the strength and resilience of such children, they are considered an especially vulnerable group. Refugee children are at high risk for severe levels of psychological distress, including depression and PTSD. Many have been exposed to extreme and multiple experiences of trauma, and studies indicate that the more traumatic events to which refugee children have been exposed, the greater the biological, psychological, and social difficulties they will experience in resettlement.

Because symptoms of the traumatic events that often befall refugee children can persist into adulthood, timely interventions for managing them are critical. Among unaccompanied refugee children,

post-traumatic stress disorder (PTSD) and depression are particularly common as results of pre-arrival trauma.

The needs of refugee children vary considerably. Studies have found that safe, supportive environments are associated with good outcomes of these children's psychological, social, and physical health. Foster care rather than group homes is considered optimal for this, particularly for younger children. In foster homes, however, cultural differences can create misunderstandings and present problems for the host families. In some cultures, for example, eye contact with an elder is considered disrespectful, and foster parents unaware of cultural differences may judge such actions as indicating impertinence. Adequate cultural preparations are therefore essential for both the families preparing to provide foster care and the children entering such care.

Although matching of the cultural backgrounds of refugee children and their foster families is recommended, older refugee children may request placement with families belonging to the dominant culture of the countries they enter, in order to gain a cross-cultural experience. For still other refugee children, particularly older children, a foster family may be too restrictive after the experiences they have already had in life, and an independent living arrangement may be more suitable. Whatever the living arrangement made for refugee children, researchers have found that many of them are determined to succeed, and that a key to becoming successful is a high level of social support and engagement in purposeful activities. For the many refugee children who have high expectations, particularly about obtaining an education, school districts with existing immigrant populations tend to be better prepared to support them.

FACTS AND FIGURES

The United Nations High Commissioner for Refugees (UNHCR) (n.d.) estimated that in 2014 there were 13 million refugees worldwide, constituting an increase over the number in 2013. An additional 4.8 million refugees are registered with the

UNHCR and currently receive assistance in 60 camps throughout the Middle East. Nearly half of all refugees reside in Asia, and 28 percent are currently in Africa (UNHCR, 2013). A study published in 2015 reported that between 4 percent and 7 percent of the applications for asylum in countries of the European Union were for unaccompanied minors (Banco, 2015). Approximately 2 million Syrian children are living as refugees in neighboring countries, and more than 8,000 children have crossed the Syrian border unaccompanied by an adult (UNICEF, n.d.).

APPLICABLE LAWS AND REGULATIONS

Under international law, countries have an obligation to protect the human rights of all refugees entering them, and must not force these individuals to return to the countries from which they have fled. Both the 1951 United Nations Convention relating to the status of refugees and the 1989 United Nations Convention on the Rights of the Child address the status of refugee children directly. The central principle of these treaties is protection of the "best interests" of the refugee child.

Social workers engaged in the adoption and foster-care placement of refugee children should begin with a thorough biological, psychological, social, and spiritual assessment in consultation with the child (Bates et al., 2005), including information on any physical, mental, environmental, cultural, and medical factors as they relate to the child and his/her family of origin. This should include the child's history of trauma and trauma-related symptoms, prior caregiving, difficulties in attachment, family history, circumstances that resulted in the child being a refugee, adjustment to placement, and psychiatric symptoms or issues that might pose a risk to the child itself or to others (e.g., suicidality, self-harm, substance abuse, aggression, child-to-parent violence, fire setting, running away, harming animals, sexual perpetration). An assessment should also be done of the child's stress-management and coping skills and level of acculturation, with the last of these being used to ensure that relevant services are provided to the child. Concurrent with this should be planning with the child for its permanent placement, with child given a voice in the decision-making process. Agencies that provide specialized refugee services should be included in the planning process. It is important to be aware that children accompanied by undocumented adults face complex and difficult legal proceedings that further compromise their well-being. Also, because refugee children arriving from West Africa have high rates of asymptomatic malaria, it is recommended that they have a complete blood count (CBC) and blood smear for malaria.

A local child welfare agency can provide information about foster care for refugee children. Links to state foster care information websites are available at the Child Welfare Information Gateway, https://www.childwelfare.gov/nfcad/ Social workers assisting refugee children can provide linkage to community medical, financial, childcare, housing, educational, and counseling services as appropriate. Information on each step in international adoption is available at the Child Welfare Information Gateway, https://www.childwelfare.gov/topics/adoption/

Host families for refugee children need specialized training in differences between these children's cultures and their own, as well as in child development and the effects of childhood trauma, and these families benefit from ongoing support. A change in the foster parents of a refugee child should not necessarily be viewed as failure, and can sometimes benefit the child. Weekly opportunities for refugee children to meet with their peers enhance overall well-being. School-based support groups led by therapists have proven successful in helping refugee children (Bates et al., 2005). The most common signs and symptoms of trauma in refugee children are depression, anxiety, re-experiencing of the traumatic event, avoidance of reminders of the trauma, hyperarousal, somatization, and behavioral problems.

Social workers should be aware of their own cultural values, beliefs, and biases, and develop specialized knowledge about the histories, traditions, and values of the children and foster-care providers with whom they work. They should use treatment methods that reflect their knowledge of the cultural diversity of the societies in which they practice.

SERVICES AND RESOURCES

Information about the foster care and adoption of refugee children is available at the following resources:
- U.S. Department of Health & Human Services, Office of Refugee Resettlement, http://www.acf.hhs.gov/programs/orr
- War Child International Network, http://www.warchild.org

- Refugees International, http://www.refugeesinternational.org
- Bridging Refugee Youth and Children's Services (BRYCS), http://www.brycs.org
- Administration for Children & Families, U.S. Department of Health & Human Services, Child Welfare Information Gateway, http://www.childwelfare.gov
- UNICEF, http://www.unicefusa.org

Written by Jan Wagstaff, MA, MSW

Reviewed by Lynn B. Cooper, D. Crim, and Laura Gale, LCSW

REFERENCES

American Psychological Association (APA). (2009). Working with refugee children and families: Update for mental health professionals. Retrieved February 10, 2016, from https://www.apa.org/pubs/info/reports/refugees-health-professionals.pdf

Ballucci, D., & Dorow, S. (2014). Constructing childhood at the boundaries of the nation: Chinese adoptee and refugee cases in Canada. *Childhood*, 39-55. doi:10.1177/0907568213482496

Banco, E. (2015, October 5). Overwhelmed by thousands of refugee children traveling alone, Europe considers adoption. Retrieved February 10, 2016, from http://www.ibtimes.com/overwhelmed-thousands-refugee-children-traveling-alone-europe-considers-adoption-2125338

Barrie, L., & Mendes, P. (2011). The experiences of unaccompanied asylum-seeking children in and leaving the out-of-home care system in the UK and Australia: A critical review of the literature. *International Social Work, 54*(4), 485-503.

Bates, L., Baird, D., Johnson, D. J., Lee, R. E., Luster, T., & Rehagen, C. (2005). Sudanese refugee youth in foster care: The "lost boys" in America. *Child Welfare, 84*(5), 631-648.

Bean, T. M., Eurelings-Bontekoe, E., & Spinhoven, P. (2007). Course and predictors of mental health of unaccompanied refugee minors in the Netherlands: One year follow up. *Social Science & Medicine, 64*(6), 1204-1215.

British Association of Social Workers. (2012). The code of ethics for social Work: statement of principles.

Retrieved February 10, 2016, from http://cdn.basw.co.uk/upload/basw_112315-7.pdf

Dettlaff, A. J. (2008). Immigrant Latino children and families in child welfare: A framework for conducting a cultural assessment. *Journal of Public Child Welfare, 2*(4), 451-469.

Donaldson Adoption Institute. (2005, April). Policy brief: Intercountry adoption in emergencies: The tsunami orphans. Retrieved April 8, 2016, from http://www.adoptioninstitute.org/old/publications/2005_Brief_ICA_In_Emergencies_April.pdf

Duerr, A., Posner, S. F., & Gilbert, M. (2003). Evidence of support of foster care during acute refugee crisis. *American Journal of Public Health, 93*(11), 1904-1909.

Geltman, P. L., Grant-Knight, W., Mehta, S. D., Lloyd-Travaglini, C., Lustig, S., Landgraf, J. M., & Wise, P. H. (2005). The lost boys of Sudan: Functional and behavioral health of unaccompanied refugee minors resettled in the United States. *Archives of Pediatrics & Adolescent Medicine, 159*(6), 585-591.

International Federation of Social Workers. (n.d.). Statement of ethical principles. Retrieved February 10, 2016, from http://ifsw.org/policies/statement-of-ethical-principles/

Lee, M. M., Lee, R. E., Troupe, F. Y., & Vennum, A. V. (2010). Voices of foster parents of Sudanese refugee youths: Affirmations and insights. *International Social Work, 53*(6), 807-821.

Luster, T., Saltarelli, A. J., Rana, M., Qin, D. B., Bates, L., Burdick, K., & Baird, D. (2009). The experiences of Sudanese unaccompanied minors in foster care. *Journal of Family Psychology, 23*(3), 386-395.

Maroushek, S. R., Aguilar, E. F., Stauffer, W., & Abd-Alla, M. D. (2005). Malaria among refugee children at arrival in the United States. *Pediatric Infectious Disease Journal, 24*(5), 450-452.

Naughton, D., & Fay, K. L. (2003). Of kin and culture: US children and international kinship care placements. *Adoption & Fostering, 27*(4), 30-37.

Wheeler, D. (2015). NASW Standards and Indicators for Cultural Competence in Social Work Practice. Retrieved February 9, 2016, from http://www.socialworkers.org/practice/standards/PRA-BRO-253150-CC-Standards.pdf

Wright, F. (2014). Social work practice with unaccompanied asylum-seeking young people facing removal. *British Journal of Social Work, 44*(4), 1027-1044. doi:10.1093/bjsw/bcs175

Xu, Q. (2005). In the "best interest" of immigrant and refugee children: Deliberating on their unique circumstances. *Child Welfare, 84*(5), 747-770.

UNHCR (n.d.). Refugee figures. Retrieved February 10, 2016, from http://www.unhcr.org/pages/49c3646c1d.html

UNHCR. (2013). UNHRC asylum trends 2013. Retrieved February 10, 2016, from http://www.unhcr.org/5329b15a9.html

UNICEF. (n.d.). Syrian children under siege. Retrieved April 6, 2016, from https://www.unicefusa.org/mission/emergencies/child-refugees/syria-crisis

U. S. Citizenship and Immigration Services. (n.d.). Immigration and Nationality Act (INA), Section 101(a)(42)(A). Retrieved February 10, 2016, from https://www.uscis.gov/iframe/ilink/docView/SLB/HTML/SLB/0-0-0-1/0-0-0-29/0-0-0-101/0-0-0-195.html

REFUGEES IN THE UNITED STATES: PSYCHOSOCIAL ISSUES

MAJOR CATEGORIES: Behavioral & Mental Health

WHAT WE KNOW

According to the United States Immigration and Nationality Act, a refugee is "a person who is outside his/her country of nationality or habitual residence; has a well-founded fear of persecution because of his/her race, religion, nationality, membership in a particular social group or political opinion; and is unable or unwilling to avail himself/herself of the protection of that country, or to return there, for fear of persecution." Individuals and families seeking asylum in the United States must meet this definition of a refugee. Refugees are supported through resettlement agencies upon arrival.

Worldwide 43 million adults and children have been forcibly displaced from their countries of origin; over 10 million are defined as refugees. The United States is one of the world's top resettlement countries for refugees. Each year Congress determines the number of refugees the United States will accept for resettlement. In 2014 the United States registered 121,200 new asylum applicants, an increase of 44 percent from 2013. Most recent data show that 58,179 refugees were granted asylum in the United States in 2012; 36.6 percent were children, 46.1 percent were women, and 38.4 percent were married.

Between 8,000 and 14,000 unaccompanied, undocumented children enter the United States each year. On arrival these children are placed in the custody of the Office of Refugee Resettlement; 77 percent of the children are males between the ages of 14 and 17. The top three countries from which children presently arrive are Guatemala (36

percent), El Salvador (25 percent), and Honduras (20 percent).

Refugees may have high levels of war-related trauma; this frequently co-occurs with forced displacement, traumatic loss, bereavement or separation, community violence, and intimate partner violence. Children with trauma histories have high levels of academic and behavioral problems.

Refugees are significantly more likely than permanent immigrants to report chronic physical and mental health problems, have high levels of depression, post-traumatic stress disorder, and anxiety. Mental health issues are prevalent in refugees many years after resettlement.

The healthcare needs of disabled refugees are not being adequately met. Some refugees have high levels of micronutrient deficiencies and are vulnerable to worsening health after resettlement. High proportions of refugees smoke and report limited understanding of the adverse health effects of smoking. Over half of refugees lack health insurance to address their healthcare needs.

Ethnic and religious communities are an important source of support to refugees; however, these communities can become socially isolating, exacerbate adjustment stress, and thwart acculturation. Resettlement is complicated by lower levels of English language proficiency among refugees than among other immigrants, which is a barrier to accessing services. Professionals who come to the United States as refugees have higher levels of underemployment and unemployment than non-refugee immigrant professionals.

WHAT CAN BE DONE

Become knowledgeable about the difficulties refugees encounter during resettlement and advocate for improved services for all refugees and their children.

Become knowledgeable about the ethnic and religious communities of refugees in the United States and encourage integration with host communities to help refugees adjust and acculturate.

Advocate for social justice, including development and implementation of community-oriented prevention that is individualized and culturally specific, such as increasing knowledge of mental health services and supporting the resettlement process by providing immediate aid, including food and shelter, job placement, and medical attention.

Learn about interventions for traumatized refugees, including narrative exposure therapy (NIT), instrumental learning (e. g., learning concrete skills such as English proficiency, problem solving), and transformative learning (e. g., working together to help reduce stressors experienced by refugees by revising the meaning of experiences), that can improve their psychological well-being.

Encourage comprehensive health screening to include screening for infectious diseases to improve preventive and curative care of refugees.

Written by Jan Wagstaff, MA, MSW

*Reviewed by Jessica Therivel, LMSW-IPR. and
Laura Gale, LCSW*

REFERENCES

Betancourt, T. S., Newnham, E. A., Layne, C. M., Kim, S., Steinberg, A. M., Ellis, H., & Birman, D. (2012). Trauma history and psychopathology in war-affected refugee children referred for trauma-related mental health services in the United States. *Journal of Traumatic Studies, 25*(6), 682-690. doi:10.1002/jts.21749

Bogic, M., Njoku, A., & Priebe, S. (2015). Long-term mental health of war-refugees: A systematic literature review. *BMC International Health & Human Rights, 15*(29), 1-41. doi:10.1186/s12914-015-0064-9

British Association of Social Workers. (2012). The code of ethics for social work. Retrieved February 12, 2016, from http://cdn. basw.co.uk/upload/basw_112315-7.pdf

Harris, J. K., Karamehic-Muratovic, A., Herbers, S. H., Moreland-Russell, S., Cheskin, R., & Lindberg, K. A. (2012). Perceptions of personal risk about smoking and health among Bosnian refugees living in the United States. *Journal of Immigrant and Minority Health, 14*(3), 413-419.

Hess, J. M., Isakson, B., Githinji, A., Roche, N., Vadnais, K., Parker, D. P., & Goodkind, J. R. (2014). Reducing mental health disparities through transformative learning: A social change model with refugees and students. *Psychological Services, 11*(3), 347-356. doi:10.1037/a0035334

Hijazi, A. M., Lumley, M. A., Ziadni, M. S., Haddad, L., Rapport, L. J., & Arnetz, B. B. (2014). Brief narrative exposure therapy for posttraumatic stress in Iraqi refugees: A preliminary randomized clinical trial. *Journal of Traumatic Stress, 27*(3), 314-322. doi:10.1002/jts.21922

International Federation of Social Workers. (2012). Statement of Ethical Principles. Retrieved February 12, 2016, from http://ifsw.org/policies/statement-of-ethical-principles/

Jamil, H., Adhalimi, A., & Arnetz, B. B. (2012). Post-displacement employment and health in professional Iraqi refugees vs. professional Iraqi immigrants. *Journal of Immigrant & Refugee Studies, 10*(4), 395-406.

Kumar, G. S., Varma, S., Saenger, M. S., Burleson, M., Kohrt, B. A., & Cantey, P. (2014). Journal of Immigrant and Minority Health, 16(5), 922-925. doi:10.1007/s10903-013-9800-1

Martin, D. C., & Yankay, J. E. (2013). Refugees and asylees: 2012. Retrieved February 12, 1970, from http://www.dhs.gov/sites/default/files/publications/ois_rfa_fr_2012.pdf

Mirza, M., & Heinemann, A. W. (2012). Service needs and service gaps among refugees with disabilities resettled in the United States. *Disability & Rehabilitation, 34*(7), 543-552.

Migration Policy Institute (MPI). (2015). Refugees and asylees in the United States. Retrieved February 12, 2016, from http://www.migrationpolicy.org/article/refugees-and-asylees-united-states

Nazzal, K. H., Forghany, M., Geevaraughese, M. C., Mahmoodi, V., & Wong, J. (2014). An innovative community-oriented approach to prevention and early intervention with refugees in the United States. *Psychological Services, 11*(4), 477-485. doi:10.1037/a0037964

Rasmussen, A., Crager, M., Baser, R. E., Chu, T., & Gany, F. (2012). Onset of posttraumatic stress disorder and major depression among refugees and voluntary migrants to the United States. *Journal of Traumatic Stress, 25*(6), 705-712. doi:10.1002/jts.21763

Redditt, V. J., Janakiram, P., Graziano, D., & Rashid, M. (2015). Health status of newly arrived refugees in Toronto, One: Part 1: Infectious diseases. *Canadian Family Physician, 61*(7), e303-e343.

Refugee Council USA. (n. d.). Unaccompanied alien children. Retrieved February 12, 2015, from http://www.rcusa.org/index.

Refugee Council USA. (n. d.). Introduction to refugees. Retrieved February 12, 2015, from http://www.rcusa.org/index.

Sienkiewicz, H. C., Mauceri, K. G., Howell, E. C., & Bibeau, D. L. (2013). Untapped resources: Refugee employment experiences in Central North Carolina. *Work, 45*(1), 17-24.

United Nations. (n. d.). Refugees. Retrieved February 12, 2015, from http://www.un.org/en/globalissues/refugees

The UN Refugee Agency (UNHCR). (2015). UNHCR asylum trends 2014. Retrieved February 22, 2016, from http://www.unhcr.org/551128679. html

U.S. Citizenship and Immigration Services. (n. d.). Act 101(a)(42) of the Immigration and Nationality Act (INA). Retrieved February 17, 2016, from https://www.uscis.gov/iframe/ilink/docView/SLB/HTML/SLB/0-0-0-1/0-0-0-29/0-0-0-101/0-0-0-195. html

U.S. Department of Health & Human Services. (n. d.). About unaccompanied children's services. Retrieved February 12, 2015, from http://www.acf.hhs.gov/programs/orr/programs/ucs/about

Wheeler, D. (2015). NASW Standards and Indicators for Cultural Competence in Social Work Practice. Retrieved from http://www.socialworkers.org/practice/standards/PRA-BRO-253150-CC-Standards.pdf

Yun, K., Fuentes-Afflick, E., & Desai, M. M. (2012). Prevalence of chronic disease and insurance coverage among refugees in the United States. *Journal of Immigrant and Minority Health, 14*(6), 933-940.

Restorative Justice Programs: Adult Offenders

Major Categories: Community

What We Know

Restorative justice (RJ) is a worldwide movement that is primarily a system of values informing social work practice within criminal justice. Crime is conceived of principally as an offense against human relationships, and restoring human dignity is therefore critical in redressing the impact of crime. It has been most widely used with juveniles but it is increasingly being used with adult offenders in a variety of forms. It seeks to restore human dignity by increasing accountability and responsibility, increasing empathy between victims and offenders, reducing recidivism, and employing reparations.

Restorative justice programs take on a variety of forms, but all are underpinned by the key principle of the restoration of human dignity. Some educational programs are offered in prisons, others support former inmates after prison, and some are designed to support a single offender upon release. In New Zealand a program has been designed to tackle elder abuse. The main aim of all these programs is to prevent recidivism and reintegrate offenders into society.

The United Nations encourages the use of restorative justice principles and practices to help developing countries build their local and national capacity for justice. Circles of support and accountability (COSA) is an RJ risk management program that was developed in Canada and now is used in the United States and the United Kingdom; it has also been deployed in limited and modified forms in Australia and New Zealand. The program links several volunteers with a single offender to provide intense social support and assistance with reintegration into society. A small number of studies are reporting promising outcomes in reducing recidivism.

The first types of RJ programs, which are still widely used, bring perpetrators of crimes and their victims together. These meetings seek to restore the emotional and psychological integrity of all those involved in an act of crime through facilitated dialogue. Meetings may take place in lieu of criminal justice proceedings or in conjunction with them.

In the United States as of March 2014, there were 32 states that had statutes on record that supported restorative justice programs in some capacity. Investigators found that the most common RJ practice was victim–offender meetings, at 68 percent, followed by victim-impact panels and classes, at 43 percent; community boards, at 18 percent; and sentencing circles (i. e., the community process to develop consensus on sentencing plans), at 11 percent. Investigators also found that there were differences in when various states used RJ. For some it was a diversionary or pretrial process, whereas other states chose to use RJ as an intermediate sanction (i. e., a punishment that is in between probation and incarceration) or as a post-sentencing process.

Various names are used to describe these meetings depending on the country and the program: "conferencing," "victim–offender mediation," "victim–offender dialogues," "circles," and "intimate abuse circles"; in England," restorative cautioning" was pioneered as a diversion from criminal justice proceedings a decade ago.

The presence of the victim and whether the offender's apology was coerced can affect the effectiveness of an RJ program. If the victim is present, there is an increased likelihood of positive changes to the victim–offender relationship and the opportunity for forgiveness as well as open dialogue between the involved parties. If the apology is an instrumental apology that is legally required of the offender, there is cognitive dissonance that results where the offender's words and actions are not in sync. Besides seeming insincere to the victim, the offender loses the opportunity for deeper change as a result of an honest apology.

RJ programs have to break through offenders' denial and self-centeredness in order to open offenders to accountability and transformation. Becoming accountable requires recognizing the harm that was done, acknowledging the impact of the harm, paying reparations, and transforming attitudes and behaviors.Reparations may be agreed upon in meetings: through reparations, the offender works toward repairing the material consequences of the crime, such as repaying the costs of any property damage, or contributing his or her time to a community project or activity as a way of making amends and restoring safety and dignity to all those involved.

Overall, victims report satisfaction with the process and outcomes of RJ meetings. Specifically, victims feel included and empowered, unlike in the criminal justice process, in which they report being marginalized.Researchers found that there was a decrease in posttraumatic stress disorder (PTSD) symptoms for survivor victims of sex crimes who went through an RJ conferencing program with their offenders. Before the conference, 82 percent of the victims met the diagnostic criteria for PTSD; that figure went down to 66 percent after the conference.

A growing body of research is reporting success with RJ programs and practices with adults; however, there remain some areas of concern. There is a lack of research to inform RJ practice with violent offenders. Gendered crimes, such as sexual assault and intimate partner violence, often are considered unsuitable for RJ. The physical safety of victims cannot be guaranteed during the process. The power imbalances that underpin some gendered crime can be intangible and difficult to mitigate, undermining the purpose of the meetings. Participant offenders may purport to be invested, but privately be uncommitted.

Research has begun to reveal racial/ethnic disparities in the application of RJ programs for adult offenders. Researchers in Arizona found that white offenders encompassed 33 percent of the police reports, 54 percent of the cases that were referred by prosecutors, and 77 percent of the cases that went through the RJ program, called RESTORE. While 25 percent of the police reports were black offenders, these offenders made only 9 percent of prosecutor referrals and 9 percent of referrals to the RESTORE program. Hispanic offenders comprised 42 percent of the police reports, 25 percent of prosecutor referrals, and 14 percent of cases that went to RESTORE. Disparities were present for the victims as well.

RJ meetings have been run in ways considered insensitive to victims, leading to feelings of disempowerment and other negative impacts on victims. The programs often prioritize rehabilitating the offender outside formal legal proceedings; while this may benefit the offender, it may not always be in the best interest of the victim.

WHAT CAN BE DONE

Learn about RJ philosophy and its broad range of practices including the RJ programs that are in use, and promote their research and evaluation to develop and broaden understanding of RJ practice.

Develop a list of resources about restorative justice for education and referrals including the following:

- International Institute for Restorative Practices, http://www.iirp.edu/.
- University of Minnesota, Center for Restorative Justice and Peacemaking, http://www.cehd.umn.edu/ssw/RJP/default. asp.
- Centre for Justice and Reconciliation, https://restorativejustice.org/.

Written by Jan Wagstaff, MA, MSW and Jessica Therivel, LMSW-IPR

Reviewed by Lynn B. Cooper, D. Crim

REFERENCES

Armour, M. P., Safe, J., Rubin, A., & Windsor, L. C. (2005). Bridges to life: Evaluation of an in-prison restorative justice intervention. *Medicine & Law, 24*(4), 831-851.

Armstrong, S., Chistyakova, Y., Mackenzie, A., & Malloch, M. (2008). Circles of support & accountability: Consideration of the feasibility of pilots in Scotland. Retrieved November 19, 2014, from http://www.sccjr. ac. uk/wp-content/uploads/2012/10/circles.pdf

Bazemore, G. (2005). Whom and how do we reintegrate? Finding community in restorative justice. *Criminology & Public Policy, 4*(1), 131-148. doi:10.1 111/j.1745-9133.2005.00011. x

British Association of Social Workers. (2012, January). *The Code of Ethics for Social Work: Statement of principles.* Retrieved November 19, 2014, from http://cdn. basw.co.uk/upload/basw_112315-7.pdf

Choi, J., Green, D., & Kapp, S. (2010). A qualitative study of victim offender mediation: Implications for social work. *Journal of Human Behavior in the Social Environment, 20*(7), 857-874. doi:10.1007/s10560-011-0238-9

Daly, K. (2002). Sexual assault and restorative justice. In H. Strang & J. Braithwaite (Eds.), *Restorative justice and family violence* (pp.62-86). Cambridge, UK: Cambridge University Press.

Grauwiler, P., & Mills, L. G. (2004). Moving beyond the criminal justice paradigm: A radical restorative justice approach to intimate abuse. *Journal of Sociology & Social Welfare, 31*(1), 49-69.

Groth, A., & Linden, R. (2011). Addressing elder abuse: The Waterloo restorative justice approach to elder abuse project. *Journal of Elder Abuse, 23*(2), 127. doi:10.1080/08946566.2011.558780

Herman, J. L. (2005). Justice from the victim's perspective. *Violence Against Women, 11*(5), 571-602. doi:10.1177/1077801205274450

Hudson, B. (2002). Restorative justice and gendered violence. *British Journal of Criminology, 42*(3), 616-634. doi:10.1093/bjc/42.3.616

International Federation of Social Workers. (2012, March 3). Statement of ethical principles. Retrieved December 6, 2015, from http://ifsw.org/policies/statement-of-ethical-principles

Kelly, E. L. (2010). Philly stands up: Inside politics and poetics of transformative justice and community accountability in sexual assault situations. *Social Justice, 37*(4), 44-57.

Koss, M. P. (2014). The RESTORE program for restorative justice for sex crimes: vision, process, and outcomes. *Journal of Interpersonal Violence, 29*(9), 1623-1660. doi:10.1177/0886260513511537

Lawson, C. L., & Katz, J. (2004). Restorative justice: An alternative approach to juvenile crime. *Journal of Socio-Economics, 33*(2), 175-188. doi:10.1016/j.socec.2003.12.018

Littlechild, B. (2009). Restorative justice, mediation and relational conflict resolution in work with young people in residential care. *Practice, 21*(4), 229-240. doi:10.1080/09503150903191704

Livingstone, N., Macdonald, G., & Carr, N. (2013). Restorative justice conferencing for reducing recidivism in young offenders (aged 7 to 21). *Cochrane Database of Systematic Reviews.* Art. No. : CD008898. doi:10.1002/14651858. CD008898. pub2

London, R. D. (2003). The restoration of trust: Bringing restorative justice from the margins to the mainstream. *Criminal Justice Studies, 16*(3), 175-195. doi:10.1080/0888431032000151844

Mills, L. G., Barocas, B., & Ariel, B. (2013). The next generation of court-mandated domestic violence treatment: A comparison study of batterer intervention and restorative justice program. *Journal of Experimental Criminology, 9*(1), 65-90. doi:10.1007/s11292-012-9164-x

Wheeler, D. (2015). NASW standards and indicators for cultural competence in social work practice. Retrieved December 6, 2015, from http://www.

socialworkers.org/practice/standards/PRA-BRO-253150-CC-Standards.pdf

Mutter, R., Shemmings, D., Dugmore, P., & Hyare, M. (2008). Family group conferences in youth justice. *Health & Social Care in the Community, 16*(3), 262-270. doi:10.1111/j.1365-2524.2008.00770. x

Presser, L., & Van Voorhis, P. (2002). Values and evaluation: Assessing processes and outcomes of restorative justice programs. *Crime & Delinquency, 48*(1), 162-188. doi:10.1177/0011128702048001007

Proietti-Scifoni, G., & Daly, K. (2011). Gendered violence and restorative justice: The views of New Zealand opinion leaders. *Contemporary Justice Review, 14*(3), 269-290. doi:10.1080/10282580.2011.589666

Rubin, P. (2003). Restorative justice in Nova Scotia: Women's experience and recommendations for positive policy development and implementation. Retrieved November 19, 2015, from www.nawl. ca/ns/en/documents/Pub_Brief_NSRestorativeJustice03_en. doc

Silva, S. M., & Lambert, C. G. (2015). Restorative justice legislation in the American states: A statutory analysis of emerging legal doctrine. *Journal of Policy Practice, 14*(2), 77-95. doi:10.1080/15588742.2015.1017687

Sualnier, A., & Sivasubraniam, D. (2015). Effects of victim presence and coercion in restorative justice: An experimental paradigm. *Law and Human Behavior, 39*(4), 378-387. doi:10.1037/lhb0000130

Umbreit, M., Coates, R., & Vos, B. (2004). Victim-offender mediation: Three decades of practice and research. *Conflict Resolution Quarterly, 22*(1/2), 279-303. doi:10.1002/crq.102

United Nations. (2002). ECOSOC Resolution 2002/12 basic principles on the use of restorative justice programmes in criminal matters. Retrieved November 19, 2014, from http://www.un.org/en/ecosoc/docs/2002/resolution percent202002-12.pdf

Van Ness, D. W. (2005). An overview of restorative justice around the world. Retrieved November 19, 2015, from https://assets. justice. vic.gov. au/njc/resources/c4518c8a-c200-4623-afd1-42e255b62cf9/01+an+overview+of+restorative+justice.pdf

van Wormer, K. (2004). Restorative justice: A model for personal and societal empowerment. *Journal of Religion & Spirituality in Social Work, 23*(4), 103-120. doi:10.1300/J377v23n04_07

Wilson, R., Cortoni, F., & McWhinnie, A. (2009). Circles of support and accountability': A Canadian national replication study of outcome findings. *Sexual Abuse: A Journal of Research & Treatment, 21*(4), 412-430.

RESTORATIVE JUSTICE PROGRAMS: CIRCLES OF SUPPORT & ACCOUNTABILITY

MAJOR CATEGORIES: Community

WHAT WE KNOW

Restorative justice (RJ) is a process in which victims, perpetrators, and members of the community come together to discuss the impact of a crime and determine what should be done to repair the harm caused by the crime. It conceives of crime principally as an offense against human relationships and therefore aims to redress the impact of the crime by restoring human dignity by increasing accountability and responsibility on the part of offenders, increasing empathy between victims and offenders, reducing recidivism, and promoting reparations.

Restorative justice has been most widely used with juveniles. It is most often used as an alternative to the juvenile justice system in the hope of diverting young people from lives of crime and incarceration.

An important feature of restorative justice practice is the act of bringing perpetrators of crimes and their victims together in dialogue.

The meetings in which victims and offenders come together have various names depending on the country and the program: *conferencing, victim–offender mediation* (VOM), *victim–offender dialogues, circles,* and *intimate abuse circles.* In England, restorative cautioning was pioneered as a diversion from criminal justice proceedings in the late 1990s. They may take place in lieu of or in conjunction with criminal justice proceedings. They seek to restore the emotional and psychological integrity of all those involved in the crime through facilitated dialogue.

Circles of support and accountability (COSA) are risk-management programs for recently released offenders. First used with sex offenders, COSA programs link several volunteers with a single offender to provide intense social support and assistance with reintegration into society.

COSA began in Canada in the 1990s and is now being used in some jurisdictions in the United States and the United Kingdom; it has also been deployed in limited and modified forms in Australia and New Zealand.

The objective of COSA is to prevent recidivism and facilitate integration into the community following incarceration. Victims are not involved in COSA. Volunteers are trained and supported in implementing the program. Offenders are screened prior to participation; some programs exclude chronic deniers, those with psychopathic personality disorder, and offenders who have either failed to complete or not participated in previous treatment programs.

Offender support includes daily contact from one of several trained volunteers, who historically have been volunteers from faith-based organizations. Offenders receive positive and meaningful social support. Volunteers may help the offender find a place to live and welcome the offender to their church. In some cases, volunteers have acted as mediators between the offender and estranged family members.

COSA describes the offender as the "core" member of the circle, with the volunteer members completing the circle. As part of their mission to promote accountability, COSA programs require the sex offender to do the following:

- recognize the harm that was done;
- acknowledge the impact of the harm;
- remit appropriate restitution;
- transform his or her attitude and behavior.

COSA group meetings challenge cognitive distortions (e. g., blaming the victim for the crime, over-personalizing other reactions) and encourage accountability while providing support; this combination is believed to be critical to the program's success.

A small number of studies report promising outcomes of COSA programs. Investigators in a Canadian study comparing 44 COSA participants with 44 similar offenders 3 years after their release from prison showed that COSA significantly reduced recidivism:

sexual assault by 83 percent and violent assault by 73 percent compared to the non-COSA participants. In a United States study comparing a COSA group of 31 recently released sex offenders with a control group of 31 recently released sex offenders, researchers reported that between their 2008 releases and 2011, none of the COSA group reoffended, whereas one of the control group had.

Recidivism in the two studies above is defined as a charge or conviction for a new offense. It does not take into account reoffending that is not caught or behavior that is described as "precursory offending," in which offenders groom potential victims, which is especially common among child sex offenders. A study of 21 COSA groups in Vermont, United States, that had been operating for 3 years found that the circles helped the offenders remain compliant with their rules of release from prison and that the offenders felt more obligation to and respect for circle members because they were volunteers rather than paid professionals. A British study of 14 offenders in a COSA program identified three participants who were involved in precursory behaviors to reoffend. Rather than this being viewed as a failure of COSA, an alternative perception is to consider it a sign of program success since the potential to offend was intercepted.

A goal of COSA is to eradicate recidivism by transforming sex offenders; intercepting offenders before they have the chance to reoffend also helps protect communities.

WHAT CAN BE DONE

Learn about the philosophy of restorative justice and its broad range of practices and consider how it might be used in your own social work practice.

Learn about restorative justice programs that are in use. Promote research into and evaluation of such programs in order to develop and broaden understanding of the practice.

Treatment methodologies should reflect the cultural values, beliefs, and biases of the individual in need of care and treatment.

Written by Jan Wagstaff, MA, MSW

Reviewed by Lynn B. Cooper, D. Crim, and Chris Bates, MA, MSW

REFERENCES

Armstrong, S., Chistyakova, Y., Mackenzie, A., & Malloch, M. (2008). Circles of support & accountability: Consideration of the feasibility of pilots in Scotland. Retrieved from http://www.sccjr. ac. uk/wp-content/uploads/2012/10/circles.pdf

Bates, A., Saunders, R., & Wilson, C. (2007). 'Doing something about it': A follow-up study of sex offenders participating in Thames Valley circles of support and accountability. *British Journal of Community Justice, 5*(1), 19-42.

Bazemore, G. (2005). Whom and how do we reintegrate? Finding community in restorative justice. *Criminology & Public Policy, 4*(1), 131-148. doi:10.1 111/j.1745-9133.2005.00011. x

British Association of Social Workers. (2012, January). The code of ethics for social workers: Statement of principles. Retrieved December 6, 2015, from http://cdn. basw.co.uk/upload/ basw_112315-7.pdf

Duwe, G. (2013). Can circles of support and accountability (COSA) work in the United States? Preliminary results from a randomized experiment in Minnesota. *Sexual Abuse: A Journal of Research & Treatment, 25*(2), 143-165. doi:10.1177/1079063212453942

Fox, K. J. (2013). Circles of support & accountability. Retrieved from http://www.doc. state. vt. us/about/reports/circles-of-support-accountability-final-report/ view

Grauwiler, P., & Mills, L. G. (2004). Moving beyond the criminal justice paradigm: A radical restorative justice approach to intimate abuse. *Journal of Sociology & Social Welfare, 31*(1), 49-69.

Hannem, S. (2013). Experiences in reconciling risk management and restorative justice: How circles of support and accountability work in the risk society. *International Journal of Offender Therapy and Comparative Criminology, 57*(3), 269. doi:10.1177/0306624X11432538

Hudson, B. (2002). Restorative justice and gendered violence. *British Journal of Criminology, 42*(3), 616-634. doi:10.1093/bjc/42.3.616

International Federation of Social Workers. (2012, March 3). Statement of ethical principles. Retrieved December 6, 2015, from http://ifsw.org/ policies/statement-of-ethical-principles

Kelly, E. L. (2010). Philly stands up: Inside politics and poetics of transformative justice and community accountability in sexual assault situations. *Social Justice, 37*(4), 44-57.

Lawson, C. L., & Katz, J. (2004). Restorative justice: An alternative approach to juvenile crime. *Journal of Socio-Economics, 33*(2), 175-188. doi:10.1016/j. socec.2003.12.018

London, R. D. (2003). The restoration of trust: Bringing restorative justice from the margins to the mainstream. *Criminal Justice Studies, 16*(3), 175-195. doi:10.1080/0888431032000151844

Mills, L. G., Barocas, B., & Ariel, B. (2013). The next generation of court-mandated domestic violence treatment: A comparison study of batterer intervention and restorative justice program. *Journal of Experimental Criminology, 9*(1), 65-90. doi:10.1007/ s11292-012-9164-x

Presser, L., & Van Voorhis, P. (2002). Values and evaluation: Assessing processes and outcomes of restorative justice programs. *Crime & Delinquency, 48*(1), 162-188. doi:10.1177/0011128702048001007

Richards, K. (2011). Is it time for Australia to adopt circles of support and accountability (COSA)? *Current Issues in Criminal Justice, 22*(3), 483-490.

United Nations. (2002). ECOSOC Resolution 2002/12 basic principles on the use of restorative justice programmes in criminal matters. Retrieved November 14, 2014, from http://www. un.org/en/ecosoc/docs/2002/resolution percent202002-12.pdf

Van Ness, D. W. (2005). An overview of restorative justice around the world. Retrieved November 20, 2014, from http://assets. justice. vic.gov. au/njc/resources/c4518c8a-c200-4623-afd1-42e255b62cf9/01+an+overview+of+restorative+ justice.pdf

van Wormer, K. (2004). Restorative justice: A model for personal and societal empowerment. *Journal of Religion & Spirituality in Social Work, 23*(4), 103-120. doi:10.1300/J377v23n04_07

Wheeler, D. (2015). NASW standards and indicators for cultural competence in social work practice. Retrieved December 6, 2015, from http://www. socialworkers.org/practice/standards/PRA-BRO-253150-CC-Standards.pdf

Wilson, R., Cortoni, F., & McWhinnie, A. (2009). Circles of support and accountability': A Canadian national replication study of outcome findings. *Sexual Abuse: A Journal of Research & Treatment, 21*(4), 412-430.

RESTORATIVE JUSTICE PROGRAMS: JUVENILE OFFENDERS

MAJOR CATEGORIES: Adolescents

WHAT WE KNOW

Restorative justice (RJ) is a global movement that affects social work practice within both the juvenile and criminal justice systems. In the value system of restorative justice, crime is conceived of principally as an offense against human relationships, and restoring human dignity is therefore critical in redressing the impact of crime.

RJ seeks to repair the damage done by criminal acts and restore safety and dignity for the victim, the perpetrator, and society.

Criminal justice emphasizes punishment and rehabilitation, yet this has proven to be ineffectual in reducing crime.

RJ seeks to transform the impact of and responses to crime through reparation, reducing recidivism, and increasing empathy among those involved.

RJ programs began in the 1970s.

RJ places priority on helping victims participate in the justice process.

In RJ crime is understood and addressed within the social context of individuals, family, and community. It may be employed to avoid official involvement of the criminal justice system, or it may be used in conjunction with the criminal justice process.

There are two main principles of RJ:

Reconciliation of victims and perpetrators through remorse, apology, and forgiveness.

Reparation through accountability and compensation.

RJ outcomes for juvenile offenders include the following:

Financial restitution to victims (Offenders may repay the costs of property damage themselves or repair property they have damaged. Informal restitution to the community by reducing financial and social costs of crime and through visible contributions such as community service. Youth may help to improve parks and other public spaces, for example.)

Persistent reductions in recidivism rates among youth (RJ strategies can prevent school expulsions and suspensions. According to a 2013 comparative study, after youth participated in RJ programs they were without offense for significantly longer periods of time than youth who participated in the juvenile court system. In another study the recidivism rate for youth in RJ programs was 3 times lower than that of youth in control groups.).

In February 2012 the U.S. Senate voted unanimously to support restorative justice for youth. It marks a departure from zero-tolerance policies, especially in school systems. Zero tolerance, or the imposition of harsh penalties for infractions, often has negative effects (e.g., expulsions, suspensions) but does not improve school safety. RJ, an alternative to the zero-tolerance approach to problems in the school setting, puts a greater emphasis on respect, accountability, and relationship building.

With juvenile offenders, victims and families report high rates of satisfaction with the process when compared to those in nonparticipating control groups.

Satisfaction levels for victims of juvenile offenders have ranged from 57 percent to 97 percent.

RJ strategies involve victim–offender mediation, family group conferencing, neighborhood accountability boards (i.e., community-based decision-making process to respond to harm) or restorative circles of community members committed to the restoration process (i.e., a community process that brings together the victim, the perpetrator, and the community to repair harm), and community reparation boards (a small, trained committee designated to facilitate the restorative justice process).

Meetings between victims and offenders often are referred to as "conferencing." In so-called restorative conferences, victims and perpetrators meet to discuss and agree on their experiences, how they can make things as right as possible, and how to increase future safety.

"Peacemaking circles" or "circle sentencing" also are used to describe conferencing. These strategies are modeled on Australian Aboriginal rituals. Victim or community panels are forums in which community members can describe their experiences with crime.

RJ interventions require the following;

- Assurance of victim safety;
- Screening to establish the perpetrator's suitability for the program;

- Admission of the crime is essential;
- Perpetrators must voluntarily attend programs;
- Perpetrators must be willing to have face-to-face dialogue with victims.

A high degree of preparation and experience is required by the mediator for the effective mediation of meetings between offenders and victims.

Mediator preparation and training is especially critical for victims of violent crime.

Mediator preparation includes meetings with individuals to gauge readiness of all parties prior to the conference.

Victims are empowered in the RJ process by choosing their level of involvement, such as determining their desired outcome from the RJ process, engaging in dialogue and reconciliation, and receiving restitution.

Victims may bring friends or family members to meetings for support.

Youth may be referred to an RJ program by advocacy groups, schools, law enforcement, county attorneys, and local courts.

Programs may operate independently from juvenile courts, including through social service agencies.

The earlier juvenile offenders participate in RJ, the greater the positive outcomes.

Although RJ is mentioned in many state codes in the United States, few states mandate its use and there is a lack of established organizations to implement it within the juvenile justice system.

Although 32 U.S. states currently support RJ in their statutes, the legislation may be a statement of support rather than official policy.

Offenders vary in their level of willingness to participate.

Incorporating RJ into the youth justice system continues to be challenging for advocates.

Some crimes, such as intimate partner violence, and some perpetrators may be unsuitable.

Youth from smaller cities have been shown to have poorer outcomes from participation in RJ programs.

Parents of juveniles do not always understand what is involved although they report supporting RJ goals.

Victims unwilling to participate can insist on formal processing through the juvenile justice system.

Financial restitution may be difficult for some youth and their families

WHAT CAN BE DONE

Become knowledgeable about the principles of RJ.

Become knowledgeable about the outcomes of RJ programs and advocate for them.

Become knowledgeable about the RJ programs in your area.

Develop an awareness of your own cultural values, beliefs, and biases and develop knowledge about the histories, traditions, and values of your clients. Adopt treatment methodologies that reflect the cultural needs of the client.

Written by Jan Wagstaff, MA, MSW

Reviewed by Lynn B. Cooper, D. Crim, and Allison Mangin, MSW

REFERENCES

Bazemore, G. (2005). Whom and how do we reintegrate? Finding community in restorative justice. *Criminology & Public Policy, 4*(1), 131-148. doi:10.1111/j.1745-9133.2005.00011.x

Bergseth, K. J., & Bouffard, J. A. (2007). The long-term impact of restorative justice programming for juvenile offenders. *Journal of Criminal Justice, 35,* 433-451. doi:10.1016/j.jcrimjus.2007.05.006

Bergseth, K. J., & Bouffard, J. A. (2013). Examining the effectiveness of a restorative justice program for various types of juvenile offenders. *International Journal of Offender Therapy and Comparative Criminology, 57*(9), 1054. doi:10.1177/0306624X12453551https://www.ncjrs.gov/pdf-files/167887.pdf

British Association of Social Workers. (2012). The code of ethics for social work: Statement of principles. Retrieved January 28, 2016, from http://cdn.basw.co.uk/upload/basw_112315-7.pdf

Council of State Government/American Probation and Parole Association. Promising Victim Related Practices in Probation and Parole Fact Sheet. (2009). *Office for Victims of Crime.*

Crime Victim Assistance. NASW Policy Paper. (2011). *Social Work Speaks.* Washington, D.C.: National Association of Social Workers.

Goren, S. (2001). Healing the victim, the young offender, and the community via restorative justice: An international perspective. *Issues in Mental Health Nursing, 22*(2), 137-149. doi:10.1080/01612840121244

International Federation of Social Workers. (2012). Statement of ethical principles. Retrieved January 28, 2016, from http://ifsw.org/policies/statement-of-ethical-principles/

Karp, D. R., Sweet, M., Kirshenbaum, A., & Bazemore, G. (2004). Reluctant participants in restorative justice? Youthful offenders and their parents. *Contemporary Justice Review, 7*(2), 199-216.

Kirby Forgays, D., & DeMilio, L. (2005). Is teen court effective for repeat offenders? A test of the restorative justice approach. *International Journal of Offender Therapy & Comparative Criminology, 49*(1), 107-118. doi:10.1177/0306624X04269411

Koss, M., & Achilles, M. (2008). Restorative justice approaches to sexual violence. Retrieved January 28, 2016, from http://www.vawnet.org/Assoc_Files_VAWnet/AR_RestorativeJustice.pdf

Lawson, C. L., & Katz, J. (2004). Restorative justice: An alternative approach to juvenile crime. *Journal of Socio-Economics, 33*(2), 175-188. doi:10.1016/j.socec.2003.12.018

London, R. D. (2003). The restoration of trust: Bringing restorative justice from the margins to the mainstream. *Criminal Justice Studies, 16*(3), 175-195. doi:10.1080/0888431032000151844

McCold, P. (2003). An experiment in police-based restorative justice: The Bethlehem (PA) project. *Police Practice & Research, 4*(4), 379-390. doi:10.1080/15614260310001631271

Mueller, J., Wade, K., Swenson, D., Miller, D., & Sager, S. (2004). An evaluation: Restorative justice programs: Milwaukee and Outagamie Counties. Retrieved January 28, 2016, from http://legis.wisconsin.gov/lab/reports/04-6full.pdf

Noll, D. E., & Harvey, L. (2008). Restorative mediation: The application of restorative justice practice and philosophy to clergy sexual abuse cases. *Journal of Child Sexual Abuse, 17*(3-4), 377-396. doi:10.1080/10538710802330021

Presser, L., & Van Voorhis, P. (2002). Values and evaluation: Assessing processes and outcomes of restorative justice programs. *Crime & Delinquency, 48*(1), 162-188. doi:10.1177/0011128702048001007

Rateliff, K. (2000). Jailed mothers: A chaplain delivers restorative justice childbirth. *Midwifery Today, 53*, 30-31.

Silva, S. M., & Lambert, C. G. (2015). Restorative justice legislation in the American states: A statutory analysis of emerging legal doctrine. *Journal of Policy Practice, 14*(2), 77-95. doi:10.1080/15588742.2015.1017687

Stahlkopf, C. (2009). Restorative justice, rhetoric, or reality? Conferencing with young offenders. *Contemporary Justice Review, 12*(3), 231-251. doi:10.1080/10282580903105756

Teasley, M. L. (2014). Shifting from zero tolerance to restorative justice in schools. *Children & Schools, 36*(3), 131-133. doi:10.1093/cs/cdu016

Umbreit, M. S., Coates, R. B., & Vos, B. (2001). Impact of restorative justice conferencing with juvenile offenders: What we have learned from two decades of victim offender dialogue through mediation and conferencing. Retrieved January 28, 2016, from http://www.cehd.umn.edu/ssw/RJP/Projects/Victim-Offender-Dialogue/Restorative_Group_Conferencing/Victim_Impact_RJC_with percent20_Juvenile_Offenders.pdf

van Wormer, K. (2004). Restorative justice: A model for personal and societal empowerment. *Journal of Religion & Spirituality in Social Work, 23*(4), 103-120. doi:10.1300/J377v23n04_07

Washington State House Democrats. (2012). Legislature approves restorative justice for juvenile offenders. Retrieved January 28, 2016, from http://housedemocrats.wa.gov/news/legislature-approves-restorative-justice-for-juvenile-offenders/

Wheeler, D. (2015). NASW standards and indicators for cultural competence in social work practice. Retrieved January 28, 2016, from http://www.socialworkers.org/practice/standards/PRA-BRO-253150-CC-Standards.pdf

RESTORATIVE JUSTICE PROGRAMS: SEXUAL ASSAULT VICTIMS & OFFENDERS

MAJOR CATEGORIES: Community

WHAT WE KNOW

Restorative justice (RJ) has been described as "an approach to achieving justice that involves, to the extent possible, those who have a stake in a specific offense or harm to collectively identify and address harms, needs, and obligations in order to heal and put things as right as possible"(p.48).

In contrast to adversarial or retributive criminal justice approaches that view crime as an offense against societal interests and emphasize punishment, RJ views crime as harm occurring within the social context of individuals, family, and community and emphasizes participation and empowerment of the parties involved, accountability for offenders, healing and restoration for victims, and a joint determination of how offenders will repair the harm they have caused.

RJ currently is implemented in over 80 countries.

RJ has grown in popularity during the past several decades, in part owing to dissatisfaction with the current criminal justice system (e.g., high rates of incarceration, racial disparities, and insensitivity to victims).

Although RJ has been described as a "social movement" during the past several decades, RJ practices are rooted in traditions of numerous cultures, including the Maori in New Zealand, Native Americans, African Americans, Latinos, and Canadian Mennonites.

In the United States, 32 states include at least one statute addressing RJ practices.

Statutes range from a single mention of RJ to structured guidelines regarding its use.

The practices most frequently cited in state statutes include victim–offender meetings (21 states) and victim impact panels and classes (12 states).

A database of RJ legislation in the United States can be accessed at http://law.gsu.edu/centers/consortium-on-negotiation-and-conflict-resolution/programs-and-research.

An important feature of RJ practice is the act of bringing perpetrators of crimes and their victims together in dialogue.

There are three predominant variations of RJ meetings:

Victim–offender mediation (VOM), which involves a trained mediator, the victim, and the offender, is one of the most common RJ practices in the United States.

Restorative justice conferences (RJC), also referred to as "family group conferences," are similar to VOM but also include family members and friends of victims and offenders, who are considered to be "secondary victims" who also are affected by the crime.

Peacemaking circles, also referred to as "sentencing circles" or "talking circles," include community members in addition to victims, offenders, family members, and friends.

In Canada "circles of support and accountability" (COSA) were introduced in the 1990s to prevent recidivism among sex offenders and facilitate their integration into society following incarceration. COSA programs are based on RJ philosophy but do not involve victim participation.

RJ meetings may take place in lieu of criminal justice proceedings or in conjunction with them.

These RJ meetings include a number of important elements.

Participation of both victims and offenders is voluntary.

Trained facilitator meets with participants prior to the meeting and prepares them for the process.

Offender acceptance of responsibility is a precondition of participation.

Adequate preparation is crucial particularly in cases of sexual assault, preparation may be extensive and take weeks or months.

Face-to-face encounters have been linked with the greatest satisfaction among participants, but victims who are not comfortable with meeting face-to-face with the offender may be represented by a "surrogate victim;" letters, videos, and video/telephone conferencing can also be used.

The victim/offender encounter is guided by facilitator and tends to follow a structured format:

The offender makes a statement regarding the crime.

The victim (and secondary victims, if included) talk about the impact of the crime.

Offender, victim, and other participants, if included, discuss how the offender can make reparations.

Written, signed restitution agreements often are used.

Through reparations, the offender works toward repairing the material consequences of the crime, such as by repaying the costs of property damage, as a way of making amends.

A protocol used in Australia, the United States, and the United Kingdom includes filing the restitution agreement with authorities to be monitored for compliance.

Overall, victims report satisfaction with the process and outcomes of RJ meetings. Specifically, victims feel included and empowered, in contrast to the conventional criminal justice process in which victims report being marginalized.

Sexual assault is understood as when an individual is coerced, threatened, or forced to engage in sexual contact of any kind.

It covers a spectrum of behaviors from forced kissing and nonpenetrative sexual contact to sexual abuse of children and rape.

Predominantly, sexual violence is perpetrated against women and children by men; it occurs in all classes and races and frequently is used as a weapon of war.

Sexual assault is reportedly high in some countries among men who have sex with men. Sexual assault often is committed in relationships in which domestic violence/intimate partner violence is present. Gender inequality and sex discrimination contribute to sexual assault. In most cases of sexual violence, the perpetrator of the assault is known to the victim.

The consequences of sexual assault may include physical, psychological, emotional, sexual, and reproductive health problems; these consequences may be lifelong. Sexual assault can increase vulnerability to HIV. In addition, the social consequences for women and girls, whether they are victims of sexual violence or not, include the restriction of spatial and social freedom.

RJ has been proposed as an alternate response to sexual assault cases, in part because of concerns that the conventional criminal justice response to sexual assault has not made society safer; there is a high rate of attrition (i.e., closing of cases without resolution) in sexual assault cases; and the legal process does not address victims' needs (e.g., to be heard, validated, have input) and may cause more harm than healing for victims of sexual assault.

A 2013 study of youth sex offenders with no prior convictions showed that those attending conferencing procedures had significantly lower recidivism rates.

A case study tentatively reported a positive outcome when an adult survivor met her childhood rapist.

A study of three men condemned to death who met relatives of the women they had sexually assaulted and murdered indicated positive outcomes for both the families of the victims and the perpetrators.

The use of RJ conferences has been examined in several recent studies.

In a systematic review and meta-analysis published in 2013, researchers were able to identify only four studies that met criteria for inclusion; the researchers did not find sufficient evidence that RJ is more effective than traditional court procedures as a means to reduce recidivism in young offenders or affect their recognition or remorse regarding their behavior. There was some indication that RJ may be associated with higher satisfaction among victims.

Researchers in a systematic review of data from 10 randomized studies found that RJ conferences were associated with reduced recidivism and victim satisfaction Subsequent meta-analysis found that 2-year recidivism was lower among offenders who participated in RJ conferences, an effect that was particularly strong for those who had committed violent crimes.

Victim contact may have more of an impact on perpetrators of violent crimes involving serious injuries.

Although there is a growing body of research in support of RJ, few studies have compared the outcomes of RJ conferencing for violent crimes versus formal criminal proceedings. Many scholars are cautious about its use in areas such as sexual assault. Concerns include that the physical safety of victims cannot be guaranteed in RJ forums.

RJ meetings have been carried out in ways that are insensitive to victims, leading to feelings of disempowerment and other negative impacts on victims.

RJ frequently prioritizes rehabilitating the offender outside formal legal proceedings over the concerns of victims; because of this, scholars are critical of its use with sexual assault offenses.

Survivors of violent crimes have sometimes expressed dissatisfaction with both restorative justice and retributive justice; one study of women survivors found that neither type of justice ensured their safety or freedom from harm.

Investigators in a recent study designed and tested a program (RESTORE) that adapted RJ for use in adult misdemeanor and felony sexual assault cases referred by prosecutors. Adaptations included forensic assessment of offenders to determine their appropriateness for participation, extensive preparation of participants, monitoring of physical and psychological safety, use of surrogate victims if face-to-face meetings were too threatening for victims, and use of a supervised redress plan for offenders.

Victims' psychological safety was assessed using the Post-Traumatic Symptoms Scale (PSS), which showed a decrease in PTSD symptoms from 82 percent of victim participants meeting criteria for PTSD at intake to only 66 percent meeting criteria for PTSD following the RJ conference.

RJ conferences were accepted by the majority of participants, with 63 percent of victims and 90 percent of offenders choosing RJ over conventional criminal justice resolution. Participants who knew each other prior to the assault were more likely than those who were strangers to choose face-to-face contact.

Participant satisfaction was high (90 percent).

The majority (80 percent) of offenders met the requirements of their redress plan.

WHAT CAN BE DONE

Learn about RJ programs in use in your area of practice and promote research and evaluation of them in order to develop and broaden understanding of RJ practice.

Learn about best practices in RJ.

The Restorative Justice Council in the UK has published the detailed *Best Practice Guidance for Restorative* Practice, which includes core competencies and guidance for practitioners, supervisors, managers, and service providers.

Learn about specific challenges in using RJ with sexual assault cases and prioritize victims' safety.

Develop an awareness of your own cultural values, beliefs, and biases and develop knowledge about the histories, traditions, and values of your clients. Adopt treatment methodologies that reflect the cultural needs of the client.

Written by Jan Wagstaff, MA, MSW

Reviewed by Lynn B. Cooper, D. Crim

REFERENCES

British Association of Social Workers. (2012, January). The Code of Ethics for Social Work: Statement of principles. Retrieved December 30, 2015, from http://cdn.basw.co.uk/upload/basw_112315-7.pdf

Choi, J., Green, D., & Kapp, S. (2010). A qualitative study of victim offender mediation: Implications for social work. *Journal of Human Behavior in the Social Environment, 20*(7), 857-874. doi:10.1007/s10560-011-0238-9

Daly, K. (2002). Sexual assault and restorative justice. In H. Strang & J. Braithwaite (Eds.), *Restorative justice and family violence* (pp. 62-86). Cambridge, UK: Cambridge University Press.

Daly, K., Bouhours, B., Broadhurst, R., & Loh, N. (2013). Youth sex offending and restorative justice: Comparing court and conference cases. *Australian & New Zealand Journal of Criminology, 46*(2), 1-27. doi:10.1177/0004865812470383

Dartnall, E., & Jewkes, R. (2013). Sexual violence against women: The scope of the problem. *Best Practice & Research Clinical Obstetrics & Gynaecology, 27*(1), 3-13. doi:10.1016/j.bpobgyn.2012.08.002

Gavrielides, T., & Artinopoulou, V. (2013). Restorative justice and violence against women: Comparing Greece and the United Kingdom. *Asian Criminology, 8*(1), 25-40. doi:10.1007/s11417-011-9123-x

Grauwiler, P., & Mills, L. G. (2004). Moving beyond the criminal justice paradigm: A radical restorative justice approach to intimate abuse. *Journal of Sociology & Social Welfare, 31*(1), 49-69.

Gumz, E. J., & Grant, C. L. (2009). Restorative justice: A systematic review of the social work literature. *Families in Society: The Journal of Contemporary Social Services, 90*(1), 119-126. doi:10.1606/1044-3894.3853

Hannem, S. (2013). Experiences in reconciling risk management and restorative justice: How circles of support and accountability work in the risk society. *International Journal of Offender Therapy and Comparative Criminology, 57*(3), 269. doi:10.1177/0306624X11432538

Herman, J. L. (2005). Justice from the victim's perspective. *Violence Against Women, 11*(5), 571-602. doi:10.1177/1077801205274450

Hopkins, C. Q., & Koss, M. P. (2005). Incorporating feminist theory and insights into a restorative justice response to sex offenses. *Violence Against Women, 11*(5), 693-723.

International Federation of Social Workers. (2012, March 3). Statement of ethical principles. Retrieved December 30, 2015, from http://ifsw.org/policies/statement-of-ethical-principles/

Koss, M. P. (2014). The RESTORE program of restorative justice for sex crimes: Vision, process, and outcomes. *Journal of Interpersonal Violence, 29*(9), 1623-1660. doi:10.1177/0886260513511537

Koss, M. P., Bachar, K. J., Hopkins, C. Q., & Carlson, C. (2004). Expanding a community's justice response to sex crimes through advocacy, prosecutorial, and public health collaboration: Introducing the RESTORE program. *Journal of Interpersonal Violence, 19*(12), 1435.

Koss, M. P., Wilgus, J. K., & Williamsen, K. M. (2014). Campus sexual misconduct: Restorative justice approaches to enhance compliance with Title IX guidance. *Trauma, Violence and Abuse, 15*(3), 242-257. doi:10.1177/1524838014521500

Livingstone, N., MacDonald, G., & Carr, N. (2013). Restorative justice conferencing for reducing recidivism in young offenders (aged 7 to 21). *Cochrane Database of Systematic Reviews,* (2), CD008898. doi:10.1002/14651858.CD008898.pub2

London, R. D. (2003). The restoration of trust: Bringing restorative justice from the margins to the mainstream. *Criminal Justice Studies, 16*(3), 175-195. doi:10.1080/0888431032000151844

McGlynn, C., Westmarland, N., & Godden, N. (2012). 'I just wanted him to hear me': Sexual violence and the possibilities of restorative justice. *Journal of Law & Society, 39*(2), 213-240. doi:10.1111/j.1467-6478.2012.00579.x

Mills, L. G., Barocas, B., & Ariel, B. (2013). The next generation of court-mandated domestic violence treatment: A comparison study of batterer intervention and restorative justice program. *Journal of Experimental Criminology, 9*(1), 65-90. doi:10.1007/s11292-012-9164-x

Wheeler, D., & McClain, A. (2015). NASW standards for cultural competence in social work practice. Retrieved December 30, 2015, from http://www.socialworkers.org/practice/standards/PRA-BRO-253150-CC-Standards.pdf

Mutter, R., Shemmings, D., Dugmore, P., & Hyare, M. (2008). Family group conferences in youth justice. *Health & Social Care in the Community, 16*(3), 262-270. doi:10.1111/j.1365-2524.2008.00770.x

Presser, L., & Van Voorhis, P. (2002). Values and evaluation: Assessing processes and outcomes of restorative justice programs. *Crime & Delinquency, 48*(1), 162-188. doi:10.1177/0011128702048001007

Restorative Justice Council. (2011). Best practice guidance for restorative practice. Retrieved December 30, 2015, from https://www.restorativejustice.org.uk/sites/default/files/resources/files/Best percent20practice percent20Guidance percent202011.pdf

Rubin, P. (2003). Restorative justice in Nova Scotia: Women's experience and recommendations for positive policy development and implementation. Retrieved December 30, 0205, from http://restorativejustice.org/rj-library/restorative-justice-in-nova-scotia-womens-experience-and-recommendations-for-positive-policy-development-and-implementation-report-and-recommendations/5570/

Sherman, L. W., Strang, H., Mayo-Wilson, E., Woods, D. J., & Ariel, B. (2015). Are restorative justice conferences effective in reducing repeat offending? Findings from a Campbell Systematic Review. *Journal of Quantitative Criminology, 31*(1), 1-24. doi:10.1007/s10940-014-9222-9

Silva, S. M., & Lambert, C. G. (2015). Restorative justice legislation in the American states: A statutory analysis of emerging legal doctrine. *Journal of Policy Practice, 14*(2), 77-95. doi:10.1080/15588742.2015.1017687

Strang, H., Sherman, L. W., Mayo-Wilson, E., Woods, D., & Ariel, B. (2013). Restorative justice conferencing (RJC) using face-to-face meetings of offenders and victims: Effects on offender recidivism and victim satisfaction. *Campbell Systematic Reviews, 9*(12), 1-59.

Umbreit, M., Coates, R., & Vos, B. (2004). Victim-offender mediation: Three decades of practice and research. *Conflict Resolution Quarterly, 22*(1/2), 279-303. doi:10.1002/crq.102

Umbreit, M., & Vos, B. (2000). Homicide survivors meet the offender prior to execution: Restorative justice through dialogue. *Homicide Studies, 4*(1), 63-87.

United Nations. (2002). ECOSOC resolution 2002/12: Basic principles on the use of restorative justice programmes in criminal matters. Retrieved December 30, 2015, from http://www.un.org/en/ecosoc/docs/2002/resolution percent202002-12.pdf

Van Ness, D. W. (2005). An overview of restorative justice around the world. Retrieved December 30, 1970, from http://assets.justice.vic.gov.au/njc/resources/c4518c8a-c200-4623-afd1-42e255b62cf9/01+an+overview+of+restorative+justice.pdf

World Health Organization. (2012). Violence against women: Intimate partner and sexual violence against women. Retrieved December 30, 2015, from http://www.who.int/mediacentre/factsheets/fs239/en/

Zehr, H. (2015). The little book of restorative justice. New York, NY: Good Books.

RESTORATIVE JUSTICE PROGRAMS: VICTIM-OFFENDER DIALOGUES

MAJOR CATEGORIES: Community

WHAT WE KNOW

Restorative justice (RJ) is a process in which victims, perpetrators, and the members of the community come together to discuss the impact of a crime and determine together what should be done to repair the harm caused by the crime. RJ conceives of crime principally as an offense against human relationships; restoring human dignity is central to redressing the impact of crime in RJ.

Restorative justice is considered an effective alternative to traditional responses to juvenile crime.

Incarceration has been found to be both expensive and ineffective in deterring recidivism among juvenile offenders.

An important feature of RJ practice worldwide is the act of bringing perpetrators of crimes and their victims together in dialogue.

Meetings are professionally facilitated; they involve the victim, the offender, and the facilitator and may also include the police, parents/guardians if there is a juvenile involved, or other individuals whom the victim or perpetrator wishes to have present.

One method of achieving restorative justice is victim–offender mediation (VOM)

The VOM process usually includes these steps: The facilitator confers separately with both parties prior to the meeting to screen them and the case for appropriateness and to explain the VOM process. Each party then completes some form of preparation before the meeting (e.g., worksheets, one-on-one meetings with the facilitator).All parties again agree that they want to participate in a meeting. The meeting is held is a safe and secure environment.

Victim–offender dialogues (VODs) is another term used to describe facilitated meetings between victims and offenders that occur after a case has been concluded in the criminal justice system. The VOD may or may not be part of the criminal justice process.

Preparation by the facilitator for meetings between victims and offenders is critically important.

Facilitators may meet with both parties more than once before the meeting is arranged to discuss the parties' expectations, concerns, and fears.

Some facilitators design questionnaires that help participants understand what they hope to gain from the meeting.

Some victims and offenders prepare statements that they then read at the beginning of the meeting.

Meeting structure and guidelines are agreed upon either prior to or at the beginning of the meeting.

Dialogues in meetings require that the facilitator understand the power dynamics between offenders and victims and avoid victim domination. In addition, for empathy to occur, a level of comfort must be cultivated between the participants. Distance between the victim and the offender may hinder the healing process.

Researchers who studied VODs in one jurisdiction showed that all victims and offenders for whom the VOD process had been instigated had some form of relationship prior to the crime; after starting the mediation process, however, most did not end up actually meeting. The VOD process was more likely to conclude with a meeting between victims and offenders with no prior relationship.

An apology from the offender to the victim can help achieve a positive outcome from meetings.

Victims who received and accepted an apology expressed satisfaction with the mediation.

Researchers found that an apology was not forthcoming at two thirds of the meetings.

Researchers caution that some meetings are carried out in ways that are insensitive to victims, leading to feelings of disempowerment and other negative impacts on victims.

Some victims report feeling pressured and rushed into meeting the offender.

Statistics gathered from a cross-section of VOM programs in North America showed that approximately 66 percent of referred cases resulted in a face-to-face meeting, 95 percent of those cases resulted in a written restitution agreement, and over 90 percent of the agreements were fulfilled within a year.

WHAT CAN BE DONE

Learn about the preparation required for meetings between victims of crime and offenders: screening to ensure that candidates are suitable and ensuring that victims are psychologically prepared are especially important.

Learn about all aspects of RJ and ensure that victims and offenders understand what the process entails before they agree to participate.

Develop a list of resources about RJ for education and referrals, such as

International Institute for Restorative Practices, http://www.iirp.edu.

University of Minnesota Center for Restorative Justice & Peacemaking, http://www.cehd.umn.edu/ssw/RJP/default.asp.

Develop an awareness of your own cultural values, beliefs, and biases and develop knowledge about the histories, traditions, and values of your clients. Adopt treatment methodologies that reflect the cultural needs of the client.

Written by Jan Wagstaff, MA, MSW

Reviewed by Lynn B. Cooper, D. Crim, and Chris Bates, MA, MSW

REFERENCES

Borton, I. (2012). Effect of time and relationships on victim-offender dialogue completion in felony cases. *Contemporary Justice Review, 15*(4), 399-412. doi:10.1080/10282580.2012.734566

British Association of Social Workers. (2012). The code of ethics for social work: Statement of principles. Retrieved December 5, 1970, from http://cdn.basw.co.uk/upload/basw_112315-7.pdf

Choi, J., Green, D., & Gilbert, M. (2011). Putting a human face on crimes: A qualitative study on restorative justice processes for youth. *Child & Adolescent Social Work Journal, 28*(5), 335-355. doi:10.1007/s10560-011-0238-9

Choi, J., Green, D., & Kapp, S. (2010). A qualitative study of victim offender mediation: Implications for social work. *Journal of Human Behavior in the Social Environment, 20*(7), 857-874. doi:10.1007/s10560-011-0238-9

Dhami, M. (2012). Offer and acceptance of apology in victim-offender mediation. *Critical Criminology, 20*(1), 45-60. doi:10.1007/s10612-011-9149-5

International Federation of Social Workers. (2012). Statement of ethical principles. Retrieved December 5, 2014, from http://ifsw.org/policies/statement-of-ethical-principles/

Restorative Justice Resources. (n.d.). Victim offender mediation or dialogue. Retrieved from http://www.restorativejustice.info/victimoffenders.html

Tsui, J. C. (2014). Breaking free of the prison paradigm: Integrating restorative justice techniques into Chicago's juvenile justice system. *Journal of Criminal Law and Criminology, 104*(3), 635.

Wheeler, D. (2015). NASW standards and indicators for cultural competence in social work practice. Retrieved December 14, 2015, from http://www.socialworkers.org/practice/standards/PRA-BRO-253150-CC-Standards.pdf

RESTORATIVE JUSTICE: INTIMATE PARTNER VIOLENCE VICTIMS & OFFENDERS

MAJOR CATEGORIES: Community

WHAT WE KNOW

Restorative justice (RJ) is a worldwide movement that informs social work practice within juvenile and criminal justice. In the value system of restorative justice, crime is conceived of principally as an offense against human relationships, and restoring human dignity is therefore critical in redressing the impact of crime.

RJ seeks to restore human dignity by increasing accountability and responsibility, increasing empathy between victims and offenders, reducing recidivism, and promoting reparations.

RJ has been most widely used with juveniles. It is most often used to circumvent the juvenile justice system in the hope of diverting young people from lives of crime and incarceration. The juvenile justice system's traditional methods of punishment are considered failures by many scholars.

An important feature of RJ practice is the act of bringing perpetrators of crimes and their victims together in dialogue.

Various names are given to RJ meetings between victims and perpetrators: "conferencing," "victim–offender mediation," "victim–offender dialogue," "circles," and sometimes "intimate abuse circles."

In England "restorative cautioning" was pioneered as a diversion from criminal justice proceedings a decade ago.

RJ meetings may take place in lieu of criminal justice proceedings or in conjunction with them. They seek to restore the emotional and psychological integrity of all those involved in the crime through facilitated dialogue.

In meetings, reparations may also be agreed upon: through reparations the offender works toward repairing the material consequences of the crime, such as by repaying the costs of property damage, as a way of making amends and restoring safety and dignity to all those involved.

Overall, victims report satisfaction with the process and outcomes of RJ meetings. Specifically, victims feel included and empowered, in contrast to the criminal justice process, in which victims report being marginalized.

Intimate partner violence (IPV),also known as *domestic violence* (DV), is understood as a human rights issue.

IPV is physical, sexual, psychological, or emotional harm inflicted on one person by another within an intimate, romantic, and/or spousal relationship that is ongoing or has ended.

It is overwhelmingly a crime against women and children by men. IPV may happen in same-sex relationships and men can be victims also.

It is described as a global public health problem that causes profound degradation in the quality of human life.

The circumstances of IPV can differ dramatically, but the relational dynamics are the same in all instances: Individual power is used to exploit and abuse victims.

Advocates of IPV victims have worked for over three decades to have the problem publicly recognized and criminalized. Many countries have adopted laws against IPV and sought prosecution against perpetrators, with some jurisdictions introducing dedicated IPV police units.

In spite of these advancements the problem of IPV has not abated; prosecution and conviction rates are persistently low.

Advocates of victims of intimate partner violence and advocates of restorative justice both are concerned with victim empowerment. Because of this, some suggest that RJ is a suitable tool for use in DV cases.

Investigators argued that RJ may be an especially useful tool in cases in which black women have been abused by black men because it circumvents the criminal justice system, in which black men are overrepresented.

Many scholars are cautious about the use of RJ with IPV cases, however. Some consider it unsuitable for several reasons. The physical and psychological safety of victims, especially women and children, cannot be guaranteed within an RJ process. The power imbalances that underpin an abusive intimate relationship can be intangible, difficult to mitigate, and perhaps impossible to prevent.

RJ meetings have been carried out in ways that are insensitive to victims, leading to feelings of disempowerment and other negative impacts on victims. There can also be the presence of double pressure wherein the victim is negatively impacted both by the violence and again by the RJ Abusers, especially men, are known to frequently apologize and express remorse as a means to manipulate victims yet continue to engage in abusive behavior.

The presence of the victim and whether the offender's apology was coerced can have an impact on the effectiveness of an RJ program. If the victim is present, there is an increased likelihood of positive changes to the victim–offender relationship and the opportunity for forgiveness and open dialogue between the involved parties. If the apology is an instrumental apology that is legally required of the offender, there is cognitive dissonance that results where the offender's words and actions are not in sync. Besides seeming insincere to the victim, the offender loses the opportunity for deeper change as a result of an honest apology.

Although there is a growing body of research on RJ, there is little research on the efficacy of RJ in cases of violent crime.

RJ concepts were developed primarily with the aim of redressing juvenile nonviolent crime.

The development of formal criminal procedures for serious crimes, especially those that have not been treated seriously in the past such as IPV, is considered important to society. RJ is seen as a diversion from established criminal justice systems; without those systems in place, RJ may lose its effectiveness.

RJ is typically a short-term intervention, and general theory on IPV argues that long-term interventions are needed to effect change.

Investigators in a 2012 study comparing the results of a court-mandated treatment program for batterers with an RJ program showed no significant difference: Both had high rates of attrition and recidivism.

Researchers conducting a study of women survivors of violent crimes found that they were not satisfied by either restorative justice or retributive justice: Neither ensured their safety or freedom from harm.

Investigators in a 2013 study found that abusers who took part in a RJ program for IPV versus a traditional batterer's intervention program had lower rates of recidivism, but those rates were not always statistically significant. Even without statistical significance, the RJ program was not worse than the traditional program so could be a potential option.

WHAT CAN BE DONE

Become knowledgeable about the complexities of intimate partner violence and how it affects the lives of victims.

Learn about the problems encountered when using RJ in IPV cases and prioritize safety.

Learn about RJ programs in use and promote research and evaluation of them to develop and broaden understanding of RJ practice in IPV situations.

Develop a list of resources about restorative justice for education and referrals, such as

International Institute for Restorative Practices, http://www.iirp.edu/.

University of Minnesota, Center for Restorative Justice & Peacemaking, http://www.cehd.umn.edu/ssw/rjp/.

Develop an awareness of your own cultural values, beliefs, and biases and develop knowledge about the histories, traditions, and values of your clients. Adopt treatment methodologies that reflect the cultural needs of the client.

Written by Jan Wagstaff, MA, MSW

*Reviewed by Lynn B. Cooper, D. Crim, and
Chris Bates, MA, MSW*

REFERENCES

Bazemore, G. (2005). Whom and how do we reintegrate? Finding community in restorative justice. *Criminology & Public Policy, 4*(1), 131-148. doi:10.1111/j.1745-9133.2005.00011.x

British Association of Social Workers. (2012). The code of ethics for social work: Statement of principles. Retrieved December 8, 2015, from http://cdn.basw.co.uk/upload/basw_112315-7.pdf

Choi, J., Green, D., & Kapp, S. (2010). A qualitative study of victim offender mediation: Implications for social work. *Journal of Human Behavior in the Social Environment, 20*(7), 857-874. doi:10.1007/s10560-011-0238-9

Curtis-Fawley, S., & Daly, K. (2005). Gendered violence and restorative justice: The views of victim advocates. *Violence Against Women, 11*(5), 603-638. doi:10.1177/1077801205274488

Drost, L., Haller, B., Hofinger, V., van der Kooij, T., Lunnermann, K., & Wolthuis, A. (2015). Restorative justice in cases of domestic violence. Retrieved November 2, 2015, from http://restorativejustice.org/rj-library/restorative-justice-in-cases-of-domestic-violence/11143/

Gavrielides, T., & Artinopoulou, V. (2013). Restorative justice and violence against women: Comparing Greece and the United Kingdom. *Asian Criminology, 8*(1), 25-40. doi:10.1007/s11417-011-9123-x

Goel, R. (2005). Sita's trousseau: Restorative justice, domestic violence, and South Asian culture. *Violence Against Women, 11*(5), 639-665. doi:10.1177/1077801205274522

Grauwiler, P., & Mills, L. G. (2004). Moving beyond the criminal justice paradigm: A radical restorative justice approach to intimate abuse. *Journal of Sociology & Social Welfare, 31*(1), 49-69.

Lawson, C. L., & Katz, J. (2004). Restorative justice: An alternative approach to juvenile crime. *Journal of Socio-Economics, 33*(2), 175-188. doi:10.1016/j.socec.2003.12.018

London, R. D. (2003). The restoration of trust: Bringing restorative justice from the margins to the mainstream. *Criminal Justice Studies, 16*(3), 175-195. doi:10.1080/0888431032000151844

Mills, L. G., Barocas, B., & Ariel, B. (2013). The next generation of court-mandated domestic violence treatment: A comparison study of batterer intervention and restorative justice program. *Journal of Experimental Criminology, 9*(1), 65-90. doi:10.1007/s11292-012-9164-x

Mutter, R., Shemmings, D., Dugmore, P., & Hyare, M. (2008). Family group conferences in youth justice. *Health & Social Care in the Community, 16*(3), 262-270. doi:10.1111/j.1365-2524.2008.00770.x

Hampton, R. L., La Tailade, J. J., Dacey, A., & Marghi, J. R. (2008). Evaluating domestic violence interventions for Black women. *Journal of Aggression, Maltreatment & Trauma, 16*(3), 330-353. doi:10.1080/10926770801925759

Herman, J. L. (2005). Justice from the victim's perspective. *Violence Against Women, 11*(5), 571-602. doi:10.1177/1077801205274450

Hudson, B. (2002). Restorative justice and gendered violence. *British Journal of Criminology, 42*(3), 616-634. doi:10.1093/bjc/42.3.616

International Federation of Social Workers. (2012, March 3). Statement of ethical principles. Retrieved December 8, 2015, from http://ifsw.org/policies/statement-of-ethical-principles

Mills, L. G., Barocas, B., & Ariel, B. (2013). The next generation of court-mandated domestic violence treatment: A comparison study of batterer intervention and restorative justice program. *Journal of Experimental Criminology, 9*(1), 65-90. doi:10.1007/s11292-012-9164-x

Pelikan, C. (2010). On the efficacy of victim-offender-mediation in cases of partnership violence in Austria, or: Men don't get better, but women get stronger: Is it still true?. *European Journal of Criminal Policy & Research, 16*(1), 49-67. doi:10.1007/s10610-010-9117-8

Presser, L., & Van Voorhis, P. (2002). Values and evaluation: Assessing processes and outcomes of restorative justice programs. *Crime & Delinquency, 48*(1), 162-188. doi:10.1177/0011128702048001007

Proietti-Scifoni, G., & Daly, K. (2011). Gendered violence and restorative justice: The views of New Zealand opinion leaders. *Contemporary Justice Review, 14*(3), 269-290. doi:10.1080/10282580.2011.589666

Rubin, P. (2003). Restorative justice in Nova Scotia: Women's experience and recommendations for positive policy development and implementation. Retrieved December 8, 2015, from www.nawl.ca/ns/en/documents/Pub_Brief_NSRestorativeJustice03_en.doc

Stubbs, J. (2007). Beyond apology? Domestic violence and critical questions for restorative justice. *Criminology and Criminal Justice, 7*(2), 169-187. doi:10.1177/1748895807075570

Sualnier, A., & Sivasubraniam, D. (2015). Effects of victim presence and coercion in restorative justice: An experimental paradigm. *Law and Human Behavior, 39*(4), 378-387. doi:10.1037/lhb0000130

Umbreit, M., Coates, R., & Vos, B. (2004). Victim-offender mediation: Three decades of practice and research. *Conflict Resolution Quarterly, 22*(1/2), 279-303. doi:10.1002/crq.102

United Nations. (2002). ECOSOC Resolution 2002/12 basic principles on the use of restorative justice programmes in criminal matters. Retrieved December 8, 2015, from http://www.un.org/en/ecosoc/docs/2002/resolution percent202002-12.pdf

Van Ness, D. W. (2005). An overview of restorative justice around the world. Retrieved December 8, 2015, from http://assets.justice.vic.gov.au/njc/resources/c4518c8a-c200-4623-afd1-42e255b62cf9/01+an+overview+of+restorative+justice.pdf

van Wormer, K. (2004). Restorative justice: A model for personal and societal empowerment. *Journal of Religion & Spirituality in Social Work, 23*(4), 103-120. doi:10.1300/J377v23n04_07

Wheeler, D. (2015). NASW standards and indicators for cultural competence in social work practice. Retrieved December 8, 2015, from http://www.socialworkers.org/practice/standards/PRA-BRO-253150-CC-Standards.pdf

World Health Organization/London School of Hygiene and Tropical Medicine. (2010). *Preventing intimate partner and sexual violence against women: Taking action and generating evidence.* Retrieved December 8, 2015, from http://whqlibdoc.who.int/publications/2010/9789241564007_eng.pdf

S

Schizoaffective Disorder

Major Categories: Behavioral & Mental Health

Description

Schizoaffective disorder is a mental disorder marked by characteristics of both schizophrenia and a major affective disorder, consisting of either a manic mood disorder or a depressive mood disorder. Whether or not schizoaffective disorder is a distinct disorder, apart from other mental disorders, is the subject of debate. Among the proposed explanations for its having symptoms of both schizophrenia and a mood disorder are that there exist two distinct groups of individuals with schizoaffective disorder, with one group meeting the diagnostic criteria for schizophrenia and incidentally having mood-related symptoms, and another group meeting the diagnostic criteria for a mood disorder and incidentally having symptoms of schizophrenia. Other explanations for schizoaffective disorder are that it represents a midpoint between schizophrenia and mood disorders on a continuum of mental disorders; that it consists of two distinct disorders occurring simultaneously; and that it is a completely distinct disorder unrelated to either schizophrenia or to mood disorders but sharing some symptoms of both.

As defined by the fifth edition of the *Diagnostic and Statistical Manual of Mental Disorders* (*DSM-5*), schizoaffective disorder is characterized by features of both schizophrenia and major episodes of either of the conditions known as a manic mood disorder or a depressive mood disorder. The criteria in the *DSM-5* for the diagnosis of schizoaffective disorder are drawn directly from the criteria in the *DSM-5* for schizophrenia and those for a major depressive or manic disorder, and require an uninterrupted period of either a major depressive or manic mood disorder accompanied by at least 2 weeks of any of the symptoms of schizophrenia, which consist of delusions, hallucinations, disorganized speech, grossly disorganized or catatonic behavior, or flattening of affect, absence of speech, or absence of motivation. The diagnosis of schizoaffective disorder in the *DSM-5* does not require the social impairment in work or in relationships that is needed for a diagnosis of schizophrenia.

The tenth revision of the *International Statistical Classification of Diseases and Related Health Problems* (*ICD-10*) also includes schizoaffective disorder, which it defines as a disorder characterized by the simultaneous presence of both an affective disorder and schizophrenialike symptoms. However, the diagnosis of a schizoaffective disorder as defined by the *ICD-10* does not require that the full criteria be met for a diagnosis of schizophrenia or either a manic or a depressive mood disorder, as is required by the *DSM-5*, but instead requires that symptoms of both schizophrenia and an affective disorder be present and prominent.

Schizoaffective disorder is particularly difficult to diagnose and treat, and its neurological and other biological characteristics are difficult to investigate. The timing of occurrence of its symptoms makes its initial diagnosis difficult, and changes in the severity and duration of its symptoms may lead to changes in its diagnosis from schizoaffective disorder to either schizophrenia or a mood disorder. Moreover, some studies do not distinguish schizoaffective disorder from schizophrenia, making it difficult to clarify etiologic factors and treatment outcomes specific to schizoaffective disorder. Differing views among individual clinicians and researchers about the nature and distinct characteristics of schizoaffective disorder further complicate its diagnosis, treatment, and investigation.

Because of the difficulty of distinguishing schizoaffective disorder from schizophrenia and mood disorders, it is the subject of research involving genetic, brain imaging, and electrophysiological studies to assist in clarifying and better defining its diagnosis. As this research continues, it may provide neurologic and other evidence for a more definitive diagnosis of schizoaffective disorder.

Although uncertainty attends the diagnosis of schizoaffective disorder as compared with that of schizophrenia and mood disorders, there is general agreement that its prognosis is usually poorer than that for mood disorders but slightly better than that for schizophrenia. Predictors of poor outcomes of schizoaffective disorder include an insidious onset (a gradual onset, in which its symptoms are well established before the diagnosis is apparent), an absence of precipitating factors for its occurrence in a particular individual, a poor level of functioning before its onset, an early age of onset, poor recovery between episodes of the disorder, and a predominance of psychotic symptoms in the disorder. There is no consensus about whether schizoaffective disorder should be treated pharmacologically with antipsychotic drugs, mood stabilizers, or antidepressant drugs, or a combination of medications belonging to one or more these three groups of agents. Education of the individual with schizoaffective disorder about adherence to a treatment regimen of medication for the disorder, and of the affected individual's family members, is recommended. Other treatments for schizoaffective disorder can include family therapy, training in social skills, and cognitive behavioral therapy (CBT).

FACTS AND FIGURES

The varying definitions of schizoaffective disorder and changes in the diagnostic criteria for it make calculations of its incidence and prevalence difficult. However, there is consensus that schizoaffective disorder is less common than schizophrenia, occurring approximately one third as often. The National Alliance on Mental Illness has stated that schizoaffective disorder occurs in approximately 0.3 percent of the population of the United States. The disorder may occur more often in women than in men, and may have a later age of onset in women than in men. Depressive features of the disorder are more common in older adults and in women.

RISK FACTORS

No risk factors have been identified that are specific for schizoaffective disorder and distinct from those for schizophrenia or mood disorders. Research into genetics and neurocognitive deficits as risk factors for schizoaffective disorder has been inconclusive. However, stressful life events (job loss, divorce, death in the family) or psychoactive drug use may trigger the onset of schizoaffective disorder.

SIGNS AND SYMPTOMS

The signs and symptoms of schizophrenia given in the *DSM-5* also apply to schizoaffective disorder, and consist of delusions, hallucinations, disorganized speech, grossly disorganized or catatonic behavior, negative symptoms (significantly reduced affect or expression of emotion, lethargy). A number of the signs and symptoms of major depressive or manic disorder given in the *DSM-5* also apply to schizoaffective disorder. Those for a major depressive disorder consist of a depressed mood during most of every day; a markedly decreased interest or pleasure in daily activities; significant weight loss; insomnia or hypersomnia; observable restlessness or lack of movement; fatigue or loss of energy; excessive feelings of worthlessness or guilt; indecisiveness; a decreased ability to concentrate; recurrent thoughts about death; and thoughts, plans, intentions, or attempts at suicide. Signs and symptoms of a manic disorder as given in *DSM-5* and which also apply to schizoaffective disorder are a distinct period of elevated, expansive, or irritable mood lasting for at least one week; grandiosity or inflated self-esteem; a decreased need for sleep; talkativeness; racing thoughts; distractibility; an increase in goal-oriented activity; and engagement in highly pleasurable and/or high-risk activities.

TREATMENT

The social worker assisting an individual in whom a diagnosis of schizoaffective disorder has been made as comorbidities should conduct a standard biological, psychological, social, and spiritual assessment of the individual, including an assessment of his or her risk for suicide and for inflicting harm on him- or herself and others. The social worker should observe the individual's functioning and demeanor during the assessment, with particular attention to distinguishing symptoms of schizophrenia and those of mood disorder from one another, and with particular attention to the timing and overlapping of symptoms of each type of disorder. The assessment should also include the collection of collateral information from the treated individual's family, friends, and co-workers, as well as evaluation of the treated individual's living situation and referrals if and as needed to appropriate sources of assistance.

Treatment of schizoaffective disorder may vary according to the prominence of different symptoms at different times. It is particularly important with schizoaffective disorder to note and report changes in symptoms and behavior in order to find an effective medication regimen. There is no consensus as to whether the disorder should be treated with antipsychotic, mood-stabilizing, or antidepressant medications, or a combination of two or more of these types of medication, but the social worker should schedule an appointment of an individual with schizoaffective disorder with a mental health professional who can prescribe the appropriate medications if and as needed. and close monitoring for side effects, changes in symptoms, and efficacy. The social worker should follow up on the adherence to any regimen of medication with the individual being treated, including discussion of the importance of adhering to prescribed dosages and times of medication and periodic assessment for any risk of suicide or other harm to the self.

Problems in the treatment of schizoaffective disorder can include nonadherence to a regimen of medication prescribed for it and a loss of family and/or peer support of the individual with the disorder. Nonadherence should be addressed by education of the affected individual about the nature of the disorder and the importance of a medication regimen prescribed for it. Loss of family/peer support should be addressed by education of the affected individual's family and peers about schizoaffective disorder, including education about its complex and changing nature, the various treatments available for it, and community resources that can provide support in cases of the disorder. This should including the teaching of stress management techniques and problem solving skills to the family, and the encouragement of self-care and mutual support within family, including the enhancement of communication skills.

Social workers assisting individuals with schizoaffective disorder and their families and peers should be aware of their own cultural values, beliefs, and biases, and develop specialized knowledge about these people's histories, traditions, and values. They should adopt treatment methods that reflect their knowledge of the cultural diversity of the communities in which they provide this assistance.

APPLICABLE LAWS AND REGULATIONS

The U.S. government and individual states have their own standards, procedures, and laws for the involuntary restraint and detention of persons who may be a danger to themselves or to others. Because the rate of attempted suicide is high among individuals with schizoaffective disorder and schizophrenia, knowledge of local requirements for involuntary detention is important. Local requirements for reporting the neglect and abuse of schizoaffective individuals should also be known.

SERVICES AND RESOURCES
- Brain & Behavior Research Foundation (formerly NARSAD), https://bbrfoundation.org/
- National Alliance on Mental Illness (NAMI), http://www.nami.org/
- National Institute of Mental Health (NIMH), http://www.nimh.nih.gov/index.shtml

Written by Chris Bates, MA, MSW

Reviewed by Jessica Therivel, LMSW-IPR, and Pedram Samghabadi

REFERENCES

American Psychiatric Association. (2013). *Diagnostic and statistical manual of mental disorders: DMS-5* (5th ed.). Arlington, VA: Author.
British Association of Social Workers. (2012, January). The code of ethics for social work: Statement of principles. Retrieved April 11, 2016, from http://cdn.basw.co.uk/upload/basw_112315-7.pdf
Feiner, J. S., & Frese, F. J. (2009). Recovery in schizophrenia. In B. J. Sadock, V. A. Sadock, & P. Ruiz (Eds.), *Kaplan & Sadocks's comprehensive textbook of psychiatry* (9th ed., Vol. 1, pp. 1582-1593). Philadelphia, PA: Wolters Kluwer Health/Lippincott Williams & Wilkins.
International Federation of Social Workers. (2012). Statement of ethical principles. Retrieved

April 11, 2016, from http://ifsw.org/policies/statement-of-ethical-principles/

Jager, M., Becker, T., Weinmann, S., & Frasch, K. (2010). Treatment of schizoaffective disorder - A challenge for evidence-based psychiatry. *Acta Psychiatrica Scandinavica, 121*(1), 22-32. doi:10.1111/j.1600-0447.2009.01424.x

Jager, M., Haack, S., Becker, T., & Frasch, K. (2011). Schizoaffective disorder - An ongoing challenge for psychiatric nosology. *European Psychiatry, 26*(3), 159-165. doi:10.1016/j.eurpsy.2010.03.010

Kantrowitz, J. T., & Citrome, L. (2011). Schizoaffective disorder: A review of current research themes and pharmacological management. *CNS Drugs, 25*(4), 317-331. doi:10.2165/11587630-000000000-00000

Lewandowski, K. E., Eack, S. M., Hogarty, S. S., Greenwald, D. P., & Keshavan, M. S. (2011). Is cognitive enhancement therapy equally effective for patients with schizophrenia and schizoaffective disorder? *Schizophrenia Research, 125*(2-3), 291-294. doi:10.1016/j.schres.2010.11.017

National Alliance on Mental Illness (NAMI). (n.d.). Schizoaffective disorder. Retrieved April 11, 2016, from https://www.nami.org/Learn-More/Mental-Health-Conditions/Schizoaffective-Disorder

Sadock, B. J., Sadock, V. A., & Ruiz, P. (2015). In *Kaplan & Sadock's synopsis of psychiatry: Behavioral sciences/clinical psychiatry* (11th ed., pp. 323-326). Philadelphia, PA: Wolters Kluwer.

Wheeler, D. (2015). NASW standards and indicators for cultural competence in social work practice. Retrieved April 11, 2016, from http://www.socialworkers.org/practice/standards/PRA-BRO-253150-CC-Standards.pdf

Yang, L. P. H. (2011). Oral paliperidone: A review of its use in the management of schizoaffective disorder. *CNS Drugs, 25*(6), 523-538. doi:10.2165/11207440-000000000-00000

SCHIZOID PERSONALITY DISORDER

MAJOR CATEGORIES: Behavioral & Mental Health

DESCRIPTION

Schizoid personality disorder (SPD) is one of ten diagnosable personality disorders that appear in the *Diagnostic and Statistical Manual of Mental Disorders*, Fifth Edition (*DSM-5*); it is grouped with paranoid personality disorder and schizotypal personality disorder to form the Cluster A personality disorders, which share the appearance of eccentricity and oddness. The *DSM-5* general criteria for all 10 personality disorders include significant variation in behavior and internal life experience from one's own cultural norms in at least two of the following areas: cognition, affectivity, interpersonal functioning, and impulse control; a long-term and consistent history across a variety of life situations apparent since at least adolescence that has caused significant disturbances in functioning in important areas of life and which could be described as an abiding pattern; and the abiding pattern is not caused by another mental health disorder, including substance use disorder(s), impact of medications, or a medical condition. The specific criteria for SPD are an absolute lack of interest or concern about social relations and a severely limited display of emotions when with people. An individual must have four of the specific criteria that enumerate examples of social detachment and emotional flatness (does not seek or enjoy close relationships, prefers a limited number of solo activities, does not have intimate relationships, seems to not care what other people think of him or her, shows little or no emotion). Also, these criteria do not occur in association with a diagnosis of schizophrenia, bipolar or depressive disorders, other psychotic disorders, or the autism spectrum. The absence of delusions and hallucinations distinguishes SPD from psychotic disorders. Individuals with SPD may appear aimless, directionless, or disinterested, behave inappropriately (by underreacting) in social situations, have a notable absence of friends and have disrupted relationships with family, and have difficulty functioning in workplaces that require interpersonal interactions. Many of the signs and symptoms of SPD overlap the negative signs and symptoms of schizophrenia.

Personality is generally agreed to refer to the internal organization and evolution of an individual's psychobiological and social inheritance and learning that enable him or her to live in, and adapt to, a constantly changing world. To make evaluation easier, personality can be broken down into three components: temperament (how one responds to outside stimuli), character (one's self-concept, motivation, and object relations), and psyche (intuitive self-awareness, consciousness, and spirit). An individual's personality is a complex arrangement (and continuous rearrangement) of elements of temperament such as harm avoidance, novelty seeking, reward dependence, and persistence; of character such as self-directedness, cooperativeness, and self-transcendence; and of psyche such as memory or recollection, awareness, hopefulness, aesthetic sense, and spirituality. To be considered disordered, the sum of these elements must be dysfunctional on both an individual level and a social level, and the personality elements usually are inflexible. Furthermore, persons with personality disorders lack awareness that there are problems in their personal or social functioning.

Controversy surrounds the personality disorders and is reflected by the inclusion in the *DSM-5* of a chapter entitled "Alternative DSM-5 Model for Personality Disorders" in Section 3, "Emerging Measures and Models." The alternative model was introduced to address shortcomings in the current model, including that many individuals simultaneously meet the criteria for several personality disorders and that the general categories of "other specified" or "unspecified" are the most often diagnosed and are uninformative about the individual. A larger question about the personality disorder diagnosis is its categorical nature (meaning either the criteria are met and there is a disorder/diagnosis, or the criteria are not met and there is no disorder/diagnosis) as opposed the dimensional nature (meaning that personality traits occur along a continuum from not present at all to having overwhelming impact) of actual human behavior and lives. The *DSM-5* personality disorders remain

categorical, yet the alternative model introduces the concept of dimensional assessment. Another issue of contention is the theory that personality disorders are actually a point on the continuum of a larger mental health disorder, usually at the less impactful end of a dimensional model. In particular, some researchers contend that SPD is the early stages of schizophrenia rather than the discrete disorder described in the *DSM*, or a stable variant of schizophrenia that does not include delusions or hallucinations.

The etiology of SPD is unresolved, with most literature attributing it to an interaction of genetically inherited traits and environmental influences. Because SPD is diagnosed in few persons, and because the diagnosis can be unreliable due to subjective and vague criteria as well as errors due to limited experience with SPD by assessors, the progression and prognosis of the disorder are not well understood. Additionally, individuals with SPD rarely seek treatment unless there is another mental health disorder present, which complicates assessment, treatment, and research into SPD. The viability of treatment for personality disorders is the subject of debate, with some literature claiming that individuals with personality disorders are unreceptive to treatment and other literature asserting that the problem with treatment lies with professionals who blame their countertransference and lack of success on the individuals with personality disorders.

FACTS AND FIGURES

Given the negative nature of many of the criteria (the criteria cite absence, lack, indifference), which makes diagnosis and measurement difficult, and the fact that individuals with SPD rarely seek treatment, there are few generally agreed-upon facts and figures about SPD. Different studies have found prevalence rates of SPD in the general population ranging from 0.5 to 7 percent. Two generally agreed-upon facts are that SPD is among the least-often diagnosed personality disorders and that when it does occur it is more often found in men. An analysis of data about 2,619 patients in the Norwegian Network of Personality-Focused Treatment Programs revealed 19 (0.7 percent) with

SPD, the second least-occurring after histrionic personality disorder; a higher rate for men (1.3 percent) than for women (0.5 percent); and only two patients with a diagnosis of SPD alone, with the paranoid and obsessive-compulsive personality disorders those most frequently co-occurring with SPD.

RISK FACTORS

As with all other aspects of SPD, risk factors are complicated by the debate around the nature of the disorder and the relatively few cases. However, there is a generally agreed-upon higher risk for individuals with first-degree relatives in whom schizophrenia or schizotypal personality disorder has been diagnosed. Various environmental factors have been researched without conclusive findings, including emotionally inadequate parenting and childhoods marked by neglect.

SIGNS AND SYMPTOMS

Signs and symptoms include a preference for solitary activities, lack of friendships or relationships of any kind with the possible exception of immediate family, social detachment, limited and restricted emotional expression, appearing distant and aloof, being difficult to engage, and a lack of awareness or concern about any of these traits.

ASSESSMENT

Professionals may perform a standard bio-psycho-social-spiritual history including risk for suicide, observe functioning and demeanor during interview, and gather collateral information from family, friends, and coworkers (especially important because individuals frequently have limited insight into the oddness of their behavior and rarely believe there is any disruption of functioning).

Care should be used with self-reporting screening tools due to the general lack of insight. These tools are not specific to SPD but are used for general measurement of personality dysfunction and may include Structured Interview for DSM-IV Personality (SIDP-IV), Personality Diagnostic Questionnaire-Revised (PDQ-R), Minnesota Multiphasic Personality Inventory (MMPI), Millon Clinical Multiaxial Inventory (MCMI), and Temperament and Character Inventory (TCI).

Tests for the presence of alcohol or other substances at levels indicating abuse may be useful.

TREATMENT

Individuals with SPD rarely seek treatment, and if they do it is likely that another mental health disorder or a need for social services has prompted them. Usually it is difficult to engage individuals in whom SPD has been diagnosed in treatment because of the nature of the disorder: an absolute lack of interest in interpersonal interactions and relationships. Also, lack of insight and concern about dysfunction further complicates engagement and progress in treatment, which may cause clinicians to lose interest in treatment. A commonly repeated myth holds that individuals with personality disorders are untreatable, or that personality disorders are inflexible and cannot be treated. In fact, research shows that progress can be made if barriers to treatment are not erected. The three most common barriers are strong and counterproductive feelings of countertransference, belief (and covert communication of that belief to the individual being treated) in the myth of untreatability, and giving direct and specific advice on social functioning or personal problems, which usually produces dependence, noncompliance, or resentment.

Countertransference during treatment with an individual with SPD may be rooted in the individual's disconnection and disinterest in personal relationships, which is directly contrary to most professional caregivers' beliefs about relationship. Clinicians may feel inadequate, incompetent, hopeless, frustrated, and pessimistic about the outcome of treatment and may feel that the person might be better off with a different clinician. A first step in treatment of SPD is collaborative goal-setting about treatment. There is no consensus on the use of medications in the treatment of SPD, although since other mental health disorders usually are present medications may be used to treat them.

Professionals may also review the medication regimen and make follow-up appointment with the agency issuing the prescription, assess the stability of employment and living situation, refer to an appropriate treatment modality, and provide referrals for support and education for family members.

Problem	Goal	Intervention
Inappropriate social interactions and difficulty in situations requiring interpersonal interactions, such as at work.	Learn social and cognitive skills to successfully interact with people.	Cognitive-behavioral and social skills training using thought recording, role-playing, group social-skills training, or cognitive-behavioral therapies (CBTs) as appropriate. All interventions for SPD will depend on initial establishment of a therapeutic relationship.
Lack of engagement in or pleasure from the daily activities of life.	Engage in daily activities and relationships and pleasure of life.	Existential therapy to engage in discussion about the meaning of life and seek insight into one's existence or psychodynamic therapy to address unresolved issues from childhood.

APPLICABLE LAWS AND REGULATIONS

Each jurisdiction (nation, state, province) has its own standards, procedures, and laws for involuntary restraint and detention of persons who may be a danger to themselves or others. Individuals with SPD generally are not at higher risk of this danger; however, because there frequently are other mental health disorders present, and some theories hold that SPD is an early stage of schizophrenia, assessment should include this danger. Local and professional reporting requirements for neglect and abuse should also be known and observed.

SERVICES AND RESOURCES

- National Alliance on Mental Illness (NAMI), http://www.nami.org/
- U.S. National Institutes of Health (NIH), http://www.nih.gov/
- U.S. National Institute of Mental Health (NIMH), http://www.nimh.nih.gov/index.shtml
- National Association of Social Workers (NASW), http://www.socialworkers.org/

FOOD FOR THOUGHT

Different cultures value different levels of engagement and interaction in social situations. In fact, in some contexts an individual displaying the traits of SPD might be considered to be at a higher state of being. For example, Buddhist monks practice meditation in part to experience freedom from emotions, attachment, and striving, all of which could be observed while assessing for SPD. Cultural as well as professional expectations about acceptable levels of interpersonal interaction and affective demonstration vary greatly.

RED FLAGS

Individuals with SPD may engender strong positive or negative feelings that may lead to countertransference.

SPD may be difficult to diagnose because it is hard to distinguish from other Cluster A personality disorders, from prodromal schizophrenia, and from avoidant personality disorder.

Written by Chris Bates, MA, MSW

Reviewed by Pedram Samghabadi

REFERENCES

Ahmed, A. O., Green, B. A., Buckley, P. F., & McFarland, M. E. (2012). Taxometric analyses of paranoid and schizoid personality disorders. *Psychiatry Research, 196*(1), 123-132. doi:10.1016/j.psychres.2011.10.010

American Psychiatric Association. (2013). Diagnostic and statistical manual of mental disorders: (DSM-5). (5th ed.). Arlington, VA: American Psychiatric Publishing.

Bockian, N. R. (2006). Depression in schizoid personality disorder. In N. R. Bockian (Ed.), *Personality-guided therapy for* (pp. 63-90). Washington, DC: American Psychological Association.

Bostrom, C. E. (2011). Personality disorders. In N. L. Keltner, C. E. Bostrom, & T. M. McGuinness (Eds.), *Psychiatric nursing* (6th ed., pp. 343-354). St. Louis, MO: Elsevier Mosby.

Cloninger, C. R., & Svrakic, D. R. (2009). Personality disorders. In B. J. Sadock, V. A. Sadock, & P. Ruiz (Eds.), *Kaplan & Sadock's comprehensive textbook of psychiatry* (9th ed., Vol. 2, pp. 2197-2240). Philadelphia, PA: Lippincott Williams & Wilkins.

Colli, A., Tanzilli, A., Dimaggio, G., & Lingiardi, V. (2014). Patient personality and therapist response: An empirical investigation. *American Journal of Psychiatry, 171*(1), 102-108. doi:10.1176/appi.ajp.2013.13020224

HUmmelen, B., Pedersen, G., Wilberg, T., & Karterud, S. (2015). Poor validity of the DSM-IV schizoid personality disorder construct as a diagnostic category. *Journal of Personality Disorders, 29*(3), 334-346. doi:10.1521/pedi_2014_28_159

Lenzenweger, M. F., & Willett, J. B. (2009). Does change in temperament predict change in schizoid personality disorder? A methodological framework and illustration from the Longitudinal Study of Personality Disorders. *Development and Psychopathology, 21*(4), 1211-1231. doi:10.1017/S0954579409990125

Mittal, V. A., Kalus, O., Bernstein, D. P., & Siever, L. J. (2007). Schizoid personality disorder. In W. O'Donohue, K. A. Fowler, & S. O. Lilienfeld (Eds.), *Personality disorders: Towards the DSM-V* (pp. 63-79). Thousand Oaks, CA: Sage Publications.

Sadock, B.J., Sadock, V.A., & Ruiz, P. (2015). Personality disorders. In *Kaplan & Sadocks Synopsis of Psychiatry: Behavioral Sciences/Clinical Psychiatry* (11th ed., pp. 746-745). Philadelphia, PA: Wolters Kluwer Health/Lippincott Williams & Wilkins.

Silverstein, M. L. (2007). Descriptive psychopathology and theoretical viewpoints: Schizoid, schizotypal, and avoidant personality disorders. In M. L. Silverstein (Ed.), *Disorders of the self: A personality-guided approach* (pp. 61-72). Washington, DC: American Psychological Association.

Silverstein, M. L. (2007). A self psychological viewpoint: Schizoid, schizotypal, and avoidant personality disorders. In M. L. Silverstein (Ed.), *Disorders of the self: A personality-guided approach* (pp. 73-94). Washington, DC: American Psychological Association.

Thylstrup, B, & Hesse, M. (2009). "I am not complaining" – ambivalence construct in schizoid personality disorder. *American Journal of Psychotherapy, 63*(2), 147-167.

Townsend, M. C. (2015). Personality disorders. In *Psychiatric Mental Health Nursing: Concepts of Care in Evidence-Based Practice* (8th ed., pp. 673-674). Philadelphia, PA: F. A. Davis Company.

SCHIZOPHRENIA & CIGARETTE SMOKING

MAJOR CATEGORIES: Behavioral & Mental Health, Substance Abuse

DESCRIPTION

The rate of tobacco use, and particularly the smoking of cigarettes, is disproportionately high among individuals with schizophrenia. The theory that smoking, as a form of self-medication, eases symptoms of schizophrenia is widely used to explain its relatively high prevalence among persons with this mental disorder, and data confirm that as compared with smokers who do not have schizophrenia, those with schizophrenia smoke more cigarettes per day, inhale more often and more deeply when smoking, have higher levels of nicotine in their blood, and spend a greater percentage of their income on cigarettes.

Among persons with schizophrenia, as among those without it, the increased smoking of cigarettes is accompanied by an increased risk of the adverse effects of smoking on health. Examples of this are the two- to threefold greater rates of lung cancer, chronic obstructive pulmonary disease (COPD), and cardiovascular disease among smokers with schizophrenia as compared with those without it. In fact, about half of all deaths of persons with schizophrenia can be attributed to tobacco-related diseases, and the effects of smoking on persons with schizophrenia may include a greater severity of akathisia (a state of motor restlessness and/or inner distress) or tardive dyskinesia (random movements of muscles of the face, jaw, and limbs) as effects of this mental disorder, an increase in its psychiatric symptoms, a reduced efficacy of psychiatric medications in treating it, and an increased risk of the use of other substances and of substance use disorder among persons with schizophrenia.

Moreover, smokers with schizophrenia face greater barriers to stopping smoking than do other smokers. These barriers include the use of cigarettes and other forms of tobacco as behavioral rewards in some settings of mental healthcare, a reduced focus on smoking cessation among healthcare professionals who treat individuals with schizophrenia, a failure to tailor smoking cessation programs to the personal characteristics and circumstances of individuals with schizophrenia, in addition to the hypothesis that smoking eases symptoms of schizophrenia.

Although the etiology of schizophrenia is unknown, several theories account for the increased rate of smoking among persons with this disorder. The most common of these is is the self-medication theory, which, as noted earlier, posits that smoking helps to relieve both positive (symptoms not normally seen in healthy people, such as delusions and hallucinations) and negative (disruptions of normal behaviors and emotions) symptoms of schizophrenia. This is based on the effect of nicotine on dopamine and other neurotransmitters in the reward pathways of the brain. Conversely, research has also and recently suggested that rather than schizophrenia prompting smoking, smoking triggers the development of schizophrenia and other disorders of mental health. In support of this have been recent clinical trials showing the success of a combination of psychotherapy and cognitive behavioral therapy (CBT) for smoking cessation. Other treatment interventions for smoking cessation in persons with schizophrenia, albeit with less successful outcomes, have included individualized nicotine replacement plans, motivational treatment and reward (monetary) systems, and intensive cessation programs.

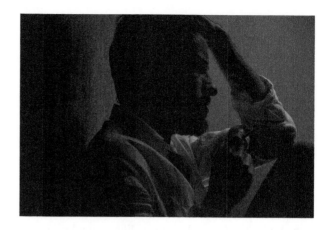

FACTS AND FIGURES

Approximately 70 to 80 percent of persons with schizophrenia smoke, as opposed to 20 to 30 percent of the overall population. Smokers with schizophrenia have twice the risk of coronary heart disease, spend more of their monthly income on tobacco, are 10 times more likely to be daily smokers, and achieve higher systemic doses of nicotine at a faster rate than smokers in the general population. Several studies have reported increased rates of abstinence among smokers with serious mental illnesses, including schizophrenia, through the combined use of CBT and varenicline, a substance that partly blocks the body's receptors for nicotine in the nervous system, thus acting to block the muscle contraction that nicotine stimulates.

RISK FACTORS

Although risk factors exist both for the development of schizophrenia and for smoking, no consensus exists about how these factors may interact with one another to promote or exacerbate each of these conditions. Furthermore, schizophrenia and smoking, in and of themselves, are considered risk factors for one another.

Biologically, risk factors for schizophrenia include a genetic predisposition to it, hyperactivity of the components of the brain and nervous system that depend on dopamine for the transmission of signals between nerves, a decreased brain size, premature birth or excessive maternal bleeding during birth, traumatic brain injury, and maternal exposure to trauma in the first trimester of pregnancy. Environmental risk factors for schizophrenia are a low socioeconomic status, family dysfunction, exposure to trauma, and birth in winter or early spring; social stigma and isolation associated with a diagnosis of schizophrenia may exacerbate its symptoms.

Risk factors for beginning and continuing cigarette smoking include peer pressure, low self-esteem, a low socioeconomic status, nicotine addiction, and discomfort upon withdrawal from the use of nicotine.

SIGNS AND SYMPTOMS

Symptoms of schizophrenia include disordered thoughts and speech; sudden stopping of speech followed by its resumption on a different topic; long pauses in speech; delusions and visual and/or auditory hallucinations; the stuporlike state known as catatonia; failure to show emotion; an inability to feel pleasure; social withdrawal; and in some cases violent behavior. Signs and symptoms of smoking may include a tobacco odor of the breath and clothing; nicotine stains on the fingers and teeth; shortness of breath; a persistent cough; and hoarseness of the voice.

TREATMENT

The social worker assisting an individual who is both a smoker and has schizophrenia should conduct a standard biological, psychological, social, and spiritual assessment of the individual, including an assessment of his or her risk for suicide and for inflicting harm on him- or herself and others. This should include a determination of the individual's current and lifetime use of cigarettes and other forms of tobacco, as well as the collection of information on any prior diagnoses of disorders other than schizophrenia. The assessment should also include a history of any smoking-related medical problems experienced by the individual, with laboratory tests ordered as appropriate for smoking-related diseases or conditions, and the collection of collateral information from the individual's family, friends, and coworkers.

Treatment for concurrent schizophrenia and nicotine addiction can follow any of several paths. Persons who lack the motivation to stop smoking despite knowing its consequences on health may benefit from motivational interviewing, which seeks to change a particular behavior, such as smoking, by helping those who exhibit it to explore and resolve ambivalent feelings that keep them tied to the habit. Alternatively, a lack of motivation to stop smoking can be treated with psychoeducation focused on the effects of smoking and the benefits of its cessation, or through personalized feedback about smoking habits, provided in person or by handheld computers or other devices on the basis of information specific to the individual being treated. Individuals with schizophrenia who have intense cravings for nicotine or are experiencing adverse effects of the interaction of nicotine and antipsychotic medications can be treated with measured, diminishing doses of nicotine delivered by patch or nasal spray and calibrated to the types and doses of medications being given to such an individual.

The approach to smoking cessation in schizophrenia known as Treatment for Addiction to Nicotine in Schizophrenia (TANS) incorporates aspects of motivational interviewing, training in social skills, nicotine replacement medication, and relapse prevention. Programs based on this approach involve six months of weekly sessions ending with abstinence from nicotine. These programs emphasize the use of nicotine replacement patches, individualized feedback, and increasing awareness, by persons with schizophrenia, of social cues that encourage them to smoke.

Persons who smoke and have schizophrenia should be referred as needed for medical care and to local support groups for schizophrenia and smoking cessation, and should also be provided with referrals as needed for support of their living situations and for their family members.

Social workers treating individuals who have both schizophrenia and a smoking habit should be aware of their own cultural values, beliefs, and biases, and develop specialized knowledge about these individuals' histories, traditions, and values. They should adopt treatment methods that incorporate knowledge of these individuals' personal and cultural attributes.

APPLICABLE LAWS AND REGULATIONS

The U. S. government and individual states have their own standards, procedures, and laws for the involuntary restraint and detention of persons who may be a danger to themselves or to others. Because persons with schizophrenia have a high rate of attempted suicide, and, albeit rarely, may be dangerous to others, familiarity with the local requirements for their involuntary detention is highly important in case this should be needed.

Many jurisdictions and facilities have laws and regulations restricting smoking. It is important to know and enforce these laws and regulations while also not alienating smokers as persons needing treatment for smoking and other disorders, such as schizophrenia, since doing so may lead them to refuse to seek treatment or to discontinue ongoing treatment.

SERVICES AND RESOURCES

- American Cancer Society, http://www.cancer.org/
- Brain & Behavior Research Foundation (formerly NARSAD), http://bbrfoundation.org/
- National Alliance on Mental Illness (NAMI), http://www.nami.org/
- U.S. National Institutes of Health (NIH), http://www.nih.gov/
- U.S. National Institute of Mental Health (NIMH), http://www.nimh.nih.gov/index.shtml
- National Association of Social Workers (NASW), http://www.socialworkers.org/

Written by Chris Bates, MA, MSW

Reviewed by Lynn B. Cooper, D Crim

REFERENCES

Ahlers, E., Hahn, E., Ta, T. M., Goudarzi, E., Dettling, M., & Neuhaus, A. H. (2014). Smoking improves divided attention in schizophrenia. *Psychopharmacology, 231*(19), 3871-3877. doi:10.1007/s00213-0143525-2

Berk, M., Henry, L. P., Elkins, K. S., Harrigan, S. M., Harris, M. G., Herrman, H., & McGorry, P. D. (2010). The impact of smoking on clinical outcomes after first episode psychosis: Longer-term outcome findings from the EPPIC 800 follow-up study. *Journal of Dual Diagnosis, 6*(3-4), 212-234.

Caponetto, P., Polosa, R., Auditore, R., Minutolo, G., Signorelli, M., Maglia, M., & Aguglia, E. (2014). Smoking cessation and reduction in schizophrenia (SCARIS) with e-cigarette: Study protocol for a randomized control trial. *Trials, 15*, 88-95. doi:10.1186/1745-6215-15-88

Cuijpers, P., Smit, F., ten Have, M., & de Graaf, R. (2007). Smoking is associated with first-ever incidence of mental disorders: A prospective population-based study. *Addiction, 102*(8), 1203-1309.

Evins, A. E., Cather, C., Pratt, S. A., Pachas, G. N., Hoeppner, S. S., Goff, D. C., ... Schoenfield, D. A. (2014). Maintenance treatment with varenicline for smoking cessation in patients with schizophrenia and bipolar disorder: A randomized clinical trial. *JAMA, 311*(2), 145-154. doi:10.1001/jama.2013.285113

Evins, A. E., Hong, L. E., & Kelly, D. L. (2014). T. Kishi and N. Iwata: Varenicline for smoking cessation in people with schizophrenia: Systematic review meta-analysis. *European Archives of Psychiatry and Clinical Neuroscience, 265*(3), 269-270. doi:10.1007/s00406-014-0556-y

Freeman, T. P., Stone, J. M., Orgaz, B., Noronha, L. A., Minchin, S. L., & Curran, H. V. (2014). Tobacco smoking in schizophrenia: Investigating the role of incentive salience. *Psychological Medicine, 44*(10), 2189-2197. doi:10.1017/S0033291713002705

International Federation of Social Workers. (2012). Statement of ethical principles. Retrieved June 16, 2014, from http://ifsw.org/policies/statement-of-ethical-principles/

Jamal, A., Agaku, I. T., O'Connor, E., King, B. A., Kenemer, J. B., & Neff, L. (2014). Current cigarette smoking among adults – United States, 2005-2013. *Morbidity and Mortality Weekly Report (MMWR), 63*(47), 1108-1112.

Lee, J., Green, M. F., Calkins, M. E., Greenwood, T. A., Gur, R. E., ... Braff, D. L. (2014). Verbal working memory in schizophrenia from the Consortium on the Genetics of Schizophrenia (COGS) Study: The moderating role of smoking status and antipsychotic medications. *Schizophrenia Research, 161*(1-3), 24-31. doi:10.1016/j.schres.2014.08.014

Martins, S. S., & Gorelick, D. A. (2011). Conditional substance abuse and dependence by diagnosis of mood or anxiety disorder or schizophrenia in the U.S. population. *Drug and Alcohol Dependence, 119*(1-2), 28-36. doi:10.1016/j.drugalcdep.2011.05.010

Mizrahi, T., & Mayden, R. W. (2001). NASW standards for cultural competence in social work practice. Retrieved June 16, 2014, from http://www.naswdc.org/practice/standards/NASWcultural-standards.pdf

Moss, T. G., Sacco, K. A., Allen, T. M., Weinberger, A. H., Vessicchio, J. C., & George, T. P. (2009). Prefrontal cognitive dysfunction is associated with tobacco dependence treatment failure in smokers with schizophrenia. *Drug and Alcohol Dependence, 104*(1-2), 94-99. doi:10.1016/j. drugalcdep.2009.04.005

Robson, D., Keen, S., & Mauro, P. (2008). Physical health and dual diagnosis. *Advances in Dual Diagnosis, 1*(1), 27-32.

Schneider, C. E., White, T., Hass, J., Geisler, D., Wallace, S. R., Roessner, V., ... Ehrlich, S. (2014). Smoking status as a potential confounder in the study of brain structure in schizophrenia. *Journal of Psychiatric Research, 50*(84). doi:10.1016/j. jpsychires.2013.12.004

Steinberg, M. L., & Williams, J. (2007). Psychosocial treatments for individuals with schizophrenia and tobacco dependence. *Journal of Dual Diagnosis, 3*(3/4), 99-112.

Strube, W., Bunse, T., Nitsche, M. A., Wobrock, T., Aborowa, R., Misewitsch, K., & Hasan, A. (2014). Smoking restores impaired LTD-like plasticity in schizophrenia: a transcranial direct current stimulation study. *Neuropsychopharmacology, 40*(4), 822-830. doi:10.1038/npp.2014.275

Tantirangsee, N., Assanangkornchai, S., & Marsden, J. (2015). Effects of a brief intervention for substance use on tobacco smoking and family relationship functioning in schizophrenia and related psychoses: A randomised controlled trial. *Journal of Substance Abuse Treatment, 51*, 30-37. doi:10.1016/j. jsat.2014.10.011

The Policy, Ethics, and Human Rights Committee, British Association of Social Workers. (2012, January). The code of ethics for social work: Statement of principles. Retrieved June 16, 2014, from http:// cdn.basw.co.uk/upload/basw_112315-7.pdf

Tidey, J. W., & Williams, J. (2007). Clinical indices of tobacco use in people with schizophrenia. *Journal of Dual Diagnosis, 3*(3/4), 79-98.

Williams, J. M., Gandhi, K. K., Karavidas, M. K., Steinberg, M. L., Lu, S. E., & Foulds, J. (2008). Open-label study of craving in smokers with schizophrenia using nicotine nasal spray compared to nicotine patch. *Journal of Dual Diagnosis, 4*(4), 355-376.

Williams, J. M., Gandhi, K. K., Lu, S. E., Kumar, S., Shen, J., Foulds, J., & Benowitz, N. L. (2010). Higher nicotine levels in schizophrenia compared with controls after smoking a single cigarette. *Nicotine & Tobacco Research, 12*(8), 855-859.

Xu, Y. M., Chenn, H. H., Li, F., Deng, F., Liu, X. B., Yang, H. C., ... Liu, T. B. (2014). Prevalence and correlates of cigarette smoking among Chinese schizophrenia inpatients receiving antipsychotic mono-therapy. *Plos One, 9*(2). doi:10.1371/ journal.pone.0088478

Ziedonis, D., Parks, J., Zimmermann, M. H., & McCabe, P. (2007). Program and system level interventions to address tobacco amongst individuals with schizophrenia. *Journal of Dual Diagnosis, 3*(3/4), 151-175.

SCHIZOPHRENIA & SUBSTANCE USE DISORDER

MAJOR CATEGORIES: Behavioral & Mental Health, Substance Abuse

DESCRIPTION

The term *comorbidity* describes concurrent diagnoses of two concurrent disorders in a particular individual within time criteria specified by the diagnostic requirements for each of the two types of disorder. The diagnosis of both schizophrenia and a substance use disorder (SUD) is an example of a comorbidity. In this context, it is important to note that both in research and clinically, the specific circumstances, diagnosis, and treatment of multiple mental health disorders occurring simultaneously are much more complex than the term *comorbidity* implies.

It is also important to note that in the fifth edition of the *Diagnostic and Statistical Manual of Mental Disorders* (*DSM-5*), the chapter on disorders related to the intake of various substances, which bears the title "Substance-Related and Addictive Disorders," divides substance-related disorders into the two groups of SUDs and substance-induced disorders (intoxication, withdrawal, and other substance-/ medication-induced mental disorders), removing the distinction between substance abuse and substance dependence that was used in describing these disorders in the fourth edition of the manual (*DSM-IV*). Instead, the *DSM-5* divides each of the types of substance-related disorders into mild, moderate, and severe subtypes.

Individually, schizophrenia and SUD are chronic, progressive disorders that may have a severe effect on an individual's daily functioning, physical health, education, employment, social and family relationships, personal well-being, safety, and happiness. The effect of the combination of the two disorders is more severe than that of either of the disorders alone, and often produces more severe and chronic symptoms. Further possible effects of this comorbidity are a decrease in adherence to prescribed regimens of medication, an increase in the side effects of medications caused by their interaction with nonprescribed medicinal or other substances or alcohol, an exacerbation of psychotic symptoms, a decreased reliability of both self-reported symptoms and substance use, a relapse of substance use, increased rehospitalizations, increased involvement in the criminal justice system, pathological impulsivity, and increased exposure to violence both as a victim and a perpetrator of it, as well as exacerbation of the effects of each of the disorders in the comorbidity.

Hostility and aggression are associated with schizophrenia, with aggression occurring more often than average in younger males who have a history of violence, and who have a SUD and do not adhere to their treatment of both schizophrenia and SUD. Recent research suggests that an individual with a comorbidity involving schizophrenia and another disorder is far more likely to engage in violent crime than is an individual with a diagnosis of schizophrenia alone.

Moreover, persons with comorbid schizophrenia and SUD experience insomnia and sleep disturbances, which may lead to depression, adverse effects of medications, and cognitive deficits. Essentially, every aspect of the situation caused by the comorbidity becomes more complicated because of the more rapid progression of each of the two comorbid disorders as a result of the presence of the other, and because of the occurrence of situations that do not occur when either disorder is present by itself.

Many theories have been advanced about the development of comorbid schizophrenia and substance use, the interaction of the two disorders, the prognosis for each disorder or both of them, and the optimal treatment for individuals with this comorbidity. A belief in one theory for some cases of comorbid schizophrenia and substance use does not necessarily mean ruling out other theories for other cases of this comorbidity. As an example of the theories that have been advanced, the self-medication theory holds that substance use is a response to underlying schizophrenia, for the purpose of relieving its symptoms. Another theory holds that SUD may precede and facilitate the development of schizophrenia and other psychiatric disorders. This theory suggests that individuals who abuse substances are more likely to develop psychiatric disorders than those who do not abuse them, although a causal relationship between substance use and the later development of a psychiatric disorder such as schizophrenia is subject to debate. Yet another theory suggests that there is a common vulnerability to both SUDs and mental health disorders, possibly as a result of individual brain biology and the highly complex pleasure or reward system of the brain, in which signaling between nerves is largely mediated by the substance known as dopamine, or that abnormalities in the development of the brain and other components of the nervous system increase the vulnerability to both substance use and schizophrenia.

Among other theories for the concurrence of substance use and schizophrenia is that the two conditions exacerbate the symptoms and effects of one another, with the result that what might have been a nonaddictive social consumption of alcohol becomes alcohol abuse, and manageable symptoms of schizophrenia become unmanageable in the presence of alcohol or other nonprescribed substances. Alternatively, it has been proposed that long-term exposure to antipsychotic medications, such as those used to treat schizophrenia, may induce changes in the brain and nervous system that increase the susceptibility to substance use, or that no causal relationship exists between substance use and schizophrenia or other psychiatric disorders, despite a correlation between the rates of substance use and these disorders.

FACTS AND FIGURES

Comorbidity of schizophrenia and substance abuse can occur at the same time or with one condition preceding the other, and with the two conditions' interactions with one another illnesses worsening the course of both. According to the Substance Abuse and Mental Health Services Administration's

(SAMHSA) national survey of drug use and health, conducted in 2008 and 2009, more than 8.9-million persons in the United States have both a mental illness and SUD. The same survey found that 7.4 percent of individuals with comorbid mental health and SUDs receive treatment for both conditions, and that 55.8 percent of individuals with such comorbidities receive no treatment at all. However, the evidence base for this population is limited because individuals with comorbid conditions are often excluded from clinical trials.

RISK FACTORS

A wide range of risk factors exist for schizophrenia and for substance abuse, but no there is no consensus about their relative effects on the comorbid occurrence of these two disorders. The two types of disorder may share risk factors for their occurrence, including overlapping genetic vulnerabilities, overlapping environmental triggers, age of onset, and involvement of similar brain regions.

SIGNS AND SYMPTOMS

Because of the complex and interwoven nature of comorbidities, signs and symptoms of concurrent schizophrenia and SUD may not appear as discretely as they would with each of these disorders as a single diagnosis.

TREATMENT

The social worker assisting an individual in whom diagnoses of schizophrenia and SUD have been made as comorbidities should conduct a standard biological, psychological, social, and spiritual assessment of the individual, including an assessment of his or her risk for suicide and for inflicting harm on him- or herself and others. This should include an in-depth history of the individual's alcohol and drug consumption, with the latter including legal, illegal, prescribed, and nonprescribed drugs, as well as the collection of information on any prior diagnoses of disorders other than schizophrenia or SUD. Testing for the presence of alcohol and drugs can be done by urine or blood analysis. The assessment should also include the collection of collateral information from the individual's family, friends, and coworkers.

The first priority of treatment for comorbid schizophrenia and SUD is to assess and stabilize the particular disorder that is currently dominant and may

disrupt treatment interventions that would otherwise ordinarily be effective. Pharmacological therapy for schizophrenia, SUD, or both can be provided by a mental health professional licensed to prescribe appropriate medications. The treating professional or the social worker should monitor the adherence of an individual to a treatment regimen of medication, including discussion of the importance of adhering to scheduled dosages and treatment times, and should monitor the treated individual for changes in behavior that accompany treatment. Alertness is essential for preventing interactions caused by the concurrent use of nonprescribed substances with prescribed medications, which can have serious adverse consequences.

Successful nonpharmacological interventions for comorbid schizophrenia and SUD include psychoeducation and cognitive behavioral therapy (CBT), which have been noted to decrease the risk of relapse (which in terms of schizophrenia implies psychiatric hospitalization). Research indicates that psychoeducation increases patients' understanding of illness and crisis management, and therefore reduces relapses of illness, while CBT focuses on learning skills for coping more effectively with stress and preventing relapse.

Other nonpharmacological interventions for comorbid schizophrenia and SUD include motivational interviewing (MI); assertive community treatment (ACT); and family intervention (FI). These methods of intervention have been noted to be part of most integrated treatment programs, which involve simultaneous interventions for substance abuse-related and mental health disorders provided by a team of professionals. MI emphasizes increasing motivation by enhancing personal choice and responsibility. ACT involves a multidisciplinary team of professionals in psychiatry, nursing, social work, and the treatment of substance abuse that provides patients with intensive services as needed on a 24-hour-per-day day, 7-day-per-week basis. FI focuses on increasing families' knowledge about the specific comorbidity affecting a family member and improving communication between these individuals and their families.

An integrated approach to treatment that addresses substance abuse and mental illness at the same time is associated with better treatment outcomes (decreased hospitalization, improved psychiatric functioning, fewer arrests).

Additionally, the social worker can assist individuals being treated for comorbid schizophrenia and SUD in finding housing or employment, with issues involving the criminal justice system, and in the attainment of a personal support system,

and can connect such individuals to recovery organizations, both for schizophrenia and for substance abuse, and refer them to appropriate agencies for housing, legal services, affordable medications, and support for family members.

Social workers assisting persons with comorbid schizophrenia and SUD should be aware of their own cultural values, beliefs, and biases, and develop specialized knowledge about the histories, traditions, and values of these persons and their families. They should adopt methods that reflect their knowledge of the cultural diversity of the societies of the individuals whom they assist, which is especially important when assessing delusions and hallucinations because what may be considered delusional in one culture (witchcraft) may be a commonly held belief in another culture. In some cultures, visual or auditory hallucinations with religious content, such as hearing the voice of a deity or an ancestor, can be a customary part of certain religious experiences.

APPLICABLE LAWS AND REGULATIONS

The United Nations recognizes the protection and treatment of people with mental disorders as a fundamental human right. The United Nations' Principles for the Protection of Persons with Mental Illness, adopted in 1991, promote access to quality healthcare services and provides a legal framework to eliminate discrimination of people with mental disabilities. Both the U. S. government and individual states have standards, procedures, and laws for the involuntary restraint and detention of persons who may be a danger to themselves or others. Because individuals with schizophrenia have a high rate of suicide attempts, it is important to become familiar with the local requirements for involuntary detention. Also, because comorbidity of schizophrenia with SUD often involves the use of illegal drugs, it is important to know local laws and reporting requirements concerning such use.

SERVICES AND RESOURCES

- National Alliance on Mental Illness (NAMI), http://www.nami.org/

- World Fellowship for Schizophrenia and Allied Disorders, http://www.world-schizophrenia.org/
- U.S. National Institute of Mental Health (NIMH), http://www.nimh.nih.gov/index.shtml
- Schizophrenia.com, http://schizophrenia.com/
- SMART Recovery, http://www.smartrecovery.org/
- Recovery.org, http://www.recovery.org/forums/
- Dual Diagnosis Anonymous World Services, http://ddaws.com/

Written by Chris Bates, MA, MSW

Reviewed by Lynn B. Cooper, D Crim, and Melissa Rosales Neff, MSW

REFERENCES

American Psychiatric Association. (2013). Diagnostic and statistical manual of mental disorders. (5th ed.). Arlington, VA: Author.

Armijo, J., Mendez, M. E., Schilling, S., Castro, A., Alvarado, R., & Rojas, G. (2013). Efficacy of community treatments for schizophrenia and other psychotic disorders: A literature review. *Frontiers in Psychiatry, 4*(116), 1-10. doi:10.3389/fpsyt.2013.00116

British Association of Social Workers. (2012). The code of ethics for social work. Retrieved October 31, 2015, from http://cdn.basw.co.uk/upload/basw_112315-7.pdf

Chung, R. K., Large, M. M., Starmer, G. A., Tattam, B. N., Paton, M. B., & Nielssen, O. B. (2009). The reliability of reports of recent psychoactive substance use at the time of admission to an acute mental health unit. *Journal of Dual Diagnosis, 5*(3-4), 392-403. doi:10.1080/15504260903176039

De Witte, N. A., Crunelle, C. L., Sabbe, B., Moggi, F., & Dom, G. (2013). Treatment for outpatients with comorbid schizophrenia and substance use disorders: A review. *European Addiction Research, 20*(3), 105-114. doi:10.1159/000355267

Fabricius, V., Langa, M., & Wilson, K. (2008). An exploratory investigation of co-occurring substance-related and psychiatric disorders. *Journal of Substance Use, 13*(2), 99-114. doi:10.1080/14659890701680877

Fazel, S., Langstrom, N., Hjern, A., Grann, M., & Lichtenstein, P. (2009). Schizophrenia, substance abuse, and violent crime. *Journal of the American Medical Association, 301*(1), 2016-2023. doi:10.1001/jama.2009.675

Feiner, J. S., & Frese, F. J. (2009). Recovery in schizophrenia. In B. J. Sadock, V. A. Sadock, & P. Ruiz (Eds.), *Kaplan & Sadocks's comprehensive textbook of psychiatry* (9th ed., Vol. 1, pp. 1582-1593). Philadelphia, PA: Wolters Kluwer Health/Lippincott Williams & Wilkins.

Fleischhacker, W. W., Arango, C., Arteel, P., Barnes, T. R. E., Carpenter, W., Duckworth, K., ... Woodruff, P. (2014). Schizophrenia: Time to commit to policy change. *Schizophrenia Bulletin, 40*(3), S165-S194. doi:10.1093/schbul/sbu006

Greenberg, G., Rosenheck, R. A., Erickson, S. K., Desai, R. A., Stefanovics, E. A., Swartz, M., & Stroup, T. S. (2011). Criminal justice system involvement among people with schizophrenia. *Community Mental Health Journal, 47*(6), 727-736. doi:10.1007/s10597-010-9362-9

Gregg, L., Haddock, G., & Barrowclough, C. (2009). Self-reported reasons for substance use in schizophrenia: A Q methodological investigation. *Mental Health & Substance Use: Dual Diagnosis, 2*(1), 24-39. doi:10.1080/17523280802593293

Horn, W. T., Akerman, S. C., & Sateia, M. J. (2013). Sleep in schizophrenia and substance use disorders: A review of the literature. *Journal of Dual Diagnosis, 9*(3), 228-238. doi:10.1080/15504263.2013.806088

International Federation of Social Workers. (2012, March 3). Statement of ethical principles. Retrieved October 31, 2015, from http://ifsw.org/policies/statement-of-ethical-principles/

Machielsen, M., der Sluis, S., & de Haan, L. (2010). Cannabis use in patients with a first psychotic episode and subjects at ultra high risk of psychosis: Impact on psychotic and pre-psychotic symptoms. *Australian & New Zealand Journal of Psychiatry, 44*(8), 721-728. doi:10.3109/00048671003689710

McRae-Clark, A. L., Verduin, M. L., Tolliver, B. K., Carter, R. E., Wahlquist, A. E., Brady, K. T., & Anderson, S. (2009). An open-label trial of Aripiprazole treatment in dual diagnosis individuals: Safety and efficacy. *Journal of Dual Diagnosis, 5*(1), 83-96. doi:10.1080/15504260802620210

Mizrahi, T., & Mayden, R. W. (2001). NASW standards for cultural competency in social work practice. Retrieved October 31, 2015, from http://www.socialworkers.org/practice/standards/NASWCulturalStandards.pdf

National Institute on Drug Abuse. (2011). Drug facts: Comorbidity: Addiction and other mental disorders. Retrieved October 31, 2015, from http://www.drugabuse.gov/publications/drugfacts/comorbidity-addiction-other-mental-disorders

Olivares, J. M., Sermon, J. H., Hemels, M., & Schreiner, A. (2013). Definitions and drivers of relapse in patients with schizophrenia: A systematic literature review. *Annals of General Psychiatry, 12*(1), 32. doi::10.1186/1744-859X-12-32

Ouzir, M. (2013). Impulsivity in schizophrenia: a comprehensive update. *Aggression and Violent Behavior, 18*(2), 247-254. doi:10.1016/j.avb.2012.11.014

Ralevski, E., O'Brien, E., Jane, J. S., Dwan, R., Dean, E., Edens, E., & Petrakis, I. (2011). Treatment with Acamprosate in patients with schizophrenia spectrum disorders and comorbid alcohol dependence. *Journal of Dual Diagnosis, 7*(1-2), 64-73. doi:10.1097/NMD.0b013e3182214297

Samaha, A. N. (2014). Can antipsychotic treatment contribute to drug addiction in schizophrenia? *Progress in Neuro-Psychopharmacology & Biological Psychiatry, 52*, 9-16. doi:10.1016/j.pnpbp.2013.06.008

Vadhan, N. P., Serper, M. R., & Haney, M. (2009). Effects of delta-THC on working memory: Implications for schizophrenia?. *Primary Psychiatry, 16*(4), 51-99.

Van Os, J., & Allardyce, J. (2009). The clinical epidemiology of schizophrenia. In B. J. Sadock, V. A. Sadock, & P. Ruiz (Eds.), *Kaplan & Sadocks's Comprehensive Textbook of Psychiatry* (9th ed., Vol. 1, pp. 1475-1587). Philadelphia: Wolters Kluwer Health/Lippincott Williams & Wilkins.

Volkow, N. (2009). Substance use disorders in schizophrenia-clinical implications of comorbidity. *Schizophrenia Bulletin, 35*(3), 469-472. doi:10.1093/schbul/sbp016

Westermeyer, J. (2006). Comorbid schizophrenia and substance abuse: A review of epidemiology and course. *The American Journal on Addictions, 15*(5), 345-355. doi:10.1080/10550490600860114

World Health Organization (WHO). (n.d.). Schizophrenia. Retrieved October 31, 2015, from http://www.who.int/mental_health/management/schizophrenia/en/

World Health Organization. (2004). The global burden of disease: 2004 update. Retrieved October 31, 2015, from http://www.who.int/healthinfo/global_burden_disease/GBD_report_2004update_full.pdf

Weinstein, J. J., & Stovall, J. G. (2014). Schizophrenia. In F. J. Domino (Ed.), *The 5-minute clinical consultant standard 2015* (23rd ed., pp. 1074-1075). Philadelphia, PA: Wolters Kluwer.

United Nations. (1991). The United Nations General Assembly 46/119; The protection of persons with mental illness and the improvement of mental health care. Retrieved October 31, 2015, from http://www.un.org/documents/ga/res/46/a46r119.htm

Substance Abuse and Mental Health Service Administration (SAMHSA). (n.d.). Co-occurring disorders. Retrieved October 31, 2015, from http://www.samhsa.gov/co-occurring/topics/data/disorders.aspx

Psychology Today. (2014). Co-occurring disorders. Retrieved October 31, 2015, from https://www.psychologytoday.com/conditions/co-occurring-disorders

SCHIZOPHRENIA IN ADULTS

MAJOR CATEGORIES: Behavioral & Mental Health

DESCRIPTION

Schizophrenia is a chronic and incapacitating mental health disorder that severely affects a person's thought processes, stimulus perception, communication, behavior, and the ability to maintain relationships and a stable living environment. Schizophrenia is characterized by positive (noticeably present) and negative (notable by their absence) symptoms. Schizophrenia shares the feature of psychosis with several other *Diagnostic and Statistical Manual of Mental Disorders*, Fifth Edition (*DSM-5*), diagnoses, including mood disorders, and therefore can be difficult to distinguish from other disorders featuring psychosis. However, schizophrenia is primarily a thought disorder versus a mood disorder.

The *Diagnostic and Statistical Manual of Mental Disorders (DSM)* is a text that guides the diagnosis of mental health disorders including schizophrenia. There have been some changes in the criteria to diagnosis schizophrenia from the fourth edition (*DSM-IV*) to the *DSM-5*. Mental health professionals must use the most current version of the *DSM* for diagnosis needs.

The *DSM-5* lists the five primary psychotic features and symptoms of schizophrenia as delusions, hallucinations, disorganized thought (thoughts and conversation are not logical, which can be inferred from speech), grossly disorganized behavior (including catatonic behavior, that is, being in a rigid position for an extended amount of time), and negative symptoms. The symptoms of schizophrenia that may be categorized as positive symptoms include exaggerated thoughts, perceptions and ideas, or behaviors that disrupt the individual's daily functioning.

Positive symptoms of schizophrenia may include hallucinations through sight, hearing, or smell (auditory hallucinations, visual hallucinations, somatic hallucinations), delusions (illogical thoughts such as persecutory delusions, believing someone will harm them; erotomanic delusions, having a strong romantic belief about another person; grandiose delusions with an exaggerated or superior sense of self; thought broadcasting, the belief others can hear their thoughts ideas of reference, believing that certain events have extra importance or reason in relation to their life); disorganized thinking as demonstrated by disorganized speech (derailment, tangentiality, word salad), and grossly disorganized or catatonic behaviors. Symptoms of schizophrenia that are categorized as negative symptoms may include apathy, withdrawal, avolition (lack of motivation), flat or restricted affect, poverty or loss of thought, and anhedonia (lack of interest or pleasure from things).

Negative symptoms, decline in thoughts and responses to stimuli, and behaviors that disrupt functioning are not as apparent as positive symptoms, and the onset of negative symptoms may be gradual and therefore not noticed or assigned appropriate significance by a mental health professional. Negative symptoms may also be confused with symptoms of other disorders, particularly mood disorders (depression). Furthermore, they may fall within cultural norms and therefore may not indicate a disorder. Cognitive symptoms, which may appear in conjunction with positive or negative symptoms, may include disruption of working memory, trouble focusing or paying attention, and poor executive functioning.

The *DSM-5* diagnostic criteria include the need for the individual to experience 6 months of symptoms. The individual must also experience at least 1 month, or less if treated successfully, of at least two core symptoms (delusion, hallucinations, disorganized thought/speech, grossly disorganized behavior, or negative symptoms), one of which must be from the first three listed (delusion, hallucinations, disorganized thought/speech) and a decreased level of functioning in at least one major area of life (work, self-care). The individual must also have a thorough differential diagnosis completed by the mental health professional completing their assessment to rule out other possible mental health diagnosis.

Onset of schizophrenia usually occurs between late adolescence and the mid-30s. Each person will follow a unique course; however, there generally are recurrent acute (short term) episodes with psychotic symptoms, which lead to further deterioration of functioning unless relapses are prevented, thus interrupting the cycle.

Symptoms, diagnosis, and course of the disease are the same for early onset (before 15 years of age) and later onset (after 45 years of age), although prognosis for patients with early onset is worse because of less-developed life skills, whereas the prognosis is better for patients with later onset because of better-developed life skills. Men tend to have their first episode of schizophrenia between ages 18 and 26, and women generally first develop symptoms between ages 26 and 40. Prevalence is the same for men and women, however, and the worldwide geographic distribution of schizophrenia is even.

The etiology and origin of schizophrenia is unknown. Current research indicates a complex interaction between inherited indicators and genes and environmental factors. Researchers are investigating numerous potential factors, including gray matter volume in the brain in specific areas such as the cerebral cortex, hippocampus, and thalamus; disruption of neurotransmitters (particularly dopamine); network level dysfunction among different systems and parts of the brain; impairment of stimulus inhibition in the brain; exposure to trauma; and maternal exposure to viruses during pregnancy. Depending on the subtype, etiology, and current phase, treatment might include involuntary detention, medication, social skills training, psychological education about schizophrenia, and referrals to community and family support services. Prognosis varies widely from complete and long-term remission, to long-term treatment with a slow and steady decrease in quality of life, to suicide.

FACTS AND FIGURES

The *DSM-5* reports the lifetime prevalence of schizophrenia to be approximately 0.3 to 0.7 percent, with the exact way the disorder is defined affecting the breakdown of prevalence by gender, location, and race/ethnicity. For example, emphasis on prevalence of long duration of symptoms and experiencing negative symptoms results in higher rates for males than for females. The *DSM-5* also reports that approximately 20 percent of individuals with schizophrenia attempt suicide at least once, and between 5 and 6 percent die by suicide. Schizophrenia accounts for up to 50 percent of long-term psychiatric hospitalizations despite its relatively low prevalence.

RISK FACTORS

Biological risk factors may include genetics, dopamine hyperactivity, decreased brain size, premature birth or excessive maternal bleeding during pregnancy, traumatic brain injury, and maternal exposure to trauma in first trimester.

Environmental risk factors may include family dysfunction, exposure to trauma, winter or early spring birth, and low socioeconomic status. Stigma and social isolation associated with diagnosis may exacerbate symptoms.

SIGNS AND SYMPTOMS

When assessing signs and symptoms of schizophrenia, the social worker or other mental health professional must note that every symptom of schizophrenia appears in at least one other mental health disorder; that signs and symptoms change over time; and that the intellectual ability, education, and cultural background of the individual may influence how he or she perceives and describes symptoms.

Social signs and symptoms of schizophrenia may include social withdrawal and a decrease in the individual's level of personal hygiene and care. Physical and observable symptoms of schizophrenia may include an inappropriate, usually flat (lacking expression of emotion), affect and rapidly changing affect.

Psychological signs and symptoms of schizophrenia may include hallucinations, frequently auditory; delusions, often persecutory or grandiose; disrupted thought processes and speech, or absence of thought and speech; and absorption with inner thoughts.

ASSESSMENT

The social worker should complete a thorough biological, psychological, social, and spiritual history of the patient and include an assessment for the risk of suicide or harm to self or others. The social worker should observe the individual's level of functioning and demeanor during the interview, with particular attention to possible negative symptoms. Collateral information from family, friends, and coworkers may be necessary to complete the assessment. Prior diagnosis of disorders other than schizophrenia, including substance abuse, are important to note.

ASSESSMENT AND SCREENING TOOLS

Social workers and other mental health professionals may use standardized assessments and screening tools when determining an individual's symptoms and assessing for needs. Appropriate standardized assessments and tools may include the Positive and Negative Syndrome Scale (PANSS) for Schizophrenia, the Scale for the Assessment of Negative Symptoms (SANS), and the Scale for the Assessment of Positive Symptoms (SAPS).

Currently, there are no laboratory tests that can detect schizophrenia; however, appropriate laboratory tests may be useful in determining the presence of alcohol or other substances to rule out other factors for the individual's symptoms.

TREATMENT

Treatments and interventions for schizophrenia aim to improve quality of life for the individual and family, decrease the number and severity of active-phase schizophrenic episodes, and strengthen family and community support. Over the course of the disorder, treatments might include hospitalization, psychopharmacology (prescribed medication), various psychological treatments (individual, group, or family therapy; social skills training; cognitive behavioral therapy), involvement in an assertive community treatment (ACT) multidisciplinary team, or community-based recovery movement programs. Because schizophrenia is a chronic disorder, treatment is a lifelong process.

Intervention

If an individual is experiencing a severe active episode of schizophrenia including psychotic features and has the possibility of harm to self or others, the social worker should assist the patient in reducing severe symptoms and maintaining safety. Possible hospitalization and provision of appropriate medications may be necessary.

If an individual is experiencing hallucinations/delusions/erratic or self-destructive behavior, the social worker should assist the patient in decreasing hallucinations or delusions, help stabilize erratic behavior, and decrease destructive behavior. The social worker may schedule an appointment with mental health professional who can prescribe appropriate medications. The social worker should follow up on medication adherence with the individual, including a discussion of the importance of adhering to prescription dosage and timing, and noting any changes in behavior to report on follow-up visits with the prescribing health professional. The social worker may also discuss possible side effects of medication and ways the individual can deal with them.

Schizophrenia may cause social withdrawal, decreased social function, and lack of self-care. The individual may need to learn how to increase necessary life skills to improve their independent function and maintain social relationships and self-care. The social worker may refer the individual to a social skills training (SST) program. SST programs vary, but generally include goal setting, role modeling, behavior rehearsal, positive reinforcement, and exercises to generalize learning to community settings.

Schizophrenia may cause a loss of family/peer support. The social worker should encourage and assist the individual to reestablish relations with family and appropriate support groups. Psychological education for the family regarding schizophrenia, including education about the nature of schizophrenia, different treatments available, and available community resources should be provided. The social worker should teach the individual and family necessary stress management techniques, appropriate communication skills, and problem solving skills. The individual and family should be encouraged to participate in self-care and encouraged to provide mutual support within the family. Referrals to a community-based recovery movement group may be made for further support.

APPLICABLE LAWS AND REGULATIONS

Each jurisdiction (nation, state, province) has its own standards, procedures, and laws for involuntary restraint and detention of persons who may be a danger to themselves or to others. Because those affected by schizophrenia have a high rate of suicide attempts, it is important for social workers and mental health professionals to become familiar with the local requirements for involuntary detention. Local laws and professional reporting requirements for abuse and safety should also be known and followed by social workers and mental health professionals.

SERVICES AND RESOURCES

- Recovery within Reach, http://www.recoverywithinreach.org
- Brain & Behavior Research Foundation (formerly NARSAD), http://bbrfoundation.org/
- National Alliance on Mental Illness (NAMI), http://www.nami.org/
- U.S. National Institutes of Health (NIH), http://www.nih.gov/
- U.S. National Institute of Mental Health (NIMH), http://www.nimh.nih.gov/index.shtml
- National Association of Social Workers (NASW), http://www.socialworkers.org/

FOOD FOR THOUGHT

Researchers studying Medicaid recipients in the United States found that adults with schizophrenia die at 3.5 times the rate of the general adult population. Individuals with schizophrenia have an increased risk for mortality from chronic obstructive pulmonary disease (COPD), diabetes mellitus, cardiovascular disease, suicide, influenza and pneumonia, lung and other cancers, and accidents. Researchers believe that smoking is a major risk factor for the development of these diseases, as approximately two thirds of individuals with schizophrenia smoke.

RED FLAGS

The social worker should assess any patient with schizophrenia for suicide risk and follow appropriate procedures or regulations (calling police or referral to a hospital) to maintain safety. The social worker should assess any patient with schizophrenia for the likelihood of harming others and follow appropriate procedures or regulations (calling police or referral to a hospital) to maintain safety.

Because symptoms of other disorders are similar to those of schizophrenia and they may overlap, social workers and mental health professionals must carefully distinguish schizophrenia from other mental health diagnoses, in particular any disorder that includes psychotic features. Incorrect diagnosis may lead to inappropriate pharmacological treatments. In children, symptoms of autism or pervasive developmental disorders, including disorganized behavior, social difficulties, and language impairment, can be confused with schizophrenia symptoms, particularly negative ones.

Loss of family and other support may lead to a decline in socioeconomic status, which may lead to increased stress that further impairs ability to function and brings on acute episodes, which may further alienate family and support.

NEXT STEPS

The social worker should review the medication regimen with the patient and help the patient make necessary follow-up appointments with the agency issuing the prescription. The social worker should discuss the importance of the medications and the importance of taking them as prescribed. Possible side effects of the medications and ways to deal with them should be discussed.

Referrals to local schizophrenia support groups, supported work, or mental health agencies may be necessary. The social worker should assess the stability of the patient's living situation and make referrals as appropriate.

Referrals for continued support to family members should be provided.

Written by Chris Bates, MA, MSW

Reviewed by Pedram Samghabadi

REFERENCES

American Psychiatric Association. (2013). Diagnostic and statistical manual of mental health disorders. (5th ed.). Arlington, VA: American Psychiatric Publishing.

Barnes, A. (2008). Race and hospital diagnoses of schizophrenia and mood disorders. *Social Work, 53*(1), 77-83. doi:10.1093/sw/53.1.77

British Association of Social Workers. (2012). The code of ethics for social work: Statement of principles. Retrieved April 18, 2016, from http://cdn.basw.co.uk/upload/basw_112315-7.pdf

Corcoran, J., & Walsh, J. (2010). *Clinical assessment and diagnosis in social work practice* (2nd ed.). New York, NY: Oxford University Press.

DeBattista, C., Eisendrath, S. J., & Lichtmacher, J. E. (2015). Psychiatric disorders. In M. A. Papadakis & S. J. McPhee (Eds.), *2015 current medical diagnosis & treatment* (54th ed., pp. 1042-1051). Philadelphia, PA: Wolters Kluwer.

International Federation of Social Workers. (2012, March 3). Statement of Ethical Principles. Retrieved April 18, 2016, from http://ifsw.org/policies/statement-of-ethical-principles/

Kay, S. K., Fiszbein, A., & Opler, L. A. (1987). The Positive and Negative Syndrome Scale (PANSS) for schizophrenia. *Schizophrenia Bulletin, 13*(2), 261-276. doi:10.1093/schbul/13.2.261

Kurtz, M. M., & Mueser, K. T. (2008). A meta-analysis of controlled research on social skills training for schizophrenia. *Journal of Consulting and Clinical Psychology, 76*(3), 491-504. doi:10.1037/0022-006X.76.3.491

Marley, J. A., & Buila, S. (2001). Crimes against people with mental illness: Types, perpetrators, and influencing factors. *Social Work, 46*(2), 115-124. doi:10.1093/sw/46.2.115

Olfson, M., Gerhard, T., Huang, C., Crystal, S., & Stroup, T. S. (2015). Premature mortality among adults with schizophrenia in the United States. *JAMA Psychiatry, 72*(12), 1172-1181. doi:10.1001/jamapsychiatry.2015.1737

Pfammatter, J., Junghan, U. M., & Brenner, H. D. (2006). Efficacy of psychological therapy in schizophrenia: Conclusions from meta-analyses.

Schizophrenia Bulletin, 32(1), S64-S80. doi:10.1093/schbul/sbl030

Sadock, B. J., Sadock, V. A., & Ruiz, P. (2015). Schizophrenia spectrum and other psychotic disorders. In *Kaplan & Sadock's synopsis of psychiatry: Behavioral sciences/clinical psychiatry* (11th ed., pp. 300-323). Philadelphia, PA: Wolters Kluwer.

Sherrer, M. V. (2011). The role of cognitive appraisal in adaptation to traumatic stress in adults with serious mental illness: A critical review. *Trauma, Violence & Abuse, 12*(3), 151-167. doi:10.1177/1524838011404254

Stein, C. H., Jaclyn, E. L., Osborn, L. A., Greenberg, S., Petrowski, C. E., Jesse, S., ... May, M. C. (2015). Mental health system historians: Adults with schizophrenia describe changes in community mental health care over time. *The Psychiatric Quarterly, 86*(1), 33-48. doi:10.1007/s11126-014-9325-3

Townsend, M. C. (2015). Schizophrenia spectrum and other psychotic disorders. In *Psychiatric mental health nursing: Concepts of care in evidence-based practice* (8th ed., pp. 419-457). Philadelphia, PA: F. A. Davis Company.

Weinstein, J. J., & Stovall, J. G. (2014). Schizophrenia. In F. J. Domino (Ed.), *The 5-minute clinical consultant standard 2015* (23rd ed., pp. 1074-1075). Philadelphia, PA: Wolters Kluwer.

Wheeler, D. (2015). NASW standards and indicators for cultural competence in social work practice. Retrieved April 18, 2016, from http://www.socialworkers.org/practice/standards/PRA-BRO-253150-CC-Standards.pdf

SCHIZOPHRENIA IN CHILDHOOD

MAJOR CATEGORIES: Behavioral & Mental Health

DESCRIPTION

Schizophrenia is a chronic and incapacitating psychiatric disorder that severely affects an individual's thought processes, stimuli perception, communication, behavior, and the ability to maintain relationships and stable living environments. When symptoms of schizophrenia manifest during childhood or adolescence, it may also disrupt, delay, or cease all aspects of expected, normal development.

Schizophrenia is characterized by positive (noticeably present) and negative (notable by their absence) symptoms. As described by the *Diagnostic and Statistical Manual of Mental Disorders,* Fifth Edition (*DSM-5*), schizophrenia shares the feature of psychosis (hallucinations and delusions) with several other *DSM-5* mental health diagnoses, including mood disorders, and therefore symptoms of schizophrenia can be difficult to distinguish from other disorders that feature psychosis. However, schizophrenia is primarily a thought disorder versus a mood disorder.

Childhood-onset schizophrenia (COS) and adolescent-onset schizophrenia (AOS) together are referred to as *early-onset schizophrenia* (EOS). COS is sometimes called *very early-onset schizophrenia* (VEOS). It is generally agreed that start of symptoms, and possibly diagnosis, of COS is prior to age 13 (some sources use age 14). AOS indicates symptoms, and possibly diagnosis, from ages 13 to 18 (some sources use age 17), and EOS indicates onset at any time before age 18 (or 17). The *DSM-5* uses the same criteria for diagnosis of schizophrenia regardless of age of onset. Generally, the younger a person is when schizophrenia is diagnosed, the more severe the lifetime course of the disorder. On average, schizophrenia is diagnosed in males at a younger age than in females and COS is diagnosed more often in males, at a rate of 2:1. COS is rare and severe.

COS cycles through four phases of symptoms, usually with increased deterioration of cognitive or behavioral functioning with each cycle. Depending on the success of treatment such as counseling or medication, the acute phases of symptoms may diminish in frequency and intensity after 10 years. The first phase of symptoms in schizophrenia is the prodromal phase, which is characterized by functional deterioration. This may include social withdrawal, unusual preoccupations, decreased self-care, and changes in appetite or sleep patterns. It is not unusual for the prodromal phase to pass unnoticed in COS. Next is the acute or active phase, which is marked by positive symptoms (behaviors or thoughts that are not normally present), including delusions (false beliefs or thoughts), hallucinations (experiencing visions, sounds, or smells that are not actually present), and a significant decrease in social and cognitive function. Intellectual functioning deteriorates and hospitalization is common during this phase. The third phase is the recovery, or recuperative, phase, which is characterized by more negative symptoms (loss of typical behavior or emotions) than positive symptoms. Negative symptoms such as withdrawal, flat affect, poor attention, and bizarre behavior may be noted during this phase. The fourth phase is the residual phase, characterized by an absence of positive symptoms, a decrease in negative symptoms and typically an increase in the individual's functioning.

Extreme caution must be used by mental health professionals and social workers when diagnosing EOS and when attempting to assign children to a specific phase of schizophrenia. An examination of 20 years of data on 3,500 referrals for EOS schizophrenia evaluations by specialists found that of the 350 persons in whom schizophrenia was provisionally diagnosed after the initial referral, 44 percent did not meet the diagnostic criteria for schizophrenia after 2–5 months of hospitalization that included continuing assessment. Because children and adolescents by their very nature are developing and changing in every aspect of their lives (physical, social, verbal, cognitive, relational, spiritual), it may be difficult for mental health professionals to discern and properly evaluate the significance of changes in behavior or developmental progress in a child as being related to symptoms of schizophrenia.

Furthermore, some symptoms of EOS may not manifest as the deterioration in already acquired social skills but as developmental delays or entirely missed developmental milestones (walking, talking, and toileting). Additionally, there may be developmental disruption that is unrelated to schizophrenia. However, given the increased severity of schizophrenia in individuals diagnosed with EOS, and particularly COS, concerning symptoms should not be ignored. The social worker or other mental health professional completing the assessment should consult with professional(s) experienced in EOS. Given the complexity of identifying symptoms of schizophrenia in children, it is important that the developmental progression of a child is taken into consideration. Additionally, it is important that mental health professionals assessing the symptoms consider possible communication barriers due to children developing self-awareness and communication skills. Consultation with professional(s) experienced in EOS is required to appropriately identify and differentiate possible symptoms of schizophrenia.

The etiology and cause of schizophrenia is unknown. Current research indicates a complex interaction between inherited indicators and environmental factors. Researchers are investigating numerous potential factors, including abnormalities in gray matter volume in the cerebral cortex, hippocampus, and thalamus; disruption of neurotransmitters (particularly dopamine); impairment of stimulus inhibition in the brain; decreased coordination and connectivity between the regions of the brain associated with sociality and cognition; exposure to trauma; and maternal exposure to viruses during pregnancy. COS is believed to be more influenced by genetics than postchildhood onset; approximately 50 percent of children with COS have at least one first-degree relative (mother, father) with schizophrenia or a schizophrenic spectrum disorder. Researchers have explored the role played by puberty in EOS, but the current consensus is that there is no correlation. Depending on the severity of symptoms and ability to maintain daily functioning, etiology, current phase of schizophrenia, and age of the individual being treated, treatment might include involuntary detention or hospitalization, medication, social skills training, psychological education about the disorder and coping skills, and referrals to community and family support services. Prognosis and expected recovery varies widely, from complete recovery of symptoms and long-term remission to long-term treatment with a slow and steady decrease in the individual's quality of life to suicide, although prognosis is inversely related to age of onset and the younger the symptoms begin, the worse the prognosis and vice versa.

FACTS AND FIGURES

Because EOS is not common and because the diagnosis frequently changes, up-to-date facts and figures about the disorder are not readily available. The *DSM-5* reports the lifetime prevalence for all cases of schizophrenia to be 0.3 to 0.7 percent. A 2012 meta-analysis of 21 studies that measured outcomes at least 1 year after diagnosis found that studies with exclusively EOS participants had worse outcomes than studies that included participants with a range of disorders that included psychotic symptoms.

RISK FACTORS

A strong biological risk factor for COS is a family history of schizophrenia. Additional risk factors for childhood schizophrenia are dopamine hyperactivity, decreased brain size, premature birth or excessive maternal bleeding, traumatic brain injury, and maternal exposure to trauma in the first trimester of pregnancy.

Environmental risk factors for childhood schizophrenia include a low socioeconomic status, family

dysfunction, exposure to trauma, and winter or early spring birth. Social stigma and isolation associated with a diagnosis of schizophrenia may exacerbate symptoms.

SIGNS AND SYMPTOMS

Signs and symptoms of childhood schizophrenia will vary with developmental age. For example, in COS delusions are more likely to center on monsters and other childish fears than more mature concerns such as government security agencies. Social workers and mental health professionals should also note that symptoms may manifest and appear as the absence of the development of skills rather than their deterioration (not speaking at all rather than loss of ability to speak).

Possible social signs and symptoms of childhood schizophrenia may include social withdrawal, poor relationships with peers, missing or delayed developmental milestones, and a decrease in level of personal hygiene and care.

Possible physical signs and symptoms of childhood schizophrenia may include inappropriate, usually flat affect (lacking physical expression of emotion), or a rapidly changing affect.

Possible psychological signs and symptoms of childhood schizophrenia may include hallucinations, frequently auditory hallucinations; delusions, which may reflect the child's developmental maturity, such as believing that monsters live under the bed; disrupted thought processes and speech, or absence of thought and speech; and an absorption with internal preoccupations and thoughts.

ASSESSMENT

The social worker should complete a thorough biological, psychological, social, and spiritual history of the child and family, including any risk for suicide and harm to self and others. The social worker should be observant of the child or adolescent's functioning and demeanor during the interview. Particular attention should be paid to possible negative symptoms and developmental progression and variations from established norms. Collateral information from family, friends, and teachers is particularly important in EOS since self-awareness, a personal sense of what is normal, and communication skills are still developing.

ASSESSMENT AND SCREENING TOOLS

Social workers may utilize standardized assessments and screening tools as part of their assessment of the child or adolescent. Appropriate assessments and screening tools may include the Positive and Negative Syndrome Scale for Children (Kiddie-PANSS), the Schedule for Affective Disorders and Schizophrenia for School-Aged Children (K-SADS), or the Brief Psychiatric Rating Scale for Children (BPRS-C).

No applicable laboratory tests currently are used in the diagnosis of schizophrenia; however, substance abuse screening and blood/urine toxicology lab tests are important to rule out general effects of a substance that may appear as symptoms of schizophrenia.

TREATMENT

Treatments and interventions for EOS aim to ensure safety and improve the child's quality of life, decrease the number and severity of active-phase episodes of schizophrenia, provide opportunities to develop life and cognitive skills, and strengthen family and community support. A multidisciplinary team approach assists in addressing the broad range of treatment needs usually present in EOS, including the need to provide support to family and caregivers. Because schizophrenia is a chronic disorder, treatment may be a lifelong process.

Intervention

If a child or adolescent with schizophrenia is experiencing symptoms of hallucinations, delusions, or erratic or self-destructive behavior, the social worker should assist in decreasing these behaviors and assist with maintaining the safety of the child/adolescent. The social worker may assist the child and family with scheduling an appointment with a mental health professional who can prescribe appropriate medications or hospitalization if appropriate.

The social worker should follow up with the child and family regarding medication adherence, including discussing the importance of adhering to the prescription dosage and specific timing and noting any changes in the child's behavior in order to report on it during the follow-up visits with the prescribing professional. Pharmacological (medication) treatment of EOS requires continual monitoring and reevaluation.

If a child or adolescent with schizophrenia is experiencing symptoms of withdrawal, a decrease in social function, or a decrease in self-care, the social worker should assist the child and family with increasing necessary life skills to improve the child/adolescent's independent function and ability to maintain social relationships and appropriate level of self-care. Social skills training (SST) may be appropriate and has varying programs, but generally includes training on age-appropriate goal setting, role modeling, appropriate behavior rehearsal, positive reinforcement, and exercises to generalize the child/adolescent's learning to appropriate peer and community settings.

If a child or adolescent with schizophrenia is experiencing a disruption or breakdown of relationship(s) with their family, community, or school, the social worker should assist the child/adolescent and family in maintaining these relationships. Social workers may identify appropriate academic supports and resources to encourage enhanced relationships and make necessary referrals. Psychological education for the child's family may be beneficial. Education about schizophrenia may include information about the nature of schizophrenia, different treatments available, and available community resources for support, including school programs. Stress management techniques, communication, and problem solving skills should be taught to the family and child. The social worker should encourage the family to practice self-care and mutual support within family.

APPLICABLE LAWS AND REGULATIONS

Each jurisdiction (nation, state, and province) has its own standards, procedures, and laws for involuntary restraint and detention of persons who may be a danger to themselves or others. Laws specific to involuntary restraint and detention concerning children may be different from those concerning adults. Because persons with schizophrenia have a high rate of suicide attempts, it is important that mental health professionals including social workers become familiar with the local requirements for involuntary detention. Other regulations to be aware of are local school district rules concerning individualized education programs and accommodations for children with EOS. Local and professional reporting requirements for neglect and abuse of children should be known and observed by all mental health professionals and social workers.

SERVICES AND RESOURCES

Enter *schizophrenia, COS, AOS,* or *EOS* in the search box to access relevant information available on each website.

- Brain & Behavior Research Foundation (formerly NARSAD), https://bbrfoundation.org/
- National Alliance on Mental Illness (NAMI), http://www.nami.org/
- U.S. National Institutes of Health (NIH), http://www.nih.gov/
- U.S. National Institute of Mental Health (NIMH), http://www.nimh.nih.gov/index.shtml
- National Association of Social Workers (NASW), http://www.socialworkers.org/

FOOD FOR THOUGHT

Working with children with EOS and particularly COS can be challenging. Research suggests that professionals should practice heightened alertness to their own reactions and preconceived ideas about severe mental illness in children. For example, it is possible that a practitioner might blame the family for the child's condition because of research that suggests that emotion expressed by family members may contribute to relapses of positive symptoms.

In one study, children of adoptive parents who were critical, constrained, or inconsistent in communications with their children had a risk of schizophrenia of 36 in 100, compared to a risk of 6 in 100 for children whose adoptive parents communicated consistently, clearly, without criticism, and with firm boundaries.

RED FLAGS

Mental health professionals and social workers must always assess a child with schizophrenia for the risk of suicide and self-harm. Because of the similarity and overlap in symptoms with other disorders, social workers and mental health professionals must carefully distinguish schizophrenia from other psychiatric diagnoses, in particular any disorder that includes psychotic features. An incorrect mental health diagnosis may lead to the child receiving incorrect pharmacologic treatments. In COS and EOS, symptoms of autism and other pervasive developmental disorders, including disorganized behavior, social difficulties, and language impairment, can be confused with schizophrenia symptoms, particularly negative ones.

Possible delays in every aspect of development should be addressed to decrease long term developmental impact. Long-term functioning with an EOS diagnosis may be severely limited if life skills and cognitive abilities are never developed. Social workers should evaluate the ability of the family to provide necessary support and care for an individual with EOS. Referral(s) should be provided as appropriate.

NEXT STEPS

All discharge planning from a hospital or mental health facility must be conducted in conjunction with parents or guardians. Ideally, the child's discharge planning will be coordinated with other professionals (medical, school, justice system) as well. Coordination of services after a hospitalization may be more challenging with teens. The social worker should review the child's medication regimen with the child and family and help the family make follow-up appointments with the agency issuing the prescription. The importance of medications, taking them as prescribed, and regular follow-up appointments with the issuing agency to monitor medications should be emphasized.

Referrals to local schizophrenia support groups, supported work programs if appropriate to age, or mental health agencies should be completed. The social worker should ascertain appropriate school placement and available school services, encourage family involvement, and make appropriate referrals. Referrals for available support services to the family members of a child with schizophrenia should be completed.

Written by Chris Bates, MA, MSW

Reviewed by Lynn B. Cooper, D Crim, and Pedram Samghabadi

REFERENCES

American Psychiatric Association. (2013). Diagnostic and statistical manual of mental health disorders (DSM-5). (5th ed.). Arlington, VA: American Psychiatric Publishing.

Berman, R. A., Gotts, S. J., McAdams, H. M., Greenstein, D., Lalonde, F., Clasen, L., ... Rapoport, J. (2015). Disrupted sensorimotor and social-cognitive networks underlie symptoms in childhood-onset schizophrenia. *BRAIN A Journal of Neurology,* 1-16.

British Association of Social Workers. (2012, January). The code of ethics for social work: Statement of principles. Retrieved December 30, 2015, from http://cdn.basw.co.uk/upload/basw_112315-7.pdf

Clemmensen, L., Vernal, D. L., & Steinhausen, H. C. (2012). systematic review of the long-term outcome of early onset schizophrenia. *BMC Psychiatry, 12*(150).

DeBattista, C., Eisendrath, S. J., & Lichtmacher, J. E. (2015). Psychiatric disorders. In M. A. Papadakis & S. J. McPhee (Eds.), *2015 current medical diagnosis & treatment* (54th ed., pp. 1042-1051). Philadelphia, PA: Wolters Kluwer.

Eggers, C., Bunk, D., & Krause, D. (2000). Schizophrenia with onset before age of eleven: Clinical characteristics of onset and course. *Journal of Autism and Developmental Disorders, 30*(1), 29-38. doi:10.1023/A:1005408010797

Greenstein, D., Kataria, R., Gochman, P., Dasgupta, A., Malley, J. D., Rapoport, J., & Gogtay, N. (2014). Looking for childhood-onset schizophrenia: Diagnostic algorithms for classifying children and adolescents with psychosis. *Journal of Child and Adolescent Psychopharmacology, 24*(7), 366-373. doi:10.1089/cap.2013.0139

Hall, S. D., & Bean, R. A. (2008). Family therapy and childhood-onset schizophrenia: Pursuing clinical and bio/psycho/social competence. *Contemporary Family Therapy, 30*(2), 61-74.

International Federation of Social Workers. (2012, March 3). Statement of Ethical Principles. Retrieved December 20, 2015, from http://ifsw.org/policies/statement-of-ethical-principles/

Kao, Y. C., & Liu, Y. P. (2010). Effects of age of onset on clinical characteristics in schizophrenia spectrum disorders. *BMC Psychiatry, 10,* 63.

Kay, S. R., Fiszbein, A., & Opler, L. A. (1987). The positive and negative syndrome scale (PANSS) for schizophrenia. *Schizophrenia Bulletin, 13*(2), 261-276. doi:10.1093/schbul/13.2.261

Kurtz, M. M., & Mueser, K. T. (2008). A meta-analysis of controlled research on social skills training for schizophrenia. *Journal of Consulting and Clinical Psychology, 76*(3), 491-504. doi:10.1037/0022-006X.76.3.491

Kyriakopoulos, M., & Frangou, S. (2007). Pathophysiology of early onset schizophrenia. *International Review of Psychiatry, 19*(4), 315-324.

Lachman, A. (2014). New developments in diagnosis and treatment update: Schizophrenia/first episode psychosis in children and adolescents. *Journal of Child and Adolescent Mental Health, 26*(2), 109-124. doi:10.2989/17280583.2014.924416

Malone Cole, J. A. (2012). Schizophrenia and other psychotic disorders. In K. M. Fortinash & P. A. Holoday Worret (Eds.), *Psychiatric mental health nursing* (5th ed., pp. 259-296). St. Louis, MO: Elsevier Mosby.

Ordonez, A. E., Sastry, N. V., & Gogtay, N. (2015). Functional and clinical insights from neuroimaging studies in childhood-onset schizophrenia. *CNS Spectrums, 20,* 442-450.

Sadock, R. J., Sadock, V. A., & Ruiz, P. (2015). Kaplan & Sadock's synopsis of psychiatry: Behavioral sciences/clinical psychiatry. In *Child psychiatry* (11th ed., pp. 1268-1305). Philadelphia, PA: Wolters Kluwer.

Skikic, M., & Stovall, J. G. (2015). Schizophrenia. In F. J. Domino (Ed.), *The 5-minute clinical consult standard 2016* (24th ed., pp. 1000-1001). Philadelphia, PA: Wolters Kluwer.

Uher, R. (2010). The genetics of mental illness: A guide for parents and adoption professionals. *Adoption & Fostering, 34*(3), 105-108. doi:10.1177/030857591003400319

SCHIZOPHRENIA IN OLDER ADULTS

MAJOR CATEGORIES: Behavioral & Mental Health

DESCRIPTION

Schizophrenia is a chronic and incapacitating psychiatric disorder that severely impairs thought processes, the perception of stimuli, communication, behavior, and the ability to maintain relationships and a stable living environment. According to the fifth edition of the *Diagnostic and Statistical Manual of Mental Disorders (DSM-5),* a diagnosis of schizophrenia requires that at least one of the symptoms consisting of delusions, hallucinations, or disorganized speech be present for a significant portion of time during a one-month period, and that this be accompanied during this same period by grossly disorganized or catatonic behavior, negative symptoms such as reduced or limited speech and anhedonia, and an inability to experience pleasure from normally enjoyable activities such as exercise, hobbies, or music. In addition, negative symptoms may be present. Negative symptoms are characterized by the absence of cognitive, emotional, social, or physical qualities that are present in those without the disorder; they may lead to a grave disability in self-care or severe disruption of activities of daily living. Schizophrenia shares the feature of psychosis with several other *DSM-5* diagnoses, including mood disorders, and therefore can be difficult to distinguish from other disorders that feature psychosis. However, schizophrenia is primarily a thought disorder.

Schizophrenia diagnosed in adults older than 40 years of age has the same diagnostic criteria, symptoms, and course as schizophrenia diagnosed at a younger age. However, when the diagnosis is made later in life, the prognosis is generally better. This may be due to the better development of life skills and more stable living circumstances (long-term employment, financial security, more mature and longer relationships, established self-care habits) of older persons. In persons older than approximately 30 years of age, schizophrenia is diagnosed more often in women than in men. Because of the later diagnosis and therefore improved prognosis for women, more older persons with schizophrenia are female than male.

Onset of schizophrenia after the age of 50 years is unusual, with 80 percent of cases diagnosed at younger ages. Therefore, most older adults with schizophrenia have been living with the disease for years. By the time these people reach older age, the chronic and disruptive nature of schizophrenia has had a profound effect on their lives. Those who have lived with schizophrenia for many years frequently fall to the bottom of the socioeconomic scale, have limited support from family and friends, and may develop concurrent mental and physical health conditions that are difficult to detect and diagnose because they are masked by the symptoms of schizophrenia. Depression is particularly common among older persons with schizophrenia, and may be difficult to differentiate from negative symptoms of schizophrenia, such as flattening or diminution of emotional expression and impoverishment of speech and language.

Suicide remains a concern in older persons with schizophrenia, and the accumulated physical, emotional, and psychological stress of living with schizophrenia may accelerate the development of medical problems (e.g., cardiovascular, respiratory, and neurological diseases; cancer; diabetes; obesity and its complications). Given that schizophrenia is primarily a thought disorder, it may amplify or accelerate the decline of cognitive abilities ordinarily associated with aging, and schizophrenia of long duration may interfere with the detection and diagnosis of neurocognitive or other disorders related to cognition.

The etiology of schizophrenia is unknown. Current research indicates that it reflects a complex interaction between inherited and environmental factors. Research continues to investigate a wide range of such factors, including the volume of gray matter in the cerebral cortex, hippocampus, and thalamus of the brain; disruption of the quantities and functions of the neurotransmitter substances (particularly dopamine) that transmit signals between nerve cells; impaired inhibition of the transmission and effect of stimuli on the brain; exposure to trauma; and maternal exposure to viruses during pregnancy. As with the etiology of schizophrenia, the reasons for the specific age of its onset in a particular individual are unknown.

Treatment of schizophrenia depends on its severity, etiology, and phase at the time of its diagnosis, and can include medication, psychotherapy, involuntary detention, medication, social skills training, education of affected individuals and their families about the nature and effects of schizophrenia, and referrals to community and family support services. The prognosis for schizophrenia in a particular individual varies widely, from complete remission, to long-term treatment with a slow and steady decrease in the quality of life, to suicide. Schizophrenia continues to evolve in older adults, with some entering remission, others regressing from remission to active signs and symptoms, and others achieving stability.

FACTS AND FIGURES

All information presented here is for the United States. In the United States, the onset of schizophrenia occurs before age 40 in approximately 67 percent of cases, between the ages of 41 and 50 in 13 percent, between the ages of 51 and 60 in 7 percent, and after age 60 in 3 percent. Most persons in whom schizophrenia is diagnosed after the age of 45 years are women. Approximately 85 percent of older adults with schizophrenia live in their communities, 13 percent live in homes, 1 percent live in hospitals, and 0.5 percent live in veterans' hospitals.

A study of persons 65 years of age and older found higher rates of medical illness in those with than in those without schizophrenia, except for cancer, the rate of which was significantly lower in persons with schizophrenia, at 31 percent and 43 percent, respectively.

By comparison, congestive heart failure was present in 45 percent of the participants who had schizophrenia and 39 percent of those who did not; chronic obstructive pulmonary disease (COPD) was present in 53 percent schizophrenia and 41 percent, respectively, of the two groups; hypothyroidism was present in 37 percent and 27 percent, respectively; and dementia was present in 64 percent and 32 percent, respectively.

RISK FACTORS

Risk factors for schizophrenia remain the same from childhood (age 13 to 14) onward. Biological risk factors for the disease include a family history of it, overactivity of the dopaminergic nervous system, decreased brain size, premature birth or excessive maternal bleeding at birth, traumatic brain injury, and maternal exposure to trauma in the first trimester of pregnancy. Environmental risk factors for schizophrenia include low socioeconomic status, family dysfunction, exposure to trauma, and birth in winter or early spring. Stigma and isolation associated with a diagnosis of schizophrenia may exacerbate symptoms of the disease.

SIGNS AND SYMPTOMS

Manifestations of schizophrenia include cognitive symptoms (disorganized thought and speech to the point of adversely affecting communication, delusions) and negative symptoms (limited expression of emotion or affect, rapid changes in emotion, lack of motivation or will, inability to speak, lack of enjoyment or pleasure, social withdrawal). Other symptoms can include hallucinations, absorption with inner thoughts, a decrease in personal hygiene and self, and catatonia (lack of responsiveness to external stimuli).

TREATMENT

The social worker assisting an individual who has schizophrenia of the disorganized subtype should conduct a standard biological, psychological, social, and spiritual assessment of the individual, including an assessment of his or her risk for suicide and for inflicting harm on him- or herself and others. This should include an assessment of the individual's level of functioning and demeanor during the interview conducted for the assessment, with particular attention to the individual's affect and cognitive symptoms, the individual's satisfaction with current daily and social activities, and the collection of information on any previous mental health disorders that have affected the individual, other than schizophrenia. The assessment should also include laboratory tests if and as needed to identify medical disorders and substance abuse; the collection of collateral information from the individual's family, friends, and coworkers; and information about any family history of schizophrenia or other disorders.

Treatments and interventions for schizophrenia are directed at improving the quality of life of the affected individual, decreasing the number and severity of active-phase episodes of the disease, and returning the affected individual to a state of stability. When possible, family members of the affected individual should be included in the treatment process, in order to build social support for him or her. Because schizophrenia is a chronic disorder, some level of treatment is a lifelong necessity.

Comprehensive treatment for schizophrenia involves a combination of medication, psychotherapeutic and psychosocial intervention, involvement of family members or other supportive individuals or systems, and inpatient care if and when needed for the management of active-phase symptoms of the disease or for acute crises. Treatment can be divided according to the acute or active phase of schizophrenia, stabilization phase, and stable phase of the disease.

Treatment in the active or acute phase of schizophrenia is directed at decreasing hallucinations or delusions, stabilizing erratic behavior, and decreasing destructive and/or aggressive behavior to reduce self-harm or harm to others by the affected individual, and can include hospitalization if safety becomes a concern. Psychotropic medication plays a major role in the treatment of schizophrenia. Antipsychotic medications substantially reduce the active symptomology of the disease and reduce the risk of relapse for individuals with stabilized disease. A psychiatrist or other medical professional can prescribe medication if needed, with cognitive behavioral therapy (CBT) or another treatment technique given in conjunction with medication to assist the affected individual in recognizing distorted thoughts and responding more appropriately to hallucinations and delusions, reducing psychosocial stressors, and creating a more calm, structured, and organized environment for the affected individual.

Treatment in the stabilization phase of schizophrenia can begin when treatment of the acute phase has brought an affected individual to a state of partial remission. The goal of treatment during the stabilization phase is to minimize the likelihood of a return of active-phase symptoms.

Treatment in the stable phase of schizophrenia begins when an individual with the disease has returned to his or her optimal level of functioning. In cases of partial remission, after negative symptoms have disappeared but with some active symptoms remaining, CBT or another form of interpersonal therapy can be continued with the goal of reducing or eliminating remaining active symptoms, reducing stress, enhancing the functioning of the affected individual within the community, and providing assistance in setting small and realistic vocational and social goals. Treatment in the stable phase of schizophrenia can include educating the affected individual and his or her family on the course of the disease and the importance of continuing its treatment for as long as needed.

Social workers assisting individuals with schizophrenia should have a working knowledge of antipsychotic medication and its potential for causing side effects, known medically as extrapyramidal effects, and must be able to weigh the benefits of such medication against these extrapyramidal effects, which can include involuntary motor movements such as tremors or muscle spasms, sedation, slurring of speech, effects on vision, weight gain, and other such effects, especially since some of these effects can become permanent. An individual taking antipsychotic medication and who develops extrapyramidal symptoms should immediately be referred to the prescribing or other responsible physician.

Individuals with schizophrenia and/or their family members should be referred to local schizophrenia support groups, supported work, or mental health agencies if and as needed. The social worker should also ascertain the stability of the individual's living situation and make referrals as appropriate. It is also important to recognize that primary caregivers

of older adults with schizophrenia may themselves develop health conditions for which they need care.

Social workers assisting older individuals who have schizophrenia should be aware of their own cultural values, beliefs, and biases, and should develop specialized knowledge about these individuals' histories, traditions, and values. Social workers should adopt treatment methods that reflect their knowledge of the cultural diversity of the communities in which these individuals live.

Applicable Laws and Regulations
The U.S. government and individual states of the United States have their own standards, procedures, and laws for the involuntary restraint and detention of persons who may be a danger to themselves or to others. Because persons with schizophrenia have a high rate of attempted suicide and may lack the ability to meet their basic personal needs for food, shelter, and clothing, it is important to become familiar with the local requirements for involuntary detention and the appropriate management of persons with grave disability. Local and professional requirements for reporting neglect and abuse should be known and observed.

Services and Resources
Enter the term *schizophrenia* in the search box to access relevant information available on each website.
- Brain & Behavior Research Foundation (formerly NARSAD), http://bbrfoundation.org/
- National Alliance on Mental Illness (NAMI), http://www.nami.org/
- U.S. National Institutes of Health (NIH), http://www.nih.gov/
- U.S. National Institute of Mental Health (NIMH), http://www.nimh.nih.gov/index.shtml
- National Association of Social Workers (NASW), http://www.socialworkers.org/

Written by Chris Bates, MA, MSW

Reviewed by Lynn B Cooper, D. Crim, and Laura Gale, LCSW

References
American Psychiatric Association. (2013). *Diagnostic and statistical manual of mental disorders* (5th ed.). Arlington, VA: American Psychiatric Publishing.

Anderson, J. S., & Stovall, J. G. (2012). Schizophrenia. In F. J. Domino (Ed.), *The 5-minute clinical consult 2012* (20th ed., pp. 1174-1175). Philadelphia, PA: Walters Kluwer Health/Lippincott Williams & Wilkins.

Bond, G. R., Drake, R. E., Mueser, K. T., & Latimer, E. (2001). Assertive community treatment for people with severe mental illness. *Disease Management & Health Outcomes, 9*(3), 141-159.

British Association of Social Workers. (2012, January). The code of ethics for social work: Statement of principles. Retrieved December 8, 2015, from http://cdn.basw.co.uk/upload/basw_112315-7.pdf

Cohen, C. I. (2003). Introduction. In *Schizophrenia into later life* (pp. xiii-xx). Washington DC: American Psychiatric Publishing.

Cohen, C. I., & Iqbal, M. (2014). Longitudinal study of remission among older adults with schizophrenia spectrum disorder. *The American Journal of Geriatric Psychiatry, 22*(5), 450-458. doi:10.1016/j.jagp.2013.09.004

Corcoran, J., & Walsh, J. (2010). *Clinical assessment and diagnosis in social work practice* (2nd ed.). New York, NY: Oxford University Press.

Cummings, S. M., & Cassie, K. M. (2008). Perceptions of biopsychosocial services needs among older adults with severe mental illness: Met and unmet needs. *Health & Social Work, 33*(2), 133-143.

Cummings, S. M., & Kropf, N. P. (2009). Formal and informal support for older adults with severe mental illness. *Aging & Mental Health, 13*(4), 619-627.

Dickerson, F. B. (2007). Women, aging, and schizophrenia. *Journal of Women & Aging, 19*(1-2), 49-61.

Eisendrath, S. J., & Lichtmacher, J. E. (2011). Psychiatric disorders. In S. J. McPhee & M. A. Papadakis (Eds.), *Lange 2011 current medical diagnosis & treatment* (50th ed., pp. 1010-1019). New York, NY: McGraw-Hill Medical.

Fow, D. S. (2010). Significance of spirituality in the lives of older adults with and without serious mental illnesses. *Social Work in Mental Health, 8*(5), 469-481. doi:10.1080/15332981003744545

Hendrie, H. C., Tu, W., Tabbey, R. P., Purnell, C. E., Ambuehl, R. J., & Callahan, C. M. (2014). Health outcomes and cost of care among older adults with schizophrenia: a 10-year study using medical records across the continuum of care. *The American Journal of Geriatric Psychiatry, 22*(5), 427-436. doi:10.1016/j.jagp.2012.10.025

International Federation of Social Workers. (2012, March 3). *Statement of ethical principles.* Retrieved March 29, 2015, from http://ifsw.org/policies/statement-of-ethical-principles/

Kay, S. R., Fiszbein, A., & Opler, L. A. (1987). The positive and negative syndrome scale (PANSS) for schizophrenia. *Schizophrenia Bulletin, 13*(2), 261-276. doi:10.1093/schbul/13.2.261

Kurtz, M. M., & Mueser, K. T. (2008). A meta-analysis of controlled research on social skills training for schizophrenia. *Journal of Consulting and Clinical Psychology, 76*(3), 491-504. doi:10.1037/0022-006X.76.3.491

Malone Cole, J. A. (2012). Schizophrenia and other psychotic disorders. In K. M. Fortinash & P. A. Holoday Worret (Eds.), *Psychiatric mental health nursing* (5th ed., pp. 259-296). St. Louis, MO: Elsevier Mosby.

Mausbach, B. T., Cardenas, V., Goldman, S. R., & Patterson, T. L. (2007). Symptoms of psychosis and depression in middle-aged and older adults with psychotic disorders: The roles of activity satisfaction. *Aging & Mental Health, 11*(3), 339-345.

Scottish Intercollegiate Guidelines Network. (2013). Management of schizophrenia (SIGN no. 131). Edinburgh, Scotland.

Wheeler, D. (2015). NASW standards and indicators for cultural competence in social work practice. Retrieved December 8, 2015, from http://www.socialworkers.org/practice/standards/PRA-BRO-253150-CC-Standards.pdf

SCHIZOPHRENIA: AN OVERVIEW

MAJOR CATEGORIES: Behavioral & Mental Health

DESCRIPTION

Schizophrenia is a chronic and debilitating psychiatric disorder that severely impacts cognitive, behavioral, and emotional functioning and is characterized by hallucinations, delusions, and thought disturbance. The *Diagnostic and Statistical Manual of Mental Disorders,* Fifth Edition (*DSM-5,*) includes schizophrenia within the category of schizophrenia spectrum and other psychotic disorders. Other disorders included in this category are delusional disorder, schizotypal disorder, brief psychotic disorder, schizophreniform disorder, schizoaffective disorder, substance/medication-induced psychotic disorder, psychotic disorder due to another medical condition, and unspecified schizophrenia spectrum and other psychotic disorders. Catatonia is also included in this category as a specifier for other related conditions.

For schizophrenia to be diagnosed, two or more of the following active-phase symptoms must be present for a significant portion of time during a 1-month period: positive symptoms of delusions, hallucinations, disorganized speech, or grossly disorganized or catatonic behavior, and/or negative symptoms such as poverty of speech or anhedonia. At least one of the two active-phase symptoms must be delusions, hallucinations, or disorganized speech. These active-phase symptoms are described in more detail below. In addition, for a significant portion of the time since onset of the disturbance, the person's level of functioning in one or more areas such as work, interpersonal relationships, or self-care must be significantly diminished from the level achieved prior to onset of the disturbance. For children and adolescents, this criterion can be met by a failure to achieve expected level of interpersonal, academic, or occupational functioning. Continuous signs of the disturbance must be present for at least 6 months for the diagnosis to be assigned. During these 6 months, at least 1 month must include active-phase symptoms, which may include signs of prodromal symptoms or residual symptoms. During these periods of prodromal or residual symptoms, the disturbance may be manifested only by negative symptoms or two or more active symptoms. During this phase, the active-phase symptoms may also exist in an attenuated form. Furthermore, the duration of these periods may be shorter than specified if treated successfully.

The *DSM-5* provides course specifiers for schizophrenia, which are only to be used after the disorder has been present for 1 year. They include the following.

First episode, currently in acute episode: An acute episode is a time period in which the full symptom criteria for diagnosis are met. This specifier is used only for a first episode of active-phase symptoms.

First episode, currently in partial remission: Partial remission refers to a state in which there has been some improvement in functioning after a previous acute episode. During this time, the diagnostic criteria are only partially met. This specifier is only to be used following the first acute episode.

First episode, currently in full remission: During full remission, no symptoms are present. This specifier is to be used only following a first acute episode and/or an acute episode in partial remission.

Multiple episodes, currently in acute episode: This specifier is used when at least two previous episodes of active-phase symptoms have been present and the individual is currently experiencing an acute episode.

Multiple episodes, currently in partial remission: This specifier is used when an individual has experienced multiple acute episodes and is currently experiencing some improvement in functioning.

Multiple episodes, currently in full remission: This specifier is assigned when an individual has had multiple acute-phase symptoms but is not currently experiencing symptoms of the disorder.

Continuous: This specifier is used when full diagnostic criteria for the disorder continue to be met for the majority of the duration of the disorder, with only brief episodes of subthreshold symptoms.

Unspecified: This specifier is used when criteria for schizophrenia are met but other specifiers are not, or during the first year of diagnosis.

The *DSM-5* includes a specifier for catatonia and optional specifiers for severity. Severity is determined by rating each of the patient's active symptoms. These symptoms are rated based on the most severe presentation within the last 7 days and are rated on a scale ranging from 0 (not present) to 4 (present and severe).

Additional associated symptoms may include inappropriate affect, depression, dysphonia (voice impairment), anxiety or anger, and disturbed sleep. Impulsivity, hostility, and aggression are often associated with schizophrenia, although they are not included in the diagnostic criteria. Neurological symptoms may also be evident, including poor motor coordination and poor sensory integration. In some cases, minor physical abnormalities may be evident in the face and/or limbs. Some individuals with schizophrenia may lack insight, and may not recognize that they have a disorder. This often persists throughout the course of the illness. This symptom is a common cause of treatment nonadherence and predicts higher rates of relapse and poorer prognosis.

The onset of schizophrenia may be sudden or gradual, with the majority of those affected slowly developing a variety of clinical symptoms that become worse over time. Many individuals with schizophrenia first identify symptoms of depression, followed by the emergence of negative symptoms.

Differential diagnosis of schizophrenia from other disorders is important. Schizoaffective and bipolar disorders with psychotic features can be ruled out if no manic or depressive episodes have occurred concurrently with the active-phase symptoms, or, if present, have been present only for a short time of the duration of the presence of the active symptoms. For children and adolescents, if there is a history of autism spectrum disorder (ASD), schizophrenia is not diagnosed unless prominent delusions or hallucinations have been present, in addition to the other criteria, for at least 1 month. Individuals with obsessive-compulsive disorder (OCD) or body dysmorphia may also experience delusions. However, these disorders are characterized by obsessions and compulsions. Posttraumatic stress disorder (PTSD) can be distinguished from schizophrenia in that the flashbacks and hallucinations experienced in PTSD are preceded and informed by a traumatic event.

In order for schizophrenia to be fully understood, it is necessary to take a closer look at the active-phase symptoms by which the disorder is characterized.

Delusions are beliefs that are strongly held despite clear evidence to the contrary. Such false beliefs are fixed in nature and are not shared by others within the person's community. Delusions may include grandiose ideas about one's own powers or influence, beliefs that one's significant other is being unfaithful, or beliefs that one is being persecuted in some way, such as being tortured, poisoned, drugged, cheated, or otherwise mistreated. Delusions may also be somatic in nature, such as when a person believes that someone has removed his or her internal organs. Some delusions contain bizarre content that is clearly implausible, whereas others may have a basis in ordinary life experiences, such as when one believes that he or she is under police surveillance. When present by themselves without other existing symptoms of schizophrenia, delusions are their own diagnostic criteria in the *DSM-5*.

Hallucinations are distorted or false sensory perceptions that are experienced as real. Hallucinations may be auditory, visual, or, less frequently, olfactory, tactile, or gustatory (related to taste). Auditory hallucinations are the most common, and may include command hallucinations, in which one or more voices tell the individual having the hallucination to carry out an act, which may include harming himself or herself or someone else. For others, the auditory hallucination may be experienced as a hissing or whistling sound, or a running commentary about their actions. Visual hallucinations involve seeing something that is not present.

Disorganized speech features frequent derailment of speech or incoherence. Speech may begin in one direction but suddenly move tangentially in another without logical connection. This may appear as rambling dialogues or disjointed speech. In extreme cases, one word in a sentence does not connect in a logical way to those around it. Disorganized speech may also appear as if the person is holding an internal dialogue with himself or herself or with an unknown or invisible person.

Negative symptoms are characterized by the absence of cognitive, emotional, social, or physical qualities that are present in those without the disorder. Negative symptoms may include alogia (dysfunction of communication or poverty of speech), blunted affect (reduced range of experienced or expressed emotion), asociality (minimal or absent social interaction or interest in social interaction), anhedonia (a reduced capacity for pleasure, or loss of interest in activities that previously were pleasurable), or avolition (a decrease in motivation or desire, or a decreased ability to start or complete everyday tasks such as personal hygiene). These negative symptoms may lead to a grave disability in self-care and severe disruption of activities of daily living (ADLs).

Catatonia is characterized by extreme motor inability. Symptoms may include stupor, mutism, catalepsy (rigid body and/or limbs, or holding a fixed position against the forces of gravity), resistance to reposturing by another person, odd mannerisms, repetitive nongoal-directed motor activity, agitation, or grimacing. Echolalia or echopraxia may also be present. Grossly disorganized behavior is activity that is extremely incongruous given the context, such as extreme silliness, aggression, or anger.

People with early-onset schizophrenia have a worse prognosis due to less developed life functioning skills, whereas prognosis is better for those with later onset as they have had the chance to develop better life skills prior to the onset of the disorder. Men tend to have their first episode in their early- to mid-20s and experience more severe symptoms, whereas women generally develop symptoms in their late 20s. Prevalence is the same for men and women, and the worldwide geographic distribution is even.

The etiology of schizophrenia is unknown. Current research indicates that a complex interaction between genetic and environmental factors contributes to the development of the disorder. Studies of identical twins indicate about an 80-percent heritability rate. Current research is exploring numerous potential factors, including decreases in gray matter volume in the cerebral cortex, hippocampus, and thalamus; disruption of neurotransmitters (particularly dopamine); and impairment of stimulus inhibition in the brain.

Culture plays a significant role in the clinical presentation of symptoms. The content of an individual's delusions and hallucinations often is culturally based. Thus a patient in the United States may believe that Barack Obama is communicating with him or her, whereas a patient in India may believe that he or she is speaking to Lord Shiva. Cultural beliefs determine what is normative, and one culture may sanction some symptoms that are considered pathological in another culture. For some cultures, communication with higher powers, spirit possession, speaking in tongues, and dissociative states are normative, and a part of religious practices, whereas other cultures find these experiences abnormal.

Cultural beliefs also influence the reactions of individuals towards persons with schizophrenia and the level of stigma persons with schizophrenia experience. Although stigma towards mental illness exists in all cultures, researchers have found that in developing countries mental illness is less stigmatized and as a result persons with schizophrenia often experience higher levels of family and community support than those in developed countries.

The onset of schizophrenia may be sudden or gradual, with the majority of individuals slowly decompensating and developing a variety of clinical symptoms that become worse over time. Many individuals with schizophrenia first identify symptoms of depression. Others first express frustration, anxiety, and an inability to cope with day-to-day activities. This leads to increasing disorganization and a loosening of accurate perceptions of reality. This prodromal phase is followed by a phase of active symptoms, when

hallucinations, delusions, and distorted thought patterns appear. When active-phase symptoms resolve, usually through the use of psychotropic medications, the individual enters a state of remission or partial remission during which optimal community functioning is attainable. Prognosis varies widely, with some individuals with schizophrenia maintaining long-term remission and others continuing to experience continuous active-phase symptoms. Most individuals with schizophrenia will experience cycling between active-phase symptoms and periods of remission or partial remission. There is no cure for schizophrenia, and most individuals continue to experience some effects of the disorder throughout life. Depending on the severity, etiology, and current presence or absence of active-phase symptoms, treatment might include involuntary psychiatric hospitalization, outpatient medication management, social skills training, psychoeducation, psychotherapy, and referrals to community and family support services.

Childhood- or adolescent-onset schizophrenia typically is referred to as early-onset schizophrenia. Childhood-onset schizophrenia, in which symptoms are present before the age of 13, is sometimes referred to as very-early-onset schizophrenia. Adolescent-onset schizophrenia indicates symptoms, and possibly diagnosis, from ages 13 to 18. The onset of symptoms usually is earlier for males, and as a result males are given a diagnosis of childhood-onset schizophrenia more often than females.

The *DSM-5* uses the same criteria for diagnosis regardless of age of onset. Generally, the earlier the onset, the more severe the lifetime course of the disorder. Childhood-onset schizophrenia cycles through four phases. Increased deterioration usually takes place with each cycle. With successful treatment, the acute phases may diminish in frequency and intensity after 10 years. The first phase is the prodromal phase, which is characterized by a subtle deterioration in functioning. Prodromal symptoms may include social withdrawal, unusual preoccupations, changes in appetite or sleep patterns, or decreased self-care. The prodromal phase may pass unnoticed in childhood-onset schizophrenia, as symptoms may be perceived as a normal reaction to environmental stressors.

Caution must be used when diagnosing early-onset schizophrenia. Children and adolescents by their very nature are growing and changing in multiple developmental domains (physical, social, verbal, cognitive, relational, spiritual). It may be difficult to discern or evaluate the significance of changes in behavior or developmental progress. Some symptoms of early-onset schizophrenia may manifest not as deterioration of already acquired social skills but as developmental delays or missed developmental milestones. Developmental disruption may be present that is related to environmental stressors, not schizophrenia. However, given the increased severity of early-onset schizophrenia, symptoms should not be ignored. Given these complexities, consultation with professional(s) experienced in early-onset schizophrenia should be sought.

For most individuals, symptoms begin between 15 and 25 years of age. Schizophrenia diagnosed later in life (after age 40) has the same diagnostic criteria, symptoms, and course as schizophrenia diagnosed at a younger age. However, the prognosis generally is better when onset is later in life. Onset of schizophrenia after age 50 is unusual, with 80 percent of cases diagnosed at a younger age. Given that the disorder usually manifests in early adulthood, the majority of older adults with schizophrenia have been living with the disease for many years. For older adults, the chronic and disruptive nature of schizophrenia will have had a profound impact on their lives. Medical problems are common in older adults with schizophrenia as a result of the accumulated physical, emotional, and psychological stress of living with the disease. Individuals who have lived with schizophrenia for many years are often of low socioeconomic status, have compromised support systems, and develop co-occurring mental or physical health conditions. These conditions may be difficult to detect and diagnose because they are often masked by the symptoms of schizophrenia. Depression is common among older persons with schizophrenia and may be difficult to differentiate from the negative symptoms of schizophrenia, such as a decrease in volition and anhedonia. All adults with schizophrenia are at risk for suicide. The accumulated physical, emotional, and psychological stress of living with schizophrenia may accelerate the development of medical problems such as cardiovascular, respiratory, and neurological diseases; cancer; diabetes; and obesity. Declines in cognitive abilities associated with aging may be accelerated or amplified, making detection and diagnosis of dementia or other disorders related to cognition more difficult.

Environmental conditions are important to the effectiveness of treatment and to the overall prognosis of schizophrenia. Many individuals with schizophrenia experience family and social rejection or job loss as a result of their disorder. Many live in social isolation. Poverty and homelessness are common, and the thought disturbances that accompany schizophrenia make navigating the social service, public housing, mental health, and healthcare systems difficult. For individuals without social support or family involvement, board and care homes or nursing homes may be the safest living environment. In the United States, an inadequate mental health system results in individuals with schizophrenia and other serious mental health disorders frequently entering the criminal justice system, usually for nonviolent offenses.

The family members of individuals with schizophrenia are profoundly affected by the disorder. Family members may experience a wide range of emotions, including isolation, sadness, loss, fear, guilt, anger, resentment, exhaustion, inadequacy, failure, frustration, and ambiguity. Family members often are the caretakers and advocates for their loved ones with schizophrenia. Because schizophrenia is chronic in nature, the family is affected for the entire postdiagnosis life of the person with schizophrenia. The cyclical nature of schizophrenia, in which individuals move through active phases and remission, reduces the stability and predictability for the family and places significant stress on the family system. Significant changes may take place in family roles and functioning. For example, parents may have to change work schedules to accommodate treatment appointments, a child may take on a caretaking role for a parent, and the whole family may have to make financial sacrifices. Family members experience disruption of various aspects of their lives, including disruptions in time due to caregiving responsibilities and finances as they take on the financial burden of caring for their loved one. For those whose caretaking role includes having the loved one with schizophrenia living with them, disruptions may also occur to their privacy and levels of self-care may decrease. Family members may also experience effects on their own health and well-being, including increased stress and increased levels of depression and anxiety, and may feel taken advantage of by both the loved one and the medical system, which often is grossly inadequate for the needs of the stressed family system and the individual with schizophrenia.

Complicating the impact on the family is the stigma associated with schizophrenia in many cultures. Research and professional assessments that attribute schizophrenia to dysfunctions in family dynamics or disturbed parent-child relationships have inadvertently added to the stigma and for some families transformed it into guilt or shame. Further exacerbating these feelings of shame and guilt are the perceived implication that the family is responsible because of the strong evidence of a genetic etiology of schizophrenia. Families in the United States report difficulty navigating the disjointed mental health system, receiving conflicting advice from professionals, and being ignored or condescended to by the multitude of professionals with whom they come into contact.

Laws and regulations related to patient/patient confidentiality also create frustrations for family members. Privacy laws and ethical practices regarding health information and the preservation of patient-therapist privilege, a hallmark of the mental health system, protect an individual's right to confidentiality, often despite indications that the individual is unable to make decisions for himself or herself, such as during active-phase symptoms of schizophrenia. While this preservation of the rights of the individual is important, it often creates barriers to family members seeking information regarding the well-being of their loved one. For family members in caretaking roles, the inability to access medical and psychiatric information can result in feeling as if they are being ignored by professionals who are following facility and legal confidentiality regulations. However, in principle, confidentiality regulations are not designed to impede healthcare services, and they are not intended to enable the clinician or treatment facility to further isolate the person from his or her family or other supports. For example, many settings obtain emergency contact details to facilitate collaboration in appropriate circumstances. Furthermore, certain settings (such as emergency rooms) are by definition unpredictable, and ethical or clinical necessity may trump privacy laws provided the intent is not malicious but rather is to deliver the appropriate service within the limitations of the setting. Finally, confidentiality is trumped in circumstances in which the person is at risk for neglect, self-harm, or homicidal ideation.

The presence of both schizophrenia and substance use disorder is a common co-occurrence. The term *dual diagnosis* is used when any mental health disorder and a substance use disorder are present at the same time and within the same time frame as specified by the *DSM-5* diagnostic requirements. Individually, schizophrenia and substance use disorder are chronic, progressive disorders that may have a severe impact on multiple facets of an individual's life. Combined, the impact of both disorders increases, complicating the identification and treatment of both. When both a substance use disorder and schizophrenia are present, there is an increased likelihood of a decrease in adherence to the prescribed medication regimen, an increase in side effects of medications as they interact with nonprescribed drugs or alcohol, an exacerbation of psychotic symptoms, and decreased reliability of self-reporting of symptoms and substance use. In addition, there is an increased risk of substance use relapse, increased involvement in the criminal justice system, higher risk of psychiatric hospitalization, and increased exposure to violence both as a victim and as a perpetrator. Persons with co-occurring schizophrenia and substance use disorder may struggle with insomnia and other sleep disturbances, which may further lead to depression, adverse medication effects, and cognitive deficits. Both disorders individually progress more rapidly due to the presence of the other disorder, and combine to generate dynamics and situations not present when only one disorder is present.

Violence and involvement in the criminal justice system both increase when a substance use disorder and schizophrenia are present. The use of controlled substances is itself frequently a crime that may lead to incarceration. Once the person is incarcerated, treatment for underlying mental health diagnoses becomes secondary, and may be overlooked in the correctional system. Recent research suggests that violent crime is substantially increased with comorbid schizophrenia and substance use disorder, whereas it is only slightly increased for those with diagnosis of schizophrenia alone. Other studies have had similar findings, shedding light on long-held beliefs about the relationship of schizophrenia and violence.

There are numerous theories about the development of the co-occurrence of schizophrenia and substance use disorder, the interaction of the two disorders, the prognosis for each disorder, and the optimal treatment course for these individuals. It is likely that there are multiple causative factors and treatment options based upon the clinical assessment of the individual. The self-medication theory holds that substance use is often a response to symptoms of an underlying mental health disorder and that the substances are used to relieve symptoms of schizophrenia. Other theorists believe that a substance use disorder is premorbid for schizophrenia. This theory posits that individuals who abuse substances are more likely to develop schizophrenia than those who do not. Another theory is that there is a common vulnerability to both substance use disorders and mental health disorders, possibly due to brain structure and dopamine circuitry, which controls the highly complex reward system in the brain. The conditions may exacerbate one another, so that what might have been nonaddictive social alcohol consumption becomes dependence, and manageable symptoms of schizophrenia become unmanageable in the presence of nonprescribed substances. It is also possible that there is no causal relationship between the two despite a correlation between rates of schizophrenia and substance use disorders.

The rate of tobacco use, in particular cigarette smoking, is disproportionately high among individuals with schizophrenia. Individuals with schizophrenia have a higher lifetime prevalence of smoking than individuals without schizophrenia. Individuals with schizophrenia smoke more cigarettes per day than smokers without schizophrenia, and the amount of nicotine in the blood, depth and frequency of inhaling while smoking, and percent of income spent on cigarettes are higher among smokers with schizophrenia. Individuals with schizophrenia have increased smoking-related negative health consequences compared to individuals who smoke but do not have schizophrenia. For example, individuals with schizophrenia who smoke have 2 to 3 times the rates of lung cancer, chronic obstructive pulmonary disease (COPD), and cardiovascular disease as smokers without schizophrenia. Approximately half of all deaths among individuals with schizophrenia can be attributed to tobacco-related illnesses. Specific to those with schizophrenia, the impact of smoking may include increased mental health medication side effects such as akathisia and tardive dyskinesia, reduced efficacy of psychiatric medications, increased active-phase symptoms of schizophrenia, and increased risk of other substance abuse and dependence.

Individuals with schizophrenia who smoke face greater barriers to stopping than smokers in the general population. Cigarettes and smoking may be used as part of behavior reward systems in mental health settings. Healthcare professionals place less focus on smoking cessation, as symptoms and behaviors related to schizophrenia take priority. Cessation programs may not be customized to the circumstances of individuals with schizophrenia, and smoking may relieve some symptoms of schizophrenia for some individuals. Relief of schizophrenia symptoms is widely reported and underlies the self-medication theory of why smoking is so prevalent among persons with schizophrenia. The self-medication theory also influences healthcare professionals to place less emphasis on smoking cessation.

There are several theories about the reasons for the elevated rates of smoking among persons with schizophrenia. The self-medication theory posits that individuals with schizophrenia obtain relief from symptoms from smoking. Research has focused on schizophrenia symptom relief provided by nicotine as it affects dopamine and other neurotransmitters in conjunction with their interaction with the reward pathways in the brain. Recently, researchers have proposed that instead of schizophrenia causing smoking, it is smoking that increases the risk of psychiatric disorders, including schizophrenia.

Smoking cessation therapy in persons with schizophrenia includes nicotine replacement, motivational interviewing, and reward (monetary) systems. Intensive cessation programs that are more individualized than those for the general population also are effective. These intensive programs include emphasis on the ubiquitous nature of smoking in the environments of those with schizophrenia.

FACTS AND FIGURES

The *DSM-5* reports a lifetime prevalence of schizophrenia of approximately 0.3 to 0.7 percent, with the specific symptomology used in defining the disorder having an impact on the breakdown by sex, location, and race/ethnicity. For example, emphasis on long duration and negative symptoms results in higher rates for males than females. Approximately 20 percent of individuals with schizophrenia attempt suicide at least once; 5 to 6 percent of individuals with schizophrenia die due to suicide.

Of the approximately 1 percent of the population with a diagnosis of schizophrenia, only 0.1 to 1 percent develop symptoms before age 10, with 4 percent developing symptoms before age 15. IQ in the majority of children with childhood-onset schizophrenia is normal, with 10 to 20 percent having IQs in the borderline intellectual functioning to intellectually disabled range. Thirty-four percent of children with childhood-onset schizophrenia exhibit motor and language abnormalities.

Schizophrenia affects approximately 1 percent of the world's population. Statistics regarding comorbidity of schizophrenia and substance use disorder fall in a wide range. This may be due to low reliability of self-reporting, lack of cooperation between mental health and substance abuse service providers, and the complexity of determining diagnosis between the two disorders.

Thirty percent of individuals with schizophrenia in 1970 reported substance abuse, increasing to 60 percent by 1990. Alcohol is the substance most often reported to be abused (43.1 to 65 percent); cannabis is next (50.8 percent), followed by cocaine (23 percent) and opiates (10 to 20 percent). Substance use disorder is 4.6 times more common among persons with schizophrenia than among the general population. Approximately 70 to 80 percent of individuals with schizophrenia smoke, versus 20 to 30 percent of the general population. Individuals with schizophrenia who smoke have twice the risk of coronary heart disease, are 10 times more likely to be daily smokers, and achieve higher systemic doses of nicotine at a faster rate than smokers in the general population.

In the United States, 14.5 percent of incarcerated men and 31 percent of incarcerated women have a serious mental health disorder, although the specific number of incarcerated individuals with schizophrenia is unknown. Research indicates that individuals with schizophrenia are 13 times more likely to commit suicide than individuals in the general population.

RISK FACTORS

Environmental risk factors include low socioeconomic status, living in an urban area at the time of birth, family dysfunction, exposure to trauma, winter or early spring birth, and maternal stress during pregnancy. Symptoms may be exacerbated by stigma and isolation associated with the diagnosis.

Biological risk factors include genetics, dopamine hyperactivity, decreased brain size, premature birth or excessive maternal bleeding during delivery, traumatic brain injury, and maternal exposure to trauma in first trimester. In childhood-onset schizophrenia, a family history of schizophrenia is a strong risk factor.

SIGNS AND SYMPTOMS

Individuals with schizophrenia may exhibit some or all of the following signs and symptoms: Social withdrawal, usually progressive; decreased level of personal hygiene and self-care; inappropriate or flat affect or rapidly changing affect; hallucinations, frequently visual or auditory; delusions, often persecutory or grandiose; slowed thought processes, loose associations, or rapidly shifting thought processes; reduced motor activity or catatonia; and bizarre appearance in dress or unkempt appearance.

In children, signs and symptoms will vary with developmental age. For example, in children, delusions are more likely to center on monsters than on government security agencies. Also note that symptoms may manifest as the absence of the achievement of developmental skills rather than their deterioration.

ASSESSMENT

Assessment is an ongoing process that should be reevaluated as new information regarding the person becomes available and as his or her symptoms move from active phase to remission.

A standard bio-psycho-social-spiritual history should be taken, with specific attention to risk of harm to self or others.

The social environment of the person can have a profound effect on adherence to and response to treatment. The social context of the person should be closely assessed to determine areas of support and vulnerabilities as it relates to treatment.

Accurate information on the response to past treatment is key to effective treatment planning, as each individual will have his or her own responses to treatment modalities and settings, medications, and psychosocial stressors.

When working with children or adolescents with schizophrenia, it is useful to use a family systems framework assessment using the ecological and strengths perspectives. Noting the positive events and positive attitudes of family members can help them identify their own strengths and resiliencies. In addition, the use of a family genogram with attention to mental health history can alert the professionals and the family to possible genetic predisposition for the disorder.

Inclusion of family members in the assessment process is advised unless the person refuses to grant permission or it is otherwise clinically contraindicated. Family members or others familiar with the person often are able to give more accurate information than the person, who may be having active symptoms at the time of assessment and be unable to accurately self-report. It is important to engage individuals with schizophrenia about their social supports and to offer collateral services during all phases of treatment, as those who may be initially opposed to such collaboration may change their minds, especially if they respond well to treatment.

The healthcare professional should be aware of the cultural attitudes towards mental illness that the family and person may hold and how these beliefs may impact social and familial support.

The healthcare professional should become knowledgeable about how religious beliefs may impact the experience of symptoms, coping mechanisms, and adherence to treatment strategies.

The healthcare professional should assess the norms of the family and determine the roles that each family member plays as they relate to the individual with schizophrenia.

An observation of functioning and demeanor during the initial interview should be made, with particular attention to possible negative symptoms.

The healthcare professional should gather collateral information from family, friends, and coworkers regarding functioning in home, work, and social settings, including any recent changes in affect or behavior.

The healthcare professional should determine any prior diagnoses other than schizophrenia, including substance use disorders and mood disorders.

The healthcare professional should assess for current and past use of cigarettes and other nicotine consumption and for a history of smoking-related medical complications.

The healthcare professional should assess for alcohol and other substance use. Such use may or may not meet the criteria for diagnosis of substance use disorder but may be significant as it may highlight patterns of self-medication.

Tools relevant to screening for symptoms or severity of symptoms of schizophrenia include the following: Social Network Questionnaire (SNQ), Positive and Negative Syndrome Scale (PANSS) for Schizophrenia, Scale for the Assessment of Negative Symptoms (SANS), and the Scale for the Assessment of Positive Symptoms (SAPS).

Tools relevant for screening children and adolescents for symptoms of schizophrenia include the following: Schedule for Affective Disorders and Schizophrenia for School-Aged Children (K-SADS) and Brief Psychiatric Rating Scale for Children (BPRS-C).

Screening tools useful for assessing smoking include the following: Fagerstrom Test for Nicotine Dependence (FTND) and Minnesota Nicotine Withdrawal Scale (MNWS).

Appropriate laboratory tests may be useful in determining presence of alcohol or other substances.

Ventricular enlargement and cortical atrophy seen on CT scan have been associated with severe cognitive impairment and poor response to antipsychotic medications.

Decreased frontal lobe activity as seen on PET scan is associated with the presence of negative symptoms.

TREATMENT

Comprehensive treatment for schizophrenia involves a combination of outpatient medication management, psychosocial interventions, involvement of family members or other support systems, and inpatient care for acute crisis intervention or management of active-phase symptoms. Many individuals with schizophrenia will be receiving services from multiple providers. Because of the importance of psychotropic medication in controlling active symptoms of schizophrenia, it is likely that a psychiatrist or other medical professional will be a part of the treatment team. In addition, the individual may be receiving assistance with housing, employment, and financial needs. It is important for professionals to take on a care coordination role as well as to provide psychological intervention.

Creating and maintaining a therapeutic alliance is essential, as it allows professionals to gain important information and allows development of trust as well as a willingness to participate in the treatment process. The individual and, when appropriate, his or her family should be included in the treatment planning process as much as possible based on cognitive impairments and level of disorganization.

Treatment can be divided into three phases: the acute treatment phase, the stabilization phase, and the stable phase. The acute treatment phase begins when the individual begins having active-phase symptoms. Active-phase symptoms often are triggered by medication noncompliance, substance abuse, or stressful life events, but they can also be a part of the ordinary course of the disorder. A thorough assessment of precipitating events should be taken to determine possible causes for the deterioration in functioning. Goals include harm reduction and returning the individual to a state of maximum functioning as quickly as possible. Harm reduction consists of assessing and managing agitation and aggression and controlling disturbed behavior. The presence of command hallucinations increases the risk of suicidal or homicidal ideation and aggression, so safety planning for possible risk of harm to self or others should take place. Psychotropic medication reevaluation may be necessary to assist with reducing the severity of the psychosis and the associated symptoms and returning the individual to a state of equilibrium as quickly as possible.

Psychosocial interventions during the acute phase of treatment may include reducing contact with overstimulating environments, reducing psychosocial stressors, and promoting a calm routine and structured environment. Tolerant, nondemanding interactions can reduce aggressive behavior. The individual should be included in treatment planning during the acute treatment phase as much as possible based on his or her level of functioning. Insight-oriented therapy during the acute phase is contraindicated because of the cognitive and perceptual distortions present during active symptoms. However, some success has been found with the use of cognitive behavioral therapy (CBT) once the acute symptoms are stabilized. This can help challenge psychotic thinking and alter responses to hallucinations and delusions.

Involving family members in the acute treatment phase can be helpful, as they often have the most complete history of the individual, know what works to de-escalate him or her, and have the most familiarity with the success of past efforts at stabilization. Family members also play an important role in treatment adherence, for individuals who often are unable to care for themselves adequately during this phase. It is important to remember that family members are often under extreme stress during active-phase symptoms and may need separate support and resources.

Upon returning to a state of partial remission, the individual enters the stabilization phase of treatment. The goal of treatment during the stabilization phase is to minimize the likelihood of a return to active-phase symptoms. This includes reducing stress, facilitating a continued reduction in symptoms, and promoting positive community functioning. Educating the individual and family members about the course of treatment, factors that influence reduction in symptoms, and the importance of treatment adherence is important during this phase. Consistent service delivery continues to be important. For individuals who were hospitalized during the acute phase, connection to outpatient treatment and ongoing medication support are imperative. CBT and family meetings continue to be important during this phase of treatment. Social skills training can be beneficial for individuals with persistent difficulties in social environments. Community functioning can be supported by assisting the individual in setting small, realistic social and vocational goals without undue pressure to perform at a level that will be stressful. Behavioral techniques such as positive reinforcements and token economies can assist with learning social skills. Psychotropic medication should continue to be evaluated by the treating psychiatrist or medical professional.

Once individuals have returned to their optimal level of functioning, they enter the stable phase of treatment. Treatment goals during this phase are to ensure that symptoms are controlled and to continue to support the maximum level of functioning. Individuals should be fully involved in the treatment planning process and should take an active role in setting social and vocational goals that they find achievable. Continued inclusion of family members is important, as they are often the first to become aware of the reemergence of active-phase symptoms or a deterioration in functioning. CBT continues to be useful in changing the individual's responses to environmental triggers. Evaluation for medication compliance and side effects continues to be important, and referrals to the treating psychiatrist or treating medical professional should be made if any concerns emerge. Vocational rehabilitation services can provide assessment, training, and job placement opportunities commensurate with the level of functioning. Housing may also be a need for those without family support, particularly those who were hospitalized during their active-phase symptoms. Choice of housing should focus on developing, improving, and utilizing personal and community resources with the goal of achieving as much autonomy as possible. When possible, housing and resource preferences should be favored, acknowledging the right of the individual to live in an environment that is as normalized as possible. Supportive service may be needed for the individual to remain in independent or assisted living.

Psychotropic medication plays a major role in the treatment of schizophrenia. Antipsychotic medications substantially reduce active symptomology and, for stabilized individuals, reduce the risk of relapse. Professionals working with individuals with schizophrenia should have a working knowledge of antipsychotic medication and potential side effects.

Antipsychotic medications, also known as neuroleptics, are used to reduce active-phase symptoms such as catatonia, hallucinations, disorganized speech, and delusions. Antipsychotic medications are divided into first-generation and second-generation agents. Commonly used first-generation antipsychotics, also known as typical antipsychotics, include chlorpromazine (Thorazine), haloperidol (Haldol), perphenazine (Trilafon), trifluoperazine (Stelazine), and fluphenazine (Prolixin). Commonly used second-generation antipsychotics, also known as atypical antipsychotics, include clozapine (Clozaril), quetiapine (Seroquel), and risperidone (Risperdal).

The benefits of medication must be weighed against the presence of or risk for extrapyramidal symptoms (EPSs) and other side effects. EPSs include tremors, dystonia, restlessness, slurred speech, sedation, sexual dysfunction, tachycardia, and weight gain. The most common EPS is akathisia, which usually occurs early in treatment and is characterized by an inability to sit or stand still and a subjective feeling of restlessness and need to be in constant motion. This may be accompanied by feelings of terror, suicidality, or anxiety. It is important to educate individuals that what they are experiencing is a side effect

and not an exacerbation of the schizophrenia itself. Individuals with akathisia should be referred back to their treating psychiatrist for an adjustment to their medication regimen.

Acute dystonia is an EPS that usually occurs in individuals who have been on neuroleptic medication for many years and in younger individuals. It is characterized by bizarre muscle spasms in the neck, head, and tongue. The use of antiparkinson medication can be helpful in alleviating symptoms, and all individuals with signs of acute dystonia should be referred back to their treating psychiatrist.

One of the most serious potential EPSs is tardive dyskinesia (TD), which may include involuntary movements of the face (grimacing), tongue (tongue thrusting), jaw (repetitive chewing), or extremities (finger movements). Early identification of TD is important, as TD can become permanent and may worsen even after suspension of the associated medication. Stopping the medication soon after the emergence of TD may cause the symptoms to reverse, so immediate referral back to the treating psychiatrist is imperative. First-generation antipsychotics pose a higher risk for movement disorders such as TD than do second-generation antipsychotics. However, because some individuals respond more positively to first-generation medications, they are still utilized. The medications that most commonly result in TD are chlorpromazine, fluphenazine, haloperidol, and trifluoperazine.

Neuroleptic malignant syndrome (NMS) is a catatonia-like state that is an uncommon but serious EPS. NMS manifests as muscle rigidity, confusion, involuntary movements, stupor, and cardiovascular instability; it may result in coma or death. Symptoms usually occur within the first 2 weeks of drug treatment, and may occur at small doses. Both typical and atypical neuroleptics can have a range of additional side effects, including dry mouth, blurred vision, urinary retention, and acute glaucoma.

Medication nonadherence is a significant barrier to successful treatment. Medication nonadherence increases the risk for the reemergence of active-phase symptoms and subsequent psychiatric hospitalization. Reasons for nonadherence are complex. Individuals may be unaware or in denial about the severity of the illness, or they may experience stigma related to taking a daily psychotropic medication. Many individuals with schizophrenia have cognitive issues or a substance use disorder that prevents or interferes with adherence to a prescribed medication regimen. Individuals with schizophrenia also report environmental barriers such as lack of access to healthcare services and an inability to pay for the medications due to poverty, unemployment, or insurance issues. Neuroleptics can have severe and debilitating side effects that discourage adherence. A multidisciplinary team approach is recommended to encourage medication adherence and assessment of adverse effects. A team approach allows for the opportunity not only to address clinical issues but also to provide assistance in navigating the healthcare system and overcoming environmental obstacles to compliance.

Working with children and adolescents with schizophrenia presents an additional set of considerations. There is limited evidence as to the efficacy of psychotropic medication in children and adolescents despite its use as a common treatment modality for these age groups. Parents or caretakers of the child or adolescent will need to be involved in the treatment process for legal as well as clinical reasons. Family interventions should be started in the acute phase of treatment and should continue throughout the treatment process. As with adults, CBT is recommended for all children and adolescents with schizophrenia. Art therapies can also be considered as adjunctive therapy for children and adolescents. Through art therapies, children and adolescents learn to express themselves, establish a sense of mastery, and develop a new way of relating to others. Family therapy is particularly relevant in the treatment of children and adolescents with schizophrenia. Children requiring psychiatric hospitalization or residential care should be placed in an environment that is appropriate to their developmental level and should be placed in a setting with others their own age. Throughout the course of treatment, attention should be given to maintaining the child's academic progress as much as possible.

Research has reported several forms of nonpharmacological interventions that have been successful with persons with both schizophrenia and a substance use disorder. Psychoeducation and CBT have been noted to decrease the risk of relapse resulting in psychiatric hospitalization. Motivational interviewing (MI), assertive community treatment (ACT), and family interventions (FI) are part of most integrated treatment, in which addiction and mental health interventions occur simultaneously by the same team of professionals. Research indicates that psychoeducational interventions increase understanding of illness and that teaching about crisis management reduces relapses. CBT focuses on establishing coping skills to deal more effectively with stress in order to prevent relapse. MI emphasizes increasing willingness to change behaviors that may be exacerbating symptoms. ACT is an approach that involves a multidisciplinary team of psychiatrists, nurses, social workers, and substance abuse counselors who provide intensive services. These services are available whenever individuals need them, 24 hours a day, 7 days a week. FI focus on increasing the family's knowledge about schizophrenia, giving them skills that can be used to assist the individual when he or she begins to decompensate, and improving communication and collaborative problem solving between the individual and his or her family.

Music therapy has been found to be an effective adjunct to traditional schizophrenia treatmen. Researchers have found that including music therapy as a treatment intervention results in more positive outcomes than standard treatment alone in improving schizophrenic symptoms. Music therapy is designed to complement an interdisciplinary approach to care and to improve quality of life; it is not intended to replace traditional treatments or medications. Music therapy involves the planned use of music to treat physical, cognitive, psychological, emotional, and social needs of individuals and groups. Music therapy is a professional discipline practiced by board-certified music therapists. Music therapy can be either active or passive. In active music therapy, the therapist and individual create music with instruments or their voices. In passive music therapy, the individual rests while the therapist plays music or has music playing. Passive music therapy may also include guided imagery. Music therapy may include listening to and discussing music with the therapist, singing or producing music using instruments, or playing or listening to music in a group setting. Although significant improvements in active-phase symptoms have not been reported in most studies, improvements in behavioral and cognitive abilities have been demonstrated with adjunctive music therapy. Supplementing standard treatment with music therapy improves the mental health of individuals with schizophrenia by engaging them in interactive activities that improve social functioning, reducing symptoms of depression and anxiety, improving their ability to adapt to the social environment, and improving their ability to cope with symptoms.

For individuals with substance use disorders, the first treatment priority is to assess and stabilize whichever disorder is currently dominant or is disrupting the possibility of any effective treatment interventions. Flexibility is important, as this may require the exclusive treatment of one or the other of the disorders, or both simultaneously.

Professionals should take into account the cultural and religious context within which symptoms take place. What may be considered delusional in one culture (belief in spirits, ghosts, or witches) may be a normative belief in another culture. Further, in some cultures visual or auditory hallucinations with religious content, such as hearing the voices of supernatural beings, or that of a supreme being in monotheistic cultures, can be an expected and welcome part of certain religious practices or personal experience. Furthermore, statements should be carefully explored, as they may use "seeing," "hearing," and other sensory labels that seem to connote hallucinations to mean something rather different, such as auditory or visual experiences during falling asleep or waking, or particularly vivid dreams and reveries.

Problem	Goal	Intervention
Active-phase symptoms are present, including disorganized thinking, hallucinations/delusions/erratic or self-destructive behavior.	Decrease hallucinations or delusions, stabilize erratic behavior, harm reduction to decrease self destructive aggressive and/or behavior.	Initiate hospitalization or involve emergency personnel if safety becomes a concern. Connect individual to psychiatrist or other medical professional for medication evaluation or reevaluation; reduce psychosocial stressors; create calm, structured, and organized environment; involve family members in the stabilization and treatment process if clinically appropriate and supported by individual. Provide CBT in conjunction with medication management to assist in recognizing distorted thoughts and beliefs, and in responding differently to hallucinations and delusions.
Partial remission, negative symptoms are present, some active symptoms remain.	Stabilization, reduce or eliminate active-phase symptoms, enhance community supports and functioning, reduce stress.	Continue use of CBT, provide psychoeducation to the individual and his or her family on the course of treatment and need for medication adherence, begin token economies and positive reinforcements to teach social skills, continue medication management, assist in setting small, realistic vocational and social goals, mobilize family and community supports.
Individual is stabilized, no active-phase symptoms present, or optimal level of functioning has been reached.	Maintain optimal level of community functioning.	Continue with CBT and medication management, refer to peer support groups and vocational rehabilitation services, maintain collaboration with family and community supports.

APPLICABLE LAWS AND REGULATIONS

Each jurisdiction (nation, state, province) has its own standards, procedures, and laws for involuntary restraint and detention of persons who may be a danger to themselves or to others, or who are gravely disabled (unable to perform basic self-care). Those with schizophrenia have a high rate of suicide attempts and grave disability during active-phase symptoms. Minor children living in the home with a parent who has schizophrenia and is experiencing active-phase symptoms or is abusing substances are at risk for abuse or neglect. Older adults with schizophrenia may be at risk for elder abuse.

SERVICES AND RESOURCES

- Brain & Behavior Research Foundation (formerly NARSAD), http://bbrfoundation.org/
- National Alliance on Mental Illness (NAMI), http://www.nami.org/
- U.S. National Institutes of Health (NIH), http://www.nih.gov/
- U.S. National Institute of Mental Health (NIMH), http://www.nimh.nih.gov/index.shtml
- National Association of Social Workers (NASW), http://www.socialworkers.org/

FOOD FOR THOUGHT

With the development of antipsychotic medications, reductions in public mental health funding, and more diverse forms of treatment, a movement started among consumers of mental health services that embraced the concept of recovery as a treatment objective for persons with schizophrenia. Recovery recognizes the importance of self-directed, individualized, and person-centered care; takes a holistic and strengths-based approach; and emphasizes peer support, respect, empowerment, responsibility, increased community integration, and hope as integral parts of the treatment of schizophrenia.

Research has been conducted on spirituality in older adults as a tool for bringing purpose to their lives as they experience decreased ability to function and profound losses often associated with aging. This research found that older adults with a serious mental illness turned to spirituality at the same rate as other older adults and that both groups increased their spiritual practice as they aged. It is recommended that mental health professionals explore issues of spirituality with older adults with a serious mental illness and assist them in making connections to sources of spiritual support if requested and appropriate.

An Austrian study measured attitudes that influence social distance towards those with schizophrenia among three groups of people: the general public, relatives of people with schizophrenia, and nonmedical mental health workers. The authors found that the general public had twice as high a level of

perceived dangerousness in interacting with individuals with schizophrenia compared to the other two groups. The authors concluded that this perception contributed to social distancing, as well as to stigma and discrimination. They also pointed out that there is no consensus among mental health professionals about whether or not there is an actual increased level of danger from individuals with schizophrenia to the general public. In contrast to public perception, according to the *DSM-5*, individuals with schizophrenia are more likely to be victims of aggression and violence than the general population.

One study found that children of adoptive parents who were critical, constrained, or inconsistent in communications with their children had a risk of schizophrenia of 36 in 100 as compared to a risk of 6 in 100 for children whose adoptive parents communicated consistently, clearly, without criticism, and with firm boundaries.

Substance use is often either underreported or overreported by persons with schizophrenia, complicating the differential diagnosis of both schizophrenia and substance use disorders and increasing the risk that the substance abuse will be left untreated. One study found that women and African Americans underreported substance use more frequently. Underreporting was also more common among the elderly, those who had been experiencing schizophrenia longer, and those with greater neurocognitive deficits. This study also found that self-reporting of substance use during an intake interview in an acute mental health unit was not accurate. The study compared information gathered using a semistructured interview to the results of an analysis of blood samples. There were discrepancies due to underreporting of substance use; however, there was also overreporting, as cannabis and opiates were not found in the blood of most of those who reported having used them. The authors propose the wider use of substance testing at admission to facilitate more accurate diagnosis and more effective treatment.

Another study found that there is a culture of acceptance among mental health workers of smoking by those with schizophrenia that makes smoking cessation especially difficult. Smoking privileges are often used as positive reinforcement or as tokens in a reward system. The use of cigarettes instead of money as currency, rationalization by both mental health workers and individuals that smoking is a form of self-medication and therefore should be accepted, and assertion of the right to smoke as an element of personal autonomy are parts of this culture that mental health workers may be reluctant to challenge. There is also camaraderie among smokers, who are limited to specific locations outdoors, as well as a fear of aggressive or disruptive behavior if smoking is banned or individuals are encouraged to stop. The culture of acceptance leads to decreased attention to smoking as a health concern and less effort by healthcare workers to encourage cessation among individuals with schizophrenia than with the general population.

A systemic review of prior research to determine the prevalence of mental heath disorders among family members of those with schizophrenia found that mood, anxiety, childhood onset, and substance use disorders were more prevalent among family members of individuals with schizophrenia. Added emphasis should be placed on assessing for and, when necessary, treating the mental health issues commonly found in family members of individuals with schizophrenia.

RED FLAGS

Due to similarity and overlap of symptoms with other disorders, it is important to distinguish schizophrenia from other mental health diagnoses, in particular any disorder that includes psychotic features. Incorrect diagnosis may lead to incorrect pharmacologic treatments. In children, symptoms of ASD, including disorganized behavior, social difficulties, and language impairment, can be confused with schizophrenia symptoms, particularly negative ones.

Possible delays in every aspect of development should be addressed in children with schizophrenia to decrease impact. Long-term functioning with a childhood-onset diagnosis may be severely limited if life skill and cognitive abilities are never developed.

Social workers should maintain cultural awareness concerning family attitudes towards schizophrenia and the stigma that may be attached to the disorder, and be aware of different cultural and religious perceptions within the family by individual family members. For example, younger or more acculturated family members may have adopted different attitudes toward mental health disorders than older family members.

Social workers should continually assess stability of the living environment when there are shifts in

responsibility for caregiving. Primary caregivers such as parents may not be able to continue to provide care as they age, or may in fact need care themselves. Referrals to assisted living or nursing home care may be indicated.

Hostility and aggression are associated with schizophrenia. Aggression is more common in younger males with a history of violence and a substance use disorder who do not adhere to the treatment regimen for either disorder.

Women with schizophrenia are more likely to have unplanned or unwanted pregnancies than women without schizophrenia. Women on psychotropic medications should be made aware of the fetal risks and should be referred to their treating psychiatrist and obstetrician to determine medication treatment during pregnancy.

Loss of family and other support is common for individuals with schizophrenia. A lack of social supports may lead to a decline in socioeconomic status, which may lead to increased stress that may further impair ability to function and bring on acute episodes. This may further alienate family members and other sources of support.

Support for families and individuals by community-based services is being reduced as resources become more limited.

Written by Laura Gale, LCSW

Reviewed by Pedram Samghabadi

REFERENCES

Abu-Akel, A. (1999). Phoricity as a measure of Clozaril's efficacy in treating disorganized schizophrenia. *Clinical Linguistics & Phonetics, 13*(5), 381-393. doi:10.1080/026992099299040

American Psychiatric Association. (2013). *Diagnostic and statistical manual of mental disorders: DSM-IV-TR* (4th ed.). Arlington, VA: Author.

Anderson, J. S., & Stovall, J. G. (2012). Schizophrenia. In F. J. Domino (Ed.), *The 5-minute clinical consult 2012* (20th ed., pp. 1174-1175). Philadelphia, PA: Walters Kluwer Health/Lippincott Williams & Wilkins.

Asmal, L., Mall, S., Kritzinger, J., Chiliza, B., Emsley, R., & Swartz, L. (2011). Family therapy for schizophrenia: Cultural challenges and implementation barriers in the South African context. *African Journal of Psychiatry, 14*(5), 367-371. doi:10.4314/ajpsy.v14i5.3

Bahorik, A. L., Newhill, C. E., Queen, C. C., & Eack, S. M. (2014). Under-reporting of drug use among individuals with schizophrenia: Prevalence and predictors. *Psychological Medicine, 44*, 61-69. doi:10.1017/S0033291713000548

Baker-Brown, S. (2006). A patient's journey: Living with paranoid schizophrenia. *BMJ, 333*(7569), 636-638. Barnes, A. (2008). Race and hospital diagnoses of schizophrenia and mood disorders. *Social Work, 53*(1), 77-83.

Berk, M., Henry, L. P., Elkins, K. S., Harrigan, S. M., Harris, M. G., Herrman, H., ... McGorry, P. D. (2010). The impact of smoking on clinical outcomes after first episode psychosis: Longer-term outcome findings from the EPPIC 800 follow-up study. *Journal of Dual Diagnosis, 6*(3-4), 212-234.

Bond, G. R., Drake, R. E., Mueser, K. T., & Latimer, E. (2001). Assertive community treatment for people with severe mental illness: Critical ingredients and impact on patients. *Disease Management & Health Outcomes, 9*(3), 141-159.

Bope, E., & Kellerman, R. (2014). *Conns Current Therapy* (7th ed.). Philadelphia, PA: Elsevier Saunders.

Bora, E., Gokcen, S., Kayahan, B., & Veznedaroglu, B. (2008). Deficits of social-cognitive and social-perceptual aspects of theory of mind in remitted patients with schizophrenia: Effect of residual symptoms. *The Journal of Nervous and Mental Disease, 196*(2), 95-99. doi:10.1097/NMD.0b013e318162a9e1

Bradshaw, W., & Roseborough, D. (2004). Evaluating the effectiveness of cognitive-behavioral treatment of residual symptoms and impairment in schizophrenia. *Research on Social Work Practice, 14*(2), 112-120. doi:10.1177/1049731503257872

British Association of Social Workers. (2012). The Code of Ethics for Social Work: Statement of Principles. Retrieved from http://cdn.basw.co.uk/upload/basw_112315-7.pdf

Carr, A. (2009). The effectiveness of family therapy and systemic interventions for adult-focused problems. *Journal of Family Therapy, 31*(1), 46-74.

Ceccato, E., Caneva, P., & Lamonaca, D. (2006). Music therapy and cognitive rehabilitation in schizophrenic patients: A controlled study. *Nordic Journal of Music Therapy, 15*(2), 111-120. doi:10.1080.080981300609478158

Chan, S. M., & Chau, Y. S. (2010). Growing up with a parent with schizophrenia: What children say they need. *Journal of Children's Services, 5*(4), 31-42.

Chung, R. K., Large, M. M., Starmer, G. A., Tattam, B. N., Paton, M. B., & Nielssen, O. B. (2009). The reliability of reports of recent psychoactive substance use at the time of admission to an acute mental health unit. *Journal of Dual Diagnosis, 5*(1), 392-403.

Cicero, D. C., & Kerns, J. G. (2010). Can disorganized and positive schizotypy be discriminated from dissociation?. *Journal of Personality, 78*(4), 1239-1270.

Corcoran, J., & Walsh, J. (2010). *Clinical assessment and diagnosis in social work practice* (2nd ed.). New York: Oxford University Press.

Cuijpers, P., Smit, F., ten Have, M., & de Graaf, R. (2007). Smoking is associated with first-ever incidence of mental disorders: A prospective population-based study. *Addiction, 102*(8), 1203-1309.

Dhossche, D. M., Wilson, C., & Wachtel, L. E. (2010). Catatonia in childhood and adolescence: Implications for the DSM-5. *Primary Psychiatry, 17*(4), 35-39.

Dixon, C. M. (2008). Management of schizophrenia symptoms: Implications for recreation therapy. *American Journal of Recreation Therapy, 7*(3), 40-46.

DynaMed. (2014, October 2). *Schizophrenia.* Ipswich, MA: EBSCO Publishing. Retrieved October 8, 2014, from http://search.ebscohost.com/login.aspx?direct=true&db=dme&AN=115234

DeVylder, J. E., & Oh, H. Y. (2014). A systematic review of the familial co-aggregation of schizophrenia with non-psychotic disorders. *Social Work in Mental Health, 12*(3), 280-301. doi:10.1080/15332985.2014.881457

Earl, T. R. (2006). Mental health care policy: Recognizing the needs of minority siblings as caregivers. *Journal of Human Behavior in the Social Environment, 14*(1-2), 51-72.

Eggers, C., Bunk, D., & Krause, D. (2000). Schizophrenia with onset before age of eleven: Clinical characteristics of onset and course. *Journal of Autism and Developmental Disorders, 30*(1), 29-38.

Eisendrath, S. J., & Lichtmacher, J. E. (2011). Psychiatric disorders. In S. J. McPhee & M. A. Papadakis (Eds.), *Lange 2011 current medical diagnosis & treatment* (50th ed., pp. 1010-1019). New York, NY: McGraw-Hill Medical.

Fazel, S., Langstrom, N., Hjern, A., Grann, M., & Lichtenstein, P. (2009). Schizophrenia, substance abuse, and violent crime. *Journal of the American Medical Association, 301*(1), 2016-2023.

Feiner, J. S., & Frese, F. J. (2009). Other psychotic disorders. In B. J. Sadock, V. A. Sadock, & P. Ruiz

(Eds.), *Kaplan & Sadock's comprehensive textbook of psychiatry* (9th ed., Vol. Vol. 1, pp. 1582-1593). Philadelphia: Lippincott Williams & Wilkins.

Fow, D. S. (2010). Significance of spirituality in the lives of older adults with and without serious mental illnesses. *Social Work in Mental Health, 8*(5), 469-481. doi:10.1080/15332981003744545

Gearing, R. E., Alonzo, D., Smolak, A., McHugh, K., Harmon, S., & Baldwin, S. (2011). Association of religion with delusions and hallucinations in the context of schizophrenia: Implications for engagement and adherence. *Schizophrenia Research, 126*(1-3), 150-163. doi:10.1016/j.schres.2010.11.005

Gonthier, M., & Lyon, M. A. (2004). Childhood onset schizophrenia: An overview. *Psychology in the Schools, 41*(7), 803-811. doi:10.1002/pits.20013

Grandon, P., Jenaro, C., & Lemos, S. (2008). Primary caregivers of schizophrenia outpatients: Burden and predictor variables. *Psychiatry Research, 158*(3), 335-343.

Grausgruber, A., Meise, U., Katschnig, H., Schony, W., & Fleischhacker, W. W. (2007). Patterns of social distance towards people suffering from schizophrenia in Austria: A comparison between the general public, relatives and mental health staff. *ACTA Psychiatrica Scandinvica, 115*(4), 310-319.

Grocke, D., Bloch, S., & Castle, D. (2008). Is there a role for music therapy in the care of the severely mentally ill? *Australasian Psychiatry, 16*(6), 442-445. doi:10.1080/10398560802366171

Hall, S. D., & Bean, R. A. (2008). Family therapy and childhood-onset schizophrenia: pursuing clinical and bio/psycho/social competence. *Contemporary Family Therapy, 30*(2), 61-74. doi:10.1007/s10591-008-9061-7

Huang, T. L. (2005). Lorazepam and diazepam rapidly relieve catatonic signs in patients with schizophrenia. *Psychiatry and Clinical Neurosciences, 59*(1), 52-55. International Federation of Social Workers. (2012, March 3). Statement of Ethical Principles. Retrieved October 8, 2014, from http://ifsw.org/policies/statement-of-ethical-principles/

Jones, D. W. (2004). Families and serious mental illness: Working with loss and ambivalence. *British Journal of Social Work, 34*(7), 961-979.

Jones, S. L. (1997). Caregiver burden: the experience of parents, children, siblings, and spouses of people with mental illness. *Psychiatric Rehabilitation Journal, 20*(4), 84-87.

Kalra, G., Bhugra, D., & Shah, N. (2012). Cultural aspects of schizophrenia. *International Review of Psychiatry, 24*(5), 441-449. doi:10.3109/09540261.2012.708649 Kao, Y. C., & Liu, Y. P. (2010). Effects of age of onset on clinical characteristics in schizophrenia spectrum disorders. *BMC Psychiatry, 10,* 63.

Kay, S. K., Fiszbein, A., & Opler, L. A. (1987). The Positive and Negative Syndrome Scale (PANSS) for schizophrenia. *Schizophrenia Bulletin, 13*(2), 261-276.

King, S. (2000). Is expressed emotion cause or effect in the mothers of schizophrenic young adults?. *Schizophrenia Research, 45*(1-2), 65-78. Kurtz, M. M., & Mueser, K. T. (2008). A meta-analysis of controlled research on social skills training for schizophrenia. *Journal of Consulting and Clinical Psychology, 76*(3), 491-504. doi:10.1037/0022-006X.76.3.491

Kyriakopoulos, M., & Frangou, S. (2007). Pathophysiology of early onset schizophrenia. *International Review of Psychiatry, 19*(4), 315-324.

Ledoux, Y., & Minner, P. (2006). Occasional and frequent repeaters in a psychiatric emergency room. *Social Psychiatry and Psychiatric Epidemiology, 41*(2), 115-121.,. doi:10.1007/s00127-005-0010-6

Lu, S. F., Lo, C. H. K., Sung, H. C., Hsieh, T. C., Yu, S. C., & Chang, S. C. (2013). Effects of group music intervention on psychiatric symptoms and depression in patient with schizophrenia. *Complementary Therapies in Medicine, 21*(6), 682-688. doi:10.1016/j.ctim.2013.09.002

Lysaker, P. H., & Lysaker, J. T. (2006). Psychotherapy and schizophrenia: An analysis of requirements of an individual psychotherapy for persons with profoundly disorganized selves. *Journal of Constructivist Psychology, 19,* 171-189.

Lysaker, P. H., Salvatore, G., Grant, M. L. A., Procacci, M., Olesek, K. L., Buck, K. D., & Dimaggio, G. (2010). Deficits in theory of mind and social anxiety as independent paths to paranoid feature in schizophrenia. *Schizophrenia Research, 124*(1-3), 81-85.

Malone Cole, J. A. (2012). Schizophrenia and other psychotic disorders. In K. M. Fortinash & P. A. Holoday Worret (Eds.), *Psychiatric mental health nursing* (5th ed., pp. 259-296). St. Louis, MO: Elsevier Mosby.

Marley, J. A., & Buila, S. (2001). Crimes against people with mental illness: Types, perpetrators, and influencing factors. *Social Work, 46*(2), 115-124.

Mizrahi, T., & Mayden, R. W. (2001). NASW standards for cultural competence in social work practice. Retrieved July 16, 2014, from http://www.

socialworkers.org/practice/standards/NASWCul-turalStandards.pdf

National Institute for Health and Care Excellence. (2013). Psychosis and schizophrenia in children and young people (nice clinical guideline no. 155). Manchester, U.K. National Guidleine Clearinghouse. (2009). *Clinical practice guideline for schizophrenia and insipient psychotic disorder (CAHTA; no. 2006/05-2).*

Rockville MD. Papadakis, M., & McPhee, S. (Eds.). (2014). *2014 Current medical diagnosis and treatment* (53rd ed.). New York: McGraw-Hill.

Pfammatter, J., Junghan, U. M., & Brenner, H. D. (2006). Efficacy of psychological therapy in schizophrenia: Conclusions from meta-analyses. *Schizophrenia Bulletin, 32*(1), S64-S80. Scottish Intercollegiate Guidelines Network. (2013). *Management of schizophrenia. (SIGN no. 131).* Edinburgh, Scotland.

Salinas, J. A., Paul, G. L., & Springer, J. R. (2008). Consensus judgments of discharge readiness based on paranoid behavior: To what are clinical staff responding? *Social Psychiatry and Psychiatric Epidemiology, 43*(5), 380-386. doi:10.1007/s00127-008-0319-z

Sherrer, M. V. (2011). The role of cognitive appraisal in adaptation to traumatic stress in adults with serious mental illness: A critical review. *Trauma, Violence & Abuse, 12*(3), 151-167. doi:10.1177/1524838011404254

Shuler, K. M. (2014). Approaches to improve adherence to pharmacotherapy in patients with schizophrenia. *Patient Preference and Adherence, 8*, 701-714.

Sikorski, K. A., & Barker, D. M. (2009). Clients with pain. In J. M. Black & J. H. Hawks (Eds.), *Medical-surgical nursing: Clinical management for positive outcomes* (8th ed., pp. 379-380). St. Louis, MO: Saunders Elsevier.

Stahl, S. M., & Buckley, P. F. (2007). Negative symptoms of schizophrenia: A problem that will not go away. *Acta Psychiatrica Scandinavica, 115*(1), 4-11. International Federation of Social Workers. (2012). Statement of Ethical Principles. Retrieved August 13, 2015, from http://ifsw.org/policies/statement-of-ethical-principles/

Steinberg, M. L., & Williams, J. (2007). Psychosocial treatments for individuals with schizophrenia and tobacco dependence. *Journal of Dual Diagnosis, 3*(3/4), 99-112.

Stompe, T., Ortwein-Swoboda, G., Ritter, K., Schanda, H., & Friedmann, A. (2002). Are we witnessing the disappearance of catatonic schizophrenia?. *Comprehensive Psychiatry, 43*(3), 167-174.

Talwar, N., Crawford, M. J., Maratos, A., Nur, U., McDermott, O., & Procter, S. (2006). Music therapy for in-patients with schizophrenia: Exploratory randomised controlled trial. *British Journal of Psychiatry, 189*, 405-409. doi:10.1192/bjp.bp.105.015073

Taylor, M. A., & Fink, M. (2003). Catatonia in psychiatric classification: A home of its own. *American Journal of Psychiatry, 160*(7), 1233-1241.

Tenhula, W. N., Bellack, A. S., & Drake, R. E. (2009). Schizophrenia: Psychosocial approaches. In B. J. Sadock, V. A. Sadock, & P. Ruiz (Eds.), *Kaplan & Sadock's comprehensive textbook of psychiatry* (9th ed., Vol. 1, pp. 1556-1572). Philadelphia, PA: Wolters Kluwer Health/Lippincott Williams & Wilkins.

Tidey, J. W., & Williams, J. (2007). Clinical indices of tobacco use in people with schizophrenia. *Journal of Dual Diagnosis, 3*(3/4), 79-98. Uher, R. (2010). The genetics of mental illness: A guide for parents and adoption professionals. *Adoption & Fostering, 34*(3), 105-108.

Ulrich, G., Houtmans, T., & Gold, C. (2007). The additional therapeutic effect of group music therapy for schizophrenic patients: A randomized study. *Acta Psychiatrica Scandinavica, 116*(5), 362-370. doi:10.1111/j.1600-0447.2007.01073.x

Weder, N. D., Muralee, S., Penland, H., & Tampi, R. R. (2008). Catatonia: A review. *Annals of Clinical Psychiatry, 20*(2), 97-107. Wiens, S. E., & Daniluk, J. C. (2009). Love, loss, and learning: The experiences of fathers who have children diagnosed with schizophrenia. *Journal of Counseling & Development, 87*(1), 339-348.

Xiang, Y. T., Wang, C. Y., Chiu, H. F., Weng, Y. Z., Bo, Q. J., Chan, S. S., & Ungvari, G. S. (2010). Socio-demographic and clinical profiles of paranoid and nonparanoid schizophrenia: A prospective, multicenter study in China. *Perspectives in Psychiatric Care, 47*(3), 126-130.

Ziedonis, D., Parks, J., Zimmermann, M. H., & McCabe, P. (2007). Program and system level interventions to address tobacco amongst individuals with schizophrenia. *Journal of Dual Diagnosis, 3*(3/4), 151-175.

U.S. National Library of Medicine. (2014, October 9). Tardive Dyskinesia. Retrieved October 10, 2014, from http://www.nlm.nih.gov/medlineplus/ency/article/000685.htm

SCHIZOPHRENIA: CATATONIC SUBTYPE

MAJOR CATEGORIES: Behavioral & Mental Health

DESCRIPTION

Schizophrenia is a mental health disorder that may include symptoms of delusions, hallucinations, and disorganized speech that effect a person in many aspects of their daily life. Schizophrenia was previously diagnosed with specified subtypes such as catatonic subtype, disorganized subtype, paranoid subtype, residual subtype, and undifferentiated subtype. A diagnosis of schizophrenia is made with meeting specific criteria as outlined in the The *Diagnostic and Statistical Manual of Mental Disorders* (*DSM*). The two most recent editions of this diagnostic manual are the fourth edition (*DSM-IV*) and the fifth edition (*DSM-5*).

The *DSM-5* retains the general description of schizophrenia as a chronic and incapacitating psychiatric disorder that severely impacts a person's thought processes, stimuli perception, communication, and behavior. It greatly affects the ability of the individual to maintain relationships and a stable living environment. The individual with schizophrenia will display positive (noticeably present, such as a repeated sound or behavior) and negative (notable by their absence, such as a loss of speech) symptoms.

Directly related to the catatonic subtype of schizophrenia in the *DSM-IV*, the *DSM-5* has broadened the application of the catatonia specifier, which can be used as a specifier with numerous disorders that appear in the manual, including schizophrenia. The criteria for the catatonia specifier in the *DSM-5* include the significant presence of 3 or more of 12 possible catatonic symptoms: stupor, catalepsy, waxy flexibility, mutism, negativism, posturing, mannerisms, stereotypes, agitation, grimacing, echolalia (repeating words and sounds), and echopraxia (repeating movements).

Schizophrenia shares the feature of psychosis (having delusions or hallucinations) with several other *DSM* diagnoses, including mood disorders, and therefore can be difficult to distinguish from other disorders featuring psychosis. However, schizophrenia is primarily a thought disorder. The etiology and cause of schizophrenia has not been pinpointed; it is believed to derive from multiple factors, including genetics, environmental influences, and imbalances in neurotransmitters.

The *DSM-5*, which was published in 2013, includes changes for the diagnosis criteria from the *DSM-IV* in the "Schizophrenia Spectrum and Other Psychotic Disorders" chapter. In addition to clarifying some of the language, the more significant changes are as follows. Two active symptoms are required for a diagnosis of schizophrenia, at least one of which is one of the core symptoms: delusions, hallucinations, or disorganized speech. The specifications about the type of delusions and hallucinations have been removed from the *DSM-5*. Course specifiers of diagnosing schizophrenia have been changed to reflect the elimination of the subtypes of schizophrenia from *DSM-IV* to *DSM-5*. All subtypes of schizophrenia, including catatonic subtype, have been eliminated in *DSM-5*.

The subtypes of schizophrenia were eliminated from the *DSM-5* because of their "limited diagnostic stability, low reliability, and poor validity." In place of the subtypes, the *DSM-5* introduces a symptoms severity tool: Clinician-Rated Dimensions of Psychosis Symptom Severity, which consists of eight symptoms that may be present in psychosis that the clinician rates using a 5-point scale, from 0 (not present) to 4 (present and severe). The goal is to measure the range and severity of symptoms to assist in planning treatment, prognosis estimates, and research. The measure may be used regularly to track changes in symptoms.

The *DSM-IV* previously used a hierarchical diagnosis method to determine the appropriate subtype of schizophrenia. Because the subtype was determined by the most prominent symptoms at the time of assessment, the diagnosed subtype was subject to change over time. Individuals with schizophrenia frequently have symptoms of more than one subtype simultaneously. To determine a single diagnostic subtype, the *DSM-IV* used this hierarchy:

The catatonic subtype was assigned whenever catatonic symptoms predominated at the time of the assessment (*DSM-5* allows for the addition of a catatonia specifier in the diagnosis). The disorganized (sometimes referred to as *hebephrenic*) subtype was assigned whenever flat or inappropriate affect (facial expression matching the person's mood) and disorganized speech and behavior were prominent at the time of the assessment (unless catatonic subtype had already been assigned).

The paranoid subtype was assigned through the *DSM-IV* when delusions or hallucinations predominated at the time of the assessment (unless catatonic or disorganized subtype had already been assigned). The undifferentiated subtype was assigned when there were prominent active-phase (active schizophrenic episode) symptoms at the time of the assessment that did not meet the criteria for catatonic, disorganized, or paranoid subtypes. The residual subtype was assigned when there were continuing symptoms of schizophrenia but criteria for an active phase were not met.

Specifically, the catatonic subtype as described by the *DSM-IV* and research based on *DSM-IV* criteria features excessive, purposeless mobility; partial immobility (waxy flexibility, in which the extremities remain in specific positions after being moved); or the complete absence of motor activity, which may manifest as total immobility. Odd gestures or movements, stereotyped behaviors, mutism, and repeating the words (echolalia) or movements (echopraxia) of others may also be present. The symptoms frequently are not congruent with the current environment. Catatonia can include rapid alteration of symptoms. Self-injury from either the extreme mobility or the lack of mobility (not eating) is possible. Onset of symptoms frequently is sudden, with an identifiable precipitating event.

Catatonic symptoms are the same in children and adolescents as in adults. Prognosis varies depending on prior functioning and support before the onset of symptoms. Depending on etiology and the current presenting phase, treatment might include involuntary detention, medication, social skills training, psychoeducation, and referrals to community and family support services.

Facts and Figures

The *DSM-5* notes that in inpatient settings catatonic features occur in 35 percent of individuals with schizophrenia. Although only approximately 1 percent of the population in the United States has schizophrenia, it accounts for up to 50 percent of all long-term hospitalizations for psychiatric disorders.

Risk Factors

Risk factors for catatonia vary with the underlying diagnosis. Among the risk factors for schizophrenia, none of the risk factors are unique and specific to the catatonic subtype.

Biological risk factors include genetics, dopamine hyperactivity, decreased brain size, premature birth or excessive maternal bleeding, traumatic brain injury, and maternal exposure to trauma in first trimester.

Environmental risk factors include low socioeconomic status, family dysfunction, exposure to trauma, and winter or early spring birth. There is a stigma associated with a diagnosis of schizophrenia that may exacerbate symptoms in an individual.

Signs and Symptoms

Physical indicators specific to the catatonic subtype of schizophrenia may include immobility or excessive motor activity, staring, stupor, rigid posture, grimacing, assuming bizarre postures, withdrawal, echolalia, echopraxia, mutism, catalepsy, and decreased sensitivity to pain.

Cognitive indicators specific to catatonic subtype of schizophrenia may include extreme negativism (resistance to all instruction or advice, and to move body parts).

Assessment

The social worker assisting an individual who may have schizophrenia, catatonic subtype, should complete a biological, psychological, social, and spiritual assessment, including an assessment of risk for suicide and harm to self and others to determine the individual's immediate needs. Close observation of the individual's functioning and demeanor during the interview, with particular attention to physical symptoms, should be made. Collateral information from family, friends, and coworkers may also be beneficial for the assessment. A history of any prior diagnosis of mental health disorders other than schizophrenia should be obtained.

Assessment and Screening Tools

A few standardized assessments and screening tools that may be helpful in further determining the individual's needs may include the Positive and Negative Syndrome Scale (PANSS) for Schizophrenia, the Scale for the Assessment of Negative Symptoms (SANS), and the Scale for the Assessment of Positive Symptoms (SAPS).

No specific tests can identify schizophrenia; however, standard tests may identify relevant medical condition(s) or substance abuse that may need to be addressed by a medical professional.

TREATMENT

Treatments and interventions for schizophrenia aim to improve quality of life, decrease the number and severity of active-phase episodes and symptoms, and strengthen family and community support. Because schizophrenia is a chronic disorder, treatment may be a lifelong process.

INTERVENTION

An active phase of schizophrenia, catatonic subtype, may affect an individual physically or cognitively. If the individual is experiencing extreme physical symptoms of catatonia, self-injury could occur. Medically supervised treatment, possibly including medications such as benzodiazepines or treatments such as electroconvulsive therapy (ECT) could alleviate physical symptoms and to provide safety.

Schizophrenia, catatonic subtype, may lead to withdrawal/decreased social function or a lack of self-care. Social skills training (SST) are programs that vary but generally include goal setting, role modeling, behavior rehearsal, positive reinforcement, and exercises to generalize individual learning needs to specific community settings. SST could increase the individual's life skills in order to increase their independent functionality and assist them in maintaining essential social relationships and self-care.

Schizophrenia, catatonic subtype, is a chronic mental health diagnosis. An individual experiencing frequent active-phase catatonic episodes and frequent hospitalizations may experience a severe decline in self-care and loss of family and peer support. The individual may become disconnected from necessary preventive clinic-based services and regularly miss necessary appointments.

Assertive community treatment (ACT) style intervention could assist the individual to become more engaged in their treatment and reduce hospitalizations. ACT style intervention may include treatment from a multidisciplinary team with professionals from various backgrounds, consistent contact in the community, assertive outreach, and individualized services with no time limit on provided services and rapid access and response to the individual's needs. Improved engagement in the individual's treatment and the community may assist the individual in gaining stabilized housing and improve their overall quality of life.

APPLICABLE LAWS AND REGULATIONS

Each jurisdiction (nation, state, and province) has its own standards, procedures, and laws for involuntary restraint and detention of persons who may be a danger to themselves or others. Because individuals with schizophrenia have a high rate of suicide attempts, it is important for professionals working with the individual to become familiar with the local requirements for involuntary detention. Some jurisdictions have laws limiting the use of ECT. Local laws pertaining to professional reporting requirements should be known and followed.

SERVICES AND RESOURCES

Enter *schizophrenia catatonic* or *catatonia* in the search box to access relevant information available on each website.

- Brain & Behavior Research Foundation (formerly NARSAD), http://bbrfoundation.org/
- National Alliance on Mental Illness (NAMI), http://www.nami.org/
- U.S. National Institutes of Health (NIH), http://www.nih.gov/
- U.S. National Institute of Mental Health (NIMH), http://www.nimh.nih.gov/index.shtml
- National Association of Social Workers (NASW), http://www.socialworkers.org/

FOOD FOR THOUGHT

According to long-term studies showing improvements in the quality of life for persons living with schizophrenia, as well as variation in the course of the disorder, some professionals in the field call into question the long-held view that schizophrenia is always a chronic condition with poor outcomes. Simultaneously, a consumer movement has developed around the concept of recovery as a valid and obtainable treatment goal. The fundamental concepts embodied in the recovery movement are self-direction; individualized and person-centered treatment; empowerment of the individual; holistic and nonlinear approaches to treatment and care; strengths-based perspective treatment; peer support; respect; responsibility; and hope. The recovery movement focuses on the person rather than the illness and emphasizes healing and choice, with multiple goals including gaining independence and fulfillment of the individual's full potential.

RED FLAGS

Side effects of medications should be monitored. Treatment with some antipsychotic medications can exacerbate catatonic symptoms. In addition, benzodiazepines, which frequently are prescribed to persons with schizophrenia, catatonic subtype, can be addictive.

There may be a stigma attached to receiving ECT. Professionals and social workers should remain alert to possible self-harm, including malnutrition, exhaustion to the point of not having the energy to feed oneself, or unintentional self-inflicted injury, as well as suicidal ideation.

Social workers should always confirm that the diagnosis of schizophrenia, catatonic subtype, is correct. Catatonic symptoms may be the result of other underlying behavioral or medical conditions; misdiagnosis of the underlying condition may lead to incorrect and potentially harmful treatment of the individual.

NEXT STEPS

Social workers assisting individuals with schizophrenia, catatonic subtype, should review and discuss the individual's medication regimen, including the importance of the medications, the importance of taking them as prescribed, and the need to report any side effects. Follow-up appointment with the agency issuing the prescription may be needed.

Referrals to local schizophrenia support groups, supported work agencies, or mental health agencies may be made. The stability of the individual's living situation should be ascertained and any necessary referrals made by the social worker as appropriate. Referrals for support to family members of the individual with schizophrenia, catatonic subtype, should be made.

Written by Chris Bates, MA, MSW

Reviewed by Lynn B. Cooper, D Crim, and Pedram Samghabadi

REFERENCES

American Psychiatric Association. (2000). *Diagnostic and statistical manual of mental disorders: DSM-IV-TR* (4th ed.). Arlington, VA: Author.

American Psychiatric Association. (2013). Diagnostic and statistical manual of mental health disorders (DSM-5). (5th ed.). Arlington, VA: American Psychiatric Publishing.

Bond, G. R., Drake, R. E., Mueser, K. T., & Latimer, E. (2001). Assertive community treatment for people with severe mental illness. *Disease Management & Health Outcomes, 9*(3), 141-159.

Corcoran, J., & Walsh, J. (2010). *Clinical assessment and diagnosis in social work practice* (2nd ed.). New York, NY: Oxford University Press.

Dhossche, D. M., Wilson, C., & Wachtel, L. E. (2010). Catatonia in childhood and adolescence: Implications for the DSM-5. *Primary Psychiatry, 17*(4), 35-39.

Feiner, J. S., & Frese, F. J. (2009). Recovery in schizophrenia. In B. J. Sadock, V. A. Sadock, & P. Ruiz (Eds.), *Kaplan & Sadocks's comprehensive textbook of psychiatry* (9th ed., Vol. 1, pp. 1582-1593). Philadelphia, PA: Wolters Kluwer Health/Lippincott Williams & Wilkins.

Huang, T. L. (2005). Lorazepam and diazepam rapidly relieve catatonic signs in patients with schizophrenia. *Psychiatry and Clinical Neurosciences, 59*(1), 52-55.

International Federation of Social Workers. (2012, March 3). Statement of Ethical Principles. Retrieved September 21, 2015, from http://ifsw.org/policies/statement-of-ethical-principles/

Kay, S. R., Fiszbein, A., & Opler, L. A. (1987). The positive and negative syndrome scale (PANSS) for schizophrenia. *Schizophrenia Bulletin, 13*(2), 261-276.

Kurtz, M. M., & Mueser, K. T. (2008). A meta-analysis of controlled research on social skills training for schizophrenia. *Journal of Consulting and Clinical Psychology, 76*(3), 491-504. doi:10.1037/0022-006X.76.3.491

Malone Cole, J. A. (2012). Schizophrenia and other psychotic disorders. In K. M. Fortinash & P. A. Holoday Worret (Eds.), *Psychiatric mental health nursing* (5th ed., pp. 259-296). St. Louis, MO: Elsevier Mosby.

Mizrahi, T., & Mayden, R. W. (2001). *NASW Standards for Cultural Competency in Social Work Practice.* Retrieved September 21, 2015, from http://www.socialworkers.org/practice/standards/NASWCulturalStandards.pdf

The Policy, Ethics, and Human Rights Committee, British Association of Social Workers. (2012, January). The Code of Ethics for Social Workers: Statements of principles. Retrieved September 21, 2015, from http://cdn.basw.co.uk/upload/basw_112315-7.pdf

Sadock, B. J., Sadock, V. A., & Ruiz, P. (2015). Schizophrenia spectrum and other psychotic disorders. In *Kaplan & Sadock's Synopsis of Psychiatry: Behavioral Sciences/Clinical Psychiatry* (11th ed., pp. 300-323). Philadelphia, PA: Wolters Kluwer.

Stompe, T., Ortwein-Swoboda, G., Ritter, K., Schanda, H., & Friedmann, A. (2002). Are we witnessing the disappearance of catatonic schizophrenia?. *Comprehensive Psychiatry, 43*(3), 167-174.

Taylor, M. A., & Fink, M. (2003). Catatonia in psychiatric classification: A home of its own. *American Journal of Psychiatry, 160*(7), 1233-1241.

Weder, N. D., Muralee, S., Penland, H., & Tampi, R. R. (2008). Catatonia: A review. *Annals of Clinical Psychiatry, 20*(2), 97-107.

Williams, N., & DeBattista, C. (2016). Psychiatric disorders. In *Current Medical Diagnosis & Treatment 2016* (55th ed., pp. 1048-1056). New York: McGraw-Hill Education.

SCHIZOPHRENIA: DISORGANIZED SUBTYPE

MAJOR CATEGORIES: Behavioral & Mental Health

DESCRIPTION

The fifth edition of the *Diagnostic Statistical Manual of Mental Disorders (DSM-5)*, published in 2013, eliminates the various subtypes of schizophrenia that were described in earlier editions of the manual, and instead describes schizophrenia as a chronic and incapacitating psychiatric disorder that has a severe impact on thought processes, stimulus perception, communication, and behavior, and which also affects the ability to maintain relationships and a stable living environment. Persons with schizophrenia may display positive (noticeably present) and negative (notable by their absence) symptoms. Because schizophrenia shares psychosis as one of its features, and psychosis is also a feature of several other psychiatric disorders whose diagnostic criteria are given in the *DSM-5*, including mood disorders, it can be difficult to distinguish schizophrenia from other disorders of which psychosis is a feature. However, schizophrenia is primarily a disorder of thought processes.

Because the diagnosis of schizophrenia of the disorganized subtype, as described in the *DSM-IV* (and also known as *hebephrenic* schizophrenia), will remain in the medical records of patients whose schizophrenia was classified as being of this subtype when it was diagnosed, even though this subtype of schizophrenia is now outdated, and because the subtype of a patient's schizophrenia in the *DSM-IV* was determined by the patient's most prominent symptoms at the time of diagnosis, it remains useful to understand what was meant by schizophrenia of the disorganized subtype as defined in the *DSM-IV*.

The disorganized subtype of schizophrenia has as its most prominent features a flat or inappropriate affect, marked by a severe reduction in emotional expressiveness, such as speaking in a monotonous voice and having an apathetic appearance, accompanied by disorganized speech and behavior. The disorganized behavior in this form of schizophrenia may prevent the performance of self-care tasks or other functions, and may severely disrupt ordinary activities of daily living. If delusions and hallucinations are present, they are not organized around a particular theme, as in some other types of schizophrenia. The disorganized subtype of schizophrenia is also associated with poor functioning of the affected individual before the beginning of the disorder, and by an earlier onset than in some other subtypes of schizophrenia. Some studies have also found that the disorganized subtype of schizophrenia may be the most heritable subtype of this disorder. with a poor prognosis for the affected individual to return to his or her level of functioning before the onset of the disorder. Depending on the etiology and phase of disorganized schizophrenia at the time of its diagnosis, its treatment may include involuntary detention, medication, social skills training, psychoeducation, and referrals to community and family support services.

FACTS AND FIGURES

Given the low reliability of the diagnosis of schizophrenia of the disorganized subtype in the context of a number of other psychiatric disorders, facts and figures associated with this diagnosis are not reliable. The *DSM-5* reports a lifetime prevalence of schizophrenia of the disorganized subtype of approximately 0.3 to 0.7 percent, with the specific definition of the disorder affecting its calculated prevalence according to gender, location, and race/ethnicity. Thus, for example, an emphasis on illness of long duration and on negative symptoms, such as a flattening of emotional expression, results in higher rates of schizophrenia of the disorganized subtype for males than for females.

RISK FACTORS

Risk factors for the disorganized subtype of schizophrenia are the same as for the other subtypes of schizophrenia described in the *DSM-IV*. Its biological risk factors are genetic factors, hyperactivity of components of the nervous system in which dopamine mediates the transmission of nerve impulses, premature birth or excessive maternal bleeding at birth, a decreased brain size, brain injury, and maternal exposure to trauma in the first trimester of pregnancy. Environmental risk factors for the disorganized subtype of schizophrenia are familial dysfunction, exposure to trauma, birth in winter or early spring, and a low socioeconomic status; stigma associated with the diagnosis of this subtype of schizophrenia may exacerbate its symptoms.

SIGNS AND SYMPTOMS

Signs and symptoms of the disorganized subtype of schizophrenia change over time, but physical signs that are specific to this disorder may include grimacing, verbal responses that are inappropriate or unrelated to the content of a conversation, poor hygiene or an unkempt appearance, inability to care for the self (bathe, eat, dress), and sexual or other behavior that is inappropriate to the affected individual's culture. Cognitive signs of the disorganized subtype of schizophrenia may include disorganized speech.

TREATMENT

The social worker assisting an individual who has schizophrenia of the disorganized subtype should conduct a standard biological, psychological, social, and spiritual assessment, including an assessment the individual's risk for suicide and for inflicting harm on him- or herself and others. This should include an assessment of the individual's level of functioning and demeanor during the interview conducted for the assessment, with particular attention to the individual's affect and cognitive symptoms and to the collection of information on any prior mental health disorders other than schizophrenia. The assessment should also include laboratory tests if and as needed to identify medical disorders and substance abuse, and the collection of collateral information from the individual's family, friends, and coworkers.

Treatments and interventions for schizophrenia are directed at improving the quality of life of the affected individual; decreasing the number and severity of active episodes of the disorder; and strengthening the affected individual's family and community support. Over the course of the disorder, the treatment of schizophrenia of the disorganized subtype may include hospitalization, medication, various psychological treatments (individual, group, or family therapy; social skills training; cognitive behavioral therapy [CBT]); and community-based recovery programs. The affected individual's adherence to a regimen of prescribed medication, which may be especially difficult for those with schizophrenia of the disorganized subtype, should be monitored. The use of electroconvulsive therapy as a long-term maintenance treatment option is being explored clinically for individuals with disorganized subtype of schizophrenia who do not respond to other treatments. Persons treated with a combination of medication for schizophrenia and psychosocial therapy tend to have better outcomes. Because schizophrenia is a chronic disorder, its treatment may be a lifelong process.

Individuals experiencing a severe active-phase episode of schizophrenia with a possible risk of harm to themselves or others should be hospitalized and treated with appropriate medication. Those exhibiting erratic or self-destructive behavior, inadequate self-care, deteriorating social relationships, or delusions or hallucinations should be seen by a mental health professional who can prescribe appropriate medication, and should be followed for adherence to their medication regimen and reporting any side effects of medications. These individuals may benefit from social skills training (SST) programs, which generally include setting of goals, role modeling, behavioral training, positive reinforcement, and learning of adaptation to community settings. Individuals with schizophrenia of the disorganized subtype who exhibit a severe decline in self-care, loss of family or peer support, frequent active episodes of illness requiring hospitalization or emergency room visits, and cessation of clinic-based services may benefit from assertive community treatment (ACT), with treatment by a multidisciplinary team of professionals, individualized assistance, assertive outreach, and rapid access to help as needed.

Extended studies showing improvements in the quality of life of persons living with schizophrenia, as well as variations in its progression, have led some professionals in the field to question the long-held view that schizophrenia is always a chronic condition with poor outcomes. Simultaneously, a consumer movement has developed around the concept of recovery from schizophrenia as a valid goal of its treatment. This movement focuses on the person rather than the illness and emphasizes healing and choice, with multiple goals including independence and the fulfillment of personal potential. The fundamental concepts embodied in this recovery movement are the self-direction and empowerment of individuals with schizophrenia; individualized and person-centered treatment for it; holistic, nonlinear, and strengths-based approaches to its treatment; and peer support, respect, responsibility, and hope for the individual with schizophrenia.

Social workers assisting persons with schizophrenia should assess their support system and the stability of their living situations. The chronic nature of the disorganized subtype of schizophrenia frequently leads to slow but steady decline in socioeconomic level and possible loss of support from an affected individual's family. Social workers should refer affected individuals to local schizophrenia support groups, supported work, or mental health agencies as needed, and provide referrals for support of their family members.

In providing this assistance, social workers should be aware of their own cultural values, beliefs, and biases, and develop specialized knowledge about the histories, traditions, and values of the individuals and families with whom they work. They should adopt treatment methods that reflect their knowledge of these factors.

APPLICABLE LAWS AND REGULATIONS

The U.S. government and individual states of the United States have their own standards, procedures, and laws for the involuntary restraint and detention of persons who may be a danger to themselves or others. Because individuals with schizophrenia have

a high rate of suicide attempts, it is important to become familiar with local requirements for their involuntary detention should this prove necessary.

AVAILABLE SERVICES AND RESOURCES

- Recovery within Reach, http://www.recoverywithinreach.org
- Brain & Behavior Research Foundation (formerly NARSAD), http://bbrfoundation.org/
- National Alliance on Mental Illness (NAMI), http://www.nami.org/
- U.S. National Institutes of Health (NIH), http://www.nih.gov/
- U.S. National Institute of Mental Health (NIMH), http://www.nimh.nih.gov/index.shtml
- National Association of Social Workers (NASW), http://www.socialworkers.org/

Written by Chris Bates, MA, MSW

Reviewed by Lynn B Cooper, D. Crim, and Pedram Samghabadi

REFERENCES

Abu-Akel, A. (1999). Phoricity as a measure of Clozaril's efficacy in treating disorganized schizophrenia. *Clinical Linguistics & Phonetics, 13*(5), 381-393. doi:10.1080/026992099299040

American Psychiatric Association. (2000). *Diagnostic and statistical manual of mental disorders* (4th Rev ed.). Arlington, VA: Author.

American Psychiatric Association. (2013). *Diagnostic and statistical manual of mental health disorders (DSM-5) (5th ed.)* (5th ed.). Arlington, VA: American Psychiatric Publishing.

British Association of Social Workers. (2012). The code of ethics for social work: Statement of principles. Retrieved April 20, 2016, from http://cdn.basw.co.uk/upload/basw_112315-7.pdf

Cicero, D. C., & Kerns, J. G. (2010). Can disorganized and positive schizotypy be discriminated from dissociation?. *Journal of Personality, 78*(4), 1239-1270.

Corcoran, J., & Walsh, J. (2010). *Clinical assessment and diagnosis in social work practice* (2nd ed.). New York, NY: Oxford University Press.

Dahan, E., Or, E., Bleich, A., & Melamed, Y. (2015). Maintenance electroconvulsive therapy for a neuroleptic-intolerant patient with disorganized schizophrenia. *Clinical Schizophrenia & Related Psychoses*, 8(4), 201-204. doi:10.3371/CSRP.DAOR.030113

DeBattista, C., Eisendrath, S. J., & Lichtmacher, J. E. (2015). Psychiatric disorders. In M. A. Papadakis & S. J. McPhee (Eds.), *2015 current medical diagnosis & treatment* (54th ed., pp. 1042-1051). Philadelphia, PA: Wolters Kluwer.

Holder, S. D., & Wayhs, A. (2014). Schizophrenia. *American Family Physician*, 90(11), 775.

Feiner, J. S., & Frese, F. J. (2009). Recovery in schizophrenia. In B. J. Sadock, V. A. Sadock, & P. Ruiz (Eds.), *Kaplan & Sadocks's comprehensive textbook of psychiatry* (9th ed., Vol. 1, pp. 1582-1593). Philadelphia, PA: Wolters Kluwer Health/Lippincott Williams & Wilkins.

International Federation of Social Workers. (2012, March 3). Statement of ethical principles. Retrieved April 20, 2016, from http://ifsw.org/policies/statement-of-ethical-principles/

Kurtz, M. M., & Mueser, K. T. (2008). A meta-analysis of controlled research on social skills training for schizophrenia. *Journal of Consulting and Clinical Psychology*, 76(3), 491-504. doi:10.1037/0022-006X.76.3.491

Malone Cole, J. A. (2012). Schizophrenia and other psychotic disorders. In K. M. Fortinash & P. A. Holoday Worret (Eds.), *Psychiatric mental health nursing* (5th ed., pp. 259-296). St. Louis, MO: Elsevier Mosby.

Sadock, B. J., Sadock, V. A., & Ruiz, P. (2015). Schizophrenia spectrum and other psychotic disorders. In *Kaplan & Sadock's synopsis of psychiatry: Behavioral sciences/clinical psychiatry* (11th ed., pp. 300-323). Philadelphia, PA: Wolters Kluwer.

Townsend, M. C. (2015). Schizophrenia spectrum and other psychotic disorders. In *Psychiatric mental health nursing: Concepts of care in evidence-based practice* (8th ed., pp. 419-457). Philadelphia, PA: F. A. Davis Company.

Weinstein, J. J., & Stovall, J. G. (2014). Schizophrenia. In F. J. Domino (Ed.), *The 5-minute clinical consult standard 2015* (23rd ed., pp. 1074-1075). Philadelphia, PA: Wolters Kluwer.

Wheeler, D. (2015). NASW standards and indicators for cultural competence in social work practice. Retrieved April 20, 2016, from http://www.socialworkers.org/practice/standards/PRA-BRO-253150-CC-Standards.pdf

SCHIZOPHRENIA: EFFECT ON THE FAMILY

MAJOR CATEGORIES: Behavioral & Mental Health

DESCRIPTION
Schizophrenia is a chronic and incapacitating mental disorder that severely affects thought processes, the perception of stimuli, communication, and behavior. It also impairs the ability to maintain social and emotional relationships and a stable living environment. Schizophrenia is characterized by positive (i.e., noticeably present) and negative (i.e., notable because of their absence) symptoms. It shares the feature of being a psychosis, or severe mental disorder marked by a loss of recognition of external reality, with several other disorders described in the Fifth Edition of the *Diagnostic and Statistical Manual of Mental Disorders* (*DSM-V*), including mood disorders, and can therefore be difficult to distinguish from other disorders of which psychosis is a characteristic. However, schizophrenia is primarily a disorder of thinking.

Two aspects of schizophrenia intensify its impact on the family. First, the chronic nature of schizophrenia means that the family is affected for the entire life of ta family member in whom a diagnosis of schizophrenia is made. Second, the increasing incapacitation of many individuals with schizophrenia as they cycle through active phases of the disorder or become less able to care for themselves financially and otherwise creates major instability and unpredictability for the families of such individuals. Additionally, the diagnosis of schizophrenia in a family member is likely to cause significant changes in the other family members' roles and functioning. Thus, for example, siblings may stop bringing friends home because of embarrassment about an affected member's illness or behavior, parents may have to change their work schedules to accommodate an affected child's treatment, a child may have to fill the role of caregiver to an affected parent, the family may have to make financial sacrifices, and all members of the family may at various times and under various circumstances have to take on the role of caregiver. Additionally, every member of an affected family may experience a wide range of complex and sometimes conflicting emotions and feelings, including sorrow, devotion, guilt, anger, inadequacy, hope, fear, failure, frustration, isolation, and ambiguity. Essentially, every member of the family will embark on a lifelong personal journey that in many ways will mirror the life course of the family member in whom schizophrenia has been diagnosed.

The effect of the care that must be given by individual family members to a schizophrenic member is referred to as the individual burden of the illness, and the sum of the care given collectively by the family is referred to as the family burden, with each type of burden divided into objective and subjective burdens. Components of the objective burden include disruption of various aspects of the caregiver's life (e.g., time, money, privacy, self-care). The subjective burden consists of the caregiver's perceived and physically and emotionally experienced effect of his or her caregiving on his or her quality of life and emotional balance (e.g., stress, depression, anxiety).

Further complicating the effect on the family of a family member's schizophrenia is the stigma that many cultures associate with this disorder. Research and professional assessments have added to this stigma and for some families have transformed it into guilt or shame by attributing the development of schizophrenia to parental behavior and/or to the inheritance of genetic susceptibility to schizophrenia to a particular parent. Further complicating the situation that schizophrenia creates for families of those it affects are difficulty in navigating the complex and multipartite mental-health system in the United States in order to obtain care for this disorder, the often conflicting advice provided by different healthcare providers and authorities, and the time, effort, and cost of obtaining the professional care needed for schizophrenia.

The etiology of schizophrenia is unknown. Current research indicates that it results from a complex interaction between inherited and environmental factors. Studies are investigating numerous potential factors among these, including the volume of gray matter in the cerebral cortex, hippocampus, and thalamus; disruption of neurotransmitter substances (particularly dopamine) involved in the transmission of signals between nerve cells in the brain; impaired inhibition of stimulation in components of the brain; exposure to trauma; and maternal exposure to viruses during pregnancy. As with the etiology of schizophrenia, the reasons for the specific age of its onset, which reaches a peak between 20 and 40 years of age, are unknown.

FACTS AND FIGURES

The *DSM-V* reports a worldwide prevalence of schizophrenia of approximately 0.3 percent to 0.7 percent, with location, gender, and race/ethnicity among the criteria influencing this figure. The ratio of the prevalence of schizophrenia in males to that in females is 1.4:1, with males having a younger average age of onset of the disorder (early to mid-20s) than females (late 20s) (Skikic & Stovall, 2015). Approximately 20 percent of individuals with schizophrenia attempt suicide at least once, and 5 percent to 6 percent die by suicide.

RISK FACTORS

The risk of a person developing schizophrenia if a relative had the disorder is 68 percent in the case of an identical twin; 9 percent in the case of a sibling; 6 percent if a parent had schizophrenia; 5 percent if a grandparent had it. Biological risk factors for the development of schizophrenia include genetic factors, hyperactivity of components of the nervous system in which dopamine mediates the transmission of nerve impulses, premature birth or excessive maternal bleeding at birth, a decreased brain size, brain injury, and maternal exposure to trauma in the first trimester of pregnancy. Environmental risk factors for schizophrenia are familial dysfunction, exposure to trauma, birth in winter or early spring, and a low socioeconomic status; stigma associated with the diagnosis of schizophrenia may exacerbate its symptoms.

SIGNS AND SYMPTOMS

Signs and symptoms of schizophrenia typically include delusions, auditory or visual hallucinations, disorganized thinking as reflected by disorganized speech, and disorganized or abnormal motor behavior, such as immobility or excessive movement, or the utterance of meaningless phrases, and odd postures. Negative symptoms, reflected by diminished or absent function, include lack of attention to personal hygiene, lack of emotion, failure to make eye contact, loss of interest in daily activities, and a lack of enjoyment of activities.

APPLICABLE LAWS AND REGULATIONS

The U.S. Government and individual states of the United States have their own standards, procedures, and laws for the involuntary restraint and detention of persons who may be a danger to themselves or others, such as some persons with schizophrenia. Also, the laws and regulations that apply to schizophrenia may differ according to the age of the affected individual. Because persons with schizophrenia have a high rate of attempted suicide, it is important to become familiar with the local requirements for their involuntary detention should this prove necessary.

The Health Insurance Portability and Accountability Act (HIPAA) Privacy Rule in the United States provides privacy rights and protections to individuals with mental health issues. In recognition of the important role that family members and friends play in the life of an individual with a mental or physical illness, healthcare providers are permitted to communicate about this with family members of such an individual if he or she does not object. Information may also be shared when the affected individual is incapacitated and/or the healthcare professional determines that it is in the best interest of the affected individual to provide family members with information that is directly related to his or her care or payment for care. In the case of notes relating to psychotherapy, the individual who was the source of the notes must provide authorization for them to be shared, unless the of information in or relating to the notes is required by law (i.e., mandated reporting of abuse, duty to warn, imminent harm).

TREATMENT

The social worker assisting the family of an individual with schizophrenia should examine the long-term course and current status of the affected individual's illness, and can use a bereavement model, based on the perceived loss of the family member to illness, to help family members in expressing and processing feelings of grief and stress about this loss. Such a model can facilitate dialogue among family members and acclimate the family to the realm of psychiatric care, medications, and treatments for schizophrenia. Counseling family members about self-care can help to address the long-term stress and fatigue of their caregiving for an individual with schizophrenia; referral of the affected member to assertive community treatment (ACT)-style intervention by a multidisciplinary team of professionals can also be helpful, as can the identification of available respite-care options for family members, or their referral to a consumer-based recovery movement.

The social worker can also conduct a family-systems framework assessment, which examines the relationships among family members and the patterns of their interactions, as a guide in helping them to cope effectively with an affected member's schizophrenic illness, behavior, and needs. A family genogram, or graphic diagram of a family tree, with particular attention to family members' patterns of inheritance of genetic and psychological factors and mental-health histories, can help in analyzing the biological and psychological relationships among individual family members. The family-systems assessment should also examine family roles, norms, and strengths, and family attitudes toward mental illness.

Whereas traditional individual psychotherapy typically addresses an individual's psyche for the purpose of generating change in it and in the individual's relationships with others and with society generally, family-systems therapy, introduced in the late 1960s after extended research into the family patterns of people with schizophrenia, is based on the concept that individuals are inseparable from the network of their relationships. According to this concept, the structure and behavior of the family- relationship system plays a part in the formation of individual character, and the way in which a family functions over time can either harm or help to normalize the behavior of its individual members. [Bowen, M (1966). The use of family theory in clinical practice. *Comprehensive Psychiatry* 7(5), 345-374].

Adjunctively or alternatively, culturally informed therapy for schizophrenia (CIT-S) can be used with family members of an individual with this illness to improve family cohesion; identify family members' spiritual beliefs, values, and practices; and provide education about common symptoms of schizophrenia, training in communication among family members of the affected individual, and the development of problem-solving skills that can help family members cope with schizophrenia and manage the challenges associated with it (e.g., medication compliance). Evidence-based family therapies, which include stress reduction, emotional processing, and cognitive reappraisal, can help reduce the risk of relapse of schizophrenia in an affected family member and can ease the burden experienced by the member's caregivers.

Care must be taken when communicating with family members of an individual with schizophrenia to avoid using language or conveying attitudes that blame them for any aspect of the illness or its course, or for the level of caregiving that specific family members choose to provide. It is also important to be aware that family members' perceptions of a member with schizophrenia may differ, with younger family members having adopted attitudes toward disorders of mental health that differ from those of older members. Equally important is continuous awareness of the ability to provide care (e.g., as they age, parents may not be able to continue to provide care for a schizophrenic son or daughter).

Social workers assisting the families of individuals with schizophrenia should be aware of their own cultural values, beliefs, and biases, and should develop specialized knowledge about the histories, traditions, and values of these families. The treatment methods that these social workers use should reflect knowledge of the cultural diversity of families affected by schizophrenia and the communities in which they live.

SERVICES AND RESOURCES

The following resources can provide information and/or assistance about schizophrenia:

- Schizophrenia.com, http://schizophrenia.com/
- World Fellowship for Schizophrenia and Allied Disorders, http://www.world-schizophrenia.org/
- Schizophrenia and Related Disorders Alliance of America (SARDAA), http://www.sardaa.org/
- Brain & Behavior Research Foundation (formerly NARSAD), https://bbrfoundation.org/
- National Alliance on Mental Illness (NAMI), http://www.nami.org/
- U.S. National Institutes of Health (NIH), http://www.nih.gov/
- U.S. National Institute of Mental Health (NIMH), http://www.nimh.nih.gov/index.shtml

- National Association of Social Workers (NASW), http://www.socialworkers.org/

Written by Chris Bates, MA, MSW

Reviewed by Lynn B. Cooper, D. Crim, and Laura McLuckey, MSW, LCSW

REFERENCES

American Psychiatric Association. (2013). Diagnostic and statistical manual of mental health disorders. (5th ed.). Arlington, VA: American Psychiatric Publishing.

Bishop, M., & Greeff, A. P. (2015). Resilience in families in which a member has been diagnosed with schizophrenia. *Journal of Psychiatric and Mental Health Nursing, 22*(7), 463-471. doi:10.1111/jpm.12230

Bond, G. R., Drake, R. E., Mueser, K. T., & Latimer, E. (2001). Assertive community treatment for people with severe mental illness. *Dis Manage Health Outcomes, 9*(3), 141-155.

Bowen, M (1966). The use of family theory in clinical practice. *Comprehensive Psychiatry* 7(5), 345-374.

British Association of Social Workers. (2012, January). The code of ethics for social work: Statement of principles. Retrieved May 19, 2016, from http://cdn.basw.co.uk/upload/basw_112315-7.pdf

Caqueo-Urízar, A., Rus-Calafell, M., Urzúa, A., Escudero, J., & Gutiérrez-Maldonado, J. (2015). The role of family therapy in management of schizophrenia: Challenges and solutions. *Neuropsychiatric Disease and Treatment, 11*(1), 145-151.

Carr, A. (2009). The effectiveness of family therapy and systemic interventions for adult-focused problems. *Journal of Family Therapy, 31*(1), 46-74.

Chan, S. M., & Chau, Y. S. (2010). Growing up with a parent with schizophrenia: What children say they need. *Journal of Children's Services, 5*(4), 31-42.

Corcoran, J., & Walsh, J. (2010). *Clinical assessment and diagnosis in social work practice* (2nd ed.). New York, NY: Oxford University Press.

Durmaz, H., & Okanli, A. (2014). Investigation of the effects of self-efficacy levels of caregiver family members of the individuals with schizophrenia on burden of care. *Archives of Psychiatric Nursing, 28*(4), 290-294. doi:10.1016/j.apnu.2014.04.004

Earl, T. R. (2006). Mental health care policy: Recognizing the needs of minority siblings as caregivers. *Journal of Human Behavior in the Social Environment, 14*(1-2), 51-72.

Williams, N., & DeBattista, C. (2016). Psychiatric disorders. In *Lange 2016 current diagnosis & treatment* (55th ed., pp. 1048-1057). New York, NY: McGraw-Hill Education.

Grandon, P., Jenaro, C., & Lemos, S. (2008). Primary caregivers of schizophrenia outpatients: Burden and predictor variables. *Psychiatry Research, 158*(3), 335-343.

Hall, S. D., & Bean, R. A. (2008). Family therapy and childhood-onset schizophrenia: Pursuing clinical and bio/psycho/social competence. *Contemporary Family Therapy, 30*(2), 61-74.

International Federation of Social Workers. (2012, March 3). Statement of ethical principles. Retrieved February 4, 2015, from http://ifsw.org/policies/statement-of-ethical-principles/

Jones, D. W. (2004). Families and serious mental illness: Working with loss and ambivalence. *British Journal of Social Work, 34*(7), 961-979.

Jones, S. L. (1997). Caregiver burden: the experience of parents, children, siblings, and spouses of people with mental illness. *Psychiatric Rehabilitation Journal, 20*(4), 84-87.

King, S. (2000). Is expressed emotion cause or effect in the mothers of schizophrenic young adults?. *Schizophrenia Research, 45*(1-2), 65-78.

Lasebikan, V. O., & Ayinde, O. O. (2013). Family burden in caregivers of schizophrenia patients: Prevalence and socio-demographic correlates. *Indian Journal of Psychological Medicine, 35*(1), 60-66.

National Association of Social Workers. (2015). Standards and indicators for cultural competence in social work practice. Retrieved May 19, 2016, from http://www.socialworkers.org/practice/standards/PRA-BRO-253150-CC-Standards.pdf

Olwit, C., Musisi, S., Leshabari, S., & Sanyu, I. (2015). Chronic sorrow: Lived experience of caregivers of patients diagnosed with schizophrenia in Butabika Mental Hospital, Kampala, Uganda. *Archives of Psychiatric Nursing, 29*(1), 43-48. doi:10.1016/j.apnu.2014.09.007

Skikic, M., & Stovall, J. G. (2015). Schizophrenia. In F. J. Domino (Ed.), *The 5-minute clinical consultant standard 2016* (24th ed., pp. 1000-1001). Philadelphia, PA: Wolters Kluwer.

Townsend, M. C. (2015). Schizophrenia spectrum and other psychotic disorders. In *Psychiatric mental health nursing: Concepts of care in evidence-based practice* (8th ed., pp. 429-439). Philadelphia, PA: F. A. Davis Company.

U.S. Department of Health & Human Services. (n.d.). HIPAA privacy rule and sharing information related to mental health. Retrieved February 4, 2015, from http://www.hhs.gov/ocr/privacy/hipaa/understanding/special/mhguidance.html

Wiens, S. E., & Daniluk, J. C. (2009). Love, loss, and learning: The experiences of fathers who have children diagnosed with schizophrenia. *Journal of Counseling & Development, 87*(1), 339-348.

SCHIZOPHRENIA: PARANOID SUBTYPE

MAJOR CATEGORIES: Behaioral & Mental Health

DESCRIPTION

Schizophrenia is a mental health disorder that may include symptoms of delusions, hallucinations, and disorganized speech that affect a person in many aspects of their daily life. Schizophrenia was previously diagnosed with specified subtypes such as catatonic subtype, disorganized subtype, paranoid subtype, residual subtype, and undifferentiated subtype. A diagnosis of schizophrenia is made with meeting specific criteria as outlined in the The *Diagnostic and Statistical Manual of Mental Disorders* (*DSM*). The two most recent editions of this diagnostic manual are the fourth edition (*DSM-IV*) and the fifth edition (*DSM-5*).

The *DSM-5* retains the general description of schizophrenia as a chronic and incapacitating psychiatric disorder that has a severe impact on thought processes, stimulus perception, communication, behavior, and the ability to maintain relationships and a stable living environment. Schizophrenia is characterized by positive (noticeably present, such as a repeated sound or behavior) and negative (notable by their absence, such as the loss of speech) symptoms. Schizophrenia shares the feature of psychosis (hallucinations and delusions) with several other *DSM-5* diagnoses, including mood disorders, and therefore can be difficult to distinguish from other disorders featuring psychosis. However, schizophrenia is primarily a thought disorder.

The *DSM-5*, which was published in 2013, includes changes in the diagnostic criteria for schizophrenia from the *DSM-IV* in the "Schizophrenia Spectrum and Other Psychotic Disorders" chapter. In addition to clarifying some of the language used, the significant diagnosis criteria changes are as follows.

At least one of the active symptoms must be one of the core symptoms of schizophrenia: delusions, hallucinations, or disorganized speech. Specifications about the type of delusions and hallucinations have been removed for the *DSM-5*. All subtypes of schizophrenia, including paranoid subtype, have been eliminated in the *DSM-5*. Course specifiers have been changed to reflect elimination of subtypes in the *DSM-5*. Standardized assessment tools for a dimensional assessment of severity of symptoms have been added in the *DSM-5*.

The subtypes of schizophrenia were eliminated because of their "limited diagnostic stability, low reliability, and poor validity." In place of the subtypes, the *DSM-5* introduces a symptoms severity tool, the Clinician-Rated Dimensions of Psychosis Symptom Severity, which consists of eight symptoms that may be present in psychosis that the clinician rates the symptoms using a 5-point scale, from 0 (not present) to 4 (present and severe). The goal is to measure the range and severity of symptoms to assist in planning treatment needs, make prognosis estimates, and research. The measure may be used regularly to track changes in the symptoms.

Because diagnoses assigned using *DSM-IV* criteria (schizophrenia, paranoid subtype) will remain in patient records, and because patients may continue to identify with the disorder that was diagnosed, it remains useful to understand the nature of the subtypes that have been eliminated from the *DSM-5*. The *DSM-IV* used a hierarchical method to determine the appropriate subtype of schizophrenia. Because the subtype was determined by the most prominent symptoms at the time of the assessment, the diagnosed subtype may have changed over time. Individuals with schizophrenia frequently have

symptoms of more than one subtype simultaneously. To determine a single diagnostic subtype, the *DSM-IV* used the following hierarchy.

The catatonic subtype was assigned whenever catatonic symptoms predominated at the time of assessment. The disorganized (sometimes referred to as *hebephrenic*) subtype was assigned whenever flat or inappropriate affect and disorganized speech and behavior predominated at the time of assessment (unless the catatonic subtype had been assigned).

The paranoid subtype was assigned when delusions or hallucinations predominated at the time of assessment (unless catatonic subtype or disorganized subtype had been assigned). The undifferentiated subtype was assigned when there were prominent active-phase symptoms that did not meet the criteria for the catatonic, disorganized, or paranoid subtype at the time of assessment. The residual (sometimes referred to as *simple*) subtype was assigned when there were continuing symptoms of schizophrenia but the specific criteria for the active phase of schizophrenia were not met at the time of assessment.

The paranoid subtype of schizophrenia, as described in the *DSM-IV* and research based on the *DSM-IV* diagnostic criteria, may include prominent delusions; hallucinations; a stilted, overly formal, or intense style of interpersonal interaction; and a superior or patronizing manner. The delusions frequently are organized around a coherent theme: primarily persecutory or grandiose, but other themes may predominate or simultaneously be present (religiosity, jealousy, somatization). Hallucinations observed for the paranoid type of schizophrenia typically are auditory and in some manner related to the individual's delusions.

Cultural awareness must be used by social workers to distinguish delusions and hallucinations from the norms of a cultural group or beliefs that may have some grounding in facts about the hallucinations or delusions. The delusions and hallucinations may be externalized as anger, anxiety, aloofness, or argumentativeness. Usually cognitive functioning remains prior to the onset of schizophrenic symptom levels, and features of the disorganized subtype do not intrude in the individual's cognitive functioning. Symptoms of the paranoid subtype can appear in numerous other diagnoses (brief psychotic disorder, delusional disorder, mood disorders, epileptic or drug-induced psychoses).

The paranoid subtype of schizophrenia does not have a cause that is distinct from those of other subtypes of schizophrenia. Onset of symptoms tends to be later and more acute (short-lasting), and some evidence suggests that the prognosis for independent living and employment is better for those with paranoid subtype than for other subtypes of schizophrenia. Depending on cause and current phase of symptoms, treatment may include involuntary detention, medication, social skills training, psychoeducation, and referrals to community and family support services.

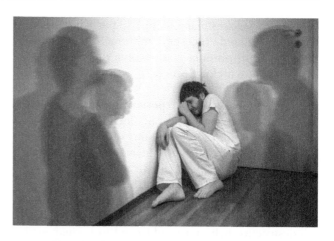

FACTS AND FIGURES

Given the stated low reliability of the diagnosis of the paranoid subtype of schizophrenia, facts and figures directly associated with it are not reliable. The *DSM-5* reports lifetime prevalence of schizophrenia at approximately 0.3 to 0.7 percent.

RISK FACTORS

Among the risk factors for schizophrenia, none are specifically unique to the paranoid subtype. Biological risk factors for schizophrenia, paranoid subtype, may include genetics, dopamine hyperactivity, decreased brain size, premature birth or excessive maternal bleeding, traumatic brain injury, or maternal exposure to trauma in first trimester.

Environmental risk factors for schizophrenia, paranoid subtype, may include a history of family dysfunction, exposure to trauma, winter or early spring birth, or a low socioeconomic status. There is a stigma associated with a diagnosis of schizophrenia and this may exacerbate an individual's symptoms.

SIGNS AND SYMPTOMS

Physical signs and symptoms of schizophrenia, paranoid subtype, may include stiff or tense body language, sudden anger, irritability, and an overly formal or intense style of interpersonal interaction.

Cognitive signs and symptoms of schizophrenia, paranoid subtype, may include delusions frequently organized around a single theme, and/or hallucinations frequently related to delusions.

SOCIAL WORK ASSESSMENT

The social worker assisting an individual who may have schizophrenia, paranoid subtype, should complete a biological, psychological, social, and spiritual assessment, including any risk for suicide and harm to self and others to determine the individual's immediate needs. Close observation of the individual's functioning and mood during the interview should be made, with particular attention to any suspected presence and themes of delusions and the nature of any noted hallucinations (auditory, visual, command, or noncommand). The social worker may gather collateral information from family, friends, and coworkers regarding the individual's behavior and history. A history of any prior diagnosis of mental health disorders other than schizophrenia should be obtained.

ASSESSMENT AND SCREENING TOOLS

Standardized assessments and screening tools that may be used in an assessment regarding schizophrenia, paranoid subtype, may include the Scale for the Assessment of Negative Symptoms (SANS) and the Scale for the Assessment of Positive Symptoms (SAPS).

There are no specific tests that can identify schizophrenia; however, the above mentioned standard tests may help identify relevant medical condition(s) or substance misuse that may need to be addressed by a medical professional.

TREATMENT

Treatments and interventions for schizophrenia aim to improve quality of life, decrease the number and severity of active-phase symptoms and episodes of schizophrenia, and strengthen the individual's family and community support. Over the course of the disorder, treatment might include hospitalization, psychopharmacology, various psychological treatments (individual, group, or family therapy; social skills training; cognitive behavioral therapy [CBT]), involvement in an assertive community treatment

(ACT) multidisciplinary team, or participation in community-based recovery movement programs. Because schizophrenia is a chronic disorder, treatment may be a lifelong process.

Intervention

An individual who is experiencing severe active-phase episodes of schizophrenia including psychotic features could have the possibility of harm to self or others. Such individuals would benefit from hospitalization and appropriate medication to reduce the severity of their symptoms and protect them from hurting themselves or others.

Symptoms of hallucinations, delusions, or erratic or self-destructive behavior would need to be managed through scheduled appointments with a mental health professional who can prescribe appropriate medications. Medications may be used to decrease hallucinations or delusions, stabilize erratic behavior, decrease destructive behavior, and increase the individual's level of personal safety. The social worker should discuss and assist the individual in medication adherence including appropriate dosage and timing. Side effects of the medications and any changes in the individual's behavior should be noted and reported on follow-up visits with their prescribing mental health professional. It is important that regular evaluations are completed for any signs of suicidality or homicidality.

Psychological education to the family regarding schizophrenia may be necessary to reestablish lost relations with family or peer support. Education may include information about the nature of schizophrenia, different treatments available, and available community resources. The social workers should teach stress management techniques, communication skills, and problem solving skills to both the individual and the family. Self-care and mutual support within the family should be encouraged. The individual may be referred to a recovery-based consumer movement support group.

Assertive community treatment (ACT) style intervention could assist the individual to become more engaged in their treatment and reduce hospitalizations and frequent emergency room (ER) visits. ACT style intervention may include treatment from a multidisciplinary team with professionals from various backgrounds, consistent contact in the community, assertive outreach, and individualized services with no time limit on provided services and rapid access and response to the individual's needs.

Improved engagement in the individual's treatment and the community may assist the individual in gaining stabilized housing, maintain adherence to their medication regimen, and improve their overall quality of life.

APPLICABLE LAWS AND REGULATIONS

Each jurisdiction (nation, state, and province) has its own standards, procedures, and laws for involuntary restraint and detention of persons who may be a danger to themselves or others. Because individuals with schizophrenia have a high rate of suicide attempts, it is important for professionals working with the individual to become familiar with the local requirements for involuntary detention. Local laws and professional reporting requirements for neglect and abuse should be known and followed.

SERVICES AND RESOURCES

Enter *schizophrenia, paranoid* or *paranoid schizophrenia* in the search box to access relevant information available on each website.

- Recovery within Reach, http://www.recoverywithinreach.org
- Brain & Behavior Research Foundation (formerly NARSAD), http://bbrfoundation.org/
- National Alliance on Mental Illness (NAMI), http://www.nami.org/
- U.S. National Institutes of Health (NIH), http://www.nih.gov/
- U.S. National Institute of Mental Health (NIMH), http://www.nimh.nih.gov/index.shtml
- National Association of Social Workers (NASW), http://www.socialworkers.org/

FOOD FOR THOUGHT

According to long-term studies showing improvements in the quality of life for persons living with schizophrenia, as well as the variation in the progress of the disorder, some professionals in the field call into question the long-held view that schizophrenia is always a chronic condition with poor outcomes. Simultaneously, a consumer movement has developed around the concept of recovery as a valid treatment goal. The fundamental concepts embodied in the recovery movement are self-direction, individualized and person-centered treatments, empowerment of the individual, holistic and nonlinear approaches to treatment and care, strengths-based perspective treatment, peer support, respect, responsibility, and hope. The recovery movement focuses on the person rather than the illness and emphasizes healing and choice, with multiple goals including gaining independence and the fulfillment of the individual's full potential.

Researchers studying Medicaid recipients in the United States found that adults with schizophrenia die at 3.5 times the rate of the general adult population. Individuals with schizophrenia have an increased risk for mortality from chronic obstructive pulmonary disease (COPD), diabetes mellitus, cardiovascular disease, suicide, influenza and pneumonia, lung and other cancers, and accidents. Researchers believe that smoking is a major risk factor for the development of these diseases, as approximately two thirds of individuals with schizophrenia smoke.

RED FLAGS

Careful investigation of delusions and hallucinations should be conducted to assess for any increased risk for self-harm or harm to others associated with the paranoid subtype of schizophrenia. Paranoid symptoms appear in several other disorders. A complete differential diagnosis should be made by a qualified mental health professional to ensure that correct treatments are selected. Some research shows a tendency for persons with the paranoid subtype to self-medicate with nonprescription drugs and an assessment should be made for any suspected nonprescription drug use.

NEXT STEPS

The social worker should review the medication regimen, including the importance of medications, and the importance of taking them as prescribed with the individual. Any side effects should be reported. Follow-up appointments with the agency issuing the prescription should be made. The individual should be referred to any local schizophrenia support groups, supported work, or mental health agencies for continued support. The stability of the individual's current living situation should be ascertained and appropriate referrals made. Referrals for support to family members should be completed.

Written by Chris Bates, MA, MSW

Reviewed by Lynn B. Cooper, D Crim, and Pedram Samghabadi

REFERENCES

American Psychiatric Association. (2000). *Diagnostic and statistical manual of mental disorders* (4th Rev ed.). Arlington, VA: Author.

American Psychiatric Association. (2013). Diagnostic and statistical manual of mental health disorders. (5th ed.). Arlington, VA: American Psychiatric Publishing.

Baker-Brown, S. (2006). A patient's journey: Living with paranoid schizophrenia. *BMJ, 333*(7569), 636-638. doi:10.1136/bmj.38968.608275.AE

British Association of Social Workers. (2012). *The code of ethics for social work: Statement of principles.* Retrieved April 18, 2016, from http://cdn.basw.co.uk/upload/basw_112315-7.pdf

Corcoran, J., & Walsh, J. (2010). *Clinical assessment and diagnosis in social work practice* (2nd ed.). New York, NY: Oxford University Press.

DeBattista, C., Eisendrath, S. J., & Lichtmacher, J. E. (2015). Psychiatric disorders. In M. A. Papadakis & S. J. McPhee (Eds.), *2015 current medical diagnosis & treatment* (54th ed., pp. 1042-1051). Philadelphia, PA: Wolters Kluwer.

Feiner, J. S., & Frese, F. J. (2009). Recovery in schizophrenia. In B. J. Sadock, V. A. Sadock, & P. Ruiz (Eds.), *Kaplan & Sadocks's comprehensive textbook of psychiatry* (9th ed., Vol. 1, pp. 1582-1593). Philadelphia, PA: Wolters Kluwer Health/Lippincott Williams & Wilkins.

International Federation of Social Workers. (2012). Statement of ethical principles. Retrieved April 18, 2016, from http://ifsw.org/policies/statement-of-ethical-principles/

Kudumija, S. M., Jukic, V., Novalic, D., Zarkovic-Paligan, T., Milosevic, M., & Rosenzweig, I. (2014). Alcohol abuse as the strongest risk factor for violent offending in patients with paranoid schizophrenia. *Croatian Medical Journal, 55*(2), 156-162. doi:10.3325/cmj.2014.55.156

Lysaker, P. H., Salvatore, G., Grant, M. L. A., Procacci, M., Olesek, K. L., Buck, K. D., & Dimaggio, G. (2010). Deficits in theory of mind and social anxiety as independent paths to paranoid feature in schizophrenia. *Schizophrenia Research, 124*(1-3), 81-85. doi:10.1016/j.schres.2010.06.019

Olfson, M., Gerhard, T., Huang, C., Crystal, S., & Stroup, T. S. (2015). Premature mortality among adults with schizophrenia in the United States. *JAMA Psychiatry, 72*(12), 1172.

Salinas, J. A., Paul, G. L., & Springer, J. R. (2008). Consensus judgments of discharge readiness based on paranoid behavior: To what are clinical staff responding? *Social Psychiatry and Psychiatric Epidemiology*, *43*(5), 380-386. doi:10.1007/s00127-008-0319-z

Schizophrenia spectrum and other psychotic disorders. (2015). In B. J. Sadock, V. A. Sadock, & P. Ruiz (Eds.), *Kaplan & Sadock's synopsis of psychiatry: Behavioral sciences/clinical psychiatry* (11th ed., pp. 300-329). Philadelphia, PA: Wolters Kluwer Health/Lippincott Williams & Wilkins.

Townsend, M. C. (2015). Schizophrenia spectrum and other psychotic disorders. In *Psychiatric mental health nursing: Concepts of care in evidence-based practice* (8th ed., pp. 419-457). Philadelphia, PA: F. A. Davis Company.

Weinstein, J. J., & Stovall, J. G. (2014). Schizophrenia. In F. J. Domino (Ed.), *The 5-minute clinical consult 2015* (23rd ed., pp. 1074-1075). Philadelphia, PA: Wolters Kluwer Health/Lippincott Williams & Wilkins.

Wheeler, D. (2015). NASW standards and indicators for cultural competence in social work practice. Retrieved April 18, 2016, from http://www.socialworkers.org/practice/standards/PRA-BRO-253150-CC-Standards.pdf

Xiang, Y. T., Wang, C. Y., Chiu, H. F., Weng, Y. Z., Bo, Q. J., Chan, S. S., & Ungvari, G. S. (2010). Socio-demographic and clinical profiles of paranoid and nonparanoid schizophrenia: A prospective, multicenter study in China. *Perspectives in Psychiatric Care*, *47*(3), 126-130. doi:10.1111/j.1744-6163.2010.00281.x

SCHIZOPHRENIA: RESIDUAL SUBTYPE

MAJOR CATEGORIES: Behavioral & Mental Health

DESCRIPTION

The fifth edition of the *Diagnostic and Statistical Manual of Mental Disorders* (*DSM-5*) retains the general description of schizophrenia given in the fourth edition of the manual (*DSM-IV*) as a chronic and incapacitating psychiatric disorder with a severe effect on thought processes, the perception of stimuli, and communication. Besides these effects, schizophrenia greatly affects behavior and the ability to maintain relationships and a stable living environment. Schizophrenia is characterized by positive (noticeably present) and negative (notable by their absence) symptoms, and shares psychosis as a feature with several other diagnoses described in the *DSM-5*, including mood disorders, which can make it difficult to distinguish this psychiatric disorder from these other disorders. However, schizophrenia is primarily a disorder of thinking.

Although the *DSM-5* has abandoned the use of subtypes of schizophrenia, the *DSM-IV* defined the residual subtype of schizophrenia as causing at least one active episode of psychotic symptoms in the month before its diagnosis. The symptoms that must be present during an active episode of schizophrenia of the residual subtype in order for this subtype of schizophrenia to be diagnosed can be can be any of the following, but at least one of them must be present:

delusions, hallucinations, disorganized speech, grossly disorganized or catatonic behavior, or negative symptoms in the form of an absence of emotion, limitation of speech, or lack of motivation. However, a diagnosis of the residual subtype of schizophrenia requires that the active phase of this disorder be absent at the time of diagnosis, and that the symptoms at the time of diagnosis instead be predominantly negative. These negative symptoms of the residual subtype of schizophrenia may include the following.

- Alogia (dysfunction of communication or poverty of speech, with minimal talking and few words);
- Blunted affect (reduced range of emotion, including expression, experience, and perception);
- Asociality (minimal or absent social interaction or interest in social interaction);
- Anhedonia (dysfunction of the capacity for pleasure, minimal or absent ability to experience pleasure, loss of interest in activities that previously were pleasurable);
- Avolition (dysfunction of motivation, minimal or absent persistence, motivation or desire, decreased ability to start or complete everyday tasks such as personal hygiene).

The residual subtype of schizophrenia does not have a cause or origin that differs from those of the other subtypes of schizophrenia described in the *DSM-IV*, but may become a lifelong disorder or may have symptoms that slowly decrease, with the disorder eventually going into full remission.

The prognosis for patients with the residual subtype of schizophrenia depends heavily on their level of functioning before the onset of this subtype of schizophrenia, and on the level(s) of their continuing family, peer, and professional support. Treatment for the residual subtype of schizophrenia may include medications, cognitive behavioral therapy (CBT), and training in social skills, among other interventions, in addition to help provided upon referrals to community and family support services.

FACTS AND FIGURES

Because the general description of schizophrenia given in the *DSM-5* supersedes the definitions of the subtypes of schizophrenia given in the *DSM-IV*, facts and figures about these subtypes may be misleading. The *DSM-5* reports a lifetime prevalence of schizophrenia as ranging from 0.3 to 0.7 percent. In a study conducted in 2015, the most common residual symptoms of individuals judged as being in remission from schizophrenia were blunted affect, conceptual disorganization, and social withdrawal.

RISK FACTORS

Apart from birth in early summer rather than in the winter or early spring, no risk factors are unique to the residual subtype of schizophrenia as compared with other subtypes of schizophrenia described in the *DSM-IV*. Biological risk factors for the residual subtype of schizophrenia are genetic factors, hyperactivity of components of the nervous system in which dopamine mediates the transmission of nerve impulses, decreased brain size, premature birth or excessive maternal bleeding at birth, traumatic brain injury, and maternal exposure to trauma in the first trimester of pregnancy. Environmental risk factors for the residual subtype of schizophrenia are a low socioeconomic status, family dysfunction, and exposure to trauma; stigma associated with the diagnosis of this type of schizophrenia may exacerbate its symptoms.

SIGNS AND SYMPTOMS

Physical signs of the residual subtype of schizophrenia may include lack of eye contact and limited communication, blunted affect, passivity and lack of initiative, limited activity, poor hygiene or an unkempt appearance, and inability to care for the self (bathe, eat, dress). Cognitive signs of the residual subtype of schizophrenia may include a lessening of the severity and frequency of hallucinations, delusions, illogical thinking, and eccentric behavior from the time at which these symptoms began. Signs and symptoms specific to the residual subtype of schizophrenia may occur simultaneously with symptoms of other subtypes of schizophrenia.

TREATMENT

The social worker assisting an individual who has schizophrenia of the disorganized subtype should conduct a standard biological, psychological, social, and spiritual assessment of the individual, including an assessment of his or her risk for suicide and for inflicting harm on him- or herself and others. This should include an assessment of the individual's level of functioning and demeanor during the interview conducted for the assessment, with particular attention to the individual's affect and cognitive symptoms and to the collection of information on any prior mental health disorders other than schizophrenia. The assessment should also include laboratory tests if and as needed to identify medical disorders and substance abuse, and the collection of collateral information from the individual's family, friends, and coworkers. Because of the possible long-term duration of the residual subtype of schizophrenia, the evaluation of persons with this subtype of schizophrenia for alcohol and substance abuse is particularly important.

The assessment should also ascertain the stability of the affected individual's living situation, with referrals if and as needed to local schizophrenia support groups, supported work services, and mental health agencies, as well as needed referrals for the individual's family members.

Treatments and interventions for schizophrenia are directed at improving the quality of life of the affected individual; decreasing the number and severity of active episodes of the disorder; and strengthening the affected individual's family and community support. Because schizophrenia is a chronic disorder, its treatment may be a lifelong process.

Treatment for the residual subtype of schizophrenia may include medication, various psychological treatments, and community-based recovery programs. A changing range and intensity of symptoms, with reduced or infrequent hallucinations, delusions, erratic or self-destructive behavior but a pronounced presence of negative symptoms, is usually treated with medication, by emphasis on adhering to medication dosage and timing, observation of changes in behavior, and reporting of impact of side effects of medication. Lack of motivation, pessimism, and the inability to set and meet goals is widely treated with CBT. The technique known as cognitive behavioral therapy for psychosis (CBTp) has been found effective in addressing residual symptoms of schizophrenia. This type of CBT is a verbal technique that seeks to reduce symptoms of the residual subtype of schizophrenia by building the affected individual's capacity to reflect on and question delusional or self-judgmental beliefs that limit the achievement of personal life goals, with guidance towards identifying new ways of responding to such beliefs.

Treatment of the negative symptoms of the residual subtype of schizophrenia, such as withdrawal, decreased social functioning, and lack of self-care, merits particular attention, because these symptoms may be overlooked during assessment or downplayed by the individuals they affect. Treatment of these negative symptoms is directed at increasing skills needed for independent functioning and maintaining social relationships and care of the self. Also used in treating schizophrenia of the residual subtype are training programs directed at improving social skills such as goal setting, role modeling, behavior rehearsal, positive reinforcement, and exercises for extending social skills to community settings.

Extended studies showing improvements in the quality of life of persons living with schizophrenia, as well as variations in its progression, have led some professionals in the field to question the long-held view that schizophrenia is always a chronic condition with poor outcomes. Simultaneously, a consumer movement has developed around the concept of recovery from schizophrenia as a valid goal of its treatment. This movement focuses on the person rather than the illness and emphasizes healing and choice, with multiple goals including independence and the fulfillment of personal potential. The fundamental concepts embodied in this recovery movement are the self-direction and empowerment of individuals with schizophrenia; individualized and person-centered treatment for it; holistic, nonlinear, and strengths-based approaches to its treatment; and peer support, respect, responsibility, and hope for the individual with schizophrenia.

Social workers assisting individuals with schizophrenia of the residual subtype should be aware of their own cultural values, beliefs, and biases, and develop specialized knowledge about the histories, traditions, and values of these individuals and their families. These social workers should adopt treatment methods that reflect their knowledge of these factors and of the communities in which they practice.

APPLICABLE LAWS AND REGULATIONS

The U.S. government and individual states of the United States have their own standards, procedures, and laws for the involuntary restraint and detention of persons who may be a danger to themselves or others, including those with the residual subtype of schizophrenia. Because individuals with schizophrenia have a high rate of attempted suicide, it is important to become familiar with local requirements for their involuntary detention if suicide becomes a risk, and also if they pose a danger to other persons.

SERVICES AND RESOURCES

- Recovery within Reach, http://www.recoverywithinreach.org
- Brain & Behavior Research Foundation (formerly NARSAD), http://bbrfoundation.org/
- National Alliance on Mental Illness (NAMI), http://www.nami.org/
- U.S. National Institutes of Health (NIH), http://www.nih.gov/
- U.S. National Institute of Mental Health (NIMH), http://www.nimh.nih.gov/index.shtml
- National Association of Social Workers (NASW), http://www.socialworkers.org/

Written by Chris Bates, MA, MSW

Reviewed by Lynn B. Cooper, D Crim, and Pedram Samghabadi

REFERENCES

American Psychiatric Association. (2000). *Diagnostic and statistical manual of mental disorders* (4th Rev ed.). Arlington, VA: Author.

American Psychiatric Association. (2013). Diagnostic and statistical manual of mental health disorders

(DSM-5). (5th ed.). Arlington, VA: American Psychiatric Publishing.

Bora, E., Gokcen, S., Kayahan, B., & Veznedaroglu, B. (2008). Deficits of social cognitive and social-perceptual aspects of theory of mind in remitted patients with schizophrenia: Effect of residual symptoms. *The Journal of Nervous and Mental Disease, 196*(2), 95-99. doi:10.1097/NMD.0b013e318162a9e1

British Association of Social Workers. (2012). The code of ethics for social work: Statement of principles. Retrieved April 20, 2016, from http://cdn.basw.co.uk/upload/basw_112315-7.pdf

Corcoran, J., & Walsh, J. (2010). *Clinical assessment and diagnosis in social work practice* (2nd ed.). New York, NY: Oxford University Press.

DeBattista, C., Eisendrath, S. J., & Lichtmacher, J. E. (2015). Psychiatric disorders. In M. A. Papadakis & S. J. McPhee (Eds.), *2015 current medical diagnosis & treatment* (54th ed., pp. 1042-1051). Philadelphia, PA: Wolters Kluwer.

Feiner, J. S., & Frese, F. J. (2009). Recovery in schizophrenia. In B. J. Sadock, V. A. Sadock, & P. Ruiz (Eds.), *Kaplan & Sadocks's comprehensive textbook of psychiatry* (9th ed., Vol. 1, pp. 1582-1593). Philadelphia, PA: Wolters Kluwer Health/Lippincott Williams & Wilkins.

Kurtz, M. M., & Mueser, K. T. (2008). A meta-analysis of controlled research on social skills training for schizophrenia. *Journal of Consulting and Clinical Psychology, 76*(3), 491-504. doi:10.1037/0022-006X.76.3.491

International Federation of Social Workers. (2012, March 3). Statement of ethical principles. Retrieved April 20, 2016, from http://ifsw.org/policies/statement-of-ethical-principles/

Sadock, B. J., Sadock, V. A., & Ruiz, P. (2015). Schizophrenia spectrum and other psychotic disorders. In *Kaplan & Sadock's synopsis of psychiatry: Behavioral sciences/clinical psychiatry* (11th ed., pp. 300-323). Philadelphia, PA: Wolters Kluwer.

Schennanch, R., Riedel, M., Obermeier, M., Spellmann, L., Musil, R., Jager, M., ... Moller, H. J. (0215). What are residual symptoms in schizophrenia spectrum disorder? Clinical description and 1-year persistence within a naturalistic trial. *European Archives of Psychiatry and Clinical Neuroscience, 265*(2), 107-116. doi:10.1007/s00406-014-0528-2

Stahl, S. M., & Buckley, P. F. (2007). Negative symptoms of schizophrenia: A problem that will not go away. *Acta Psychiatrica Scandinavica, 115*(1), 4-11. doi:10.1111/j.1600-0447.2006.00947.x

Townsend, M. C. (2015). Schizophrenia spectrum and other psychotic disorders. In *Psychiatric mental health nursing: Concepts of care in evidence-based practice* (8th ed., pp. 419-457). Philadelphia: F. A.: Davis Company.

Westcott, C., Waghorn, G., McLean, D., Statham, D., & Mowry, B. (2015). Role functioning among adults with schizophrenia. *British Journal of Occupational Therapy, 78*(3), 158-165. doi:10.1177/0308022615573372

Wheeler, D. (2015). NASW standards and indicators for cultural competence in social work practice. Retrieved April 20, 2016, from http://www.socialworkers.org/practice/standards/PRA-BRO-253150-CC-Standards.pdf

Wykes, T. (2014). Cognitive-behaviour therapy and schizophrenia. *Evidence-Based Mental Health, 17*(3), 67-68. doi:10.1136/eb-2014-101887

SCHIZOPHRENIFORM DISORDER

MAJOR CATEGORIES: Behavioral & Mental Health

DESCRIPTION

As defined by the Fifth Edition of the *Diagnostic and Statistical Manual of Mental Disorders* (*DSM-5*), *schizophreniform disorder* is a mental disorder that has the same symptoms as schizophrenia, with the two significant differences that its symptoms last for more than 1 month unless successfully treated and for less than 6 months in any case, and that there is no requirement for impairment of social or occupational functioning, as there is for schizophrenia. The *International Statistical Classification of Diseases and Related Health Problems, 10th Revision* (*ICD-10*), includes a disorder conceptually similar to schizophreniform disorder but called *acute schizophrenia-like psychotic disorder*, which requires that the criteria for schizophrenia in the *ICD-10* be met, but for the much shorter duration of less than 1 month in total as compared with the less than 6 months duration of schizophreniform disorder specified in the *DSM-V*, and also requires that the symptoms of the disorder must have an acute onset, which is not required for the diagnosis of schizophreniform disorder in the *DSM-V*.

The diagnosis of schizophreniform disorder in the *DSM-V* can be assigned either during the window of time between 1 and 6 months after the onset of symptoms of the disorder, in which case the qualifying term "provisional" can be added to the diagnosis until the 6-month mark has passed. If symptoms of the disorder resolve within 6 months after their onset, the qualifying "provisional" can be removed, with the diagnosis simply becoming "schizophreniform disorder." However, if symptoms persist beyond 6 months, the diagnosis of schizophreniform disorder must be changed to some other diagnosis. Impaired social or occupational functioning may be present in schizophreniform disorder as defined in the *DSM-V*, but is not usually present in this disorder and is not required for the diagnosis of schizophreniform disorder as it is for schizophrenia. Briefly, the criteria for schizophrenia that may also apply to schizophreniform disorder are as follows:

- Delusions.
- Hallucinations.
- Disorganized speech.
- Grossly disorganized or catatonic behavior.
- Negative symptoms.
- Exclusion of schizoaffective and mood disorders with psychotic features.
- Exclusion of a general medical condition or effects of a substance as the cause.
- Schizophrenia is primarily a thought disorder rather than a mood disorder.

Schizophreniform disorder has a rapid onset, with symptoms appearing within 4 weeks of the first noticeable change in persons with the disorder, and consisting of emotional turmoil and confusion. These symptoms, a rapid onset, good functioning before the onset of the disorder, and a full range of affect or emotion are often indicators of a good prognosis and eventual removal of the qualifying "provisional" term from the disorder in patients who recover completely from it. Schizophreniform disorder usually also lacks the negative symptoms seen with schizophrenia, consisting of flattening of affect or emotional

responsiveness, lack of motivation, inability to experience pleasure, and impaired attention, which if they persist for 6 months are indicators of a poor prognosis and usually lead to a change of diagnosis from schizophreniform disorder to schizophrenia.

The study of schizophreniform disorder is particularly difficult because the etiology of schizophreniform disorder is not distinct from that of schizophrenia, and because diagnosis of the disorder is essentially retroactive and can be confirmed only after there is full recovery. Because of this, studies of schizophreniform disorder cannot be initiated with a population known to have the disorder, but must be done with subjects carefully selected from study populations consisting chiefly of individuals whose disorder has been been diagnosed as schizophrenia.

FACTS AND FIGURES

Accurate facts and figures for schizophreniform disorder are hard to establish because of the essentially retroactive nature of the diagnosis, made after recovery from it within 6 months after its onset. According to the *DSM-5*, approximately 33 percent of persons with an initial provisional diagnosis of schizophreniform disorder recover within the 6-month period and meet the diagnostic criteria for schizophreniform disorder as a final diagnosis. Most of the remaining 67 percent eventually receive a diagnosis of schizophrenia or schizoaffective disorder.

RISK FACTORS

Ordinarily, studies of risk factors for psychotic disorders do not differentiate schizophreniform disorder from schizophrenia or vice versa. Studies done with brain imaging have tentatively associated enlargement of the fluid-filled spaces in the brain known as the *ventricles* with an initial diagnosis that progresses to schizophrenia, leading to a tentative conclusion that this ventricular enlargement is a risk factor for both schizophreniform disorder and schizophrenia, which because of the frequent provision of the former to the latter disorder may also be present in schizophreniform disorder, include genetic factors, hyperactivity of components of the nervous system in which dopamine mediates the transmission of nerve impulses, decreased brain size, premature birth or excessive maternal bleeding at birth, traumatic brain injury, and maternal exposure to trauma in first trimester of pregnancy as biological risk factors.

Environmental risk factors for schizophreniform disorder are a low socioeconomic status, family dysfunction, exposure to trauma, and borth in winter or early spring birth.

Signs and Symptoms

Signs and symptoms of schizophreniform disorder can include any of the following:

- A rapid onset of symptoms; hallucinations; delusions; emotional turmoil and confusion;
- disrupted thought processes and speech, or absence of thought and speech; inappropriate and usually flat affect or rapidly changing affect; disorganized behavior or catatonia;
- negative symptoms similar to those seen in schizophrenia (although these are unusual in schizophreniform disorder); a typically good premorbid level of functioning; a rapid onset of symptoms.

Applicable Laws and Regulations

The U.S. Government and individual states of the United States have their own standards, procedures, and laws for the involuntary restraint and detention of persons who may be a danger to themselves or others, including those with the residual subtype of schizophrenia. Because individuals with schizophrenia have a high rate of attempted suicide, it is important to become familiar with local requirements for their involuntary detention if suicide becomes a risk, and also if they pose a danger to other persons.

Local and professional requirements for reporting the neglect and abuse of such individuals should also be known and observed.

Treatment

The social worker assisting an individual who has schizophrenia of the disorganized subtype should conduct a standard biological, psychological, social, and spiritual assessment of the individual, including an assessment of his or her risk for suicide and for inflicting harm on him- or herself and others. This should include an evaluation of the affected individual's premorbid level of functioning and a detailed history of the onset of symptoms of the individual's disorder, including their timing and the rapidity and intensity of their onset. The individual's level of functioning and demeanor should be evaluated during the interview conducted for the assessment, with particular attention to the individual's affect and

cognitive symptoms and to the collection of information on any prior mental-health disorders and any history of substance use. The assessment should also include laboratory tests if and as needed to identify medical disorders and substance abuse, and the collection of collateral information from the individual's family, friends, and co-workers.

Treatment of schizophreniform disorder requires flexibility, especially because of the frequent change in diagnosis to that of schizophrenia if symptoms persist beyond the 6-month limit for duration of the disorder. The treatment of schizophreniform disorder may include medication, involuntary detention, and educational and supportive psychotherapy. Essential goals of treatment are to decrease hallucinations or delusions, stabilize erratic behavior, and decrease destructive behavior. This should be done through appointments of the affected individual with mental-health professionals who can prescribe appropriate medications and provide psychotherapy. Follow-up should be done regularly on the treated individual's adherence to prescribed regimens of medication, and should include discussion of the importance of such adherence, and observation for any changes in behavior on follow-up visits. Referral of the treated individual to care-coordination services should be made if and as indicated to increase adherence to treatment.

Essential goals of treatment of schizophreniform disorder are to decrease hallucinations or delusions, stabilize erratic behavior, and decrease destructive behavior. This should be done through appointments of the affected individual with mental-health professionals who can prescribe appropriate medications and provide psychotherapy. Follow-up should be done regularly on the treated individual's adherence to prescribed regimens of medication, and should include discussion of the importance of such adherence, and observation for any changes in behavior on follow-up visits. Referral of the treated individual to care-coordination services should be made if and as indicated to increase adherence to treatment.

Individuals in whom psychotic symptoms create confusion and distress because of psychotic symptoms should have educational and supportive psychotherapy focused on managing their daily problems, coping with the stress of their illness, and understanding its symptoms and their origins. These individuals' families should also be provided with therapy and psychoeducation as needed, and with contact information for the local office of the National Alliance on Mental Illness (NAMI) or similar support groups for additional support.

Social workers should be aware of their own cultural values, beliefs, and biases and develop specialized knowledge about the histories, traditions, and values of their clients. Social workers should adopt treatment methodologies that reflect their knowledge of the cultural diversity of the communities in which they practice.

SERVICES AND RESOURCES

The following resources can provide information about schizophreniform disorder or schizophrenia. Enter "schizophreniform disorder" or "schizophrenia" in the search box to access relevant information available on each website.

- Brain and Behavior Research Foundation (formerly NARSAD), http://bbrfoundation.org/
- National Alliance on Mental Illness (NAMI), http://www.nami.org/
- U.S. National Institutes of Health (NIH), http://www.nih.gov/
- U.S. National Institute of Mental Health (NIMH), http://www.nimh.nih.gov/index.shtml/
- National Association of Social Workers (NASW), http://www.socialworkers.org/

Written by Chris Bates, MA, MSW

Reviewed by Lynn B. Cooper, D. Crim, and Pedram Samghabadi

REFERENCES

American Psychiatric Association. (2013). Diagnostic and statistical manual of mental health disorders (DSM-5). (5th ed.). Arlington, VA: American Psychiatric Publishing.

British Association of Social Workers. (2012). The code of ethics for social work: Statement of principles. Retrieved October 21, 2015, from http://cdn.basw.co.uk/upload/basw_112315-7.pdf

Crespo-Facorro, B., Roiz-Santianez, R., Perez-Iglesias, R., Tordesillas-Gutierrez, D., Mata, I., Rodriguez-Sanchez, J. M., & Vazquez-Barquero, J. L. (2009). Specific brain structural abnormalities in first-episode schizophrenia. A comparative study with patients with schizophreniform disorder, non-schizophrenic non-affective psychoses, and healthy volunteers. *Schizophrenia Research, 115*(1), 191-201. doi:10.1016/j.schres.2009.09.007

Fochtmann, L. J., Mojtabai, R., & Bromet, R. J. (2009). Other psychotic disorders. In B. J. Sadock, V. A. Sadock, & P. Ruiz (Eds.), *Kaplan & Sadocks's comprehensive textbook of psychiatry* (9th ed., Vol. 1, pp. 1605-1628). Philadelphia, PA: Wolters Kluwer Health/Lippincott Williams & Wilkins.

International Federation of Social Workers. (2012). Statement of ethical principles. Retrieved October 21, 2015, from http://ifsw.org/policies/statement-of-ethical-principles

Kahn, R. S., Fleischhacker, W. W., Boter, H., Davidson, M., Vergouwe, Y., Keet, I. P., & Grobbee, D. E. (2008). Effectiveness of antipsychotic drugs in first-episode schizophrenia and schizophreniform disorder: An open randomised clinical trial. *Lancet, 371*(9618), 1085-1097. doi:10.1016/S0140-6736(08)60486-9

Mizrahi, T., & Mayden, R. W. (2001). NASW standards for cultural competency in social work practice. Retrieved October 21, 2015, from http://www.socialworkers.org/practice/standards/NASWCulturalStandards.pdf

Sadock, B. J., Sadock, V. A., & Ruiz, P. (2015). Schizophrenia spectrum and other psychotic disorders. In *Kaplan and Sadock's synopsis of psychiatry: Behavioral sciences/clinical psychiatry* (11th ed., pp. 327-329). Philadelphia, PA: Wolters Kluwer.

Takeuchi, J. (2000). Treatment of a biracial child with schizophreniform disorder: Cultural formulation. *Cultural Diversity & Ethnic Minority Psychology, 6*(1), 93-101. doi:10.1037/1099-9809.6.1.93

SCHIZOTYPAL PERSONALITY DISORDER

MAJOR CATEGORIES: Behavioral & Mental Health

DESCRIPTION

Schizotypal personality disorder (SPD) is one of 10 diagnosable personality disorders that appear in the *Diagnostic and Statistical Manual of Mental Disorders,* Fifth Edition (*DSM-5*); it is grouped with paranoid personality disorder and schizoid personality disorder to form the Cluster A personality disorders, which share the appearance of eccentricity and oddness. The *DSM-5* general criteria for all 10 personality disorders include significant variation in behavior and internal life experience from one's own cultural norms in at least 2 of the areas of cognition, affectivity, interpersonal functioning, and impulse control; a long-term and consistent history across a variety of life situations apparent since at least adolescence that has caused significant disturbances in functioning in important areas of life and that could be described as an abiding pattern; and the abiding pattern is not caused by another mental health disorder, including substance use disorder(s), impact of medications, or a medical condition.

The specific criteria for SPD are a pattern of perceptual and cognitive disturbances, behaviors outside cultural norms, and significantly decreased ability to form and maintain close personal relationships, including notable uneasiness if they are formed. For an individual to meet the criteria for diagnosis, 5 (or more) of 9 specific behaviors/cognitive habits must be demonstrated: reduced or inappropriate affect, magical thinking, paranoia or suspiciousness, distorted or unusual thinking and speech, behavior or appearance significantly outside cultural norms, absence of friends, extreme discomfort in social situations that remains over time, perceiving things to be about self when they are not, and out-of-the-ordinary perceptions of events. Also, these criteria do not occur only in association with active episodes of schizophrenia, bipolar disorder, depressive disorder with psychotic features, or other psychotic disorders or in conjunction with the autism spectrum. Psychotic symptoms such as delusions and hallucinations may occur, but last only minutes to hours. If psychotic symptoms persist, then another diagnosis such as brief psychotic disorder or schizophreniform disorder may be appropriate. Individuals with SPD may exhibit discomfort or even anxiety when relating to others that may increase rather than decrease during the interaction; feelings and insights of unhappiness because of the social anxiety; beliefs that they can control others with their thinking; speech that is hard to follow and does not make sense, yet also accurately reflects thinking; inattention to social norms of dress and social interaction; beliefs that events unrelated to them are about them; suspiciousness and paranoia; and culturally unusual affect, normally constrained. Many of the signs and symptoms of SPD overlap with the signs and symptoms of schizophrenia.

Personality is generally agreed to refer to the internal organization and evolution of an individual's psychobiological and social inheritance and learning that enable one to live in, and adapt to, a constantly changing world. The five-factor model (FFM) divides and measures personality using five traits: openness to experience, conscientiousness, extraversion, agreeableness, and neuroticism. Each trait is measured using a continuum (for agreeableness, a continuum from friendly/compassionate to cold/unkind). To be considered disordered, the personality created by the sum of these elements must be dysfunctional on both an individual level and a social level, and is usually inflexible and outside of the norms of the individual's culture. Furthermore, individuals with SPD usually lack awareness that there are problems in their personal or social functioning.

Controversy surrounds the personality disorders and is reflected by the inclusion in the *DSM-5* of a chapter entitled "Alternative DSM-5 Model for Personality Disorders" in Section 3, "Emerging Measures and Models." The alternative model was introduced to address shortcomings in the current model, including the fact that many individuals meet the criteria for several personality disorders and that the general categories of "other specified" or "unspecified" are the most often diagnosed and are uninformative. A larger question about the personality disorder diagnosis is its categorical nature (meaning either the criteria are met and there is a disorder/diagnosis, or the criteria are not met and there is no disorder/diagnosis) as opposed to the dimensional nature of actual human behavior and lives (meaning that personality traits occur along a continuum from not present at all to having overwhelming impact). The *DSM-5* personality disorders remain categorical; however, the alternative model introduces the concept of dimensional assessment. Another issue of contention is the theory that personality disorders are actually a point on the continuum of another mental health disorder. In particular, the relationship between SPD and schizophrenia continues to be investigated, with increasing numbers of studies indicating that SPD is at one end of a gradation with severe schizophrenia at other end. Specifically, studies are finding overlaps between the disorders in the areas of genetics, cognition, and neurobiology.

The etiology of SPD is unresolved, with most literature attributing it to an interaction of genetically inherited traits and environmental influences. Research shows that there is likely a genetic predisposition and also shows a strong correlation between childhood trauma and development of SPD. Personality disorders are by definition stable: once established, they usually do not progress, although the individual's socioeconomic and occupational status may decline due to inability to function effectively. The effectiveness of treatment for personality disorders is the subject of debate, with some literature claiming that individuals with personality disorders are unreceptive to treatment and some asserting that the problem with treatment lies with professionals who blame their countertransference and lack of success on the individuals with personality disorders.

FACTS AND FIGURES
Researchers using data from the Wave 2 National Epidemiologic Survey on Alcohol and Related Conditions found a lifetime prevalence of SPD of 3.9 percent (4.2 percent men, 3.7 percent women). African American women; individuals in the three lowest income brackets; and those never married, separated, divorced, or widowed all had statistically significant greater rates of SPD. The rates of SPD among survey participants with mood, anxiety, and substance abuse disorders were 17.2 percent, 13.7 percent, and 8.2 percent, respectively.

RISK FACTORS
Risk factors include having a first-degree relative with schizophrenia or SPD; trauma, neglect, or abuse during childhood; and lower socioeconomic status. In males, environmental factors such as prenatal

exposure to certain diseases such as influenza in the sixth month of pregnancy are also risk factors.

SIGNS AND SYMPTOMS
Physical symptoms include a possible decreased volume of temporal lobe gray matter.

Psychological signs include odd or magical thinking, unusual perceptual experiences that may include bodily illusions, inappropriate affect, suspiciousness or paranoid ideation, or childlike fears and fantasies.

Social/behavioral problems include lack of close friends, extreme social anxiety and notable discomfort in social situations, odd or eccentric appearance or behavior, or being aloof or emotionally distant.

ASSESSMENT
Professionals should obtain a standard bio-psycho-social-spiritual history with attention to cultural norms of behavior, including risk for suicide, observe functioning and demeanor during interview, and collect collateral information from family, friends, and coworkers (especially important because individuals may have limited insight into the oddness of their behaviors).

Care should be used with self-reporting screening tools because of possible lack of insight. The first four tools are not specific to SPD, but are general measures of personality dysfunction. Screening tools include Structured Interview for DSM-IV Personality Disorders (SIDP-IV), Personality Diagnostic Questionnaire-Revised (PDQ-R), Minnesota Multiphasic Personality Inventory (MMPI), Millon Clinical Multiaxial Inventory (MCMI), Five-Factor Schizotypal Inventory (FFSI), and Schizotypal Personality Questionnaire-Brief (SPQ-B).

Tests for the presence of alcohol or other substances necessary to rule out the possibility that symptoms are the result of a substance ingestion rather than SPD may be performed.

TREATMENT
Individuals with SPD most often seek treatment for co-occurring disorders or symptoms of depression and/or anxiety rather than for SPD. Other reasons to seek treatment include application for or maintenance of Social Security Insurance/Social Security Disability or other social service benefits, or as required—for example, by supported mental health housing programs. Unlike those with other personality disorders,

individuals with SPD may have insight into their disorder by virtue of being unhappy about their discomfort in social situations. A commonly repeated myth holds that individuals with personality disorders are untreatable, or that personality disorders are inflexible and cannot be treated. Yet research shows that progress can be made if barriers to treatment are not erected. The three most common barriers are strong and counterproductive feelings of counter transference, belief (and covert communication of that belief to the individual being treated) in the myth of untreatability, and giving direct and specific advice on social functioning or personal problems, which usually produces dependence, noncompliance, or resentment. A first step in treatment of SPD is collaborative goal setting about treatment. There is no consensus on the use of medications in the treatment of SPD, although because other mental health disorders usually are present, medications may be used to treat them.

Professionals may also review the medication regimen and make follow-up appointment with the agency issuing the prescription, assess the stability of the employment and living situation, refer to an appropriate treatment modality, and provide referrals for support and education for family members.

Problem	Goal	Intervention
Depression and/or anxiety in association with dysfunction because of difficulty with social relations.	Decrease depression and/or anxiety to allow for participation in other forms of treatment.	Schedule appointment with mental health professional who can prescribe appropriate medications. Follow up on medication adherence and effectiveness, including discussion with family and caregivers on importance of adhering to prescription dosage and timing.
Dysfunction in social and occupational settings because of inability to read social cues and signals.	Increased ability to read social cues and signals.	Social and behavior skills training and therapy, either individually or in a group setting, focused on reading and responding to social cues and signals in appropriate ways.
Dysfunction in social and occupational settings because of distorted cognition and thought patterns.	Reduction in distorted cognition and thought patterns.	Discover and restructure cognitive dysfunction and thought patterns to better function within cultural norms. Cognitive therapy, either individual or group, aimed at uncovering and changing cognitive distortions.
Limited support system and need for participation of support network in treatment.	Improved support system that participates in treatment.	Family therapy, including educational component. Engage support network, usually family members, in treatment. Educate family about SPD.

APPLICABLE LAWS AND REGULATIONS

Each jurisdiction (nation, state, province) has its own standards, procedures, and laws for involuntary restraint and detention of persons who may be a danger to themselves or others. Individuals with SPD are not generally at higher risk; however, because they frequently have diagnoses of other mental health disorders and some theories hold that SPD is an early stage of schizophrenia, assessment should include these dangers. Local and professional reporting requirements for neglect and abuse should also be understood and observed.

AVAILABLE SERVICES AND RESOURCES

- National Alliance on Mental Illness (NAMI), http://www.nami.org/
- U.S. National Institutes of Health (NIH), http://www.nih.gov/
- U.S. National Institute of Mental Health (NIMH), http://www.nimh.nih.gov/index.shtml

- National Association of Social Workers (NASW), http://www.socialworkers.org/

FOOD FOR THOUGHT

Individuals with SPD frequently have not been prescribed antipsychotic medications, and as a result they are often the subject of studies of brain function and how it relates to disorders on the schizophrenia spectrum. One study focused on the role of the neurotransmitter dopamine in cognitive function in individuals with an exclusive diagnosis of SPD. After 4 weeks of treatment with a medication (pergolide) that acts on brain receptors related to dopamine, the study participants "showed an improved performance on a number of neuropsychological assessments.... in particular, processing speed, executive function/working memory, and verbal learning and memory."

Another study found that gray matter volume in the brain's temporal lobe and measures of spatial-working memory provided "good detection" of SPD.

SPD is frequently co-occurring with other mental health disorders. Researchers found that 13.6 percent of clients meeting criteria for obsessive-compulsive disorder (OCD) also had SPD. This study population also more frequently showed signs and symptoms of bipolar disorder, behavior compulsivity, and more severe depression than those participants with OCD and borderline personality disorder (BPD) or only OCD.

SPD in childhood has been an area of little research even though SPD can be associated with psychosis. The Melbourne Assessment of Schizotypy in Kids (MASK) is a 57-item interview that is semistructured and gathers information from the child, the parents, and the involved clinician. This tool can also distinguish these children from those who are on the autism spectrum.

RED FLAGS

Individuals with SPD have high rates of comorbidity with major depressive disorder, anxiety disorders, and posttraumatic stress disorder (PTSD) as well as traits of other personality disorders, and therefore may require simultaneous treatment for different disorders.

People with SPD may be misdiagnosed over time with attention-deficit/hyperactivity disorder-inattentive type, social anxiety disorder, being on the autism spectrum, or dysthymia.

Care should be exercised not to consider and treat SPD as an automatic precursor to schizophrenia because treatments for the two, particularly medication, differ significantly.

Written by Chris Bates, MA, MSW

Reviewed by Pedram Samghabadi

REFERENCES

American Psychiatric Association. (2013). Diagnostic and Statistical Manual of Mental Disorders DSM-5. In (5th ed., pp. 50-59). Washington, DC: American Psychiatric Publishing.

Berenbaum, H., Thompson, R. J., Milanak, M. E., Boden, M. T., & Bredemeier, K. (2008). Psychological trauma and schizotypal personality disorder. *Journal of Abnormal Psychology, 117*(3), 502-519. doi:10.1037/0021-843X.117.3.502

Cloninger, C. R., & Svrakic, D. R. (2009). Personality disorders. In B. J. Sadock, V. A. Sadock, & P. Ruiz (Eds.), *Kaplan & Sadock's comprehensive textbook of psychiatry* (9th ed., Vol. II, pp. 2197-2240). Philadelphia: Lippincott, Williams & Wilkins.

Edmundson, M., Lynam, D. R., Miller, J. D., Gore, W. L., & Widiger, T. A. (2011). A five-factor measure of schizotypal personality traits. *Assessment, 18*(3), 321-334. doi:10.1177/1073191111408228

Ettinger, U., Meyhofer, I., Steffens, M., Wagner, M., & Koutsouleris, N. (2014). Genetics, cognition, and neurobiology of schizotypal personality: A review of the overlap with schizophrenia. *Frontiers In Psychiatry, 5*(18). doi:10.3389/fpsyt.2014.00018

Hazlett, E. A., Goldstein, K. E., & Kolaitis, J. C. (2012). A review of structural MRI and diffusion tensor imaging in schizotypal personality disorder. *Current Psychiatry Reports, 14*(1), 70-78. doi:10.1007/s11920-011-0241-z

Hazlett, E. A., Lamade, R. V., Graff, F. S., McClure, M. M., Kolaitis, J. C., Goldstein, K. E., ... Moshier, E. (2014). Visual-spatial working memory performance and temporal gray matter volume predict schizotypal personality disorder group membership. *Schizophrenia Research, 152*(2-3), 350-357. doi:10.1016/j.schres.2013.12.006

Lentz, V., Robinson, J., & Bolton, J. M. (2010). Child-hood adversity, mental disorder comorbidity, and suicidal behavior in schizotypal personality disorder. *Journal of Nervous and Mental Disease, 198*(11), 795-801. doi:10.1097/NMD.0b013e3181f9804c

McClure, M. M., Harvey, P. D., GOodman, M., Triebwasser, J., New, A., Koenigsberg, H. W., ... Siever, L. J. (2010). Pergolide treatment of cognitive deficits associated with schizotypal personality disorder: Continued evidence of the importance of the dopamine system in the schizophrenia spectrum. *Neuropsychopharmacology, 35*(6), 1356-1362. doi:10.1038/npp.2010.5

Otruno-Sierra, J., Badoud, D., Knecht, F., Paino, M., Eliez, S., Fonseca-Pedrero, E., ... Debbane, M. (2013). Testing measurement invariance of the schizotypal personality questionnaire-brief scores across Spanish and Swiss adolescents. *Plos One, 8*(12), 1-7. doi:10.1371/journal.pone.0082041

Pulay, A. J., Stinson, F. S., Dawson, D. A., Goldstein, R. B., Chou, S. P., Huang, B., ... Grant, B. F. (2009). Prevalence, correlates, disability, and comorbidity of DSM-IV schizotypal personality disorder:

Results from the Wave 2 National Epidemiologic Survey on Alcohol and Related Conditions. *Primary Care Companion to the Journal of Clinical Psychiatry, 11*(2), 53-67.

Powers, A. D., Thomas, K. M., Ressler, K. J., & Bradley, B. (2011). The differential effects of child abuse and posttraumatic stress disorder on schizotypal personality disorder. *Comprehensive Psychiatry, 52*(4), 438-445. doi:10.1016/j.comppsych.2010.08.001

Silverstein, M. L. (2007). Descriptive psychopathology and theoretical viewpoints: Schizoid, schizotypal, and avoidant personality disorders. In M. L. Silverstein (Ed.), *Disorders of the self: A personality-guided approach* (pp. 61-72). Washington, DC: American Psychological Association.

Silverstein, M. L. (2007). A self psychological viewpoint: Schizoid, schizotypal, and avoidant personality disorders. In M. L. Silverstein (Ed.), *Disorders of the self: A personality-guided approach* (pp. 73-94). Washington, DC: American Psychological Association.

SEX EDUCATION OF BLACK YOUTH: IMPROVING PROGRAM RELEVANCY

MAJOR CATEGORIES: Community

WHAT WE KNOW

It is projected that by 2020 black adolescents will make up approximately 15 percentof adolescents in the United States. No sex education strategy can be effective if it is not specifically relevant to this large segment of the population.

The results of the 2013 Youth Risk Surveillance survey by the Centers for Disease Control and Prevention (CDC) found that black youths have sexual intercourse before age 13 at a greater rate—14 percent (males 24 percent, females 4.9 percent), than Hispanic (6.4 percent: males 9.2 percent, females 3.8 percent) and white (3.3 percent: males 4.4 percent, females 2.1 percent) youths.

The same CDC survey found the overall rate for high school students of ever having sexual intercourse was 60.6 percent for black students (68.4 percent for males, 53.4 percent for females); 49.2 percent for Hispanic students (51.7 percent for males, 46.9 percent for females); and 43.7 percent for white students (42.2 percent for males, 45.3 percent for females).

Sexually transmitted infections (STIs, also referred to as sexually transmitted diseases [STDs]) and HIV/AIDS disproportionately affect black youth.

Black persons have the highest rate of HIV/AIDS in the United States; black youths represent more than half of all new HIV infections among persons ages 13–24.

The rate of new infections among black male youths is 11 times higher than that among white male youths and 4 times higher than among Hispanic male youths.

The rate of new infections among black female youths is 20 times higher than that among white female youths and 6 times higher than among Hispanic female youths.

Black youths are disproportionately poor.

Teenagers in families living below the poverty threshold are more likely to experience racial discrimination, lack of access to healthcare, and incarceration.

How black youths assess the consequences of having unprotected intercourse and make decisions about handling unintended pregnancies is influenced by perceived present and future options for employment, education, social mobility, marriage, safety, and health.

Adolescents make decisions based on perceived available options and on values, beliefs, and attitudes that are based in their cultural, social, and economic circumstances. Research and observation have documented the following characteristics of black clients related to sexual education and reproductive health:

Many black men learn to measure their masculinity by their level of risk-taking; their drive for money, power, and sex; and their non-submission to all behaviors perceived to be female.

Black males are more likely than other males to try to prove their masculinity by engaging in risky sexual encounters, such as having many sexual partners or fathering children.

Black clients exhibit a greater tolerance for sexual intercourse outside of marriage and rate the state of marriage as less important than do members of other groups. They may tolerate and show less disapproval for births taking place before marriage or outside of marriage.

Black clients are more likely than clients of other racial or ethnic minority groups to think that birth control is less effective than it actually is and to believe that it may be dangerous.

When youths engage with their communities in new ways, forming relationships with mentors and valuing their ability to contribute to society, they choose to take greater measures to prevent pregnancy.

Sex education is provided most often to young persons in school settings. It usually covers information on sex and sexuality, abstinence, STIs, HIV/AIDS, contraception, reproduction, and safer sex practices. Because the federal government has allocated a significant amount of funding to education that promotes abstinence until marriage, school-based sex education focuses primarily on abstinence.

In a 2013 study that interviewed black youths in focus groups, the youths stated they desired a more comprehensive sex education curriculum which would include information beyond abstinence. To find out more about sex they looked beyond school sex education to support networks such as peers, family members, and healthcare providers.

They wanted to learn more about less risky sexual behavior, emotional aspects of sexuality, and practicalities of condom use.

Another study reported that black youths utilize a broad range of persons in their sexual education process. Some of these social networks include siblings, extended family, peers, parents of friends, and romantic partners.

The black youths reported that they use these social networks to learn about family values, facts about sex and sexuality, and the social aspects of sexuality (e.g., appropriate dating behavior).

Members of these networks play several functional roles: teacher, guide, challenger, confidant, chaperone, role model, and provider of access to reproductive services.

A study of black females supported the use of educational interventions which involve trusted adults from the community to help young women make contraceptive decisions.

Girls have reported that they would like to be able to discuss sexual health with peers and trained facilitators in an all-female environment.

Involving parents of black youths in sexual education interventions can delay the age of first intercourse and promote lower-risk sexual behavior.

Research states that black youths are more receptive to and trusting of information about sex that is presented to them in a church setting, since faith communities are important community resources for black youth. Some congregations, however, believe that providing sexual education in the church contradicts some of their faith values.

WHAT CAN BE DONE

Develop an awareness of our own cultural values, beliefs, and biases and develop knowledge about the histories, traditions, and values of our clients. Adopt treatment methodologies that reflect the cultural needs of the client.

Become knowledgeable about sexual education of black youths in the United States; share this knowledge with your colleagues.

Conduct focus groups with black youth to identify their specific needs regarding sexual education.

Develop relevant programs for black youth that educate them about abstinence as well as offer strategies for reducing risks associated with sexual activity.

In order for sexuality education, pregnancy prevention, and HIV/AIDS programs to be effective they must be culturally relevant, which includes acknowledging and meeting the needs specific to black youth. These include the following areas, which need to be presented in a manner that reflects cultural competence:

- Contraceptive education.
- STI and HIV risk education.
- Opportunities for open and honest discussions.
- Exploration of attitudes, beliefs, and values.
- Challenging teens' ambivalent notions about themselves and their present and future options.
- Abstinence.
- Target elementary-school-aged and middle-school-aged children with messages about the importance of staying in school and completing their education
- Include the family to increase the possibilities for developing:
- Self-esteem.
- Interpersonal and communication skills.
- Education, employment, career, and child-bearing options.
  To ensure quality of care, social workers should:
- Provide sex/contraceptive education.
- Provide referrals to health services.
- Provide access to community supports.
- Consistently monitor clients' progress.

Written by Tricia Peneku, MS, PPS

Reviewed by Jessica Therivel, LMSW-IPR, and Melissa Rosales Neff, MSW

REFERENCES

Centers for Disease Control and Prevention. (2011). HIV among youth. Atlanta, GA: Centers for Disease Control and Prevention.

Centers for Disease Control and Prevention. (2013). Youth risk behavior surveillance - United States, 2013. *Morbidity and Mortality Weekly Report, 63*(4), 24-30.

Centers for Disease Control and Prevention. (2014). *HIV among African American youth.* Atlanta, GA: Centers for Disease Control and Prevention.

Fact Sheet on Demographics: Adolescents. (2003). *National Adolescent Health Information Center.* San Francisco, CA: Author, University of California, San Francisco.

George, A., Abatemarco, D., Terry, M., Yonas, M., Butler, J., & Akers, A. (2013). A qualitative exploration of the role of social networks in educating urban African American adolescents about sex.

Ethnicity & Health, 18(2), 168-189. doi:10.1080/13557858.2012.708915

Hodgson, E., Collier, C., Hayes, L., Curry, L. A., & Fraenkel, L. (2013). Family planning and contraceptive decision-making by economically disadvantaged, African-American women. *Contraception, 88*(2), 289-296. doi:10.1016/j.contraception.2012.10.011

Kimmel, A., Williams, T. T., Veinot, T. C., Campbell, B., Campbell, T. R., Valacak, M., & Kruger, D. J. (2013). "I make sure I am safe and I make sure I have myself every way possible": African-American youth perspectives on sexuality education. *Sex Education, 13*(2), 172-185.

Lightfoot, A. F., Taggart, T., Woods-Jaeger, B. A., Riggins, L., Jackson, M., & Eug, E. (2014). Where is the faith? Using a CBPR approach to propose adaptations to an evidence-based HIV prevention intervention for adolescents in African American faith settings. *Journal of Religion & Health, 53*(4), 1223-1235. doi:10.1007/s10943-014-9846-y

Mizrahi, T., & Mayden, R. W. (2001). NASW standards for cultural competence in social work practice. Retrieved March 3, 2016, from http://www.socialworkers.org/practice/standards/NASWCulturalStandards.pdf

Morrison-Beedy, D., Passmore, D., & Carey, M. (2013). Exit interviews from adolescent girls who participated in a sexual risk reduction intervention: Implications for community-based health education promotion for adolescents. *Journal of Midwifery & Women's Health, 58*(3), 313-320. doi:10.1111/jmwh.12043

Pittman, K. J., Wilson, P. M., Adams-Taylor, S., & Randolph, S. (1992). Making sexuality education and prevention programs relevant for African-American youth. *Journal of School Health, 62*(7), 339-44. doi:10.1111/j.1746-1561.1992.tb01253.x

The Policy, Ethics, and Human Rights Committee, British Association of Social Workers. (2012, January). The code of ethics for social work: Statement of principles. Retrieved March 3, 2016, from http://cdn.basw.co.uk/upload/basw_112315-7.pdf

Sisson, G. (2012). Finding a way to offer something more: Reframing teen pregnancy prevention. *Sexuality Research & Social Policy, 9*(1), 57-69. doi:10.1007/s13178-011-0050-5

Statement of Ethical Principles. (2012, March 3). *International Federation of Social Workers.* Retrieved

March 3, 2016, from http://ifsw.org/policies/statement-of-ethical-principles/

Weekes, C. V., Haas, B. K., & Gosselin, K. P. (2014). Expectations and self-efficacy of African American parents who discuss sexuality with their adolescent sons: An intervention study. *Public Health Nursing,* *31*(3), 253-261. doi:10.1111/phn.12084

SEXUAL ASSAULT IN PRISON: VICTIMS—ASSESSMENT & INTERVENTION

MAJOR CATEGORIES: Incarceration/Probation, Violence

WHAT WE KNOW

Sexual assault typically is defined as any type of sexual activity that is non-consensual (including when the victim is unable to provide consent), whether physical, verbal, visual (e.g., being forced to view pornographic images), or any other type of unwanted sexual contact or attention.

Examples include the following:

- rape within marriage or dating relationships;
- rape by acquaintances or strangers, gang rape (i.e., rape involving two or more perpetrators);
- systematic rape (common during armed conflicts);
- unwanted sexual advances;
- inappropriate touching;
- voyeurism (i.e., when someone watches private sexual acts);
- exhibitionism (i.e., when someone exposes him/herself in public);
- incest (i.e., sexual contact between family members); and
- sexual harassment.

Ascertaining the prevalence of sexual assault within the U.S. prison system is extremely difficult. Incidents of sexual assault in prisons often are undetected and unreported. Male victims report less often than female victims.

Studies indicate that approximately 4.5 percent of male and female inmates (in both federal and state institutions) report that they were sexually victimized in the previous 12 months. In actuality, however, this number is assumed to be greater because of underreporting.

According to one study the three most commonly given reasons for underreporting of sexual assault in prison are embarrassment, fear of harassment, and fear of retaliation by other inmates.

Possible psychosocial and physical effects of sexual assault in prison include feelings of fear of a subsequent sexual assault and post-traumatic stress disorder (PTSD).

In one study 44.9 percent of inmates who had been sexually assaulted in prison reported being highly distressed after the assault. They began to distrust others and became nervous and fearful in group situations.

Sexually transmitted diseases (STDs) such as human immunodeficiency virus (HIV), hepatitis B, chlamydia, genital warts, herpes, syphilis, and rectal and pharyngeal gonorrhea.

Male victims of assault who identify as heterosexual may wonder if they are homosexual if they experience an erection during a sexual assault. Homosexual males may feel as if the crime committed against them is a punishment for their sexual orientation.

In a study of inmate-on-inmate sexual assault, 53.1 percent of victims reported feeling depressed after the sexual assault. Suicide is reported as the second leading cause of death in prison (following illness/natural causes). Research indicates that inmate rape, along with overcrowding and brutality on the part of other prisoners and staff, strongly contributes to inmate suicide.

The Prison Rape Elimination Act (PREA) was enacted in 2003 to establish a zero-tolerance standard of incidence for prisoner rape in the United States and to develop national standards for prevention of, reduction of, and punishment for prisoner rape.

The American Bar Association's standards on the treatment of prisoners require that every prisoner who is a victim of sexual assault should have medical treatment, STD testing, and psychological counseling immediately available.

Correctional officials should ensure that confidentiality is upheld: only those persons who are involved in the prisoner's immediate care should know about the incident (e.g., healthcare staff, therapist, law enforcement).

When a prisoner has been sexually assaulted, he or she should be assessed in a four-phase process.

Immediately upon disclosure of an assault. The victim should be assessed immediately for any life-threatening injuries. Attention should be given to any bleeding, head trauma, gagging, anal or vaginal tears or fissures, or suicidality.

Within 72 hours of an assault. Whether in a prison medical facility or a hospital emergency room, a sexual assault examination (SAE) should be completed. The goals of the sexual assault exam are treatment of injuries, prophylactic treatment to prevent pregnancy and infection, crisis intervention, safety planning, and evidence collection

Evidence collection is time sensitive: it must take place no more than 72-96 hours after an assault because of the potential loss of forensic evidence (e.g., pubic hair, bodily fluids, bruising, lacerations). The sexual assault examination is performed by a sexual assault forensic examiner (SAFE) and/or a sexual assault nurse examiner (SANE). Pregnancy tests as well as tests for sexually transmitted diseases are administered as part of the exam.

A mental health assessment is completed. Suicide risk is carefully assessed. If medically necessary, the victim may be admitted into the prison medical facility or local hospital.

Short-term intervention. The victim should receive follow-up medical care as needed (e.g., medications, changes of dressings for any wounds received during the assault).

The victim should be given the results of pregnancy and STD tests. Tests for STDs should be readministered 2 months and 4 months after the assault. Supportive counseling and education about STDs and HIV should be offered if applicable. The victim should have access to a mental health professional on prison grounds. Prisons should have a mental health professional on staff or arrange for a mental health professional to come to the prison on a regular basis to visit and treat the victim.

Long-term intervention. STD/HIV tests should be administered 6 months after the assault and up to 18 months after the assault, in addition to the 2- and 4-month retesting. The victim should continue to see a mental health professional to address any symptoms of PTSD, questions of sexual identity, or coping skills responses. Follow-up referrals should be made for all inmates who have been sexually assaulted during their time in prison upon release to the community.

Each prison has its own protocol for addressing the medical needs of victims of sexual assault. Large jails and state prisons tend to have well-equipped and staffed medical facilities which are capable of responding to a sexual assault emergency. Small prisons or jails usually are not equipped with medical staff. Therefore the victim will need to be transported to a local hospital emergency room.

Transporting a prisoner who is a victim of sexual assault from prison to a local hospital calls for strict security measures because of the high incidence of inmates attempting or completing escapes from hospitals.

WHAT CAN BE DONE

Learn about sexual assault in prison and appropriate assessment and intervention strategies; share this information with your colleagues.

Use your knowledge to accurately assess your client's individual characteristics and health education needs.

Develop an awareness of your own cultural values, beliefs, and biases and develop knowledge about the histories, traditions, and values of your clients. Adopt treatment methodologies that reflect the cultural needs of the client.

Work in collaboration with prison staff (e.g., administrators, guards). Advocate for all staff to receive PREA training and to understand the zero-tolerance policy toward sexual assault.

Ensure that all inmates who have experienced sexual victimization have access to the specialized services they may need.

If in a clinical setting, use treatment interventions (e.g., cognitive behavioral therapy) to address PTSD, depression, or any other mental health issues resulting from sexual assault. Teach relaxation and meditation methods as well as coping skills. Carefully inquire about and assess for suicidal ideation on a regular basis.

Tailor interventions specifically to inmates. For example, an individual in the community who is a victim of sexual assault can employ methods of coping such as going for a run, having dinner with a friend, and participating in a hobby. Inmates who are victims of sexual assault do not have these options. Work with prisoner victims on journaling, guided imagery, or breathing techniques as possible ways to cope.

If the victim is transferred from one prison to another, try to continue treatment with victim if at all possible. Continuity of care is important for sexual assault victims.

Explain importance of being tested for HIV and other STDs at 2, 4, and 6 months after an assault. Ensure that inmate has access to continued medical attention in prison.

If following up with inmate in person is not possible, be creative and flexible. Communicate through letters sent via confidential legal mail, for example. Use simple and clear language.

Provide a written list of community resources for sexual assault victims upon the inmate's release from prison.

Written by Melissa Rosales Neff, MSW

Reviewed by Laura Gale, LCSW

REFERENCES

International Federation of Social Workers. (2012, March). Statement of ethical principles. Retrieved January 15, 2015, from http://ifsw.org/policies/statement-of-ethical-principles/

Wheeler, D. (2015). *NASW standards for cultural competency in social work practice.* Retrieved March 3, 2015, from http://www.socialworkers.org/practice/standards/PRA-BRO-253150-CC-Standards.pdf

British Association of Social Workers. (2012, January). The code of ethics for social work: Statement of principles. Retrieved October 11, 2015, from http://cdn.basw.co.uk/upload/basw_112315-7.pdf

American Bar Association. (2013). Standards of treatment of prisoners. Retrieved from http://www.americanbar.org/publications/criminal_justice_section_archive/crimjust_standards_treatment-prisoners.html#23-5.3

California Coalition Against Sexual Assault. (2010). Survivors behind bars: Supporting survivors of prison rape and sexual assault. Retrieved from http://www.prearesourcecenter.org/sites/default/files/library/survivors-behind-bars.pdf

Department of Justice. (2008). Report on rape in jails in the U.S. : Findings and best practices. Retrieved from http://ojp.gov/reviewpanel/pdfs/prea_finalreport_081229.pdf

Dumond, R. W. (2001, October). The impact and recovery of prisoner rape. Paper presented at the conference "Not Part of the Penalty": Ending Prisoner Rape, Washington, D.C.

Dumond, R. W., & Dumond, D. A. (2002). The treatment of sexual assault victims. C. Hensley (Ed.), *Prison sex: Practice and policy.* Boulder, CO: Lynne Rienner Publishers.

Just Detention International. (2010). Hope behind bars: An advocate's guide to helping survivors of sexual abuse in detention. Retrieved from http://www.justdetention.org/en/SART-Toolkit/Advocates_Manual_FINAL.pdf

Miller, K. L. (2010). The darkest figure of crime: Perceptions of reasons for male inmates to not report sexual assault. *Justice Quarterly, 27*(5), 692-712. doi:10.1080/07418820903292284

Office on Women's Health, U.S. Department of Health and Human Services. (2009). Sexual assault: Frequently asked questions. Retrieved October 11, 2015, from https://www.womenshealth.gov/publications/our-publications/fact-sheet/sexual-assault.html

Office on Violence Against Women. (2013). Recommendations for administrators of prisons, jails, and community confinement facilities for adapting the U.S. Department of Justice's. *A national protocol for sexual assault medical forensic examinations, adults/adolescents.* Retrieved from http://www.ovw.usdoj.gov/docs/confinement-safe-protocol.pdf

Prison Rape Elimination Act of 2003, 108 U.S.C § 79. (2003).

Schneider, K., Richters, J., Butler, T., Yap, L., Richards, A., Grant, L.,... Donovan, B. (2011). Psychological distress and experience of sexual and physical assault among Australian prisoners. *Criminal Behavior and Mental Health, 21*(5), 333-349. doi:10.1002/cbm.816

Wolff, N., & Shi, J. (2009). Contextualization of physical and sexual assault in male prisons: Incidents and their aftermath. *Journal of Correctional Health Care, 15*(1), 58-77. doi:10.1177/1078345808326622

World Health Organization (WHO). (2012). Understanding and addressing violence against women: Sexual violence. Retrieved from http://apps.who.int/iris/bitstream/10665/77434/1/WHO_RHR_12.37_eng.pdf?ua=1

SEXUAL ASSAULT IN PRISON: VICTIMS—PSYCHOSOCIAL EFFECTS

MAJOR CATEGORIES: Incarceration/Probation, Violence

WHAT WE KNOW

Sexual assault typically is defined as any type of sexual activity that is non-consensual (including when the victim is unable to provide consent), whether physical, verbal, visual (e.g., being forced to look at pornographic images), or any other type of unwanted sexual contact or attention.

Examples include the following:

- rape within marriage or dating relationships;
- rape by acquaintances or strangers, gang rape (i.e., rape involving two or more perpetrators);
- systematic rape (common during armed conflicts);
- unwanted sexual advances;
- inappropriate touching;
- voyeurism (i.e., when someone watches private sexual acts);
- exhibitionism (i.e., when someone exposes him/herself in public);
- incest (i.e., sexual contact between family members); and
- sexual harassment.

Ascertaining the prevalence of sexual assault within the U.S. prison system is extremely difficult. Incidents of sexual assault in prisons often are undetected and unreported.

Research studies have reported that approximately 4.5 percent of male and female inmates (in both federal and state institutions) have stated that they were sexually victimized in the previous 12 months. However, it is assumed that this number actually is greater because of underreporting.

The author of a study stated that the three most likely reasons for underreporting of sexual assault in prison are embarrassment, fear of harassment, and fear of retaliation by other inmates.

In a study of 6,964 male inmates, 201 (3 percent) reported that they had been victims of assault by another inmate that involved attempted, coerced, or physically forced anal or oral sex.

In a study of 1,788 male inmates in seven Midwestern prisons, 21 percent reported that they had been sexually targeted or assaulted during their time in prison.

In a study of 174 male inmates, 14 percent reported that they had been sexually assaulted by another inmate during their time in prison.

In a study of 142 male inmates, 8.5 percent reported that they had been sexually assaulted by another inmate during their time in prison.

Investigators who conducted a study on psychological distress among inmates in Australia reported that it is difficult to distinguish between psychological distress stemming from traumatic life events that occurred before individuals entered prison (specifically, abuse in childhood or as an adult) versus that resulting from traumatic events occurring after entering prison.

Because of underreporting, little is known about prison sexual assaults. However, based on incidents that have been reported it is known that

- white inmates are targets of sexual assault in prison more often than inmates of other races;
- men and women who are young (under age 24) and physically attractive are more likely to be targets of sexual assault in prison;
- male and female inmates older than age 25 rarely are sexually assaulted;
- inmates with mental disorders prior to entering prison are more likely to be targets of sexual assault;
- inmates who identified as other than heterosexual reported higher rates of sexual assault than their heterosexual counterparts;
- transgender inmates are at an especially high risk of being sexually assaulted in prison; and
- inmate-on-inmate sexual assault is most likely to occur between 6 p.m. and midnight, and in inmate cells and bathrooms.

Possible psychosocial and physical effects of sexual assault in prison include

Feelings of fear and/or anxiety. (In a study 44.9 percent of inmates who had been sexually assaulted in prison reported being highly distressed after the assault. They began to distrust others and became nervous and fearful in social situations. Results of a study in Australia indicated that the Kessler Psychological Distress Scale was an effective screening tool with the

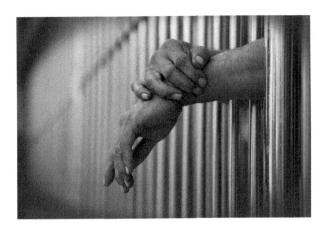

prisoner population to identify inmates in need of treatment and care. Victim inmates may live in daily fear of a subsequent sexual assault. Others may feel helpless and fearful as they experience repetitive assaults from a particular inmate.

Sexually transmitted diseases. Inmates tend to have higher-risk lifestyles and behaviors before prison and therefore higher rates of sexually transmitted diseases. Because of this, sexual assault in prison often results in the spread of sexually transmitted diseases. Inmate victims are at risk of acquiring human immunodeficiency virus (HIV), hepatitis B, chlamydia, genital warts, herpes, syphilis, and rectal and pharyngeal gonorrhea.

Post-traumatic stress disorder (PTSD). PTSD is a mental health disorder that can occur following the experience of a traumatic event (e.g., natural disaster, combat, sexual assault). A victim of sexual assault who experiences PTSD has feelings of anxiety, stress, and fear that last for more than a month. The victim continually relives the sexual assault in his or her mind. He or she may avoid places or events that remind him or her of the assault, which is more difficult to do when incarcerated. He or she also may experience hyperarousal, which is characterized by being easily startled and having angry outbursts.

The most effective treatments for PTSD are cognitive-behavioral therapy (CBT), which helps the individual identify unhealthy beliefs and behaviors and replace them with positive ones, and eye movement desensitization and reprocessing (EMDR), which is guided eye movement that helps process traumatic memories. Psychotherapy also is used to treat PTSD. These treatments help with symptom reduction.

Rape trauma syndrome (RTS). RTS is a medical term for the response of survivors to rape. The symptoms of RTS and PTSD often overlap. RTS indentifies three phases of response to rape: acute, adjustment, and resolution.

It is important to note that most, but not all, rape victims experience these effects in this predictable pattern.

Acute phase: this phase occurs within days or weeks of the sexual assault and may consist of open emotions (crying spells, anxiety attacks, hysteria), closed emotions (calmness, behaving as if nothing happened), and/or shocked disbelief (victim becomes disoriented and is unable to do daily tasks or recall the assault accurately).

Outward adjustment phase: in this phase the victim resumes normal day to day activities and may appear outwardly to have recovered from the trauma, but is simultaneously experiencing inner turmoil (e.g., analyzing the assault to determine if it was his or her fault, using escape mechanisms, experiencing depression, rage, fear).

Resolution phase: During this phase the victim no longer views the assault as being the center of his or her life.

Sexual confusion: Inmate victims may experience confusion regarding their sexual identity after an assault. Heterosexual male victims of assault may wonder if they are gay if they experienced an erection during the rape. Homosexual males may feel as if the crime committed against them is a punishment for their sexual orientation.

Depression and suicidal tendencies: In a study of inmate-on-inmate sexual assault, 53.1 percent of victims reported feeling depressed after the sexual assault. Suicide is reported as the second leading cause of death in prison (following illness/natural causes). Results of studies indicate that inmate rape, along with overcrowding and brutality on the part of other prisoners and staff, strongly contributes to inmate suicide.

Sleep disturbances: In a study of inmate-on-inmate sexual assault, 49 percent of sexual assault victims reported difficulty sleeping and nightmares.

WHAT CAN BE DONE

Learn about prison sexual assault, including its psychosocial effects; share this information with your colleagues.

Use this knowledge to accurately assess your client's individual characteristics, mental health needs, and health education needs.

Develop an awareness of your own cultural values, beliefs, and biases and develop knowledge about the histories, traditions, and values of your clients. Adopt treatment methodologies that reflect the cultural needs of the client.

If in a clinical setting, use treatment interventions (CBT, EMDR, psychotherapy) to address PTSD, depression, or any other mental health issues resulting from assault. Teach relaxation and meditation methods as well as coping skills. If not in a clinical setting, make referrals as needed.

If in clinical setting, carefully inquire about and assess for suicidal ideation on a regular basis with victim inmate.

Explain importance of being tested for HIV and other STDs at 2, 4, and 6 months after the assault. Ensure that inmate has access to medical attention in prison.

Written by Melissa Rosales Neff, MSW

Reviewed by Jessica Therivel, LMSW-IPR

REFERENCES

Drummond, R. W. (2001). The impact and recovery of prisoner rape. A paper presented at the National Conference "Not Part of the Penalty": Ending Prisoner Rape, Washington DC October 19, 2001.

Felson, R. B., Cundiff, P., & Painter-Davis, N. (2012). Age and sexual assault in correctional facilities: A blocked opportunity approach. *Criminology, 50*(4), 887-911.

Hensley, C., Koscheski, M., & Tewksbury, R. (2005). Examining the characteristics of male sexual assault targets in a Southern maximum-security prison. *Journal of Interpersonal Violence, 20*(6), 667-679.

Hensley, C., Tewksbury, R., & Castle, T. (2003). Characteristics of prison sexual assault targets in male Oklahoma correctional facilities. *Journal of Interpersonal Violence, 18*(6), 595-606. doi:10.1177/0886260503251132

International Federation of Social Workers. (2012, March 3). Statement of Ethical Principles. Retrieved May 21, 2014, from http://ifsw.org/policies/statement-of-ethical-principles/

Mair, J. S., Frattaroli, S., & Teret, S. P. (2003). New hope for victims of prison sexual assault. *Journal of Law, Medicine & Ethics, 31*(4), 602-606.

Miller, K. L. (2010). The darkest figure of crime: Perceptions of reasons for male inmates to not report sexual assault. *Justice Quarterly, 27*(5), 692-712. doi:10.1080/07418820903292284

Mizrahi, T., & Mayden, R. W. (2001). NASW standards for cultural competence in social work practice. Retrieved from http://www.socialworkers.org/practice/standards/NASWCulturalStandards.pdf

Rape, Abuse, and Incest National Network (RAINN). (2014). Rape trauma syndrome. Retrieved May 21, 2014, from https://ohl.rainn.org/online/resources/how-long-to-recover.cfm

Office on Women's Health. (2012, July 16). Sexual assault: Frequently asked questions. Retrieved May 21, 2014, from https://www.womenshealth.gov/publications/our-publications/fact-sheet/sexual-assault.html

Schneider, K., Richters, J., Butler, T., Yap, L., Richards, A., Grant, L.,... Donovan, B. (2011). Psychological distress and experience of sexual and physical assault among Australian prisoners. *Criminal Behavior and Mental Health, 21*(5), 333-349. doi:10.1002/cbm.816

Struckman-Johnson, C., & Struckman-Johnson, D. (2000). Sexual coercion rates in seven mid-western prison facilities for men. *The Prison Journal, 80*, 368-378.

The Policy, Ethics, and Human Rights Committee, British Association of Social Workers. (2012, January). The Code of Ethics for Social Work: Statement of principles. Retrieved May 21, 2014, from http://cdn.basw.co.uk/upload/basw_112315-7.pdf

Wolff, N., & Shi, J. (2009). Contextualization of physical and sexual assault in male prisons: Incidents and their aftermath. *Journal of Correctional Health Care, 15*(1), 58-77. doi:10.1177/1078345808326622

World Health Organization (WHO). (2002). World report on violence and health: Sexual violence. Retrieved October 11, 2015, from http://www.who.int/violence_injury_prevention/violence/global_campaign/en/chap6.pdf?ua=1

World Health Organization (WHO). (2012). Understanding and addressing violence against women: Sexual violence. Retrieved from http://apps.who.int/iris/bitstream/10665/77434/1/WHO_RHR_12.37_eng.pdf?ua=1

SEXUAL ASSAULT: ADULT FEMALE VICTIMS—AFTERCARE

MAJOR CATEGORIES: Violence

WHAT WE KNOW

Sexual assault is any type of sexual activity that is non-consensual (including when one is unable to provide consent), including physical, verbal, visual (e.g., being forced to view pornography), or any other type of unwanted sexual contact or attention. Sexual assault includes inappropriate touching, voyeurism (i.e., when someone watches private sexual acts), exhibitionism (i.e., when someone exposes him/herself in public), incest (i.e., sexual contact between family members), unwanted sexual advances (i.e., unwelcome sexual gestures, requests for sexual favors), and rape (i.e., nonconsensual vaginal, anal, or oral penetration).Sexual assault includes acts perpetrated within marriage or dating relationships, acts perpetrated by acquaintances or strangers, gang rape (i.e., rape involving two or more perpetrators), and systematic rape (i.e., mass rapes that occur during armed conflicts).

Sexual assault is both a criminal and a public health problem.

Lifetime prevalence rates of sexual assault vary from country to country, ranging from 4.2 percent in Singapore to 38.9 percent in Mexico. Approximately 1 in 5 women in Australia, the United States, and the United Kingdom experience sexual assault at some point in their lives.

A 2012 study by the U.S. Centers for Disease Control and Prevention (CDC) on sexual assault in the United States reported that.

1 in 5 women reported experiencing rape at some time in their lives

1 in 20 women experienced sexual violence other than rape (such as sexual coercion or unwanted sexual contact)

37.4 percent of female rape victims were first raped between ages 18 and 24

The majority of sexual assault victims know their attacker. In a United States study that investigated subtypes of sexual assault, researchers found that:.

27 percent of high-violence assaults, 18 percent of alcohol-related assaults, and 46 percent of moderate-severity assaults were committed by intimate partners

33 percent of high-violence assaults, 55 percent of alcohol-related assaults, and 32 percent of moderate-severity assaults were committed by acquaintances

19 percent of high-violence assaults, 15 percent of alcohol-related assaults, and 4 percent of moderate-severity assaults were committed by strangers

Women's decisions to report and/or seek care after a sexual assault are influenced by a variety of personal and environmental factors.

Personal factors include emotional states (i.e., shame, embarrassment, humiliation, and self-blame); fear of negative consequences of reporting (i.e., not being believed, retaliation, lack of confidentiality, poor treatment by law enforcement, public exposure, stigma, and unfair treatment); being assaulted by someone known to the victim (i.e., intimate partner, family member, acquaintance); and lack of knowledge (i.e., not knowing what services are available and how they are paid for).

Investigators in a 2014 study also found that posttraumatic stress disorder (PTSD) symptomatology was linked with likelihood of reporting sexual assault; re-experiencing and hyperarousal symptoms were associated with increased likelihood of reporting whereas avoidance symptoms were associated with decreased likelihood of reporting an assault.

Environmental factors include organizational and structural barriers (i.e., limited services, services that are difficult to access, inadequate funding, staff who are inexperienced or uncomfortable with sexual assault cases) and societal myths (i.e., biases based on race, gender, and sexual orientation, doubts about the authenticity of sexual assault).

The effects of sexual assault on women are well documented in research, including:.

physical effects: pregnancy, chronic pelvic pain, migraines, gynecological complications, pain;

psychological effects: shock, denial, fear, guilt, depression, PTSD, sleep disturbances, attempted suicide;

social effects: strained relationships with family members and friends, decreased contact with family members and friends, lower likelihood of marriage; and

health effects: engaging in high-risk behaviors (e.g., unprotected sex, trading sex for food or money), substance use, unhealthy diet-related behaviors (e.g., overeating, abusing diet pills, fasting, self-induced vomiting).

The impacts of sexual assault vary among survivors based in part on factors such as preexisting personality characteristics, history of childhood sexual abuse, and characteristics of the assault.

In a United States study, researchers found that women who experienced severe, forceful assault experienced higher levels of trauma symptoms, depression, and anxiety than women who experienced contact assault or attempted rape, or women who were incapacitated by intoxication rather than by violence.

Researchers in a longitudinal study in the United States found that women who experienced severe violence or alcohol-related assaults had more PTSD symptoms than those who experienced moderately severe assault. Victims who experienced severe violence initially had the highest level of PTSD symptoms, but victims of alcohol-related assaults experienced an increase in PTSD symptoms over time, which was attributed in part to self-blame and negative social reactions.

Certain risk factors may predispose women to react to sexual assault in specific ways; for instance, women who tend to act more impulsively when distressed have been found to have higher levels of externalizing dysfunction (e.g., increased alcohol and/or drug use) following sexual assault, whereas those with a predisposition to depression and anxiety have higher levels of internalizing dysfunction.

Self-stigma, or perceiving oneself in a negative light based on perception of social stereotypes of sexual assault victims, is associated with more severe trauma symptoms.

Sexual assault victims who have a history of childhood sexual abuse are at higher risk of PTSD and depression, in part as a result of having maladaptive coping strategies and difficulties with emotional regulation.

Emergency assessments and interventions generally take place immediately for sexual assault victims who report sexual assault to police or go to an emergency room setting. These address the victim's injuries and usually include a forensic sexual assault exam, a medical evaluation of the individual who has been raped to collect information and forensic evidence for potential use in a law-enforcement investigation.

The goals of the sexual assault exam include the treatment of injuries, prophylactic treatment to prevent pregnancy and infection, crisis intervention, and safety planning. Sexual assault exams usually are conducted in the emergency department of a hospital and are time sensitive: they must take place no more than 72-96 hours after the rape because of the potential loss of forensic evidence (e.g., pubic hair, bodily fluids, bruising, lacerations).

A sexual assault response team (SART) is responsible for timely response to a victim of rape, including completion of a sexual assault exam. A SART is a collaborative effort of personnel including a victim service provider/advocate, sexual assault forensic examiner (SAFE) and/or a sexual assault nurse examiner (SANE), law enforcement officer, crime laboratory specialist, and the prosecutor. As a result of the creation of sexual assault response teams at the initial point of care (emergency departments of hospitals), most rape victims now receive prompt medical treatment, forensic evidence collection, thorough documentation of the sexual assault, crisis counseling, and safety planning.

Most victims of sexual assault need further support, known as aftercare. Crisis centers, individual or group therapy, and support groups can provide support and therapeutic interventions.

Crisis hotline services often are utilized by sexual assault victims. These hotlines usually are accessible 24 hours a day. The goals of crisis hotlines are to help the caller cope effectively with the crisis, to educate the caller on facts of sexual assault as well as possible short- and long-term impacts, and to inform the caller of safety resources as well as possible medical and legal resources.

The crisis-line provider should be nonjudgmental, use active listening skills, help the victim identify and clarify her feelings, help the victim explore all of her options, provide empathic responses, and provide referrals to community resources for ongoing support.

Victims may seek individual therapy after a sexual assault. Several therapeutic interventions have been noted to be beneficial for individuals who have experienced the trauma of sexual assault.

Psychodynamic therapy (also known as insight-oriented therapy) targets the client's avoidance symptoms and resolution of any inner conflicts. The therapist helps the client to understand the conscious and unconscious meanings of the symptoms she may be experiencing as a result of the trauma of sexual assault.

Eye-movement desensitization and reprocessing (EMDR) is a treatment often used within psychodynamic therapy. The therapist asks the client to produce images, thoughts, and feelings related to the sexual assault and to evaluate their distressing qualities. The client is then asked to generate alternative pleasing thoughts and images while using specific eye movements to follow the therapist as he or she waves his or her finger rapidly in front of the client's face.

Cognitive behavioral therapy (CBT) is a type of psychotherapy in which the client and therapist work together to examine the relationship between the client's thoughts, feelings, and behaviors. There are several subtypes of CBT:.

In *exposure therapy* (also known as flooding) the client repeatedly confronts fearful images and thoughts of the traumatic sexual assault in order to lessen her fear and anxiety. It is believed to be the most effective of the CBT treatments for victims of sexual assault.

Stress inoculation therapy involves the therapist teaching the client concrete skills to manage anxiety and fear as they relate to the incident of sexual assault.

Multiple channel exposure therapy educates the client on panic and trauma and uses breathing exercises to help in reducing panic and anxiety.

Cognitive processing therapy (CPT) helps victims process the sexual assault by confronting cognitive distortions and maladaptive beliefs concerning the sexual trauma (e.g., No one will ever love me now that I have been raped). CPT for sexual assault survivors usually consists of 12 weekly hour-and-a-half long sessions. One study reported that at the conclusion of CPT treatment none of the participants in the study, all of whom had a diagnosis of PTSD, met the full criteria for PTSD; this was maintained at 6 months following treatment.

Psychopharmacological treatment may also be utilized to treat symptoms of depression and PTSD.

Researchers have examined the benefits of therapy for sexual assault victims, who were not victims of intimate partner violence, that includes their spouse or partner.

One study used CBT not only to address the PTSD diagnosis of the sexual assault victim but also to improve the support offered by the victim's spouse. Results at the conclusion of treatment and 3-month follow-up indicated that the victims no longer met the criteria for PTSD and that all reported significant improvement in the ways they were receiving support from their spouse as well as increased satisfaction in their overall relationship.

In another study investigators examined the use of solution-oriented therapy (SOT) (also called solution-focused therapy) with sexual assault survivors and their spouses/partners who had both disclosed negative impacts on their sexual functioning as a result of the sexual assault. The research suggests that SOT empowers the victim as well as the partner to regain a sense of control, improves mutual sexual functioning, and decreases the victim's PTSD symptoms.

SOT is brief (several sessions only), goal oriented, and is focused on solutions rather than problems or symptoms. SOT uses "the miracle question" (How would your future look different if the problem was no longer present?), scaling questions, coping questions, and problem-free talk (in which the client talks about problem-free areas of her life). These types of questions are intended to help the victim envision what she wants to change in her life and then use those desired changes as goals to work on in therapy.

Sexual assault group therapy is another effective therapeutic intervention for victims of sexual assault. Groups provide a sense of normalcy for victims as well as a safe place in which they may experience and share empathy and encouragement.

A study of a psychoeducational group model of therapy for sexual assault victims in a university setting in the Midwestern United States reported that participants experienced a decrease in PTSD symptoms and a lessening of their initial sense of isolation.

In this model the group is closed (i.e., no new members are accepted after the group is formed), consists ideally of 7-10 participants, and lasts 10-12 weeks. Goals of the group include empowerment, reduced isolation, increased self-esteem, learning about and modeling healthy relationships, and participants regaining a sense of control over their lives.

These goals are attained through group discussion as well as hands-on activities (e.g.,an imagined older version of oneself writing a letter to one's current self that shares what the current self can and will overcome; sharing a meaningful song or piece of poetry with the group).

A controlled trial of psychotherapy for survivors of sexual violence in the Democratic Republic of Congo indicated that the improvements experienced by participants in group therapy were far greater than those experienced by participants in individual therapy. After 6 months of treatment, only 9 percent of the group therapy participants met the criteria for anxiety and/or depression versus 42 percent of the participants in individual counseling.

Researchers have found that many victims of sexual assault do not receive needed services.

In a study in London, approximately half of sexual assault victims followed through with recommended medical care following the initial sexual assault exam, and only 33 percent of victims who were prescribed HIV preventive treatment completed the regimen.

Researchers in a United States study found that 43.5 percent of sexual assault victims utilized mental health services at 1.5 months after the assault, decreasing to only 31.4 percent at 6 months post-assault. Victims who had received previous mental health services and victims who abused alcohol were more likely to participate in mental health services following sexual assault.

WHAT CAN BE DONE

Learn about sexual assault dynamics, aftercare, and interventions; share this information with your colleagues.

Use this knowledge to accurately and sensitively assess your client's individual characteristics and mental and physical health education needs.

Develop an awareness of your own cultural values, beliefs, and biases and develop knowledge about the histories, traditions, and values of your clients. Adopt treatment methodologies that reflect the cultural needs of the client.

Conduct a biopsychosocialspiritual assessment, making sure to ask about any history of sexual violence.

Encourage clients who are victims of sexual assault to follow through with recommended medical and mental health treatment; provide support as needed.

Use appropriate therapeutic interventions to address anxiety, depression, and PTSD symptoms, if applicable (e.g., CBT, solution-focused therapy, psychodynamic therapy).

Help victim build or increase social support system.

Listen, encourage, validate, provide resources, and normalize victim's reactions to sexual assault.

Educate victim about legal procedures she may experience or pursue.

Be familiar with both local and state policies regarding sexual assault.

Practice with awareness of, and adherence to, the social work principles of respect for human rights and human dignity, social justice, and professional conduct as described in the International Federation of Social Workers (IFSW) Statement of Ethical Principles. Become knowledgeable of the IFSW ethical standards as they apply to victims of sexual assault, and practice accordingly(1).

Refer to online resources for additional information National Sexual Violence Resource Center, http://www.nsvrc.org/.

Rape, Abuse & Incest National Network (RAINN), https://rainn.org/, 1-800-656-HOPE.

Womenshealth.gov, https://www.womenshealth.gov/publications/our-publications/fact-sheet/sexual-assault.html.

Written by Melissa Rosales Neff, MSW

Reviewed by Laura Gale, LCSW, and Chris Bates, MA, MSW

REFERENCES

British Association of Social Workers. (2012). *The code of ethics for social work: Statement of principles.* Retrieved May 9, 2016, from http://cdn.basw.co.uk/upload/basw_112315-7.pdf

Bass, J. K., Annama, J., Murray, S. M., Kaysen, D., Griffiths, S., Cetinoglu, T.,... Bolton, P. (2013). Controlled trial of psychotherapy for Congolese survivors of sexual violence. *The New England Journal of Medicine, 368*(23), 2182-2191. doi:10.1056/NEJMoa1211853

Beckerman, N. L., & Pass, J. (2008). After the assault: Cognitive Trauma Therapy with a single event trauma survivor. *Clinical Social Work Journal, 36*(3), 255-263. doi:10.1007/s10615-008-0145-5

Billette, V., Guay, S., & Marchand, A. (2008). Posttraumatic Stress Disorder and social support in female victims of sexual assault: The impact of spousal involvement on the efficacy of cognitive-behavioral therapy. *Behavior Modification, 32*(6), 876-896. doi:10.1177/0145445508319280

Centers for Disease Control and Prevention. (2012). Sexual violence: Facts at a glance. Retrieved May 9, 2016, from http://www.cdc.gov/violenceprevention/pdf/sv-datasheet-a.pdf

Centers for Disease Control and Prevention. (2014). Sexual violence: Consequences. Retrieved May 9, 2016, from http://www.cdc.gov/violenceprevention/sexualviolence/consequences.html

Combs, J. L., Jordan, C. E., & Smith, G. T. (2014). Individual differences in personality predict externalizing versus internalizing outcomes following sexual assault. *Psychological Trauma: Theory, Research, Practice, and Policy, 6*(4), 375-383. doi:10.1037/a0032978

Deitz, M. F., Williams, S. L., Rife, S. C., & Cantrell, P. (2015). Examining cultural, social, and self-related aspects of stigma in relation to sexual assault and trauma symptoms. *Violence Against Women, 21*(5), 598-615. doi:10.1177/1077801215573330

International Federation of Social Workers. (2012, March). Statement of ethical principles. Retrieved May 9, 2016, from http://ifsw.org/policies/statement-of-ethical-principles/

Jonas, D. E., Cusack, K., Forneris, C. A., Wilkins, T. M., Sonis, J., Middleton, J. C.,... Gaynes, B. N. (2013). Psychological and pharmacological treatments for adults with posttraumatic stress disorder (PTSD). Comparative Effectiveness Review No. 92. Retrieved from https://www.ncbi.nlm.nih.gov/books/NBK137702/

Lee, J., Willis, L., Newman, D., Hazan, A., Kurobe, A., Giordano, L.,... Shah, K. (2014). Are sexual assault victims presenting to the emergency department in a timely manner? *Social Work, 60*(1), 29-33. doi:10.1093/sw/swu051

Macy, R., Giattina, M., Sangster, T., Crosby, C., & Montijo, N. J. (2009). Domestic violence and sexual assault services: inside the black box. *Aggression and Violent Behavior, 14*(5), 359-373.

Masters, N. T., Stappenbeck, C. A., Kaysen, D., Kajumulo, K. F., Davis, K. C., George, W. H.,... Heiman, J. R. (2015). A person-centered approach to examining heterogeneity and subgroups among survivors of sexual assault. *Journal of Abnormal Psychology, 124*(3), 685-696. doi:10.1037/abn0000055

Morgan, L., Brittain, B., & Welch, J. (2015). Medical care following multiple perpetrator sexual assault: A retrospective review. *International Journal of STD & AIDS, 26*(2), 86-92.

Munro, M. L. (2014). Barriers to care for sexual assault survivors of childbearing age: An integrative review. *Women's Healthcare, 2*(4), 19-29.

National Association of Social Workers. (2015). NASW standards and indicators for cultural competence in social work practice. Retrieved May 9, 2016, from http://www.socialworkers.org/practice/standards/PRA-BRO-253150-CC-Standards.pdf

A national protocol for sexual assault medical forensic examinations: Adults/adolescents. Second edition. (2013). *U. S. Department of Justice, Office on Violence Against Women.* Retrieved May 9, 2016, from http://www.ncjrs.gov/pdffiles1/ovw/241903.pdf

Office for Victims of Crime. (2013). Sexual assault. Retrieved May 9, 2016, from https://www.ovcttac.gov/downloads/views/TrainingMaterials/NVAA/Documents_NVAA2011/ResourcePapers/Color_Sexual percent20Assault percent20Resource percent20Paper_2012_final percent20percent20508c_9_13_2012.pdf

Office on Women's Health. (2009). Sexual assault: Frequently asked questions. Retrieved May 9, 2016, from https://www.womenshealth.gov/publications/our-publications/fact-sheet/sexual-assault.html

Parcesepe, A. M., Martin, S. L., Pollock, M. D., & Garcia-Moreno, C. (2015). The effectiveness of mental health interventions for adult female survivors of sexual assault: A systematic review. *Aggression & Violent Behavior, 25*(A), 15-25. doi:10.1016/j.avb.2015.06.004

Peter-Hagene, L. C., & Ullman, S. E. (2015). Sexual assault-characteristics effects on PTSD and psychosocial mediators: A cluster-analysis approach to sexual assault types. *Psychological Trauma: Theory, Research, Practice, and Policy, 7*(2), 162-170. doi:10.1037/a0037304

Price, M., Davidson, T. M., Ruggiero, K. J., Acierno, R., & Resnick, H. S. (2014). Predictors of using mental health services after sexual assault. *Journal of Traumatic Stress, 27*(3), 331-337. doi:10.1002/jts.21915

Resick, P. A., & Schnicke, M. K. (1992). Cognitive processing therapy for sexual assault victims. *Journal of Consulting and Clinical Psychology, 60*(5), 748-756.

Tambling, R. (2012). Solution-oriented therapy for survivors of sexual assault and their partners. *Contemporary Family Therapy, 34*(3), 391-401. doi:10.1007/s10591-012-9200-z

Ullman, S. E., Peter-Hagene, L. C., & Relyea, M. (2014). Coping, emotion regulation, and self-blame as mediators of sexual abuse and psychological symptoms in adult sexual assault. *Journal of Child Sexual Abuse, 23*(1), 74-93. doi:10.1080/10538712.2014.864747

United Nations Statistics Division. (2015). The World's Women 2015 Trends and Statistics. Retrieved May 9, 2016, from http://unstats.un.org/unsd/gender/worldswomen.html

VanDeusan, K., & Carr, J. L. (2004). Group work at the university: A psychoeducational sexual assault group for women. *Social Work with Groups, 27*(4), 51-63.

Walsh, R. M., & Bruce, S. E. (2014). Reporting decisions after sexual assault: The impact of mental health variables. *Psychological Trauma: Theory, Research, Practice & Policy,* 6(6), 691-699. doi:10.1037/a0036592

World Health Organization. (2012). Understanding and addressing violence against women: Sexual violence. Retrieved May 9, 2016, from http://www.who.int/reproductivehealth/topics/violence/vaw_series/en

World Health Organization. (2013). Global and regional estimates of violence against women: Prevalence and health effects of intimate partner violence and non-partner sexual violence. Retrieved from http://www.who.int/reproductivehealth/publications/violence/9789241564625/en

SEXUAL ASSAULT: ADULT FEMALE VICTIMS—EMERGENCY ASSESSMENT & INTERVENTION

MAJOR CATEGORIES: Violence

WHAT WE KNOW

Sexual assault is any type of sexual activity that is nonconsensual (including when one is unable to provide consent), including physical, verbal, visual (e.g., being forced to view pornography), or any other type of unwanted sexual contact or attention.

Examples include rape within marriage or dating relationships, rape by acquaintances or strangers, gang rape (i.e., rape involving two or more perpetrators), systematic rape (i.e., mass rapes that occur during armed conflicts); and inappropriate touching, voyeurism (i.e., when someone watches private sexual acts), exhibitionism (i.e., when someone exposes him-/herself in public), incest (i.e., sexual contact between family members), unwanted sexual advances (e.g., unwelcome sexual gestures, requests for sexual favors).

In 2013 the United States Federal Bureau of Investigation began using a more inclusive definition of rape (formerly defined as "the carnal knowledge of a female forcibly and against her will"): "the penetration, no matter how slight, of the vagina or anus with any body part or object, or oral penetration by a sex organ of another person, without consent of the victim."

Sexual assault is a global criminal and public-health problem.

According to the World Health Organization (WHO),in 2013 the lifetime prevalence of sexual assault by an intimate partner reported by women ages 15 to 49 years old ranged from 6 percent in Japan to 59 percent in Ethiopia. Rates in other countries included 46.7 percent in Peru, 28.9 percent in Thailand, and 14.3 percent in Brazil. WHO reported that 0.3 percent–12 percent of women reported being forced after age 15 to have sexual intercourse or perform a sexual act with someone other than their partners. The wide range is due to the variance from country to country of reported rapes.

A 2012 study by the U.S. Centers for Disease Control and Prevention (CDC) on sexual assault in the United States reported that.

1 in 5 women experienced rape at some time in their lives

1 in 20 women experienced sexual violence other than rape (such as sexual coercion or unwanted sexual contact)

37.4 percent of female rape victims were first raped between ages 18 and 24

A literature review of 12 articles and 4 national surveys about barriers to seeking care after a sexual assault in the United States identified personal and environmental factors.

Personal factors included emotional states (i.e., shame, embarrassment, humiliation, and self-blame),fear of negative consequences of reporting (i.e., not being believed, retaliation, lack of confidentiality, poor treatment by law enforcement, public exposure, stigma, and unfair treatment), and lack of knowledge (i.e., not knowing what services are available and how they are paid for).

Environmental factors included organizational and structural barriers (i.e., limited services, services that were difficult to access, inadequate funding, staff members who are inexperienced or uncomfortable with sexual assault cases) and societal myths (i.e., biases based on race, gender, and sexual orientation; doubts about the authenticity of sexual assault).

The effects of sexual assault on women are well documented in research, including:

physical effects: pregnancy, chronic pelvic pain, migraines, gynecological complications, back pain, facial pain;

psychological effects: shock, denial, fear, guilt, depression, posttraumatic stress disorder, sleep disturbances, attempted suicide;

social effects: strained relationships with family members and friends, decreased contact with family members and friends, lower likelihood of marriage; and

health effects: engaging in high-risk behavior (e.g., unprotected sex, trading sex for food or money), substance use, unhealthy diet-related behaviors (e.g., overeating, abusing diet pills, fasting, self-induced vomiting).

A forensic sexual assault exam is a medical evaluation of an individual who has been raped. Information and forensic evidence are collected in the exam for potential use in a law enforcement investigation.

The goals of the sexual assault exam are treatment of injuries, prophylactic treatment to prevent pregnancy and infection, crisis intervention, and safety planning. Sexual assault exams typically are conducted in the emergency department of a hospital and are time-sensitive: They must take place no more than 72–96 hours after the rape because of potential loss of forensic evidence (e.g., pubic hair, bodily fluids, bruising, lacerations).

A sexual assault response team (SART) is a support team responsible for timely response to a victim of rape, including completion of a sexual assault exam. A SART is a collaborative effort of personnel including a victim service provider/advocate, a sexual assault forensic examiner (SAFE) and/or sexual assault nurse examiner (SANE), a law enforcement officer, a crime laboratory specialist, and the prosecutor who is assigned to the case at the time. As a result of the creation of sexual assault response teams at the initial point of care (emergency departments of hospitals), most rape victims now receive prompt medical treatment, forensic evidence collection, thorough documentation of the sexual assault, crisis counseling, and safety planning.

A primary goal of the SART is to provide victim-centered care throughout the entire sexual assault examination process. This process consists of:

giving sexual assault victims priority care in the hospital emergency department. The longer a victim waits, the greater the potential for loss of evidence and the greater possible emotional and physical trauma;

providing necessary means of ensuring victims' privacy. Victims should not be left in the main emergency department waiting room, but should be given a private room in which to wait for the sexual assault exam;

accommodating victims' requests to have a relative, friend, or other personal support person present during the exam (unless considered harmful by staff);

accommodating victims' requests for staff of a specific gender throughout the exam; and

providing information that is easy for victims to understand, in lay terms and in their native language. An interpreter should be used if needed.

Although SART evidence-collection protocols may vary slightly from place to place, they typically include:

- a history in which the victim is questioned about the following aspects of the assault. It is important for the entire sexual assault response team to be present so that the victim need share this information only once, to prevent further possible trauma;
- circumstances of the assault (date, time, location);
- physical description of the alleged perpetrator;
- areas of trauma (specifically, details of oral, vaginal, or anorectal contact or penetration);
- condom use or ejaculation (absence or presence of);
- presence of bleeding in victim or perpetrator;
- recent consensual sexual activity prior to the assault;
- whether the victim has showered, bathed, or changed clothes since the assault;
- physical examination performed by a sexual assault forensic examiner or a sexual assault nurse examiner.

This exam can take 3-6 hours to complete. The exam includes:

physical examination of entire body. Individuals who have experienced assault can feel revictimized by the exam. It is vital to allow the victim to have control whenever possible during the exam (e.g., to control who is in the room); and

forensic evaluation and treatment. A sexual assault evidence collection kit is used that contains necessary items for specimen collection based on evidence requirements of the local crime laboratory.

Samples of vaginal or cervical secretion, anal secretion, pubic hair, blood, and urine are taken from the victim. Clothing (if unchanged after the event) samples also are taken.

Once complete, the forensic examiner or nurse examiner must complete, sign, and date the sexual assault evidence collection kit form, which indicates that the examination is complete and sealed.

Gonorrhea and chlamydia testing is recommended for all victims; human immunodeficiency virus (HIV), hepatitis B, and syphilis tests also are recommended.

Retesting is recommended at 6 weeks, 3 months, and 6 months after the assault.

Pregnancy risk is estimated to be 5 percent per rape in women ages 12–45.

Emergency contraception should be offered in all cases.

WHAT CAN BE DONE

Learn about sexual assault and emergency assessment and interventions; share this information with your colleagues.

Use your knowledge to accurately and sensitively assess your clients' individual characteristics and their mental health and physical health education needs.

Develop an awareness of your own cultural values, beliefs, and biases and develop knowledge about the histories, traditions, and values of your clients. Adopt treatment methodologies that reflect the cultural needs of the client.

Victim advocates, often social workers, are integral members of sexual assault response teams; they are valuable assets to the victim before, during, and after the sexual assault exam.

Before the exam is conducted, the victim advocate may

- serve as an information resource for the victim by explaining the role of law enforcement in the process; explaining the value of medical and evidence-collection procedures; and explaining

treatment options for STDs, HIV, and pregnancy (if applicable);

- assist in the coordination of transportation to and from the sexual assault exam site (home to hospital or police station to hospital);

- provide crisis intervention: short-term counseling to help the victim identify options and resources so that she is able to make informed decisions when needed (e.g., whether to make a formal report of rape);

- during the exam, communicate the victim's wishes to the rest of the sexual assault response team;

- provide replacement clothing and toiletries when clothing is retained for evidence; and

- help victim identify possible support persons in her life, such as family members, friends, employers, and spiritual counselors.

- After the exam is complete, the victim advocate may

- address the victim's physical comfort needs;

- help the victim make a safety plan: Where will she go after she is discharged? Who will she go with? Does she need an emergency shelter option? Would she like to file a restraining order?;

- explain what victim should expect in terms of how SART members (prosecutor, law enforcement) will be following up with her as well as the need to follow up with STD and pregnancy retests; and

- explain and provide contact information for mental health services and other community resources that are available to victim.

Written by Melissa Rosales Neff, MSW

Reviewed by Laura Gale, LCSW, and Chris Bates, MA, MSW

REFERENCES

British Association of Social Workers. (2012, January). The code of ethics for social work: Statement of principles. Retrieved October 11, 2015, from http://cdn.basw.co.uk/upload/basw_112315-7.pdf

Centers for Disease Control and Prevention. (2012). Sexual violence: Facts at a glance. Retrieved October 11, 2015, from http://www.cdc.gov/violenceprevention/pdf/SV-DataSheet-a.pdf

Chisolm, S. L. (2014). Sexual assault. In F. F. Ferri (Ed.), *2014 Ferri's clinical advisor: 5 books in 1* (16th ed., p. 1010). Philadelphia, PA: Elsevier Mosby.

Federal Bureau of Investigation. (2013). Frequently asked questions about the change in the UCR definition of rape. Retrieved October 11, 2015, from http://www.fbi.gov/about-us/cjis/ucr/recent-program-updates/new-rape-definition-frequently-asked-questions

Holleran, R. S. (2009). Sexual assault examination. In J. A. Proehl (Ed.), *Emergency nursing procedures* (4th ed., pp. 894-900). St. Louis, MO: Saunders Elsevier.

International Federation of Social Workers. (2012, March). Statement of ethical principles. Retrieved January 15, 2015, from http://ifsw.org/policies/statement-of-ethical-principles/

Wheeler, D. (2015). *NASW standards for cultural competency in social work practice*. Retrieved March 3, 2015, from http://www.socialworkers.org/practice/standards/PRA-BRO-253150-CC-Standards.pdf

Munro, M. L. (2014). Barriers to care for sexual assault survivors of childbearing age: An integrative review. *Women's Healthcare, 2*(4), 19-29.

Office on Women's Health, U.S. Department of Health and Human Services. (2009). Sexual assault: Frequently asked questions. Retrieved October 11, 2015, from https://www.womenshealth.gov/publications/our-publications/fact-sheet/sexual-assault.html

Office for Victims of Crime. (2013). Sexual assault. Retrieved October 11, 2015, from https://www.ovcttac.gov/downloads/views/TrainingMaterials/NVAA/Documents_NVAA2011/ResourcePapers/Color_Sexual percent20Assault percent20Resource percent20Paper_2012_final percent20- percent20508c_9_13_2012.pdf

Sexual violence: Consequences. (2014). *Centers for Disease Control and Prevention*. Retrieved October 11, 2015, from http://www.cdc.gov/violenceprevention/sexualviolence/consequences.html

World Health Organization (WHO). (2012). Understanding and addressing violence against women: Sexual violence. Retrieved October 11, 1970, from http://apps.who.int/iris/bitstream/10665/77434/1/WHO_RHR_12.37_eng.pdf?ua=1

(2013). Sexual assault examination. In E. Eckman (Ed.), *Lippincott's nursing procedures and skills* (6th ed., pp. 648-650). Philadelphia, PA: Wolters Kluwer Health/Lippincott Williams & Wilkins.

U. S. Department of Justice, Office on Violence Against Women. (2013). A national protocol for sexual assault medical forensic examinations: Adults/adolescents. Second edition. Retrieved October 11, 2015, from http://www.ncjrs.gov/pdffiles1/ovw/241903.pdf

World Health Organization (WHO). (2002). World report on violence and health: Sexual violence. Retrieved October 11, 2015, from http://www.who.int/violence_injury_prevention/violence/global_campaign/en/chap6.pdf?ua=1

World Health Organization. (2013). Global and regional estimates of violence against women: Prevalence and health effects of intimate partner violence and non-partner sexual violence. Retrieved October 11, 2015, from http://www.who.int/reproductivehealth/publications/violence/9789241564625/en

SEXUAL ASSAULT: ADULT MALE VICTIMS—EMERGENCY ASSESSMENT & INTERVENTION

MAJOR CATEGORIES: Violence

WHAT WE KNOW

Sexual assault is any type of sexual activity that is nonconsensual (including when one is unable to provide consent), whether physical, verbal, visual (e.g., forcing someone to look at pornography), or any other type of unwanted sexual contact or attention.

Examples include rape within marriage or dating relationships, rape by acquaintances or strangers, gang rape (i.e., rape involving two or more perpetrators), systematic rape (i.e., mass rapes that occur during armed conflicts); and

inappropriate touching, voyeurism (i.e., when someone watches private sexual acts), exhibitionism (i.e., when someone exposes him/herself in public), incest (i.e., sexual contact between family members), unwanted sexual advances (e.g., unwelcome sexual gestures, requests for sexual favors).

In 2013 the United States Federal Bureau of Investigation began using a more inclusive definition of rape (formerly defined as "the carnal knowledge of a female forcibly and against her will"): "the penetration, no matter how slight, of the vagina or anus with any body part or object, or oral penetration by a sex organ of another person, without consent of the victim."

Sexual assault of males is both a criminal and a public-health problem.

Although 10–20 percent of female victims of sexual assault in the United States report the crime, the percentage of males who disclose sexual assault and file a report is much lower.

Retrospective studies in the United States of sexual assault of males indicate that 3–7 percent of men report that they have experienced sexual assault in adulthood, usually taking place in their 20s and 30s.

Rape, Abuse, and Incest National Network (RAINN) reports that approximately 10 percent of sexual assault victims in the United States are males.

Investigators for the most recent national study on sexual assault by the U.S. Centers for Disease Control and Prevention (CDC) in 2012 reported that:

- 1 in 71 men (1.4 percent) reported experiencing rape at some time in their lives
- 1 in 20 men experienced sexual violence other than rape (such as sexual coercion or unwanted sexual contact)
- 4.8 percent of men reported that they were forced to penetrate someone else at some point in their lives

Researchers conducting a chart review for a Boston hospital found that 4 percent of the sexual assault cases that were in the emergency department involved male victims.

In South Africa, researchers found that for the emergency department of a hospital there, 12.7 percent of the victims were male. 47.6 percent of the men reported physical injury and 81 percent knew the perpetrator.

In London, researchers studying multiple-perpetrator sexual assaults found that 4 percent (or 6 individuals) of the victims were men. All of the men reported violence in addition the sexual assault itself and that the perpetrators were strangers to them.

Although most perpetrators of sexual assault of males are male, it is important to note that females can sexually assault males as well.

Researchers studying males in the United States reported that male victims of sexual assault were more likely to be assaulted by groups (two or more perpetrators) than by individuals.

The effects of sexual assault on males can be extensive. They include the following:.

Physical effects: sexually transmitted diseases (STDs), such as human immunodeficiency virus (HIV) and rectal or pharyngeal gonorrhea from unprotected anal sex (which can cause anal tearing and abrasions) or oral sex.

Psychological effects: shock, denial, fear, guilt (some men believe that they somehow gave the perpetrator permission or feel guilty if they experienced an erection during the assault), depression, posttraumatic stress disorder, sleep disturbances, attempted suicide, confusion about sexual orientation.

Social effects: strained relationships with family members and friends, decreased contact with family members and friends, inability to form close and trusting relationships with other men.

Health effects: engagement in high-risk behavior (e.g., unprotected sex, trading sex for food or money) and substance use.

A forensic sexual assault exam is a medical evaluation of an individual who has been raped. Information and forensic evidence is collected in the exam for potential use in a law enforcement investigation.

The goals of the sexual assault exam are the treatment of injuries, prophylactic treatment to prevent infection, crisis intervention, and safety planning. Sexual assault exams typically are conducted in the emergency department of a hospital and are time sensitive: they must take place no more than 72–96 hours after the assault because of potential loss of forensic evidence (e.g., pubic hair, bodily fluids, bruising, lacerations).

A sexual assault response team (SART) is a support team responsible for timely response to a victim of rape, including completion of a sexual assault exam. A sexual assault response team is a collaborative effort of personnel including a victim service provider/advocate, a sexual assault forensic examiner (SAFE) and/or a sexual assault nurse examiner (SANE), a law enforcement officer, a crime laboratory specialist, and the prosecutor who is assigned to the case at the time. As a result of the creation of sexual assault response teams at the initial point of care (emergency departments of hospitals),many rape victims now receive prompt medical treatment, forensic evidence collection, thorough documentation of the sexual assault, crisis counseling, and safety planning.

A primary goal of the sexual assault response team is to provide victim-centered care throughout the entire sexual assault examination process. This process consists of the following:

Victims of sexual assault are given priority care in the hospital emergency department. The longer a victim waits, the greater the potential for loss of evidence and the greater potential emotional and physical trauma.

Providing necessary means to ensure the victim's privacy. Victims should not be left in the main emergency department waiting room, but should be given a private room in which to wait for the sexual assault exam.

Accommodating the victim's request to have a relative, friend, or other personal support person present during the exam (unless considered harmful by staff).

Accommodating the victim's request for staff of a specific gender throughout the exam.

Providing information that is easy for the victim to understand, in lay terms and in his native language. Use an interpreter if needed.

Although evidence-collection protocols may vary slightly from place to place, they typically include the following:

- history in which the victim is questioned about the following aspects of the assault. It is important for the entire sexual assault response team to be present so that the victim need share this information only once, to prevent further trauma;
- circumstances of the assault (date, time, location);
- physical description of the alleged perpetrator;
- areas of trauma (specifically, details of oral or ano-rectal contact or penetration).
- condom use or ejaculation (absence or presence of);
- presence of bleeding in victim or perpetrator;
- recent consensual sexual activity prior to the assault; and
- whether the victim has showered, bathed, or changed clothes since the assault.

Physical examination performed by a sexual assault forensic examiner or a sexual assault nurse examiner. This exam can take 3–6 hours to complete. The exam includes the following:

physical examination of entire body. Males who have been sexually assaulted often experience more extensive physical injuries than females, Individuals who have experienced assault can feel revictimized by the exam. It is vital to allow the victim to have control whenever possible during the exam (e.g., who is in the room);

forensic evaluation and treatment. A sexual assault evidence collection kit is used that contains necessary items for specimen collection based on the evidence requirements of the local crime laboratory.

Samples of penile secretion, anal secretion, pubic hair, blood, and urine are taken from victim. Clothing (if unchanged after the event) samples also are taken.

Once the sexual assault evidence-collection process is complete, the forensic examiner or nurse examiner must complete, sign, and date the kit form, which indicates that the examination is complete and sealed.

Gonorrhea and chlamydia testing is recommended for all victims; human immunodeficiency virus (HIV), hepatitis B, and syphilis tests also are recommended.

Retesting is recommended at 2 months, 4 months, and 6 months after the assault.

Although rare, it is important to note that if the victim is a transgender male who still has a uterus and ovaries, he can become pregnant from a sexual assault despite taking testosterone.

WHAT CAN BE DONE

Learn about male sexual assault emergency assessment and interventions; share this information with your colleagues.

Use this knowledge to accurately and sensitively assess your client's individual characteristics as well as his healthcare and education needs.

Develop an awareness of your own cultural values, beliefs, and biases and develop knowledge about the histories, traditions, and values of your clients. Adopt treatment methodologies that reflect the cultural needs of the client.

Victim advocates, often social workers, are integral members of sexual assault response teams; they are valuable assets to the victim before, during, and after the sexual assault exam.

Before, during, and after the exam is conducted, the victim advocate may

- serve as an information resource for the victim by explaining the role of law enforcement in the process, explaining the value of medical and evidence-collection procedures, and explaining treatment options for STDs and HIV;
- assist in the coordination of transportation to and from the sexual assault exam site (home to hospital or police station to hospital);
- provide crisis intervention (short-term counseling to help victim identify options and resources so that he is able to make informed decisions when needed [e.g., whether to make a formal report of rape]);
- communicate the victim's wishes to the rest of the sexual assault response team during the exam;
- provide replacement clothing and toiletries when clothing is retained for evidence; and
- help the victim identify possible support people in his life, such as family members, friends, employers, and spiritual counselors.
- After the exam is complete, the victim advocate may
- address the victim's physical comfort needs;
- help the victim make a safety plan: Where will he go after he is discharged? Who will he go with? Does he need an emergency shelter option? Would he like to file a restraining order?;
- explain what the victim should expect in terms of how sexual assault response team members (prosecutor, law enforcement) will be following up with victim and emphasize the need to follow up with STD re-tests; and
- explain and provide contact information for mental health services and other community resources (e.g., Male Survivor at http://www.male-survivor.org/) that are available to him.

Ask agencies if they provide services specifically for male victims.

Written by Melissa Rosales Neff, MSW

Reviewed by Laura Gale, LCSW

REFERENCES

Adefolalu, A. O. (2014). Fear of the perpetrator: A major reason why sexual assault victims delayed presenting at hospital. *Tropical Medicine & International Health, 19*(3), 342-347. doi:10.1111/tmi.12249

British Association of Social Workers. (2012, January). The code of ethics for social workers: Statement of principles. Retrieved March 24, 2016, from http://cdn.basw.co.uk/upload/basw_112315-7.pdf

Bullock, C. M., & Beckson, M. (2011). Male victims of sexual assault: Phenomenology, psychology, and physiology. *Journal of American Academy Psychiatry Law, 39*(2), 197-205.

Centers for Disease Control and Prevention. (2012). Sexual violence: Facts at a glance. Retrieved March 24, 2016, from http://www.cdc.gov/ViolencePrevention/pdf/sv-datasheet-a.pdf

Chisholm, S. L. (2016). Sexual assault. In F. F. Ferri (Ed.), *2016 Ferri's clinical advisor: 5 books in 1* (18th ed., pp. 1118-1119). Philadelphia, PA: Elsevier Mosby.

Eckerman, M. (Ed.). (2016). Sexual assault examination. In *Lippincott's nursing procedures and skills* (18th ed., pp. 690-692). Philadelphia, PA: Wolters Kluwer Health/Lippincott William & Wilkins.

Federal Bureau of Investigation. (2014). Frequently asked questions about the change in the UCR definition of rape. Retrieved March 24, 2016, from http://www.fbi.gov/about-us/cjis/ucr/recent-program-updates/new-rape-definition-frequently-asked-questions

International Federation of Social Workers. (2012). Statement of ethical principles. Retrieved March 24, 2016, from http://ifsw.org/policies/statement-of-ethical-principles/

Lee, J., Willis, L., Newman, D., Hazan, A., Kurobe, A., Giordano, L.,... Kaushal, S. (2015). Are sexual assault victims presenting to the emergency department in a timely manner? *Social Work, 60*(1), 29-33. doi:10.1093/sw/swu051

McLean, I., Balding, V., & White, C. (2005). Further aspects of male-on-male rape and sexual assault in Greater Manchester. *Medical Science Law, 45*(3), 225-232. doi:10.1258/rsmmsl.45.3.225

Mizrahi, T., & Mayden, R. W. (2001). NASW standards for cultural competency in social work practice. Retrieved June 19, 2015, from http://www.

socialworkers.org/practice/standards/NASWCul-turalStandards.pdf

Morgan, L., Brittain, B., & Welch, J. (2015). Medical care following multiple perpetrator sexual assault: A retrospective review. *International Journal of STD & AIDS, 26*(2), 86-92.

New York City Alliance Against Sexual Assault. (1997). Factsheets: Male rape. Retrieved March 24, 2016, from http://www.svfreenyc.org/survivors_factsheet_38.html

Office for Victims of Crime, Office of Justice Programs. (2013). Sexual assault. Retrieved March 24, 2016, from https://www.ovcttac.gov/downloads/views/TrainingMaterials/NVAA/Documents_NVAA2011/ResourcePapers/Color_Sexual percent20Assault percent20Resource percent20Paper_2012_final percent20- percent20508c_9_13_2012.pdf

Office on Women's Health, U.S. Department of Health and Human Services. (2015, May 21). Sexual assault fact sheet. Retrieved March 24,

2016, from https://www.womenshealth.gov/publications/our-publications/fact-sheet/sexual-assault-factsheet.pdf

Rape, Abuse & Incest National Network (RAINN). (2014). Male sexual assault. Retrieved October 11, 1970, from http://www.rainn.org/get-information/types-of-sexual-assault/male-sexual-assault

U.S. Department of Justice, Office on Violence Against Women. (2013, April). A national protocol for sexual assault medical forensic examinations: Adults/adolescents. Retrieved March 24, 2016, from http://www.ncjrs.gov/pdffiles1/ovw/241903.pdf

World Health Organization (WHO). (2012). Understanding and addressing violence against women: Sexual violence. Retrieved March 24, 2016, from http://apps.who.int/iris/bitstream/10665/77434/1/WHO_RHR_12.37_eng.pdf?ua=1

SEXUAL ASSAULT: ADULT MALE VICTIMS—AFTERCARE ASSESSMENT & INTERVENTION

MAJOR CATEGORIES: Violence

WHAT WE KNOW

Sexual assault is any type of sexual activity that is nonconsensual (including when one is unable to provide consent), including physical, verbal, visual (e.g., being forced to look at pornography), or any other type of unwanted sexual contact or attention.

Examples include rape within marriage or dating relationships, rape by acquaintances or strangers, gang rape (rape involving two or more perpetrators), systematic rape (i.e., mass rapes that occur during armed conflicts); and inappropriate touching, voyeurism (i.e., when someone watches private sexual acts), exhibitionism (i.e., when someone exposes him/herself in public), incest (i.e., sexual contact between family members), unwanted sexual advances (e.g., unwelcome sexual gestures, requests for sexual favors).

In 2013 the United States Federal Bureau of Investigation began using a more inclusive definition of rape (formally defined as "the carnal knowledge of a female forcibly and against her will"): "the penetration,

no matter how slight, of the vagina or anus with any body part or object, or oral penetration by a sex organ of another person, without consent of the victim."

Sexual assault is both a criminal and a public-health problem.

Retrospective studies in the United States of male sexual assault indicate that 3 percent–7 percent of men report that they have experienced sexual assault in adulthood, usually taking place in their 20s or 30s.

Rape, Abuse, and Incest National Network (RAINN) reports that approximately 10 percent of sexual assault victims in the United States are males.

A 2012 national study by the U.S. Centers for Disease Control and Prevention (CDC) on sexual assault reported that.

1 in 7 men experienced rape at some time in their lives

1 in 20 men experienced sexual violence other than rape (such as sexual coercion or unwanted sexual contact)

4.8 percent of men reported that they were forced to penetrate someone else at some point in their lives

Although 10 percent–20 percent of female victims of sexual assault in the United States report the crime, the percentage of males who disclose sexual assault and file a report is much lower.

Although most perpetrators of sexual assault of males are male, it is important to note that women can sexually assault males as well.

The U.S. Department of Defense (DOD) produces an annual report on sexual assault and sexual assault prevention in the military. For fiscal year 2012, research indicated that 1.2 percent of men in the military reported experiencing unwanted sexual contact. The DOD has acknowledged that sexual assault in the military is underreported: It estimated that the actual rate of sexual assault of males in the military could be 15 times greater.

It is important to note that there is little empirical research focused specifically on male victims of sexual assault. The majority of research is focused on female victims.

A study reported that male victims of sexual assault are more likely to be assaulted by groups (two or more perpetrators), rather than by individuals.

The effects of sexual assault on males can be extensive, including:

physical effects: sexually transmitted diseases (STDs) such as human immunodeficiency virus (HIV) as well as rectal and pharyngeal gonorrhea from unprotected anal sex (which can cause anal tearing and abrasions) or oral sex;

psychological effects: shock, denial, fear, guilt (some men believe that they somehow gave the perpetrator permission or feel guilty if they experienced an erection during the assault), depression, posttraumatic stress disorder (PTSD), sleep disturbances, attempted suicide, confusion about sexual orientation;

social effects: strained relationships with family members and friends, decreased contact with family members and friends, inability to form close and trusting relationships with other men; and

health effects: engaging in high-risk behavior (e.g., unprotected sex, trading sex for food or money) and substance use.

Emergency assessments and interventions take place immediately for sexual assault victims who report the assault. These usually include a forensic sexual assault exam (SAE), a medical evaluation of an individual who has been raped in which information and forensic evidence are collected for potential use in a law enforcement investigation.

The goals of the sexual assault exam for male victims are the treatment of injuries, prophylactic treatment to prevent infection, crisis intervention, and safety planning. Sexual assault exams typically are conducted in the emergency department of a hospital and are time-sensitive: They must take place no more than 72–96 hours after the rape because of potential loss of forensic evidence (e.g., pubic hair, bodily fluids, bruising, lacerations).

A sexual assault response team (SART) is responsible for timely response to a victim of rape, including completion of a sexual assault exam. A SART is a collaborative effort of personnel including a victim service provider/advocate, a sexual assault forensic examiner (SAFE) and/or sexual assault nurse examiner (SANE), a law enforcement officer, a crime laboratory specialist, and the prosecutor who will prosecute the case. As a result of the creation of sexual assault response teams at the initial point of care (emergency departments of hospitals), most rape victims now receive prompt medical treatment, forensic evidence collection, thorough documentation of the sexual assault, crisis counseling, and safety planning.

Most victims of sexual assault require continued support after the sexual assault exam is completed. Crisis hotlines, individual or group therapy, and support groups can provide support and therapeutic interventions. Victims most often utilize these services when experiencing symptoms of PTSD.

Crisis hotline services may be utilized by victims of sexual assault.

These hotlines usually are accessible 24 hours a day. The goals of a crisis hotline are to help the caller cope effectively with the crisis, to educate the caller on facts of sexual assault as well as possible short- and long-term impacts, and to inform the caller of safety resources as well as possible medical and legal resources.

The crisis-line counselor should be nonjudgmental, use active listening skills, help the victim identify and clarify his feelings, help the victim explore all of his options, and provide empathic responses.

Researchers have found that these hotlines can be invaluable in helping victims navigate the complex medical and legal systems after their assault.

RAINN reports that males tend to find it easier to talk about their sexual assault with an anonymous person answering a crisis hotline than with a family member or friend. Talking to a crisis-line operator who listens well and is helpful may help male victims feel more comfortable telling a family member or friend about the sexual assault at a later time.

Male victims also might seek out individual therapy after a sexual assault. Several therapeutic interventions have been noted to be beneficial for individuals who have experienced the trauma of sexual assault.

Psychodynamic therapy (also known as insight-oriented therapy) targets the client's avoidance symptoms and resolution of any inner conflicts. The therapist helps the client understand the conscious and unconscious meanings of the symptoms he may be experiencing as a result of the trauma of sexual assault.

A case study of a male victim of sexual assault reported that the victim's distress and PTSD symptoms improved significantly through psychodynamic therapy sessions.

Eye movement desensitization and reprocessing (EMDR) is a treatment often used with victims of trauma. The therapist asks the client to produce images, thoughts, and feelings related to the sexual assault and to evaluate their distressing qualities. The client is then asked to generate alternative pleasing thoughts and images while using specific eye movements to follow the therapist as he or she waves his or her finger rapidly in front of the client's face.

In cognitive behavioral therapy (CBT), the client and therapist work together to examine the relationship between the client's thoughts, feelings, and behaviors. There are several subtypes of CBT.

In exposure therapy (also known as flooding), the client repeatedly confronts fearful images and thoughts of the traumatic sexual assault to lessen his fear and anxiety. Exposure therapy is believed to be the most effective of the CBT treatments for victims of sexual assault.

Stress inoculation therapy involves the therapist teaching the client concrete skills to manage anxiety and fear as they relate to the incident of sexual assault.

Multiple channel exposure therapy educates the client on panic and trauma and uses breathing exercises that help in reducing panic and anxiety.

Cognitive processing therapy (CPT) helps the victim process the sexual assault by confronting cognitive distortions and maladaptive beliefs concerning the sexual trauma (e.g., no one will ever love me now that I have been raped).

CPT for sexual assault survivors usually consists of 12 weekly hour-and-a-half-long sessions.

One study reported that at the conclusion of CPT treatment, none of the participants in the study, all of whom had a diagnosis of PTSD, met the full criteria for PTSD; this was maintained at 6 months following treatment.

Adlerian art therapy incorporates visual, linguistic, symbolic, and sensory expressions. Victims who feel detached or numb often begin to experience a connection to their trauma as they use different areas of their brains in the process of creating art.

Research has examined the benefits for sexual assault victims of therapy that includes their spouses or partners.

A study researched the use of solution-oriented therapy (SOT) (also called solution-focused therapy) with sexual assault survivors and their spouses/partners who had both disclosed negative impacts on their sexual functioning as a result of a sexual assault. The research suggests that SOT empowers the victim as well as the partner to regain a sense of control, improves mutual sexual functioning, and decreases the victim's PTSD symptoms.

SOT is brief (several sessions only), goal oriented, and focused on solutions rather than problems or symptoms.

SOT uses the miracle question (How would your future look different if the problem were no longer present?), scaling questions, coping questions, and problem-free talk (in which the client talks about problem-free areas of his life). These types of questions are intended to help the victim envision what he wants to change in his life and then use those desired changes as goals to work on in therapy.

A Canadian descriptive study of the use of services by male victims of sexual assault reported that men valued and benefited from services such as crisis counseling, medical treatment, HIV counseling, and safety planning. The study also pointed to the need for gender-sensitive services rather than female-centered services.

A 2013 study examined differences between male and female victims of sexual assault in their recovery from PTSD.

Women in the study had higher levels of guilt and shame than men did, and men reported higher levels of anger. Both reported similar levels of depression at the outset of the study.

Through CPT sessions, both the males and females reported a significant decrease in PTSD symptoms at the end of the study as well as at the follow-up.

However, the symptom that did not decrease for the majority of men was anger. Further studies should focus on how to specifically address anger issues in treatment of male victims of sexual assault.

What Can Be Done

Learn about assessment of and interventions for male victims of sexual assault; share this information with your colleagues.

Use this knowledge to accurately and sensitively assess your clients' individual characteristics and mental and physical health education needs.

Develop an awareness of your own cultural values, beliefs, and biases and develop knowledge about the histories, traditions, and values of your clients. Adopt treatment methodologies that reflect the cultural needs of the client.

If in a clinical setting, conduct a biopsychosocial-spiritual assessment, making sure to ask about any history of sexual violence. Use treatment interventions (cognitive behavioral therapy, psychotherapy, eye movement desensitization) to address PTSD, depression, and anxiety. Teach relaxation and meditation methods as well as coping skills. If not in a clinical setting, make referrals as needed.

Listen, encourage, validate, provide resources, and normalize the client's reactions to sexual assault. Educate client about medical and legal procedures should he choose to pursue those. Be extremely familiar with both local and state policies regarding sexual assault.

Assess for suicidality and make safety plan and referrals as appropriate.

If applicable, collaborate with hospital staff and law enforcement (if client decides to file a report).

Encourage the client to attend local rape support groups and use crisis hotlines (e.g., MaleSurvivor at http://www.malesurvivor.org) as appropriate. Ask agencies if they provide services specifically for male victims. Advocate for services for male victims if not available.

When applicable, explain the plan for all follow-up appointments and provide details in writing.

Explain the importance of having HIV and other STD tests done at 2, 4, and 6 months after the assault.

Help the client build or increase his social support system.

Written by Melissa Rosales Neff, MSW

Reviewed by Jessica Therivel, LMSW-IPR

References

International Federation of Social Workers. (2012, March). Statement of ethical principles. Retrieved January 15, 2015, from http://ifsw.org/policies/statement-of-ethical-principles/

Wheeler, D. (2015). *NASW standards for cultural competency in social work practice.* Retrieved March 3, 2015, from http://www.socialworkers.org/practice/standards/PRA-BRO-253150-CC-Standards.pdf

British Association of Social Workers. (2012, January). The code of ethics for social work: Statement of principles. Retrieved October 11, 2015, from http://cdn.basw.co.uk/upload/basw_112315-7.pdf

Abbas, A., & Macfie, J. (2013). Supportive and insight-oriented psychodynamic psychotherapy for posttraumatic stress disorder in an adult male survivor of sexual assault. *Clinical Case Studies, 12*(2), 145-156. doi:10.1177/1534650112471154

Beckerman, N. L., & Pass, J. (2008). After the assault: Cognitive trauma therapy with a single even trauma victim. *Clinical Social Work Journal, 36*(3), 255-263. doi:10.1007/s10615-008-0145-5

Bullock, C. M., & Beckson, M. (2011). Male victims of sexual assault: Phenomenology, psychology, and physiology. *Journal of American Academy Psychiatry Law, 39*(2), 197-205.

Centers for Disease Control and Prevention. (2012). Sexual violence: Facts at a glance. Retrieved June 18, 2014, from http://www.cdc.gov/ViolencePrevention/pdf/sv-datasheet-a.pdf

Department of Defense. (2013). Fiscal year 2012. *Department of Defense annual report on sexual assault in the military.* Washington, DC: Author.

Du Mont, J., Macdonald, S., White, M., & Turner, L. (2013). Male victims of adult sexual assault: A descriptive study of survivors' use of sexual assault treatment services. *Journal of Interpersonal Violence, 28*(13), 2676-2694. doi:10.1177/0886260513487993

Federal Bureau of Investigation. (2013). Frequently asked questions about the change in the UCR definition of rape. Retrieved October 11, 2015, from http://www.fbi.gov/about-us/cjis/ucr/recent-program-updates/new-rape-definition-frequently-asked-questions

Galovsky, T., Blain, L., Chappuis, C., & Fletcher, T. (2013). Sex differences in recovery from PTSD in male and female interpersonal assault survivors. *Behaviour Research and Therapy*, *51*(6), 247-255. doi:10.1016/j.brat.2013.02.002

Macy, R., Giattina, M., Sangster, T., Crosby, C., & Montijo, N. J. (2009). Domestic violence and sexual assault services: Inside the black box. *Aggression & Violent Behavior*, *14*(5), 359-373.

McLean, I., Balding, V., & White, C. (2005). Further aspects of male-on-male rape and sexual assault in greater Manchester. *Medicine, Science, and the Law*, *45*, 225-232. doi:10.1258/rsmmsl.45.3.225

National Center for Victims of Crime. (1997). Fact sheets: Male rape. Retrieved October 11, 2015, from http://www.svfreenyc.org/survivors_factsheet_38.html

Office for Victims of Crime. (2013). Sexual assault. Retrieved October 11, 2015, from https://www.ovcttac.gov/downloads/views/TrainingMaterials/NVAA/Documents_NVAA2011/ResourcePapers/Color_Sexual percent20Assault percent20Resource percent20Paper_2012_final percent20- percent20508c_9_13_2012.pdf

Office on Women's Health, U.S. Department of Health and Human Services. (2009). Sexual assault: Frequently asked questions. Retrieved October 11, 2015, from https://www.womenshealth.gov/publications/our-publications/fact-sheet/sexual-assault.html

Rape, Abuse & Incest National Network (RAINN). (2014). Male sexual assault. Retrieved October 11, 1970, from http://www.rainn.org/get-information/types-of-sexual-assault/male-sexual-assault

Rosen-Saltzman, M., Matic, M., & Marsden, E. (2013). Adlerian art therapy with sexual abuse and assault survivors. *The Journal of Individual Psychology*, *69*(3), 223-241.

Resick, P. A., & Schnicke, M. K. (1992). Cognitive processing therapy for sexual assault victims. *Journal of Consulting and Clinical Psychology*, *60*(5), 748-756.

Tambling, R. (2012). Solution-oriented therapy for survivors of sexual assault and their partners. *Contemporary Family Therapy*, *34*(3), 391-401. doi:10.1007/s10591-012-9200-z

U. S. Department of Justice, Office on Violence Against Women. (2013). A national protocol for sexual assault medical forensic examinations: Adults/adolescents. Second edition. Retrieved October 11, 2015, from http://www.ncjrs.gov/pdffiles1/ovw/241903.pdf

World Health Organization (WHO). (2012). Understanding and addressing violence against women: Sexual violence. Retrieved October 11, 1970, from http://apps.who.int/iris/bitstream/10665/77434/1/WHO_RHR_12.37_eng.pdf?ua=1

SEXUAL ASSAULT: FACTORS IMPACTING THE PROSECUTION OF PERPETRATORS

MAJOR CATEGORIES: Incarceration/Probation, Violence

WHAT WE KNOW

Sexual assault is any type of sexual activity that is nonconsensual (including when the victim is unable to provide consent), whether physical, verbal, visual (e.g., being forced to view pornographic images), or any other type of unwanted sexual contact or attention.

Examples include

- rape within marriage or dating relationships;
- rape by acquaintances or strangers;
- gang rape (i.e., rape involving two or more perpetrators);
- unwanted sexual advances
- systematic rape (common during armed conflicts);
- inappropriate touching;
- voyeurism (i.e., when someone watches private sexual acts);
- exhibitionism (i.e., when someone exposes him/herself in public); and incest (i.e., sexual contact between family members).

In 2013 the United States Federal Bureau of Investigation began using a more inclusive definition of rape (formally defined as "the carnal knowledge of a female forcibly and against her will"): "the penetration, no matter how slight, of the vagina or anus with any body part or object, or oral penetration by a sex organ of another person, without consent of the victim."

Sexual assault is a crime that has implications for public health.

In 2012, investigators for a study by the U.S. Centers for Disease Control and Prevention (CDC) on sexual assault in the United States reported.

- 1 in 5 women reported experiencing rape at some time in their lives
- 37.4 percent of female rape victims were first raped between ages 18 and 24
- 1 in 7 men reported experiencing rape at some time in their lives
- 4.8 percent of men reported that they were made to penetrate someone else at some point in their lives

Sexual assault is one of the most underreported crimes. The Rape, Abuse & Incest National Network (RAINN) reports that of every 100 rapes in the United States, only 40 are reported to the police. Of those 40 reports, 10 lead to an arrest. From those 10 arrests, 8 alleged perpetrators are prosecuted. Of those 8 perpetrators, 3 will be convicted of a felony and be incarcerated.

The U.S. Bureau of Justice reported that from 2006 to 2010, rape or sexual assault was one of the most underreported crimes in the United States: 65 percent of victimizations were not reported.

Posttraumatic stress disorder (PTSD) symptomatology can affect the reporting behavior of a sexual assault victim. Investigators found that when victims had symptoms related to re-experiencing the trauma or hyperarousal, those victims were more likely to report the assault. When victims had symptoms related to avoidance, those victims were less likely to report.

Reporting behavior for victims of sexual assault may differ for victims from Western nations versus those from non-Western nations. Researchers found that Western victims were more likely in general to report being a victim of sexual assault to the police. In non-Western nations, sexual assault victims living in urban areas were less likely than those in rural areas to report victimization to the police. This is the opposite of tendencies in Western nations.

Individuals with intellectual disabilities are more likely to be the victims of sexual assault and have higher rates of underreporting than individuals without intellectual disabilities.

In interacting with the justice system, victims of sexual assault with intellectual disabilities are more likely to have difficulty communicating testimony in a way that can result in a suspect's being identified and charged and can face more challenges with communication if the case gets to a courtroom setting.

After an alleged perpetrator of sexual assault in the United States has been arrested, the judicial system must decide whether to indict the individual or to dismiss the case. Charges are less likely to be filed in sexual assault cases if:

- the victim does not report the incident right away(e.g., victim reports assault to the police 6 months after it takes place);
- the victim's statements about what he or she experienced are inconsistent;
- there are questions about the victim's moral character or conduct(e.g., criminal record, DUIs);
- the victim is unwilling to cooperate with the investigation; and
- the suspect is a stranger rather than an acquaintance of the victim (a stranger is harder to track down and arrest than an acquaintance).

If the investigation finds sufficient information to support the filing of a criminal case, charges are filed and the suspect is arrested. The prosecutor's office then decides whether to actually take the case to court

In a study of 465 sexual assault cases handled by a large metropolitan police department in the U.S. Midwest, only 35.2 percent of the cases resulted in an arrest. Only 45 of the 465 cases (9.7 percent) were approved for felony charges by the prosecutor's office.

Factors leading to a perpetrator's being found guilty of a sexual assault can be divided into three categories: victim characteristics, the involvement of a sexual assault nurse examiner (SANE), and forensic evidence

Characteristics of victims play a role in determining whether alleged perpetrators of sexual assault are charged with a crime

In a study of 666 sexual assault cases that resulted in an arrest, the following victim characteristics were identified as influencing prosecutors' decisions: whether the victim had a prior criminal record, whether the victim had been using substances (alcohol and/or drugs) prior to the assault, and whether the victim had voluntarily invited the alleged perpetrator into his or her home.

In another study researchers found that a victim's ability to articulate the details of an assault affects whether the perpetrator is prosecuted. The same study found that whether the victim engaged in risk-taking behavior (such as drug or alcohol use) either in the present case or in the past influences whether the alleged perpetrator is prosecuted.

SANEs practicing in rural settings may face more challenges than those in urban settings. Researchers found that in a rural medical setting, the SANE frequently had fewer resources, came up against local legal experts who were less familiar with SANEs, and, in rural settings with more limited exposure to sexual assault, dealt with legal entities that may be less inclined to prosecute.

The involvement of a SANE can affect prosecution of a perpetrator.

In the 1970s the sexual assault nurse examiner specialty was created by the nursing profession to staff emergency rooms with nurses specifically trained to provide first-response care to sexual assault victims. These nurses have received training in the dynamics of sexual assault, the assessment of victims, the elements of a forensic interview, DNA testing, and therapeutic communication.

Researchers conducting a longitudinal study reported that more cases of sexual assault resulted in a conviction after the development of SANE programs than before SANE programs. Because they facilitate the successful collection of forensic evidence, SANE programs appear to be an important factor in addressing the problem of low rates of prosecution of sexual assault cases.

In another study, investigators reported that SANEs aid the prosecution of perpetrators of sexual assault by serving as fact witnesses and expert witnesses during sexual assault trials. Their testimony often leads to successful prosecution of a sexual assault perpetrator.

Alleged perpetrators of sexual assault are more likely to be charged and convicted if forensic evidence is collected from victims

Investigators studying 821 sexual assaults found that the factor most associated with successful prosecution of a perpetrator was the presence of physical evidence of body trauma, genital trauma, or both. The authors of the study stated that the presence of trauma evidence establishes the veracity of the incident and can be compelling to the jury and judge.

Researchers for another study of 888 sexual assault cases found a high correlation between cases in which there was forensic evidence of anogenital trauma and conviction of the perpetrator of sexual assault.

Despite the positive correlation between severe body or genital trauma and successful prosecution of a sexual assault perpetrator, it is important to note that when testifying in court, forensic examiners must educate the judge and jury that the absence of dramatic forensic evidence should not discount the victim's claim. In cases of assault, it is possible that physical trauma may not be identified or semen not be found (perhaps because the victim delayed going to the hospital or bathed after the assault).

WHAT CAN BE DONE

Learn about factors that affect the prosecution of perpetrators of sexual assault; share this information with your colleagues.

Use your knowledge to accurately and sensitively assess your clients' individual characteristics and mental health and physical health education needs.

Develop an awareness of your own cultural values, beliefs, and biases and develop knowledge about the histories, traditions, and values of your clients. Adopt treatment methodologies that reflect the cultural needs of the client.

Educate your clients on the police and legal process of filing charges of sexual assault and court proceedings.

Educate your clients on the factors that influence the prosecution of perpetrators of sexual assault so that they may be more willing to submit to a forensic examination.

Connect your clients with local resources such as rape crisis centers and support groups for sexual assault victims.

Written by Melissa Rosales Neff, MSW

Reviewed by Laura Gale, LCSW, and Chris Bates, MA, MSW

REFERENCES

Alderden, M. A., & Ullman, S. E. (2012). Creating a more complete and current picture: examining police and prosecutor decision-making when processing sexual assault cases. *Violence Against Women, 18*(5), 525-551. doi:10.1177/1077801212453867

Annan, S. L. (2015). "We desperately need some help here" – The experience of legal experts with sexual assault and evidence collection in rural communities. *Rural & Remote Health, 14*(4), 1-13.

Antaki, C., Richardson, E., Stokoe, E., & Willott, S. (2015). Can people with intellectual disability resist implications of fault when police question their allegations of sexual assault and rape? *Intellectual and Developmental Disabilities, 53*(5), 346-357. doi:10.1352/1934-9556-53.5.346

Beichner, D., & Spohn, C. (2012). Modeling the effects of victim behavior and moral character on prosecutors' charging decisions in sexual assault cases. *Violence & Victims, 27*(1), 3-24. doi:10.1891/0886-6708.27.1.3

British Association of Social Workers. (2012). The code of ethics for social work: Statement of principles. Retrieved April 17, 2016, from http://cdn.basw.co.uk/upload/basw_112315-7.pdf

Bureau of Justice Statistics, Office of Justice Programs, U.S. Department of Justice. (2012). National crime victimization survey: Victimizations not reported to the police, 2006-2010. Retrieved April 17, 2016, from http://www.bjs.gov/content/pub/pdf/vnrp0610.pdf

Campbell, R., Patterson, D., & Bybee, D. (2012). Prosecution of adult sexual assault cases: a longitudinal analysis of the impact of a sexual assault nurse examiner program. *Violence Against Women, 18*(2), 223-244. doi:10.1177/1077801212440158

Centers for Disease Control and Prevention. (2012). Sexual violence: Facts at a glance. Retrieved April 17, 2016, from http://www.cdc.gov/violenceprevention/pdf/sv-datasheet-a.pdf

Chon, D. S. (2014). Police reporting by sexual assault victims in Western and in non-Western countries. *Journal of Family Violence, 29*(8), 859-868. doi:10.1007/s10896-014-9644-z

Federal Bureau of Investigation. (2014, December 11). Frequently asked questions about the change in the UCR definition of rape. Retrieved April 17, 2016, from http://www.fbi.gov/about-us/cjis/ucr/recent-program-updates/new-rape-definition-frequently-asked-questions

Gray-Eurom, K., Seaberg, D. C., & Wears, R. L. (2002). The prosecution of sexual assault cases: Correlation with forensic evidence. *Annals of Emergency Medicine, 39*(1), 39-46. doi:10.1067/mem.2002.118013

International Federation of Social Workers. (2012, March 3). Statement of ethical principles. Retrieved April 17, 2016, from http://ifsw.org/policies/statement-of-ethical-principles/

Maier, S. L. (2012). Sexual assault nurse examiners' perceptions of their relationship with doctors, rape victim advocates, police, and prosecutors. *Journal of Interpersonal Violence, 27*(7), 1314-1340. doi:10.1177/0886260511425242

McGregor, M. J., DuMont, J., & Myhr, T. L. (2002). Sexual assault forensic medical examination: Is evidence related to successful prosecution? *Annals of Emergency Medicine, 39*(6), 639-647.

Wheeler, D. (2015). NASW standards and indicators for cultural competence in social work practice. Retrieved April 17, 2016, from http://www.socialworkers.org/practice/standards/PRA-BRO-253150-CC-Standards.pdf

Office on Women's Health, U.S. Department of Health and Human Services. (2015). Sexual assault. Retrieved April 17, 2016, from https://www.womenshealth.gov/publications/our-publications/fact-sheet/sexual-assault.html

Ort, J. A. (2002). The sexual assault nurse examiner: a nurse who is crucial to treating victims and prosecuting assailants. *American Journal of Nursing, 102*(9), 24-26.

Rape, Abuse, & Incest National Network. (2014). Reporting rates. Retrieved April 17, 2016, from https://www.rainn.org/get-information/statistics/reporting-rates

Spohn, C., & Holleran, D. (2001). Prosecuting sexual assault: A comparison of charging decisions in sexual assault cases involving strangers, acquaintances, and intimate partners. *Justice Quarterly, 18*(3), 651-688. doi:10.1080/07418820100095051

Walsh, R. M., & Bruce, S. E. (2014). Reporting decisions after sexual assault: The impact of mental health variables. *Psychological Trauma: Theory, Research, Practice & Policy, 6*(6), 691-699. doi:10.1037/a0036592

Wiley, J., Sugar, N., Fine, D., & Eckert, L. (2003). Legal outcomes of sexual assault. *American Journal of Obstetrics and Gynecology, 188*(6), 1638-1641. doi:10.1067/mob.2003.396

World Health Organization (WHO). (2012). Understanding and addressing violence against women: Sexual violence. Retrieved April 17, 2016, from http://www.who.int/reproductivehealth/topics/violence/vaw_series/en

SEXUAL ASSAULT: PSYCHOSOCIAL EFFECTS ON ADULT MALE VICTIMS

MAJOR CATEGORIES: Incarceration/Probation, Violence

WHAT WE KNOW

Sexual assault is any type of sexual activity that is nonconsensual (including activity that occurs when one is unable to provide consent), whether physical, verbal, visual (e.g., forcing someone to look at pornography), or any other type of unwanted sexual contact or attention.

Examples include the following:
- rape within marriage or dating relationships;
- rape by acquaintances or strangers, gang rape (i.e., rape involving two or more perpetrators);
- systematic rape (common during armed conflicts);
- unwanted sexual advances;
- inappropriate touching;
- voyeurism (i.e., when someone watches private sexual acts);
- exhibitionism (i.e., when someone exposes him/herself in public);
- incest (i.e., sexual contact between family members); and
- sexual harassment.

In 2013 the United States Federal Bureau of Investigation began using a more inclusive definition of rape (formerly defined as "the carnal knowledge of a female forcibly and against her will"): "the penetration, no matter how slight, of the vagina or anus with any body part or object, or oral penetration by a sex organ of another person, without consent of the victim."

More specifically, rape of a male is any kind of sexual assault that involves forced penetration of the anus or mouth by a penis, finger, or any other object.

Sexual assault is a criminal and a public health problem.

Retrospective studies in the United States of male sexual assault indicate that 3–7 percent of men report that they have experienced sexual assault in adulthood, usually taking place in their 20s or 30s.

The Rape, Abuse, and Incest National Network (RAINN) reports that approximately 10 percent of sexual assault victims in the United States are males.

A 2011 national survey by the U.S. Centers for Disease Control and Prevention (CDC) on sexual assault found that.
- 6.7 percent of men reported experiencing rape at some time in their lives; and
- 5.8 percent of men experienced sexual coercion and 10.8 percent of men experienced unwanted sexual contact.

Although 10–20 percent of female victims of sexual assault in the United States report the crime, the percentage of males who disclose and file a report is much lower.

Although most perpetrators of sexual assault of males are male, it is important to note that women can sexually assault males.

In a study it was reported that male victims were more likely to be assaulted by groups (two or more perpetrators), rather than by individuals.

The effects of sexual assault on men have not been researched extensively. Sexual assault in men is underreported. However, male victims of sexual assault who have been interviewed and cases that have been investigated indicate that men experience negative psychosocial effects as a result of sexual assault. It is important to note that men may experience none, some, or many of the following effects. Effects(s) of sexual assault are influenced by the victim's relationship with the perpetrator, the duration of the assault, and the response of family members and friends to the assault.

The following are well-documented possible effects of sexual assault on men:

Guilt/blame. Some male victims blame themselves for the sexual assault, feeling that they somehow gave permission to the perpetrator or were at fault for not being able to physically defend themselves.

Male victims can also feel guilt or blame if they experienced an erection or ejaculated during the assault, giving the impression that they enjoyed the experience. Research indicates that increased anxiety, fear, and other intense emotions can cause involuntary arousal and ejaculation for male sexual assault victims.

Sexually transmitted diseases. Male victims are at risk of acquiring human immunodeficiency virus (HIV) as well as rectal and pharyngeal gonorrhea from unprotected anal sex (which can cause anal tearing and abrasions) or oral sex. Six-month follow-up tests for these conditions are recommended.

Confusion about sexual orientation. Male victims may be confused about their sexual identity after an assault by another male. Heterosexual males may wonder if they are gay if they experienced an erection during the rape.

Mistrust of men (if assaulted by a male). Male victims may experience an inability to form close and trusting relationships with other males.

Mood disturbances/suicide. Male victims may experience loss of appetite, changes in sleep patterns, anger, anxiety, depression, suicidal ideations, and mood swings.

Posttraumatic stress disorder (PTSD). PTSD is a mental health disorder that can occur following the experience of a traumatic event (such as a natural disaster, combat, or a sexual assault). A victim of sexual assault with PTSD has feelings of anxiety, stress, and fear that last for more than a month. The victim continually relives the sexual assault in his mind. He may also avoid places or events that remind him of the assault. He may experience hyperarousal, in which he is easily startled and may have angry outbursts.

The most effective treatments for PTSD are cognitive behavioral therapy (CBT), which helps the client identify unhealthy beliefs and behaviors and replace them with positive ones, and eye movement desensitization and reprocessing (EMDR), in which guided eye movement is used to help process traumatic memories. Research indicates that these treatments help reduce symptoms of PTSD.

Male victims can be slower to seek out counseling services than females. Of 115 male victims of sexual assault in one study, the mean amount of time that elapsed from the attack to when they sought counseling services was 16 years.

It has been documented that there are few resources that are focused on helping male victims of sexual assault, as opposed to female victims.

In a survey of 30 different agencies (medical facilities, mental health agencies, community rape crisis centers) that advertised themselves as rape crisis or sexual assault service providers, 11 indicated that they did not provide services to male victims. Ten stated that they could theoretically provide services to males but had never done so. Nine had dealt with at least one male in the past year.

WHAT CAN BE DONE

Learn about male sexual assault and its possible psychosocial effects; share this information with your colleagues.

Use your knowledge to accurately and sensitively assess your client's individual characteristics as well as his healthcare and health education needs.

Develop an awareness of your own cultural values, beliefs, and biases and develop knowledge about the histories, traditions, and values of your clients. Adopt treatment methodologies that reflect the cultural needs of the client.

Practice with awareness of, and adherence to, the social work principles of respect for human rights and human dignity, social justice, and professional conduct as described in the International Federation of Social Workers (IFSW) Statement of Ethical Principles as well as the ethical standards and principles of social work associations in the United States, Great Britain, and Australia. Become knowledgeable of the IFSW ethical standards as they apply to victims of sexual assault, and practice accordingly.

If in a clinical setting, use treatment interventions (cognitive behavioral therapy, psychotherapy, eye movement desensitization and reprocessing) to address PTSD, depression, and anxiety. Teach relaxation and meditation methods as well as coping skills. If not in a clinical setting, make referrals as needed.

Make referrals to peer-based support groups or other community resources (e.g., MaleSurvivor at http://www.malesurvivor.org).

Assess for suicidality and make a safety plan and referrals as appropriate.

If applicable, collaborate with hospital staff and law enforcement (if victim decides to file a report).

Encourage client to join local rape support groups and call crisis hotlines, as appropriate. Ask agencies whether they provide services specifically for male victims.

When applicable, explain the plan for all follow-up appointments and provide details in writing.

Explain the importance of having HIV or other STD tests done at 2, 4, and 6 months after an assault.

Written by Melissa Rosales Neff, MSW

Reviewed by Laura Gale, LCSW

REFERENCES

Boyd, C. (2011). Australian Center for the Study of Sexual Assault: The impacts of sexual assault on women. Retrieved April 23, 2016, from https://aifs.gov.au/publications/impacts-sexual-assault-women

British Association of Social Workers. (2012, January). The code of ethics for social work: Statement of principles. Retrieved April 23, 2016, from http://cdn.basw.co.uk/upload/basw_112315-7.pdf

Bullock, C. M., & Beckson, M. (2011). Male victims of sexual assault: Phenomenology, psychology, and physiology. *Journal of American Academy Psychiatry Law, 39*(2), 197-205.

Centers for Disease Control and Prevention. (2014). Sexual violence: Facts at a glance. Retrieved April 21, 2016, from http://www.cdc.gov/violenceprevention/pdf/sv-factsheet.pdf

Federal Bureau of Investigation. (2014). Frequently asked questions about the change in the UCR definition of rape. Retrieved April 23, 2016, from http://www.fbi.gov/about-us/cjis/ucr/recent-program-updates/new-rape-definition-frequently-asked-questions

International Federation of Social Workers. (2012, March 3). Statement of ethical principles. Retrieved April 23, 2016, from http://ifsw.org/policies/statement-of-ethical-principles/

King, M., & Woollett, E. (1997). Sexually assaulted males: 115 men consulting a counseling service. *Archives of Sexual Behavior, 26*(6), 579-588. doi:10.1023/A:1024520225196

McLean, I., Balding, V., & White, C. (2005). Further aspects of male-on-male rape and sexual assault in greater Manchester. *Medicine, Science, and the Law, 45*, 225-232. doi:10.1258/rsmmsl.45.3.225

McLean, I. A. (2013). The male victim of assault. *Best Practice & Research. Clinical Obstetrics and Gynaecology, 27*(1), 39-46. doi:10.1016/j.bpobgyn.2012.08.006

Office on Women's Health. (2012, July 16). Sexual assault: Frequently asked questions. Retrieved April 23, 2016, from http://www.womenshealth.gov/publications/our-publications/fact-sheet/sexual-assault.html

National Association of Social Workers. (2015). Standards and indicators for cultural competence in social work practice. Retrieved March 2, 2016, from http://www.socialworkers.org/practice/standards/PRA-BRO-253150-CC-Standards.pdf

New York City Alliance Against Sexual Assault. (2014). Factsheets: Male rape. Retrieved May 21, 2014, from http://www.svfreenyc.org/survivors_factsheet_38.html

Rape, Abuse & Incest National Network (RAINN). (2014). Sexual assault of men and boys. Retrieved June 29, 2015, from http://www.rainn.org/get-information/types-of-sexual-assault/male-sexual-assault

SEXUAL HARASSMENT AT WORK: SUPPORTING VICTIMS

MAJOR CATEGORIES: Community

WHAT WE KNOW

Sexual harassment is unwanted verbal or physical conduct of a sexual nature that results in feelings of humiliation, embarrassment, or intimidation in another person.

Legally, there are two types of sexual harassment in the U.S. workplace: *quid pro quo* sexual harassment, in which sexual cooperation is required in return for employment or promotion, and hostile environment sexual harassment, in which unwelcome sexual conduct from a harasser creates an uncomfortable environment in the workplace. The former constitutes 5 percent of sexual harassment cases and the latter 95 percent of reported instances of sexual harassment in the United States. Instances of sexual harassment in the workplace are known to be significantly underreported for fear of job loss or retaliation.

Examples of sexual harassment in the workplace include:

- unwelcome comments about a person's physical characteristics or sexual behavior;
- whistling or other sexually suggestive sounds or gestures;
- obscene jokes told to coworkers or employees;
- asking about private matters or asking for dates repeatedly after the victim has refused;
- sending inappropriate email messages from work computers or text messages during work hours;
- showing any pictures of a sexual nature, such as pornography, in the workplace;
- speculating about a person's sexual orientation or asking him or her directly about his or her sexual behaviors; and
- physically touching another person in the workplace in a way that makes him or her feel uncomfortable.

Perpetrators and victims of sexual harassment in the workplace can be men or women, and the victim and the perpetrator may be of the same sex. However, the majority of victims of workplace sexual harassment are women and the majority of harassers are men.

Female victims of sexual harassment tend to be vulnerable (e.g., divorced or separated women, women who live alone, young women, women with financial problems, women who have recently experienced domestic violence, women with disabilities, lesbians, non-white women).

In a study of Mexican immigrant farm workers in Oregon,researchers found that the workplace environment for farm workers is a place of increased vulnerability to sexual harassment for women due to low social status, poverty, cultural issues(e.g., traditional societal norms and acceptance of harassment), and isolation (e.g., for women who only know indigenous languages and do not know Spanish).

In another study researchers found that teenage girls who are employed and sexually harassed develop negative attitudes toward work and tend to withdraw from academics.

Male victims of sexual harassment tend to be gay men or young men.

Researchers in a study highlighted that even female executives in high-power positions are sexually harassed by male subordinates and often feel powerless. These victims report feeling a loss of control over their bodies, a destruction of their gender identity, and an increased desire to quit their jobs.

The harasser in a workplace may be a supervisor, a co-worker, a subordinate, or a non-employee (e.g., a customer).

The U.S. Equal Employment Opportunity Commission (EEOC) investigates allegations of sexual harassment in workplaces. In its investigations both the circumstances of the alleged harassment (i.e., the nature of the sexual conduct) and the context in which the alleged incident occurred are examined.

In 2014 the EEOC received 6,862 complaints of sexual harassment in the workplace. Males filed 17.5 percent of the complaints; females filed 84.5 percent.

Results from a study of nurses and midwives in a hospital setting in Australia indicated that 34.4 percent of the nurses and midwives had been sexually harassed in their workplace, a hospital which has zero-tolerance policies regarding aggression.

In a study of 265 female hospital personnel in Italy, 54 percent stated that they had been sexually harassed at work in the previous 12 months.

Results from a quantitative review of 136 journal articles worldwide indicated that 25 percent of nurses had been exposed to sexual harassment in the workplace.

The psychosocial impact of sexual harassment on victims can be extensive and debilitating. Emotional and physical reactions to harassment include poor concentration at work, stress on personal relationships, self-blame, fear, anxiety, depression, increased absenteeism, and post-traumatic stress disorder (PTSD).

Researchers of a Norwegian longitudinal study found that sexual harassment in the workplace contributed significantly to psychological distress for female victims.

Results of another study indicated that sexual harassment in the workplace was a strong predictor of alcohol and drug use and other mental health issues for victims.

Researchers have reported that sexual harassment is consistently associated with PTSD symptoms as well as PTSD diagnosis.

Researchers found that sexual harassment combined with racial harassment negatively impacts the psychological well-being of victims.

Results of a meta analysis of 49 studies indicate that sexual harassment leads to adverse job-related outcomes (e.g., less job satisfaction, lower job performance), physical outcomes (e.g., headaches, sleep disturbances, gastrointestinal disorders), and psychological outcomes (e.g., distress, depression, lower self-esteem).

Male victims of sexual assault often report higher levels of shock and surprise following sexual harassment than female victims because their own perceptions of their gender (i.e., that men are strong and should not be vulnerable to sexual harassment) increase their feelings of self-blame (i.e., that they should not have allowed themselves to be sexually harassed).

The impact of sexual harassment on the workplace itself can be extensive. Sexual harassment may tarnish a company's reputation, increase payouts of sick leave and medical leave for victims, increase legal costs, lower staff productivity, and contribute to poor staff morale and impaired teamwork.

An integral part of supporting a victim of sexual harassment is knowing the policies and procedures regarding sexual harassment in the workplace. In the United States many of these policies are determined by state law. It is vital for the victim and any advocates to be familiar with the laws.

Most workplaces have adopted the Employment Equity Act or other sexual harassment policies that define prohibited behaviors and detail the steps that will be taken by the employer if sexual harassment occurs. All employees, particularly victims of harassment, should familiarize themselves with these policies.

If he or she feels safe doing so, it is important for the victim to confront the harasser. Research indicates that ignoring sexual harassment, avoiding the harasser, or making a joke about the harassment does little to stop the harasser from continuing to harass.

Confronting a harasser can increase a victim's self-esteem and help him or her feel that he or she is gaining control of the situation. The victim should tell the harasser that he or she does not appreciate the harasser's comments or actions and that the harasser needs to stop. The victim should be specific and name the behavior that he or she wants the harasser to stop. If the victim decides to confront the harasser in writing rather than face to face, he or she should keep a copy of the document for his or her records.

The victim should document all incidents of harassment. The victim should keep a log in which each incident of sexual harassment is noted, including the time and place it occurred and the names of any witnesses to the incident. The victim should include as much detail as possible and keep the log in a safe place such as his or her home.

The victim should also document any of his or her own negative reactions a result of the workplace sexual harassment.

The victim has the option to begin a grievance procedure process. The employee handbook should lay out the procedure for beginning this process in the victim's particular workplace.

If the victim meets with managers to inform them of the harassment, he or she should document who was at the meeting, what was said, and what actions were agreed upon.

The victim should also contact the workplace's head of human resources to inform him or her of the sexual harassment.

In the United States, the victim also may file a formal complaint with the Equal Employment Opportunity Commission.

Victims in the United States may want to contact a lawyer who is familiar with the employer's obligations under Title VII of the Civil Rights Act of 1964, which prohibits discrimination in employment on the basis of sex, race, color, national origin, and religion.

The victim can seek support for the negative impacts of harassment by:

- understanding that the behavior he or she experienced constituted harassment and that it was not his or her fault. Self-blame is one of the most common psychosocial effects of sexual harassment;
- joining a support group of others who have experienced sexual harassment in the workplace;
- strengthening his or her support network; and
- attending therapy if symptoms of sexual harassment become debilitating or if he or she would like to process the incident(s) with someone other than a friend or family member.

Conclusions from a study of PTSD resulting from sexual harassment indicated that high levels of self-blame were negatively related to recovery and fear of future harassment. Therefore, it is important for victims to address self-blame in therapy.

WHAT CAN BE DONE

Become knowledgeable about sexual harassment in the workplace so you can accurately assess your client's personal characteristics and health education needs; share this information with your colleagues.

Develop an awareness of your own cultural values, beliefs, and biases and develop knowledge about the histories, traditions, and values of your clients. Adopt treatment methodologies that reflect the cultural needs of the client.

Prevention is vital. Education about sexual harassment can help in prevention. Collaborate with management in workplaces to ensure that sexual harassment policies are in place and are widely disseminated and help with any sexual harassment training.

Support client and assist him or her in identifying grievance procedures in the workplace; support client in the decision whether to make a formal grievance or pursue litigation.

If in a clinical setting:

- Listen carefully to the client without judgment.
- Conduct a biopsychosocialspiritual assessment, making sure to ask about any history of sexual violence.
- Consider using behaviorally worded questions: ask specific questions about the behaviors that occurred during the alleged incident rather than asking, "Were you sexually harassed?" The term "sexual harassment" often should be avoided because some victims (especially male victims) are unlikely to define what they have experienced as sexual harassment.
- Use appropriate therapeutic interventions to address anxiety, depression, sleep disturbances, and PTSD symptoms, if applicable (e.g., cognitive behavioral therapy, solution-focused therapy, psychotherapy).

If not in a clinical setting, make referrals to mental health agencies as needed.

Written by Melissa Rosales Neff, MSW

Reviewed by Lynn B. Cooper, D. Crim, and Laura Gale, LCSW

REFERENCES

American Association of University Women. (2012). Know your rights: Workplace sexual harassment. Retrieved from http://www.aauw.org/what-we-do/legal-resources/know-your-rights-at-work/workplace-sexual-harassment/

Bridges, G. (2011). Dealing with sexual harassment in the workplace. *Dental Nursing, 7*(3), 157-159.

Buchanan, N., & Fitzgerald, L. (2008). Effects of racial and sexual harassment on work and the psychological well-being of African American women. *Journal of Occupational Health Psychology, 13*(20), 137-151.

Chan, D., Lam, C., Chow, S., & Cheung, S. (2008). Examining the job-related, psychological, and physical outcomes of workplace sexual harassment: a meta-analytic review. *Psychology of Women Quarterly, 32*, 362-376.

Demir, D., & Rodwell, J. (2012). Psychological antecedents and consequences of workplace aggression for hospital nurses. *Journal of Nursing Scholarship, 44*(4), 376-384. doi:10.1111/j.15475069.2012.01472.x

Fayankinnu, E. (2012). Female executives' experiences of contra-power sexual harassment from male subordinates in the workplace. *Bangladesh Journal of Sociology, 9*(2), 40-56.

Fielden, F., Davidson, M., Woolnoughm, H., & Hunt, C. (2010). A model of racialized sexual harassment of women in the UK workplace. *Sex Roles, 62*, 20-34.

Fineran, S., & Gruber, J. (2009). Youth at work: adolescent employment and sexual harassment. *Child Abuse & Neglect, 33*(8), 550-559.

Hibino, Y., Ogino, K., & Inagaki, M. (2006). Sexual harassment of female nurses by patients in Japan. *Journal of Nursing Scholarship, 38*(4), 400-405.

How to recognize and respond to sexual harassment in the workplace. (2010, January). *Massachusetts Nurse Advocate*, 20.

International Federation of Social Workers. (2012, March 3). Statement of ethical principles. Retrieved December 1, 1970, from http://ifsw.org/policies/statement-of-ethical-principles/

Larsen, S. E., & Fitzgerald, L. F. (2011). PTSD symptoms and sexual harassment: The role of attributions and perceived control. *Journal of Interpersonal Violence, 26*(13), 2555-2567. doi:10.1177/0886260510388284

McDonald, P. (2012). Workplace sexual harassment 30 years on: A review of the literature. *International Journal of Management Reviews, 14*(1), 1-17. doi:10.1111/j.1468-2370.2011.00300.x

Murphy, J., Samples, J., Morales, M., & Shadbeh, N. (2014). "They talk like that, but we keep working": sexual harassment and sexual assault experiences among Mexican indigenous farmworker women in Oregon. *Center for Minority Public Health*.

Nielsen, M. B., & Einarsen, S. (2012). Prospective relationships between workplace sexual harassment and psychological distress. *Occupational Medicine, 62*(3), 226-228. doi:10.1093/occmed/kqs010

The Policy, Ethics, and Human Rights Committee, British Association of Social Workers. (2012, January). The Code of Ethics for Social Work: Statement of principles. Retrieved December 1, 2014, from http://cdn.basw.co.uk/upload/basw_112315-7.pdf

Rape, Abuse, & Incest National Network (RAINN). (2014). Sexual harassment in the workplace. Retrieved December 16, 2015, from https://www.rainn.org/get-information/types-of-sexual-assault/sexual-harassment

Romito, P., Ballard, T., & Maton, N. (2004). Sexual harassment among female personnel in an Italian hospital: Frequency and correlates. *Violence Against Women, 10*(4), 386-417. doi:10.1177/1077801204263505

Rospenda, K. M., Richman, J. A., & Shannon, C. A. (2009). Prevalence and mental health correlates of harassment and discrimination in the workplace: Results from a national study. *Journal of Interpersonal Violence, 24*(5), 819-843. doi:10.1177/0886260508317182

Saunders, K. A., & Senn, C. Y. (2009). Should I confront him? Men's reactions to hypothetical confrontations of peer sexual harassment. *Sex Roles, 61*(5/6), 399-415.

Sexual harassment. (2012). *Nursing Update, 37*(6), 44-45.

Spector, P., Zhou, Z., & Che, X. (2014). Nurse exposure to physical and nonphysical violence, bullying, and sexual harassment: a quantitative review. *International Journal of Nursing Studies, 51*(1), 72-84. doi:10.1016/j.ijnurstu.2013.01.010

Street, A. E., Gradus, J. L., Stafford, J., & Kelly, K. (2007). Gender differences in experiences of sexual harassment: Data from a male-dominated environment. *Journal of Consulting and Clinical Psychology, 75*(3), 464-474.

Varone, C. (2009). Sexual harassment in the fire service: policies, training help ensure a safe & healthy work environment. *Firehouse, 34*(7), 52-54.

U.S. Equal Employment Opportunity Commission. (2015). Charges alleging sexual harassment FY2010–FY2014. Retrieved December 1, 2015, from http://www.eeoc.gov/eeoc/statistics/enforcement/sexual_harassment_new.cfm

Wheeler, D. (2015). NASW Standards and Indicators for Cultural Competence in Social Work Practice. Retrieved November 23, 2015, from http://www.socialworkers.org/practice/standards/PRA-BRO-253150-CC-Standards.pdf

SEXUAL HARASSMENT AT WORK: WORKING WITH PERPETRATORS

MAJOR CATEGORIES: Community

WHAT WE KNOW

Sexual harassment is unwanted conduct of a sexual nature, either physical or verbal, that results in feelings of humiliation, embarrassment, or intimidation in another person.

There are two legal terms used to describe types of sexual harassment in the workplace: *quid pro quo* sexual harassment, in which cooperation is required in return for employment or promotion; and hostile environment sexual harassment, in which unwelcome sexual conduct from a harasser creates an uncomfortable environment in the workplace. The former constitutes 5 percent of sexual harassment incidents, and the latter constitutes 95 percent.

Types of sexual harassment in the workplace include:
- unwelcome comments about a person's physical characteristics or sexual behavior;
- obscene jokes told to coworkers or employees;
- asking about private matters or asking for dates;
- sending inappropriate email messages from work computers or inappropriate text messages;
- showing any pictures of a sexual nature, such as pornography, in the workplace;
- speculating about a person's sexual orientation or asking him or her directly about his or her sexual behaviors; and
- physically touching another person in the workplace in a way that makes him or her feel uncomfortable.

Perpetrators and victims of sexual harassment in the workplace can be men or women, and the victim and perpetrator may be the same sex. However, the majority of victims of workplace sexual harassment are women, and the majority of harassers are men.

A study of nurses and midwives in a hospital setting in Australia revealedthat 34.4 percent of the nurses and midwives had been sexually harassed in their workplace, a hospital which has zero-tolerance policies toward aggression.

In a study of 265 female hospital personnel in Italy, 54 percent stated that they had been sexually harassed at work in the previous 12 months.

Certain factors make some female victims more vulnerable to sexual harassment (e.g., victims may be divorced or separated women, women who live alone, young women, women with financial problems, women who have recently experienced domestic violence, women with disabilities, lesbians, or non-white women).

Male victims often are young and/or gay.

The harasser may be a supervisor, a co-worker, or a non-employee (e.g., a customer).

The U.S. Equal Employment Opportunity Commission (EEOC) investigates allegations of sexual harassment in workplaces. In its investigations both the circumstances of the alleged harassment (i.e., the nature of the sexual conduct) and the context in which the alleged incidents occurred are examined.

Sexual harassment is known to be significantly underreported; however, in 2014, the EEOC received 6,862 complaints of sexual harassment in the workplace. Males filed 17.5 percent of the complaints; females filed 82.5 percent.

Research has identified common characteristics of sexual harassers.

Sexual harassers tend to be males.

One study reveals that individuals with highly authoritarian personalities (i.e., people who display rigid adherence to cultural traditions, traditional gender roles, and hypermasculinity) are more likely to sexually harass others. This study posited that individuals with authoritarian personalities tended to have had punitive childhood experiences, which led to negative emotions such as anger, shame, or terror.

Another study shows that male sexual harassers tend to overanalyze or infer criticism or rejection in women's thoughts and feelings, which can lead to hostile and aggressive sexual harassment as a response.

Other studies have indicated that sexual harassers lack social consciousness and engage in immature, irresponsible, manipulative, and exploitative behaviors in addition to sexually harassing behaviors.

Sexual harassers come from all social strata, occupations, and age categories.

Sexual harassers tend to lack impulse control and feelings of empathy.

Because sexual harassment cases are heard in civil court (as opposed to criminal court for crimes such as sexual assault and rape), individuals who are convicted of sexual harassment are less likely to receive court-ordered treatment, to be held accountable for completing any treatment ordered, or to receive probation or parole.

If evidence exists to support a claim of sexual harassment, managers will determine disciplinary action depending on the type and severity of the harassment. Discipline may take the form of issuing a written reprimand that notes details of the claim and warns of the measures that will be taken if a future incident occurs, referring the perpetrator for sexual harassment counseling and education, suspension of employment, or termination of employment.

If an alleged incident is investigated and there is no evidence of harassment, the victim can either contact an attorney to determine whether he or she has a legal claim based on what has happened or the victim can continue to document any ongoing harassment issues and resubmit a complaint to the management of the company or to the EEOC.

There is little research on which treatments for sexual harassers are most effective. More empirical data are needed to determine if the treatments that are most commonly used are effective and are leading to a decrease in sexual harassment in the workplace.

The following methods are used to treat persons who have engaged in sexual harassment:.

If the sexual harasser's offense was minor, the most common intervention is a general psychoeducation approach: reviewing with the perpetrator the definition of sexual harassment, the company policy on sexual harassment, and the legal aspects of sexual harassment; and having the individual watch a video on workplace harassment and/or review any pertinent readings about sexual harassment and its consequences.

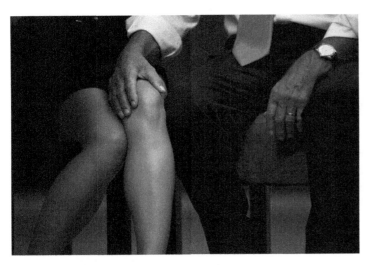

For more serious incidents of sexual harassment, counseling and treatment is recommended.

Treatment should incorporate a biopsychosocialspiritual assessment, a focus on the presenting problem (sexual harassment offense), setting of goals (e.g.,preventing future incidents of sexual harassment), and interventions (e.g., relapse prevention, cognitive behavioral therapy, motivational interviewing, support group meetings).

An integral piece of sexual harassment counseling is homework for the perpetrator. In addition to attending therapy sessions, the harasser usually is asked to work on various skills and interventions outside of the sessions. The homework can range from worksheets to completing assigned activities in the workplace or at home.

After the general psychoeducation on workplace sexual harassment is complete, the harasser usually is asked to write down in detail the incident in the workplace of which he or she was accused. This will help reveal the harasser's perception of the situation and indicate if denial and minimization need to be addressed in the therapeutic setting.

The sexual harasser may have deficits in social skills which need to be addressed. Basic social skills include identifying friendly people, offering friendly interactions, greeting people, initiating conversation, balancing listening and talking, sharing appropriate information about oneself, offering opinions in an appropriate way, responding to criticism openly, using humor appropriately, and learning how to accept when someone says no to one. These skills are most effectively learned and practiced through role

play between the harasser and the person conducting treatment.

Interventions should include having the sexual harasser work to develop empathy for the victim of the harassment. It is argued that if the perpetrator were to be aware of the impact his or her behavior had on the victim, he or she would be less likely to harass again.

The sexual harasser should spend time identifying potential high-risk situations for him or her, such as being alone in the copy room with a co-worker whom he or she may harass. The sexual harasser can work on avoidance and coping skills as well as increased self-monitoring to prevent a relapse of sexual harassment.

Toward the end of treatment, a formal relapse prevention plan can be developed to incorporate all of the aspects discussed and practiced during treatment.

WHAT CAN BE DONE

Learn about sexual harassment in the workplace so we can accurately assess our clients' personal characteristics and health education needs; share this information with our colleagues.

Develop an awareness of our own cultural values, beliefs, and biases, and develop knowledge about the histories, traditions, and values of our clients. Adopt treatment methodologies that reflect the cultural needs of the client.

Collaborate with workplace or company personnel to ensure that sexual harassment policies are in place and are widely disseminated, and help with any sexual harassment training.

Encourage and assist in the creation of organizational culture that discourages sexual harassment by examining normalized behaviors for policy violations.

If in a clinical setting, use appropriate therapeutic interventions to address accountability for perpetrator's behavior, enhance appropriate social skills, improve impulse control, and develop relapse prevention (e.g., psychoeducation, role play, cognitive behavioral therapy).

If not in a clinical setting, make referrals to treatment services as needed.

Written by Melissa Rosales Neff, MSW

Reviewed by Jessica Therivel, LMSW-IPR

REFERENCES

American Association of University Women. (2012). Know your rights: Workplace sexual harassment. Retrieved from http://www.aauw.org/what-we-do/legal-resources/know-your-rights-at-work/workplace-sexual-harassment/

Begany, J. J., & Milburn, M. A. (2002). Psychological predictors of sexual harassment: Authoritarianism, hostile sexism, and rape myths. *Psychology of Men & Masculinity, 3*(2), 119-126. doi:10.1037/1524-9220.3.2.119

Sexual harassment. (2002). *Behavioral Medicine Institute of Atlanta.* Retrieved October 8, 2015, from http://www.bmiatlanta.com/sexualharassment.html

Bridges, G. (2011). Dealing with sexual harassment in the workplace. *Dental Nursing, 7*(3), 157-159.

Brunswig, K. A., & O'Donohue, W. (2002). Relapse prevention as an appropriate model for the treatment of sexual harassers. In *Relapse prevention for sexual harassers* (pp. 5-7). New York, NY: Kluwer Academic/Plenum Publishers.

Brunswig, K. A., & O'Donohue, W. (2002). Treatment modules. In *Relapse Prevention for Sexual Harassers* (pp. 15-108). New York, NY: Kluwer Academic/Plenum Publishers.

Demir, D., & Rodwell, J. (2012). Psychosocial antecedents and consequences of workplace aggression for hospital nurses. *Journal of Nursing Scholarship, 44*(4), 376-384. doi:10.1111/j.1547-5069.2012.01472.x

Hibino, Y., Ogino, K., & Inagaki, M. (2006). Sexual harassment of female nurses by patients in Japan. *Journal of Nursing Scholarship, 38*, 4. doi:10.1111/j.1547-5069.2006.00134.x

International Federation of Social Workers. (2012, March 3). Statement of ethical principles. Retrieved May 22, 2014, from http://ifsw.org/policies/statement-of-ethical-principles/

McDonald, P. (2012). Workplace sexual harassment 30 years on: A review of the literature. *International Journal of Management Reviews, 14*(1), 1-17. doi:10.1111/j.1468-2370.2011.00300.x

National Association of Social Workers. (2001). NASW standards for cultural competence in social work practice. Retrieved October 8, 2015, from http://www.socialworkers.org/practice/standards/NASWCulturalStandards.pdf

Pina, A., Gannon, T. A., & Saunders, B. (2009). An overview of the literature on sexual harassment: Perpetrator, theory, and treatment issues. *Aggression and Violent Behavior, 14*(2), 126-138. doi:10.1016/j.avb.2009.01.002

Sexual harassment. (2009). *Rape, Abuse, & Incest National Network (RAINN).* Retrieved October 8, 2015, from https://www.rainn.org/get-information/types-of-sexual-assault/sexual-harassment

Romito, P., Ballard, T., & Maton, N. (2004). Sexual harassment among female personnel in an Italian hospital: Frequency and correlates. *Violence Against Women, 10*(4), 386-417. doi:10.1177/1077801204263505

Schweinle, W. E., Cofer, C., & Schatz, S. (2009). Men's empathic bias, empathic inaccuracy, and sexual harassment. *Sex Roles, 60*(1-2), 142-150. doi:10.1007/s11199-008-9507-2

The Policy, Ethics, and Human Rights Committee, British Association of Social Workers. (2012, January). The code of ethics for social work: Statement of principles. *The Policy, Ethics and Human Rights Committee, British Association of Social Workers.* Retrieved October 8, 2015, from http://cdn.basw.co.uk/upload/basw_112315-7.pdf

Facts about sexual harassment. (2002). *U.S. Equal Employment Opportunity Commission.* Retrieved October 8, 2015, from http://www.eeoc.gov/facts/fs-sex.html

Charges alleging sexual harassment EEOC: FY 2010-FY 2014 [Table]. (2014). *U.S. Equal Employment Opportunity Commission.* Retrieved October 8, 2015, from http://www.eeoc.gov/eeoc/statistics/enforcement/sexual_harassment_new.cfm

SEXUAL HARASSMENT: PEER HARASSMENT IN MIDDLE & HIGH SCHOOL

MAJOR CATEGORIES: Adolescents, Emotional Abuse

DESCRIPTION

In the past 25 years research on sexual harassment has extended from investigations of sexual harassment in the workplace to sexual harassment in schools, particularly secondary schools and universities. Although students can be sexually harassed by teachers or other school staff, sexual harassment by peers is much more common. Perpetrators and victims can be of the opposite sex or the same sex.

In 1997 the U.S. Department of Education formulated the following definition for school sexual harassment:

Sexual harassment is defined as unwelcome sexual advances, requests for sexual favors, and other verbal, nonverbal, or physical conduct of a sexual nature by an employee, by another student, or by a third party that is sufficiently severe, persistent, or pervasive to limit a student's ability to participate in or benefit from an education program or activity, or to create a hostile or abusive educational environment.

It is important to note that even though bullying and sexual harassment can overlap, they are distinct actions and are addressed by different policies and laws. Although bullying is repeated unwanted behavior that involves an imbalance of power and intention to harm, it is not sexual in nature; it may take the form of physical aggression (e.g., hitting, pushing, spitting) or name-calling, teasing, or social exclusion. Peer sexual harassment takes many forms. Students report other students making sexual comments, telling "dirty" jokes, making inappropriate gestures, or spreading sexual rumors about them. Other students report that they have been shown sexual pictures, called gay or lesbian pejoratively, have been shown someone's private parts, or have been grabbed in a sexual way. Finally, sexual harassment can take place by electronic means, such as text, email, and social media. Researchers agree that sexual harassment is about power. It is a way for someone to intimidate and assert dominance over another, creating a power imbalance between the perpetrator and the victim.

The goal of all schools should be to have a safe school climate in which rules are unambiguous, students feel that they are treated fairly, and students feel safe. A large national study recommended that all schools appoint a coordinator who is assigned to receive all complaints of sexual harassment and that schools make this person known to the student body(AAUW, 2011). Students will be more likely to approach the identified staff member rather than

keeping incidents of sexual harassment to themselves because they do not know whom they can talk to.

Researchers have found that educators need more training in how to identify and handle sexual harassment in their classrooms. When they see inappropriate behavior, teachers should address the behavior directly and state that it must stop immediately. They should educate their students on what is appropriate and inappropriate behavior. Most importantly, they need to follow through with school discipline and report the perpetrator to the school administration so that actions can be taken according to the school's sexual harassment policy (e.g., suspension, expulsion). Schools can hold workshops or assemblies for the student body to raise awareness about what sexual harassment is, what to do if students witness it, and how to respond if they are harassed. Schools should teach students assertive methods with which to respond appropriately and effectively to sexual harassment on school campuses and electronically. (Generally speaking, schools are considered liable for any electronic harassment that occurs on school grounds during school hours. Parents are liable for any that occurs after school hours.)

FACTS AND FIGURES

The American Association of University Women (AAUW) published a national study in 2011 that reported that among students in grades 7–12, 56 percent of the girls and 40 percent of the boys had experienced sexual harassment in school. Of those, 87 percent reported that the harassment affected them negatively (AAUW, 2011). In another study, 130 adolescents who self-identified as lesbian, gay, bisexual, or questioning their sexuality were interviewed with a group of their heterosexual peers. The questioning and sexual minority youth reported higher rates of sexual harassment than their heterosexual peers (National Sexual Violence Resource Center, 2012). Researchers of a 2012 study of middle-school (grades 5–8) students in the U.S. Midwest reported that 28 percent of the girls and 34 percent of the boys reported perpetrating sexual harassment (Espelage et al., 2012).

In a large population-based study of 18,090 students from 26 different high schools, 30 percent of the students disclosed that they had been victims of sexual harassment at school (37 percent were females, 21 percent were males) and 8.5 percent disclosed that they had perpetrated sexual harassment at school (Clear et al., 2014).

Results from a study of 12–18-year-olds indicated that 59 percent of the participants had been sexually harassed. The majority were girls. Furthermore, the researchers found a correlation between being sexually harassed and psychological impairment, especially for girls (Eom et al., 2015). Researchers in another study found that boys are overwhelmingly the perpetrators of sexual harassment in high school, but that boys and girls have similar rates of sexual harassment victimization (Gruber & Fineran, 2016).

Risk Factors

Attending a school with a hostile climate is a risk factor for experiencing sexual harassment. The majority of sexual harassment between students takes place in classrooms, hallways, gyms, parking lots, and cafeterias. Therefore, if a student attends a school in which sexual harassment policies are absent or are not taken seriously, an environmental risk factor is present. Gender is also a risk factor: boys are much more likely to perpetrate sexual harassment. Therefore, being a girl is a risk factor.

Signs and Symptoms

The psychosocial impact of sexual harassment for victims can be extensive and debilitating. The negative effects reported include depression, heightened anxiety, loss of appetite, sleep disturbance, feelings of being sad, afraid, or embarrassed, low self-esteem (effects on self-esteem are reported by girls more often than boys), negative educational outcomes (i.e., participating less in class, receiving lower grades, skipping class, getting in trouble with school authorities, difficulty studying). Girls also report lowered hopes and expectations for the future as a result of sexual harassment. Girls who are sexually harassed are more likely than boys who are harassed to attempt suicide (Clear et al., 2014).

Assessment

Conduct a complete biopsychosocialspiritual assessment

Acquire as much information as possible regarding the sexual harassment incident, both from the alleged perpetrator and the victim

Determine if school authorities were informed and what the school's response to the incident was

Assessments and Screening Tools

Beck Depression Inventory-II: a 21-item instrument for detecting depression that can be completed by adolescents 13 years and older

Children's Depression Inventory: a 28-item scale to assess depressive symptoms in children and adolescents

Laboratory and Diagnostic Tests of Interest to the Social Worker

There are no applicable laboratory tests

Treatment

Social workers should be aware of their own cultural values, beliefs, and biases and develop specialized knowledge about the histories, traditions, and values of their clients. Social workers should adopt treatment methodologies that reflect their knowledge of the cultural diversity of the communities in which they practice

An important way to support victims of sexual harassment in schools is to provide an environment in which victims feel safe disclosing what happened to them. Victims often fail to report an incident of sexual harassment out of the belief that nothing will change, that the situation will get worse, or that the incident was not severe enough to report. If a student does disclose a sexual harassment incident to a social worker, he or she should respond in supportive ways. The social worker should listen to the student respectfully, letting the student know that he or she is being heard. The social worker should affirm that the incident was not the student's fault (since many victims blame themselves for how they dressed or something that they said or did). The social worker should advise the student of his or her rights and options and help the student navigate the process of filing a complaint if the student wishes. The social worker should use appropriate therapeutic interventions to address anxiety, depression, sleep disturbances, and academic problems if applicable (e.g., cognitive behavioral therapy [CBT], solution-focused therapy)

Problem	Goal	Intervention
Student has experienced sexual harassment at school and is unsure of the sexual harassment complaint process	Clarity	Validate what the student reports and address any potential blame student is placing on him- or herself. Explain the complaint process and potential outcomes. Answer any further questions
Student is fearful of another sexual harassment incident	Decrease fear	Role-play with student and teach appropriate assertiveness skills to build the student's confidence and address the student's fear of what he or she will do in the possible case of a future sexual harassment incident. Establish a safety plan with the student victim to help victim feel safe. This could be a route change, schedule change, or an assigned friend to accompany victim at different points in the day
Student is complaining of anxiety and sleep disturbances after sexual harassment incident	Decrease anxiety and improve sleep	Work on stress management and coping skills. Teach relaxation methods which may help with sleep disturbances. Use CBT as appropriate
Student sexually harassed another student	Address the sexual harassment offense and prevent it from happening again	Provide psychoeducation about sexual harassment. Address accountability for his or her behavior and impulse control

LAWS AND REGULATIONS

Each country has its own standards for cultural competency and diversity in social work practice. Social workers must be aware of the standards of practice set forth by their governing body (National Association of Social Workers, British Association of Social Workers, etc.) and practice accordingly

Title IX of the Education Amendments of 1972 states that "no person in the United States shall, on the basis of sex, be excluded from participation in, be denied the benefits of, or be subjected to discrimination under any educational program or activity receiving federal financial assistance." Sexual harassment is considered a form of discrimination within the education system

SERVICES AND RESOURCES

- American Association of University Women: http://www.aauw.org/tag/sexual-harassment/
- National Sexual Violence Resource Center: www.nsvrc.org

FOOD FOR THOUGHT

Comprehensive sex education classes in schools enable students to discuss sexuality in a healthy, age-appropriate way and to address unwanted and unwelcome sexual experiences, such as sexual harassment

Parents often are unaware of the prevalence of sexual harassment in schools. Parents as well as students should be educated about this problem

RED FLAGS

In a study of 270 teachers the only sexual harassment training teachers received was reported to be a video about workplace or teacher-to-student sexual harassment, as opposed to student-on-student sexual harassment. This left teachers unprepared to handle sexual harassment at their schools. Many teachers do not know how to distinguish sexual harassment from bullying, which are treated differently by the legal system (Charmaraman et al., 2013).

Research indicates that sexual harassment occurs more often in high school than middle school.

If a girl reports an incident of sexual harassment to a school employee and is told that the boy likely is teasing her because he likes her, then it instills the idea at an early age that violence is a part of love.

Researchers found that experiencing sexual harassment can erode school attachment and academic performance for high school students more than experiencing bullying (Gruber & Fineran, 2016).

NEXT STEPS
Ensure that client feels supported and has access to information and resources

Follow through with the school to ensure that if a complaint was filed, an investigation is underway

Written by Melissa Rosales Neff, MSW

Reviewed by Laura Gale, LCSW

REFERENCES
British Association of Social Workers. (2012, January). The code of ethics for social workers: Statement of principles. Retrieved October 11, 2015, from http://cdn.basw.co.uk/upload/basw_112315-7.pdf

Becker, J. V., & Hunter, J. A., Jr. (1998). Understanding and treating child and adolescent sexual offenders. *Advances in Clinical Child Psychology, 19*, 177-197.

Charmaraman, L., Jones, A. E., Stein, N., & Espelage, D. L. (2013). Is it bullying or sexual harassment? Knowledge, attitudes, and professional development experiences of middle school staff. *The Journal of School Health, 83*(6), 438-444. doi:10.1111/josh.12048

Clear, E., Coker, A., Cook-Craig, P., Bush, H., Garcia, L., Williams, C., ... Fisher, B. (2014). Sexual harassment victimization and perpetration among high school students. *Violence Against Women, 20*(10), 1203-1219. doi:10.1177/1077801214551287

deLara, E. W. (2008). Developing a philosophy about bullying and sexual harassment: Cognitive coping strategies among high school students. *Journal of School Violence, 7*(4), 72-96.

Eom, E., Restaino, S., Perkins, A., Neveln, N., & Harrington, J. (2015). Sexual harassment in middle and high school children and effects on physical and mental health. *Clincial Pediatrics, 54*(5), 430-438.

Espelage, D. L., Basile, K. C., & Hamburger, M. E. (2012). Bullying perpetration and subsequent sexual violence perpetration among middle school students. *Journal of Adolescent Health, 50*(1), 60-65. doi:10.1016/j.jadohealth.2011.07.015

Gadin, K. G. (2012). Sexual harassment of girls in elementary school: A concealed phenomenon within heterosexual romantic discourse. *Journal of Interpersonal Violence, 27*(9), 1762-1779. doi:10.1177/0886260511430387

Gruber, J., & Fineran, S. (2016). Sexual harassment, bullying and school outcomes for high school girls and boys. *Violence Against Women, 22*(1), 112-113.

International Federation of Social Workers. (2012). Statement of Ethical Principles. Retrieved March 8, 2016, from http://ifsw.org/policies/statement-of-ethical-principles/

Lichty, L. F., Torres, J. M., Valenti, M. T., & Buchanan, N. T. (2008). Sexual harassment policies in K-12 schools: Examining accessibility to students and content. *The Journal of School Health, 78*(11), 607-614. doi:10.1111/j.1746-1561.2008.00353.x

Mumford, E. A., Okamoto, J., Taylor, B. G., & Stein, N. (2013). Middle school sexual harassment, violence and social networks. *American Journal of Health Behavior, 37*(6), 769-779. doi:10.5993/AJHB.37.6.6

National Association of School Psychologists. (2010). *Sexual harassment.* Bethesda: National Association of School Psychologists. National Sexual Violence Resource Center. (2012). Sexual harassment and bullying of youth: Sexual violence & individuals who identify as LGBTQ. Retrieved March 8, 2016, from http://www.nsvrc.org/sites/default/files/Publications_NSVRC_Guides_Sexual-Harassment-Bullying-Youth.pdf

Rahimi, R., & Liston, D. (2011). Race, class, and emerging sexuality: Teacher perceptions and sexual harassment in schools. *Gender and Education, 23*(7), 799-810.

U.S. Department of Education, Office of Civil Rights. (1997). Sexual harassment guide: Harassment of students by school employees, other students, or third parties. *Federal Register, 62*(49), 12034-12051.

United States Department of Labor. (2014). Title IX, Education Amendments of 1972. Retrieved March 8, 2016, from http://www.dol.gov/oasam/regs/statutes/titleix.htm

Wheeler, D. (2015). *NASW Standards and Indicators for Cultural Competence in Social Work Practice.* Retrieved February 23, 2016, from http://www.socialworkers.org/practice/standards/PRA-BRO-253150-CC-Standards.pdf

SEXUAL HARASSMENT: PEER HARASSMENT IN SCHOOL—SUPPORTING VICTIMS

MAJOR CATEGORIES: Adolescents, Emotional Abuse

WHAT WE KNOW

In 1997 the U.S. Department of Education formulated the following definition for school sexual harassment:

Sexual harassment is defined as unwelcome sexual advances, requests for sexual favors, and other verbal, nonverbal, or physical conduct of a sexual nature by an employee, by another student, or by a third party, that is sufficiently severe, persistent, or pervasive to limit a student's ability to participate in or benefit from an education program or activity, or to create a hostile or abusive educational environment.

Title IX of the Education Amendments of 1972 states that "no person in the United States shall, on the basis of sex, be excluded from participation in, be denied the benefits of, or be subjected to discrimination under any educational program or activity receiving federal financial assistance."

Research over the past 20 years has extended from investigations of sexual harassment in the workplace to sexual harassment in schools, specifically peer harassment in middle and high schools.

The American Association of University Women published a national study in 2011 indicating that among 7th- to 12th-grade students, 56 percent of the girls and 40 percent of the boys reported experiencing sexual harassment in school. Of those, 87 percent reported that it affected them negatively.

In a recent population-based study of 18,090 students from 26 different high schools, 30 percent of the students disclosed that they had been victims of sexual harassment at school (37 percent were females, 21 percent were males) and 8.5 percent disclosed that they had perpetrated sexual harassment at school.

Lesbian, gay, bisexual, transgender, and questioning (LGBTQ) students are significantly more likely than straight students to experience harassment from their peers in school.

Sexual harassment in schools manifests in varied ways.

Students report that other students make sexual comments, sexual jokes, and inappropriate gestures and spread sexual rumors about them.

Others report that they have been shown sexual pictures or have been called gay or lesbian in hateful ways.

Students report being told inappropriate sexual information via the Internet or cellphone (e-mail, text, Facebook, etc.).

Researchers examining online harassment found that 36 percent of girls and 24 percent of boys reported experiencing cyber harassment.

These students reported that they had received text messages, e-mail messages, or posts on social media sites such as Facebook containing unwelcome sexual jokes or inappropriate pictures.

Twelve percent of the students reported that they were called gay or lesbian in a negative way via Facebook, e-mail, or text.

The most extreme reported form of sexual harassment is being touched or grabbed in a sexual manner. Students who are victims of peer harassment at school can often be perpetrators of peer harassment themselves.

The psychosocial impact of sexual harassment for victims can be extensive and debilitating.

A national study of students in grades 7–12 reported the following emotional consequences of being harassed sexually.

- 32 percent of the victims reported that they did not want to go to school.
- 31 percent of the victims reported that they felt sick to their stomachs because of the sexual harassment.
- 30 percent reported that they had a difficult time studying.
- 19 percent reported that they had a hard time sleeping.
- 10 percent reported that they started to get into trouble at school after they were sexually harassed.
- 9 percent reported that they began to take a different route to and from school to avoid the perpetrator.

Other studies reported mental health concerns of victims such as lower self-esteem, depression, heightened anxiety, and feeling alone or afraid. It has been noted that girls who are sexually harassed are more likely than boys who are sexually harassed to attempt suicide.

In a study of 12- to 18-year-olds, 124 out of 210 participants (59 percent) disclosed that they had experienced sexual harassment at school. The majority who had experienced sexual harassment were females (69 percent). Researchers of the study stated that there was a direct correlation between experiencing sexual harassment and psychological impairment in adolescents, especially in females.

Fostering a safe school environment through public policies and staff training is vital to supporting victims of sexual harassment and protecting others from harassment.

A safe school is one in which rules are unambiguous, students feel that they are treated fairly, and students feel safe.

By law, sexual harassment policies must be written to include a definition of sexual harassment, explain explicitly what actions are inappropriate, and then explain the procedure that is followed when complaints are investigated. Legally, sexual harassment policies must be made public and easily accessible online and in school facilities.

Researchers are noting that it can reduce the hostility of a school's climate for students to witness peers intervening when another peer is being harassed. Youth-led interventions with peer networks may be effective in decreasing peer harassment in the schools.

One means to ensure a safe school environment is mandating that all those who are in contact with children be specifically trained in sexual harassment cessation and prevention. Training is lacking in many schools.

In a study of 270 teachers, the sexual harassment training they received was reported to consist of a video about workplace or teacher-to-student sexual harassment, as opposed to peer sexual harassment. This left teachers unprepared to handle sexual harassment at their schools.

An important way to support victims of sexual harassment in schools is to provide an environment in which victims feel safe disclosing what happened to them.

A study reported that of students who reported being sexually harassed, 50 percent did nothing in response, including not telling anyone. Another 40 percent told a friend or family member. Only 9 percent reported the incident to a school administrator, teacher, or guidance counselor.

Victims indicate that they do not report incidents of sexual harassment because they think nothing will change, that the situation will get worse, or that the incident was not severe enough to report.

Once a student does disclose a sexual harassment incident to an administrator, guidance counselor, social worker, or educator at the school, these adults need to respond in supportive ways.

School personnel should

- listen to the student respectfully, letting the student know that he or she is being heard;
- affirm that the incident was not the student's fault (since many victims blame themselves for how they dressed or something that they said or did);
- advise the student of his or her rights and options;
- encourage the student to write down the incident, including as much detail as possible, along with names of others who may have witnessed the incident; and
- help the student navigate the process of filing a complaint per school policy.

Guidance counselors and school social workers can work with victims of sexual harassment individually to support them.

Role-play may be beneficial for victims of sexual harassment. Role-play teaches appropriate assertive skills to build the child's confidence and address what he or she will do in the event of possible future sexual harassment.

Help the victim find ways to confront the harasser and ask him or her to stop the offending behavior.

Establish a safety plan with the student victim to help him or her feel safe. This could be a route change, a schedule change, or an assigned friend to accompany the victim at different points in the day.

What Can Be Done

Learn about peer sexual harassment in schools so you can accurately assess your clients' personal characteristics and health education needs; share this information with your colleagues.

Practice with awareness of and adherence to the NASW Code of Ethics core values of service, social justice, dignity and worth of the person, importance of human relationships, integrity, and competence. Become knowledgeable of the NASW ethical standards as they apply to working with victims of peer harassment in the school system, and practice accordingly.

Develop an awareness of your own cultural values, beliefs, and biases and develop knowledge about the histories, traditions, and values of your clients. Adopt treatment methodologies that reflect the cultural needs of the client.

Collaborate with school staff to ensure that policies are public and visible; help with any sexual harassment training.

Encourage administrators and educators to include in their curriculum classes that teach civil rights, diversity,and tolerance in order to foster discussions about respectful behavior.

Use appropriate therapeutic interventions to address anxiety, depression, sleep disturbances, and academic problems, if applicable (e.g., cognitive behavioral therapy, solution-focused therapy).

Help establish a culture of intolerance of sexual harassment within the school environment.

Written by Melissa Rosales Neff, MSW

Reviewed by Laura Gale, LCSW

REFERENCES

American Association of University Women (AAUW). (2011). *Crossing the line: Sexual harassment at school.* Washington, DC: American Association of University Women.

Charmaraman, L., Jones, A. E., Stein, N., & Espelage, D. L. (2013). Is it bullying or sexual harassment? Knowledge, attitudes, and professional development experiences of middle school staff. *The Journal of School Health, 83*(6), 438-444. doi:10.1111/josh.12048

Clear, E., Coker, A., Cook-Craig, P., Bush, H., Garcia, L., Williams, C.,... Fisher, B. (2014). Sexual harassment victimization and perpetration among high school students. *Violence Against Women, 20*(10), 1203-1219. doi:10.1177/1077801214551287

Eisenberg, M., Gower, A., McNorris, B., & Bucchianeri, M. (2015). Vulnerable bullies: Perpetration of peer harassment among youths across sexual orientation, weight, and disability status. *American Journal of Public Health, 105*(9), 1784-1791. doi:10.2105/AJPH.2015.302704

Eom, E., Restaino, S., Perkins, A., Neveln, N., & Harrington, J. (2015). Sexual harassment in middle and high school children and the effects on physical and mental health. *Clinical Pediatrics, 54*(5), 430-438.

Gadin, K. G. (2012). Sexual harassment of girls in elementary school: A concealed phenomenon within heterosexual romantic discourse. *Journal of Interpersonal Violence, 27*(9), 1762-1779. doi:10.1177/0886260511430387

Hillard, P., Love, L., Franks, H., Laris, B., & Coyle, K. (2014). "They were only joking": Efforts to decrease LGBTQ bullying and harassment in Seattle public schools. *Journal of School Health, 84*(1), 1-9. doi:10.1111/josh.12120

International Federation of Social Workers. (2012). Statement of ethical principles. Retrieved April 21, 2016, from http://ifsw.org/policies/statement-of-ethical-principles/

National Sexual Violence Resource Center. (2012). Sexual harassment and bullying of youth: Sexual violence & individuals who identify as LGBTQ. Retrieved April 21, 2016, from http://nsvrc.org/sites/default/files/Publications_NSVRC_Guides_Sexual-Harassment-Bullying-Youth.pdf

The Policy, Ethics, and Human Rights Committee, British Association of Social Workers. (2012, January). The Code of Ethics for Social Work: Statement of principles. Retrieved April 21, 2016, from http://cdn.basw.co.uk/upload/basw_112315-7.pdf

U.S. Department of Education, Office of Civil Rights. (1997). Sexual harassment guide: Harassment of students by school employees, other students, or third parties. *Federal Register, 62*(49), 12034-12051.

United States Department of Labor. (2014). Title IX, Education Amendments of 1972. Retrieved April 21, 2016, from http://www.dol.gov/oasam/regs/statutes/titleix.htm

National Association of Social Workers. (2008). Code of ethics. Retrieved April 4, 2016, from http://www.socialworkers.org/pubs/code/code.asp

Wernick, L., Kulick, A., & Inglehart, M. (2014). Influences of peers, teachers, and climate on students' willingness to intervene when witnessing anti-transgender harassment. *Journal of Adolescence, 37*(6), 927-935. doi:10.1016/j.adolescence.2014.06.008

Wheeler, D. (2015). NASW standards and indicators for cultural competence in social work practice. Retrieved March 2, 2016, from http://www.socialworkers.org/practice/standards/PRA-BRO-253150-CC-Standards.pdf

Young, E., Ashbaker, B., & Young, B. (2010). Sexual harassment: A guide for school personnel. Bethesda, MD: National Association of School Psychologists.

SEXUAL HARASSMENT: PEER HARASSMENT IN SCHOOL—WORKING WITH PERPETRATORS

MAJOR CATEGORIES: Adolescents, Emotional Abuse

WHAT WE KNOW

In 1997, the U.S. Department of Education formulated the following definition for school sexual harassment:

Sexual harassment is defined as unwelcome sexual advances, requests for sexual favors, and other verbal, nonverbal, or physical conduct of a sexual nature by an employee, by another student, or by a third party that is sufficiently severe, persistent, or pervasive to limit a student's ability to participate in or benefit from an education program or activity, or to create a hostile or abusive educational environment.

Title IX of the Education Amendments of 1972 states that "no person in the United States shall, on the basis of sex, be excluded from participation in, be denied the benefits of, or be subjected to discrimination under any educational program or activity receiving federal financial assistance." Sexual harassment in an education setting is considered discrimination.

Sexual harassment in schools takes multiple forms.

Students report that peers make sexual comments, tell "dirty" jokes, make inappropriate gestures, or spread sexual rumors about them.

Others report that they have been shown sexual pictures, called gay or lesbian pejoratively, or received messages containing inappropriate sexual content via the Internet or phone (email, text, Facebook, etc.).

The most extreme reported form of sexual harassment is being touched or grabbed in a sexual manner.

The prevalence of peer harassment in schools is well researched.

In a national U.S. study 16 percent of students in grades 7–12 admitted that they had sexually harassed another student, either in person or through texting, email, or Facebook.

Results from this national study also indicated that there is not always a clear distinction between victims and perpetrators of peer sexual harassment. Of the 16 percent of students who reported harassing other students, 92 percent stated that they had been sexually harassed themselves.

Researchers of this national study concluded that it is likely that over the course of the school year many students will be both harassed and harassers.

Results from a study of four schools in Illinois indicated that 24 percent of the students sexually harassed peers. Of those, 32 percent of boys and 22 percent of girls reported making sexual comments to other students, 5 percent of boys and 7 percent of girls reported spreading sexual rumors, and 4 percent of boys and 2 percent of girls reported pulling on another student's clothing.

Researchers of a 2011 study of Midwestern U.S. schools reported that 28 percent of girls and 34 percent of boys in grades 5–8 reported perpetrating sexual harassment within that school year. The study also stated that the incidence of sexual harassment increases through middle school into high school.

In a recent large population-based study of 18,090 students from 26 different U.S. high schools, 30 percent of the students disclosed that they had been victims of sexual harassment at school (37 percent were females, 21 percent were males) and 8.5 percent disclosed that they had perpetrated sexual harassment at school.

Results from one study indicated that male and female students with discordant sexual orientation (i.e., they self-identify as heterosexual but have same-gender sexual partners) had the highest prevalence of sexually harassing peers.

Researchers of a Swedish study reported that boys sexually harass to assert their masculinity over girls and other boys. Boys often use homophobic language when harassing other boys).

When a report of sexual harassment at school is made, it is important that it be taken seriously. This is an opportunity for intervention with perpetrators.

School sexual harassment policies vary from school to school, but should have the following components: school-specific examples of harassing behavior to help define sexual harassment (e.g., sexual graffiti on bathroom stalls, groping another student);a description of the investigation process;a statement prohibiting retaliation by the alleged perpetrator; disciplinary consequences of harassment; and a list of educational and counseling resources, both for the victim and for the perpetrator.

School personnel should listen to both the victim and perpetrating student respectfully, letting the students know that they are being taken seriously.

The harasser as well as the harassed student should be interviewed individually.

The perpetrator should be advised of his or her rights and options.

The student victim and perpetrator should be encouraged to describe the incident in writing, including as much detail as possible,and also to provide the names of others who may have witnessed the incident.

Objectivity and fairness must be maintained during the investigation process.

Disciplinary actions may include suspension or expulsion as well as referral to counseling.

It is necessary for there to be disciplinary consequences for the perpetrator. Once the punishment is complete, however, the National Association of School Psychologists asserts that it is vital to move into a constructive phase in which appropriate behavior is explained and taught to the perpetrator. The social worker can work with the student on learning positive social skills in the school environment.

Although much information is available on how to support victims of school sexual harassment, there is little information on how to work with and support student perpetrators of sexual harassment. The initial steps used in treatment of adolescent sexual offenders may provide some guidance, since sexual harassment is a type of sexual offense, albeit a lesser offense than sexual violence or abuse.

Most programs for adolescent sexual offenders use the following interventions: psychoeducation, cognitive behavioral therapy, family therapy, and relapse prevention.

The first step in all these interventions is for the perpetrator to accept responsibility for his or her actions.

Another topic in treatment should be teaching the perpetrator how to develop and sustain healthy relationships with peers as well as learn skills for impulse control.

A new social theory called Bully–Sexual Violence Pathway theory suggests that bullying and

homophobic teasing in adolescence, if not addressed or redirected, can escalate to sexual harassment perpetration as well as sexual violence perpetration.

WHAT CAN BE DONE

Learn about working with student perpetrators of sexual harassment so you can accurately assess your client's personal characteristics and health education needs; share this information with your colleagues.

Develop an awareness of your own cultural values, beliefs, and biases and develop knowledge about the histories, traditions, and values of your clients. Adopt treatment methodologies that reflect the cultural needs of the client.

Collaborate with teachers and school administrators to ensure that sexual harassment policies are in place and are clearly communicated to students;help with any sexual harassment training.

Encourage administrators and educators to include topics of civil rights, diversity,and tolerance in the curriculum to provide the opportunity for discussions about respectful behavior.

Use appropriate therapeutic interventions (e.g., cognitive behavioral therapy, psychoeducation) to address accountability for the perpetrator's behavior, appropriate social skills, impulse control, or any academic problems.

Written by Melissa Rosales Neff, MSW

Reviewed by Laura Gale, LCSW

REFERENCES

American Association of University Women (AAUW). (2011). Crossing the line: Sexual harassment at school. Washington, DC: American Association of University Women.

Becker, J. V., & Hunter, J. A., Jr. (1998). Understanding and treating child and adolescent sexual offenders. *Advances in Clinical Child Psychology, 19,* 177-197.

British Association of Social Workers. (2012). The code of ethics for social work: Statement of principles. Retrieved December 1, 2015, from http://cdn.basw.co.uk/upload/basw_112315-7.pdf

Charmaraman, L., Jones, A. E., Stein, N., & Espelage, D. L. (2013). Is it bullying or sexual harassment? Knowledge, attitudes, and professional development experiences of middle school staff. *The Journal of School Health, 83*(6), 438-444. doi:10.1111/josh.12048

Clear, E., Coker, A., Cook-Craig, P., Bush, H., Garcia, L., Williams, C.,... Fisher, B. (2014). Sexual harassment victimization and perpetration among high school students. *Violence Against Women, 20*(10), 1203-1219. doi:10.1177/1077801214551287

Eisenberg, M., Gower, A., McNorris, B., & Bucchianeri, M. (2015). Vulnerable bullies: Perpetration of peer harassment among youths across sexual orientation, weight, and disability status. *American Journal of Public Health, 105*(9), 1784-1791. doi:10.2105/AJPH.2015.302704

Eom, E., Restaino, S., Perkins, A., Neveln, N., & Harrington, J. (2015). Sexual harassment in middle and high school children and effects on physical and mental health. *Clincial Pediatrics, 54*(5), 430-438.

Gadin, K. G. (2012). Sexual harassment of girls in elementary school: A concealed phenomenon within heterosexual romantic discourse. *Journal of Interpersonal Violence, 27*(9), 1762-1779. doi:10.1177/0886260511430387

International Federation of Social Workers. (2012). Statement of ethical principles. Retrieved December 1, 1970, from http://ifsw.org/policies/statement-of-ethical-principles/

Mumford, E. A., Okamoto, J., Taylor, B. G., & Stein, N. (2013). Middle school sexual harassment, violence and social networks. *American Journal of Health Behavior, 37*(6), 769-779. doi:10.5993/AJHB.37.6.6

National Center for Injury Prevention and Control. (n.d.). The bully-sexual violence pathway in early adolescence. Retrieved December 1, 2015, from http://www.cdc.gov/violenceprevention/pdf/asap_bullyingsv-a.pdf

United States Department of Labor. (2014). Title IX, Education Amendments of 1972. Retrieved December 1, 2014, from http://www.dol.gov/oasam/regs/statutes/titleix.htm

U.S. Department of Education, Office of Civil Rights. (1997). Sexual harassment guide: Harassment of students by school employees, other students, or third parties. *Federal Register, 62*(49), 12034-12051.

Wheeler, D. (2015). NASW standards and indicators for cultural competency in social work practice. Retrieved December 1, 2015, from http://www.cdc.gov/violenceprevention/pdf/asap_bullyingsv-a.pdf

Young, E., Ashbaker, B., & Young, B. (2010). Sexual harassment: A guide for school personnel. Bethesda, MD: National Association of School Psychologists.

Sexually Transmitted Diseases in Adolescents: Risk Factors for Gonorrhea & Chlamydia

Major Categories: Adolescents, Medical & Health

What We Know

Sexually transmitted diseases (STDs) are a major health problem for adolescents throughout the world. Worldwide, approximately 1 of every 4 adolescents will be infected with an STD each year. Chlamydia and gonorrhea are the two most common bacterial STDs worldwide. In the United States, among chlamydia cases reported to the CDC in 2013, 28 percent were in those aged 15–19 and 39 percent in those aged 20–24. Among gonorrhea cases reported to the CDC in 2013, 22 percent were in those aged 15–19 and 34 percent in those aged 20–24. Serious complications can develop if chlamydia or gonorrhea is left untreated, which is common because the majority of cases are asymptomatic and therefore the individual is not aware of their infection or need for treatment.

Potential complications of both chlamydia and gonorrhea include cervicitis, epididymis, ectopic pregnancy, pelvic inflammatory disease, and infertility. Coinfection with chlamydia has been reported in 20 percent–60 percent of gonorrhea cases. Perinatal infection with either disease can result in neonatal pneumonia and/or conjunctivitis in the infant.

Certain behavioral, social, and biological factors increase the risk of contracting gonorrhea and chlamydia in adolescents. Behavioral factors that increase risk include having first sexual intercourse before age 15, having a new sexual partner in the previous 60 days, having more than 2 concurrent sexual partners, having sex with a partner who is symptomatic of infection with an STD (which increases the risk of transmission of the STD), having more than 5 lifetime sexual partners, inconsistent condom use, use of drugs or alcohol, history of frequent douching in women, and serial monogamy, which increases the risk of inconsistent condom use.

Social factors that increase the risk for contracting gonorrhea or chlamydia in adolescents include a low socioeconomic status, low levels of parental supervision, being a victim of abuse, rape, or incest, lack of choice as to whether to have intercourse, incarceration, meeting one's sexual partner outside of school, being unmarried, and homelessness. A study found that homeless adolescent girls were at greater risk for STDs than homeless adolescent boys were, with homeless adolescent girls less likely to use condoms and more likely to have a sexual partner who was an injection drug user.

A study of high school students in Philadelphia, Pennsylvania, reported that where adolescents met their sex partners was consistently associated with chlamydia and gonorrhea infection rates in both males and females. Meeting the partner at their own school was protective against these STDs, whereas meeting the partner at another school or outside of school altogether increased the risk for both STDs.

Regular screening for STDs is widely recommended for all adolescents. The U.S. Preventive Services Task Force recommends routine screening for those at high risk for infection (e.g., those who are less than 25 years old, have history of an STD, have multiple sexual partners, engage in inconsistent condom use, exchange sex for money, use drugs, reside in a high-risk community). The American Medical Association (AMA) Guidelines for Adolescent Preventive Services (GAPS) recommend yearly screenings for both gonorrhea and chlamydia for all sexually active adolescents. The United Kingdom's Royal Institute of Public Health recommends yearly chlamydia screening for both adolescent and young adult women. In Norway, health authorities recommend yearly chlamydia testing for both males and females under age 25.

Adolescents' "probability judgment" (estimate of the probability of being currently infected) may be a useful tool to clinicians in estimating the adolescents'

risk of having chlamydia. Investigators found that the probability judgment of a sample of sexually active female adolescents having chlamydia was positively correlated with testing positive for the disease. Probability judgments may be more reliable than self-reports of sexual activity in establishing risk levels.

Adolescents who have an STD are at an increased risk for HIV infection, with the risk going up as the number of STDs goes up for that adolescent. Adolescent girls were at a 2.6 incidence rate ratio of HIV infections, and adolescent boys were at a 2.3 incidence rate ratio. Many adolescents avoid screening for STDs because of concerns about receiving counseling for STDs. Adolescents avoid screening for STDs due to possible stigma and anxiety regarding the testing including the perceived stigma associated with STDs, anxiety related to discovering potential infertility, anxiety related to partner's reaction if an STD is diagnosed, anxiety related to confidentiality of the testing and parental reaction to an STD diagnosis.

WHAT CAN BE DONE

Social workers can learn about the risk factors for gonorrhea and chlamydia in adolescents so to accurately assess adolescent clients' personal, medical and health education needs, support and referrals. Social workers should encourage adolescent clients who are sexually active to undergo regular STD testing/screening. Education for adolescent clients may include discussions that diagnosis and treatment for STDs is confidential and that parental consent is not required in any of the 50 states in the United States or the District of Columbia. Social workers can provide education and resources to adolescent clients on where they can obtain diagnosis and treatment. They can also discuss the importance of encouraging their partner to complete testing/screening and seek treatment if needed.

Social workers may research the availability of expedited partner therapy in the state they practice, which would allow the client to obtain a prescription for a partner without the partner's having to see a physician. Social workers and medical professionals should instruct infected adolescents to abstain from sex until the infection is medically cleared by the treating clinician and to adhere to the drug regimen for the length of time prescribed. Written information on STDs (including HIV) should be provided, if available, to reinforce verbal education that is provided to the adolescent client.

Social workers may complete counseling with adolescents on strategies for reducing their risk for STDs, including practicing safer sex with regular and correct use of condoms. Social workers and medical professionals working with adolescents should become familiar with state and local laws governing the age of consent for sex and follow facility protocols for mandated reporting of criminal activity such as forced sexual activity, if indicated.

Written by Carita Caple, RN, BSN, MSHS

Reviewed by Jessica Therivel, LMSW-IPR

REFERENCES

Anschuetz, G. L., Beck, J. N., Asbel, L., Goldberg, M., Salmon, M. E., & Spain, C. V. (2009). Determining risk markers for gonorrhea and chlamydial infection and reinfection among adolescents in public high schools. *Sexually Transmitted Diseases, 36*(1), 4-8.

Bretl, D., Vukovich, M., Schroeder, J., & Mao, J. (2007). Chlamydia and gonorrhea reoccurrence in an adolescent correctional facility. *Journal of Adolescent Health, 40*(2: Supplement), S17.

Centers for Disease Control and Prevention. (2013, September 27). Legal status of expedited partner therapy (EPT). *Sexually Transmitted Diseases.* Retrieved October 5, 2015, from http://www.cdc.gov/std/ept/legal/default.htm

Centers for Disease Control and Prevention. (2014). Reported STDs in the United States: 2013 national data for chlamydia, gonorrhea, and syphilis. CDC Fact Sheet, December 2014. Retrieved October 5, 2015, from http://www.cdc.gov/nchhstp/newsroom/docs/factsheets/std-trends-508.pdf

Cashman, C. (2014). Chlamydial sexual transmitted diseases. In F. J. Domino (Ed.), *The 5-minute clinical consult standard 2015* (23rd ed., pp. 228-229). Philadelphia, PA: Wolters Kluwer Health.

Claire-Newbern, E., Anschuetz, G. L., Eberhart, M. G., Salmon, M. E., Brady, K. A., De los Reyes, A., ... Schwarz, D. F. (2013). Adolescent sexually transmitted infections and risk for subsequent HIV. *American Journal of Public Health, 103*(10), 1874-1881. doi:10.2105/AJPH.2013.301463

de Bruin, W. B., Downs, J. S., Murray, P., & Fischhoff, B. (2010). Can female adolescents tell whether they will test positive for Chlamydia infection?. *Medical Decision Making, 30*(2), 189-193.

DynaMed. (2014, March 20). Chlamydia genital infection. Ipswich, MA: EBSCO Publishing. Retrieved October 5, 2015, from http://search.ebscohost.com/login.aspx?direct=true&db=dme&AN=114223

Fine, D., Dicker, L., Mosure, D., & Berman, S. (2008). Increasing chlamydia positivity in women screened in family planning clinics: Do we know why? *Sexually Transmitted Diseases, 35*(1), 47-52. doi:10.1097/OLQ.0b013e31813e0c26

Gerlt, T., & Starr, N. B. (2009). Gynecologic conditions. In C. E. Burns, M. A. Brady, A. M. Dunn, N. B. Starr, & C. G. Blosser (Eds.), *Pediatric primary care* (4th ed., pp. 906-937). St. Louis, MO: Saunders Elsevier.

Lewis, M. T., Newman, D. R., Anschuetz, G. L., Mettey, A., Asbel, L., & Salmon, M. E. (2014). Partner meeting place is significantly associated with gonorrhea and chlamydia in adolescents participating in a large high school sexually transmitted disease screening program. *Sexually Transmitted Diseases, 41*(10), 605-610.

McDonnell, D. D., Levy, V., & Morton, T. J. (2009). Risk factors for chlamydia among young women in a northern California juvenile detention facility: Implications for community intervention. *Sexually Transmitted Diseases, 36*(Suppl. 2), S29-S33. doi:10.1097/OLQ.0b013e31815dd07d

McMunn, V. A., & Caan, W. (2007). Chlamydia infection, alcohol and sexual behaviour in women. *British Journal of Midwifery, 15*(4), 221-224.

Mizrahi, T., & Mayden, R. W. (2001). NASW standards for cultural competence in social work practice. Retrieved October 5, 2015, from http://www.socialworkers.org/practice/standards/NASWCulturalStandards.pdf

Orr, D. P., & Blythe, M. J. (2006). Sexually transmitted diseases. In J. A. McMillan (Ed.), *Oski's pediatrics: Principles & practice* (4th ed., pp. 584-592). Philadelphia, PA: Wolters Kluwer Health/Lippincott Williams & Wilkins.

Paul, K. J., Garcia, P. J., Giesel, A. E., Holmes, K. K., & Hitti, J. E. (2009). Generation C: Prevalence of and risk factors for Chlamydia trachomatis among adolescents and young women in Lima, Peru. *Journal of Women's Health, 18*(9), 1419-1424.

Skjeldestad, F. E., Marsico, M. A., Sings, H. L., Nordbo, S. A., & Storvold, G. (2009). Incidence and risk factors for genital chlamydia trachomatis infection: A 4-year prospective cohort study. *Sexually Transmitted Diseases, 36*(5), 273-279. doi:10.1097/OLQ.0b013e3181924386

International Federation of Social Workers. (2012, March 3). Statement of Ethical Principles. Retrieved October 5, 2015, from http://ifsw.org/policies/statement-of-ethical-principles/

The Policy, Ethics, and Human Rights Committee, British Association of Social Workers. (2012,

January). The Code of Ethics for Social Work: Statements of principles. Retrieved October 5, 2015, from http://cdn.basw.co.uk/upload/basw_112315-7.pdf

Valente, A. M., & Auerswald, C. L. (2013). Gender differences in sexual risk and sexually transmitted infections correlate with gender differences in social networks among San Francisco homeless youth. *Journal of Adolescent Health, 53*(4), 486-491. doi:10.1016/j.jadohealth.2013.05.016

SEXUALLY TRANSMITTED DISEASES: CHLAMYDIA — RISK FACTORS

MAJOR CATEGORIES: Medical & Health

WHAT WE KNOW

Chlamydia is an infectious disease caused by the bacterium *Chlamydia trachomatis*. It spreads primarily by vaginal, anal, and oral sex, and is the most common bacterial sexually transmitted disease (STD; also called sexually transmitted infection) in the United States. The World Health Organization (WHO) estimates that there are 92 million new cases of chlamydia worldwide each year. In the United States, in 2013, 1,401,906 cases of chlamydia were reported to the Centers for Disease Control and Prevention (CDC).

The true disease burden is likely to be much higher. In 2012, the CDC estimated that 2,291,000 noninstitutionalized U.S. citizens aged 14–39 have chlamydia. Chlamydia is called a "silent" disease because many individuals who become infected do not experience symptoms of the disease. Seventy-five percent of infected females and 95 percent of infected males have no signs or symptoms. Of those who do experience symptoms, a yellow purulent discharge and a burning sensation while urinating are common characteristics of the disease. Left untreated, chlamydia can result in a multitude of complications.

In females, complications of untreated infection include pelvic inflammatory disease (PID), ectopic pregnancy, endometriosis, infertility, and chronic pelvic pain. Untreated chlamydia also may increase the risk of HIV infection and cervical cancer. In males, complications of untreated chlamydia include epididymitis (i.e., inflammation of the testicles) and possibly infertility, as well as an increased risk for HIV infection. Lack of treatment allows for persistent infection and possible transmission to sexual partners.

Chlamydia occurs most commonly in individuals under the age of 26.

The probability of infection in this age group is 5–8 times higher than in people aged 30–35. Among the possible explanations for the high rates of chlamydia in young people is the fact that the cervix of adolescent females is not fully matured, making it more susceptible to infection. The CDC found that 28 percent of the chlamydia cases reported in 2013 occurred among 15- to 19-year-olds and 39 percent occurred among 20- to 24-year-olds.

In the United States, non-white ethnicity is associated with an increased risk of chlamydia. The rate of chlamydia among Blacks is over 8 times higher than that among Whites. The CDC recommends that all non-pregnant, sexually active women aged 25 or younger and older non-pregnant women who are at an increased risk due to a new sexual partner or multiple sexual partners be screened for chlamydia regularly. The U.S. Preventive Services Task Force specifically recommends screening for chlamydia and gonorrhea for all females aged 24 or younger who are sexually active. The English National Chlamydia Screening Programme recommends annual testing, or with every new sex partner, for all 16- to 24-year-olds.

Social workers and other medical professionals treating the client should provide them education on the necessity of partner notification of the infection.

It is possible that clients may be able to have their healthcare providers anonymously advise the clients' prior or current sexual contacts that they should be tested for chlamydia.

A number of behavioral and social risk factors for chlamydia have been identified, including inconsistent use of barrier devices (e.g., condoms) during sex, a higher number of lifetime partners, having more than one current sexual partner, urban residence, lower education level, being single, younger age at first sexual intercourse, and having a partner with urogenital symptoms/complaints.

An Australian study found that women who were accessing emergency contraception at a pharmacy were at high risk for contracting chlamydia. Out of the women studied, 100 percent met the risk factor of inconsistent use of barrier devices, were at risk due to age, were at risk due to a history of younger age at first sexual intercourse, and/or were at risk due to the number of sexual partners. The study reported that 72 percent of the women said they would be willing to accept a chlamydia screening test from the pharmacy which would provide an opportunity for screening high-risk women who may not visit a medical professional.

WHAT CAN BE DONE

Social workers should learn about the risk factors for chlamydia to accurately assess the client's personal, medical, and health education, support, and resource needs. The social worker should assess the client's anxiety level and provide emotional support for the diagnosis of chlamydia and for partner notification needs. When providing support to clients who have been diagnosed with chlamydia, social workers should keep in mind the three themes of concern that were found in women after diagnosis with chlamydia: uncertainty about their reproductive health, perception of stigma related to STD infection, and anxiety over partner's reaction to chlamydia diagnosis.

If client is having extreme anxiety regarding his or her reproductive health, the social worker can help advocate for him or her to receive an ultrasound or further testing for damage. Social workers and medical professionals should follow facility infection-control protocols (e.g., use of standard precautions) to prevent further spread of disease. Social workers and medical professionals should advise abstinence from

sex until the chlamydia infection is medically cleared by the treating clinician.

Clients should be educated about the importance of strict adherence to the prescribed drug regimen to ensure treatment efficacy. Social workers and medical professionals should encourage clients that test positive for chlamydia that their current or previous sexual partner(s) need to be tested for chlamydia and treated, if necessary.

Social workers should encourage STD screening in adolescents who, because of limited access to healthcare, use emergency departments when they need medical attention (STDs can be missed in the emergency department due to lack of screening). Written materials on chlamydia risk factors, including the risk for HIV infection may be provided for further information and support. Instructions on safe sex, including consistent use of condoms and other barrier methods should be provided by the social worker or medical professional to encourage prevention of further infections. The social worker may assist clients in connecting with community health services to help obtain condoms if necessary. Treating professionals should be aware of and follow facility protocols for mandated reporting of infectious disease.

Written by Renee Matteucci, MPH, and Tanja Schub, BS

Reviewed by Jessica Therivel, LMSW-IPR

REFERENCES

Al-Tayyib, A. A., Miller, W. C., Rogers, S. M., Leone, P. A., Law, D. C. G., Ford, C. A., & Rothman, R. E. (2008). Evaluation of risk score algorithms for detection of chlamydial and gonococcal infections in an emergency department setting. *Academic Emergency Medicine, 15*(2), 126-135. doi:10.1111/j.1553-2712.2008.00027.x

Centers for Disease Control and Prevention. (2014). Reported STDs in the United States: 2013 national data for chlamydia, gonorrhea, and syphilis [Fact sheet]. Retrieved September 22, 2015, from http://www.cdc.gov/nchhstp/newsroom/docs/STD-Trends-508.pdf

Centers for Disease Control and Prevention. (2014, June 23). Chlamydia – CDC fact sheet. Retrieved

September 22, 2015, from http://www.cdc.gov/std/chlamydia/stdfact-chlamydia.htm

Donegan, N. (2013). Management of patients with infectious diseases. In S. C. Smeltzer, B. G. Bare, J. L. Hinkle, & K. H. Cheever (Eds.), *Brunner & Suddarth's textbook of medical-surgical nursing* (13th ed., Vol. 2, pp. 2145-2146). Philadelphia: Wolters Kluwer Health/Lippincott Williams & Wilkins.

Fine, D., Dicker, L., Mosure, D., & Berman, S. (2008). Increasing chlamydia positivity in women screened in family planning clinics: Do we know why? *Sexually Transmitted Diseases, 35*(1), 47-52. doi:10.1097/OLQ.0b013e31813e0c26

Geisler, W. M. (2007). Management of uncomplicated Chlamydia trachomatis infections in adolescents and adults: Evidence reviewed for the 2006 Centers for Disease Control and Prevention sexually transmitted diseases treatment guidelines. *Clinical Infectious Diseases, 44*(Suppl. 3), S77-S83. doi:10.1086/5114215000018069

SEXUALLY TRANSMITTED DISEASES: RISK FACTORS

MAJOR CATEGORIES: Medical & Health

WHAT WE KNOW

Many factors can increase a person's risk of acquiring a sexually transmitted disease (STD), including both individual characteristics or behaviors and broader environmental conditions. Younger age is a recognized risk factor for STDs. Nearly 50 percent of the 19 million new STD cases in the United States each year occur in 15- to 24-year-olds. Individuals in this age group are more likely to engage in risky sexual behaviors, to be less comfortable negotiating condom use or discussing sexual matters with partners, and to lack the self-confidence needed to refuse to have unprotected intercourse. Initiation of anal sex before age 18 was associated with later subsequent risky behaviors (which were defined in the study as having multiple sex partners, being paid for sex, and engaging in increased use of recreational drugs) in a study of 10,826 men in East Asia who have sex with men. Being in an age-discordant relationship (specifically, a relationship between a younger adolescent female and an older adult male) is also a risk factor for adolescent STD infection.

There are racial and ethnic disparities in rates of STDs among female young adults. Black females between the ages of 15 and 24 are 8.7 times more likely to contract chlamydia and 20.5 times more likely to contract gonorrhea when compared to white females of the same age. Hispanic females are twice as likely as whites in this age category to acquire gonorrhea or chlamydia.

Certain sexual behaviors increase the risk of acquiring STDs. These include lack of condom use/unprotected sex; having multiple sex partners; concurrent sexual relationships; anonymous sex partners; engaging in sex in exchange for money; engaging in anal intercourse, with receptive anal sex carrying the highest risk for acquiring HIV; having unprotected sex with a partner who has unhealed lesions or a known STD; serosorting, or engaging in unprotected anal sex with partners thought to have the same HIV status; and having forced sexual intercourse.

Environmental and social factors that have been associated with an increased risk of acquiring STDs include a history of substance and/or alcohol use, which lowers a person's decision making skills and inhibitions and can lead to risky sexual behavior. It is estimated that binge drinkers are 77 percent more likely than non-binge drinkers to report engaging in high-risk sexual behaviors. Intravenous drug use and the sharing of needles can cause STD transmission. In addition, having unprotected sex with an intravenous drug user is associated with an increased risk for STD infection. Unprotected sexual intercourse and the sharing of needles are estimated to both take place in approximately 29 percent of relationships in which both partners are injection drug users.

Lower socioeconomic status increases the risk of acquiring STDs because of the greater likelihood of inadequate preventive care or education on reducing STD risk. The lack of appropriate preventive care or education regarding STD risk is especially common among homeless persons. Homelessness is associated with increased risk for sexual victimization and with survival sex (i.e., trading sexual acts in exchange for shelter or food), which may expose the victim to STDs.

Homeless young women have been found to be at greater risk for STDs than homeless young men are. Having been in foster care is associated with increased risk for STDs in young adulthood. A history of exposure to sexual, verbal, and physical abuse increases the chances that an individual will experience anxiety, depression, and posttraumatic stress disorder (PTSD), all of which may increase the risk for unsafe sexual behavior. Victims of intimate partner abuse also are at increased risk for STD infection.

Childhood sexual abuse survivors report higher rates of unprotected sex and STDs than do individuals who were not abused. Relationships that lack an equal distribution of power can render individuals unable to negotiate for safe sex practices or without the perceived right to refuse to have unprotected intercourse. Male-to-female transgender persons who experienced gender abuse (i.e., abuse related to their transgender status) and had depressive symptoms were found to be more likely to engage in high-risk sexual behaviors and had a higher incidence rate of HIV and other STDs. Men who perpetrate sexual coercion or rape are less likely to routinely wear condoms than are men who do not engage in aggressive sexual behavior.

Individuals with mental illness diagnosis and symptoms are at increased risk of acquiring STDs. Presence of STDs have been associated with mental health disorders such as schizophrenia, bipolar disorder, psychotic disorder, depression, and anxiety disorder among indigent, homeless, publicly insured, and institutionalized populations. Clients with mental health problems often display poor judgment and impulsive behavior, leading to risky sexual behaviors. Low self-esteem accompanying mental illness is a barrier to taking responsibility for behavior and taking care of personal health needs.

Cultural values and accepted behaviors among various ethnic and cultural groups regarding healthcare, drug and alcohol use, and sexual behavior can place individuals at risk for STDs. For example, Hispanic adolescents are less likely than black or white adolescents to use condoms during sex. Lack of regular healthcare due to poverty, mental illness, or cultural beliefs may contribute to a lack of education regarding safe sex practices.

Psychological barriers to STD screening and treatment can increase risk for STD infection and lead to advanced disease progression or death. These include mistrust of the healthcare system, lack of culturally or linguistically appropriate treatment or education, stigma and shame related to STDs and STD care, and social pressures. Misinformation and misunderstandings about STD screening can increase risk for STD infection. Approximately one quarter of subjects across three samples were found to have an incorrect understanding of the purpose of a Pap smear, for instance. The Pap smear tests for cervical cancer, yet 82 percent to 91 percent of study subjects believed it tested for human papillomavirus (HPV), 76 percent to 92 percent thought it tested for vaginal infections, 65 percent to 86 percent thought it tested for yeast infections, 55 percent to 81 percent thought it tested for gonorrhea, 53 percent to 80 percent thought it tested for herpes, 22 percent to 59 percent thought it tested for HIV/AIDS, and 17 percent to 38 percent thought it was a pregnancy test. Such beliefs may lead women with negative Pap smears to think that they do not have an STD.

WHAT CAN BE DONE

Social workers can learn about the risk factors for STDs and use this knowledge to fully assess individual clients and their healthcare and educational needs. Social workers should provide respectful and empathic client care and avoid negative, judgmental attitudes that can alienate clients and reduce the likelihood they will pursue follow-up care for STD treatment.

Social workers can encourage a multidisciplinary approach to sexual health treatment and prevention by requesting referrals to various specialist services (e.g., mental health clinicians, drug and alcohol treatment programs, primary care clinicians, licensed social workers).

Social workers may provide behavioral counseling and prevention education to all sexually active adolescents and adults who are at increased risk of contracting an STD. Social workers should screen clients for abusive relationships and, if appropriate, provide counseling and information on community resources for safety and STD prevention. Social workers and medical professionals treating sexually active adolescents should become familiar with state and local laws governing the age of consent and reporting of abuse and neglect. Facility and professional protocols for mandated reporting of criminal activity and abuse and neglect should be followed.

Social workers should inform adolescent clients that testing and treatment for STDs is confidential and parental consent for treatment is not required in the United States. Medical professionals should provide routine screening for STDs to all sexually active clients and their partners and, if necessary, refer for treatment.

Written by Carita Caple, RN, BSN, MSHS, and Tanja Schub, BS

Reviewed by Jessica Therivel, LMSW-IPR, and Chris Bates, MA, MSW

REFERENCES

Ahrens, K. R., Richardson, L. P., Courtney, M. E., McCarty, C., Simoni, J., & Katon, W. (2010). Laboratory-diagnosed sexually transmitted infections in former foster youth compared with peers. *Pediatrics, 126*(1), e97-e103. doi:10.1542/peds.2009-2424

Chen, Y. H., McFarland, W., & Raymond, H. F. (2014). Risk behaviors for HIV in sexual partnerships of San Francisco injection drug users. *AIDS Care, 26*(5), 554-558. doi:10.1080/09540121.2013.841840

Cheung, D. H., Suharlim, C., Guadamuz, T. E., Lim, S. H., Koe, S., & Wei, C. (2014). Earlier anal sexarche and co-occurring sexual risk are associated with current HIV-related risk behaviors among an online sample of men who have sex with men in Asia. *AIDS & Behavior, 18.* doi:10.1007/s10461-014-0821-0

Daley, E., Perrin, K., Vamos, C., Hernandez, N., Anstey, E., Baker, E., ... Ebbert, J. (2013). Confusion about Pap smears: Lack of knowledge among high-risk women. *Journal of Women's Health, 22*(1), 67-74. doi:10.1089/jwh.2012.3667

Eaton, L. A., Kalichman, S. C., O'Connell, D. A., & Karchner, W. D. (2009). A strategy for selecting sexual partners believed to pose little/no risks for HIV: Serosorting and its implications for HIV transmission. *AIDS Care, 21*(10), 1279-1288. doi:10.1080/09540120902803208

Elkington, K. S., Bauermeister, J. A., & Zimmerman, M. A. (2010). Psychological distress, substance use, and HIV/STI risk behaviors among youth. *Journal of Youth and Adolescence, 39*(5), 514-527. doi:10.1007/s10964-010-9524-7

International Federation of Social Workers. (2012, March 3). Statement of ethical principles. Retrieved October 6, 2015, from http://ifsw.org/policies/statement-of-ethical-principles/

Jarama, S. L., Stultz, N. A., Parillo, K. M., Snyder, F. R., & Young, P. A. (2011). Development of an HIV/STD screening index to measure HIV/STD risk in adolescents. *Journal of HIV/AIDS & Social Services, 10*(3), 230-247. doi:10.1080/15381501.2011.596766

Marshall, B. D., Kerr, T., Shoveller, J. A., Patterson, T. L., Buxton, J. A., & Wood, E. (2009). Homelessness and unstable housing associated with an increased risk of HIV and STI transmission among street-involved youth. *Health and Place, 15*(3), 753-760. doi:10.1016/j.healthplace.2008.12.005

Mizrahi, T., & Mayden, R. W. (2001). NASW standards for cultural competence in social work practice. Retrieved October 6, 2015, from http://www.socialworkers.org/practice/standards/NASWCulturalStandards.pdf

Mosack, K. E., Randolph, M. E., Dickson-Gomez, J., Abbott, M., Smith, E., & Weeks, M. R. (2010). Sexual risk-taking among high-risk urban women with and without histories of childhood sexual abuse: Mediating effects of contextual factors. *Journal of Child Sexual Abuse, 19*(1), 43-61. doi:10.1080/10538710903485591

Nuttbrock, L., Bockting, W., Rosenblum, A., Hwahng, S., Mason, M., Macri, M., & Becker, J. (2013). Gender abuse, depressive symptoms, and HIV and other sexually transmitted infections among male-to-female transgender persons: A three year prospective study. *American Journal of Public Health, 103*(2), 300-307. doi:10.2105/AJPH.2011.300568

Peterson, Z. D., Janssen, E., & Heiman, J. R. (2010). The association between sexual aggression and HIV risk behavior in heterosexual men. *Journal of Interpersonal Violence, 25*(3), 538-556. doi:10.1177/0886260509334414

Pflieger, J. C., Cook, E. C., Niccolai, L. M., & Connell, C. M. (2013). Racial/ethnic differences in patterns of sexual risk behavior and rates of sexually transmitted infections among female young adults. *American Journal of Public Health, 103*(5), 903-909. doi:10.2105/AJPH.2012.301005

Rosenthal, L., & Levy, S. R. (2010). Understanding women's risk for HIV infection using social dominance theory and the four bases of gendered power. *Psychology of Women Quarterly, 34*(1), 21-35. doi:10.1111/j.1471-6402.2009.01538.x

Roye, C. F., Krauss, B. J., & Silverman, P. L. (2010). Prevalence and correlates of heterosexual anal intercourse among Black and Latina female adolescents. *Journal of the Association of Nurses in AIDS Care, 21*(4), 291-301. doi:10.1016/j.jana.2009.12.002

Talou-Shams, M., Feldstein Ewing, S. W., Tarantino, N., & Brown, L. K. (2010). Crack and cocaine use among adolescents in psychiatric treatment: Associations with HIV risk. *Journal of Child and Adolescent Substance Abuse, 19*(2), 122-134. doi:10.1080/10678281003634926

The Policy, Ethics, and Human Rights Committee, British Association of Social Workers. (2012, January). The Code of ethics for social work: Statement of principles. Retrieved October 6, 2015, from http://cdn.basw.co.uk/upload/basw_112315-7.pdf

Valente, A. M., & Auerswald, C. L. (2013). Gender differences in sexual risk and sexually transmitted infections correlate with gender differences in social networks among San Francisco homeless youth. *Journal of Adolescent Health, 53*(4), 486-491. doi:10.1016/j.jadohealth.2013.05.016

Villar-Loubet, O., Jones, D., Waldrop-Valverde, D., Bruscantini, L., & Weiss, S. (2011). Sexual barrier acceptability among multiethnic HIV-positive and at risk women. *Journal of Women's Health, 20*(3), 365-373.

Wen, X.-J., Balluz, L., & Town, M. (2012). Prevalence of HIV risk behaviors between binge drinkers and non-binge drinkers aged 18- to 64-years in US, 2008. *Journal of Community Health, 37*(1), 72-79. doi:10.1007/s10900-011-9418-y

Workowski, K. A., & Berman, S. (2010). Sexually transmitted diseases treatment guidelines, 2010. *MMWR. Morbidity and Mortality Weekly Report. Recommendations and Reports, 59*(RR-12), 1-110.

Wu, E. S., Rothbard, A., & Blank, M. B. (2011). Using psychiatric symptomatology to assess risk for HIV infection in individuals with severe mental illness. *Community Mental Health Journal, 47*(6), 672-678. doi:10.1007/s10597-011-9402-0

SEXUALLY TRANSMITTED DISEASES: SYPHILIS—RISK FACTORS

MAJOR CATEGORIES: Medical & Health

WHAT WE KNOW

Syphilis is an infectious bacterial disease caused by the bacterium *Treponema pallidum*. Syphilis is spread through contact of bodily fluids and is primarily contracted by sexual intercourse. The risk factors for syphilis include poverty in urban areas, illegal drug use, exchange of sex for drugs, unprotected oral sex, not using condoms, multiple sex partners, anonymous sex partners, HIV infection, incarceration, and exposure to infected body fluids such as blood. Newborns may be at risk for congenital syphilis as a result of untreated syphilis infections in their mothers. A newborn may also be at risk for syphilis through vertical transmission of the infection during passage through the birth canal of an infected mother.

Syphilis has three distinct clinical stages: primary, secondary, and latent (also called tertiary). Primary syphilis, the initial stage, is characterized by the appearance of a primary chancre (i.e., a painless lesion at the site of the infection) on the genitalia, anus, lips, tongue or elsewhere in the mouth, or tonsils. The chancre tends to be ulcerated and painless and usually heals without treatment within a few weeks. If the chancre are left untreated, primary syphilis progresses to secondary syphilis, which is characterized by a maculopapular (i.e. red spots) rash on the trunk, extremities, soles, and palms of the individual. Latent syphilis develops from untreated secondary syphilis and is divided into two stages of latency, early latent and late latent stages.

In the early latent stage (having syphilis less than a year), the individual usually is asymptomatic (does not have any symptoms). Late latent stage syphilis (having syphilis longer than a year) manifests as cardiovascular syphilis (i.e., infection of the heart and blood vessels with *T. pallidum*), neurosyphilis (i.e., infection of the brain or spine with *T. pallidum*), or gummatous syphilis (i.e., granulomatous lesions that affect the mucous membranes, skin, bones, and internal organs).

If syphilis is left untreated, complications resulting in additional medical conditions can develop, including cardiovascular disease, central nervous system disease, hepatitis, arthritis, periostitis, membranous glomerulonephritis, meningitis, hypertrophic gastritis, patchy proctitis, ulcerative colitis, rectosigmoid mass, and irreversible organ damage.

Other complications include severe ocular problems such as optic neuritis, retinitis pigmentosa syndrome, papillary abnormalities, iritis, and uveitis.

In its latent stage, untreated syphilis can result in irreversible blindness, paralysis, heart disease, dementia, chronic bone and joint inflammation, and eventually death.

Ulcerated STDs, such as syphilis in its primary stage with sores, increase the risk of acquiring and transmitting HIV. According to the CDC, in the United States in 2000, the rate of reported primary and secondary syphilis cases per 100,000 adults was 2.1. In 2005, it was 2.9; in 2008, it was 4.4; and in 2013, it was 5.3. For women, in 2005, the rate was 0.9; in 2008, it was 1.5; and in 2013, it was 0.9 again. For men, in 2005, the rate was 5.1; in 2008, it was 7.5; and by 2013, it had grown to 9.8. Rates of syphilis infection are highest in men 25–29 years of age.

Syphilis rates remain high among high-risk groups such as men who have sex with men (MSM), commercial sex workers, individuals who exchange sex for drugs, prison inmates, and certain minority groups, especially U.S. Blacks and Hispanics.

WHAT CAN BE DONE

Social workers should become knowledgeable about syphilis, including risk factors, signs and symptoms, treatment options, and possible psychological ramifications that an individual may experience if they are infected. Social workers and medical professionals assisting clients with syphilis should use standard universal precautions including wearing gloves, masks, or gowns in all client care to help prevent the spread of the disease. Social workers and medical professionals can encourage clients, especially those who are HIV-positive, to be tested for STDs in order to identify healthcare needs early.

Social workers should educate clients to have a medical exam if they have lesions to determine the cause of the lesions since primary syphilis chancres may resemble ulcerated lesions caused by other sources such as the herpes simplex virus, chancroid, granuloma inguinale, carcinoma, trauma, lichen planus, fungal infections, or drug eruptions. The rash of secondary syphilis can be similar to rashes caused by pityriasis rosea, psoriasis, drug eruptions, lichen planus, scabies, or other acute febrile rashes.

Other symptoms of secondary syphilis can mimic illnesses such as mononucleosis or hepatitis infections.

Social workers and medical professionals should advise clients with syphilis to abstain from sex until completion of the prescribed drug regimen and until the infection has cleared, as evidenced by laboratory test results interpreted by the treating clinician. Clients should be educated about the need for their sexual partner(s) to have an examination and receive medical treatment if the client is positive for syphilis. Clients should be encouraged to comply with the drug regimen and educated about the importance of completing their treatment to ensure treatment efficacy and prevent further complications.

Social workers can advocate for clients to make sure they are able to obtain the necessary medications to complete their drug regimen. Advocating may include discussing coverage options with insurance companies or seeking financial support from the community. Social workers and treating medical professionals should provide clients with educational material on syphilis and the potential for HIV and other STDs.

Written information, if available, on safe sex, including the use of condoms and other barrier methods may be helpful for further education about prevention techniques.

Social workers may assist clients in accessing community health services that can provide condoms or other materials related to safe sex.

Social workers should encourage clients to follow reporting practices for partner notification of the client's positive STD test results. The social worker and medical professionals should be aware of and follow facility protocols for mandatory reporting of infectious disease.

Written by Renee Matteucci, MPH, and
Sara Richards, MSN, RN

Reviewed by Jessica Therivel, LMSW-IPR

REFERENCES

Badowski, M., & Patel, M. C. (2014). Syphilis. In F. J. Domino, R. A. Baldor, J. A. Grimes, & J. Golding (Eds.), *The 5-minute clinical consult standard 2015* (23rd ed., pp. 1152-1153). Philadelphia, PA: Wolters Kluwer Health/Lippincott Williams & Wilkins.

Bellis, M. A., Cook, P., Clark, P., Syed, Q., & Hoskins, A. (2002). Re-emerging syphilis in gay men: A case-control study of behavioral risk factors and

HIV status. *Journal of Epidemiology and Community Health, 56*(3), 235-236. doi:10.1136/jech.56.3.235

Centers for Disease Control and Prevention (CDC). (2014). Primary and secondary syphilis – United States, 2005-2013. *Morbidity and Mortality Weekly Report (MMWR), 63*(18), 402-406.

Centers for Disease Control and Prevention. (2014, July 8). Syphilis – CDC fact sheet. Retrieved October 8, 2014, from http://www.cdc.gov/std/syphilis/STDFact-Syphilis.htm

Chen, J. L., Callahan, D. B., & Kerndt, P. R. (2002). Syphilis control among incarcerated men who have sex with men: Public health response to an outbreak. *American Journal of Public Health, 92*(9), 1473-1474. doi:10.2105/ajph.92.9.1473

Corner, H. L., Couldwell, D. L., & Bourne, C. P. (2009). Bug breakfast in the bulletin: Syphilis. *NSW Public Health Bulletin, 20*(7-8), 130-131. doi:10.1071/nb09004

Doherty, L., Fenton, K. A., Jones, J., Paine, T. C., Higgins, S. P., Williams, D., & Palfreeman, A. (2002). Syphilis: Old problem, new strategy. *BMJ (Clinical research ed.), 325*(7356), 153-156. doi:10.1136/bmj.325.7356.153

Hook, E. W., III. (2012). Syphilis. In L. Goldman & A. I. Schafer (Eds.), *Goldman's Cecil medicine* (24th ed., pp. 1922-1929). Philadelphia, PA: Elsevier Saunders.

International Federation of Social Workers. (2012, March 3). Statement of ethical principles. Retrieved September 21, 2015, from http://ifsw.org/policies/statement-of-ethical-principles

Koumans, E. H., Farley, T. A., Gibson, J. J., Langley, C., Ross, M. W., MacFarlane, M., ... St Louis, M. E. (2001). Characteristics of persons with syphilis in areas of persisting syphilis in the United States: Sustained transmission associated with concurrent partnerships. *Sexually Transmitted Diseases, 28*(9), 497-503. doi:10.1097/00007435-200109000-00004

National Association of Social Workers. (2001). NASW standards for cultural competence in social work practice. Retrieved September 21, 2015, from http://www.socialworkers.org/practice/standards/NASWCulturalStandards.pdf

Peterman, T. A., & Furness, B. W. (2007). The resurgence of syphilis among men who have sex with men. *Current Opinion in Infectious Diseases, 20*(1), 54-59. doi:10.1097/qco.0b013e32801158cc

Pletcher, S. D., & Cheung, S. W. (2003). Syphilis and otolaryngology. *Otolaryngologic Clinics of North America, 36*(4), 595-605, vi.

The Policy, Ethics, and Human Rights Committee, British Association of Social Workers. (2012, January). The code of ethics for social work: Statement of principles. Retrieved September 21, 2015, from http://cdn.basw.co.uk/upload/basw_112315-7.pdf

Rich, J. D., Hou, J. C., Charuvastra, A., Towe, C. W., Lally, M., Spaulding, A., ... Rompalo, A. (2001). Risk factors for syphilis among incarcerated women in Rhode Island. *AIDS Patient Care and STDs, 15*(11), 581-585. doi:10.1089/108729101753287676

Ruan, Y., Li, D., Li, X., Qian, H. Z., Shi, W., Zhang, X., ... Shao, Y. (2007). Relationship between syphilis and HIV infections among men who have sex with men in Beijing, China. *Sexually Transmitted Diseases, 34*(8), 592-597. doi:10.1097/01.olq.0000253336.64324.ef

Seña, A. C., Muth, S. Q., Heffelfinger, J. D., O'Dowd, J. O., Foust, E., & Leone, P. (2007). Factors and the sociosexual network associated with a syphilis outbreak in rural North Carolina. *Sexually Transmitted Diseases, 34*(5), 280-287. doi:10.1097/01.olq.0000237776.15870.c3

Sugihantono, A., Slidell, M., Syaifudin, A., Pratjojo, H., Utami, I. M., Sajimin, T., & Mayer, K. H. (2003). Syphilis and HIV prevalence among commercial sex workers in Central Java, Indonesia: Risk-taking behavior and attitudes that may potentiate a wider epidemic. *AIDS Patient Care and STDs, 17*(11), 595-600. doi:10.1089/108729103322555980

Taylor, M. M., Aynalem, G., Smith, L. V., Montoya, J., & Kerndt, P. (2007). Methamphetamine use and sexual risk behaviors among men who have sex with men diagnosed with early syphilis in Los Angeles County. *International Journal of STD & AIDS, 18*(2), 93-97. doi:10.1258/095646207779949709

U.S. Preventive Services Task Force. (2004). Screening for syphilis infection: Recommendation statement. *Annals of Family Medicine, 2*(4), 362-365. doi:10.1370/afm.215

Wolfe, M. I., Xu, F., Patel, P., O'Cain, M., Schillinger, J. A., St. Louis, M. E., & Finelli, L. (2001). An outbreak of syphilis in Alabama prisons: Correctional health policy and communicable disease control. *American Journal of Public Health, 91*(8), 1220-1225. doi:10.2105/ajph.91.8.1220

Zetola, N. M., & Klausner, J. D. (2007). Syphilis and HIV infection: An update. *Clinical Infectious Diseases, 44*(9), 1222-1228. doi:10.1086/513427

SHARED PSYCHOTIC DISORDER

MAJOR CATEGORIES: Behavioral & Mental Health

DESCRIPTION

The Fifth Edition of the *Diagnostic and Statistical Manual of Mental Disorders* (*DSM-V*) eliminated *shared psychotic disorder* as a distinct diagnosis. Instead, the concept of shared psychotic disorder appears in the *DSM-V* as a specifier, or extension of a diagnosis, that clarifies the features of the disorder to which the diagnosis applies (i.e., delusional symptoms in a partner of an individual who has a delusional disorder) within the category of diseases belonging to the schizophrenia spectrum and other psychotic disorders (*DSM-5*, p. 122). The specifier states that a dominant individual with a delusional disorder may provide the delusional material for someone with whom he or she is in a relationship but who does not meet the other criteria for having a delusional disorder.

As defined by the Fourth Edition of the *Diagnostic and Statistical Manual of Mental Disorder* (*DSM-IV*), the primary features of shared psychotic disorder (also called *folie à deux* in the *DSM-IV*) are the presence of a delusion that occurs in an individual who is in a close relationship with someone who already has an established delusion. The shared delusion is identical or similar to the established delusion of the originally affected individual, and is not better identified as constituting any other psychotic disorder, or constituting a mood disorder with psychotic features, a general medical condition, or the effects of a substance. In the *International Statistical Classification of Diseases and Related Health Problems, 10th Revision* (*ICD-10*), the disorder comparable to what is called "shared psychotic disorder" in the *DSM-IV* is called *induced delusional disorder* (which the *ICD-10* also calls "folie à deux," just as it is called in the *DSM-IV*). As defined in the *ICD-10*, this disorder requires that those in whom it is diagnosed share the same delusion or delusional system with one another and support each other in their belief(s), that the two who share the delusion have an unusually close relationship, and that there is evidence that the shared delusion was induced in the passive partner by the active partner.

The features of a shared psychotic disorder, as defined in the *DSM-V*, also appear in the disorders known as *folie à trois* (in which three individuals share

a delusion), *folie à quatre* (in which four individuals share a delusion), folie en famille (with all members of a nuclear family sharing a delusion), and folie à plusieurs (with many individuals sharing a delusion). All manifestations of this disorder feature a dominant, also called a primary, inducer, or principal individual, who has the delusion and is the most dominant member of the relationship or group. The individual who develops a shared psychotic disorder is called the passive, secondary, acceptor, or associate member of the relationship or group. In any case, the primary individual is the more dominant individual in the relationship, and gradually imposes his or her delusion on the less dominant member(s) of the relationship. In addition to the dominant/passive nature of the relationship in which a delusion is shared in a shared psychotic disorder, the individuals who share the delusion usually live together and are socially and physically isolated from the wider world. In many cases the delusion and the behavior directly associated with it are the only signs of a shared psychotic disorder, and the individual who passively shares the psychotic disorder is less severely impaired by it than is the dominant individual.

Because shared psychotic disorder is rare, and according to the *DSM-IV* goes unrecognized in some cases, little is known about its course and etiology. As noted earlier, the onset of the disorder requires a long-term intimate relationship with someone who has a delusion, although the age and rapidity of the onset of the disorder appear to be variable. Unless the relationship with the dominant or primary member of a relationship involving a shared psychotic disorder is disrupted, its course is usually chronic and remains untreated until the primary member receives treatment for it. Even with disruption of this relationship, the course of the disorder for the secondary member is unpredictable.

FACTS AND FIGURES

Because shared psychotic disorder is rare, and according to the *DSM-IV* some cases of it go unrecognized, few undisputed facts and figures are available about it. Some evidence exists that shared psychotic disorder is diagnosed more often in women than in men, and that the primary members of the relationships in which the disorder exists often have schizophrenia.

RISK FACTORS

The primary risk factor for shared psychotic disorder is being the more passive member(s) of an excessively close relationship that tends to be physically and socially isolated and in which the more dominant member has a delusion.

SIGNS AND SYMPTOMS

The primary sign of shared psychotic disorder is a delusion or delusional system that the more passive member of a relationship shares with the more dominant member of the relationship. If the shared delusion does not cause behavior that brings attention to itself, the disorder often lacks other signs or symptoms of its existence.

APPLICABLE LAWS AND REGULATIONS

Both the United States Government and individual states have their own standards, procedures, and laws for the involuntary restraint and detention of persons who may be a danger to themselves or to others. Because persons in whom delusional symptoms are diagnosed may harm themselves or others, it is important to become familiar with the local requirements for involuntary detention. Attempted physical separation from the dominant member of a relationship in which shared psychotic disorder exists may have legal consequences if the persons involved in the relationship are married or if minor children or vulnerable adults are involved. Local and professional reporting requirements for the neglect and abuse of an individual who may have a shared psychotic disorder should be known and observed.

TREATMENT

The social worker assisting an individual in whom a diagnosis of brief psychotic disorder has been made should conduct a standard biological, psychological, social, and spiritual assessment of the individual, including an assessment of his or her risk for suicide and harming him- or herself and others. This should include observation of the individual's behavior and demeanor during the assessment, and the collection of collateral information from the individual's family, friends, and co-workers, which is especially important because of the typically sudden onset of brief psychotic disorder and the need to verify the presence of external stressor(s) as factors triggering its occurrence. The individual undergoing assessment should be referred for medical tests done to eliminate a medical condition as the cause of the disorder, and for tests done to eliminate the intake of substances that may cause the symptoms of the disorder.

If the passive member has adopted the delusion of the dominant member of a relationship in which shared psychotic disorder exists, a professional effort should be made to separate the dominant and passive members both physically and psychologically, to diminish the influence of the former on the latter. The technique used for achieving psychological separation of the two members will depend on the nature of the relationship, and must be carefully designed to accommodate the bond between them. In some cases physical separation is all that is needed to diminish the delusion of the passive member of the relationship; however, care must be used to mininmize possible negative consequences of this separation because members of such relationships may depend on each other for vital resources such as housing, and the passive member of such a relationship may be using the relationship to cope with or compensate for another mental illness or other problem.

Legal and ethical considerations may come into play if the pair sharing a delusion is married or if the relationship involves minor children or vulnerable adults. If the dependent member of the relationship in which there is a shared psychotic disorder is a minor or a vulnerable adult, the appropriate protective agency should be called upon to effect the separation, and reporting requirements for the separation should be fulfilled. In cases in which separation is not possible or desirable, the psychiatric treatment or other procedure that is least disruptive to all the individuals affected by the disorder should be used.

Social workers assisting individuals with a shared psychotic disorder should be aware of their own cultural values, beliefs, and biases, and develop specialized knowledge about the histories, traditions, and values of these individuals. They should adopt treatment methodologies best suited and least disruptive to the individuals with a shared psychotic disorder, and should refer the members of a relationship with a shared psychotic disorder to available resources and supports outside of the relationship if this is indicated or needed.

Written by Chris Bates, MA, MSW

Reviewed by Lynn B. Cooper, D. Crim

REFERENCES

American Psychiatric Association. (2000). *Diagnostic and statistical manual of mental disorders* (4th ed.). Washington, DC: Author.

American Psychiatric Association. (2013). Diagnostic and statistical manual of mental health disorders. (5th ed.). Arlington, VA: American Psychiatric Publishing.

British Association of Social Workers. (2012, January). The code of ethics for social work: Statement of principles. Retrieved April 11, 2016, from http://cdn.basw.co.uk/upload/basw_112315-7.pdf

Daniel, E., & Srinivasan, T. N. (2004). Folie à famille: Delusional parasitosis affecting all the members of a family. *Indian Journal of Dermatology, Venereology, and Leprology, 70*(5), 296-297.

International Federation of Social Workers. (2012, March 3). Statement of Ethical Principles. Retrieved April 11, 2016, from http://ifsw.org/policies/statement-of-ethical-principles/

Mentjox, R., van Houten, C. A., & Kooiman, C. G. (1993). Induced psychotic disorder: Clinical aspects, theoretical considerations, and some guidelines for treatment. *Comprehensive Psychiatry, 34*(2), 120-126.

Mergui, J., Jaworowski, S., Greenberg, D., & Lerner, V. (2010). Shared obsessive-compulsive disorder: Broadening the concept of shared psychotic disorder. *Australian and New Zealand Journal of Psychiatry, 44*(9), 859-862.

National Association of Social Workers. (2015). Standards and Indicators for Cultural Competence in Social Work Practice. Retrieved April 11, 2016, from http://www.socialworkers.org/practice/standards/PRA-BRO-253150-CC-Standards.pdf

Sanjurjo-Hartman, T., Weitzner, M. A., Santana, C., Devine, C., & Grendys, E. (2001). Cancer and folie à deux: Case report, treatment, and implications. *Cancer Practice, 9*(6), 290-294.

SIBLING MALTREATMENT

MAJOR CATEGORIES: Child & Family

DESCRIPTION

Sibling maltreatment is the most common yet least researched form of family violence. Similar to other forms of maltreatment, sibling maltreatment may be physical, psychological, or sexual in nature. The siblings may be biological siblings (i.e., sharing biological parents), half siblings (i.e., sharing one parent), stepsiblings (i.e., related through marriage), adoptive siblings or foster siblings (i.e., related through a shared home), or fictive siblings (i.e., not biologically related but considered a sibling). There is lack of consensus among researchers regarding how to define sibling maltreatment. Distinguishing normal developmental behavior between siblings from abusive interactions between siblings often is challenging for both parents and professionals. Sibling maltreatment is not the same as sibling rivalry or sibling conflict, which are characterized by isolated incidents that are age-appropriate. Sibling rivalry is reciprocal between siblings and obvious to others observing the behavior. The goal of sibling rivalry is receiving recognition from their parents and a feeling of significance, not harm and domination. When determining if an interaction between siblings is abusive, it is important that professionals and parents consider the developmental appropriateness of behaviors, the frequency, severity and intent of the aggression, whether it is mutual or unilateral, and the emotional impact of the act on the aggressor and his or her victim.

For the purpose of professional assessment and treatment, sibling physical maltreatment can be defined as one sibling habitually taking the role of aggressor and acting intentionally to cause physical harm and/or injury to another sibling. Physical maltreatment may take the form of hitting, slapping, kicking, biting, pinching, pushing, choking, or hair pulling. Severe cases of maltreatment may involve the use of implements or weapons to inflict injury, such as sticks, belts, rubber hoses, broom handles, scissors, razors, broken glass, or guns. Physical violence between siblings may be proactive (i.e., violence used in an intentional manner to dominate or control) or reactive (i.e., impulsive, angry reaction to threat or perceived provocation). Aggression is more prevalent in younger children and tends to decrease as children mature, whereas aggression perpetrated by older children is more likely to result in injury. The motivation for sibling abusive behavior varies based on the aggressor's age. Children younger than 8 years typically use aggression with other siblings to settle conflicts over possessions, whereas violence in children between the ages of 9 and 13 is more likely to occur over spatial boundaries, and in teens 14 years and older physical violence between siblings is more likely to be precipitated by conflict over responsibilities and social obligations. Psychological or emotional sibling maltreatment is defined as the use of nonphysical tactics intended to harm or incite fear or emotional distress in a sibling in order to assert control and power over him or her. Sibling emotional maltreatment may be in the form of intimidation, belittling, provocation, threats, destruction of possessions, and/or torture.

Sibling sexual maltreatment is sexual behavior with a sibling that typically involves deceit or coercion, is not developmentally appropriate, and is motivated by sexual gratification. Sexual maltreatment can include intercourse, masturbation, oral sex, fondling, forcing a sibling to view pornography, and making unwanted sexual advances. Sexual abuse is distinguished from consensual sexual exploration, which is transient and mutual, and involves siblings that are close in age and motivated by developmentally appropriate curiosity rather than sexual gratification. The nature of sexual behaviors often differs as well. For instance, exploratory touch, looking at each other's genitals, or "playing doctor" are within developmental norms for young children, whereas preoccupation with sexual behaviors and acts that mimic adult sexual activities such as simulated intercourse or penetration is not.

Sibling maltreatment typically starts in childhood and may continue into adulthood; most research and treatment modalities are focused on sibling maltreatment in the age 18-and-under population.

Sibling maltreatment that is left unaddressed often continues throughout childhood, subjecting victims of sibling maltreatment to long-term physical and/ or psychological harm. There is a likelihood that continued violent behavior in siblings can manifest in adulthood as physical and emotional disorders, dating and domestic violence, and substance abuse. Victims of sibling maltreatment are at an increased risk of experiencing symptoms of depression, anxiety, trauma symptoms, adjustment problems, low self-esteem, academic deficits, relationship/intimacy problems, sexual dysfunction, eating disorders, substance abuse, and self-injurious behaviors.

Treatment of sibling maltreatment is based on a multidimensional approach that focuses on assessing and treating the entire family, not just the siblings, in order to address the needs of each family member as well as systemic family issues (e.g., lack of supervision, intimate partner violence, and combative interactions).

FACTS AND FIGURES

Sibling aggression is not uncommon. In recent studies of sibling maltreatment in Portugal, the United Kingdom, and the United States, researchers have found that 35 percent–95 percent of respondents reported perpetrating and/or being the victim of at least one act of sibling aggression (e.g., shouting, swearing, pushing, grabbing) per year. In a United States study involving youth admitted to psychiatric hospitals, researchers found that 76 percent had perpetrated sibling violence and 22 percent had been victims of sibling violence; perpetrating sibling violence was also associated with violence towards peers, mothers, teachers, and themselves.

Children who experience maltreatment and neglect by a parent/caregiver are 4 times more likely to experience emotionally abusive and physically violent sibling interactions than children from a nonabusive home. Children who are victims of sibling maltreatment are subject to a higher frequency of abusive incidents than children who are victimized by peers. Sibling maltreatment occurs most frequently in children 6–9 years of age; cases involving injuries and weapons most often occur in teens 14–17 years of age.

In a United States study based on data retrieved from the 2000–2005 database of the National Incident-Based Reporting System (NIBRS), researchers found that males were perpetrators of sibling violence more often than females and were more likely to victimize a female sibling. NIBRS data show that over 13,000 incidents of sibling sexual abuse were reported to law enforcement agencies in an 8-year period; perpetrators of sibling sexual abuse were an average of 5.5 years older than the victims. The majority of cases (67 percent) involved brother-sister dyads (e.g., interactions), whereas 25 percent of cases involved brother-brother dyads. The majority (92–94 percent) of sibling sexual abuse perpetrators are male; the majority (71 percent) of sibling sexual abuse victims are female. Approximately 55 percent of cases of sibling sexual abuse involved forcible fondling and 40 percent involved rape or sodomy. Researchers in a Canadian study found that siblings were identified as the alleged perpetrators in 10 percent of all sexual abuse reports made to child protection agencies.

RISK FACTORS

Sibling maltreatment is strongly influenced by family relationships. Children are at a significant risk of maltreatment if their parents/caregivers engage in intimate partner violence and/or child maltreatment. Poor quality parent-child relationships, harsh parenting styles, and low parental warmth towards the children are associated with increased chances of sibling maltreatment. Children are also at a greater risk for sibling maltreatment if their parents are unwilling or unable to help them resolve sibling-to-sibling conflict or if they promote sibling rivalry by playing favorites. A parent may condone the ongoing sibling maltreatment by minimizing or ignoring the maltreatment, blaming the victim for the maltreatment he/she experienced, encouraging the victim to fight back, or responding inappropriately by abusing the perpetrator for the maltreatment to their sibling. The risk of maltreatment increases with a decrease in parental supervision and availability. Family stressors such as marital conflict, parental separation, divorce, or incarceration of a parent increase the risk of sibling maltreatment. Children who are abusive toward their sibling(s) are at risk of developing conduct disorders and antisocial behaviors. Children may be predisposed to engage in sibling violence if they have a conduct disorder, mood disorder, or attention-deficit/hyperactivity disorder. Offenders of sibling maltreatment also have develop a higher rate of alcohol and substance abuse in comparison to non-offending

siblings. Victims of sibling maltreatment are at a greater risk of being involved in other abusive relationships during their lifetime than those who are not maltreated by a sibling.

SIGNS AND SYMPTOMS

Psychological signs and symptoms of sibling maltreatment may include victims experiencing symptoms of fear, anger, shame, humiliation, and guilt. Both victims and perpetrators of sibling maltreatment may experience low self-esteem and suffer from depression and anxiety. Victims of sexual abuse from a sibling may experience symptoms of grief, anger, and feelings of helplessness.

Behavioral signs and symptoms of sibling maltreatment may include the victims expressing fear due to the maltreatment in the form of anxiety, nightmares, or phobias. A victim of sibling maltreatment may avoid the offending sibling. Children may develop eating difficulties, display aggressive behavior (in the case of the victim), act out sexually, or engage in alcohol/substance abuse, self-injurious behaviors, or delinquent activities.

Developmental signs and symptoms of sibling maltreatment may include both victims and perpetrators of sibling maltreatment experiencing developmental delays in cognitive functioning, language development, and motor coordination.

Social signs and symptoms of sibling maltreatment may include the victims of sibling maltreatment refusing to attend school or experiencing academic difficulties and may isolate himself or herself. Adolescents may run away from home, engage in delinquent behavior, or withdraw from family and peers.

Physical signs and symptoms of sibling maltreatment may include the victims having physical signs of maltreatment including bruises, welts, cuts, scratches, bite marks, burns, stab wounds, and missing patches of hair or having internal injuries (e.g., head trauma, internal bleeding, broken bones).Victims of sibling maltreatment may have physical signs of sexual abuse including bruises on the thighs or arms; bleeding, swelling, pain, or itching of the vagina, anus, mouth, and/or throat; odorous vaginal discharge; cuts and bruises; urinary tract infection; and difficulty walking or sitting. Victims may have somatic complaints such as stomach pains, headaches, elimination problems, eating difficulties, and sleep disturbances.

Assessment

The social worker should complete a comprehensive biological, psychological, social and spiritual assessment of the siblings and family to include information on physical, mental, environmental, social, financial, and medical factors as they relate to the children's care and immediate safety concerns. The social worker should ask about sibling relationships, including physical/psychological aggression and sexual behaviors noticed between siblings. The assessment should include information about the history of any family history of alcohol/substance abuse, history and perception of the parent-child relationships, history of child maltreatment, intimate partner violence history, and history of mental health disorders. The social worker should ask about the children's medical, developmental, and behavioral history, prior hospitalizations and injuries, history of self-harm, history of suicidal thoughts and attempts, history of aggression, history of fire setting behavior, history of physical/sexual/emotional abuse or neglect, and history of any exposure to violence or other traumatic events.

If sibling maltreatment is disclosed during the assessment, the social worker should explore the nature, intensity, severity, frequency, chronicity, and pervasiveness of the sibling maltreatment and include the developmental stage the maltreatment took place along with any buffering influences.

The level of available supervision of children in the home, the parents' awareness of the sibling abuse and their response to it including what safety measures parents have taken to protect the victim should be assessed. It should be determined if parents are able to appropriately recognize sibling maltreatment and provide necessary intervention to protect the victim of the maltreatment. The social worker should be mindful of the abusive sibling's status as a child as well as an offender of abuse and assist parents in makings appropriate intervention plans that address both children's needs.

General questions should be asked to screen for possible sexual abuse. If indicated, enough information should be obtained to facilitate an assessment of the child's immediate safety (e.g., perpetrator's access to child, protective parent), but social workers generally should refrain from detailed questioning about sexual abuse and instead contact CPS or refer the child to a child advocacy center. Interviews regarding sexual abuse should be conducted by trained forensic interviewers using established protocols. Additional information regarding appropriate forensic interviewing techniques is available through the American Academy of Child and Adolescent Psychiatry and American Professional Society on the Abuse of Children (APSAC), the National Institute of Child Health and Human Development (NICHD) Investigative Interview Protocol, Washington State Child Interview Guide, and Gunderson National Child Protection Center's Child First forensic interviewing protocol. In the case of sibling sexual abuse, it is important that the social worker assess if the offending sibling has also been a victim of sexual abuse.

Assessments and Screening Tools

Social workers may utilize standardized assessments and tools during the screening and assessment process. Appropriate assessments and tools that may be used include The Sibling Abuse Interview (SAI) which is a comprehensive administered interview used to evaluate individual children, sibling relationships, and parents, caregivers, and the family unit. The Revised Conflict Tactics Scales Sibling Version (CTS2-SP) may be used and is a clinician-administered 78-item tool used to assess the type and frequency of violent interactions between siblings.

Treatment

The ecological perspective focuses on the complex interactions of individual, social, and transpersonal factors (e.g., factors outside of the person) that impact children and their families. Sibling maltreatment should be viewed in the context of broader problematic family dynamics and interactions that may contribute to abuse. A complete assessment of the family situation is essential to understanding the nature, extent, and impacts of sibling maltreatment, as well as the development of an individualized treatment plan to establish an environment that provides for the physical safety and emotional well-being of each family member.

Treatment for children who have been maltreated often includes education about trauma, creating a trauma narrative, cognitive restructuring, and positive coping skills. Through treatment, children learn to recognize what specific stimuli trigger memories of trauma and to develop skills to calm themselves, as well as negative thought patterns that perpetuate trauma-related symptoms. Interventions can include trauma-focused cognitive behavioral therapy (TF-CBT), prolonged exposure therapy for adolescents (PE-A), and eye movement desensitization and reprocessing (EMDR).

Treatment for children who have maltreated siblings should include processing of abusive behaviors, understanding and accepting responsibility for the impacts of physical, psychological, and/or sexual maltreatment, developing the ability to manage feelings or motivations that contributed to sibling maltreatment, addressing behavioral issues such as aggression, and building skills in communication and conflict resolution.

Psychologically educational interventions are important in helping parents recognize and respond to sibling maltreatment and understand the effects of trauma. Parents may need counseling to support them in managing their emotional responses to sibling maltreatment so that they are able to provide emotional support to their children while holding the aggressor responsible for his or her behavior. Parent training or other interventions can also be utilized to help parents gain knowledge and skills to prevent reoccurrence of abuse (e.g., appropriate supervision, family rules, reinforcing positive behaviors, mediating sibling conflicts). Family issues such as harsh discipline, poor parent-child relationships, and history of intimate partner violence can contribute to sibling maltreatment and should also be addressed. Programs that may be considered for parents and/or families include multidimensional family therapy (MDFT), Triple P Positive Parenting Program, and the Incredible Years parent training program.

INTERVENTION

If sibling maltreatment is suspected, the social worker should complete a thorough assessment to identify the presence of maltreatment and assist the family to minimize the risk of reoccurrence. The social worker should complete an interview with the victim in a safe, private setting. Standardized assessments and tools, such as the SAI or CTS2-SP, may be utilized. Rapport with family members should be built through support and validation of feelings regarding the maltreatment. The social worker should ensure the victim's safety by developing a safety plan with the family. If available information meets statutory criteria that may need legal prosecution, the social worker must make a report to CPS and/or law enforcement.

When sibling maltreatment is confirmed, the social worker should assist the family to minimize further risk of maltreatment and help resolve any high-risk safety issues. A safety plan should be in place to address immediate safety needs of the victim. The social worker should utilize psychologically educational approaches to identify inappropriate sibling behavior to teach and help the family practice appropriate adaptive behaviors and conflict-resolution strategies. The victim of the sibling maltreatment should be assessed for trauma and/or other mental health issues and referred for evidence-based treatment services. The perpetrator of sibling maltreatment should be assessed for trauma-related issues and other issues contributing to the maltreatment behavior and referred for evidence-based treatment services. The social worker should provide support to the family and children. Psychological education regarding sibling maltreatment and abuse, and counseling to the parents may be indicated. Psychological education may also help the parents build a better understanding of the dynamics between sibling maltreatment, dysfunctional family dynamics and the parent's protective capacity.

APPLICABLE LAWS AND REGULATIONS

Various countries have mandatory reporting laws that require specified professionals to report suspicions of child maltreatment to the designated authority. Social workers are guided by the legal definitions of child maltreatment in the country in which they practice.

In the United States, the Child Abuse Prevention and Treatment Act (CAPTA) establishes the federal minimum definition of child abuse and neglect, and states often enact civil and criminal status that expand on that definition. Statutory definitions of child maltreatment generally refer to that perpetrated by parents/caregivers rather than minor siblings; however, parents' failure to provide adequate supervision or protection may constitute child neglect.

If the age difference between a victim of sibling sexual abuse and the perpetrator meets state or federal regulations for mandated reporting, then the sexual abuse needs to be reported to the agency responsible for investigating suspected maltreatment (e.g., local law enforcement, child protective services [CPS]).

SERVICES AND RESOURCES

- California Evidence-Based Clearinghouse for Child Welfare, http://www.cebc4cw.org
- Stop Abuse for Everyone (SAFE), http://stopabuseforeveryone.org/
- Sibling Abuse Survivors' Information and Advocacy Network (SASIAN), www.sasian.org

FOOD FOR THOUGHT

Children are more likely to fight with the sibling closest to them in age. Marital stress and/or discord has been shown to affect how children cope with conflict.

RED FLAGS

Abuse or maltreatment between siblings is reportable to law enforcement and CPS and reporting is required of all mandated reporters. Children who abuse siblings also are more likely to bully peers.

Written by Nikole Seals, MSW, ACSW, and Jennifer Teska, MSW

Reviewed by Lynn B. Cooper, D. Crim

REFERENCES

Bowes, L., Wolke, D., Joinson, C., Lereya, S. T., & Lewis, G. (2014). Sibling bullying and risk of depression, anxiety, and self-harm: A prospective cohort study. *Pediatrics, 134*(4), e1032. doi:10.1542/peds.2014-0832

British Association of Social Workers. (2012). *The code of ethics for social work: Statement of principles.* Retrieved March 22, 2016, from http://cdn.basw.co.uk/upload/basw_112315-7.pdf

Button, D. M., & Gealt, R. (2010). High risk behaviors among victims of sibling violence. *Journal of Family Violence, 25*(2), 131-140.

Chambliss, R. B., & McLeer, S. V. (2009). Relational problems. In B. J. Sadock, V. A. Sadock, & P. Ruiz (Eds.), *Kaplan & Sadock's comprehensive textbook of psychiatry* (9th ed., Vol. 2, pp. 2476-2478). Philadelphia, PA: Wolters Kluwer Health/Lippincott Williams & Wilkins.

Collin-Vezina, D., fast, E., Helie, S., Cyr, M., Pelletier, S., & Fallon, B. (2014). Young offender sexual abuse cases under protection investigation: Are sibling cases any different? *Child Welfare, 93*(4), 91-111.

Eriksen, S., & Jensen, V. (2006). All in the family? Family environmental factors in sibling violence. *Journal of Family Violence, 21*(8), 497-507.

Finkelhor, D., Turner, H., & Ormrod, R. (2006). Kid's stuff: The nature and impact of peer and sibling violence on younger and older children. *Child Abuse and Neglect, 30*(12), 1401-1421.

Horne, A., & Sayger, T. (1990). *Treating conduct and oppositional defiant disorders in children.* New York: Penguin Press.

International Federation of Social Workers. (2012, March 3). Statement of ethical principles. Retrieved March 22, 2016, from http://ifsw.org/policies/statement-of-ethical-principles/

Keane, M., Guest, A., & Padbury, J. (2013). A balancing act: A family perspective to sibling sexual abuse. *Child Abuse Review, 22*(4), 246-254. doi:10.1002/car.2284

Kiselica, M. S., & Morrill-Richards, M. (2007). Sibling maltreatment: The forgotten abuse. *Journal of Counseling & Development, 85*(2), 148-160.

Krienert, J. L., & Walsh, J. A. (2011). My brother's keeper: A contemporary examination of reported sibling violence using national level data, 2000-2005. *Journal of Family Violence, 26*(5), 331-342.

Krienert, J. L., & Walsh, J. A. (2011). Sibling sexual abuse: An empirical analysis of offender, victim, and event characteristics in national incident-based reporting system (NIBRS) data, 2000-2007. *Journal of Child Sexual Abuse, 20*(4), 353-372. doi:10.1080/10538712.2011.588190

Mathis, G., & Mueller, C. (2015). Childhood sibling aggression and emotional difficulties and aggressive behavior in adulthood. *Journal of Family Violence, 30*(3), 315-327. doi:10.1007/s10896-015-9670-5

McDonald, C., & Martinez, K. (2016). Parental and others' responses to physical sibling violence: A descriptive analysis of victims' retrospective accounts. *Journal of Family Violence, 31*(3), 401-410. doi:10.1007/s10896-015-9766-y

Michalski, R. L., Russell, D. P., Shackelford, T. K., & Weekes-Shackelford, V. A. (2007). Siblicide and genetic relatedness in Chicago 1870-1930. *Homicide Studies, 11*(3), 231-237.

Morrill, M. (2014). Sibling sexual abuse: An exploratory study of long-term consequences for self-esteem and counseling considerations. *Journal* of Family Violence, 29(2), 205-213. doi:10.1007/s10896-013-9571-4

National Association of Social Workers. (2015). Standards and indicators for cultural competence in social work practice. Retrieved March 14, 2016, from http://www.socialworkers.org/practice/standards/PRA-BRO-253150-CC-Standards.pdf

Phillips, D. A., Bowie, B. H., Wan, D. C., & Yukevich, K. W. (2016). Sibling violence and children hospitalized for serious mental and behavioral health problems. Journal of Interpersonal Violence, 1-21. Advance online publication. doi:10.1177/0886260516628289

Rapoza, K. A., Cook, K., Zaveri, T., & Malley-Morrison, K. (2010). Ethnic perspectives on sibling abuse in the United States. Journal of Family Issues, 31(6), 808-829.

Relva, I. C., Fernandes, O. M., & Mota, C. P. (2013). An exploration of sibling violence predictors. Journal of Aggression, Conflict and Peace Research, 5(1), 47-61. doi:10.1108/17596591311290740

Sadock, B. J., Sadock, V. A., & Ruiz, P. (2015). Chapter 25: Other conditions that may be a focus of clinical attention. In Synopsis of Psychiatry: Behavioral Sciences/Clinical Psychiatry (pp. 822-823). Philadelphia, PA: Wolters Kluwer.

Shadik, J. A., Perkins, N. H., & Kovacs, P. J. (2013). Incorporating discussion of sibling violence in the curriculum of parent intervention programs for child abuse. Heath & Social Work, 38(1), 53-57. doi:10.1093/hsw/hls066

Stutey, D., & Clemens, E. V. (2014). Hidden abuse within the home: Recognizing and responding to sibling abuse. Professional School Counseling, 18(1), 206-216. doi:10.5330/1096-2409-18.1.206

Tippett, N., & Wolke, D. (2015). Aggression between siblings: Associations with the home environment and peer bullying. Aggressive Behavior, 41(1), 14-24. doi:110.1002/ab21557

Tucker, C. J., Cox, G., Sharp, E. H., Van Gundy, K. T., Rebellon, C., & Stracuzzi, N. F. (2013). Sibling proactive and reactive aggression in adolescence. Journal of Family Violence, 28(3), 299-310. doi:10.1007/s10896-012-9483-8

Tucker, C. J., Finkelhor, D., Shattuck, A. M., & Turner, H. (2013). Prevalence and correlates of sibling victimization types. Child Abuse & Neglect, 37(4), 213-223. doi:10.1016/j.chiabu.2013.01.006

Tucker, C. J., Finkelhor, D., Turner, H., & Shattuck, A. M. (2014). Family dynamics and young children's sibling victimization. Journal of Family Psychology, 28(5), 625-633. doi:10.1037/fam0000016

Wolke, D., Tippett, N., & Dantchev, S. (2015). Bullying in the family: Sibling bullying. The Lancet Psychiatry, 2(10), 917-929. doi:10.1016/S2215-0366(15)00262-X

SICKLE CELL DISEASE: HEALTHCARE COSTS

MAJOR CATEGORIES: Medical & Health

WHAT WE KNOW

Sickle cell disease (SCD) is a group of inherited conditions characterized by defective hemoglobin (Hgb), which causes deformed (sickle-shaped) red blood cells (RBCs) that carry inadequate amounts of oxygen and become easily trapped and destroyed in normal circulation, resulting in hemolysis (i.e., rupturing of RBCs with a release of the cell contents into surroundings), anemia, and ischemia (i.e., restriction in blood supply to tissues).

RBC blockages in blood vessels and organs and a shortened RBC lifespan result in a range of clinical issues, including sickle cell crisis (i.e., an episode of intense pain caused by sudden occlusion of blood vessels), infection, and acute chest syndrome (i.e., occlusion of the pulmonary blood vessels that is characterized by cough, fever, and hypoxemia).

In addition to the burden of the disease, patients with SCD have increased risk for treatment-related complications (e.g., iron overload caused by multiple transfusions).

The healthcare costs associated with the management of patients with SCD are substantial

Persons with SCD have significantly higher healthcare rates and costs than persons without SCD.

Blood transfusions and procedures that reduce the iron overload associated with frequent transfusions (e.g., iron chelation therapy) increase the cost of treatment of patients with SCD

A 2009 study estimated the lifetime cost of SCD for one patient in the United States to be $460,000.

A study in England found that for the 6,077 admissions to the hospital for SCD between 2010 and 2011, the total cost was £18,798,255.

In Nigeria, the average cost per hospitalization for children with SCD was $132.67, and the average number of hospitalizations per year was 2.5. One third of caregivers had to spend at least 10 percent of their annual income on hospitalizations.

An investigation of more than 3,000 children aged 1–17 years enrolled in Medicaid and private insurance revealed that SCD-related medical costs totaled about $335 million in 2005. (All amounts are in USD).

In the United States, publicly insured pediatric patients with SCD have higher healthcare rates but lower healthcare costs than privately insured pediatric patients.

In 2005, median annual total healthcare costs per publicly insured (Medicaid) pediatric patient (birth to age 18 years) with SCD were $11,075 (versus $14,722 per privately insured pediatric patient).

There were 0.91 hospital admissions per publicly insured patient (versus 0.79 admissions per privately insured patient).

There were 1.36 emergency department visits per publicly insured patient (versus 0.91 visits per privately insured patient).

There were 12.6 outpatient visits per publicly insured patient (versus 11.5 visits per privately insured patient).

During the period 2004–2007, average annual total healthcare costs per low-income pediatric patient (birth to age 18 years) with SCD enrolled in the Texas Children's Health Plan were approximately $30,434 (versus $8,926 for children without SCD).

Hospitalization accounted for annual costs of $27,760 per patient with SCD (versus $7,466 per patient without SCD).

Emergency department usage accounted for annual costs of $1,097 per patient with SCD per year (versus $636 per patient without SCD).

During the period 2001–2005, average annual total healthcare costs per patient with SCD enrolled in the Florida Medicaid program were $23,352.

Average annual healthcare costs per patient for care related to SCD were $12,096.

Hospitalization related to SCD accounted for $9,677 per patient per year.

Emergency department usage related to SCD accounted for $387 per patient per year.

Physician visits related to SCD accounted for $109 per patient per year.

Prescription medications for SCD accounted for $435 per patient per year.

Other care (including home healthcare) accounted for $1,415 per patient per year.

In England between 2010 and 2011, there were 6,077 hospital admissions associated with SCD, at an estimated total cost of £17.1 million

Healthcare costs for patients with SCD increase with age

WHAT CAN BE DONE

Learn about healthcare costs for SCD so that you can maximize resources; share this knowledge with your friends and family

Educate yourself about the disease, its management, and common misconceptions

Keep accurate records of medications so it is clear to the emergency department during a crisis what works for pain management

Explore alternative coping skills for pain, such as distraction techniques, to reduce emergency department visits

Address the psychological and emotional pain that the person with SCD may be experiencing and that may be exacerbating their physical pain, especially depression and anxiety related to their illness

Written by Sharon Richman, MSPT

Reviewed by Jessica Therivel, LMSW-IPR

REFERENCES

Adegoke, S. A., Abioye-Kuteyi, E. A., & Orji, E. O. (2014). The rate and cost of hospitalization in children with sickle cell anaemia and its implications in a developing economy. *African Health Sciences, 14*(2), 475-480. doi:10.4314/ahs.v14i2.27

Amendah, D. D., Mvundura, M., Kavanagh, P. L., Sprinz, P. G., & Grosse, S. D. (2010). Sickle cell disease-related pediatric medical expenditures in the U.S. *American Journal of Preventive Medicine, 38*(4 Suppl.), S550-S556. doi:10.1016/j.amepre.2010.01.004

Blinder, M. A., Duh, M. S., Sasane, M., Trahey, A., Paley, C., & Vekeman, F. (2015). Age-related emergency department reliance in patients with sickle cell disease. *Journal of Emergency Medicine, 49*(4), 513-522.e1. doi:10.1016/j.jemermed.2014.12.080

British Association of Social Workers. (2012, January). The Code of Ethics for Social Work: Statement of Principles. Retrieved December 16, 2015, from http://cdn.basw.co.uk/upload/basw_112315-7.pdf

Dunlop, R. J., & Bennett, K. C. L. B. (2006). Pain management for sickle cell disease in children and adults. Cochrane Database of Systematic Reviews. Art. No.: CD003350. doi:10.1002/14651858.CD003350.pub2.

DynaMed. (2014, November 24). Sickle cell disease in adults and adolescents. Ipswich, MA: EBSCO Information Services.

International Federation of Social Workers. (2012, March 3). Statement of Ethical Principles. Retrieved December 16, 2015, from http://ifsw.org/policies/statement-of-ethical-principles/

Kauf, T. L., Coates, T. D., Huazhi, L., Mody-Patel, N., & Hartzema, A. G. (2009). The cost of health care for children and adults with sickle cell disease. *American Journal of Hematology, 84*(6), 323-327. doi:10.1002/ajh.21408

Wheeler, D. (2015). NASW standards and indicators for cultural competency in social work practice. Retrieved December 16, 2015, from http://www.socialworkers.org/practice/standards/PRA-BRO-253150-CC-Standards.pdf

Mvundura, M., Amendah, D., Kavanagh, P. L., Sprinz, P. G., & Grosse, S. D. (2009). Health care utilization and expenditures for privately and publicly insured children with sickle cell disease in the United States. *Pediatric Blood and Cancer, 53*(4), 642-646. doi:10.1002/pbc.22069

Pizzo, E., Laverty, A. A., Phekoo, K. J., Aljuburi, G., Green, S. A., Bell, D., & Majeed, A. (2015). A retrospective analysis of the cost of hospitalizations for sickle cell disease with crisis in England, 2010/11. *Journal of Public Health (Oxford, Engalnd), 37*(3), 529-539. doi:10.1093/pubmed/fdu026

Raphael, J. L., Dietrich, C. L., Whitmire, D., Mahoney, D. H., Mueller, B. U., & Giardino, A. P. (2009). Healthcare utilization and expenditures for low income children with sickle cell disease. *Pediatric Blood and Cancer, 52*(2), 263-267. doi:10.1002/pbc.21781

Robinson, N. (n.d.). Sickle cell disease pain control with children. *Help Starts Here*. Retrieved January 16, 2015, from http://www.helpstartshere.org/health-and-wellness/living-with-illness/sickle-cell-disease-pain-control-with-children.html

Zhang, B., Donga, P. Z., Corral, M., Sasane, M., Miller, J. D., & Pashos, C. L. (2011). Pharmacoeconomic considerations in treating iron overload in patients with B-thalassaemia, sickle cell disease and myelodysplastic syndromes in the US: A literature review. *PharmacoEconomics, 29*(6), 461-474.

SMOKING CESSATION & PREGNANCY

MAJOR CATEGORIES: Substance Abuse

WHAT WE KNOW

Smoking during pregnancy is associated with significant health risks for both the mother and fetus, including increased risk for low birth weight, intrauterine growth retardation, sudden infant death syndrome (SIDS), ectopic pregnancy, premature birth, and miscarriage. Smoking during pregnancy is associated with development of major health problems in infants and children, including asthma, bronchitis, and impaired development.

Smoking during pregnancy exposes the fetus to toxic chemicals, including nicotine, carbon monoxide, and lead. When a pregnant woman smokes, the fetus is exposed to nicotine concentrations that are approximately equal to those in the mother's body, reducing the amount of nutrients and oxygen that are able to reach the fetus.

There is a relationship between how much a pregnant woman smokes and how much her baby will weigh at birth. Light smoking and heavy smoking are associated with an increase in the risk of low birth weight of 53 percent and 130 percent, respectively.

If all pregnant women quit smoking during pregnancy and maintained nonsmoking status for the duration of their pregnancies, there would be an 11 percent reduction in stillbirths and a 5 percent reduction in neonatal deaths. Most pregnant women know that smoking is bad for their baby. Historically, pregnant women underreport any current smoking, although some physicians may have in-office saliva testing for more accurate results.

Smoking cessation interventions for pregnant women can reduce the rate of maternal smoking and consequently reduce smoking-related morbidity and mortality. For example, infants of women who quit smoking during the first trimester tend to have weight and body measurements comparable to those of infants born to nonsmokers. Prenatal smoking cessation programs have decreased the incidence of intrauterine growth retardation and preterm births.

Women who quit smoking early in pregnancy (for example, during the first trimester) produce significant healthcare cost savings by decreasing the number of low birth weight babies. Although quitting smoking early in pregnancy offers the greatest benefit to both mother and fetus, significant benefits can still be achieved when mothers quit later in pregnancy.

Despite high rates of women who go back to smoking after their baby is born, supporting smoking reduction and cessation in pregnant women remains worthwhile and effective. Informal smoking cessation interventions during pregnancy are effective, but more intensive interventions are even more effective. The exception to this is group-based intensive interventions. Group interventions tend to be poorly attended and are less effective than individual intervention strategies

Smoking cessation interventions include cognitive behavioral therapy, motivational programs that offer incentives (such as financial rewards, either cash or gift cards, tied to specified behavior such as attending cessation meetings or testing nicotine-free), motivational interviewing, nicotine replacement therapy (NRT), and giving pregnant women the opportunity to experience real-time ultrasound feedback of fetal health status. According to researchers, providing incentives is the most effective intervention.

Teenage pregnant smokers had an increased interest in cessation and in getting help with cessation after utilizing an online tool that was specific to adolescent pregnant smokers. The participants

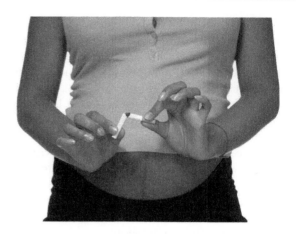

stated that the tool increased their awareness of the dangers associated with smoking while pregnant and increased their motivation to quit.

Smoking with a partner or with family or friends can be a social interaction. Partner or family member participation in cessation attempts is critical for the long-term success of smoking cessation interventions in pregnant women. It is important to provide an opportunity for the partner to learn about smoking cessation if he or she is a smoker.

Although NRT increases the likelihood of successful smoking cessation by 50–70 percent, research results differ on the effectiveness of NRT in pregnancy. Results of clinical studies suggest that the use of NRT by pregnant women increases the risk of preterm and low birth weight births. It is unclear whether these findings are related to NRT being prescribed to heavier smokers, who may already have been at risk for fetal health concerns, or if NRT itself adversely affects the developing fetus.

Researchers who analyzed a trial of NRT in pregnancy to determine factors associated with cessation found that women who are better educated and have lower pretreatment cotinine (the predominant metabolite in nicotine) concentrations were more likely to stop smoking with the NRT treatment.

60 percent of pregnant smokers continue to smoke past their first prenatal visit. For these women, interventions that are not pharmacologically based have smoking cessation rates that usually are less than 20 percent. These interventions have almost no impact on heavier smokers, who tend to be poor and undereducated and whose social networks are filled with smokers.

Women who smoke are 30 percent less likely than nonsmokers to breastfeed their infants. Researchers who studied women who smoked during the post-partum period but had previously quit smoking found that the longer a women quit smoking during pregnancy, the more likely she was to at least begin breastfeeding her baby.

Vouchers with monetary value and a free breast pump are likely the most effective incentives for women to quit smoking while pregnant and to breast-feed after their child is born (and continue to not smoke). Other effective parts of cessation programs are support through having a "quitting pal" as well as initial daily text/telephone support.

Although 20–40 percent of female smokers stop smoking during pregnancy, they are vulnerable to relapse. Up to 60 percent of mothers who quit smoking during pregnancy resume smoking within 6 months of giving birth, and 80–90 percent do so within 12 months. Risk factors for smoking relapse after delivery include intending to quit smoking only for the duration of the pregnancy, not breastfeeding, using smoking as a way to cope with stress, lack of social support, and living with smokers. Researchers have found that a low-intensity smoking cessation program combined with relapse prevention can improve the quit rates in pregnant women and lead to smoking abstinence of up to one year postpartum.

WHAT CAN BE DONE

Learn about the risks of smoking during pregnancy and about smoking cessation techniques; share this knowledge with your friends and neighbors.

Encourage anyone you know who becomes pregnant to learn about the benefits of smoking cessation and the risks of cigarette smoking to themselves and their babies.

Find out about smoking cessation programs specifically designed for pregnant women in your area, such as the Smoking Cessation and Reduction in Pregnancy Treatment (SCRIPT) Program so you can tell friends about these types of programs.

Written by Jessica Therivel, LMSW-IPR, and
Chris Bates, MA, MSW

Reviewed by Lynn B. Cooper, D. Crim, and
Tanja Schub, BS

REFERENCES

Association of Women's Health, Obstetric & Neonatal Nursing. (2010). AWHONN position statement. Smoking and women's health. *JOGNN: Journal of Obstetric, Gynecologic & Neonatal Nursing, 39*(5), 611-613. doi:10.1111/j.1552-6909.2010.01178.x

Bailey, B. A., McCook, J. G., Clements, A. D., & Mc-Grady, L. (2011). Quitting smoking during pregnancy and birth outcomes: Evidence of gains following cessation by third trimester. *JOGNN: Journal of Obstetric, Gynecologic & Neonatal Nursing, 40*(Suppl. 1), S98-S99.

Collins, B. N., DiSantis, K. I., & Nair, U. S. (2011). Longer previous smoking abstinence relates to successful breastfeeding initiation among underserved smokers. *Breastfeeding Medicine, 6*(6), 385-391. doi:10.1089/bfm.2011.0076

Crossland, N., Thomson, G., Morgan, H., Dumbrowski, S., & Hoddinott, P. (2015). Incentives for breastfeeding and for smoking cessation in pregnancy: an exploration of types and meanings. *Social Science & Medicine, 128,* 10-17. doi:10.1016/j.socscimed.2014.12.019

Dias-Dame, J., & Cesar, J. (2015). Disparities in prevalence of smoking and smoking cessation during pregnancy: a population based study. *BioMed Research International, 345430.* doi:10.1155/2015/345430

Fitzgerald, E. M. (2012). Evidence-based tobacco cessation strategies with pregnant Latina women. *Nursing Clinics of North America, 47*(1), 45-54.

Flemming, K., Graham, H., McCaughan, D., Angus, K., & Bauld, L. (2015). The barriers and facilitators to smoking cessation experienced by women's partners during pregnancy and the post-partum period: a systematic review of qualitative research. *BMC Public Health, 15*(849), 1-10.

Gyllstrom, M. E., Hellerstedt, W. L., & Hennrikus, D. (2012). The association of maternal mental health with prenatal smoking cessation and postpartum relapse in a population-based sample. *Maternal and Child Health Journal, 16*(3), 685-693.

International Federation of Social Workers. (2012). Statement of Ethical Principles. Retrieved March 2, 2015, from http://ifsw.org/policies/statement-of-ethical-principles/

Lee, M., Miller, S., Wen, K. Y., Hui, S. K., Roussi, P., & Hernandez, E. (2015). Cognitive-behavioral intervention to promote smoking cessation for pregnant and postpartum inner city women. *Journal of Behavioral Medicine, 38*(6), 932-943. doi:10.1007/s10865-015-9669-7

Lumley, J., Chamberlain, C., Dowswell, T., Oliver, S., Oakley, L., & Watson, L. (2009). Interventions for promoting smoking cessation during pregnancy. Cochrane Database of Systematic Reviews. Art. No.: CD001055. doi:10.1002/14651858. CD001055.pub3.

Montalto, N. J., & Wells, W. O. (2007). Validation of self-reported smoking status using saliva cotinine: a rapid semiquantitative dipstick method. *Cancer Epidemiology, Biomarkers & Prevention, 16*(9), 1858-1862.

Morgan, H., Hoddinott, P., Thomson, G., Crossland, N., Farra, S., Yi, D., & Campbell, M. (2015). Benefits of Incentives for Breastfeeding and smoking cessation in pregnancy (BIBS): A mixed-methods study to inform trial design. *Healthy Technology Assessment, 19*(30), 1-300. doi:10.3310/hta19300

National Association of Social Workers. (2015). *Standards and Indicators for Cultural Competence in Social Work Practice.* Retrieved February 23, 2016, from http://www.socialworkers.org/practice/standards/PRA-BRO-253150-CC-Standards.pdf

Olaiya, O., Sharma, A., Tong, V., Dee, D., Quinn, C., Agaku, I.,... Satteri, G. (2015). Impact of the 5As brief counseling on smoking cessation among pregnant clients of Special Supplemental Nutrition Program for Women, Infants, and Children (WIC) clinics in Ohio. *Preventive Medicine, 81,* 438-443. doi:10.1016/j.ypmed.2015.10.011

Parrish, D. E., von Sternberg, K., Velasquez, M. M., Cochran, J., Sampson, M., & Mullen, P. D. (2012). Characteristics and factors associated with the risk of a nicotine exposed pregnancy: Expanding the CHOICES preconception counseling model to tobacco. *Maternal and Child Health Journal, 16*(6), 1224-1231.

Phelan, S. (2014). Smoking cessation in pregnancy. *Obstetrics & Gynecology Clinics of North America, 41*(2), 255-266. doi:10.1016/j.ogc.2014.02.007

Polanska, K., Hanke, W., Sobala, W., Lowe, J. B., & Jaakkola, J. J. (2011). Predictors of smoking relapse after delivery: Prospective study in central Poland. *Maternal and Child Health Journal, 15*(5), 579-586.

Shipton, D., Tappin, D. M., Vadivelo, T., Crossley, J. A., Aitken, D. A., & Chalmers, J. (2009). Reliability of self reported smoking status by pregnant women for estimating smoking prevalence: a retrospective, cross sectional study. *British Medical Journal, 339*(b43347). doi:10.1136/bmj.b4347

Stotts, A. L., Groff, J. Y., Velasquez, M. M., Benjamin-Garner, R., Green, C., Carbonari, J. P., & DiClemente, C. C. (2009). Ultrasound feedback and motivational interviewing targeting smoking cessation in the second and third trimesters of pregnancy. *Nicotine and Tobacco Research, 11*(8), 961-968. doi:10.1093/ntr/ntp095

Vaz, L., Leonardi-Bee, J., Aveyard, P., Cooper, S., Grainfe, M., & Coleman, T. (2013). Factors associated with smoking cessation in early and late pregnancy in the Smoking, Nicotine, and Pregnancy trial: A trial of nicotine replacement therapy. *Nicotine & Tobacco Research, 16*(4), 381-389. doi:10.1093/ntr/ntt156

Warland, J., & McCutcheon, H. (2011). The 'quit' smoker and stillbirth risk: A review of contemporary literature in the light of findings from a case-control study. *Midwifery, 27*(5), 607-611. doi:10.1016/j.midw.2010.05.007

Windsor, R., Clark, J., Cleary, S., Davis, A., Thorn, S., Abroms, L., & Wedeles, J. (2014). Effectiveness of the Smoking Cessation and Reduction in Pregnancy Treatment (SCRIPT) dissemination project: A science to prenatal care practice partnership. *Maternal and Child Health Journal, 18*(1), 180-190. doi:10.1007/s10995-013-1252-7

Windsor, R., Woodby, L., Miller, T., & Hardin, M. (2011). Effectiveness of Smoking Cessation and Reduction in Pregnancy Treatment (SCRIPT) methods in Medicaid-supported prenatal care: Trial III. *Health Education & Behavior, 38*(4), 412-422. doi:10.1177/1090198110382503

SMOKING CESSATION IN ADOLESCENCE

MAJOR CATEGORIES: Adolescents, Substance Abuse

WHAT WE KNOW

Every day in the United States approximately 3,800 adolescents smoke their first cigarette, and 2,100 adolescents become daily cigarette smokers. Smoking is the leading preventable cause of morbidity and mortality in the United States. Smoking has carcinogenic effects and adverse cardiovascular and pulmonary effects and compromises life expectancy at all ages.

More than 80 percent of regular smokers began smoking before age 18. In 2014 the National Youth Tobacco Survey (NYTS) found that 24.6 percent students in grades 9 to 12 (20.9 percent of females, 28.3 percent of males) in the United States had used some kind of tobacco product at least once during the last 30 days; the three most used were electronic cigarettes (13.4 percent), hookahs (9.4 percent), and conventional cigarettes (9.2 percent). In grades 6 to 8, 7.7 percent of students (6.6 percent of females, 8.8 percent of males) had used some kind of tobacco product; the three most used were electronic cigarettes (3.9 percent), hookahs (2.5 percent), and cigarettes (2.5 percent)

According to the U.S. Centers for Disease Control and Prevention (CDC), smoking during adolescence is associated with increased risk for alcohol use, drug use, and sexual behavior during adolescence. Most adolescents who are regular smokers believe that most adolescents smoke, do not believe they are addicted to nicotine, and believe that smoking controls weight (a predominantly female perception).

Risk factors for smoking during adolescence include availability of tobacco, low socioeconomic status, low academic achievement, the perception that tobacco use is common, lack of parental involvement or support, having a parent or guardian who is a smoker, advertising, social approval of tobacco use, peer pressure, decreased self-esteem/self-image, lack of self-efficacy to refuse tobacco, not having plans to attend a 4-year college, stress, psychiatric disorders, antisocial behavior, believing that tobacco use has functional benefits such as improved concentration or weight control, and early menarche in female adolescents.

Tobacco use patterns among adolescents are changing: Use of cigarettes declined from 2011 to 2014 among students in grades 6-8 from 4.3 percent to 2.5 percent, and among those in grades 9 to 12 from 15.8 percent to 9.2 percent; electronic cigarette use increased from 0.6 percent to 3.9 percent and 1.5 percent to 13.4 percent, respectively, and hookah use increased from 1.0 percent to 2.5 percent and 4.1 percent to 9.4 percent, respectively. According to the National Youth Tobacco Survey (NYTS), the use of e-cigarettes among youth in the United States grades 6 through 12 doubled from 3.3 percent to 6.8 percent between 2011 and 2012.

Electronic cigarettes (e-cigarettes) are heavily marketed on the radio, on television, and through electronic communications such as internet advertising. Various flavors that appeal to youth such as candy, fruit, and chocolate can be purchased. E-cigarettes deliver nicotine or other substances into the lungs in the form of a vapor. Use of e-cigarettes is currently unregulated and increasing in popularity among adolescent youth. E-cigarettes are marketed as a cessation aid and touted as being healthier than tobacco cigarettes. However, e-cigarette use contributes to addiction to nicotine and among adolescents is associated with increased likelihood of ever smoking cigarettes and becoming a daily smoker.

For every 3 young smokers, only 1 will be likely to quit smoking in his or her lifetime. Although the harmful effects associated with smoking typically do not become apparent until midlife, it is estimated that if the current rate of smoking among youth continues, about 1 in 13 Americans currently younger than 17 will die early because of smoking-related illness. The desire to stop smoking and first attempts to stop typically begin 1–3 months after smoking on a regular basis begins. Adolescents who are depressed or play sports are more likely to try to stop smoking; adolescents who engage in high-risk sexual activity and abuse substances other than alcohol and marijuana are less likely to attempt to quit smoking.

Smoking cessation efforts targeting adolescents include community-based interventions, pharmacotherapy, formal smoking cessation programs, and media campaigns. Most studies on adolescent smoking find a low participation rate in smoking cessation programs, a high level of attrition from the programs, and a low quit rate for stopping smoking. Pharmacologic, behavioral, and combination smoking cessation strategies are considered moderately effective at 6 months of regular smoking but significantly less effective by 12 months. Smoking cessation by a parent or peer positively affects adolescent smoking cessation. Healthcare providers can play a key role by providing information about the dangers of smoking and by promoting smoking and tobacco abstinence among adolescents. School cessation programs have shown some promise in helping adolescents quit or reduce the use of smoking and tobacco.

There is insufficient evidence to universally support the use of nicotine replacement therapy (NRT) for adolescents. NRT was found to be effective in assisting with smoking cessation among adolescents who scored higher levels of agreeableness and conscientiousness and lower levels of extraversion on the Quick Big Five Inventory of personality traits.

Psychoactive medication, such as bupropion, commonly used to support adult smoking cessation efforts, is not approved for adolescent use. Pharmacotherapy with varenicline, a nicotinic receptor partial agonist, is being tested for adolescent use. In a recent study, a brief image-based intervention targeting social images and self-images resulted in reductions in frequency and quantity of cigarette smoking in high-school-age adolescents. Other interventions to prevent and reduce smoking in adolescents include smoking bans and smoke-free zones at schools, increasing the price of and taxes on tobacco products, mass media campaigns, and legislation prohibiting online cigarette sales to minors.

Motivational interviewing can be a powerful technique with adolescents since it does not focus on confrontation, promotes self-efficacy, and works to help the person who smokes arrive at his or her own conclusions about the best way to make behavior changes. The nonconfrontational approach can be disarming when adolescents are expecting a lecture from an authority figure.

The Not on Tobacco (N-O-T) smoking cessation intervention, supported by the American Lung Association, can be effective in helping adolescents quit smoking. Adding exercise as part of the program has significantly increased smoking cessation rates among males. In the United States, the Project EX school cessation program utilizes talk show and game modalities to improve coping skills, motivation, and personal commitment.

Learning new coping strategies is a powerful tool for adolescents trying to quit smoking. Behavioral and cognitive strategies have been found to help adolescents quit smoking. Behavioral coping strategies include keeping busy, avoiding smoking opportunities, and substituting food, drink, gum, and toothpicks for a cigarette. Cognitive coping strategies include telling oneself that smoking is not permitted and thinking about the risks of smoking, the long-term benefits of abstinence, or a relative or friend who died as a result of smoking-related disease.

Another approach to smoking cessation is harm reduction. This model aims to minimize the negative consequences associated with smoking by using alternative sources of nicotine (e.g., smokeless tobacco products). The model promote changes in behavior that will decrease harm to the adolescent who continues to smoke and use tobacco.

Proponents believe that reducing the number of cigarettes smoked per day is desirable for adolescents who do not want to quit entirely.

WHAT CAN BE DONE

Learn about smoking cessation so you can give accurate information to your friends who smoke.

Recommend counseling to friends who smoke to help them quit.

Help your friends discover triggers (for example, stress) for smoking and help them find ways to minimize or avoid those triggers.

Provide emotional support to friends who smoke by recognizing and acknowledging that quitting smoking is difficult and may require multiple attempts.

Learn and share information about community programs for adolescents on stress management, peer pressure, self-efficacy, appropriate methods of weight control, and support of abstinence and smoking cessation efforts

Provide resources for information about smoking cessation, such as Quit Now, 1-800-784-8669; SFT, http://teen.smokefree.gov/; N-O-T Not Tobacco, http://www.youthtobaccocessation.org/resources/

programs.html ; CDC, http://www.cdc.gov/tobacco/quit_smoking/index.htm; BeTobaccoFree.gov, http://betobaccofree.hhs.gov/quit-now/index.html

Written by Jessica Therivel, LMSW-IPR, and Leonard Buckley, BS, MD

Reviewed by Lynn B. Cooper, D. Crim, and Laura Gale, LCSW

REFERENCES

Abrantes, A. M., Lee, C. S., MacPherson, L., Strong, D. R., Borrelli, B., & Brown, R. A. (2009). Health risk behaviors in relation to making a smoking quit attempt among adolescents. *Journal of Behavioral Medicine, 32*(2), 142-149. doi:10.1007/s10865-008-9184-1 R

Brinker, T. J., Stamm-Balderjahn, S., Seeger, W., & Groneberg, D. A. (2014). Education Against Tobacco (EAT): A quasi-experimental prospective evaluation of a programme for preventing smoking in secondary schools delivered by medical students: a study protocol. *BMJ Open, 4*(7), e004909. Retrieved from http://bmjopen.bmj.com/content/4/7/e004909.full?g=w_tc_open_tab, doi:10.1136/bmjopen-2014-004909

Cengelli, S., O'Loughlin, J., Lauzon, B., & Cornuz, J. (2012). A systematic review of longitudinal population-based studies on the predictors of smoking cessation in adolescent and young adult smokers. *Tobacco Control, 21*(3), 355-362. doi:10.1136/tc.2011.044149

Centers for Disease Control and Prevention. (2014, February 14). Youth and tobacco use. Retrieved January 22, 2016, from http://www.cdc.gov/tobacco/data_statistics/fact_sheets/youth_data/tobacco_use/index.htm

Centers for Disease Control and Prevention (CDC). (2013). Notes from the Field: Electronic cigarette use among middle and high school students in the United States, 2011-2012. *Morbidity and Mortality Weekly Report (MMWR).* Retrieved January 22, 2016, from http://www.cdc.gov/mmwr/preview/mmwrhtml/mm6235a6.htm

Dutra, L. M., & Glantz, S. A. (2014). Electronic cigarettes and conventional cigarette use among U.S. adolescents: A cross-sectional study. *JAMA, 168*(7), 610-617. doi:10.1001/jamapediatrics.2013.5488

Faessel, H., Rawa, P., & Williams, K. (2009). Pharmacokinetics, safety, and tolerability of varenicline in healthy adolescent smokers: A multicenter, randomized, double-blind, placebo-controlled, parallel-group study. *Clinical Therapeutics, 31*(1), 177-189. doi:10.1016/j.clinthera.2009.01.003

Fritz, D. J., Wider, L. C., Hardin, S. B., & Horrocks, M. (2008). Program strategies for adolescent smoking cessation. *Journal of School Nursing: Official Publication of the National Association of School Nurses, 24*(1), 21-27. doi:10.1177/10598405080240010401

International Federation of Social Workers. (2012, March 3). Statement of ethical principles. Retrieved January 22, 2016, from http://ifsw.org/policies/statement-of-ethical-principles

Jaszyna-Gasior, M., Schroeder, J. R., Thorner, E. D., Heishman, S. J., Collins, C. C., Lo, S., & Moolchan, E. T. (2009). Age at menarche and weight concerns in relation to smoking trajectory and dependence among adolescent girls enrolled in a smoking cessation trial. *Addictive Behaviors, 34*(1), 92-95. doi:10.1016/j.addbeh.2008.08.001

Kim, M. J., Fleming, C. B., & Catalano, R. F. (2009). Individual and social influences on progression to daily smoking during adolescence. *Pediatrics, 124*(3), 895-902. doi:10.1542/peds.2008-2015

Klein, J. D. (2014). Delivering tobacco control interventions in adolescent health care visits: time for action. *Pediatrics, 134*(3), 600-601. doi:1-.1542/peds.2014-1925

Kleinjan, M., Engels, R. C., van Leeuwe, J., Brug, J., van Zundert, R. M., & den Eijnden, R. J. (2009). Mechanisms of adolescent smoking cessation: Roles of readiness to quit, nicotine dependence, and smoking of parents and peers. *Drug and Alcohol Dependence, 99*(1-3), 204-214. doi:10.1016/j.drugalcdep.2008.08.002

Minor, M., & Sondike, S. (2014). Adolescent smoking cessation methods: A review article. *The West Virginia Medical Journal, 110*(4), 16-20.

Myhre, K. E., & Adelman, W. (2013). Motivational interviewing: Helping teenaged smokers to quit. *Contemporary Pediatrics, 30*(10), 18-23.

O'Loughlin, J., Gervais, A., Dugas, E., & Meshefedjian, G. (2009). Milestones in the process of cessation among novice adolescent smokers. *American Journal of Public Health, 99*(3), 499-504. doi:10.2105/AJPH.2007.128629

Pbert, L., Flint, A. J., Fletcher, K. E., Young, M. H., Druker, S., & DiFranza, J. R. (2008). Effect of a pediatric practice-based smoking prevention and cessation intervention for adolescents: A randomized, controlled trial. *Pediatrics, 121*(4), e738-e747. doi:10.1542/peds.2007-1029

Rosen, I. M., & Maurer, D. M. (2008). Reducing tobacco use in adolescents. *American Family Physician, 77*(4), 483-490.

Schauer, G. L., Agaku, I. T., King, B. A., & Malarcher, A. M. (2014). Health care provider advice for adolescent tobacco use: results from the 2011 National Youth Tobacco Survey. *Pediatrics, 134*(3), 446-455. doi:10.1542/peds.2014-0458

Scherphof, C. S., Eijnden, R. J. J. M., Lugtig, P., Engels, R. C. M. E., & Vollebergh, W. A. M. (2014). Adolescents' use of nicotine replacement therapy for smoking cessation: Predictors of compliance trajectories. *Psychopharmacology, 231*(8), 1743-1752. doi:10.1007/s00213-014-3511-8

Scherphof, C. S., van den Eijnden, R. J., Engels, R. C., & Vollebergh, W. A. (2014). Long-term efficacy of nicotine replacement therapy for smoking cessation in adolescents: A randomized controlled trial. *Drug and Alcohol Dependence, 140*, 217-220. doi:10.1016/j.drugalcdep.2014.04.007

Sussman, S., McCuller, W. J., Zheng, H., Pfingston, Y. M., Miyano, J., & Dent, C. W. (2004). Project EX: A program of empirical research on adolescent tobacco use cessation. *Tobacco Induced Diseases, 2*(3), 119-132. doi:10.1186/1617-9625-2-3-119

Thrul, J., Stemmler, M., Buhler, A., & Goecke, M. (2014). The role of participants' self-selected future smoking goals in adolescent smoking cessation interventions. *Drug and Alcohol Dependence, 141*(1), 118-123. doi:10.1016/j.drugalcdep.2014.05.016

U.S. Department of Health and Human Services. (2012). Preventing tobacco use among youth and young adults: A report of the Surgeon General, 2012. Retrieved January 22, 2016, from http://www.surgeongeneral.gov/library/reports/preventing-youth-tobacco-use/

U.S. Department of Health and Human Services. (2014). Helping smokers quit: A guide for clinicians. Retrieved January 22, 2016, from http://www.ahrq.gov/professionals/clinicians-providers/guidelines-recommendations/tobacco/clinicians/references/clinhlpsmkqt/index.html

U.S. Department of Health and Human Services. (n.d.). Treatment for tobacco use and dependence. Retrieved January 22, 2016, from http://www.surgeongeneral.gov/library/reports/50-years-of-progress/sgr50-chap-14-app14-4.pdf

Werch, C. E., Bian, H., Diclemente, C. C., Moore, M. J., Thombs, D., Ames, S. C., & Pokorny, S. (2010). A brief image-based prevention intervention for adolescents. *Psychology of Addictive Behaviors: Journal of the Society of Psychologists in Addictive Behaviors, 24*(1), 170-175. doi:10.1037/a0017997

Wheeler, D. (2015). NASW standards and indicators for cultural competence in social work practice. Retrieved January 22, 2016, from http://www.socialworkers.org/practice/standards/PRA-BRO-253150-CC-Standards.pdf

World Health Organization. (2009). WHO Study Group on Tobacco Product Regulation: Report on the scientific basis of tobacco product regulation: Third report of a WHO study group. Retrieved from http://whqlibdoc.who.int/publications/2009/9789241209557_eng.pdf?ua=1PFR

SOCIAL MEDIA: PSYCHOSOCIAL IMPLICATIONS FOR ADOLESCENTS

MAJOR CATEGORIES: Adolescents, Community, Behavioral & Mental Health

WHAT WE KNOW

Adolescence is a time when adolescents are learning how to manage their emotions, building relationships, and developing life skills. This period involves the development of self-identity and the formation of peer relationships. Many adolescents experience an interconnectedness between the need for personal identity and a simultaneous need and desire for powerful group affiliations. They push for independence while still requiring social connections. Social media offers both challenges and opportunities for adolescents engaging in its use.

Adolescents are more limited in their ability to self-regulate and more vulnerable to peer pressure than adults.

Today's adolescent clients have never lived in a time without the Internet, and technology tends to amplify emotions, both positive and negative.

"Social media" refers to any website that allows social interactions, including but not limited to social networking sites (e.g., Facebook, Instagram, Twitter, Snapchat), gaming sites and virtual worlds (e.g., Second Life, Minecraft, Sims), video sites (e.g., YouTube), and blogs.

Social media sites wax and wane in popularity over time, with new sites constantly coming into use as the market and demands change. Social workers need to stay current on the social media sites that are popular with adolescents.

A significant number of adolescents access all of their social media via their phones, which means a much higher rate of unsupervised access.

The Pew Research Center conducted a study in 2015 to study trends among teens with social media and technology. The researchers found that 92 percent of adolescents between the ages of 13 to 17 went online daily, with 24 percent of adolescents stating that they were online "almost constantly." Only 12 percent reported once-a-day online use, 6 percent weekly online use, and 2 percent more infrequent use than that.

Almost 75 percent of adolescents reported having a smartphone, which allows for more frequent online access.

Black and Hispanic youth reported Internet use that was more frequent than that of white youth.

Seventy-one percent of adolescents reported using more than one social networking site.

According to their self-reports, 71 percent of adolescents use Facebook, 52 percent use Instagram, 41 percent use Snapchat, 33 percent use Twitter, 33 percent use Google+, 24 percent use Vine, 14 percent use Tumblr, and 11 percent use a different social media site.

The Pew Research Center conducted a study in 2013 on teens ages 12 to 17 and their relationship to social media and privacy. This study showed that many adolescents are sharing more personal information on social media than in the past. Only 60 percent of adolescents kept their profiles private on Facebook. Only 9 percent reported being very concerned about third-party access to their information, whereas 81 percent of parents expressed that they were either very concerned or somewhat concerned about third-party access.

- 91 percent had posted a personal photo, up from 79 percent in 2006.
- 71 percent had posted the name of their school, up from 49 percent in 2006.

- 71 percent had posted the name of their city or town, up from 61 percent in 2006.
- 20 percent had posted a cell number, up from 2 percent in 2006.
- 33 percent are Facebook friends with people they have never met in person.
- 39 percent admitted to lying about their age to access a website or sign up for an account.

There are varying hypotheses and theories on social media use in adolescence and how use of social media affects adolescents' identity development and ability to connect to others.

The stimulation hypothesis theorizes that adolescents may have an easier time with online self-disclosure than with in-person communication. Since self-disclosure leads to closer relationships, adolescents may be able to form close, high-quality friendships through social media communication.

The rich-get-richer hypothesis theorizes that it is only the more social adolescents who will benefit from online communication, whereas those adolescents with poorer social skills will not be able to develop high-quality connections and are therefore at an increased risk for depression.

In contrast, the social compensation hypothesis theorizes that those adolescents who are uncomfortable with in-person peer relationships can develop relationships and meet their social needs online.

The media practice model posits that adolescents choose and will interact with media based on not only who they are but also who they want to be. When adolescents choose to explore certain behaviors or experiences, they may receive reinforcement that will then push them toward further engagement in that behavior choice (e.g., an adolescent who is thinking about experimenting with alcohol use may be influenced by viewing social media that shows peer endorsement of that behavior).

The Facebook influence model outlines four concepts related to Facebook and its influences on self-identity, social norms, and connectedness to others. These are:.

Connection – Facebook both provides and improves peer communication, connection, and networking.

Comparison – Facebook takes the always-present concept of peer comparison and uses actual information, photos, stated preferences, and other elements to provide a point of comparison while also giving adolescents the option of commenting on one another's material. When a post or photo is not generating as many comments as a peer's post or photo, this is another point of comparsion.

Identification – The user can develop an online identity and receive feedback on that identity, providing a multimedia self-view.

Immersive experience – Facebook features create a fully immersive experience.

Use of social media in adolescence can have positive effects by helping the adolescent with identity development, self-disclosure, and forming affiliations.

Many adolescents use social media to extend relationships that are found in other parts of their lives.

Use of social media can allow adolescents to both provide and receive virtual empathy (e.g., taking part in an online fundraiser, receiving supportive comments and messages after posting about an ill loved one).

This support may include support for adolescents who are otherwise marginalized by sexual orientation, illness, disability, or shyness.

Social media allows adolescents to reach out for health information on topics that might otherwise be hard to talk about (e.g., substance use, sexual health).

Some challenges and concerns do arise with adolescent use of social media.

Social comparison is common on most social media sites. This can provide some positive feedback with responses to a posting but can also end up making adolescents feel inadequate, whereupon their self-esteem may suffer. Adolescents may also post misleading or inaccurate information to present an idealized version of themselves.

Many social media sites have measuring tools such as "likes" or "friends" that are collected, and adolescents may let these measures influence their sense of self-worth. An adolescent may also feel that if a picture or comment is not getting enough feedback from the adolescent's circle of friends,then it should be shared with a wider audience.

Adolescents are vulnerable to the online disinhibition effect in which people tend to share personal details and more private information in a social media format than in face-to-face interactions because of feeling more anonymous and disassociated online than in the real world.

This phenomenon is also referred to as "public intimacy," where the adolescent's perception is

that the content is private because ofhis or her own privacy settings when in reality the information is still public (e.g., can be hacked, accessed by IT employees, tagged by a friend who does not have a private profile, data mined by data collection companies).

Adolescents can be impulsive in behavior decisions, and this, coupled with how rapidly information can spread on social media, can have major negative implications that may personally affect teens.

Adolescents are not often thinking about the digital footprint that is left through social media use. Adolescents can post impulsively and do not fully consider privacy issues. Adolescents are often not forward thinking enough to realize that any public information on social media may be accessed by higher education institutes or future employers.

Risk-taking behavior (e.g., alcohol use, substance use, high-risk sexual behaviors) is often promoted by adolescents within their social media profiles and postings.

Some of these behaviors can result in legal consequences, especially when related to the sending and receiving of nude pictures of adolescents to other adolescents. In many jurisdictions, these exchanges are being classified as the transmission of child pornography and resulting in criminal charges.

Cyberbullying is online aggression or harassment and is a concern with adolescent social media use. The attackers' ability to remain anonymous can result in harsher attacks than those that would take place with in-person bullying.

Adolescents are engaging in sexting, the receiving or sending of images, video, or text messages with sexually explicit content, at increasing rates. Some researchers believe that sexting can lead to more high-risk sexual behaviors.

Social workers need to recognize the impact of social media and ensure that questions about social media and Internet use are incorporated into assessments. The HEEADSSS 3.0 interview, an adolescent psychosocial interview, now includes questions on social media use.

Media-related depression, also referred to as "Facebook depression," is a debated phenomenon that is supported by some researchers and dismissed by others.

Researchers in 2014 conducted a study that documented a deterioration of mood after Facebook use; what's more, the longer a subject's Facebook use session, the more his or her mood deteriorated. The researchers hypothesized that users perceived that being on Facebook was a waste of time, which led to the decrease in mood. Subjects were making a forecasting error, thinking the time on Facebook would improve their mood, and instead it made their mood worse.

The marketing that takes place over the Internet is largely unregulated, and adolescents may be exposed to alcohol and tobacco marketing, which is more restricted on television.

In 2013, 30 percent of online adolescents stated that they had received online advertising that was "clearly inappropriate" for their age.

Adolescence is a time when good judgment and decision making are still developing and not yet fully formed, which indicates a need for parental oversight. Social workers may want to follow the physician recommendations from the American Academy of Pediatrics and use the screening questions asking how much time an adolescent spends with screen/social media and if the adolescent has a device in his or her bedroom that affords Internet access.

Parents need to be informed that in the United States, 13 years old is considered the minimum age for legal use of most social media sites as a result of the Children's Online Privacy Protection Act (COPPA), which prohibits websites from collecting information on users younger than 13 without parental permission.

WHAT CAN BE DONE

Become knowledgeable about the psychosocial implications of social media for adolescents so you can accurately assess your clients' personal characteristics and mental health and health education needs; share this information with your colleagues.

Develop an awareness of your own cultural values, beliefs, and biases and develop knowledge about the histories, traditions, and values of your clients. Adopt treatment methodologies that reflect the cultural needs of the client.

Stay informed on any developing trends in social media technology and the Internet so that you will be aware of how adolescents may be using them and any connected risks.

Identify adolescent clients who are at risk for social media misuse or vulnerable to social media exploitation.

Ask adolescent clients how much they use social media and what they are doing online in order to assess for a lack of parental control or connection, avoidance behaviors, or any behavior that indicates problematic use or addiction..

Encourage parents of adolescent clients to establish rules and limits for technology use both in the home and in outside environments.

Written by Jessica Therivel, LMSW-IPR

Reviewed by Lynn B. Cooper, D. Crim

REFERENCES

American Academy of Pediatrics. (2013). Children, adolescents, and the media. Retrieved October 6, 2015, from http://elf2.library.ca.gov/pdf/AAP.pdf

British Association of Social Workers. (2012, January). Code of ethics for social work. Retrieved October 6, 2015, from http://cdn.basw.co.uk/upload/basw_112315-7.pdf

Barth, F. D. (2015). Social media and adolescent development: Hazards, pitfalls, and opportunities for growth. *Journal of Clinical Social Work, 43*, 201-208. doi:10.1007/s10615-014-0501-6

Brown University Child and Adolescent Behavior Letter. (2014). Social media use and adolescents: A guide for parents. *Child Adolescent Behavior Letter, 30*, I-II. doi:10.1002/cbl.20208

Cookingham, L. M., & Ryan, G. L. (2015). The impact of social media on the sexual and social wellness of adolescents. *Journal of Pediatric and Adolescent Gynecology, 28*(1), 2-5.

International Federation of Social Workers. (2012). Statement of ethical principles. Retrieved October 6, 2015, from http://ifsw.org/policies/statement-of-ethical-principles/

Klein, D. A., Goldenring, J. M., & Adelman, W. P. (2014, January 1). HEEADSSS 3.0: The psychosocial interview for adolescents updated for a new century fueled by media. *Contemporary Pediatrics.* Retrieved from http://contemporarypediatrics.modernmedicine.com/contemporary-pediatrics/content/tags/adolescent-medicine/heeadsss-30-psychosocial-interview-adolesce

Mizrahi, T., & Mayden, R. W. (2001). NASW standards for cultural competence in social work practice. Retrieved October 6, 2015, from http://www.

socialworkers.org/practice/standards/NASWCul-
turalStandards.pdf

Moreno, M. A., & Whitehill, J. M. (2014). Influence
of social media on alcohol use in adolescents and
young adults. *Alcohol Research: Current Reviews,
36*(1), 91-100.

O'Keeffe, G. S., & Clarke-Pearson, K. (2011). Clinical
report – The impact of social media on children,
adolescents, and families. *Pediatrics, 127*(4), 800-804.

Pew Research Center. (2013, May 21). Teens, social
media and privacy. Retrieved October 6, 2015,
from http://www.pewinternet.org/2013/05/21/
teens-social-media-and-privacy/

Pew Research Center. (2015, April 9). Teens, social media &
technology overview 2015. Retrieved October 6, 2015,
from   http://www.pewinternet.org/2015/04/09/
teens-social-media-technology-2015/

Raffia, M., Carson, N. J., & DeJong, S. M. (2014).
Adolescents and the Internet: What mental health
clinicians need to know. *Child and Adolescent Disorders, 16*, 472.

Rosen, L. D. (2011, August 4). Poke me: How social
networks can both help and harm our kids. Paper
presented at American Psychological Association
119th Annual Convention, Washington, D.C.

Shapiro, L. A., & Margolin, G. (2014). Growing up
wired: Social networking sites and adolescent psychosocial development. *Clinical Child and Family
Psychological Review, 17*, 1-18.

Sagioglouc, C., & Greitemeyer, T. (2014). Facebook's
emotional consequences: Why Facebook causes a
decrease in mood and why people still use it. *Computers and Human Behavior, 35*, 359-363.

Spiritual Needs of Hospitalized Patients

Major Categories: Behavioral & Mental Health, Cultural Competency

What We Know

Although the concept of spirituality is highly individualized and thus defined by patients in a variety of
ways, religious beliefs and values exert a deep influence on how many patients perceive illness, make decisions, cope with the burden of disease, and adhere
to treatment.

Spirituality often is defined as the personal quality
of being concerned with religion or the human spirit;
a set of beliefs that sustain the individual through
times of difficulty; the search for meaning and hope;
one's conception of the purpose of life; or the nature
1of one's relationship with oneself, others, nature, or
God (as defined by the individual).

It is important to know that the concept of spirituality does not always equate with a religious affiliation.

Many patients consider spirituality and structured
participation in an organized religion to be synonymous; other patients believe that spirituality is contained within oneself and has little to do with identifying oneself with one particular religion.

Hospitalization can cause existential conflicts
for patients. They may grapple with concerns related to morbidity, mortality, grief, loss, and uncertainty. These internal conflicts can result in a greater
spiritual need that may require assistance to explore
and address during hospitalization.

There is increasing evidence that religious beliefs
and/or spirituality help patients to cope with the
fear and anxiety caused by illness. In particular, patients who are at the end of life or experiencing severe illness often express a need to find meaning in
life and in death, make peace with themselves and
with loved ones, and reconstruct beliefs or spiritual
practices.

Patients who are ill may request the assistance of
a clergy member (e.g., priest, minister, rabbi, imam)
for rituals and customs such as prayer, a spiritual
blessing, reading of a holy book (e.g., Bible, Torah,
Qur'an), or confession of sins.

Hospital-based clergy report assisting patients to
cope not only with their religious/spiritual concerns
but also with feelings of loneliness, despair, anger,
frustration, guilt and shame, physical pain and suffering, and with issues surrounding familial discord.

Hospital workers commonly request the help of
hospital-based clergy in assisting patients with decision-making, for emotional crisis intervention, and
for bereavement support for families of patients who
have died.

Research has suggested that spiritual well-being can directly impact physical and emotional/psychological outcomes and is of great importance to patients.

Multiple studies have demonstrated that attending to a patient's spiritual needs is associated with improvement in psychosocial and physiological variables, and even decreases in mortality.

Studies confirm that hospital patients rank spiritual care as a priority in their recovery, and see good spiritual care as very important to their overall satisfaction with care during hospitalization.

Several models have been proposed to assess the patient's spirituality and religious beliefs with regard to healthcare, including the HOPE model (sources of Hope, Organized religion, Personal spiritual practices, and Effects of these behaviors on healthcare), the BELIEF model (Belief system, Ethics of values, Lifestyle, Involvement in religious community, Education, and Future events), and Fowler's stages of faith model.

The spiritual distress assessment tool (SDAT) is a useful clinical instrument to evaluate negative feelings and thoughts associated with spiritual and religious beliefs of hospitalized older patients.

Providing optimal, total care requires respect for and support their patients' spiritual beliefs.

Showing respect for patients' spiritual beliefs helps build rapport and trust between the hospital workers and the patient and allows the patient to openly discuss spiritual concerns with his or her caregivers.

Respect for each patient's spirituality means to recognize that each patient has his/her own distinctive values and life plans, which may differ from the hospital workers it also refers to the caregiver's willingness to learn about the spiritual needs, resources, and preferences of the patient.

Respect for a patient's spiritual needs is not prescribing a specific spiritual practice or urging a patient to relinquish his or her religious beliefs in exchange for those of the caregiver(s).

It is important to incorporate a spiritual discharge plan as needed for patients who are discharging from the hospital, since spiritual needs that come up during hospitalization may not be addressed during a brief hospital stay. This plan may include information on connecting with community religious advisors, finding spiritual support groups, or helping the patient connect with his or her existing congregation/parish for assistance after discharge.

Patients of different cultures may have different spiritual needs or issues that need to be recognized and addressed by hospital workers or caregivers.

For many Native American patients, spirituality is not a separate dimension in life but is incorporated into the mental and physical dimensions, with spiritual issues being represented in physical and mental illnesses.

Black patients are less likely than white patients to be asked about spiritual concerns while in the hospital.

Asian patients may belong to one of as many as 30 ethnic subgroups in the United States, with correspondingly varied spiritual needs. Social workers should become familiar with some of the common spiritual practices for various groups.

Even if there has not been specially training in providing spiritual care it is still important to provide spiritual support by inquiring about and actively listening to patients' spiritual concerns, observing for and facilitating adherence to their religious preferences, and providing a peaceful environment for reflection.

When discussing spirituality with patients, hospital or mental health workers should encourage open communication by using open-ended questions (e.g., How do you express your spirituality? How can I support you in your religious and/or spiritual needs while you are in the hospital?) and actively listening to patients' responses.

Hospital workers should assess for religious restrictions that may affect the patient's medical care or diet (e.g., Jehovah's Witnesses do not accept blood transfusions, food eaten by Jews who "keep kosher" must be prepared in accordance with Jewish dietary laws, Muslims follow halal dietary laws), and be especially mindful of these beliefs, recognizing that violations of religious practices can result in deep psychological distress for the patient.

Document and verbally communicate the patient's beliefs with the medical team to ensure the patient's preferences are respected. Adhering to the patient's beliefs will reassure the patient that he or she does not have to violate his or her beliefs while hospitalized and that his or her dignity will be maintained.

Create an environment that will allow for spiritual reflection by honoring the patient's dignity at all times, providing physical comfort (e.g., pain/symptom relief), and eliminating noisy distractions.

WHAT CAN BE DONE

Learn about the importance of spirituality in order to respectfully understand and care for the spiritual needs of hospitalized patients and to accurately conduct biopsychosocial and spiritual assessments.

Remain aware and accepting of variations in spiritual expression, be empathetic and respectful of the spiritual and/or religious needs of all patients, and observe for unspoken spiritual preferences.

Offer and provide access to hospital and/or local community spiritual resources (e.g., chaplain, spiritual mentor, rabbi, folk healer).

Be observant for the spiritual preferences of patients and, if appropriate and available, provide patients with spiritual books (e.g., religious scriptures), videos (e.g., guided imagery), music (e.g., religious hymns, nature sounds, chanting), and access to places of worship (e.g., hospital chapels) or facility-based religious support groups.

Utilize active listening skills in order to better assess patients' spiritual needs.

Ensure that hospitalized patients with spiritual needs leave the hospital with a spiritual discharge plan.

Establish a multidisciplinary quality improvement team to research, implement, and measure the effectiveness of resources and interventions used to address issues of spirituality.

Attend and/or set up ongoing in-service education sessions that focus on discussion of spiritual and religious needs and appropriate interventions that can be used to support patients.

Written by Penny March, PsyD, and Carita Caple, RN, BSN, MSHS

Reviewed by Lynn B. Cooper, D. Crim, and Melissa Rosales Neff, MSW

REFERENCES

Delaney, C., & Barrere, C. (2008). Blessings: The influence of a spirituality-based intervention on the psychospiritual outcomes in a cardiac population. *Holistic Nursing Practice, 22*(4), 210-219. doi:10.1097/01.hnp.0000326004.57687.74

Dzul-Church, V., Cimino, J. W., Adler, S. R., Wong, P., & Anderson, W. G. (2010). "I'm sitting here by myself ...": Experiences of patients with serious illness at an urban public hospital. *Journal of Palliative Medicine, 13*(6), 695-701. doi:10.1089/jpm.2009.0352

Hilbers, J., Haynes, A. S., & Kivikko, J. G. (2010). Spirituality and health: An exploratory study of hospital patients' perspectives. *Australian Health Review, 34*(1), 3-10. doi:10.1071/AH09655

Hodge, D. R., Boninifas, R. P., Sun, F., & Wolosin, R. J. (2014). Developing a model to address African Americans' spiritual needs during hospitalization. *Clinical Gerontologist, 37*(4), 386-405. doi:10.1080/07317115.2014.907593

Hodge, D. R., Sun, F., & Wolosin, R. J. (2014). Hospitalized Asian patients and their spiritual needs: Developing a model of spiritual care. *Journal of Aging & Health, 26*(3), 380-400. doi:10.1177/0898264313516995

Hodge, D. R., & Wolosin, R. (2014). Spiritual needs and satisfaction with service provision: Mediating pathways among a national sample of hospital inpatients. *Social Work Research, 38*(3), 135-143. doi:10.1093/swr/svu009

Hodge, D. R., & Wolosin, R. J. (2014). American Indians and spiritual needs during hospitalization: Developing a model of spiritual care. *The Gerontologist, 26*(3), 380-400. doi:10.1177/0898264313516995

Hollywell, C., & Walker, J. (2009). Private prayer as a suitable intervention for hospitalised patients: A critical review of the literature. *Journal of Clinical Nursing, 18*(5), 637-651. doi:10.1111/j.1365-2702.2008.02510.x

International Federation of Social Workers. (2012, March 3). Statement of ethical principles. Retrieved September 27, 2015, from http://ifsw.org/policies/statement-of-ethical-principles

Jolley, D., & Moreland, N. (2011). Dementia care: Spiritual and faith perspectives. *Nursing and Residential Care, 13*(8), 388-391. doi:10.12968/nrec.2011.13.8.388

Monod, S. M., Rochat, E., Bula, C. J., Jobin, G., Martin, E., & Spencer, B. (2010). The spiritual distress assessment tool: An instrument to assess spiritual distress in hospitalised elderly persons. *BMC Geriatrics, 10*(88). doi:10.1186/1471-2318-10-88

Montoyne, M., & Calderone, S. (2010). Pastoral interventions and the influence of self-reporting: A preliminary analysis. *Journal of Health Care Chaplaincy*, *16*(1-2), 65-73. doi:10.1080/08854720903519976

National Association of Social Workers. (2001). NASW standards for cultural competency in social work practice. Retrieved September 27, 2015, from http://www.socialworkers.org/practice/standards/NASWCulturalStandards.pdf

Neuman, M. E. (2011). Addressing children's beliefs through Fowler's stages of faith. *Journal of Pediatric Nursing*, *26*(1), 44-50. doi:10.1016/j.pedn.2009.09.002

Onslow, L. (2009). End-of-life care for older people in the acute hospital setting. *End of Life Care*, *3*(3), 26-29.

Policy, Ethics, and Human Rights Committee, British Association of Social Workers. (2012, January). The code of ethics for social work: Statement of principles. Retrieved September 27, 2015, from http://cdn.basw.co.uk/upload/basw_112315-7.pdf

Rushton, L. (2014). What are the barriers to spiritual care in a hospital setting?. *British Journal of Nursing*, *23*(7), 370-374. doi:10.12968/bjon.2014.23.7.370

Sulmasy, D. P. (2009). Spirituality, religion, and clinical care. *Chest*, *135*(6), 1634-1642. doi:10.1378/chest.08-2241

STROKE REHABILITATION: TAKING CARE OF THE CAREGIVER

MAJOR CATEGORIES: Caregivers, Medical & Health

WHAT WE KNOW

Worldwide, in 2012, strokes were responsible for 6.7 million deaths worldwide and were the second leading cause of death and a primary source of disability. In the United States, in 2013, 6.8 million people were living after having experienced a stroke.

In the United States there are 34.2 million unpaid, nonprofessional caregivers (e.g., family, friends) providing care to an adult over the age of 50. Nearly 1 in 10 of these caregivers is over the age of 75. 23 percent of the caregivers are providing more than 40 hours of care a week. These nonprofessional caregivers are often the primary caregiver for individuals who have had a stroke.

An individual who has experienced a stroke will typically move from having 24-hour medical care and an intensive therapy program to being at home with little or no professional support and the expectation that family or friends will provide any needed supportive care. These nonprofessional caregivers will often describe the experience of a transition to home as being difficult or traumatic.

Preparing caregivers (e.g., in using medical equipment, providing mouth care, feeding, managing medication) before the stroke survivor is discharged from the hospital helps prepare them to deal with the physical, emotional, and cognitive needs of the stroke survivor and improves the caregiver's self-efficacy.

In recognition that excessive caregiver burden can affect not only stroke survivors but also the caregivers' quality of life (QOL), increasing attention has been drawn to the needs of nonprofessional caregivers, or individuals who care for disabled individuals.

Because stroke often results in persistent functional and cognitive deficits, survivors often require comprehensive assistance from caregivers. Individuals who become caregivers may find their social lives, occupational and financial situations, and emotional health threatened by their new roles and responsibilities.

The majority of caregivers (62 percent) are nonprofessional caregivers (typically the spouse and other family members) who lack medical or nursing experience yet provide challenging physical care for stroke survivors who need day-to-day assistance with eating, bathing, dressing, ambulation, and transfer from one place to another (e.g., bedroom, bathroom, doctor's appointments).Caregivers may also face the burden of handling their loved one's financial and legal matters.

Because stroke is a sudden, unanticipated event, caregivers are thrust into their new roles with little preparation, training, or support. As a result, caregivers often face high levels of stress, burden, and feelings of helplessness and hopelessness.

The impact of stroke reaches beyond functional outcomes for affected clients. Caregivers report feeling particularly overwhelmed by emotional, cognitive, and behavioral changes that may persist after the stroke client regains physical functionality.

Stroke survivors typically need the most assistance during their first year of recovery; thus, caregivers often are most burdened during this time period.

An early hospital discharge poststroke is associated with improved functional ability in clients but may result in increased caregiver burden.

There are specific factors that can influence the success of care at home and ease the stress on the caregiver. These include the strength of the caregiver–client relationship, the caregiver's understanding of and willingness to provide care, the caregiver's preexisting health issues, pre-stroke roles and responsibilities, accessibility of the home, availability of informal support resources for the caregiver, financial resources, pre-stroke caregiver experiences, a sustained ability to provide care over the long term, and having strategies for self-care (35).

The ability of caregivers to adapt to and cope with their caregiving role is important to both their own well-being and the well-being of the stroke survivor.

An active coping style, or using problem solving and information gathering to deal with a stressful life event, is associated with positive outcomes for the caregiver.

Passive coping, also referred to as avoidance or escape coping, is a negative predictor of caregiver QOL.

Formal interventions for caregivers often include structured courses on improving coping ability; assistance with daily tasks, including housekeeping, meal preparation, and grocery shopping; respite for the caregiver; and emotional support via telephone, the Internet, nurse-led support groups and/or nurse home visits, and psychological counseling.

Investigators who processed a systematic review found that psychosocial interventions alone often failed to reduce the burden on caregivers because the impact on the caregiver is physical, emotional, social, and financial.

For persons newly assuming the role and responsibilities of caregiver, the Internet has become a primary means of education and informal help and support.

Internet discussion groups, blogs, message boards, social networking sites, and educational websites have become widely used resources that provide avenues for caregivers to share their feelings, glean practical advice, and receive social support, which has been cited by caregivers as their greatest need.

There are various conceptual theories and models that are related to caregiver stress and stroke survivors and affect the interventions that are provided.

Family systems theory presumes that a change in any part of the family system alters the entire system. Therefore, the changes experienced by the stroke survivor have an impact on all the members of the family, especially the caregiver.

The stress and coping theory suggests that stressful events will trigger a coping process to try to restore balance. This theory also incorporates the concept of contextual factors (e.g., background, socioenvironmental factors, illness) that can affect coping processes and outcomes.

The psychoeducational model will combine providing information on stroke and caregiving while also taking a psychological approach to any survivor or caregiver stress.

Although caregivers face numerous challenges in providing care and assistance for stroke survivors, evidence shows that most caregivers are less likely than survivors to be depressed or to focus on the survivors' functional deficits (e.g., limited mobility, difficulty with self-care, speech).

Stroke survivors often exhibit emotional, behavioral, and cognitive impairment that can alter the relationship between themselves and their caregivers. Yet evidence shows that although survivors tend to perceive a loss of intimacy with their caregivers, caregivers tend to perceive their relationship as strengthened despite increasing challenges.

Stroke survivors tend to feel uncomfortable with their need for assistance and may equate dependence with inadequacy. Conversely, caregivers generally are comfortable in their role and are willing to provide more assistance with tasks than care recipients are willing to accept.

Researchers in the Netherlands found that when stroke survivors were anxious and had lower life satisfaction, there was an increase in the strain on the caregivers.

Research indicates that the QOL of the care recipient is in part dependent upon the QOL of the caregiver. Depression in caregivers is associated with poor stroke survivor function, communication, and social participation.

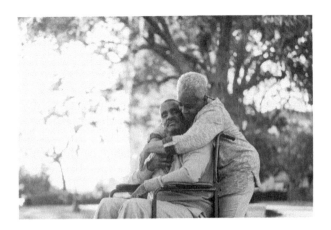

In Canada, the healthcare community has released guidelines for physicians, nurses, and any other allied health professionals to screen for depression for all clients who are living with stroke and those clients' caregivers.

If the caregivers have high levels of mastery in their caregiving skills, are in good physical health, and provide higher levels of assistance to the survivor, they typically report improved mental health and quality of life. These caregivers may feel needed and appreciated and sense that there is a positive outcome to providing care.

WHAT CAN BE DONE

Learn about the challenges faced by caregivers to better evaluate their needs and provide support; share this information with your colleagues.

Develop an awareness of your own cultural values, beliefs, and biases and develop knowledge about the histories, traditions, and values of your clients. Adopt treatment methodologies that reflect the cultural needs of the client.

Provide a family-centered approach that includes the caregiver as a client; schedule a conference with a multidisciplinary team, the patient, caregivers, and family members to discuss goal planning; provide education to help caregivers feel competent in the caregiving role.

Social work professionals need to identify conflicts within the family and gaps in services during the ongoing assessment and provide better transitions of care and care coordination.

Provide support to caregivers by
- recognizing and acknowledging the emotional, physical, and financial stress of caring for a loved one who has experienced a stroke;
- evaluating the extent and quality of available social support;
- taking sufficient time to assess the individual needs of each client and caregiver by listening actively and answering their questions;
- offering practical advice on how best to provide assistance with activities of daily living and other day-to-day care activities (e.g., transportation);
- encouraging the caregiver to resume involvement in his or her own hobbies, activities, and spiritual practices.

Based on the needs of the individual client and caregiver, request referrals to a licensed clinical social worker, vocational and rehabilitation counselor, physical and/or occupational therapist, and state or federal disability programs.

Recognize the link between the well-being of caregivers and care recipients. Assess caregivers for depression and request a referral to a mental health clinician, if indicated.

Encourage caregivers to obtain more information about stroke from the American Stroke Association at http://www.strokeassociation.org, the Stroke Network at http://www.strokenetwork.org/, and the Stroke Association at http://www.stroke.org.uk/.

Written by Laura McLuckey, MSW, LCSW

Reviewed by Lynn B. Cooper, D. Criminology

REFERENCES

Ang, J. Y. H., Chow, Y. L., & Poon, E. W. H. (2013). Literature review: Coping strategies of family caregivers caring for stroke survivors. *Singapore Nursing Journal, 40*(2), 19-27.

Bowman, L. (2009). Management of clients with stroke. In J. M. Black & J. H. Hawks (Eds.), *Medical-surgical nursing: Clinical management for positive outcomes* (8th ed., pp. 1843-1848). St. Louis, MO: Saunders Elsevier.

British Association of Social Workers. (2012, January). The code of ethics for social work: Statement of principles. Retrieved October 24, 2015, from http://cdn.basw.co.uk/upload/basw_112315-7.pdf

Cameron, J. I., Stewart, D. E., Streiner, D. L., Coyte, P. C., & Cheung, A. M. (2014). What makes family caregivers happy during the first 2 years post stroke? *Stroke*, *45*(4), 1084-1089. doi:10.1161/STROKEAHA.113.004309

Canadian Stroke Network. (2013, March 19). Depression screening essential for caregivers, people living with stroke, new national guidelines say. Retrieved October 24, 2015, from http://www.heartandstroke.com/site/apps/nlnet/content2.aspx?c=ikIQLcMWJtE&b=3485819&ct=13046441&printmode=1

Centers for Disease Control and Prevention. (2015, March 24). Stroke facts. Retrieved October 24, 2015, from http://www.cdc.gov/stroke/facts.htm

Cheng, H. Y., Chair, S. Y., & Chau, J. P. -C. (2014). The effectiveness of psychosocial interventions for stroke family caregivers and stroke survivors: A systematic review and meta-analysis. *Patient Education and Counseling*, *95*, 30-44. doi:10.1016/j.pec.2014.01.005

Cramm, J. M., Strating, M. M. H., & Nieboer, A. P. (2012). Satisfaction with care as a quality-of-life predictor for stroke patients and their caregivers. *Quality of Life Research*, *21*(10), 1719-1725. doi:10.1007/s11136-011-0107-1

Creasy, K. R., Lutz, B. J., Young, M. E., Ford, A., & Martz, C. (2013). The impact of interactions with providers on stoke caregivers' needs. *Rehabilitation Nursing*, *38*(2), 88-98. doi:10.1002/rnj.69

Forster, A., Young, J., Green, J., Patterson, C., Wanklyn, P., Smith, J., & Lowson, K. (2009). Structured re-assessment system at 6 months after a disabling stroke: A randomised controlled trial with resource use and cost study. *Age and Ageing*, *38*(5), 576-583. doi:10.1093/ageing/afp095

Go, A. S., Mozaffarian, D., Roger, V. L., Benjamin, E. J., Berry, J. D., Borden, W. B., ... Bravata, D. M. (2014). Heart disease and stroke statistics – 2013 update: A report from the American Heart Association. *Circulation*, *127*(1), e6-e245. doi:10.1161/CIR.0b013e31828124ad

Gonzalez, C., & Bakas, T. (2013). Factors associated with stroke survivor behaviors as identified by family caregivers. *Rehabilitation Nursing*, *38*(4), 202-211. doi:10.1002/rnj.85

Green, T. L., & King, K. M. (2010). Functional and psychosocial outcomes 1 year after mild stroke. *Journal of Stroke and Cerebrovascular Diseases*, *19*(1), 10-16. doi:10.1016/j.jstrokecerebrovasdis.2009.02.005

International Federation of Social Workers. (2012, March 3). Statement of ethical principles. Retrieved October 24, 2015, from http://ifsw.org/policies/statement-of-ethical-principles/

Kim, J., & Moon, S. (2007). Needs of family caregivers caring for stroke patients: Based on the rehabilitation treatment phase and the treatment setting. *Social Work in Health Care*, *45*(1), 81-97. doi:10.1300/J010v45n01_06

King, R. B., Hartke, R. J., Lee, J., & Raad, J. (2013). The stroke caregiver unmet resource needs scale: development and psychometric testing. *Journal of Neuroscience Nursing: Journal of the American Association of Neuroscience Nurses*, *45*(6), 320-328. doi:10.1097/JNN.0b013e3182a3ce40

Klinedinst, N. J., Gebhardt, M. C., Aycock, D. M., Nichols-Larsen, D. S., Uswatte, G., Wolf, S. L., & Clark, P. C. (2009). Caregiver characteristics predict stroke survivor quality of life at 4 months and 1 year. *Research in Nursing and Health*, *32*(6), 592-605. doi:10.1002/nur.20348

Krevers, B., & Oberg, B. (2011). Support/services and family carers of persons with stroke impairment: Perceived importance and services received. *Journal of Rehabilitation Medicine*, (43:3), 204-209. doi:10.2340/16501977-0649

Libert, D., & Bumby, N. (2001). Emotional problems: Evaluation and treatment in stroke rehabilitation. *Loss, Grief & Care*, *9*(1/2), 107-118. doi:10.1300/J132v09n01_08

Lutz, B., Young, M., Cox, K., Martz, C., & Creasy, K. (2011). The crisis of stroke: Experiences of patients and their family caregivers. *Topics in Stroke Rehabilitation*, *18*(6), 786-797. doi:10.1310/tsr1806-786

Lynch, E. B., Butt, Z., Heinemann, A., Victorson, D., Nowinski, C. J., Perez, L., & Cella, D. (2008). A qualitative study of quality of life after stroke: The importance of social relationships. *Journal of Rehabilitation Medicine*, *40*(7), 518-523. doi:10.2340/16501977-0203

Mizrahi, T., & Mayden, R. W. (2001). NASW standards for cultural competence in social work practice. Retrieved October 24, 2015, from http://www.socialworkers.org/practice/standards/NASWCulturalStandards.pdf

National Alliance for Caring and the AARP Public Policy Institute. (2015). Caregiving in the U.S. – 2015. Retrieved October 24, 2015, from http://www.caregiving.org/wp-content/uploads/2015/05/2015_CaregivingintheUS_Final-Report-June-4_WEB.pdf

Oi-Wah, E. C. (2013). Responding to lives after stroke: Stroke survivors and caregivers going on narrative journeys. *International Journal of Narrative Therapy & Community Work, 4,* 1-7.

Oosterveer, D. M., Mishre, R. R., van Oort, A., Bodde, K., & Aerden, L. A. (2014). Anxiety and low life satisfaction associate with high caregiver strain early after stroke. *Journal of Rehabilitation Medicine, 46*(2), 139-143. doi:10.2340/16501977-1250

O'Sullivan, S. B. (2007). Stroke. In S. B. O'Sullivan & T. J. Schmitz (Eds.), *Physical rehabilitation* (5th ed., pp. 723-736). Philadelphia, PA: F.A. Davis Company.

Pierce, L. L., Steiner, V. L., Khuder, S. A., Govoni, A. L., & Horn, L. J. (2009). The effect of a Web-based stroke intervention on carers' well-being and survivors' use of healthcare services. *Disability and Rehabilitation, 31*(20), 1676-1684. doi:10.1080/09638280902751972

Pierce, L. L., Thompson, T. L., Govoni, A. L., & Steiner, V. (2012). Caregivers' incongruence: Emotional strain in caring for persons with stroke. *Rehabilitation Nursing, 37*(5), 258-266. doi:10.1002/rnj.35

Reinhard, S. C., Given, B., Petlick, N. H., & Bernis, A. (2008). Supporting family caregivers in providing care. In R. G. Hughes (Ed.), *Patient safety and quality: An evidence-based handbook for nurses* (Vol. 1, pp. 341-404). Rockville, MD: Agency for Healthcare Research and Quality.

Stone, K. (2013). Enhancing preparedness and satisfaction of caregivers of patients discharged from an inpatient rehabilitation facility using an interactive website. *Rehabilitation Nursing, 39*(2), 76-85. doi:10.1002/rnj.123

Visser-Meily, A., Post, M., de Port, I., Mass, C., Forstberg-Warleby, G., & Lindeman, E. (2009). Psychosocial functioning of spouses of patients with stroke from initial inpatient rehabilitation to 3 years poststroke: Course and relations with coping strategies. *Stroke, 40*(4), 1399-1404. doi:10.1161/STROKEAHA.108.516682

Winkel, A., Ekdahl, C., & Gard, G. (2008). Early discharge to therapy-based rehabilitation at home in patients with stroke: A systematic review. *Physical Therapy Reviews, 13*(3), 167-187. doi:10.1179/174328808X252091

World Health Organization. (2014, May). The top 10 causes of death: Fact sheet N310. Retrieved October 24, 2015, from http://www.who.int/mediacentre/factsheets/fs310/en/

Young, M. E., Lutz, B. J., Creasy, K. R., Cox, K. J., & Martz, C. (2015). A comprehensive assessment of family caregivers of stroke survivors during inpatient rehabilitation. *Disability and Rehabilitation, 36*(22), 1892-1902. doi:10.3109/09638288.2014.881565

STROKE: RISK & PROTECTIVE FACTORS

MAJOR CATEGORIES: Medical & Health

WHAT WE KNOW

Stroke is a medical emergency that occurs as a result of cerebral ischemia (i.e., insufficient blood flow to the brain as a result of clots or events such as heart attacks) or cerebral hemorrhage (i.e., bleeding inside the brain), both of which lead to permanent damage to brain cells. Stroke is the fourth leading cause of death in the United States and a leading cause of disability.

Approximately 6.8 million American adults have had a stroke, and 795, 000 new or recurrent strokes occur each year.

Ischemic stroke is more common than hemorrhagic stroke, occurring in about 80 percent of stroke cases. By 2030 it is projected that an additional 3.4 million adults will have a stroke, which is a 20.5 percent increase in prevalence.

Numerous factors have been identified that increase an individual's risk for stroke. Risk factors for a stroke include nonmodifiable risk factors (those that cannot be changed), modifiable lifestyle factors (those that can be changed), cardiovascular and metabolic conditions, and certain biomarkers.

Nonmodifiable risk factors for stroke include gender, age, and ethinicity/race. In general, men are more likely to have a stroke than women are. The exceptions are women between the ages of 45 and 54, who are more than 2 times more likely than men in the same age range to have a stroke, and women over age 85, who have a higher risk for stroke than do men of the same age. The risk for stroke doubles every 10 years after age 55 with an esstimated 20 percent of deaths from stroke occuring after age 65.

Worldwide, rates of stroke are higher among Blacks, Hispanics, and Native Americans than among Whites. This discrepancy is likely due to the greater incidence of diabetes mellitus and hypertension in these groups.

Modifiable lifestyle factors include tobacco use, unhealthy diets, lack of physical activity, alcohol or drug abuse, the use of oral contraceptives.

Tobacco use doubles the risk for stroke. Diets low in fruits and vegetables and high in saturated or trans fat, cholesterol, and sodium are associated with an increased risk for stroke. Physical inactivity increases the risk for stroke by 50 percent. Alcohol and drug abuse can increase blood pressure (BP), thereby increasing the risk for stroke. The use of oral contraception has been linked to an increase in risk for ischemic stroke but not hemorrhagic stroke.

Cardiovascular, metabolic, and other medical conditions that may increase an individual's risk for stroke include a history of hypertension and diabetes.

Hypertension (i.e., BP > 140/90 mmHg) increases the risk for stroke twofold. Clients with both diabetes mellitus and hypertension have a risk for stroke that is increased approximately fourfold.

Pregnancy-related stroke from hypertensive disorders during pregnancy has increased dramatically. From 1994–1995 to 2010–2011, pregnancy-related stroke increased almost 65 percent. Diabetes mellitus increases stroke risk 1.8-fold in clients older than 75 years and 5.6-fold in those aged 30–44 years. Obesity, usually defined by a body mass index (BMI; i.e., a measurement of body fat based on height and weight) of >30, can be a risk factor for stroke. Ischemic stroke risk is increased twofold in people with a BMI of > 32 kg/m. Benign paroxysmal positional vertigo (BPPV) is a common type of vertigo that results from changes in head position. Investigators found in a recent study that risk for ischemic stroke was increased for clients with BPPV. Individuals who have had a transient ischemic attack (TIA) or prior stroke have a 10 percent–12 percent increased risk for stroke, especially within the first 90 days after the initial event. Sleep apnea has been found to increase risk of ischemic stroke in men. Sleep duration, both too short and too long, can increase stroke risk. The underlying mechanisms as to how sleep is related to the risk of stroke have not been clearly defined, but research has indicated that sleep duration should be included as behavioral risk factor for stroke.

Atrial fibrillation(i.e., an irregular rapid heartbeat)is responsible for approximately 20 percent of all strokes and increases an individual's stroke risk fivefold. Other cardiovascular conditions that increase stroke risk include coronary artery disease, history of myocardial infarction, left atrial enlargement, heart failure, and carotid or peripheral artery disease. A parental history of ischemic stroke can result in a threefold increase in stroke risk for adult children; the risk increases as the adult child ages. Chronic kidney disease also increases risk of stroke. Septicemia, which is infection throughout the body, creates systemic inflammation. Both infection and inflammation are associated with higher stroke risk. Clients under age 45 with a history of septicemia are at the greatest risk. Risk for stroke is highest in the first 6 months after the septicemia occurs and the stroke risk may decrease over time.

Clients who have had a stroke in the past and also have had cancer have an increased risk for recurrent stroke and a cardiovascular mortality. A study found that clients who had cancer and a stroke history had recurrent strokes at a rate of 13.94 percent a year, whereas study participants with stroke history but no cancer had recurrent strokes at a rate of only 4.65 percent a year.

Biomarkers for increased stroke risk include cholesterol levels.

Abnormal cholesterol levels are associated with an increased risk for stroke, particularly ischemic stroke. Specifically, high levels of low-density lipoprotein (LDL, "bad cholesterol") and low levels of high-density lipoprotein (HDL, "good cholesterol") increase the risk for stroke

Other risk factors for stroke include sickle cell disease; use of hormone replacement therapy (HRT), which increases ischemic stroke risk by 44 percent; a high number of births of live children; and migraine headaches, which are associated with a doubling of ischemic stroke risk.

Protective factors include medication and lifestyle modifications.

Treatment of high BP with antihypertensive medications (e.g., angiotensin-converting enzyme [ACE] inhibitors, angiotensin receptor antagonists), treatment of high cholesterol with statins (e.g., lovastatin), and treatment of coronary heart disease or atrial fibrillation with antithrombotic medications (e.g., clopidogrel [Plavix], warfarin [Coumadin]) are associated with a significant reduction in the risk for stroke. Treatment of hypertension can reduce stroke risk by up to 50 percent. Statin therapy has been shown to reduce the risk for a fatal stroke or a hemorrhagic stroke but may increase the risk for stroke in clients who have had a renal transplant, undergo regular dialysis treatment, or have already experienced a TIA or stroke, so this therapy needs to be considered carefully.

Warfarin therapy is associated with a 70 percent decrease in stroke risk in clients with atrial fibrillation. Although warfarin is highly effective, it has numerous limitations (e.g., narrow therapeutic window, drug–food interactions) that have led researchers to develop alternative agents for long-term oral anticoagulant therapy; oral direct thrombin inhibitors (e.g., dabigaran) and factor Xa inhibitors (e.g., rivaroxaban) may prove to be suitable alternatives.

Cessation of smoking, weight loss if overweight, avoidance of HRT, and avoidance of excess consumption of alcohol can significantly decrease the risk for stroke. Routine physical exercise can reduce stroke risk. Authors of a meta-analysis of 43 clinical studies found that physical exercise protects against all types of stroke but that the reduction of risk is statistically significant only for men. Researchers who evaluated the effects of walking as physical exercise found that, especially for older adults, it was the total time spent exercising more than the intensity of the activity that was important for stroke prevention.

What Can Be Done

Social workers can learn more about stroke, including the prevalence, incidence, signs, symptoms, prevention, and treatment options available. Social workers and treating medical professionals can actively discuss the prevention of stroke with clients. Education about prevention should include encouraging clients to monitor BP levels by scheduling regular checkups and adhere to their antihypertensive medication regimen, if prescribed; avoid smoking tobacco and limit alcohol consumption to fewer than 2 drinks per day; exercise (e.g., walk, run) about 30 minutes each day; if diabetic, request a referral to an endocrinologist; adhere to the diet and medications prescribed to maintain control of blood sugar levels;

eat a diet low in cholesterol (for individuals without heart disease, < 300 mg a day) and low in saturated and trans fat. If applicable, clients should be directed to take lipid-lowering drugs, as prescribed. If postmenopausal, social workers should encourage clients to talk with the treating clinician about HRT-related stroke risk.

Social workers may complete referrals for clients to the appropriate programs to help them with lifestyle modifications. Social workers may assess the client's available support systems for clients to be successful with lifestyle modifications. Referrals to hospice may be appropriate for those clients who have had a catastrophic stroke and are in need of palliative care.

More information about stroke can be obtained from the American Stroke Association at www.stroke-association.org and the Stroke Association at www.stroke.org.uk

Written by Carita Caple, RN, BSN, MSHS, and Tanja Schub, BS

Reviewed by Jessica Therivel, LMSW-IPR

References

British Association of Social Workers. (2012, January). The code of ethics for social work: Statement of principles. Retrieved October 7, 2015, from http://cdn.basw.co.uk/upload/basw_112315-7.pdf

Clayville, L. R., Anderson, K. V., Miller, S. A., & St. Onge, E. L. (2011). New options in anticoagulation for the prevention of venous thromboembolism and stroke. *P & T, 36*(2), 86-88, 93-99.

DynaMed. (2015, September 7). Risk factors for stroke or transient ischemic attack. Ipswich, MA: EBSCO Information Services. Retrieved October 7, 2015, from http://search.ebscohost.com/login.aspx?direct=true&db=dme&AN=361037

Enninful-Eghan, H., Moore, R. H., Ichord, R., Smith-Whitely, K., & Kwiatkowski, J. L. (2010). Transcranial Doppler ultrasonography and prophylactic transfusion program is effective in preventing overt stroke in children with sickle cell disease. *Journal of Pediatrics, 157*(3), 479-484. doi:10.1016/j.jpeds.2010.03.007

Furie, K. L., Kasner, S. E., Adams, R. J., Albers, G. W., Bush, R. L., Fagan, S. C., ... Wentworth, D. (2011). Guidelines for the prevention of stroke in patients with stroke or transient ischemic attack:

A guideline for healthcare professionals from the American Heart Association/American Stroke Association. *Stroke, 42*(1), 227-276. doi:10.1161/STR.0b013e3181f7d043

Ge, B., & Guo, X. (2015). Short and long sleep durations are both associated with increased risk of stroke: A meta-analysis of observational studies. *World Stroke Oraganization, 10*, 177-184. doi:10.1111/ijs.12398

Go, A. S., Mozaffarian, D., Roger, V. L., Benjamin, E. J., Berry, J. D., Blaha, M. J., ... Turner, M. B. (2014). Heart disease and stroke statistics–2014 update: A report from the American Heart Association. *Circulation, 129*(3), e28-e292. doi:10.1161/01.cir0000441139.02102.80

International Federation of Social Workers. (2012, March 3). Statement of ethical principles. Retrieved October 7, 2015, from http://ifsw.org/policies/statement-of-ethical-principles/

Jefferis, B. J., Whincup, P. H., Papacosta, O., & Wannamethee, S. G. (2014). Protective effect of time spent walking on risk of stroke in older men. *Stroke: A journal of Cereberal Circulation, 45*(1), 194-199. doi:10.1161/STROKEAHA.113.002246

Jung, S.-Y., Bae, H.-J., Park, B.-J., & Yoon, B.-W. (2010). Parity and risk of hemorrhagic strokes. *Neurology, 74*(18), 1424-1429. doi:10.1212/WNL.0b013e3181dc13a5

Kao, C.-L., Cheng, Y.-Y., Leu, H.-B., Chen, T.-J., Ma, H.-I., Chen, J.-W., & Chan, R.-C. (2014). Increased risk of ischemic stroke in patients with benign paroxysmal positional vertigo: A 9-year follow-up nationwide population study in Taiwan. *Frontiers in Aging Neuroscience, 6*(105), 1-7. doi:10.3389/fnagi.2014.00108

Lau, K. K., Wong, Y. K., Teo, K. C., Chang, R. S. K., Hon, S. F. K., Chan, K. H., ... Siu, C. W. (2014). Stroke patients with a past history of cancer are at increased risk of recurrent stroke and cardiovascular mortality. *PLoS One, 9*(2), e88283. doi:10.1371/journal.pone.0088283

Lee, J. T., Chung, W. T., Lin, J. D., Peng, G. S., Muo, C. H., Lin, C. C., ... Hsu, C. Y. (2014). Increased risk of stroke after septicaemia: A population-based longitudinal study in Taiwan. *PLoS One, 9*(2), e89386. doi:10.1371./journal.pone.0089386

Leffert, L. R., Clancy, C. R., Bateman, B. T., Bryant, A. S., & Kuklina, E. V. (2015). Hypertensive disorders and pregnancy-related stroke: Frequency, trends, risk factors, and outcomes. *Obstatrics & Gynecology, 125*(1), 124-131. doi:10.1097/AOG.0000000000000590

Mizrahi, T., & Mayden, R. W. (2001). NASW standards for cultural competence in social work practice. Retrieved October 7, 2014, from http://www.socialworkers.org/practice/standards/NASWCulturalStandards.pdf

Meyer, D. (2009). Antiplatelets and stroke outcomes: State of the science. *Critical Care Nursing Clinics of North America, 21*(4), 517-528. doi:10.1016/j.ccell.2009.07.016

Prinz, V., & Endres, M. (2011). Statins and stroke: Prevention and beyond. *Current Opinion in Neurology, 24*(1), 75-80. doi:10.1097/WCO.0b013e3283424c53

Reimers, C. D., Knapp, G., & Reimers, A. K. (2009). Exercise as stroke prophylaxis. *Deutsches Ärzteblatt International, 106*(44), 715-721. doi:10.3238/arztebl.2009.0715

Roger, V. L., Go, A. S., Lloyd-Jones, D. M., Adams, R. J., Berry, J. D., Brown, T. M., ... Wylie-Rosett, J. (2011). Heart disease and stroke statistics—2011 update: A report from the American Heart Association. *Circulation, 123*(4), e18-e209.

Schwartz, N. E., & Albers, G. W. (2010). Dabigatran challenges warfarin's superiority for stroke prevention in atrial fibrillation. *Stroke, 41*(6), 1307-1309. doi:10.1161/STROKEAHA.110.584557

Spector, J. T., Kahn, S. R., Jones, M. R., Jayakumar, M., Dalal, D., & Nazarian, S. (2010). Migraine headache and ischemic stroke risk: An updated meta-analysis. *American Journal of Medicine, 123*(7), 612-624. doi:10.1016/j.amjmed.2009.12.021

Strauss, M. H., & Hall, A. (2009). Angiotensin receptor blockers should be regarded as first-line drugs for stroke prevention in both primary and secondary prevention settings: No. *Stroke, 40*(9), 3161-3162. doi:10.1161/STROKEAHA.109.559062

Wang, W., & Zhang, B. (2014). Statins for the prevention of stroke: A meta-analysis of randomized controlled trials. *PLoS One, 9*(3), e92388. doi:10.1371.journal.pone.0092388

Zomorodi, M. (2014). Nursing management: Stroke. In S. L. Lewis, S. R. Dirksen, M. M. Heitkemper, L. Bucher, & M. M. Harding (Eds.), *Medical-surgical nursing: Assessment and management of clinical problems* (9th ed., pp. 1388-1412). St. Louis, MO: Elsevier Mosby.

SUBSTANCE ABUSE & ADOLESCENTS: TREATMENT

MAJOR CATEGORIES: Adolescents, Substance Abuse

WHAT WE KNOW

Substance use disorder refers to a pattern of continued use of a substance (e.g., alcohol, cannabis, opioids, sedatives) that causes cognitive, physiological, and behavioral symptoms, resulting in problems in various areas of functioning. The pattern of use is pathological. The individual may experience impaired behavioral control, continued use despite risks to him or her, and social impairment. There also may be tolerance and withdrawal. This problematic pattern of use must take place for at least 12 months for substance use disorder to be diagnosed.

The *Diagnostic and Statistical Manual of Mental Disorders, 5th Edition (DSM-5)*, was published in 2013, replacing the *DSM-IV*. The *DSM-IV* chapter on "Substance-Related Disorders" included substance dependence, substance abuse, substance intoxication, and substance withdrawal, and then discussed specific substances (e.g., alcohol, amphetamines). The *DSM-5* divides these disorders into two categories: substance use disorders (SUD) and substance-induced disorders (intoxication, withdrawal, and other substance/medication-induced mental disorders). *DSM-5* removes the distinction between abuse and dependence that appeared in *DSM-IV*, and instead provides three specifiers, mild, moderate, or severe, depending on how many symptoms are present. Drug craving has been added as a criterion for substance use disorder, whereas "recurrent legal problems" has been removed. In the *DSM-5*, substance abuse and substance dependence are referred to as SUD or substance dependence, whereas in treatment settings and research literature the terms substance abuse and dependence still are commonly used.

Adolescence is a time of transition and change as the individual moves from childhood to adulthood; it is also a time of increased risk for substance abuse. The manifestation of substance use is significantly different in adolescents than it is in adults, necessitating treatment programs designed specifically for adolescents.

Compared to adults adolescents are more likely to take part in binge and opportunistic use of substances, have more difficulty recognizing that they have a problem, are more susceptible to negative peer influences, focus on immediate concerns and needs, and have higher rates of comorbidity with mental health disorders.

Adolescents may be referred to treatment via the school system, the criminal justice system, family intervention, family physicians, or social service programs.

Out of approximately 13,000 substance abuse treatment programs in the United States surveyed, only approximately 18 percent had a significant adolescent census (at least 10 adolescents in treatment at the time of the survey).

Only 50 percent of the programs serving adolescents had separate programs to address comorbidities (e.g., depression, anxiety, post-traumatic stress disorder) and only 50 percent performed any mental health testing.

Substance use disorders are present in the adolescent population in the United States at rates that have decreased slightly in the last 10 years.

In 2012 6.1 percent of adolescents between 12 and 17 met criteria for substance abuse and/or dependence.

In the 12- to 17-year-old age group comparable rates of abuse and dependence are found between males and females. For males 18 and over, the rate of abuse and dependence typically is double that of females.

In 2012 white, black, and Hispanic adolescents had comparable rates of abuse and dependence, ranging from 8.7 percent to 8.9 percent, whereas Asian and Pacific Islander adolescents had lower rates of 3.2 percent and 5.4 percent, respectively, and Native Americans had the highest rate, approximately 21 percent.

In 2012 1 million adolescents were found to need treatment for illicit drug use, of whom 121,000 actually received treatment; 889,000 adolescents needed treatment for alcohol use and 76,000 actually received treatment.

There are behavioral standards in adult substance abuse treatment that do not work well for adolescent substance abuse treatment. Usually, adult treatment will have a demand or focus on total and immediate abstinence. This expectation does not work well for adolescents who have been mandated to treatment by either parents or the legal system.

The adolescent brain is not fully developed, especially the area of the brain that controls behavioral planning and higher reasoning, so adolescent treatment may need a concrete cognitive focus (i.e., very specific goals, cognitions, behaviors).

The most commonly researched and utilized theories and models for substance abuse treatment are disease models, psychological models, motivation and change theories, transtheoretical/stages of change theory, strengths models, multisystemic therapy (MST),and harm reduction (i.e., the public health model).

The disease model is most commonly associated with Alcoholics Anonymous (AA) and other 12-step programs, in which substance use is viewed as a disease rather than a faulty personal choice. This theory recognizes the influence of biological, environmental, behavioral, and genetic factors in substance abuse.

The psychological models focus on the cognitive and behavioral perspectives on why individuals abuse substances. Strategies for change incorporate these perspectives by identifying high-risk environments and situations and having the client utilize coping strategies to reduce or eliminate substance use.

Addictive behaviors and traits are viewed as habits that can be studied and changed. Relapses are considered likely occurrences that can be beneficially used as part of the treatment process.

Successful cognitive behavioral treatment can reduce the likelihood of suicide attempts in adolescents with alcohol use disorder.

The motivation and change theory perspectives place emphasis on examining the individual's motivation for change and the nature and mechanics of change itself while working to establish a collaborative relationship between the social worker and the client.

Motivational interviewing (MI) focuses on why people make changes in behavior.

MI has been found to be an effective model with the adolescent population and is combined in some programs with contingency management (i.e., payment or rewards for participation).

The transtheoretical theory/stages of change model outlines five stages of change for any behavior:

precontemplation, contemplation, preparation, action, and maintenance.

The three key tenets of this model are that the change process can start no matter which stage the client is in, that relapse is a likely occurrence, and that interventions should match the stage the client is in (e.g., a client in the precontemplation stage is not ready for action-oriented interventions).

Strengths-based treatment teaches adolescents the importance of strengths, has adolescents identify their own strengths, helps others identify the adolescents' strengths, and works on developing personal strengths.

Multisystemic therapy is commonly used in adolescent treatment if conduct disorder is present. In MST, the determinants of the adolescent's antisocial behavior are assessed and treated with a focus on family preservation. School, peer, and community systems also are addressed.

Harm reduction programs and policies aim to reduce harm to individuals who abuse alcohol or other substances. Examples range from designated driver programs and sex education to needle exchange, methadone programs, and making naloxone widely available to counteract opiate overdoses. Harm reduction does not focus on abstinence but instead meets clients where they are relative to their use of alcohol and substances.

Family-based treatment is common when working with adolescents in treatment for substance abuse.

The family environment (e.g., families without structure, families in which parents abuse substances or are absent)may increase the risk of adolescents developing drug or alcohol problems.

Obstacles to engaging families in treatment include parental incarceration, parental addiction, parental indifference or absence (e.g., both parents working full time),and termination of parental rights.

Group work can be an option for adolescents, but the risk of an iatrogenic effect is higher (i.e., where the target behavior is compounded by the treatment):adolescents may learn negative behaviors from other group members (e.g., how to hide signs and symptoms of use, how to obtain substances). Clinicians need to be aware of this risk and protect against it.

Group therapy has more success when there is strong group cohesion.

Regardless of model, most adolescent treatment programs have core treatment elements: working toward either reducing or abstaining from substance use, psychoeducation related to substance use, and offering services and referrals for any additional issues or problems (e.g., comorbid mental health disorders, medical problems, social problems).

Clinicians need to try to find the least restrictive but most appropriate intervention for adolescent clients.

There is a history of aggressive admitting practices by parents and physicians for adolescents with substance use and/or psychiatric issues.

Hospital/facility statistics may indicate that admissions are voluntary, but because a parent or guardian can provide consent to treatment even if the adolescent is not in agreement, some admissions may in fact be involuntary, which may impact treatment success.

Successful treatment programs for adolescents need to have a strong focus on engaging the adolescent client.

Adolescents may fail to complete treatment or treatment may not be successful for a number of reasons.

Barriers to treatment retention may be related to the population, program design, and relationship and communication.

Population (i.e., adolescents) barriers may include problems related to family, language, culture, homelessness, or attending the program as an alternative to jail but without personal motivation.

Program design barriers may include transportation problems, staffing issues, program location, or program rules.

Relationship and communication barriers may include lack of trust, parent relationship issues, parent communication issues, poor parent involvement, lack of inclusion of the adolescent in treatment planning or negative relationships between staff and adolescents.

Risk factors that can derail recovery include the presence of substance users in the adolescent's social network and the presence of negative activities (e.g., school truancy, illegal activities ranging from acquiring illegal drugs to stealing cars).

Adolescents are more likely to not complete treatment if they have comorbid mental health disorders, a family history of substance use disorders, greater severity of addiction, lower socioeconomic status, younger age at time of treatment, criminal justice system involvement, prior admissions, less education, and a history of physical or sexual abuse.

In one residential treatment program studied, out of 160 participants only 30 percent completed treatment.

WHAT CAN BE DONE

Learn about substance abuse treatment for adolescents so you can accurately assess your client, including mental health needs; share this information with your colleagues.

Develop an awareness of your own cultural values, beliefs, and biases and develop knowledge about the histories, traditions, and values of your clients. Adopt treatment methodologies that reflect the cultural needs of the client

For adolescents, this includes understanding the developmental abilities and tasks of adolescence, knowing the psychosocial and emotional phases of adolescence, and being able to recognize inappropriate behaviors and attitudes.

Respect the confidentiality and self-determination needs of adolescent clients.

Encourage self-empowerment in adolescent clients by encouraging the client and his or her family to take an active role in the treatment process.

If facilitating group therapy, ensure strong group cohesion to increase treatment results.

Encourage adolescent clients to develop positive peer supports.

Written by Jessica Therivel, LMSW-IPR

Reviewed by Laura Gale, LCSW

REFERENCES

American Psychiatric Association. (2013). Substance-related and addictive disorders. *Diagnostic and Statistical Manual of Mental Disorders (DSM-5).* Arlington, VA: American Psychiatric Association.

Anastas, J. W., & Clark, E. J. (2012). Adolescent and young adult health. In C. Y. Bradley, S. Lowman, J. Cassels, & L. J. Holtzinger (Eds.), *Social Work Speaks* (9th ed., pp. 3-7). Washington, D.C.: NASW Press.

Engle, B., McGowan, M. J., Wagner, E. F., & Amrhein, P. C. (2010). Markers of marijuana use outcomes within adolescent substance abuse group treatment. *Research on Social Work Practice, 20*(3), 271-282.

Engstrom, M., Mahoney, C. A., & Marsh, J. C. (2012). Substance use problems in health social work practice. In S. Gehlert & T. Arthur Browne (Eds.), *Handbook of health social work* (2nd ed., pp. 426-427). Hoboken, NJ: Wiley.

Esposito-Smythers, C., Spirito, A., Kahler, C. W., Hunt, J., & Monti, P. (2011). Treatment of co-occurring substance abuse and suicidality among adolescents: A randomized trial. *Journal of Consulting and Clinical Psychology, 79*(6), 728-739. doi:10.1037/a0026074

Gangi, J., & Darling, C. A. (2012). Adolescent substance-use frequency following self-help group attendance and outpatient substance abuse treatment. *Journal of Child & Adolescent Substance Abuse, 21*(4), 293-309. doi:10.1080/1067828X.2012.702937

Gogel, L. P., Cavaleri, M. A., Gardin, J. G., II, & Wisdom, J. P. (2010). Retention and ongoing participation in residential substance abuse treatment: Perspectives from adolescents, parents, and staff on the treatment process. *Journal of Behavioral Health Services & Research, 38*(4), 488-496. doi:10.1007/s11414-010-9226-7

Harris, N., Brazeau, J., Clarkson, A., Brownlee, K., & Rawana, E. P. (2012). Adolescents' perspectives on strengths-based group work and group cohesion in residential treatment for substance abuse. *Journal of Social Work Practice in the Addictions, 12*(4), 333-347.

Hogue, A., & Liddle, H. A. (2009). Family-based treatment for adolescent substance abuse: Controlled trials and new horizons in services research. *Journal of Family Therapy, 13*(2), 126-154.

Mark, T. L., Song, X., Vandivort, R., Duffy, S., Butler, J., Coffey, R., & Schabert, V. F. (2006). Characterizing substance abuse programs that treat adolescents. *Journal of Substance Abuse Treatment, 31*(1), 59-65. doi:10.1016/j.jsat.2006.03.017

Mason, M. (2009). Social network characteristics of urban adolescents in brief substance abuse treatment. *Journal of Child & Adolescent Substance Abuse, 18*(1), 72-84. doi:10.1080/15470650802544123

National Association of Social Workers. (2003). NASW standards for the practice of social work with adolescents. Washington, D.C.: Author.

Neumann, A., Ojong, T. N., Yanes, P. K., Tumiel-Berhalter, L., Daigler, G. E., & Blondell, R. D. (2010). Differences between adolescents who complete and fail to complete residential substance abuse treatment. *Journal of Addictive Diseases, 29*(4), 427-435. doi:10.1080/10550887.2010.509276

Orr-Brown, D. E., & Siebert, D. C. (2007). Resistance in adolescent substance abuse treatment: A literature synthesis. *Journal of Social Work Practice in the Addictions, 7*(3), 5-28.

Rieckmann, T., Fussell, H., Doyle, K., Ford, J., Riley, K. J., & Henderson, S. (2011). Adolescent substance abuse treatment: Organizational change and quality of care. *Journal of Addictions & Offender Counseling, 31*(2), 80-93.

Ruiz, B. S., Korchmaros, J. D., Greene, A., & Hedges, K. (2011). Evidence-based substance abuse treatment for adolescents: Engagement and outcomes. *Practice: Social Work in Action, 23*(4), 215-233.

Schwartz, I. M. (1989). Hospitalization of adolescents for psychiatric and substance abuse treatment: Legal and ethical issues. *Journal of Adolescent Health Care, 10*(6), 473-478.

Spas, J., Ramsey, S., Paiva, A. L., & Stein, L. A. R. (2012). All might have won, but not all have the prize: Optimal treatment for substance abuse among adolescents with conduct problems. *Substance Abuse: Research and Treatment, 6*, 141-155.

Stevens, S. J., Schwebel, R, & Ruiz, B. (2007). The seven challenges: An effective treatment for adolescents with co-occurring substance abuse and mental health problems. *Journal of Social Work Practice in the Addictions, 7*(3), 29-49. doi:10.1300/J160v07n03_03

Substance Abuse and Mental Health Services Administration. (2013). Results from the 2012 National Survey on Drug Use and Health: Summary of national findings. NSDUH series H-46, HHS publication no. (SMA) 13-4794. Rockville, MD: Substance Abuse and Mental Health Services Administration.

Winters, K. C., Botzet, A. M., & Fahnhorst, T. (2011). Advances in adolescent substance abuse treatment. *Current Psychiatry Reports, 13*(5), 416-421. doi:10.1007/s11920-011-0214-2

SUBSTANCE ABUSE & BIPOLAR DISORDER

MAJOR CATEGORIES: Behavioral & Mental Health, Substance Abuse

WHAT WE KNOW

Substance use disorder (SUD) as described in the *Diagnostic and Statistical Manual of Mental Disorders*, fifth edition (DSM-5), refers to a pattern of continued use of a substance (e.g., alcohol, cannabis, opioids, sedatives) that causes cognitive, physiological, and behavioral symptoms, resulting in problems in various areas of functioning. It is a common co-occurrence with bipolar disorder (BD). In SUD the pattern of use is pathological. The individual may experience impaired behavioral control, continued use even when there are risks to him or her, and social impairment. There also may be tolerance and withdrawal. This problematic pattern of use must take place for at least 12 months to be diagnosed as an SUD.

The *DSM-5* was published in 2013, replacing the *DSM-IV*. The *DSM-IV* chapter on substance-related disorders included substance dependence, substance abuse, substance intoxication, and substance withdrawal, and then discussed specific substances (e.g., alcohol, amphetamines). The *DSM-5* divides these disorders into two categories: substance use disorders (SUD) and substance-induced disorders (intoxication, withdrawal, and other substance/medication-induced mental disorders). Thus, it removes the distinction between abuse and dependence and instead assigns a level of severity (i.e., mild, moderate, or severe) depending on the number of criteria that are fulfilled. Drug craving has been added as a criterion for substance use disorder, whereas "recurrent legal problems" has been removed. In the *DSM-5*, *substance use disorder* is the term used, whereas in the research literature and clinical settings *substance abuse* or *substance dependence* may still be used.

Bipolar disorder (BD) is a chronic mental health disorder with a typical onset in the late teens for bipolar I disorder (BD I) and the mid-twenties for bipolar II disorder (BD II). BD is characterized by repeated episodes of alternating mania and depression. Commonly the episodes persist for a week or more and occur at least 4 times a year.

BD I is characterized by at least one manic or mixed episode (i.e., with symptoms of both depression and mania) and usually also an episode of major depression; it has a prevalence in the United States of 0.6 percent.

BD II is characterized by at least one episode of major depression with one or more episodes of hypomania (i.e., a milder form of mania in which the individual can still function at normal or close to normal levels); it has a prevalence in the United States of 0.8 percent.

Signs and symptoms of depression may include a loss of interest in pleasurable activities, daily sadness, tearfulness, weight loss, insomnia or hypersomnia, fatigue, guilt, trouble concentrating, and/or recurrent thoughts related to death or suicide.

Signs and symptoms of mania may include an elevated or irritable mood accompanied by increased energy or activity, a decreased need for sleep, distractibility, poor judgment, difficulty controlling temper, talkativeness, racing thoughts, lack of self-control, and engaging in risk-taking behaviors.

Psychotic features may be present during a manic episode or major depressive episode, but if present during a hypomanic episode, the episode becomes a manic episode.

There is a high prevalence of substance use disorders among clients with BD. Between 33 percent and 60 percent of individuals in the United States with BD abuse substances.

Over half of the individuals who meet the criteria for diagnosis with BD1 have an alcohol use disorder. In a sample of patients hospitalized for BD, 50.3 percent met criteria for BD and a substance abuse diagnosis. Of subjects with co-occurring substance abuse, 56.8 percent were male and 43.2 percent were female, whereas in the BD-only sample 44.7 percent were male and 55.3 percent were female.

Clients with BD have higher rates of substance use disorders than individuals with other psychiatric conditions. A study of 12- to 20-year-old adolescents experiencing a first episode of mania who were diagnosed with BD1 found that 48 percent also had a SUD, with cannabis being the most common substance abused (84 percent). A high percentage of adults who received a diagnosis of BD in childhood, approximately 35 percent, developed substance use issues before age 18.

Polysubstance abuse is very common among clients with BD. Alcohol is the most commonly abused substance. Other commonly abused substances among clients with BD are cannabis, cocaine, and stimulants.

There are multiple theories to account for the increased prevalence of substance abuse in the BD population. There may be common risk factors that increase vulnerability to both disorders. The misuse of substances may trigger the initial manifestation of BD in those individuals who are at an increased risk for BD or may cause relapse in individuals in whom BD has already been diagnosed. Individuals may use substances to self-medicate the distressing symptoms of BD, including depression and stress.

Since substance abuse rules out participation in research studies for many clients with BD, there is a lack of evidence-based research related to substance abuse and bipolar disorder.

BD is already difficult to diagnose and frequently is misdiagnosed. This can be further aggravated by the co-occurrence of substance use. If a substance-abusing client mistakenly receives a diagnosis of BD, inappropriate pharmacotherapy may be prescribed.

A study of individuals with a history of substance abuse who were currently substance-free found that only 32.9 percent of those who previously had received a *DSM-IV* diagnosis of BD still met the criteria.

Since BD is a lifelong disorder, a thorough history is needed to ensure that substance abuse is not responsible for the manic state. Intoxication can result in euphoria, disrupted thinking, and risk-taking, which are common in BD; withdrawal can result in fatigue, sleep issues, and depressed mood, mimicking the signs and symptoms of a depressed episode in BD.

There are negative consequences for those with BD and concurrent substance abuse. Individuals with BD and concurrent substance use are more likely to have an earlier onset of BD, an increase in suicide attempts, more completed suicides, more severe depression and mania, more mixed and cycling episodes, poorer physical health, poorer psychosocial functioning, and more nonadherence to treatment.

Past or current substance use may not cause a longer recovery time from BD-related depression but can increase the risk of switching to a manic, mixed, or hypomanic state before recovery when compared to BD clients without substance use disorders.

Treatment nonadherence is more prevalent with co-occurring BD and substance use. There is an increased risk for relapse in this client population.

There is an increased risk for violence and violent crime for individuals with comorbid substance use and BD. The prevalence of convictions for violent crimes among individuals with bipolar disorder and substance use disorders was found in one study to be 21.3 percent, 6 times higher than in the general population.

There has been little research on concurrent treatment of BD and substance use disorders. Often the substance use excludes individuals from studies on BD. Most evidence-based treatments for substance abuse have not been carried out with subjects who have BD, so carryover effectiveness is unclear.

Risperidone, an antipsychotic, is showing some promise as a medication option for this population, with 56 percent of study subjects showing improved overall functioning on the Clinical Global Impressions Scale.

One study found that individuals with BD and co-occurring substance use disorder who took antidepressants had higher switch rates. It is theorized that substances may affect the brain in such a way that the individual is more vulnerable to the mood-destabilizing effects of antidepressants or may have an inhibited response to mood stabilizers.

Some treatment options have been explored, but social workers need to be aware that the substance use may increase a client's impulsivity and decrease his or her ability to engage in treatment.

Some clients may have treatment that separates the two disorders, whereas others may pursue integrated interventions.

Integrated group therapy (IGT) is being explored for this population. Based on a cognitive-behavioral model, IGT focuses on relapse prevention, with the therapist educating the client on the connections between BD and his or her substance use and teaching skills for coping with depression that do not include using substances. In a study, the subjects who received IGT had more significant reductions in substance use than those who received manual-based counseling (i.e., the therapists had the group participants follow a written manual).

In a 5-year study in Dublin, Ireland, of 205 people with co-occurring major depression or bipolar disorder and substance use disorder (alcohol) who participated in an integrated substance abuse and mental health treatment program, researchers found that earlier and greater reductions in alcohol consumption predicted longer-term reductions. Also, over the course of the study the mania and depression symptoms of those receiving integrated treatment lessened. The authors suggested early focus in integrated treatment on the SUD aspects of the co-occurring disorder.

An integrated inpatient program may look to first detoxify the client and stabilize mood before moving on to therapy, psychoeducation, and group treatment with a focus on relapse prevention.

Cognitive behavioral therapy can be used to examine the thoughts and behaviors that are underlying both the mood problems and substance issues.

Motivational interviewing (MI) for this population will have a focus on the positive and negative aspects of change and will examine the relationship between the client's mental health and his or her substance use.

WHAT CAN BE DONE

Learn about co-occurring SUD and bipolar disorder; share this information with your colleagues.

Use your knowledge to accurately assess your clients' individual characteristics and mental health education needs.

Develop an awareness of your own cultural values, beliefs, and biases and develop knowledge about the histories, traditions, and values of your clients. Adopt treatment methodologies that reflect the cultural needs of the client.

Practice with awareness of, and adherence to, the social work principles of respect for human rights and human dignity, social justice, and professional conduct as described in the International Federation of Social Workers (IFSW) Statement of Ethical Principles. Become knowledgeable of the IFSW ethical standards as they apply to substance abuse and mental health disorders, and practice accordingly.

Assess and monitor clients for any suicidal ideation or risk of violence.

Educate the client and any appropriate family members on both BD and substance use disorders.

Locate appropriate resources for client to address substance use and/or co-occurring BD, which may include support groups, 12-step programs, inpatient treatment, or specialized counseling.

Educate client on the importance of treatment adherence and the potential negative pharmaceutical interactions that can occur between BD medications and substances.

Written by Jessica Therivel, LMSW-IPR

Reviewed by Melissa Rosales Neff, MSW, and Chris Bates, MA, MSW

REFERENCES

Albanese, M. J., Suh, J. J., Lefebvre, R., Clodfelter, R. C., Jr, & Ghaemi, S. N. (2008). Effectiveness of risperidone in comorbid bipolar disorder and substance abuse: An observational study. *Journal of Dual Diagnosis, 4*(2), 186-196. doi:10.1080/15504260802067164

American Psychiatric Association. (2013). *Diagnostic and statistical manual of mental disorders: DSM-5* (5th ed.). Washington, DC: American Psychiatric Publishing.

British Association of Social Workers. (2012). *The code of ethics for social work: Statement of principles.* Retrieved April 20, 2016, from http://cdn.basw.co.uk/upload/basw_112315-7.pdf

Farren, C. K., Murphy, P., & McElroy, S. (2014). A 5-year follow-up of depressed and bipolar patients with alcohol use disorder in an Irish population. *Alcoholism: Clinical and Experimental Research, 38*(4), 1049-1058. doi:10.1111/acer.12330

Fazel, S., Lichtenstein, P., Grann, M., Goodwin, G. M., & Langstrom, N. (2010). olar disorder and violent crime: New evidence from population-based longitudinal studies and systematic review. *Archives of General Psychiatry, 67*(9), 931-938. doi:10.1001/archgenpsychiatry.2010.97

Gaudiano, B. A., Weinstock, L. M., & Miller, I. W. (2011). Improving treatment adherence in patients with bipolar disorder and substance abuse: Rationale and initial development of a novel psychosocial approach. *Journal of Psychiatric Practice, 17*(1), 5-20. doi:10.1097/01.pra.0000393840.18099.d6

Geller, B., Tillman, R., Bolhofner, K., & Zimerman, B. (2008). Child bipolar I disorder: Prospective continuity with adult bipolar I disorder; characteristics of second and third episodes; predictors of 8-year outcome. *Archives of General Psychiatry, 65*(10), 1125-1133. doi:10.1001/archpsyc.65.10.1125

Goldberg, J. F. (2008). Optimizing treatment outcomes in bipolar disorder under ordinary conditions. *Journal of Clinical Psychiatry, 69*(Suppl 3), 11-19.

Goldberg, J. F., Garno, J. L., Callahan, A. M., Kearns, D. L., Kerner, B., & Ackerman, S. H. (2008). Over-diagnosis of bipolar disorder among substance use disorder inpatients with mood instability. *Journal of Clinical Psychiatry, 69*(11), 1751-1757. doi:10.4088/JCP.v69n1110

Gummattira, P., Cowan, K. A., Averill, K. A., Malkina, S., Reilly, E. L., Krajewski, K.,... Averill, P. M. (2010). A comparison between patients diagnosed with bipolar disorder with versus without comorbid substance abuse. *Addictive Disorders & Their Treatment, 9*(2), 53-63. doi:10.1097/ADT.0b013e3181af1289

International Federation of Social Workers. (2012). Statement of ethical principles. Retrieved April 20, 2016, from http://ifsw.org/policies/statement-of-ethical-principles/

Liberman, D. Z., Kolodner, G., Massey, S. H., & Williams, K. P. (2009). Antidepressant-induced mania with concomitant mood stabilizer in patients with comorbid substance abuse and bipolar disorder. *Journal of Addictive Diseases, 28*(4), 348-355. doi:10.1080/10550880903182994

Ostacher, M. J. (2011). Bipolar and substance use disorder comorbidity: Diagnostic and treatment considerations. *Focus, 9*(4), 428-434. doi:10.1176/foc.9.4.foc428

Ostacher, M. J., Perlis, R. H., Nierenberg, A. A., Calabrese, J., Stange, J. P., Salloum, I.,... Sachs, G. S. (2010). Impact of substance use disorders on recovery from episodes of depression in bipolar disorder patients: Prospective data from the Systematic Treatment Enhancement Program for Bipolar Disorder (STEP-BD). *American Journal of Psychiatry, 167*(3), 289-297. doi:10.1176/appi.ajp.2009.09020299

Prisciandaro, J. J., & Myrick, D. H. (2010). Co-morbid bipolar and alcohol use disorders: A treatment-focused review. *Journal of Dual Diagnosis, 6*(2), 171-188. doi:10.1080/15504261003701858

Richardson, T. H. (2013). Substance misuse in depression and bipolar disorder: A review of psychological interventions and considerations for clinical practice. *Mental Health & Substance Use: Dual Diagnosis, 6*(1), 76-93. doi:10.1080/17523281.2012.680485

Shalini Theodore, R., Ramirez Basco, M., & Biggan, J. R. (2012). Diagnostic disagreements in bipolar disorder: The role of substance abuse comorbidities. *Depression Research and Treatment, 2012,* 435486. doi:10.1155/2012/435486

Stephens, J. R., Heffner, J. L., Adler, C. M., Blom, T. J., Anhenelli, R. M., Fleck, D. E.,... Delbello, M. P. (2014). Risk and protective factors associated with substance use disorder in adolescents with first-episode mania. *Journal of the American Academy of Child and Adolescent Psychiatry, 53*(7), 771-779. doi:10.1016/j.jaac.2014.04.018

Swann, A. C. (2005). Bipolar disorder and substance abuse: Two disorders or one?. *Journal of Dual Diagnosis, 1*(3), 9-23. doi:10.1300/J374v01n03_03

Weiss, R. D., Griffin, M. L., Kolodziej, M. E., Greenfield, S. F., Najavits, L. M., Daley, D. C.,... Hannen, J. A. (2007). A randomized trial of integrated group therapy versus group drug counseling for patients with bipolar disorder and substance dependence. *American Journal of Psychiatry, 164*(1), 100-107. doi:10.1176/appi.ajp.164.1.100

Wheeler, D. (2015). NASW standards and indicators for cultural competence in social work practice. Retrieved April 20, 2016, from http://www.socialworkers.org/practice/standards/PRA-BRO-253150-CC-Standards.pdf

SUBSTANCE ABUSE & WOMEN: TREATMENT

MAJOR CATEGORIES: Substance Abuse

WHAT WE KNOW

The *Diagnostic and Statistical Manual of Mental Disorders,* fifth edition (*DSM-5*), was published in 2013, replacing the *DSM-IV*. The *DSM-IV* chapter

"Substance-Related Disorders" included substance dependence, substance abuse, substance intoxication, and substance withdrawal and then discussed specific substances (e.g., alcohol, amphetamines).

COMMUNITY & FAMILY HEALTH ISSUES

The*DSM-5* divides these disorders into two categories: substance use disorders and substance-induced disorders (intoxication, withdrawal, and other substance- or medication-induced mental disorders). Thus,it removes the distinction between abuse and dependence and instead divides each disorder into mild, moderate, and severe subtypes. Drug craving has been added as a criterion for substance use disorder, whereas "recurrent legal problems" has been removed. In the *DSM-5*, substance abuse is referred to as *substance use disorder* or *substance dependence,* whereas in the research literature it is still commonly referred to as *substance abuse.* When there is a pattern of continued use of a substance (e.g., alcohol, cannabis, opioids, sedatives) that cause cognitive, physiological, and behavioral symptoms, resulting in problems in various areas of functioning, that use may be classified as moderate(i.e., 4 to 5 symptoms) to severe (i.e., 6 or more symptoms). The pattern of use is pathological. The individual may experience impaired behavioral control, continued use even in the face of risks to the self, and social impairment. There also may be tolerance and withdrawal. This problematic pattern of use must take place for at least 12 months to be classified as substance use.

In 2013, the Substance Abuse and Mental Health Services Administration (SAMHSA)determined that 24.6 million people over the age of 12 estimated that 24.6 million people over the age of 12 were current users of illicit drugs; 21.6 million people over the age of 12 in the United States were classified as being dependent on substances or meeting the *DSM-IV* criteria for substance abuse.

- 2.6 million met the criteria for both alcohol and illicit drug dependence or abuse (e.g., marijuana; cocaine; heroin; hallucinogens; inhalants; and the nonmedical use of prescription-type pain relievers, tranquilizers, stimulants, and sedatives).
- 4.3 million met the criteria for illicit drug dependence or abuse alone.
- 14.7 million met the criteria for alcohol dependence or abuse alone.

Rates of substance dependence and substance use vary by gender: in 2013, 10.8 percent of men over the age of 12 in the United States met the criteria for substance use or dependence, whereas 5.8 percent of women over age 12 did.

Nationwide, women made up approximately 32 percent of the population in treatment for substance use. Only 6 percent of substance use treatment facilities in the United States in 2012were for women only.

There is a general disparity between the number of people needing treatment and the number of people receiving treatment. Women seeking substance use treatment often are experiencing multiple issues(e.g., intimate partner violence, financial issues, childcare needs)that increase their vulnerability to substance use and will have an impact on their treatment.

In 2013, only 2.5 million people received specialty substance use treatment out of the 22.7 million who needed treatment. Some 908,000 respondents reported needing treatment but did not receive treatment. The most common reason given for not receiving treatment was being uninsured or unable to afford treatment at 37.3 percent,and not wanting to stop using accounted for 24.5 percent.

Women can be reluctant to recognize that their substance use is problematic; professionals (e.g., physicians, social workers, nurses) may be more reluctant to screen female clients for substance use.

Women who become pregnant while using substances are more likely to delay their first healthcare visit because of their substance use.

There is significant evidence for a connection between trauma exposure/trauma history and substance use disorders, which can be difficult to treat systemically.

Researchers found that approximately 50 percent of a sample of women who had completed a community substance use program reported childhood abuse, 87 percent reported psychological victimization by an intimate partner, 79 percent reported physical abuse by an intimate partner, and 47 percent reported physical victimization by a stranger.

Sixty-two percent of these women reported at least one symptom from each of the clusters for posttraumatic stress disorder (PTSD).

Researchers for a second study found similar results, with 51 percent of women in a substance treatment program reporting sexual abuse and 69 percent reporting physical abuse.

Dual substance dependence can further increase risk for PTSD. Participants in a study who had lifetime comorbidities of alcohol and cocaine dependence had a higher number of traumatic events in their trauma histories, were more likely to have experienced violence, and were more likely to have PTSD.

Abuse may increase the risk of substance use and addiction if the client is using substances to relieve emotional pain. There may be a higher risk for relapse if any underlying trauma is not addressed during treatment.

Childcare, child custody, and parenting issues may strongly influence the commitment and ability of substance-abusing women to undergo treatment. As a result, a stepped care model may be the most appropriate where the lowest-intensity/least invasive option is offered first and if that level of care is not sufficient, the client is stepped up to the next level.

Social support networks are critical for women seeking treatment for substance use. Such networks provide both emotional and informational support and the practical help (e.g., with childcare, financial assistance, housing) that women often need in order to complete treatment.

Researchers found that women in residential treatment had less supportive environments and more substance users in their personal networks than women in outpatient treatment did.

Substance-abusing women may report a greater severity of problems as a result of addiction and develop severe problems with addiction more quickly than men do, which is referred to as the telescoping effect (i.e., acceleration in the progression from substance use to substance use).

Depression and anxiety are common comorbidities with substance use in women. Researchers found that all of the women in a community-based treatment sample reported a history of depression, and approximately 80 percent were currently using antidepressant medication.

Researchers also found that women with high psychiatric symptom severity made greater reductions in their substance use after 12 weeks of single-gender, women-focused group therapy treatment than did participants who were in mixed-gender group drug counseling. The women assigned to single-gender treatment also had more continued improvement at 6-month follow-up than those in mixed-gender treatment did.

Conceptual models that attempt to explain why substance use develops advocate and outline interventions and desired outcomes that fit those models. Social workers need to be aware of the interventions and outcomes related to the theoretical basis for treatments that they choose to use.

The most commonly researched and utilized models are the disease model, psychological model, motivation and change theories, transtheoretical model/stages of change, and harm reduction (i.e., the public health model).

The *disease model* is most commonly associated with Alcoholics Anonymous (AA) and other 12-step programs that view substance use and substance use as a disease rather than a moral failing. The theory that substance use is a medical condition recognizes the influence of biological, environmental, behavioral, and genetic factors in addiction.

The *psychological models* focus on the cognitive and behavioral reasons individuals use substances and advocate strategies for change that incorporate these perspectives. Addictive behaviors and traits are viewed as habits that can be studied and changed. Relapses are considered to be a likely occurrence and are not considered an abject failure on the part of the client.

Motivation and change theories emphasize examining the client's motivation for change and the nature and mechanics of change itself while working to establish a collaborative relationship between social worker and client. Motivational interviewing (MI) focuses on why people make changes in behavior.

According to the *transtheoretical model/stages of change*, behavior change typically proceeds through five stages: precontemplation, contemplation, preparation, action, and maintenance. This model has three key tenets: The change process can start even if the client has not started with a stage of precontemplation, relapse is a likely occurrence, and interventions must match the client's stage (e.g., a client in precontemplation is not ready for action-oriented interventions). In the last 10 years, studies of the effectiveness of this model and interventions based on it have shown mixed results.

Harm reduction does not dismiss abstinence as a goal if it is desired but prioritizes improvement over complete cessation of use.

Successful substance use treatment programs designed for women should incorporate prenatal care and childcare. They must also recognize and address the influence of gender roles on the physical and emotional health of the client.

Many women who are in treatment for substance use have a history of childhood use and sexual victimization, so single-sex treatment with a focus on empowerment may help them feel safe and comfortable to explore that history and its role in their addiction.

Women's needs may not be met in traditional treatment models that rely on confrontational interventions, demand strict attendance at 12-step meetings (which may be dominated by men), emphasize the individual's powerlessness, focus on substance use to the exclusion of psychiatric needs, and focus solely on abstinence.

Barriers to treatment that are internal (e.g., denial, shame, guilt, self-blame) and external (e.g., poverty, limited treatment options) are experienced by both men and women who use substances, but women face a higher number of external barriers, many of which are gender-specific.

The lack of childcare in treatment programs has a more significant effect on women; many women fear they will lose custody of their children if they enter residential treatment. Nationally, only 13 percent of substance use treatment facilities have childcare programs. Only 12 percent of substance use treatment facilities offer prenatal care.

Having an insufficient number of female staff members in a treatment program can alienate female clients and make establishing trust more difficult, especially for victims of trauma.

An emphasis on traditional models of treatment that were developed for male clients results in a scarcity of gender-specific treatments.

Some female clients fear that their male partner will leave them if they enter treatment because they will be absent from the home.

Women who live in rural areas face more barriers to treatment: They may have to travel greater distances for treatment, rural populations typically experience poorer health, and rural communities are more likely to be poor.

Women with children who are involved in the child welfare system may be caught in a conflict between the timeframe of the child welfare agency and that of substance use treatment: Treatment and recovery from addiction may take months or years, but child welfare agencies may terminate parental rights before treatment and recovery are concluded.

Substance use treatment programs and child welfare agencies may also view relapse differently: child welfare agencies often view relapse as evidence of treatment failure and grounds to remove the child from the parent's care, whereas most substance use treatment programs see relapse as a common occurrence in treatment and not a failure but an opportunity for learning and personal growth.

WHAT CAN BE DONE

Learn about the treatment of women with substance use disorder so you can accurately assess your client's personal characteristics and health education needs; share this information with your colleagues.

Screen substance-using clients for trauma. If trauma history is present, incorporate counseling interventions that address the vulnerabilities of victims of trauma.

Develop an awareness of your own cultural values, beliefs, and biases and develop knowledge about the histories, traditions, and values of your clients. Adopt treatment methodologies that reflect the cultural needs of the client.

Recognize the importance of the client's role as a mother if children are involved and include parenting skills training, family therapy, childcare, or residential treatment with on-site childcare.

Operate from a strengths-based perspective rather than a deficits model.

Enhance the social networks of the client to improve her support system and recognize elements of the social network that are actively discouraging the client's recovery and treatment.

Address any internal and external barriers to treatment as these barriers present themselves.

Advocate for an increase in single-gender treatment to better address the needs of female clients.

Provide interventions that follow the model and theory of practice used by you, your agency, or your facility.

Maintain education and awareness of current best evidence-based practices.

Include assessments for suicidal ideation and risk of suicide because of their frequent comorbidity with mental health disorders in women who have substance use disorders.

Written by Jessica Therivel, LMSW-IPR

Reviewed by Megan Rabin, MEd

REFERENCES

American Psychiatric Association. (2013). Substance-related and addictive disorders. *Diagnostic and Statistical Manual of Mental Disorders, fifth edition (DSM-5).* Arlington, VA: American Psychiatric Publishing.

Brady, T. M., & Ashley, O. S. (Eds.). (2005). Women in substance abuse treatment: Results from the Alcohol and Drug Services Study (ADSS). (DHHS Publication No. SMA-04-3968, Analytic Series A-26). Rockville, MD: Substance Abuse and Mental Health Services Administration, Office of Applied Studies.

British Association of Social Workers. (2012). The code of ethics for social work: Statement of principles. Retrieved December 6, 2015, from http://cdn.basw.co.uk/upload/basw_112315-7.pdf

Brown, C. G., & Stewart, S. H. (2008). Exploring perceptions of alcohol use as self-medication for depression among women receiving community-based treatment for alcohol problems. *Journal of Prevention & Intervention in the Community, 35*(2), 33-47.

Carlson, B. E. (2006). Best practices in the treatment of substance-abusing women in the child welfare system. *Journal of Social Work Practice in Addictions, 6*(3), 97-115.

Cosden, M., Larsen, J. L., Donahue, M. T., & Nylund-Gibson, K. (2015). Trauma symptoms for men and women in substance abuse treatment: a latent transition analysis. *Journal of Substance Abuse Treatment, 50,* 18-25. doi:10.1016/j.jsat.2014.09.004

Engstrom, M., Mahoney, C. A., & Marsh, J. C. (2012). Substance use problems in health social work practice. In S. Gehlert & T. Arthur Browne (Eds.), *Handbook of health social work* (2nd ed., pp. 426-427). Hoboken, NJ: Wiley.

Golder, S., & Logan, T. K. (2010). Lifetime victimization and psychological distress: Cluster profiles of out of treatment drug-involved women. *Violence and Victims, 25*(1), 62-83.

Greenfield, S. F., Potter, J. S., Lincoln, M. F., Popuch, R. E., Kuper, L., & Gallop, R. J. (2008). High psychiatric symptom severity is a moderator of substance abuse treatment outcomes among women in single vs. mixed gender group treatment. *American Journal of Drug and Alcohol Abuse, 34*(5), 594-602.

Haug, N. A., Duffy, M., & McCaul, M. E. (2014). Substance abuse treatment services for pregnant women. *Obstetrics and Gynecology Clinics of North America, 41,* 267-296. doi:10.1016/j.ogc.2014.03.001

Hecksher, D., & Hesse, M. (2009). Women and substance use disorders. *Mens Sana Monographs, 7*(1), 50-62. doi:10.4103/0973-1229.42585

International Federation of Social Workers. (2012). Statement of ethical principles. Retrieved December 6, 2015, from http://ifsw.org/policies/statement-of-ethical-principles/

Jackson, A., & Shannon, L. (2012). Examining barriers to and motivations for substance abuse treatment among pregnant women: Does urban-rural residence matter? *Women & Health, 52*(6), 570-586. doi:10.1080/03630242.2012.699508

Johnson, S. D., Cottler, L. B., O'Leary, C. C., & Ben Abdallah, A. (2010). The association of trauma and PTSD with the substance use profiles of alcohol and cocaine dependent out-of-treatment women. *American Journal on Addictions, 19*(6), 490-495. doi:10.1111/j.1521-0391.2010.00075.x

Krejci, J., Margolin, J., Rowland, M., & Wetzell, C. (2008). Integrated group treatment of women's substance abuse and trauma. *Journal of Groups in Addiction and Recovery, 3*(3-4), 263-283.

Lafave, L., Desportes, L., & McBride, C. (2009). Treatment outcomes and perceived benefits: A qualitative and quantitative assessment of a women's substance abuse treatment program. *Women & Therapy, 32*(1), 51-68.

Littell, J. H., & Girvin, H. (2002). Stages of change: A critique. *Behavior Modification, 26*(2), 223-273.

Min, M. O., Tracy, E. M., & Park, H. (2015). Personal networks of women in residential and outpatient substance abuse treatment. *Counselor: The Magazine for Addiction Professionals, 16*(4), 66-71.

Panchanadeswaran, S., & Jayasundara, D. (2012). Experiences of drug use and parenting among women in substance abuse treatment: An exploratory study. *Journal of Human Behavior in the Social Environment, 22*(8), 971-987. doi:10.1080/10911359.2012.707943

Substance Abuse and Mental Health Services Administration. (2013). Results from the 2012 National Survey on Drug Use and Health: Summary of national findings. NSDUH series H-46, HHS publication no. (SMA) 13-4794. Rockville, MD: Substance Abuse and Mental Health Services Administration.

Tracy, E. M., Munson, M. R., Peterson, L. T., & Floersch, J. E. (2010). Social support: A mixed blessing for women in substance abuse treatment. *Journal of Social Work Practice in the Addictions, 10*(3), 257-282.

Wheeler, D. (2015). NASW standards for cultural competency in social work practice. Retrieved December 6, 2015, from http://www.socialworkers.org/practice/standards/NASWCulturalStandards.pdf

Substance Abuse & Child Maltreatment

Major Categories: Child & Family, Substance Abuse

Description

The *Diagnostic and Statistical Manual of Mental Disorders, Fifth Edition* (*DSM-5*), was published in 2013, replacing the *DSM-IV*. The *DSM-IV* chapter on "Substance-Related Disorders" included substance dependence, substance abuse, substance intoxication, and substance withdrawal, and then discussed specific substances (e.g., alcohol, amphetamines). The *DSM-5* divides these disorders into two categories: substance use disorders and substance-induced disorders (intoxication, withdrawal, and other substance/medication-induced mental disorders). Changing from distinguishing between abuse and dependence and instead divides each disorder into mild, moderate, and severe subtypes. Drug craving has been added as a criterion for substance use disorder, whereas "recurrent legal problems" has been removed. In the *DSM-5*, substance abuse is referred to as substance use disorder or substance dependence, whereas in the research literature it is still commonly referred to as substance abuse.

Substance abuse and the maltreatment of children frequently co-occur within families, social networks, and communities. Child maltreatment, including neglect, physical abuse, sexual abuse, and psychological maltreatment, is broadly defined as an action or inaction by a parent or caregiver that results in harm, or imminent risk of harm, to a child. Substance abuse places children at increased risk of maltreatment in multiple ways, including impaired parental ability (e.g., mental functioning, attention, judgment, nurture, and protection), lowered inhibitions, heightened irritability and violence, lowered financial resources, and increased likelihood of living in dangerous environments in which children are exposed to drugs, drug paraphernalia, violence, criminal activity, and other hazardous conditions. Substance abuse and the maltreatment of children often take place within families experiencing poverty, unemployment, dysfunctional relationships, and intimate partner violence (IPV). Researchers have also found that neighborhoods with higher amounts of liquor stores or bars have a higher incidence of child neglect (Morton et al., 2014). These neighborhoods are often deprived and overcrowded, increasing the stresses of those who live in them. Combined, these factors create complex, difficult situations for social workers to address.

Parental substance abuse and the maltreatment of children create lasting negative effects. The impact of maltreatment on children includes a range of mental health problems, including depression, anxiety, difficulty with emotional regulation, attachment issues, and post-traumatic stress disorder (PTSD). Maltreated children have higher rates of teen pregnancy, suicide attempts, delinquency, truancy, and poor academic achievement. Those maltreated by substance-abusing caregivers are themselves particularly susceptible to substance use disorders. Children of alcoholic parents are 4 to 10 times more likely to abuse alcohol themselves. Adults who were maltreated in childhood have a higher lifetime risk of mental health disorders, including major depression, anxiety disorders, PTSD, and personality disorders. They tend to have more severe symptoms, higher rates of multiple issues, and fare more poorly in treatment than adults who do not have a history of childhood abuse. They are more likely to experience feelings of anger, worthlessness, and helplessness. Adults who were maltreated as children also are more likely to become victims of sexual assault and intimate partner violence, and/or to perpetrate violence and engage in criminal activities.

Maltreatment can result in developmental delays, cognitive delays, and learning difficulties. Substance abuse and maltreatment may both contribute to poor attendance and difficulty progressing in school. The medical consequences of maltreatment in childhood can include poor health, severe dental decay, malnutrition, impaired brain development, injuries such as bruises, lacerations, and burns, permanent disability, and death. The toxins from substances abused during pregnancy can damage developing organs. Fetal alcohol syndrome causes medical complications and mental retardation.. Adults who experienced maltreatment in childhood are more likely to develop allergies, arthritis, asthma, bronchitis, hypertension, and ulcers.

The most important first step in helping these families is ensuring the I safety of the child. The safety of the child can be assessed and determined by the involvement of child protective services (CPS). Initial steps may include removing the child from the home. Substance abuse interventions include group therapies and individual sessions for the parent to address substance abuse as well as other mental or emotional struggles. Home visitation programs that educate parents about their responsibilities, supervise their parental behaviors and monitor families, combined with education classes to address deficits in parenting skills, can help prevent child maltreatment. Childcare during these education and emotional programs is especially important because it helps parents attend sessions. Children should be screened for mental health, developmental, educational, and medical issues and referred for services as indicated.

FACTS AND FIGURES

Substance use has found to be a contribuiting i factor in one third to two thirds of child maltreatment cases (Goldman etal., 2003). It is estimated that 1 in 8 children suffer maltreatment during their childhoods; non-White children experience a higher rate of maltreatment than White children, with 1 in 5 Black children suffering maltreatment (Wildeman et al., 2014). Neglect makes up the majority of reported cases (78.3 percent), followed by physical abuse (18.3 percent), sexual abuse (9.3 percent), and psychological maltreatment (78.5 percent) (Children's Bureau, 2013). The perpetrator is most likely to be a parent (81.5 percent). Children under the age of 1 year have the highest rates of victimization (at 21.9 per 1,000).

RISK FACTORS

Children under age 5 years are at greater risk for maltreatment. There is an elevated risk of maltreatment when parents are younger, single, and living in extreme poverty with little social support. Children in families in which male domination and sexist belief systems are present can also be at heightened risk. Children in families with histories of substance abuse, IPV, or any maltreatment are at risk. Physical or mental disability and illness in a child or the caregiver increases risk.

SIGNS AND SYMPTOMS

The signs and symptoms of neglect and psychological, emotional, physical, and/or sexual abuse in a child can vary substantially, this creates a challenge in detecting child maltreatment. Behaviors or signs to look for include,the child may be watchful, anxious, overly compliant and withdrawn, or defiant and aggressive. Indicators of possible maltreatment include behavioral regression (acting younger than they are), frequent absences or truancy, problems in school, begging for and/or hoarding food, stealing, a pattern of poor hygiene and wearing clothes that are not appropriate for the weather, and expressed fear of parents or of going home. Sleep and eating disorders, substance abuse, suicidal ideation, and self-harm may also be symptoms. Changes in a child's behavior can be a sign of maltreatment. Physical signs in younger children include unexplained injuries, particularly those that are unlikely to have occurred accidentally. Head and abdominal injuries are particularly serious. Physical symptoms of abuse may not be visible, which can be particularly problematic in sexual abuse cases. Injuries from physical maltreatment are often attributed to household accidents.

Signs of substance abuse in adults can also vary dramatically depending on the individual and the substance. When exploring substance abuse in parents, always treat the safety of the child with the upmost importance. Parents may confirm or deny their substance abuse, however concerning symptoms in children should be reported to CPS immediately.

If you are suspicions that a child may being maltreatment you should contact a helping professional immediately. These helping professionals may include doctors, social workers, teachers or coaches. When helping professionals are assessing for substance abuse and maltreatment an extensive assessment exploring risk factors is necessary. Asking about history of physical/sexual/emotional abuse or neglect, exposure to violence or other trauma, history of mental health symptoms or issues that may pose risk to self or others (e.g., suicide ideation/attempts, aggression), alcohol and drug history, child's medical and educational history, involvement with other systems (e.g., school, child welfare, corrections), and family and community supports. To further explore the parent-child relationship, ask the parent to describe the child, what things they like about her or him, and what things they enjoy sharing. Questions about parental approaches to solving conflict and disobedience may be useful.

Child protective workers may find it helpful to interview the child without the caregiver or suspected abuser present. Training in interviewing children is advisable, particularly if there is suspicion of sexual abuse. If you are untrained, seek professional assistance to ensure the safety of the child. Professionals will work to provide a safe, private, and comfortable environment and use age-appropriate, open-ended, non-leading questions and the child's colloquial language.

ASSESSMENTS AND SCREENING TOOLS

These are some commonly used screening tools to assess for child abuse. A medical examination may be required. In cases of sexual abuse, a forensic examination conducted by a medical provider with specialized training is recommended.

The Child Abuse Potential Inventory (CAPI), which consists of 160 questions, can help assess for increased risk of physical maltreatment. It can also be used to measure post-intervention risk

The National Institute on Alcohol Abuse and Alcoholism (NIAAA),http://www.niaaa.nih.gov/, has a guide on screening for heavy drinking and alcohol disorders

The Addiction Severity Index (ASI) can be downloaded from http://www.tresearch.org/tools/download-asi-instruments-manuals/

The National Child Traumatic Stress Network maintains a database of tools for assessing trauma and related mental health issues in children, which can

be accessed online at www.nctsnet.org/resources/online-research/measures-review

TREATMENT

Treatment needs to be tailored to individual families. Substance abuse treatment may be delivered in inpatient, residential, or outpatient settings, and may involve individual, family, and/or group therapy depending on the focus of the program and the parent's individual needs. Behavioral interventions commonly address the individual's readiness for change, skills necessary to maintain abstinence, constructive activities that can take the place of substance use, building peer support and healthy relationships, and strengthening problem-solving skills (NIDA, 2012). Medication may be needed to support detoxification or to address mental health disorders. Treatment is enhanced by a holistic approach that addresses the individual's mental health, medical, social, spiritual, vocational, and legal needs. It is important to recognize that recovery is a process that takes time and frequently involves one or more relapses. Scheduled or random drug testing is often used to monitor recovery and may serve to support abstinence (Welsh et al., 2008). Given the strong association between childhood maltreatment and substance abuse, a trauma-informed perspective is helpful in treating both adults and children.

Interventions for child maltreatment have emphasized prevention through home visitation programs that include parenting skills training (Guterman et al., 2005). Success was shown in a home visitation program that combined regular cell phone contact with parenting classes. It involved weekly visits, regular calls and text messages twice a day to "prompt and reinforce" the training (Bigelow et al., 2008). Interventions involving the children and/or the entire family can have positive outcomes (Oliver et al., 2009). Spirituality and religiosity can also offer "protective effects" in some child maltreatment cases (Stewart et al., 2006). Families in which substance abuse and maltreatment occur have complex coexisting problems and require a range of services and support from various agencies. Children who have experienced parental substance abuse and maltreatment may have a range of needs. Interventions may include trauma-focused cognitive-behavioral therapy, play therapy, substance abuse education or treatment, and early intervention services.

Applicable Laws and Regulations
Federal and state mandatory reporting laws require that professionals involved in the care of children and adolescents report suspicions of maltreatment to the child protection agency for assessment and follow-up. Details of state's statutes can be found at the U.S. Department of Health and Human Services website, http://www.childwelfare.gov/systemwide/laws_policies/state/

Services and Resources
- Administration for Children and Families, http://www.acf.hhs.gov
- Centers for Disease Control and Prevention (CDC), http://www.cdc.gov/ViolencePrevention/childmaltreatment/
- Child Welfare Information Gateway, http://www.childwelfare.gov/
- National Institute On Drug Abuse (NIDA), http://www.nida.nih.gov/NIDAHome.html
- Guides for interviewing children available at http://www.childwelfare.gov/responding/iia/investigation/interviewing.cfm
- National Institute on Alcohol Abuse and Alcoholism (NIAAA) guide for screening,http://pubs.niaaa.nih.gov/publications/Practitioner/pocket-guide/pocket_guide.htm
- Reports on the maltreatment of children in the United States are available at http://www.acf.hhs.gov/programs/cb/stats_research/index.htm#can
- National Resource Center for Permanency and Family Connections, http://www.nrcpfc.org/
- Futures Without Violence, http://www.futureswithoutviolence.org/
- Substance Abuse and Mental Health Services Administration, http://www.samhsa.gov/

Food for Thought
It is important to involve mental health professionals in both the assessment, intervention and treatment of substance abusing adults and maltreated children.

Ensuring the child is safe while treatment is taking place should be the number one concern.

Recovery from substance abuse is a long-term process, requiring an multi-faceted approach treating all struggles from detoxing, avoiding relapse, mental health treatment, self-care, and increasing supports.

Childcare while parents seek treatment is extremely important.

There is an overrepresentation of certain racial and ethnic groups within the child welfare system: most significantly Blacks are overrepresented.

It has been found that often the treatment focuses on the substance abusing parent or the maltreated child. It is extremely important that both the parent and child seek treatment in order to heal and create a safe and loving family environment.

Written by Jan Wagstaff, MA, MSW, and Jennifer Teska, MSW

Reviewed by Lynn B. Cooper, D. Crim

References
Bigelow, K. M., Carta, J. J., & Lefever, J. B. (2008). Txt u ltr: using cellular phone technology to enhance a parenting intervention for families at risk for neglect. *Child Maltreatment, 13*(4), 362-367.

Brook, J., & McDonald, T. P. (2007). Evaluating the effects of comprehensive substance abuse intervention on successful reunification. *Research on Social Work Practice, 17*(6), 664-673.

Child Welfare Information Gateway. Mandatory Reporters of Child Abuse and Neglect: Summary of State Laws. (2010). Retrieved August 9, 2014, from http://www.childwelfare.gov/responding/mandated.cfm

Farmer, E. (2014). Improving reunification practice: Pathways home, progress and outcomes for children returning from care to their parents. *British Journal of Social Work, 44*(2), 348-366.

Goldman, J., Salus, M. K., Wolcott, D., & Kennedy, K. Y. (2003). A coordinated response to child abuse and neglect: The foundation for practice. Retrieved August 9, 2014, from https://www.childwelfare.gov/pubs/usermanuals/foundation/index.cfm

Guterman, N. B., & Taylor, C. A. (2005). Prevention of physical child abuse and neglect. In G. P. Mallon, & P. McCartt Hess (Eds.), *Child welfare for the twenty-first century: A handbook of practices, policies, and programs* (pp. 270-289). New York, NY: Columbia University Press.

Humphreys, C. (2008). Problems in the system of mandatory reporting of children living with domestic violence. *Journal of Family Studies, 14*(2-3), 228-239.

Johnson, C. F. (2007). Chapter 36: abuse and neglect of children. In R. M. Kliegman, R. E. Behrman, H. B. Jenson, & B. F. Stanton (Eds.), *Nelson textbook of pediatrics* (18th ed., pp. 171-183). Philadelphia, PA: Saunders Elsevier.

Laslett, A., Room, R., & Dietze, P. (2014). Substance misuse, mental health problems and recurrent child maltreatment. *Advances in Dual Diagnosis, 7*(1), 15-23. doi:10.1108/ADD-11-2013-0026

Merchant, L., & Toth, P. (2007). Child interview guide. Retrieved August 9, 2014, from http://www.childwelfare.gov/responding/iia/investigation/interviewing.c fm

Mizrahi, T., & Mayden, R. W. (2001). NASW standards for cultural competence in social work practice. Retrieved October 7, 2014, from http://www.socialworkers.org/practice/standards/NASWCulturalStandards.pdf

Morton, C. M., Simmel, C., & Peterson, N. A. (2014). Neighborhood alcohol outlet density and rates of child abuse and neglect: Moderating effects of access to substance abuse services (Abstract). *Child Abuse & Neglect, 38*(5), 952-961. doi:10.1016/j.chiabu.2014.01.002

National Institute On Drug Abuse (NIDA). NIDA Infofacts: drug related hospital emergency room visits. Retrieved August 9, 2014, from http://www.nida.nih.gov/infofacts/hospitalvisits.html

National Institute On Drug Abuse (NIDA). (2012, December). Principles of drug addiction treatment: A research-based guide, third edition. Retrieved August 9, 2014, from http://www.drugabuse.gov/sites/default/files/podat_1.pdf

Oliver, J., & Washington, K. T. (2009). Treating perpetrators of child physical abuse: A review of interventions. *Trauma, Violence & Abuse, 10*(2), 115-124.

Quas, J. A., Davis, E. L., Goodman, G. S., & Myers, J. E. (2007). Repeated questions, deception, and children's true and false reports of body touch. *Child Maltreatment, 12*(1), 60-67.

Reinarman, C., & Levine, H. G. (2004). Crack in the rearview mirror: Deconstructing drug war mythology. *Social Justice, 31*(1-2), 182-199.

Roditti, M. G. (2005). Understanding communities of neglectful parents: Child caregiving networks and child neglect. *Child Welfare, 84*(2), 277-298.

Small, E., & Kohl, P. L. (2012). African American caregivers and substance abuse in child welfare: Identification of multiple risk profiles. *Journal of Family Violence, 27*(5), 415-426. doi:10.1007/210896-012-9442-4

Staton-Tindall, M., Sprang, G., Clark, J., Walker, R., & Craig, C. D. (2013). Caregiver substance use and child outcomes: A systematic review. *Journal of Social Work Practice in the Addictions, 13*(1), 6-31. doi:10.1080/1533256X.2013.752272

Stewart, C., & Mezzich, A. C. (2006). The effects of spirituality and religiosity on child neglect in substance use disorder families. *Journal of Family Social Work, 10*(2), 35-57.

Street, K., Whitlingum, G., Gibson, P., Cairns, P., & Ellis, M. (2008). Is adequate parenting compatible with maternal drug use? A 5-year follow up. *Child Care Health and Development, 34*(2), 204-206.

Teicher, M. H., & Samson, J. A. (2013). Childhood maltreatment and psychopathology: A case for ecophenotypic variants as clinically and neurobiologically distinct subtypes. *American Journal of Psychiatry, 170*(10), 1114-1133. Retrieved from http://www.ncbi.nlm.nih.gov/pmc/articles/PMC3928064/pdf/nihms546876.pdf

U.S. Department of Health and Human Services, Administration for Children and Families, Administration on Children, Youth and Families, Children's Bureau. (2013). Child Maltreatment 2012. Retrieved August 9, 2014, from http://www.acf.hhs.gov/programs/cb/resource/child-maltreatment-2012

Walker, C. A., & Davies, J. (2010). A critical review of the psychometric evidence base of the child abuse potential inventory. *Journal of Family Violence, 25*(2), 215-227.

Welsh, J., Precey, G., & Lambert, P. (2008). Parents of children at risk - a multi-agency initiative to address substance misuse amongst parents whose children are at risk of neglect. *Child Abuse Review, 17*(6), 454-462.

Wildeman, C., Emanuel, N., Leventhal, J. M., Putnam-Hornstein, E., Waldfogel, J., & Lee, H. (2014). The prevalence of confirmed maltreatment among US children, 2004 to 2011 (Abstract).

JAMA Pediatrics, 168(8), 706-713. doi:10.1001/jamapediatrics.2014.410

World Health Organization. Alcohol and violence: child maltreatment and alcohol. Retrieved August 9, 2014, from http://www.who.int/violence_injury_prevention/violence/world_report/factsheets/fs_child.pdf

Long-term consequences of child abuse and neglect. (2013). Washington, D.C.: U. S. Department of Health and Human Services, Children's Bureau. Retrieved August 9, 2014, from http://www.childwelfare.gov/pubs/factsheets/long_term_consequences.cfm

(2013). What is child abuse and neglect? Recognizing the signs and symptoms. *Child Welfare Information Gateway.* Washington, DC: U.S. Department of Health and Human Services, Children's Bureau.

Statement of Ethical Principles. (2012, March 3). *International Federation of Social Workers.* Retrieved January 16, 2014, from http://ifsw.org/policies/statement-of-ethical-principles/

The Policy, Ethics, and Human Rights Committee, British Association of Social Workers. (2012, January). The Code of Ethics for Social Work: Statement of principles. Retrieved October 7, 2014, from http://cdn.basw.co.uk/upload/basw_112315-7.pdf

SUBSTANCE ABUSE IN ADOLESCENCE: RISK & PROTECTIVE FACTORS

MAJOR CATEGORIES: Adolescents, Substance Abuse

WHAT WE KNOW

Substance use disorder (SUD) is a group of cognitive, behavioral, and physiological symptoms which demonstrate the continued use of a substance despite an individual experiencing significant social, emotional, or physical impairment or distress caused or exacerbated by the effects of the substance. In the *Diagnostic and Statistical Manual of Mental Disorders,* fifth edition (*DSM-5*), which is used to diagnose substance use disorders, SUD combines the *DSM-IV* categories of substance abuse and substance dependence into a single disorder. In the previous version of the DSM, the *DSM-IV*, substance abuse was considered a mild or early phase and substance dependence was a more severe manifestation of the condition.

SUD among adolescents is a significant public health concern. More than 50 percent of adolescents in the United States have used alcohol or tobacco, and almost as many have tried marijuana or other illicit drugs. Substances commonly abused by adolescents, youth aged 12–17 years, include alcohol, tobacco, marijuana, y-hydroxybutyrate (GHB), phencyclidine hydrochloride (PCP), methamphetamine, cocaine, heroin, inhalants (e.g., paint thinners, glue, gasoline), and prescription drugs (e.g., Ritalin, Valium, Xanax, oxycodone).

Surveys in the United States and United Kingdom have shown that the average age of onset of alcohol and tobacco use disorder is 11–16 years old.

SUD often co-occurs and shares risk factors with other health risk behaviors. SUD among teens has been associated with deterioration of physical and mental health; risky sexual behaviors; automobile accidents; participation in crime; developmental impairment; problems at school (e.g., truancy, poor grades, suspension, expulsion), home (e.g., family conflict), and work (e.g., job loss); and lifelong dependency.

Younger age at onset of substance use is associated with a greater risk for lifetime dependency of the substance. For example, the prevalence of lifetime alcohol dependence is over 40 percent for children who begin drinking at age 12 or younger.

Risk factors for SUD in adolescents include individual factors, familial factors, mental illness, racial/ethnic factors, peer influence, genetic and biological factors, media influence, and social/community factors.

Evidence shows that teens with a history of physical or sexual abuse start using drugs and alcohol earlier than peers with no history of abuse. Research has consistently shown that a parental history of SUD is a major risk factor for adolescent SUD. Lack of family cohesion and lack of secure attachment to a parent or caregiver increases the risk for SUD. A permissive parental attitude toward substance use can increase drug use risk among adolescents, whereas strong parental enforcement of household rules against substance abuse can discourage this behavior.

SUD is closely associated with certain mental illnesses, including conduct disorder, attention deficit hyperactivity disorder, depression, anxiety disorder, bulimia, and schizophrenia. The link between mental illness and teen SUD is reciprocal meaning teens with mental illness are more likely to use drugs and teens who use drugs are more likely to exhibit psychological problems and to commit suicide. Greater incidence of adolescent SUD has been found among adolescents who have a history of head injury, with these teens being more likely to take risks and less capable of impulse control.

In Monitoring the Future, a U.S. survey on drug use among students in 8th, 10th, and 12thgrades, Black adolescents report lower rates of use for most substances than White or Hispanic teens. Hispanic students reported the highest use of most classes of drugs in the 8th grade and continued to have the highest prevalence of use at 12th grade for many substances, including marijuana, inhalants, cocaine, and methamphetamine.

Peer influence is one of the strongest risk factors for adolescent SUD. Adolescents with substance-using friends are more likely to use substances than those with friends who do not use substances. Peer disapproval of drug and alcohol use reduces risk for SUD and is more influential than parental disapproval. Negative peer relationships during childhood are also a risk factor for adolescent SUD. Victims of childhood bullying are at greater risk for cigarette and marijuana use in adolescence, and association with antisocial peers in childhood is linked with higher risk of polysubstance use in adolescence. Fatalistic attitudes (i.e., expectations of early death) among friends are also associated with increased drug use.

Compared to adults, teens may be more susceptible to inherited tendencies toward SUD. Adolescent twin studies have demonstrated that for adolescents, the magnitude of genetic predisposition toward substance use was greater than the influence of environmental factors.

Advertisements aimed at youth that depict substance use as appealing and normative increase the risk for teen substance abuse. Conversely, advertisement campaigns designed to discourage adolescent substance abuse and related risky behaviors (e.g., drinking and driving) are less effective, particularly when the characters and social situations in these ads are perceived by teens as unrealistic or unrelatable.

Community patterns of drug abuse affect adolescent drug use. Teens living in neighborhoods where drug use is common and where drugs are accessible and affordable are at increased risk for SUD.

Several family characteristics have been found to serve as protective factors. Living in a two-parent rather than a single-parent household may offer greater protection against SUD because of the likelihood of greater parental supervision. Adolescents who communicate regularly with their parents are less at risk for SUD than those who do not. Similarly, high family cohesiveness is protective, whereas a lack of family cohesion increases risk.

Frequent family meals have been associated with lower rates of adolescent SUD when adolescents perceive the mealtime environment as positive and cohesive. However, research findings about family meals are not consistent. Analysis of data from the 1997 National Longitudinal Survey of Youth did not find that family dinners affect the adolescent's initiation of substance use or use of cigarettes or alcohol and found only a modest association with frequency of marijuana use.

Living with a family member and spending after-school time with parents rather than with friends are linked with less substance use behaviors.

Family obligation values are associated with lower levels of substance use and may be a cultural protective factor for some youth, including those of Mexican origin. Adolescents who feel a strong sense of respect and responsibility for their families are less likely to associate with negative peers and more likely to communicate with their parents regarding their activities. A related value, family assistance (i.e., the youth's responsibility for helping with child care or other tasks), may act as a protective factor in low-conflict homes or as a risk-factor in high-conflict homes. Researchers in one study found that attachment to God or religiosity can be a protective factor for SUD among adolescents, whether Jewish, Muslim, or Christian (the 3 religions studied). The Muslim religion and its prohibition of alcohol and drug use could be a part of this protective factor.

WHAT CAN BE DONE

Social workers, mental health and medical professionals who treat adolescents should learn about risk and protective factors for adolescent SUD. Accurate assessments of adolescent clients' social, behavioral, medical, and mental health needs should be completed to identify any substance abuse disorders or needs.

The American Academy of Pediatrics encourages pediatricians and other healthcare professionals who care for adolescents to become knowledgeable about adolescent SUD through structured training programs and/or continuing medical education, discuss the effects of drugs and alcohol with both parents and adolescents, screen for SUD by obtaining a complete family medical history and by recognizing risk factors during health supervision visits, and inform adolescent patients about the rules of patient confidentiality prior to discussing their use of drugs and prevention strategies.

Social workers can encourage parents to strongly advise children and adolescents against substance use; be positive role models; limit accessibility of potentially abused substances (e.g., alcohol, cigarettes, inhalants); spend time together as a family, especially at meals; and monitor their children's whereabouts. Social workers may provide addicted adolescents with local resources for age-appropriate treatment options and support services. Prevention programs that emphasize life skills and address multiple health-risk behaviors have been found to have positive effects on adolescent substance use as well as other associated health-related behaviors.

More information about adolescent substance abuse may be obtained from the Substance Abuse and Mental Health Services Administration (SAMHSA) at http://store.samhsa.gov/home

Written by Tanja Schub, BS, and
Jennifer Teska, MSW

Reviewed by Jessica Therivel, LMSW-IPR

REFERENCES

American Academy of Pediatrics. Committee on Substance Abuse. (2010). Policy statement: Alcohol use by youth and adolescents: A pediatric concern. *Pediatrics, 125*(5), 1078-1087. doi:10.1542/peds.2010-0438

American Psychiatric Association. (2013). *Diagnostic and Statistical Manual of Mental Disorders* (5th ed.). Arlington, VA: American Psychiatric Publishing.

Badr, L., Taha, A., & Dee, V. (2014). Substance abuse in Middle Eastern adolescents living in two different countries: Spiritual, cultural, family and personal factors. *Journal of Religion & Health, 53*(4), 1060-1074. doi:10.1007/s10943-013-9694-1

Bramstetter, S. A., Low, S., & Furman, W. (2011). The influence of parents and friends on adolescent substance use: A multidimensional approach. *Journal of Substance Use, 16*(2), 150-160. doi:10.3109/14659891.2010.519421

British Association of Social Workers. (2012). NASW standards and indicators for cultural competence in social work practice. Retrieved December 22, 2015, from http://cdn.basw.co.uk/upload/basw_112315-7.pdf

Hale, D. R., Fitzgerald-Yau, N., & Viner, R. M. (2014). A systematic review of effective interventions for reducing multiple health risk behaviors in adolescence. *American Journal of Public Health, 104*(5), e19-e41. doi:10.2105/AJPH.2014.301874

Haynie, D., Soller, B., & Williams, K. (2014). Anticipating early fatality: Friends', schoolmates' and individual perceptions of fatality on adolescent risk behaviors. *Journal of Youth & Adolescence, 43*(2), 175-192. doi:10.1007/s10964-013-9968-7

International Federation of Social Workers. (2012). Statement of ethical principles. Retrieved December 22, 1970, from http://ifsw.org/policies/statement-of-ethical-principles

Hernandez, L., Eaton, C. A., Fairlie, A. M., Chun, T. H., & Spirito, A. (2010). Ethnic group differences in substance use, depression, peer relationships, and parenting among adolescents receiving brief alcohol counseling. *Journal of Ethnicity in Substance Abuse, 9*(1), 14-27.

Hicks, B., Johnson, W., Durbin, E., Blonigen, D., Iacono, D., & McGue, M. (2014). Delineating selection and mediation effects among childhood personality and environmental risk factors in the development of adolescent substance abuse. *Journal of Abnormal Child Psychology, 42*(5), 845-859. doi:10.1007/s10802-013-9831-z

Hoffman, J. P., & Warnick, E. (2013). Do family dinners reduce the risk for early adolescent substance use? A propensity score analysis. *Journal of Health & Social Behavior, 54*(3), 335-352. doi:10.1177/0022146513497035

Johnston, L. D., O'Malley, P. M., Miech, R. A., Bachman, J. G., & Schulenberg, J. E. (2014). Monitoring the Future national survey results on drug use: 1975-2013. 2013 overview, key findings on adolescent drug use. Ann Arbor: Institute for Social Research, The University of Michigan.

Lamont, A., Woodlief, D., & Malone, P. (2014). Predicting high-risk versus higher-risk substance use during late adolescence from early adolescent risk factors using latent class analysis. *Addiction Research and Theory, 22*(1), 78-89. doi:10.3109/16066359.2013.772587

Myers, L. (2013). Substance use among rural African American adolescents: Identifying risk and protective factors. *Child & Adolescent Social Work Journal, 30*(1), 79-93. doi:10.1007/s10560-012-0280-2

Nasim, A., Belgrave, F. Z., Corona, R., & Townsend, T. G. (2009). Predictors of tobacco and alcohol refusal efficacy for urban and rural African-American adolescents. *Journal of Child and Adolescent Substance Abuse, 18*(3), 221-242.

National Insititue on Drug Abuse. (2014). Drug facts: High school and youth trends. Retrieved December 22, 2015, from http://www.drugabuse.gov/publications/drugfacts/high-school-youth-trends

Pinkleton, B. E., Austin, E. W., & de Vord, R. (2010). The role of realism, similarity, and expectancies in adolescents' interpretation of abuse-prevention messages. *Health Communication, 25*(3), 258-265.

Schindler, A., & Broning, S. (2015). A review on attachment and adolescent substance abuse: Empirical evidence and implications for prevention and treatment. *Substance Abuse, 36*(3), 304-313. doi:10.1080/08897077.2014.983586

Stevens, A., Coulton, S., O'Brien, K., Butler, S., Gladstone, B., & Tonkin, J. (2014). RisKit: The participatory development and observational evaluation of a multi-component programme for adolescent risk behaviour reduction. *Drugs: Education, Prevention & Policy, 21*(1), 24-34. doi:10.3109/09687637.2013.787526

Talou-Shams, M., Feldstein Ewing, S. W., Tarantino, N., & Brown, L. K. (2010). Crack and cocaine use among adolescents in psychiatric treatment: Associations with HIV risk. *Journal of Child and Adolescent Substance Abuse, 19*(2), 122-134. doi:10.1080/10678281003634926

Telzer, E., Gonzales, N., & Fuligni, A. (2014). Family obligation values and family assistance behaviors: Protective and risk factors for Mexican-American adolescents' substance use. *Journal of Youth & Adolescence, 43*(2), 270-283. doi:10.1007/s10964-013-9941-5

Thoma, R. J., Hill, D. E., Tonigan, J. S., Kuny, A. V., Vermont, L. N., & Lewine, J. D. (2010). Adolescent self-reported alcohol/other drug use consequences: Moderators of self- and parent agreement. *Alcoholism Treatment Quarterly, 28*(2), 101-110.

Wheeler, D. (2015). *NASW standards and indicators for cultural competence in social work practice.* Retrieved December 22, 2015, from http://www.socialworkers.org/practice/standards/PRA-BRO-253150-CC-Standards.pdf

White, J., & Halliwell, E. (2010). Alcohol and tobacco use during adolescence: The importance of the family mealtime environment. *Journal of Health Psychology, 15*(4), 526-532.

SUBSTANCE ABUSE IN OLDER ADULTS

MAJOR CATEGORIES: Senior Care/Abuse (Gerontology), Substance Abuse

WHAT WE KNOW

Substance abuse refers to a pattern of continued use of a substance (e.g., alcohol, cannabis, opioids, sedatives) that causes cognitive, physiological, and behavioral symptoms, resulting in problems in various areas of functioning. The pattern of use is pathological. The individual may experience impaired behavioral control, continued use even when there are risks to him or her, and social impairment. There also may be tolerance and withdrawal. This problematic pattern of use must take place for at least 12 months to be classified as substance abuse.

The *Diagnostic and Statistical Manual of Mental Disorders, 5th Edition* (*DSM-5*), was published in 2013, replacing the *DSM-IV*. The *DSM-IV* chapter on "Substance-Related Disorders" included substance dependence, substance abuse, substance intoxication, and substance withdrawal, and then discussed specific substances (e.g., alcohol, amphetamines). The *DSM-5* divides these disorders into two categories: substance use disorders and substance-induced disorders (intoxication, withdrawal, and other substance/medication-induced mental disorders). Thus it removes the distinction between abuse and dependence and instead divides each disorder into mild, moderate, and severe subtypes. Drug craving has been added as a criterion for substance use disorder, whereas "recurrent legal problems" has been removed. In the *DSM-5* substance abuse is referred to as substance use disorder or substance dependence whereas in the research literature it is still commonly referred to as substance abuse.

Substance abuse among older adults is a growing health concern, particularly in developed countries.

Prevalence rates for substance abuse among older adults have been increasing due to the large size of the baby boom cohort (persons born between 1946 and 1964, who are now beginning to be classified as older adults), an increase also evident in higher prevalence rates of adults seeking treatment.

The age range indicated by the term "older adult" is not uniform across studies; some studies use 50 and older, others 55, 60, etc. Chronological age also may not accurately represent biologic age if chronic illnesses and health problems are present.

The first of the baby boomers began turning 65 in 2011. By 2030 there will be more than 70 million Americans over the age of 65.

Alcohol use among older Americans declines with age, with 53.1 percent of respondents between 60 and 64 reporting regular use and this number falling to 41.2 percent for those 65 and over.

Among the 60–64-year-old respondents, 14.3 percent reported binge drinking (i.e., drinking 5 or more drinks on one occasion at least once in the past 30 days) and 4.3 percent reported heavy alcohol consumption (i.e., 5 or more days of binge drinking during the past 30 days), compared to 8.2 percent of those 65 and over reporting binge drinking and 2 percent reporting heavy alcohol consumption.

Research has shown that birth cohorts that had higher rates of illicit (i.e., illegal drugs or prescription drugs used for nonmedical purposes) drug use as young adolescents or young adults will have higher rates of use as the cohort ages

The 2012 National Survey on Drug Use and Health found that rates of illicit drug use among adults between ages 55 and 59 increased from the 2002 survey: from 1.9 percent to 6.6 percent.

Rates of past-year marijuana use ranged from 2.8 percent for older adults born between 1943 and 1947 to 8.0 percent of those born between 1958 and 1962.

Researchers in one study found an increased proportion of older adults entering substance abuse treatment for the first time and found an increase in illicit drug use in older adult admissions.

In 1992 87.6 percent of older adults admitted for substance abuse treatment abused only alcohol; by 2009, this figure had declined to 58.0 percent. The proportion of older adults admitted for treatment for both alcohol and drugs increased from 12.4 percent to 40 percent.

In 2009 females over age 50 made up 22.2 percent of admissions for alcohol treatment whereas men over age 50 made up 77.8 percent.

Older adult substance abusers, including those who abuse alcohol, fall into three categories.

Early-onset users begin their use early in life and are at high risk as older adults for the health problems that may result from a lifetime of substance or alcohol use.

Late-onset users may be reacting to stressors or life events that have taken place in later life (e.g., loss of spouse, retirement, loss of purpose).

Intermittent or episodic users tend to use only occasionally but when they do use it is to excess. This use among older adults still is problematic and also may make it hard for professionals or family members to recognize that a problem is present.

Substance abuse among older adults most commonly involves alcohol use. A major complication for older adults who abuse alcohol is the interaction that can occur between alcohol and prescription or over-the counter (OTC) medications. Older adults also may have maladaptive use of illicit drugs as well.

Older adults are at high risk for prescription and OTC drug misuse because these medications are easily available.

Many older adults take multiple medications, many of which may interact negatively with alcohol or with other medications, resulting in negative consequences for the individual. Seventy percent of older adults take OTC medications.

Illicit drug use is an often overlooked problem with older adults. Marijuana is the most common illicit drug used, followed by the nonmedical use of prescription medications.

In 2011, 4.8 million adults over age 50 reported illicit drug use in the past year.

Nine percent of 50-to-59-year-olds and 2.3 percent of those 60 and older had used an illicit drug.

Male respondents age 50 and older used illicit drugs at a higher rate than female respondents of the same age. However, when nonmedical use of prescription medication was considered, the rates were almost equal.

Among these respondents, 45.2 percent had used only marijuana, 31.5 percent had used only prescription drugs nonmedically, and 5.6 percent had used other illicit drugs (e.g., cocaine, heroin, hallucinogens, inhalants).

Use of marijuana was more common than nonmedical prescription use for older adults ages 50–59 but for those 60 and older nonmedical prescription use was as common as marijuana use.

Problematic use of alcohol is associated with past-year use of illicit or nonmedical drugs, nicotine dependence, major depression, lower income, and stressful life events.

In a study of older adults aged 50 years and over living in public housing, researchers found that 23 percent drank in excess of National Institute on Alcohol Abuse and Alcoholism(NIAAA) guidelines. Higher prevalence of problematic alcohol use was found among Black men, and those who were unemployed and lacked housing stability. Illicit drug use and smoking were also associated with higher levels of alcohol use.

Older adults may have a significantly different experience with substance use and abuse than younger persons.

Older adults may be more sensitive to the effects of alcohol and other drugs due to inefficiencies in organ functions in aging body systems and decreased lean body mass and may experience more severe and more prolonged withdrawal.

The criteria developed to identify substance abuse have tended to underestimate the prevalence of potentially harmful alcohol use among older adults, due to older adults not reporting the same consequences as younger adults (e.g., problems at work) and having a lower threshold of consumption before experiencing adverse effects.

NIAAA and Substance Abuse and Mental Health Services Administration (SAMHSA) guidelines for adults ages 60 and over recommend that older adults consume no more than 1 drink per day and 7 drinks per week. They define binge drinking as 4 or more drinks for men and 3 or more drinks for women on a single occasion.

Older adults who are engaged in substance abuse are at a higher risk for psychiatric comorbidities such as depression and dementia.

Binge drinking is associated with increased psychological distress in older adults.

Aging and alcohol use both increase the risk of cognitive impairment, ranging from short-term memory deficits to difficulty carrying out routine activities independently; however, cognitive impairment among older people with alcohol problems frequently is undiagnosed.

Alcohol use may contribute to worsening chronic medical conditions or adversely impact their management.

In a study of alcohol use among adults 65 years and older with seven identified medical conditions (hypertension, diabetes, chronic obstructive pulmonary disease, heart failure, stroke, Alzheimer's disease, and depression), 30.9 percent of respondents acknowledged using alcohol during the past year and 6.9 percent reported drinking that exceeded NIAAA guidelines. Substance abuse in the older adult population may be difficult for primary care physicians and other professionals (e.g., nurses, social workers) to recognize.

Dementia, comorbid mental health issues, and medical problems that mimic the side effects of substance abuse make it harder to identify substance abuse.

Professionals may not have awareness of substance abuse among older adults and may think of it as a problem only for younger adults.

There may be an increased stigma surrounding substance abuse for older adults so they may go to greater lengths to hide their use and its effects or be in denial about having a problem.

Family and friends may enable the older adult's substance abuse by rationalizing that the older adult's age entitles him or her to the substance use.

Many screening tools were standardized using younger populations and may not be as relevant for older adults.

The frequency and consumption levels used in these tools were determined using younger drinkers or substance users. Older adults can become impaired on smaller amounts due to aging (e.g., organs not clearing toxins as quickly, presence of dementia, decreased lean body mass).

The CAGE Questionnaire and Michigan Alcoholism Screening Test-Geriatric may be appropriate choices but have not yet been tested with all age populations.

Older adults have particular vulnerabilities that may lead to substance abuse and may make substance abuse harder to treat.

Cognitive impairment, if present, may interfere with the older person's ability to remember appointments, give accurate history, and progress in treatment; adaptations to screening and treatment may be needed.

Older adults often are socially isolated and/or homebound, which makes them vulnerable to substance abuse. Social isolation and the frequent losses of later life may lead to grief and depression, which increases the likelihood that an older adult will turn to substance use.

Because transportation issues with older adults may impede access to treatment, they may be referred by healthcare providers for residential treatment. Yet the severity of their substance abuse may not be high enough to match the treatment program's protocol, resulting in a poor fit.

The psychoeducation needs of older adults are different from those of younger persons for a variety of reasons: differences in physical response to substances, different family configurations (e.g., older adults are more likely to be geographically distant from family; they may have lost their spouses), different cognitions related to drugs and alcohol (e.g., the social acceptance of daily alcohol use versus the social taboos of drug use for this age group).

Differences in values and life experiences between older and younger adults experiencing substance abuse may create obstacles to open communication in mixed-age settings.

Traditional self-help groups or 12-step programs may be a poor fit for older adults with limited mobility and transportation.

It is likely that older substance-abusing adults the social worker encounters are not yet feeling a need for change, do not view their use as a problem, and are not looking to make any changes. This is an opportunity for the social worker to begin the education process.

Motivational interviewing (MI) is common in substance abuse treatment but has not always been supported by strong empirical evidence. The general structure may work well with the older-adult population. The practice strategies include showing empathy, providing choices to the client, removing barriers, providing feedback, and clarifying the client's goals. MI techniques for the social worker include open-ended questions, reflective listening, and avoiding direct confrontation.

In one study of the effectiveness of MI with drug users researchers found that it improved treatment retention but did not have a noticeable impact on outcomes.

Treatment programs specific to older adults can address the depression, isolation, and health problems that may be central components of substance abuse in this age group.

Social bonding with same-age peers can improve compliance and outcomes.

WHAT CAN BE DONE

Become knowledgeable about substance abuse in older adults so you can accurately assess your patient's/client's personal characteristics and health education needs; share this information with your colleagues.

Develop an awareness of your own cultural values, beliefs, and biases and develop knowledge about the histories, traditions, and values of your clients. Adopt treatment methodologies that reflect the cultural needs of the client.

Educate primary care providers on the need to screen all older individuals for substance abuse and educate family members and caregivers on its signs and symptoms.

Annual screening is recommended, as well as re-screening when the older adult experiences a significant life event such as the death of a spouse.

Screening tools widely used with older adults include the Alcohol Use Disorders Identification Test (AUDIT) and the Short Michigan Alcoholism Screening Test–Geriatric Version (SMAST-G).

Screening for cognitive impairment, depression, and suicide risk should also be considered given their high rate of co-occurrence with substance abuse in older adults.

Screen all older clients for substance abuse but frame the conversation around recognizing the challenges and difficulties of aging to reduce chance of alienating client; it can also be helpful to incorporate substance-abuse related questions in health-related screenings rather than conducting a separate substance use screening, which may be offensive to some older adults(30) Advocate for an increase in research and funding of research to explore substance abuse in the older-adult age cohort.

Work with your clients on establishing positive social support systems, recognizing that these support networks can diminish with age; promote the continued use of existing supports and explore an expansion of supports.

Recognize that clients using illicit drugs may be dealing with pain management issues that need to be addressed to improve outcomes.

Educate clients about the increased sensitivity to alcohol that accompanies aging, the impact of alcohol use on specific medical conditions, and interactions between alcohol and medications.

Educate older clients on importance of following instructions on any prescription and OTC medications. Determine if they need assistance setting up a medication management system to reduce unintentional errors.

Refer to appropriate substance abuse treatment program and/or community programs (e.g., home-delivered meals, transportation help, financial assistance).

Brief intervention and treatment strategies have been found to be effective with older adults.

Refer to online resources for additional resources and educational materials.

Substance Abuse and Mental Health Services Administration (SAMHSA), http://www.samhsa.gov/, offers a toolkit for professionals working with older adults, as well as educational materials for consumers.

National Institute on Aging (NIA), http://www.nia.nih.gov/, has resources for professionals and consumers. A 24-page booklet, *Older Adults and Alcohol*, is available online at http://www.nia.nih.gov/sites/default/files/older_adults_and_alcohol.pdf.

Written by Jessica Therivel, LMSW-IPR

Reviewed by Chris Bates, MA, MSW, and Jennifer Teska, MSW

REFERENCES

American Psychiatric Association. (2013). Diagnostic and statistical manual of mental disorders. (5th ed.). Arlington, VA: Author.

Andrews, C. (2008). An exploratory study of substance abuse among Latino older adults. *Journal of Gerontological Social Work, 51*(1-2), 87-107.

Arndt, S., Clayton, R., & Schultz, S. K. (2011). Trends in substance abuse treatment 1998-2008: Increasing older adult first-time admissions for illicit drugs. *American Journal of Geriatric Psychiatry, 19*(8), 704-711. doi:10.1097/JGP.0b013e31820d942b

Blazer, D. G., & Wu, L. (2011). The epidemiology of alcohol use disorders and subthreshold dependence on in a middle-aged and elderly community sample. *American Journal of Geriatric Psychiatry, 19*(8), 685-694. Retrieved from http://www.ncbi.nlm.nih.gov/pmc/articles/PMC3144522/

Bryant, A. N., & Kim, G. (2013). The relation between frequency of binge drinking and psychological distress among older adult drinkers. *Journal of Aging & Health, 25*(7), 1243-1257. doi:10.1177/0898264313499933

Carroll, K. M., Ball, S. A., Nich, C., Martino, S., Frankforter, T. L., Farentinos, C., ... Woody, G. E. (2006). Motivational interviewing to improve treatment engagement and outcome in individuals seeking treatment for substance abuse: A multisite effectiveness study. *Drug Alcohol Depend, 81*(3), 301-321. doi:10.1016/j.drugalcdep.2005.08.002

Christie, M. M., Bamber, D., Powell, C., Arrindell, T., & Pant, A. (2013). Older adult problem drinkers: Who presents for alcohol treatment? *Aging and Mental Health, 17*(1), 24-32. doi:10.1080/13607863.2012.696577

Cooper, L. (2012). Combined motivational interviewing and cognitive-behavioral therapy with older adults drug and alcohol abusers. *Health & Social Work, 37*(3), 173-179. doi:10.1093/hsw/hls023

Cummings, S. M., Bride, B., & Rawlins-Shaw, A. M. (2006). Alcohol abuse treatment for older adults: A review of recent empirical research. *Journal of Evidence-Based Social Work, 3*(1), 79-99.

Cummings, S. M., Cooper, R. L., & Johnson, C. (2013). Alcohol misuse among older adult public housing residents. *Journal of Gerontological Social Work, 56*(5), 407-422. doi:10.1080/01634372.2013.790868

Farkas, K.J., & Drabble, L. (2008). Prevalence of alcohol, tobacco, and other drug use and problems among older adults. S. Diwan (Ed.), *Substance use and older adults resource review*. Alexandria, VA: CSWE Gero-Ed Center Master's Advanced Curriculum Project.

Hanson, M., & Gutheil, I. A. (2004). Motivational strategies with alcohol-involved older adults: Implications for social work practice. *Social Work, 49*(3), 364-372. doi:10.1093/sw/49.3.364

Jensen, C. J., Lukow, H. R., & Heck, A. L. (2012). Identifying barriers to care for older adults with substance use disorders and cognitive impairments. *Alcoholism Treatment Quarterly, 30*(2), 211-223. doi:10.1080/07347324.2012.663302

Kalapatapu, R. K., & Sullivan, M. A. (2010). Prescription use disorders in older adults. *American Journal on Addictions, 19*(6), 515-522. doi:10.1111/j.1521-0391.2010.00080.x

Lay, K., King, L. J., & Rangel, J. (2008). Changing characteristics of drug use between two older adult cohorts: Small sample speculations on baby boomer trends to come. *Journal of Social Work Practice in the Addictions, 8*(1), 116-126.

Memmott, J. L. (2003). Social work practice with the elderly substance abuser. *Journal of Social Work Practice in the Addictions, 3*(2), 85-103. doi:10.1300J160v03n02_06

Wheeler, D. (2015). NASW standards and indicators for cultural competence in social work practice. Retrieved December 8, 2015, from http://www.socialworkers.org/practice/standards/PRA-BRO-253150-CC-Standards.pdf

Naegle, M. (2008). Substance misuse and alcohol use disorders. In E. Capezuti, D. Zwicker, M. Mezey, & T. Fulmer (Eds.), *Evidence-based geriatric nursing; Protocols for best practice* (3rd ed., pp. 649-676). New York, NY: Springer.

Older Americans Behavioral Health Issue Brief 2: Alcohol Misuse and Abuse Prevention. (2012). *Substance Abuse and Mental Health Services Administration*. Rockville, MD: Author.

Reed, M. J. (2011). Substance abuse. In S. M. Meiner (Ed.), *Gerontologic nursing* (4th ed., pp. 307-321). St. Louis, MO: Elsevier Mosby.

Ryan, M., Merrick, E. L., Hodgkin, D., Horgan, C. M., Garnick, D. W., Panas, L., ... Saitz, R. (2013). Drinking patterns of older adults with chronic medical conditions. *JGIM: Journal of General Internal Medicine, 28*(10), 1326-1332. doi:10.1007/s11606-013-2409-1

Sacco, P., Bucholz, K. K., & Harrington, D. (2014). Gender differences in stressful life events, social support, perceived stress, and alcohol use among older adults: Results from a national survey. *Substance Use & Misuse, 49*(4), 456-465. doi:10.3109/10826084.2013.846379

Schonfeld, L., King-Kallimanis, B. L., Duchene, D. M., Etheridge, R..L., Herrera, J. R., Barry, K. L., & Lynn, N. (2010). Screening and brief intervention for substance misuse among older adults: The Florida BRITE project. *American Journal of Public Health, 100*(1), 108-114. doi:10.2105/AJPH.2008.149534

Smith, M. L., & Rosen, D. (2009). Mistrust and self-isolation: Barriers to social support for older adult methadone clients. *Journal of Gerontological Social Work, 52*(7), 653-667. doi:10.1080/01634370802609049

Statement of Ethical Principles. (2012, March 3). *International Federation of Social Workers*. Retrieved December 8, 2015, from http://ifsw.org/policies/statement-of-ethical-principles/

Substance Abuse and Mental Health Services Administration. (2001). Summary of findings from the 2000 National Household Survey on Drug Abuse. *NHSDA Series: H-13, DHHS Publication No. SMA 01-3549*. Rockville, MD: Author.

Substance Abuse and Mental Health Services Administration. (2013). *Results from the 2012 National Survey on Drug Use and Health: Summary of National Findings, NSDUH Series H-46, HHS Publication (SMA) 13-4795*. Rockville, MD: Author.

Substance Abuse and Mental Health Services Administration, Center for Behavioral Health Statistics and Quality. (2011). *The NSDUH Report: Illicit Drug Use among Older Adults*. Rockville, MD: Author.

Substance Abuse and Mental Health Services Administration, Center for Behavioral Health Statistics and Quality. (2011). *The TEDS Report: Older Adult Admissions Reporting Alcohol as a Substance of Abuse: 1992 and 2009*. Rockville, MD: Author.

White, J. B., Duncan, D. F., Nicholson, T., Bradley, D., & Bonaguro, J. (2011). Generational shift and drug abuse in older Americans. *Journal of Social, Behavioral, and Health Sciences, 5*(1), 58-66. doi:10.5590/JSBHS.2011.05.1.06

British Association of Social Workers. (2012, January). The code of ethics for social work: Statement of principles. Retrieved December 8, 2015, from http://cdn.basw.co.uk/upload/basw_112315-7.pdf

Wadd, S., Randall, J., Thake, A., Edwards, K., Galvani, S., McCabe, L., & Coleman, A. (2013). Alcohol misuse and cognitive impairment in older people.

UK: Substance Misuse & Ageing Research Team. Retrieved December 8, 2015, from http://alcoholresearchuk.org/downloads/finalReports/FinalReport_0110.pdf

Wang, Y., & Andrade, L. H. (2013). Epidemiology of alcohol and drug use in the elderly. *Curr Opin Psychiatry*, *26*(4), 343-348. doi:10.1097/YCO.0b013e328360eafd

SUBSTANCE ABUSE IN PREGNANCY

MAJOR CATEGORIES: Substance Abuse

DESCRIPTION

Abuse of substances, including alcohol, illicit drugs, and prescription drugs taken for non-medical reasons, during pregnancy has serious implications for both the mother and fetus. In 2013 the fifth edition of the *Diagnostic and Statistical Manual of Mental Disorders* (*DSM-5*) was published, replacing the *DSM-IV*. The DSM-IV chapter on "Substance-Related Disorders" included substance dependence, substance abuse, substance intoxication, and substance withdrawal, and then discussed specific substances (e.g., alcohol, amphetamines). The *DSM-5* instead separates these disorders into two categories: substance use disorders and substance-induced disorders (intoxication, withdrawal, and other substance/medication-induced mental disorders). Thus it removes the distinction between abuse and dependence and instead divides each disorder into mild, moderate, and severe subtypes. Drug craving was added as a criterion for substance use disorder, whereas "recurrent legal problems" was removed. Substance use disorders refer to a pattern of continued use of a substance (e.g., alcohol, cannabis, opioids, sedatives) that causes cognitive, physiological, and behavioral symptoms, resulting in problems in various areas of functioning. The substance may be illegal (e.g., cannabis, cocaine, heroin), legal (e.g., alcohol), or prescription medications used for purposes (i.e., recreational use) other than for which they were prescribed. The pattern of use is pathological. The individual may experience impaired self-control and may continue to use even when risks are present. There also may be tolerance and withdrawal (APA, 2013).

Abuse of substances during pregnancy has effects on the mother; effects on the course of pregnancy, including delivery; and effects on the fetus, newborn, and/or developing child. Substances abused during pregnancy cross the placenta and can affect the fetus directly or indirectly, as when abuse during pregnancy leads to poor maternal nutrition and sleep deprivation.

Alcohol is a teratogen (i.e., a substance that can cause birth defects); the use of alcohol during pregnancy, particularly heavy or binge drinking, has been identified as the leading preventable cause of intellectual disability and is associated with an array of physical, cognitive, and behavioral issues that fall under the umbrella term fetal alcohol spectrum disorder (FASD) (Grant et al., 2013). (For more information about the effects of alcohol abuse during pregnancy, see *Quick Lesson About ...Alcohol Abuse and Pregnancy* .) The use of stimulants (e.g., nicotine, cocaine, methamphetamine) and/or repeated episodes of withdrawal can reduce blood supply to the fetus, causing fetal growth restriction, spontaneous termination, neurological abnormalities, premature birth and its associated morbidity, and low birth weight (NIDA, 2011). Chronic opiate use during pregnancy has been linked with smaller head circumference (Visconti et al., 2015). Substance abuse in pregnancy can continue to cause problems for the neonate after birth as well. Neonatal abstinence syndrome (NAS), a condition in which babies develop physical dependence on narcotic drugs in utero and experience withdrawal symptoms after delivery, may cause irritability, feeding issues, tremors, increased muscle tension (i.e., hypertonia), vomiting, diarrhea, seizures, and respiratory problems. Most infants with NAS require care in a neonatal intensive care unit (NICU), which is expensive and frequently is stressful for parents (Patrick et al., 2012). Prenatal substance exposure is associated with a heightened risk of long-term cognitive, language, and behavioral issues, although lasting effects may be subtle and difficult to differentiate from psychosocial issues that often accompany maternal substance abuse (e.g., poverty, unstable living situations, inadequate nutrition and care, maternal mental illness).

Treatment barriers for pregnant women who are abusing substances can be categorized into four types: accessibility, acceptability, availability, and affordability

(Jackson & Shannon, 2012b). Accessibility may include issues with transportation, employment, child care, family responsibilities, social support, and incarceration. Acceptability refers to fears of stigmatization, self-denial, and fear of loss of custody. Availability refers to whether the client qualifies for treatment, if the program accepts women or pregnant women, and whether there is a waiting list. Affordability refers to financial and insurance issues that may prevent treatment.

In some cases pregnancy provides an opportunity to motivate women who abuse substances to begin treatment. Pregnant women already in treatment should be encouraged to pursue good prenatal care. A multidisciplinary approach that includes medical support for the mother as well as addiction treatment and supportive counseling may be the most effective. Women who are coping with substance abuse in pregnancy often feel stigmatized by society and by the healthcare professionals they may be seeing for prenatal care. Treatment must be approached nonjudgmentally and supportively. Treatment may include psychiatric or psychological counseling (cognitive-behavioral therapy, psychodynamic therapy), pharmacotherapy (e.g., methadone, buprenorphine), residential treatment, and/or support groups.

Facts and Figures

Substance abuse is more common in adolescents and younger adults; younger pregnant women report higher rates of substance abuse than older pregnant women. Alcohol is the most commonly used substance during pregnancy: 9.4 percent of pregnant women between ages 15 and 44 report alcohol use (SAMHSA, 2014). Maternal binge drinking may cause preterm birth and low birth weight: a study found that women ages 40 to 44 had the highest binge-drinking rates and the highest rate of preterm births (Truong et al., 2013). In the United States, prevalence rates for substance-affected live births decreased for cocaine from 1999 to 2008, but increased for narcotics and hallucinogens (Pan & Yi, 2013). The increase in narcotic use during pregnancy is believed largely to be due to non-medical use of prescription opioids (et al., 2015). Marijuana is the most commonly used illicit drug during pregnancy. One United States study found that although the rate of women being admitted to substance abuse treatment during pregnancy remained fairly stable from 1992 to 2012, at approximately 4 percent of

all female admissions, there has been a significant increase in women who report marijuana use upon admission (from 29 percent to 43 percent) and who report that marijuana is their primary substance (from 6 percent to 20 percent) (Martin et al., 2015). Approximately 15 percent of pregnant women between ages 15 and 17 use illicit drugs, with this number decreasing to 9 percent of pregnant women ages 18 to 25 and to 3 percent of pregnant women ages 26 to 44 (SAMHSA, 2014). An estimated 6 percent of pregnant women reported using an opioid analgesic at some point during pregnancy, of which only 20 percent had a current or lifetime medical condition that might require treatment with opioids (Smith et al., 2015).

In 2009 NAS was diagnosed in 3.39 per 1,000 U.S. births (Patrick et al., 2012). These newborns were more likely to have breathing issues, low birth weight, feeding problems, and seizures. Pregnant women in detoxification programs who live in rural areas have been found to have higher rates of illicit drug use than pregnant women in detoxification programs who are from urban areas (Shannon et al., 2010). In one study of rural women who were pregnant and abusing substances, researchers found that 83 percent of the respondents had experienced a barrier to treatment, with respondents reporting two barriers each on average (Jackson & Shannon, 2012a). Higher rates of family discord, often including violence, were associated with greater drug use in a study of pregnant women entering substance use treatment (Denton et al., 2014).

Risk Factors

Substance abuse in pregnancy occurs across all races, ethnicities, and socioeconomic statuses, but the highest risk is found among women who are extremely poor; have high levels of stress; have poor self-esteem and coping skills; have comorbid mental health issues, including depression; have histories of physical, sexual, or interpersonal violence; have lower levels of education; and have inadequate access to healthcare and social services. Youth increases the risk for substance abuse during pregnancy, as stated above. A past history before pregnancy of using substances increases risk for substance abuse during pregnancy.

Signs and Symptoms

Signs and symptoms will vary depending on the specific substance being used or consumed.

Psychological: mood swings, feelings of sadness and hopelessness, worry, irritability, memory problems, anxiety, paranoia, euphoria, anger, guilt, loneliness.

Behavioral: panic attacks, disorientation, suicidal ideation or suicide attempts, sedation, inebriation, frequent falls, problems at school or work, driving while impaired, periods of violence.

Physical: dilated pupils, rapid eye movement, tremors, track marks or infected injection sites, inflamed nasal passages, increased pulse rate and blood pressure, hair loss, gum disease, skin conditions, weight loss, frequent hospitalizations.

Social: withdrawal from family, friends, and other social supports, self-isolation.

ASSESSMENT

Screen clients for substance abuse; reassess at every visit, as clients may not disclose use until a trusting relationship has been established.

Obtain complete biopsychosocialspiritual history,including the following dimensions identified by the American Society of Addiction Medicine (ASAM, 2015):

- Current use and/or withdrawal potential;
- Current health and medical history;
- Cognitive, behavioral, and/or mental health conditions;
- Readiness to change;
- Potential for continued use or relapse;
- Current living situation and relationships;
- Assess for suicidal ideation;
- Screen client for intimate partner violence, which has been associated with substance abuse.

The TWEAK Problem Drinking Questionnaire is a 5-question tool designed for pregnant women. TWEAK is an acronym for Tolerance, Worried, Eye opener, Amnesia, "Kut" down.

The CAGE questionnaire is a short screening tool consisting of four questions relating to alcohol use; a positive answer to two or more questions indicates clinical significance.

TICS is a 2-item conjoint screening that inquires about alcohol and drug use.

The Addiction Severity Index (ASI) is a semi-structured interview that addresses seven problem areas: medical status, employment and support, drug use, alcohol use, legal status, family/social status, and mental health status.

The T-ACE is a four-item tool designed specifically for pregnant women; the acronym, used to direct the questions, stands for Tolerance, Annoyed, Cut down, Eye opener.

The AUDIT is a 10-item instrument for adults designed to measure consumption, dependence, and consequences of drinking. This tool can detect patterns in use which can help the clinician design appropriate interventions.

The 5 P's is a screening tool that assesses parents, peers, partner substance use, and past and present use.

Many of the above screens are designed to screen for moderate or heavy use. Pregnant women are encouraged not to drink at all, so an initial screening question to assess any current drinking should be utilized. The Centers for Disease Control and Prevention's Behavioral Risk Factor Surveillance System uses one question: "During the past 30 days, how many days per week or per month did you have at least one drink of any alcoholic beverage such as beer, wine, a malt beverage, or liquor?" This question has not been validity tested for pregnant women, however.

Any urine toxicology screen that indicates substance use will be relevant to the social worker.

A nutrition screening may be indicated to determine if client is nutritionally deficient as a result of substance abuse, which is important to discover when client is pregnant.

TREATMENT

For any pregnant client who is using alcohol or illicit substances, a reduction in use is imperative, with abstinence preferred in most situations if possible. Pregnant clients should be informed about the risks of substance use during pregnancy; the process of asking detailed questions about substance use may itself raise the client's awareness of risks and prompt her to reduce or cease use (WHO, 2014). Screening all clients for substance abuse is recommended but universal urine testing is not. Social workers often employ the transtheoretical stages of change model when approaching clients who are abusing substances. In this model there are five stages involved in making changes in behavior: precontemplation, contemplation, preparation, action, and maintenance (Engstrom et al., 2012). If a client is in the precontemplation stage, in which she is unaware that a problem exists and has no plans to change her behavior, the social worker will approach counseling differently from counseling the client who is actively taking action to change. In the contemplation stage the individual is beginning to recognize that a problem exists and is starting to think about making changes. In the preparation stage the client is starting to make small steps, whereas the action stage involves more overt modifications. The maintenance stage is also referred to as relapse prevention.

From a health perspective abstinence is the preferred approach for pregnant clients. For clients who cannot be successfully abstinent, a harm reduction approach can be appropriate. Social workers employing harm reduction look for underlying issues, encourage the client to keep track of substance use, try to reduce frequency of use and amount used, encourage avoidance of substance-using peers, and help the client plan for the future.

Treatment approaches vary widely in intensity; care should be individualized based on comprehensive assessment of the pregnant client. Twelve-step approaches conceptualize substance abuse as a disease and focus on abstinence, socialization, and enhancing self-efficacy (Engstrom et al., 2012). Motivational interviewing focuses positively on why an individual changes behavior, not why he or she does not. This approach uses collaboration and empathy to engage the client in change, and often is used in combination with other treatment approaches (Engstrom et al., 2012). Psychodynamic therapy techniques examine underlying trauma and conflicts, stress and negative emotions resulting from which the client copes with through substance abuse. Cognitive-behavioral therapy helps individuals identify and change the dysfunctional thoughts and behaviors that are leading to substance abuse in order to gain control and make changes. More intensive treatment (e.g., day treatment, residential treatment, inpatient treatment) may be indicated for women who have severe substance abuse and/or mental health issues and/or an unsupportive living situation. Pregnant women have complex treatment needs and are most successful in programs that are comprehensive (e.g., include child care and offer assistance with employment, education, and housing), designed for women, and culturally sensitive. Opioid maintenance treatment often is recommended for pregnant women who are dependent on opioids; medical support may be required for initial detoxification and stabilization depending on the substance(s) involved (e.g., benzodiazepines, alcohol).

Problem	Goal	Intervention
Pregnant client is exhibiting signs and symptoms of substance abuse	Client will reduce or discontinue substance use while pregnant	Educate client on the risks and consequences of substance abuse during pregnancy. Evaluate client's support system and try to build up deficient areas. Provide counseling interventions or refer client to an addictions specialist to aid in recovery. Provide a safe, supportive, non-judgmental environment for client
Client who is pregnant and abusing substances is encountering barriers preventing her from receiving treatment	Barriers will be removed and client will be able to access treatment	Have client share what barriers she is facing (e.g., accessibility, availability, acceptability, affordability). Advocate for client and try to broker appropriate services. Provide a non-judgmental environment to reduce feelings of stigma. Assist client in finding child care or other supports that are needed for her to receive treatment
Client has limited access to services	Increase services and program availability for pregnant women with substance abuse issues	Advocate for an increase in pregnancy-specific treatment programs. Advocate with the state legislature and/or the agency/facility for policies and laws regarding substance abuse in pregnancy that decriminalize substance abuse and encourage treatment versus punishment. Educate the local physician communities on how to avoid judgment in practice to foster trust and decrease stigma

LAWS AND REGULATIONS

In the United States there has been a trend to criminalize substance abuse during pregnancy, with 18 states classifying substance abuse during pregnancy as child abuse under their child-welfare statutes and 3 states allowing for involuntary commitment of pregnant women to mental health or substance abuse facilities. One state, Tennessee, recently enacted a law that makes women who use certain substances while pregnant eligible to be charged with assault (Guttmacher Institute, 2015). This trend has raised concerns that incarceration or the threat of incarceration is not an effective method of reducing substance abuse, and may instead lead to women avoiding prenatal care if they are worried about incarceration, involuntary commitment, custody loss, or housing loss. Criminalization treats substance abuse as a moral failing rather than as a sign of the biological and behavioral disorder of addiction. Social workers need to become knowledgeable regarding the rules and legislation of their state and nation to ensure that they can safeguard their clients' rights without breaking the law.

In 2001 the U.S. Supreme Court heard the case *Ferguson et al. v. City of Charleston*, which arose from the practice of nurses testing pregnant women for cocaine use without consent and sending positive results to the Charleston police for those women to be prosecuted. The Supreme Court ruled that women could not be tested by a hospital without a warrant or their expressed consent (Kang, 2003).

SERVICES AND RESOURCES

- Alcoholics Anonymous, www.aa.org
- Narcotics Anonymous, www.na.org
- Harm Reduction Coalition, www.harmreduction.org
- World Health Organization (WHO), http://www.who.int/topics/substance_abuse/en/
- National Institute on Alcohol Abuse and Alcoholism (NIAAA), www.niaaa.nih.gov
- National Institute on Drug Abuse, www.drugabuse.gov
- Substance Abuse and Mental Health Services Administration (SAMHSA), www.samhsa.gov
- Canadian Centre on Substance Abuse, http://www.ccsa.ca/

FOOD FOR THOUGHT

Universal screening of all women for risk of substance use and dependence is recommended in healthcare settings beginning in adolescence, ideally before conception.

Many controversies surround the testing of pregnant women for substance use. There are concerns about biased selection of women to be tested versus the expense of testing all pregnant women, about the limitations of testing in terms of contributing meaningful information to the care of the child, and concerns that possible legal consequences will prevent women from seeking care during pregnancy.

Members of impoverished and ethnic and racial minority populations are screened more often for drug and alcohol use in pregnancy than members of other populations (Carter, 2002).

Very few addiction treatment programs are equipped to specifically manage substance abuse and pregnancy. Only 19 U.S. states have substance abuse treatment programs specifically for pregnant women (Guttmacher, 2015). Often the drug treatment facilities that do accept pregnant women are expensive and unable to help with childcare arrangements, which precludes them as an option for some clients (American College of Obstetricians and Gynecologists, 2011).

In one study the fathers and fathers-to-be in couples in which both partners were abusing substances (binge drinking, using marijuana) did not significantly reduce use during their partner's pregnancy and the mothers returned quickly to the same behaviors of drinking and marijuana use after giving birth (Bailey et al., 2008).

A study found that the majority of women who were pregnant and using drugs or who had recently delivered after using drugs during pregnancy felt that health and social care professionals were critical, unsupportive, or adversarial. These women often felt that because of their drug use history they were not afforded choices during pregnancy or delivery (Stengel, 2014).

Preconception counseling (i.e., providing medical knowledge to women of childbearing age with a chronic disorder) is recommended for women of childbearing age who are attending addiction treatment centers (Rose et al., 2013).

RED FLAGS

Many of the substance abuse screening tools are validated on adults, so if the social worker is working with pregnant adolescents who are abusing substances he or she needs to be aware of possible effects on validity and reliability due to age differences.

Women who deliver babies exposed to drugs in utero frequently have histories of physical and sexual abuse. Researchers in one study found that 80 percent reported having experienced physical violence, 63 percent reported having experienced forced sexual activity, and 48 percent reported having experienced sexual abuse in childhood (Belcher et al., 2005).

The social worker needs to be aware of his or her country's/state's statutes regarding mandatory reporting of prenatal substance abuse or substance exposure in newborns, as well as any mandatory reporting regulations at the facility or agency that employs him or her.

Universal screening is recommended, but even when this is in place clients may not be honest in their reporting of substance use. In a study investigators found that 4.6 percent of the study population reported using illicit drugs during pregnancy yet 20 percent of the study population had positive urine drug screens (Jimerson& Musick, 2013).

Postpartum pain management needs to be considered for clients with a past or present substance use history. One option may be for the physician to order opioids immediately postpartum while the patient is in the hospital but not to discharge the patient with an opioid prescription (Gopman, 2014).

Next Steps

Educate the client on the risks and consequences of substance abuse in pregnancy and educate on available resources for health.

Enhance client's self-efficacy by empowering client and helping her strengthen her social network, especially helping the client find non-substance-using supports.

Address the needs of clients with both a psychiatric disorder and a substance abuse problem by making sure any existing mental health needs are being met along with addiction treatment.

If client gives permission, include client's obstetrician in care planning to help client reduce or abstain from substance use during the pregnancy.

Follow any agency or facility protocol regarding reporting of substance abuse in pregnancy.

If the prospective father is continuing to use during the partner's pregnancy, educate and counsel him on the importance of reducing his use to benefit his partner and newborn child.

Refer client to appropriate peer-support group.

Recognize that the postpartum period is a time of high risk for relapse and assist in arranging close follow-up after delivery State Policies in Brief: Substance abuse during pregnancy.

Written by Jessica Therivel, LMSW-IPR

Reviewed by Pedram Samghabadi

References

Alcoholism & Drug Abuse Weekly. (2014, May 5). Tennessee governor signs bill making it a crime to use drugs while pregnant. *Alcoholism & Drug Abuse Weekly, 26*(18), 1-3. doi:10.1002/adaw

American College of Obstetricians and Gynecologists. (2011, January). Substance abuse reporting and pregnancy: The role of the obstetrician-gynecologist. *Committee on Health Care for Underserved Women: Committee Opinion, 473,* 200-201.

American Psychiatric Association. (2013). *Diagnostic and statistical manual of mental disorders: DSM-5* (5th ed.). Washington, DC: American Psychiatric Publishing.

American Society of Addiction Medicine (ASAM). (2015). What is the ASAM criteria?. Retrieved July 18, 2015, from http://www.asam.org/publications/the-asam-criteria/about/

Azmitia, E. C. (2001). Impact of drugs and alcohol on the brain through the life cycle: Knowledge for social workers. *Summit on Social Work and the Neurobiology of Addictions hosted by the School of Social Work at the University of Texas at Austin on June 11-13, 2000. Journal of Social Work Practice in the Addictions, 1*(3), 41-63.

Bailey, J. A., Hill, K. G., Hawkins, J. D., Catalano, R. F., & Abbott, R. D. (2008). Men's and women's patterns of substance use around pregnancy. *Birth, 35*(1), 50-59. doi:10.1111/j.1523-536X.2007.00211.x

Bandstra, E. S., & Accornero, V. H. (2011). Infants of substance-abusing mothers. In R. J. Martin, A. A. Fanaroff, & M. C. Walsh (Eds.), *Fanaroff and Martin's neonatal-perinatal medicine: Diseases of the fetus and infant* (9th ed., pp. 735-757). St. Louis, MO: Elsevier Mosby.

Behnke, M., Smith, V. C., & Committee on Substance Abuse, and Committee on Fetus and Newborn. (2013). Prenatal substance abuse: Short- and long-term effects on the exposed fetus. *Pediatrics, 131*(3), e1009-e1024. doi:10.1542/peds.2012-3931

Belcher, H. M. E., Butz, A. M., Wallace, P., Hoon, A. H., Reinhardt, E., Reeves, S. A., & Pulsifer, M. B. (2005). Spectrum of early intervention services for children with intrauterine drug exposure. *Infants and Young Children: An Interdisciplinary Journal of Special Care Practices, 18*(1), 2-15.

Brandon, A. R. (2014). Psychosocial interventions for substance use during pregnancy. *Journal of Perinatal & Neonatal Nursing, 28*(3), 169-177. doi:10.1097/JPN.0000000000000041

Carter, C. S. (2002). Prenatal care for women who are addicted: Implications for gender-sensitive practice. *Affilia: Journal of Women & Social Work, 17*(3), 299-313.

Denton, W. H., Adinoff, B. H., Lewis, D., Walker, R., & Winhusen, T. (2014). Family discord is associated with increased substance use for pregnant substance users. *Substance Use & Misuse, 49*(3), 326-332. doi:10.3109/10826084.2013.840002

Engstrom, M., Mahoney, C. A., & Marsh, J. C. (2012). Substance use problems in health social work practice. In S. Gehlert & T. Arthur Browne (Eds.), *Handbook of health social work* (2nd ed., pp. 426-427). Hoboken, NJ: Wiley.

Goodman, D. J., & Wolff, K. B. (2013). Screening for substance abuse in women's health: A public health imperative. *Journal of Midwifery & Women's Health, 58*(3), 278-287. doi:10.1111/jmwh.12035

Gopman, S. (2014). Prenatal and postpartum care of women with substance use disorders. *Obstetrics and Gynecology Clinics of North America, 41*(2), 213-228. doi:10.1016/j.ogc.2014.02.004

Grant, T. M., Brown, N. N., Dubovsky, D., Sparrow, J., & Ries, R. (2013). The impact of prenatal alcohol exposure on addiction treatment. *Journal of Addiction Medicine, 7*(2), 87-95. doi:10.1097/ADM.0b013e31828b47a8

Jackson, A., & Shannon, L. (2012). Barriers to receiving substance abuse treatment among rural pregnant women in Kentucky. *Maternal and Child Health Journal, 16*(9), 1762-1770. doi:10.1007/s10995-011-0923-5

Jackson, A., & Shannon, L. (2012). Examining barriers to and motivations for substance abuse treatment among pregnant women: Does urban-rural residence matter? *Women & Health, 52*(6), 570-586. doi:10.1080/03630242.2012.699508

Jimerson, S. D., & Musick, S. (2013). Screening for substance abuse in pregnancy. *Journal of the Oklahoma State Medical Association, 106*(4), 133-134.

Kang, H. (2003). Comparative analysis of state statutes: Reporting, assessing, and intervening with prenatal substance abuse. *Social Policy Journal, 2*(4), 71-86.

Knudsen, A., Skogen, J., Ystrome, E., Sivertsen, B., Tell, G., & Torgersen, L. (2014). Maternal pre-pregnancy risk drinking and toddler behavior problems: The Norwegian Mother and Child Cohort Study. *European Child & Adolescent Psychiatry, 23*(10), 901-911. doi:10.1007/s00787-014-0588-x

Kotria, K., & Martin, S. (2009). Fetal alcohol spectrum disorders: A social worker's guide for prevention and intervention. *Social Work in Mental Health, 7*(5), 494-507. doi:10.1080/15332980802466565

Martin, C. E., Longinaker, N., Mark, K., Chisolm, M. S., & Terplan, M. (2015). Recent trends in treatment admissions for marijuana use during pregnancy. *Journal of Addiction Medicine, 9*(2), 99-104. doi:10.1097/ADM.0000000000000095

Matkins, P. P. (2008). Substance abuse. In P. J. A. Hillard (Ed.), *The 5-minute obstetrics and gynecology consult* (1st ed., pp. 314-315). Philadelphia: Wolters Kluwer/Lippincott Williams & Wilkins.

Narkowicz, S., Plotka, J., Polkowska, Z., Biziuk, M., & Namiesnik, J. (2013). Prenatal exposure to substance of abuse: a worldwide problem. *Environment International, 54*, 141-163. doi:10.1016/j.envint.2013.01.011

National Institute on Drug Abuse (NIDA). (2011, May). Prenatal exposure to drugs of abuse: A research update from the National Institute on Drug Abuse. *Topics in Brief: NIDA*. Retrieved July 18, 2015, from http://www.drugabuse.gov/sites/default/files/prenatal.pdf

O'Brien, P. (2014). Performance measurement: A proposal to increase use of SBIRT and decrease alcohol consumption during pregnancy. *Maternal & Child Health Journal, 18*(1), 1-9. doi:10.1007/s10995-013-1257-2

Pan, I. J., & Yi, H. Y. (2013). Prevalence of hospitalized live births affected by alcohol and drugs and parturient women diagnosed with substance abuse at liveborn delivery: United States, 1999-2008. *Maternal and Child Health Journal, 17*(4), 667-676. doi:10.1007/s10995-012-1046-3

Patrick, S. W., Schumacher, R. E., Benneyworth, B. D, Krans, E. E., McAllister, J. M., & Davis, M. M. (2012). Neonatal abstinence syndrome and associated health care expenditures, United

States, 2000-2009. *JAMA, 307*(18), 1934-1940. doi:10.1001/jama.2012.3951

Pilkinton, M. W. (2014). Correlates of race and substance abuse with religious support systems: a study of pregnant substance abusers. *Journal of Human Behavior in the Social Environment, 24*(3), 390-398. doi:10.1080/10911359.2014.875336

Reinsperger, I., Winkler, R., & Piso, B. (2015). Identifying sociomedical risk factors during pregnancy: Recommendations from international evidence-based guidelines. *Journal of Public Health, 23*(1), 1-13. doi:10.1007/s10389-015-0652-0

Rose, J., Rolland, B., Subtil, D., Vaiva, G., Jardri, R., & Cottencin, O. (2013). The need for developing preconception counseling in addiction medicine. *Archives of Women's Mental Health, 16*(5), 433-434. doi:10.1007/s00737-013-0374-7

Shannon, L. M., Havens, J. R., & Hays, L. (2010). Examining differences in substance use among rural and urban pregnant women. *The American Journal on Addictions/American Academy of Psychiatrists in Alcoholism and Addictions, 19*(6), 467-473. doi:10.1111/j.1521-0391.2010.00079.x

Smith, M., Costello, D., & Yonkers, K. (2015). Clinical correlates of prescription opioid analgesic use in pregnancy. *Maternal & Child Health Journal, 19*(3), 548-556. doi:10.1007/s10995-014-1536-6

Söderström, K. (2012). Mental preparation during pregnancy in women with substance addiction: A qualitative interview-study. *Child & Family Social Work, 17*(4), 458-467. doi:10.1111/j.1365-2206.2011.00803.x

Stengel, C. (2014). The risk of being "too honest": Drug use, stigma, and pregnancy. *Health, Risk & Society, 16*(1), 36-50. doi:10.1080/13698575.2013.868408

Substance Abuse and Mental Health Services Administration (SAMHSA). (2014). Results from the 2013 National Survey on Drug Use and Health: Summary of national findings, NSDUH Series H-48, HHS Publication No. (SMA) 14-4863. Rockville, MD: Author.

Sun, A. (2004). Principles for practice with substance-abusing pregnant women: A framework based on the five social work intervention roles. *Social Work, 49*(3), 383-394.

Truong, K., Reifsnider, O., Mayorga, M., & Spitler, H. (2013). Estimated number of preterm births and low birth weight children born in the United States due to maternal binge drinking. *Maternal & Child Health Journal, 17*(4), 677-688. doi:10.1007/s10995-012-1048-1

Visconti, K. C., Hennessy, K. C., Towers, C. V., & Howard, B. C. (2015). Chronic opiate use in pregnancy and newborn head circumference. *American Journal of Perinatology, 32*(1), 27-31. doi:10.1055/s-0034-1374817

Washington State Department of Health. (2012). Substance abuse during pregnancy: Guidelines for screening. *Washington State Department of Health: Office of Healthy Communities.* Olympia: Author. Guidelines for the identification and management of substance use and substance use disorders in pregnancy. Geneva: Author. (2014).

World Health Organization (WHO). Retrieved July 18, 2015, from http://apps.who.int/iris/bitstream/10665/107130/1/9789241548731_eng.pdf?ua=1

State policies in brief: Substance abuse during pregnancy. (2015). *Guttmacher Institute.* Retrieved July 18, 2015, from https://www.guttmacher.org/statecenter/spibs/spib_SADP.pdf

SUBSTANCE ABUSE IN THE MILITARY

MAJOR CATEGORIES: Military & Veterans, Substance Abuse

DESCRIPTION

Substance abuse has been a longtime problem within the U.S. military. Military personnel and combat veterans have higher rates of substance abuse than civilians of the same age (Larson et al., 2012). Widespread drug use during the Vietnam era resulted in the Department of Defense (DOD) adopting a "zero tolerance" policy in the mid-1980s with regard to use of illegal substances by both active-duty and non-active-duty personnel. Under this policy any report by self or others regarding illegal drug use could result in administrative discharge from the military and/or criminal prosecution. Since the enactment of this policy and mandatory urinalysis testing, there has been a decline in the use of illegal substances. However, abuse of alcohol and prescription medications has escalated and has resulted in more service members experiencing problems with or dependence on narcotics, benzodiazepines, and other prescription medications (Army Suicide Prevention Task Force, 2010). Some military personnel do not seek treatment for fear that it could result in a delay returning home, criminal prosecution, or dishonorable discharge.

The DOD and individual military branches—Air Force, Army, Navy, Marines, National Guard, and reserves—are responsible for creating and implementing substance abuse policies and programs designed to assess, treat, and discipline members of the military. The health mission of these organizations is to enforce discipline, to maintain force readiness, and to promote resilience, optimal health, and well-being of service members. Alcohol and prescription medications are the only substances identified as legal for service members to consume. The Veterans Affairs (VA)/DOD Clinical Practice Guidelines for Management of Substance Use Disorders are the guidelines used by healthcare providers for treatment and rehabilitation of both active service members and veterans (i.e., those separated from the military under an honorable or general discharge). These evidence-based guidelines and interventions were adopted to address substance use disorder (SUD), a term that encompasses a range of substance use problems, from hazardous use to dependence, and a range of substances, including alcohol, tobacco, and illicit drugs. Although each branch of the military has different programs to address SUDs, their protocols for handling misuse and abuse share the same three components: 1) commander/supervisor involvement, 2) treatment and rehabilitation, and 3) the requirement that a decision be made regarding whether a service member with a SUD will remain in military service or be discharged from duty.

There is considered to be substantial unmet need in the military for SUD treatment. The majority of military personnel and their spouses are covered by TRICARE health insurance, which does not cover intensive outpatient treatment services, office-based outpatient services, or some evidence-based pharmacological therapies that are considered standard elements of care in civilian practice. In addition, SUD services are restricted to certified facilities, resulting in an overutilization of expensive, inpatient hospital treatment when outpatient or office-based treatment would be more appropriate.

Despite the standards and procedures adopted by the military, alcohol and substance use in the armed forces continues to rise and to pose a risk to the readiness and psychological fitness of military troops. The most significant spike is the increase in alcohol abuse by military personnel returning from Operation Iraqi Freedom and Operation Enduring Freedom (Afghanistan). The rising number of cases of SUD maybe attributed to the increased number of deployments, the duration of deployments, increase in traumatic brain injuries, post-traumatic stress, increase in sexual assault trauma, moral injuries in combat veterans (i.e., trauma from witnessing or committing an act that goes against one's morals), and the fact that more soldiers are surviving and living with serious physical injuries and disabilities.

The Institute of Medicine's 2012 report *Substance Use Disorders in the U.S. Armed Forces* proposed several recommendations to improve prevention and treatment. It identified barriers to treatment, including inadequate substance abuse treatment program availability, gaps in insurance, lack of coverage, stigma, fear of negative consequences, and lack of confidential services. The Army's Confidential Alcohol Treatment and Education Project has created a way for service members to receive confidential treatment. Prevention efforts such as reducing the number of outlets on base that sell alcohol and restricting the amount of alcohol that can be purchased were noted in the report as ways to curb easy access and enforce the prohibition of underage drinking. Structural changes such as routine screenings for unhealthy alcohol use, mandating prescribers to check local drug-monitoring programs before dispensing medications with high abuse potential, and training healthcare professionals in the identification of medication-seeking behavior are seen as methods to improve the way in which SUDs are screened for and treated.

FACTS AND FIGURES

Deployment is associated with increased rates of alcohol consumption and problem drinking. Service members report significantly more problems during their third and fourth deployments than during their first and second deployments.

In 2008 nearly half of active-duty service members reported binge drinking (IOM, 2012).

There is an increased risk for substance use disorders for active-duty personnel who have deployed to Afghanistan or Iraq when compared to non-deploying military personnel (Shen et al., 2013).

Thirty-nine percent of veterans who participated in Operation Enduring Freedom or Operation Iraqi Freedom had positive screens for likely alcohol abuse and 3 percent for likely drug use, both of which are higher percentages than are found in the general population (Eisen et al., 2013).

The most recent DOD study on health behaviors of active-duty military personnel was published in 2013 and based on 2011 data. The next study is underway for 2015 and will be completed and published in the fall of 2016. The 2013 study found: (Barlas et al., 2013).

- 39.6 percent of current drinkers reported binge drinking at least once in the past 30 days;
- 8.4 percent of current drinkers reported being heavy drinkers, which was defined as more than 14 drinks per week for males and more than 7 drinks per week for females;

Over half of the heavy drinkers had an AUDIT score (i.e., common screening tool for alcohol disorders) that indicated that they were at risk for alcohol problems and 11.3 percent had an AUDIT score that indicated their drinking was hazardous:

Over 10 percent indicated not being familiar with military treatment options;

Less than 1 percent reported drug use in the last 30 days whereas 27.5 percent reported lifetime use.

Marijuana was the most common illicit substance used, followed by hallucinogens, cocaine, and MDMA.

Results from a research study of substance use in the military indicate that use of synthetic cannabis is more prevalent among military personnel than civilians (Walker et al., 2014).

In the past year, 24.9 percent of active-duty personnel reported prescription drug use, with 1.3 percent reporting misuse of prescription drugs. Misuse rates are lower than in the civilian population, but this may be due to increased monitoring in the military, including more frequent drug testing, and to messages that are presented to deter use.

Military personnel report using alcohol as a way to cope with stress, boredom, and loneliness.

Women who report sexual trauma while serving in the military are 2 to 3 times more likely to meet the screening criteria for alcohol abuse than women in the military who have not experienced sexual trauma.

Afghanistan is the leading producer of opium and heroin in the world, increasing service members' exposure to opium and the accessibility of the drug (United Nations Office on Drugs and Crime, 2016).

Military physicians wrote nearly 3.8 million prescriptions for pain medications in 2009, more than quadruple the number of such prescriptions written in 2001 (IOM, 2012).

The inpatient residential treatment facility at Eisenhower Army Medical Center in Georgia, which has 22 beds for inpatient treatment of 28 days, has been in operation since 2009. A study of 108 patients found that 80 percent had alcohol dependence, 8 percent narcotic dependence, 3 percent stimulant dependence, and 9 percent dependence on another substance. Thirty-four percent of the study population had diagnoses of co-existing depression, other mood disorder, anxiety disorder, or posttraumatic stress disorder (PTSD) (Mooney et al., 2014).

Outcome data for the program indicate that 87 percent of participants successfully complete the program, which is a completion rate 3 times higher than that for civilian programs; this likely is due to the military control and command structure. More than half of participants were able to maintain continuous sobriety for more than 6 months post-completion.

RISK FACTORS

Reserve and National Guard personnel and younger service members who are exposed to combat are at increased risk of new-onset heavy weekly drinking, binge drinking, and other alcohol-related problems. Persons with the highest risk for abusing alcohol are those who are young, White, non-Hispanic, Marines, and/or current smokers. Women may be at a higher risk for alcohol use disorders due to the stress of working in a traditionally male-dominated environment. A service member's cultural background may impact his or her views on substance use and increase his or her risk if the culture condones use of substances as an appropriate coping mechanism. Younger service members' risk of substance abuse increases with the number and length of deployments; younger service members who seek treatment have a higher chance of recovery than do older veterans with more longstanding histories. Men and women who serve in the military are at the highest risk for PTSD, which in turn increases their risk of experiencing substance abuse issues. Results from one study indicated that the odds of having a previous PTSD diagnosis were 28 times higher for service members who used opiates compared to those who did not use opiates (Dabbs et al., 2014). Researchers of another study indicated that military service members use cannabis to cope with PTSD symptoms,including reducing anxiety and insomnia (Betthauser, 2015).

SIGNS AND SYMPTOMS

Psychological: distorted sensory perception, impaired cognition, impaired motor skills; anxiety, moodiness, lethargy, or prolonged periods of high energy; symptoms of PTSD in the form of anxiety, depression, guilt, nightmares, flashbacks, suicidal ideations, and exaggerated reactions to stimuli.

Behavioral: Client may seem easily agitated or experience intense anger or psychological numbness; may have a legal prescription but take more than the recommended dosage; may create reasons for needing narcotic analgesics (this is often referred to as "medication seeking"); may engage in disassociation by attempting to avoid places, persons, feelings, thoughts, conversations, and activities associated with trauma (these may serve as triggers); may be more likely to engage in intimate partner violence or experience marital discord; may have disordered sleep or appetite.

Physical: Client may have a medical condition, have sustained painful physical injuries, or have a traumatic brain injury and use alcohol or drugs as a means of self-medicating; addiction often is characterized by a physical dependence on the drug, an increased tolerance of the drug, and/or withdrawal symptoms upon cessation of use.

Social: Client may withdraw and isolate him- or herself from family; may have limited friendships, poor social support, and reduced emotional intimacy; may not discuss use with military comrades for fear of being reported to supervisor; performance in duties may decline.

ASSESSMENT

Conduct preliminary assessment to determine if client may require detoxification and if client would best benefit from inpatient or outpatient treatment; determine if there is a need for emergency care.

Engage client and build trust by discussing reasons for joining the military and benefits of serving; address the stigmas associated with seeking treatment by identifying mental healthcare as a routine aspect of healthcare.

Learn about client's past and recent deployments, the number of deployments and time between deployments, and the range of combat experience; note physical findings, overall presentation, and level of functioning; do not force client to recount traumatic details of combat—flashbacks may occur and result in further trauma.

Identify barriers to treatment that are specific to substance use (e.g., noncompliance, denial, manipulation) and those that are specific to the military (e.g., fear of discharge, fear substance use may prevent career advancement, fear that seeking of treatment may be viewed as a sign of weakness, possible reprimand).

Assess for history of psychiatric treatment, childhood maltreatment, suicide, homicide, and any exposure to violence.

Conduct a biopsychosocialspiritual interview that assesses physical health, spiritual health, mental health, pre-military substance use, recent substance use, the function of substance use (e.g., sleep aid, social functioning, avoidance, numbing), intimate partner violence, social supports, coping strategies, strengths, and environmental, social, and financial factors as they relate to client's treatment.

Identify treatment goals; discuss the level of confidentiality, extent of supervisor involvement, and date of return to duty.

ASSESSMENTS AND SCREENING TOOLS

Alcohol Use Disorders Identification Test (AUDIT) may be used to provide accurate information about a client's substance use

Alcohol, Smoking, and Substance Involvement Screening Test (ASSIST) may be used to provide accurate information about a client's substance use

Drinker's Check-up is an Internet-based tool that allows service members to take a self-test and identify the presence of symptoms of abuse or dependence

Drug Abuse Screening Test (DAST) is a 20-item self-report test used to identify aspects of drug use that can be problematic

The Timeline Follow-Back Interview (TLFB) is a semistructured interview that is episodically based and assesses for substance use including alcohol

Drug toxicology screen via a urine sample can detect the presence of drugs and alcohol.

TREATMENT

Systems theories have proven to be an effective treatment modality when working with military personnel with SUDs. This approach is based on the importance of recognizing that a client's problems cannot be understood or addressed in isolation; rather, there is a complex interactive relationship between the client and his or her environment. This is especially critical when working with military service members, since many aspects of military culture may affect help-seeking and utilization of services. Unlike for civilian clients, treatment services for members of the military often are determined by military leadership, who decide when a problem needs to be evaluated, when someone will receive help, if treatment is needed, and when a service member needs to return to duty. As a result, harm reduction models may not be used or be appropriate in military treatment.

Cognitive behavioral therapy (CBT) can be used to address distorted thoughts and maladaptive behaviors while assisting clients in the development of healthy coping skills and behavior management techniques. Group therapy provides a safe environment for clients to share experiences, offer support, and confront stigmas that often are associated with seeking help in the military community. Group therapy has proven especially effective with military personnel, who are used to working as a unified group to achieve a common goal.

A relapse prevention program is vital in helping the client to maintain sobriety and minimize risk of relapse. Knowledge about military organizations and culture is important for good treatment outcomes. Social workers must also advocate on behalf of military members by communicating to commanders the needs and benefits of treatment, which is not always aligned with the military commander's need for the service member to return to regular duties.

Social workers should be aware of their own cultural values, beliefs, and biases and develop specialized knowledge about the histories, traditions, and values of their clients. Social workers should adopt treatment methodologies that reflect their knowledge of the cultural diversity of the communities in which they practice

Problem	Goal	Intervention
Client has symptoms of substance use disorder	Determine immediate needs	Conduct a preliminary assessment to determine misuse, abuse, or dependence; assess need for detoxification, inpatient or outpatient care
Client meets the criteria for substance use disorder	Maintain sobriety if this is the mandated goal by military command, reduce negative effects of symptoms, and improve coping skills	Conduct biopsychosocialspiritual interview; utilize systems approach to address barriers to treatment, identify negative stigmas, determine strengths, and incorporate supportive components of military culture
Client is at risk for relapse due to exposure to triggers	Develop relapse prevention plan and build support network	Work collaboratively with military supervisors, military healthcare system, and VA to address military protocol and any confidentiality conflicts; utilize CBT to address underlying issues of use and help client to develop new coping mechanisms

LAWS AND REGULATIONS

Public Law 92-129 entitles each branch of the armed forces to establish its own substance abuse treatment programs and policies.

The National Defense Authorization Act (2008) entitles combat veterans separated from active military service on or after January 28, 2003, to 5 years of VA enrollment eligibility and free healthcare services (Larson et al., 2012).

Military policies such as the Air Force's Alcohol and Drug Prevention and Treatment (ADAPT) program and the Army Substance Abuse Program (ASAP) delineate practices for management and intervention of misuse of alcohol and drugs.

Social workers should practice with awareness of and adherence to the NASW Code of Ethics core values of service, social justice, dignity and worth of the person, importance of human relationships, integrity, and competence; and become knowledgeable of the NASW ethical standards as they apply to the military population and practice accordingly.

SERVICES AND RESOURCES

- VA Substance Use Disorder Program Locator, http://www.va.gov/directory/guide/SUD.asp
- Department of Veterans Affairs, www.va.gov/
- Make the Connection – shared experiences and support for veterans, http://maketheconnection.net/
- Iraq and Afghanistan Veterans of America, http://iava.org/
- Wounded Soldier and Family Hotline, 1-800-984-8523
- VA National Caregiver Support Line, 1-855-260-3274

FOOD FOR THOUGHT

Behavioral health military personnel such as psychotherapists and social workers are deployed in combat support units at the ratio of one behavioral health professional for every 700 soldiers (Hoge, 2011).

The VA is the primary healthcare provider for discharged veterans and consists of a network of hospitals, clinics, and community-based outpatient clinics.

The VA is one of the largest providers of substance abuse services: it can provide medications, counseling for substance abuse/dependence, and relapse prevention programs.

Military service members adopt the values of the "warrior ethos," which is a professional code of conduct that involves putting the mission before personal needs, never accepting defeat, never quitting, and being loyal, respectful, selfless, and courageous. The acknowledgment of sickness, mental illness, or dependence is in direct contradiction to this mindset and idealized self-image. Seeking help may feel like an acknowledgment of weakness and set the client apart from the collective military identity.

RED FLAGS

Personnel nearing the end of deployment may be resistant to disclosing substance abuse out of fear that it may delay their return home.

Military discharges due to misconduct render service members ineligible for VA benefits.

When a report of substance abuse is made by someone other than the service member, it is often the result of positive urinalysis, criminal behavior, traffic violations, or punitive administrative action; if referred by military commander, client confidentiality will be limited.

Suicide is a major concern for veterans and military personnel with SUDs. Many veterans and military personnel who commit suicide are found to have recently been seen at the VA. Researchers found that 26 percent of the male VA patients who committed suicide had seen a VA provider within 1 week of the suicide and 56 percent had seen a VA provider within 1 month of the suicide (Ilgen et al., 2013). These statistics expose that there are possible missed opportunities for screening for suicidal ideations.

In a study, more than 1 in 10 HIV-infected male U.S. veterans who have sex with men (MSM) reported long-term abuse of alcohol (Marshall et al., 2015).

Results of research indicate that children who have a parent who serves in the military are at higher risk for emotional and behavioral issues (e.g., alcohol use disorder, harassment, physical violence, carrying a weapon to school) than their peers from non-military families (Sullivan et al., 2015; Creech et al., 2014).

A "designer" drug called methoxetamine is particularly alluring to active-duty military personnel because it is not detected in standard urine drug tests; active-duty military are subject to random urine tests throughout the year. Methoxetamine is primarily inhaled in powder form but can also be taken orally, intravenously, and rectally (Craig & Loeffler, 2014).

NEXT STEPS

Work collaboratively with military supervisors to ensure client receives appropriate treatment and to address any confidentiality conflicts.

Help client to locate a military-based support group or civilian support group that will provide more anonymity.

Provide client with hotline information and emergency contacts to use during time of crisis.

Educate client's family members on the risk factors and signs of substance use disorders so they are equipped to lend support and seek help (if client has allowed for family involvement).

Written by Nikole Seals, MSW, ACSW

Reviewed by Jessica Therivel, LMSW-IPR

REFERENCES

Army Suicide Prevention Task Force. (2010). *Army health promotion, risk reduction and suicide prevention report.* Arlington, VA: U.S. Department of Defense.

Aronson, K., Perkins, D., & Olson, J. (2014). Epidemiology of partner abuse within military families. *Journal of Family Social Work, 17*(4), 379-400. doi:10.1080/10522158.2014.921880

Barlas, F. M., Higgins, W. B., Pflieger, J. C., & Diecker, K. (2013). 2011 Health Related Behaviors Survey of Active Duty Military Personnel. Fairfax, VA: Department of Defense. Betthauser, K., Pilz, J., & Vollmer, L. (2015). Use and effects of cannabinoids in military veterans with posttraumatic stress disorder. *American Journal of Health-System Pharmacy, 72*(15), 1279-1284. doi:10.2146/ajhp140523

British Association of Social Workers. (2012, January). The Code of Ethics for Social Work: Statement of principles. Retrieved April 5, 2016, from http://cdn.basw.co.uk/upload/basw_112315-7.pdf

Craig, C. L., & Loeffler, G. H. (2014). The ketamine analog methoxetamine: A new designer drug to threaten military readiness. *Military Medicine, 179*(10), 1149-1157. doi:10.7205/MILMED-D-13-00470

Creech, S. K., Hadley, W., & Borsari, B. (2014). The impact of military deployment and reintegration on children and parenting: A systematic review.

Professional Psychology: Research and Practice, 45(6), 452-464.

Dabbs, C., Watkins, E., Fink, D., Eick-Cost, A., & Millikan, A. (2014). Opiate-related dependence/abuse and PTSD exposure among active-component U.S. military, 2001 to 2008. *Military Medicine, 179*(8), 885-890. doi:10.7205/MILMED-D-14-00012

Eisen, S. V., Schultz, M. R., Vogt, D., Glickman, M. E., Elwy, A. R., Drainoni, M. L., ... Martin, J. (2013). Mental and physical health status and alcohol and drug use following return from deployment to Iraq or Afghanistan. In *Veteran suicide: A public health imperative* (pp. 199-221). Washington, DC: American Public Health Association.

Hoge, C. W. (2011). Supporting resilience in a deployment context: Public health strategies and treatment of service members and veterans with combat-related mental health problems. In A. B. Adler, P. D. Bliese, & C. A. Castro (Eds.), *Deployment psychology: Evidence-based strategies to promote mental health in the military* (pp. 17-34). Washington, DC: American Psychology Association.

Holleran-Steiker, L., McCarthy, M., & Downing, A. (2012). Substance abuse in the military: An interview with Michael McCarthy and Alexander Downing. *Journal of Social Work Practice in the Addictions, 12*(1), 11-16. doi:10.1080/1533256X.2012.649211

Ilgen, M. A., Conner, K. R., Roeder, K. M., Blow, F. C., Austin, K., & Valenstein, M. (2013). Patterns of treatment utilization before suicide among male veterans with substance use disorders. In R. M. Bossarte (Ed.), *Veteran suicide: A public health imperative* (pp. 261-274). Washington, DC: American Public Health Association.

Institute of Medicine (IOM). (2012). Substance use disorders in the U.S. Armed Forces. Washington, DC: National Academy of Sciences. International Federation of Social Workers. (2012, March 3). Statement of Ethical Principles. Retrieved April 6, 2016, from http://ifsw.org/policies/statement-of-ethical-principles/

Kruze, M. I., Steffen, L. E., Kimbrel, N. A., & Gulliver, S. B. (2011). Co-occurring substance use disorder. In B. A. Moore & W. E. Penk (Eds.), *Treating PTSD in military personnel: A clinical handbook* (pp. 217-238). New York, NY: The Guilford Press.

Larson, M., Wooten, N. R., Adams, R. S., & Merrick, E. L. (2012). Military combat deployments and substance use; Review and future directions. *Journal of Social Work Practice in the Addictions, 12*(1), 6-27.

Marshall, B., Operario, D., Bryant, J., Cook, R., Edelman, E., Gaither, J., ... Fiellin, D. (2015). Drinking trajectories among HIV-infected men who have sex with men: A cohort study of United States veterans. *Drug and Alcohol Dependence, 148*(69-76). doi:10.1016/j.drugalcdep.2014.12.023

Mooney, S. R., Horton, P. A., Trakowski, J. H., Jr, Lenard, J. H., Barron, M. R., Nave, P. V., ... Lott, H. D. (2014). Military inpatient residential treatment of substance abuse disorders: The Eisenhower Army Medical Center experience. *Military Medicine, 179*(6), 674-678. doi:10.7205/MILMED-D-13-00308

National Association of Social Workers. (2008). Code of ethics. Retrieved April 5, 2016, from https://www.socialworkers.org/pubs/code/code.asp

National Association of Social Workers. (2012). NASW Standards for Social Work Practice with Service Members, Veterans, and Their Families. Retrieved April 5, 2016, from http://www.socialworkers.org/practice/military/documents/MilitaryStandards2012.pdf

Shen, Y. C., Arkes, J., & Williams, T. V. (2012). Effects of Iraq/Afghanistan deployments on major depression and substance use disorder: Analysis of active duty personnel in the US military. *American Journal of Public Health, 102*(S1), S80-S87. doi:10.2105/AJPH.2011.300425

Skidmoore, W. C., & Roy, M. (2011). Practical considerations for addressing substance use disorders in veterans and service members. *Social Work in Health Care, 50*(1), 85-107. doi:10.1080/00981389.2010.522913

Sullivan, K., Capp, G., Gilreath, T., Benbenishty, R., Roziner, I., & Astor, R. (2015). Substance abuse and other adverse outcomes for military-connected youth in California. *JAMA Pediatrics, 169*(10), 922-928. doi:10.1001/jamapediatrics.2015.1413

United Nations Office of Drugs and Crime. (2016). Afghanistan Opium Survey 2015. Retrieved April 6, 2016, from https://www.unodc.org/documents/crop-monitoring/Afghanistan/Afghanistan_opium_survey_2015_socioeconomic.pdf

Walker, D., Neighbors, C., Walton, T., Pierce, A., Mbilinyi, L., Kaysen, D., & Roffman, R. (2014). Spicing up the military: use and effects of synthetic cannabis in substance abusing army personnel. *Addictive Behaviors, 39*(7), 1139-1144. doi:10.1016/j.addbeh.2014.02.018

Wheeler, D. (2015). NASW standards and indicators for cultural competence in social work practice. Retrieved March 2, 2016, from http://www.socialworkers.org/practice/standards/PRA-BRO-253150-CC-Standards.pdf

SUBSTANCE ABUSE: PRENATAL

MAJOR CATEGORIES: Substance Abuse

WHAT WE KNOW

The use of illicit drugs, alcohol, tobacco, and prescription drugs other than as prescribed during pregnancy has negative ramifications for both mothers and their unborn children and is a significant public health concern.

The *Diagnostic and Statistical Manual of Mental Disorders*, 5 edition (*DSM-5*), replaced the terminology used in the *DSM-IV* (i.e., substance dependence and substance abuse) with substance use disorder (SUD), the severity of which (i.e., mild, moderate, or severe) is determined by the number of criteria that are endorsed. In research, and clinical and treatment settings, the language used to describe problematic consumption of substances changes over time, and varies greatly. Many terms have no specific definition, or may have different meanings in different settings (e.g., addiction in a medical setting might refer to the potential for physical withdrawal, whereas in a 12-step meeting addiction would have a unique meaning for each person in the meeting).

The 2013 National Survey on Drug Use and Health found that among pregnant women in the United States ages 15-44, 9.4 percent reported current alcohol use, 5.4 percent reported current use of illicit drugs, and 15.4 percent reported tobacco use within the past month. Although substantial, these rates are lower than those of non-pregnant females in the same age range, of whom 55.4 percent reported current alcohol use, 11.4 percent reported current use of illicit drugs, and 24.0 percent reported tobacco use within the past month.

Polysubstance abuse is common among women who use substances during pregnancy, including concurrent use of legal substances such as alcohol and tobacco that are potentially the most harmful to the developing fetus.

Data from the Infant Development, Environment, and Lifestyle Study (IDEAL), a longitudinal study of infants whose mothers used methamphetamine during pregnancy, have shown that:

Among women who used methamphetamine during pregnancy, the highest number (84.3 percent) reported using during the first trimester compared to 56.0 percent reporting use during the second trimester and 42.4 percent during the third trimester. 25.7 percent of women used at low to moderate levels throughout the pregnancy, 29.3 percent maintained consistently high levels of use, 35.6 percent reduced usage over the course of the pregnancy, and 9.4 percent showed an increase in use.

Almost 75 percent of women who used methamphetamine while pregnant met criteria for substance dependence, now identified in the fifth edition of the *DSM* as substance use disorder.

Ninety percent of the women reported using from one to five substances in addition to methamphetamine.

Women who continue using substances during pregnancy have been found to have higher levels of depression, anxiety, and novelty-seeking than those who stop using.

Women who abuse substances are widely recognized as having an array of psychosocial issues and often have more complex treatment needs than men who abuse substances.

Although substance use patterns among women vary globally, studies from several countries have found that women seeking treatment tend to have lower levels of education, employment, and income and more health, family, and social problems than men seeking treatment and are more likely than men to have substance-using partners, family histories of substance abuse, and personal histories of physical and sexual abuse. The majority also have co-occurring, untreated mental health issues.

Substance abuse among women is also associated with intimate partner violence, incarceration, homelessness, sexually transmitted diseases, and unplanned pregnancies.

Social disadvantage, including low levels of education and employment and not living with a spouse or partner, is associated with higher levels of psychosocial stress, substance use, and medical issues during pregnancy, such as low birth weight and early births.

Detrimental effects of prenatal substance exposure have been documented during fetal development, at birth, and in infancy; however, outcomes vary widely among individual children depending in part on the type and amount of substance(s) used, the stage(s) of pregnancy during which use occurred, and other factors related to substance use such as exposure to violence and inadequate maternal nutrition and prenatal care.

Prenatal substance exposure is associated with increased risk of medical complications such as placental abruption; intrauterine growth restriction, prematurity, and low birth weight; and increased risk of both maternal and child mortality.

Some drugs, in particular alcohol, may cause birth defects during the embryonic and fetal stages.

Substance-exposed newborns may have difficulty with orientation (e.g., difficulty responding to auditory and visual stimuli) and autonomic regulation (e.g., heart rate, breathing); and may have abnormal muscle tone (e.g., rigid or limp), poor alertness, increased startle response, tremors, and irritability.

Neonatal abstinence syndrome, in which babies are born dependent on drugs and withdrawal must be medically managed, is noted in the majority of infants who have been exposed to opiates and benzodiazepines.

Infants with signs of neonatal abstinence syndrome require special care including minimizing light, noise, and handling; swaddling; and small, frequent feedings.

Extended hospitalization may interfere with bonding between mother and child.

Fetal alcohol spectrum disorders (FASD) encompass a group of conditions resulting from prenatal alcohol exposure.

The use of alcohol during pregnancy has been identified as the leading preventable cause of mental retardation.

Although individual outcomes among infants vary and are influenced by an array of factors, maternal binge drinking (i.e., over 3 drinks at a time) is associated with particularly high risk.

Fetal alcohol syndrome (FAS) is diagnosed when three conditions are present in conjunction with a history of prenatal alcohol exposure: growth deficiency (i.e., at or below 10th percentile), characteristic facial abnormalities (e.g., smaller eye openings, smooth philtrum [the surface between the nose and the upper lip], thin upper lip), and central nervous system dysfunction (e.g., seizures, deficits in cognition, communication, memory, adaptive behavior, social skills, attention, academic achievement).

Prenatal substance exposure is associated with a heightened risk of long-term cognitive, language, and behavioral issues, school difficulties, and substance abuse among exposed children, although lasting effects may be subtle and difficult to differentiate from associated psychosocial issues.

Higher rates of prenatal cocaine exposure were associated with higher rates of attention-deficit/hyperactivity disorder in a sample of 5-year-old children, but no association was found with oppositional defiant disorder or separation anxiety disorder.

Prenatal substance exposure was associated with rates of behavior problems that were slightly higher than those among non-exposed youth in the California Long-Range Adoption Study, but this difference did not increase with age.

A review of 27 studies examining the effects of prenatal cocaine exposure on adolescents showed that the majority demonstrated small to medium effects on multiple areas of development that persisted from childhood but did not increase in adolescence.

A large, matched cohort study of children under the age of 3 years found associations between prenatal cocaine exposure and deficits in mental development and between opiate exposure and deficits in psychomotor development, but these differences were not significant once birth weight and other risk factors were controlled for.

Environmental risk factors associated with prenatal substance exposure such as poverty, low educational level, unemployment, homelessness or transient living situations, inadequate nutrition and healthcare, poor parenting, intimate partner violence, parental incarceration, and child maltreatment contribute to negative outcomes among children with a history of prenatal substance exposure.

Variability in the effects of prenatal substance exposure is strongly associated with the level of care the child receives following birth. The quality of the home environment plays a pivotal role in achieving positive developmental outcomes for children with a history of substance exposure.

A study of children with a history of prenatal cocaine exposure found that developmental outcomes at age 2 were predicted by the children's living situation and not prenatal exposure to cocaine. Those children in non-parental, non-kin care had more favorable outcomes and their homes scored higher on measures of caregiving environment.

The combination of traumatic stress combined with prenatal alcohol exposure has been found to have a significant impact on children's development, intelligence scores, and behavior.

Genetic factors may also play a role in that parents with substance use disorders also have higher rates of mental health disorders (e.g., attention-deficit/hyperactivity disorder, bipolar disorder, major depression, anxiety disorders), which are heritable and may affect children's functioning.

The United States Keeping Children and Families Safe Act of 2003 amended the Child Abuse Prevention & Treatment Act to require states to implement requirements that medical staff report children identified with prenatal exposure to substances to child protective services (CPS) and that plans be developed to ensure their safety.

Social workers should be aware of their state's statutes regarding mandatory reporting of newborns with prenatal substance exposure. Many, but not all, states have enacted laws that address substance use during pregnancy. Seventeen states include prenatal substance abuse in child welfare statutes and fifteen states mandate that suspected prenatal exposure be reported to child protective services.

Prenatal substance exposure alone does not determine the disposition of a CPS report, but the child welfare agency is mandated to complete a comprehensive assessment of the family's situation and implement safety planning as needed to ensure the child's safety.

As many as 21-50 percent of prenatal cocaine-exposed children are in nonparental care by the age of 2 years.

Substance use during pregnancy may be identified through screening and maternal self-report or through biological drug testing (i.e., urine, hair, or meconium), but under-identification is common with either approach.

Many controversies surround the testing of pregnant women for drug use. There are concerns about biased selection of women to be tested versus the expense of testing all pregnant women, about the limitations of testing in terms of contributing information meaningful to the care of the child, and concerns that possible legal consequences will prevent women from seeking care during pregnancy.

Universal screening of all women for risk of substance use and abuse is recommended in healthcare settings beginning in adolescence, before women become pregnant.

The Screening, Brief Intervention, and Referral for Treatment (SBIRT) protocol developed by the U.S. Substance Abuse and Mental Health Services Administration (SAMHSA) is used in many primary healthcare settings in the United States.

Several brief questionnaires have shown potential as screening tools, including T-ACE, T-ACER3, AUDIT-C, and TWEAK. T-ACE is noted as highly sensitive with all races, whereas TWEAK is less sensitive with races other than white.

Pregnancy can be a critical period for engaging women in treatment, building on motivating factors such as concern for the developing fetus and social pressures experienced as women become visibly pregnant.

Brief interventions such as motivational interviewing may be useful to assist women to resolve ambivalence about abstinence and to engage in treatment

Motivational interviewing, a directive counseling approach that seeks to facilitate behavioral change by exploring and resolving ambivalence about substance use and building on the individual's intrinsic motivation and commitment, has demonstrated effectiveness both as a freestanding intervention and in conjunction with other treatment.

Comprehensive, women-specific, culturally sensitive outpatient or residential treatment programs are recommended in order to address the complex service needs of pregnant and/or parenting women.

Programs should incorporate screening and treatment for issues commonly associated with substance abuse, including mental health conditions and intimate partner violence.

A survey of women entering substance abuse treatment within a year of pregnancy reported high rates

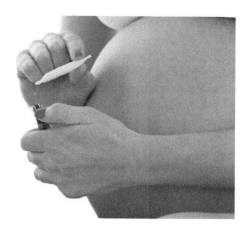

of mental health disorders (78 percent), past-year victimization (66 percent), and criminal justice system involvement (64 percent).

Medical support may be required for initial detoxification and stabilization when physical dependency on a substance is involved.

Treatment may not include total abstinence. Current practice for women who are dependent on opioids (e.g., heroin, oxycodone, morphine) is a maintenance program using carefully monitored levels of methadone or buprenorphine accompanied by counseling.

Potential clinical issues include shame and guilt regarding substance use during pregnancy and potential effects on the child; self-efficacy; and relationship issues, including the positive or negative impact of the woman's partner, rebuilding family relationships, and building a network of non-using supports.

Children's developmental and behavioral needs should be monitored on an ongoing basis. Children with prenatal substance exposure may need early intervention and other supportive services to address treatment of withdrawal, self-regulation, secure attachment, and attainment of developmentally appropriate motor, cognitive, speech, and language skills.

WHAT CAN BE DONE

Become knowledgeable about the impact of prenatal substance use, approaches for engaging women in treatment during pregnancy, and service needs of the substance-exposed child so you can accurately assess your client's unique characteristics and health education needs; gather information on local resources available for both mother and child.

Share information about prenatal substance use and local resources with your colleagues.

Ensure that parents and caregivers receive education regarding the effects of prenatal substance use on maternal nutrition and fetal development, the association of substance use with unplanned pregnancies and sexually transmitted diseases, and the needs of substance-exposed infants and children.

Develop an awareness of your own cultural values, beliefs, and biases and develop knowledge about the histories, traditions, and values of your clients. Adopt treatment methodologies that reflect the cultural needs of the client.

Assess safety, including risk for postpartum depression and suicidality. Follow state statutes regarding reporting procedures for infants who show evidence of prenatal substance exposure at birth and refer to child protective services when indicated. Up-to-date, state-by-state information about reporting requirements is available at http://www.guttmacher.org/statecenter/spibs/spib_SADP.pdf.

Provide factual information to pregnant women in a nonjudgmental manner. Refer to online resources for fact sheets and other educational materials

- Canadian Centre on Substance Abuse, http://www.ccsa.ca/eng/Pages/default.aspx.
- U.S. Centers for Disease Control and Prevention (CDC), http://www.cdc.gov/ncbddd/actearly/index.html.
- FAS aware UK, http://www.fasaware.co.uk/.
- Fetal Alcohol Spectrum Disorders Center for Excellence, content available in English and Spanish, http://fascenter.samhsa.gov/.
- Medline Plus, http://www.nlm.nih.gov/medlineplus/pregnancyandsubstanceabuse.html.
- National Organization on Fetal Alcohol Syndrome, http://www.nofas.org/.
- National Institute on Alcohol Abuse and Alcoholism, http://www.niaaa.nih.gov/.
- National Institute on Drug Abuse, http://www.drugabuse.gov/.

Written by Jennifer Teska, MSW

REFERENCES

American Psychiatric Association. (2013). Diagnostic and statistical manual of mental disorders: DSM-5. (5th ed.). American Psychiatric Publishing: Author.

Behnke, M., Smith, V. C., & Committee on Substance Abuse, and Committee on Fetus and Newborn. (2013). Prenatal substance abuse: Short- and long-term effects on the exposed fetus. *Pediatrics, 131*(3), e1009-e1024. doi:10.1542/peds.2012-3931

Brown, J. V., Bakeman, R., Coles, C. D., Platzman, K. A., & Lynch, M. E. (2004). Prenatal cocaine exposure: A comparison of 2-year-old children in parental and non-parental care. *Child Development, 75*(4), 1282-1295.

Buckingham-Howes, S., Berger, S. S., Scaletti, L. A., & Black, M. M. (2013). Systematic review of prenatal cocaine exposure and adolescent development. *Pediatrics, 131*(6), e1917-e1936. doi:10.1542/peds.2012-0945

Burns, E., Gray, R., & Smith, L. A. (2010). Brief screening questionnaires to identify problem drinking during pregnancy: A systematic review. *Addiction, 105*, 601-614. doi:10.1111/j.1360-0443.2009.02842.x

(n.d.). Improving treatment for drug-exposed infants (1993). *Center for Substance Abuse Treatment.* Rockville, MD: Substance Abuse and Mental Health Services Administration Treatment Improvement Protocol (TIP) Series, No. 5.

Chasnoff, I. J., McGourty, R. F., Bailey, G. W., HUtchins, E., Lightfoot, S. O., Pawson, L. L.,... Campbell, J. (2005). The 4P's Plus Screen for Substance Use in Pregnancy: Clinical application and outcomes. *Journal of Perinatology, 25*(6), 368-374.

Coleman-Cowger, V. H. (2012). Mental health treatment need among pregnant and postpartum women/girls entering substance abuse treatment. *Psychology of Addictive Behaviors, 26*(2), 345-350. doi:10.1037/a0025355

Crea, T. M., Guo, S., Barth, R. P., & Brooks, D. (2008). Behavioral outcomes for substance-exposed adopted children: Fourteen years postadoption. *American Journal of Orthopsychiatry, 78*(1), 11-19. doi:10.1037/0002-9432.78.1.11

Derauf, C., LaGasse, L. L., Smith, L. M., Grant, P., Smith, R., Arria, A.,... Lester, B. M. (2009). Demographic and psychosocial characteristics of mothers using methamphetamine during pregnancy: Preliminary results of the infant development, environment, and lifestyle study (IDEAL). *American Journal of Drug and Alcohol Abuse.* Retrieved from http://www.ncbi.nlm.nih.gov/pmc/articles/PMC2737408/pdf/nihms-118905.pdf

Gavin, A. R., Nurius, P., & Logan-Greene, P. (2012). Mediators of adverse birth outcomes among socially disadvantaged women. *Journal of Women's Health, 21*(6), 634-642. doi:10.1089/jwh.2011.2766

Goodman, D. J., & Wolff, K. B. (2013). Screening for substance abuse in women's health: A public health imperative. *Journal of Midwifery & Women's Health, 58*(3), 278-287. doi:10.1111/jmwh.12035

Grant, T. M., Brown, N. N., Dubovsky, D., Sparrow, J., & Ries, R. (2013). The impact of prenatal alcohol exposure on addiction treatment. *Journal of Addiction Medicine, 7*(2), 87-95. doi:10.1097/ADM.0b013e31828b47a8

Grotta, S. D., LaGasse, L. L., Arria, A. M., Derauf, C., Grant, P., Smith, L. M.,... Lester, B. M. (2009). Patterns of methamphetamine use during pregnancy: Results from the infant development, environment, and lifestyle (IDEAL) study. *Maternal and Child Health Journal, 14*(4), 519-527. doi:10.1007/s10995-009-0491-0

State policies in brief: Substance use during pregnancy. (2014). *Guttmacher Institute*. Retrieved November 8, 2015, from http://www.guttmacher.org/statecenter/spibs/spib_SADR.pdf

Hamilton, G. (2012). Neonatal abstinence syndrome as a consequence of prescription opioid use during pregnancy. *International Journal of Childbirth Education, 27*(3), 69-72.

Henry, J., Sloane, M., & Black-Pond, C. (2007). Neurobiology and neurodevelopmental impact of childhood traumatic stress and prenatal alcohol exposure. *Language, Speech, and Hearing Services in Schools, 38*(2), 99-108.

Statement of ethical principles. (2012). *International Federation of Social Workers*. Retrieved November 8, 2015, from http://ifsw.org/policies/statement-of-ethical-principles/

Jones, H. E. (2006). Drug addiction during pregnancy: Advances in maternal treatment and understanding child outcomes. *Current Directions in Psychological Science, 15*(3), 126-130. doi:10.1111/j.0963-7214.2006.00421.x

Jones, T. B., Bailey, B. A., & Sokol, R. J. (2013). Alcohol use in pregnancy: Insights in screening and intervention for the clinician. *Clinical Obstetrics and Gynecology, 56*(1), 114-123. doi:10.1097/GRF.0b013e31827957c0

Massey, S. H., Lieberman, D. Z., Reiss, D., Leve, L. D., Shaw, D. S., & Neiderhiser, J. M. (2010). Association of clinical characteristics and cessation of tobacco, alcohol, and illicit drug use during pregnancy. *The American Journal on Addictions, 20*(2), 143-150. doi:10.1111/j.1521-0391.2010.00110.x

Messinger, D. S., Bauer, C. R., Das, A., Seifer, R., Lester, B. M.,... Poole, W. K. (2004). The maternal lifestyle study: Cognitive, motor, and behavioral outcomes of cocaine-exposed and opiate-exposed infants through three years of age. *Pediatrics, 113*(6), 1677-1685.

Milligan, K., Niccols, A., Sword, W., Thabane, L., Henderson, J., & Smith, A. (2011). Birth outcomes for infants born to women participating in integrated substance abuse treatment programs: A meta-analytic review. *Addiction Research and Theory, 19*(6), 542-555. doi:10.3109/16066359.2010.545153

Mizrahi, T., & Mayden, R. W. (2001). NASW standards for cultural competency in social work practice. Retrieved November 8, 2015, from http://www.socialworkers.org/practice/standards/NASWCulturalStandards.pdf

Morrow, C. E., Accornero, V. H., Xue, L., Manjunath, S., Culbertson, J. L., Anthony, J. C., & Bandstra, E. S. (2009). Estimated risk of developing selected DSM-IV disorders among 5-year old children with prenatal cocaine exposure. *Journal of Child & Family Studies, 18*(3), 356-364. doi:10.1007/s10826-008-9238-6

Price, A., Bergin, C., Luby, C., Watson, E., Squires, J.,... Little, C. (2012). Implementing Child Abuse Prevention and Treatment Act (CAPTA) requirements to serve substance-exposed newborns: Lessons from a collective case study of four program models. *Journal of Public Child Welfare, 6*(2), 149-171. doi:10.1080/15548732.2012.667730

Substance Abuse and Mental Health Services Administration. (2013). Results from the 2013 national survey on drugs and health: Summary of national findings. NSDUH Series H-48, HHS Publications No. (SMA) 14-4863. Rockville, MD: Substance Abuse and Mental Health Services Administration. Retrieved from http://www.samhsa.gov/data/NSDUH/2012SummNatFindDetTables/NationalFindings/NSDUHresults2012.pdf

Sun, A. (2004). Principles for practice with substance-abusing pregnant women: A framework based on the five social work intervention roles. *Social Work, 49*(3), 383-394.

British Association of Social Workers. (2012). The code of ethics for social workers: Statement of principles. Retrieved November 8, 2015, from http://cdn.basw.co.uk/upload/basw_112315-7.pdf

Substance abuse treatment and care for women: Case studies and lessons learned. (Chapter 1: Women, gender and substance use problems, pp. 5-16). NY: United Nations Publication, Sales No. E04.XI.24. (2004). *United Nations Office on Drugs and Crime.* Retrieved from http://www.unodc.org/pdf/report_2004-08-30_1.pdf

Mittal, L. (2014). Buprenorphine for the treatment of opioid dependence in pregnancy. *Journal of Perinatal & Neonatal Nursing, 28*(3), 178-184.

Brocato, C. L. (2015). Managing opioid addiction in pregnancy. *The Clinical Advisor, 18*(10), 28-35.

American Psychiatric Association. (2013). Diagnostic and statistical manual of mental health disorders (DSM-5). (5th ed.). Arlington, VA: American Psychiatric Publishing.

SUBSTANCE ABUSE: CLUB DRUGS—ECSTASY

MAJOR CATEGORIES: Substance Abuse

DESCRIPTION

Club drugs are a group of recreational drugs used primarily by teenage persons and young adults, often at bars, nightclubs, concerts, and all-night dance parties called *raves*. The U.S. Office of National Drug Control Policy identifies four specific club drugs, known respectively as 3,4-methylenedioxymethamphetamine (MDMA; Ecstasy), gamma-hydroxybutyrate (GHB), ketamine, and flunitrazepam (Rohypnol). Ecstasy, one of the most popular club drugs, is illegal in the United States, where it is classified according to the Controlled Substances Act of 1970 as a Schedule I drug, meaning that it has the potential for abuse and is not accepted for medical use. It is a synthetic drug that has both stimulant and hallucinogenic properties, and produces feelings of increased energy and euphoria, as well as distortions in the senses of time and perception, and enhanced pleasure from physical experiences. Chemically, Ecstasy is similar to the stimulant drug methamphetamine and to the hallucinogenic drug mescaline. Street names for Ecstasy include XTC, E, X, Adam(s), and beans, and Ecstasy is also called the "hug" drug, the "love" drug, and the "feel-good" drug. Ecstasy is commonly called "Molly," which is a slang term for "molecular" and refers to the pure crystalline form of MDMA (National Institute on Drug Abuse, 2016).

Ecstasy is distributed almost exclusively in the form of tablets or pills, but is also available in capsule, liquid, and powder form. Tablets of Ecstasy vary in color and are often stamped with emblems, such as cartoon characters, and with words. Until recently, Ecstasy was produced primarily in Western Europe, but the primary source of its production is now Canada, from which it is smuggled into the United States by mail and in cargo, luggage, and body carriers.

The effects of Ecstasy are both physical and psychological. It increases the activity of the substances known as serotonin, dopamine, and norepinephrine, which act in the brain and other parts of the nervous system as neurotransmitters, conveying signals between nerve cells (National Institute on Drug Abuse, 2016). In doing this, Ecstasy primarily affects the parts of the brain and nervous system in which serotonin acts as the sole or primary neurotransmitter, also known as the serotoninergic nervous system. Ecstasy exerts its effects by inducing the release of serotonin by nerve cells and blocking their reuptake of this neurotransmitter substance. The serotoninergic system in which Ecstasy chiefly exerts its effects plays an important role in regulating sleep, mood, aggression, sensitivity to pain, and sexual activity.

An increased release of dopamine, which is another effect of Ecstasy, accompanying its effect on serotonin, causes euphoria and increased energy, while a surge in the release of of norepinephrine, also caused by Ecstasy, increases the heartbeat or rate of pumping of blood by the heart and therefore raises the body's blood pressure. The effects of Ecstasy may be intensified by the concurrent ingestion of alcohol and other drugs. Acute dangers of Ecstasy include coma and death from a sharp increase in body temperature (hyperthermia) combined with dehydration, resulting in liver, kidney, and heart failure. The use of Ecstasy also poses a serious risk of addiction and of permanently damaging the serotoninergic nervous system, and is associated with effects that include loss of appetite, depressed mood, fatigue, and difficulty in concentration.

The Fifth Edition of the *Diagnostic and Statistical Manual of Mental Disorders* (*DSM-V*) classifies Ecstasy as a hallucinogenic drug or hallucinogen. A clinical diagnosis of hallucinogen use disorder (HUD) according to the *DSM-5* requires a recurrent pattern of use of such a drug, within a 12-month period, that adversely affects personal functioning. The criteria for an HUD include a problematic pattern of use of a hallucinogen for at least 12 months that causes significant distress or impairment and includes at least two of the following standards: consumption of a hallucinogen in larger amounts and over a longer period than was intended; a desire or unsuccessful attempts to reduce or control one's use of it; the spending of large periods of time on activities related to obtaining, using, and recovery from its effects; cravings for it; inability to meet obligations at home, work, or school as a consequence of its use; its continued use in the face of social or interpersonal problems; the abandonment of social, recreational, or occupational activities as an effect of it; and its continued use even when this causes physical or psychological problems (American Psychiatric Association, 2013). Successful management of an HUD includes a medical evaluation, detoxification, treatment for substance abuse, recovery from drug abuse, participation in a recovery support group, and cognitive behavioral therapy (CBT).

Ecstasy is considered a public-health concern because it is associated with aggressive behavior, impaired operation of a motor vehicle, and risky sexual behavior. Ecstasy is often used together with other drugs such as ketamine, GHB, and with drugs for correcting erectile dysfunction such as sildenafil citrate (Viagra). Its use is associated with increased sexual activity because it enhances the release of neurotransmitters linked to pleasure, and effects including an increased sense of confidence, decreased inhibition, and compromised decision-making have strongly correlated the use of Ecstasy with the sexual transmission of human immunodeficiency virus (HIV) (National Institute on Drug Abuse, 2005).

FACTS AND FIGURES

Data from the 2014 National Survey on Drug Use and Health indicate that in 2014, approximately 0.2 percent of adolescents aged from 12 to 17 years in the United States used Ecstasy, as did 0.8 percent of young adults aged 18 to 25 years and 0.1 percent of adults aged 26 or older (Substance Abuse and Mental Health Services Administration, 2015). According to the 2015 Monitoring the Future survey, conducted by the Institute for Social Research at the University of Michigan, 0.9 percent of 8th-grade, 2.3 percent of 10th-grade, and 3.6 percent of 12th-grade students in the United States used Ecstasy during 2015 (National Institute on Drug Abuse, 2015). According to the Drug Abuse Warning Network (DAWN), created and operated until 2011 by the U.S. Substance Abuse and Mental Health Services Administration (SAMHSA), the period from 2005 to 2011 saw a 128 percent increase in emergency department visits involving Ecstasy among Americans younger than 21 years old, with approximately 33 percent of these visits also involving alcohol (Substance Abuse and Mental Health Services Administration, 2013).

RISK FACTORS

Risk factors for the use of Ecstasy include psychological distress, delinquency, previous drug use, low educational attainment, and being a male who has sex with other males.

SIGNS AND SYMPTOMS

Physical effects of Ecstasy begin within 20 to 40 minutes of its consumption and last for up to 8 hours. They include heightened sensory awareness, a decreased appetite, dilation of the pupils, sweating, mild psychomotor restlessness, hypertension, hyperthermia, sleep disturbance, tremors, liver toxicity, nausea, muscle cramping, blurred vision, chills, and involuntary clenching of the jaws, and Ecstasy users often suck on lollipops or pacifiers to relieve tension in their jaws. Psychological effects of Ecstasy include euphoria, a positive mood, anxiety, depression, agitation, paranoia, and irritability. Behavioral effects of Ecstasy increased impulsivity and energy, and aggression, and its social effects include increased empathy, self-confidence, feelings of connectedness with others, and friendliness. Although Ecstasy increases the sensuality of sexual experience and the desire for sex, it creates difficulty in achieving sexual arousal and orgasm.

APPLICABLE LAWS AND REGULATIONS

The pharmacological and medical name for Ecstasy, 3,4-Methylenedioxymethamphetamine (MDMA), was patented by the Merck corporation in 1914 in Darmstadt, Germany (Shulgin, 1986), to be used as a blood-clotting agent, but was never approved for public release (Bernschneider-Reif & Freudenmann, 2006). In the 1950s and 1960s, psychiatrists used MDMA to facilitate communication with patients in the formation of therapeutic relationships, but this was done without the approval of MDMA by the U.S. Food and Drug Administration or the investigation of its properties in controlled clinical trials. In the United States MDMA was legal until July 1, 1985, when it was made a Schedule I drug under the U.S. Controlled Substances Act of 1970, on the basis of its lacking tbherapeutic value and having a high potential for abuse (U.S. Department of Justice, n.d.). In 2015 the U.S. Drug Enforcement Administration (DEA) approved the first clinical trial of MDMA in combination with psychotherapy to treat anxiety among persons with life-threatening illnesses, in an attempt to obtain FDA approval for MDMA as a prescription medication by 2021 (Lewis, 2015).

TREATMENT

The social worker of an individual with a known or suspected HUD involving Ecstasy should conduct a complete biological, developmental, psychological, emotional, and medical, mental-health, social, and spiritual assessment of the individual and of his or her family. This is essential for an accurate diagnosis, appropriate case management, and successful treatment of an HUD, and should include a thorough history of the individual's use of drugs, including prescription medications, illicit drugs, and alcohol; an evaluation for risk factors associated with the use of Ecstasy; and a medical/mental health history of the individual's family. The social worker should explore whether the individual considers his or her drug use problematic, and ask the individual about mood fluctuations, irritability, depression, feelings of worthlessness, and suicidal ideation. It is also important that the social worker explore possible barriers to treatment (e.g., housing, health insurance, transportation, expenses) and provide referrals to ease such barriers.

An individual undergoing assessment and who meets the criteria for having an HUD should be referred for drug testing, medical evaluation, and a drug treatment protocol in which a multidisciplinary team provides comprehensive treatment for the individual's HUD. However, because MDMA is rapidly excreted in urine and not easily detected in the blood, routine toxicology screening tests may not be helpful in establishing its recent use.

Skills training can help individuals with an HUD to cope with stress, and a 12-step recovery group, harm-reduction treatment, or motivational enhancement therapy can also help toward recovery from an HUD. Cognitive behavioral interventions in substance abuse disorder (SUD) and HUD are designed to modify an affected individual's behaviors, thinking, and expectancies related to his or her drug use, and training in alternative coping skills and CBT addressing deficits in coping skills can help an individual who is engaging in risk-taking behavior and exhibiting poor judgment.

Motivational interviewing (MI), a treatment technique defined as a "collab-orative, person-centered form of guiding to elicit and strengthen motivation for change" may also be helpful for individuals with an HUD (Miller & Rollnick, 2009). This technique is based on collaboration with such and individual, as opposed to confrontation; the drawing out of the individual's ideas about change, as opposed to the imposition of ideas on the individual; and emphasis on the individual's autonomy. Motivation enhancement therapy (MET) is a specific application of MI that can be effective in the treatment of SUDs. It focuses on helping the individual with an SUD to acknowledge and accept his or her responsibility to change the behavior that contributes to the SUD and uses a variety of approaches to increase social support of the individual's abstinence, including the improvement of social interactional patterns to reinforce and promote sobriety.

Social workers assisting individuals with an HUD should be aware of their own cultural values, beliefs, and biases, and develop specialized knowledge about the histories, traditions, and values of these individuals. They should adopt treatment methods that reflect their knowledge of the cultural diversity of the communities in which these individuals live.

SERVICES AND RESOURCES

The following resources can provide information about Ecstasy:

- National Institute on Drug Abuse (enter ecstasy, Molly, etc. in the search box), 1-877-643-2644, https://www.drugabuse.gov/
- Teen Drug Abuse, http://www.teens.drugabuse.gov
- Secular Organizations for Sobriety (SOS), http://www.cfiwest.org/sos/index.htm
- Harm Reduction Coalition, http://harmreduction.org
- Club Drug Clinic, http://clubdrugclinic.cnwl.nhs.uk/

Written by Laura McLuckey, MSW, LCSW, and Melissa Rosales Neff, MSW

Reviewed by Lynn B. Cooper, D. Crim, and Chris Bates, MA, MSW

REFERENCES

American Psychiatric Association. (2013). Substance-related and addictive disorders. *Diagnostic and Statistical Manual of Mental Disorders* (5th ed.). Arlington, VA: Author.

Bernschneider-Reif, S., & Freudenmann, R. W. (2006). The origin of MDMA ("ecstasy") – separating the facts from the myth. *Pharmazie, 61*(11), 966-972.

Boone, M. R., Cook, S. H., & Wilson, P. (2013). Substance use and sexual risk behavior in HIV-positive men who have sex with men: An episode-level analysis. *AIDS Behavior, 17*(5), 1883-1887. doi:10.1007/s10461-012-0167-4

British Association of Social Workers, & British Association of Social Workers. (2012, January). The Code of Ethics of Social Work. Retrieved June 21, 2016, from http://cdn.basw.co.uk/upload/basw_112315-7.pdf

Britt, G., & McCance-Katz, E. (2005). A brief overview of the clinical pharmacology of "club drugs". *Substance Use and Misuse, 40*(9-10), 1189-1201.

Downey, L. A., Sands, H., Jones, L., Clow, A., Evans, P., Stalder, T., & Parrott, A. C. (2015). Reduced memory skills and increased hair cortisol levels in recent Ecstasy/MDMA users: Significant but independent neurocognitive and neurohormonal deficits. *Human Psychopharmacology, 30*(3), 199-207.

Engstrom, M., Mahoney, C. A., & Marsh, J. C. (2012). Substance use problems in health social work practice. In S. Gehlert & T. Arthur Browne (Eds.), *Handbook of health social work* (2nd ed., pp. 426-427). Hoboken, NJ: Wiley.

Gripenberg-Abdon, J., Elgan, T. H., Wallin, E., Shaafati, M., Beck, O., & Andreasson, S. (2012). Measuring substance use in the club setting: A feasibility study using biochemical markers. *Substance Abuse Treatment Prevention Policy, 7*, 7. doi:10.1186/1747-597X-7-7

Hibell, B., Guttormsson, U., Ahlstrom, S., Balakireva, O., Bjarnason, A., & Kraus, L. (2011). The 2011 ESPAD report: Substance use among students in 36 European countries.

International Federation of Social Workers. (2012, March 3). Statement of ethical principles. Retrieved June 21, 2016, from http://ifsw.org/policies/statement-of-ethical-principles/

Johnston, L. D., O'Malley, P. M., Miech, R. A., Bachman, J. G., & Schulenberg, J. E. (2014). Monitoring the Future national results on drug use 1975-2013: Overview Key Findings on Adolescent Drug Use. Ann Arbor, MI: Institute for Social Research, The University of Michigan.

Koesters, S. C., Rogers, P. D., & Rajasingham, C. R. (2002). MDMA ('ecstasy') and other 'club drugs.' The new epidemic. *Pediatric Clinics of North America, 49*(2), 415-433.

Legislation.gov.uk. Misuse of drugs act 1971. Retrieved June 22, 2016, from http://www.legislation.gov.uk/ukpga/1971/38/contents

Lewis, R. (2015). DEA approves study using MDMA for anxiety in seriously ill patients. Retrieved June 22, 2016, from http://america.aljazeera.com/articles/2015/3/17/clinical-trial-approved-for-mdma-psychotherapy.html

Matthews, A. J., Bruno, R., Dietze, P., Butler, K., & Burns, L. (2014). Driving under the influence among frequent ecstasy consumers in Australia: Trends over time and the role of risk perceptions. *Drug and Alcohol Dependence, 144*(1), 218-224. doi:10.1016/j.drugalcdep.2014.09.015

McDowell, D. (2006). Club drugs and their treatment. *Psychiatric Times, 23*(1), 83-87.

McGinn, C. (2005). Close calls with club drugs. *New England Journal of Medicine, 352*(26), 2671-2672. doi:10.1056/NEJMp058107

McKetin, R., Copeland, J., Norberg, M., Bruno, R., Hides, L., & Khawar, L. (2014). The effect of the ecstasy 'come-down' on the diagnosis of ecstasy dependence. *Drug and Alcohol Dependence, 139*(1), 26-32. doi:10.1016/j.drugalcdep.2014.02.697

Miller, E. R., & Rollnick, S. (2009). Ten things that Motivational Interviewing is not. *Behavioural and Cognitive Psychotherapy, 37*(2), 129-140. doi:10.1017/S1352465809005128

Mizrahi, T., & Mayden, R. W. (2001). NASW standards for cultural competency in social work practice. Retrieved October 17, 2015, from http://www.socialworkers.org/practice/standards/NASWCulturalStandards.pdf

National Association of Social Workers. (2008). Code of ethics. Retrieved June 21, 2016, from https://www.socialworkers.org/pubs/code/code.asp

National Institute on Drug Abuse (NIH). (2005). Learn the link – Drugs and HIV. Retrieved June 21, 2016, from https://www.drugabuse.gov/news-events/public-education-projects/learn-link-drugs-hiv

National Institute on Drug Abuse. (2015). Monitoring the future 2015 survey results. Retrieved July 6, 2016, from https://www.drugabuse.gov/related-topics/trends-statistics/infographics/monitoring-future-2015-survey-results

National Institute on Drug Abuse (NIH). (2016). Drug facts: MDMA (Ecstasy/Molly). Retrieved June 21, 2016, from https://www.drugabuse.gov/publications/drugfacts/mdma-ecstasymolly

Substance Abuse and Mental Health Services Administration (SAMHSA). (2015). Behavioral health trends in the United States: Results from the 2014 national survey on drug use and health

Norber, M. M., Hides, L., Olivier, J., Khawar, L., McKetin, R., & Copeland, J. (2014). Brief interventions to reduce ecstasy use: A multi-site randomized controlled trial. *Behavior Therapy, 45*(6), 745-759. doi:10.1016/j.beth.2014.05.006

Office of National Drug Control Policy. (2013). A 21st century drug policy. Retrieved June 21, 2016, from https://www.whitehouse.gov/sites/default/files/ondcp/policy-and-research/2013_strategy_fact_sheet.pdf

Office of National Drug Control Policy. (2013). Countering the spread of synthetic drugs- MDMA/Ecstasy. Retrieved June 21, 2016, from http://www.whitehouse.gov/ondcp/synthetic-drugs

Office for National Statistics. (2015). Crime in England and Wales: Year ending March 2015. Retrieved June 22, 2016, from http://www.ons.gov.uk/peoplepopulationandcommunity/crimeandjustice/bulletins/crimeinenglandandwales/2015-07-16

Office for National Statistics. (2015). Deaths related to drug poisoning in England and Wales, 2014 registrations. Retrieved June 22, 2016, from http://webarchive.nationalarchives.gov.uk/20160105160709/http://www.ons.gov.uk/ons/dcp171778_414574.pdf

Pathania, R. (2015). Therapeutic potential of psychedelic agents. *Journal of Mental Science, 206*(5), 433-436.

Roberts, C. A., Wetherell, M. A., Fisk, J. E., & Montgomery, C. (2014). Differences in prefrontal blood oxygenation during an acute multitasking stressor in ecstasy polydrug users. *Psychological Medicine, 45*(2), 395-406. doi:10.1017/S0033291714001500

Scott, R. M., Hides, L., Allen, J. S., & Lubman, D. I. (2013). Coping style and ecstasy use motives as predictors of current mood symptoms in ecstasy users. *Addictive Behaviors, 38*(10), 2465-2472. doi:10.1016/j.addbeh.2013.05.005

Smirnov, A., Najman, J. M., Hayatbakhsh, R., Wells, H., Legosz, M., & Kemp, R. (2013). Young adults' recreational social environment as a predictor of ecstasy use initiation: Findings of a population-based prospective study. *Addiction, 108*(10), 1809-1817. doi:10.1111/add.12239

Substance Abuse and Mental Health Services Administration. (2013). Drug abuse warning network, 2011: National estimates of drug-related emergency department visits. HHS Publication 13-4760, DAWN Series D-39. *HHS Publication 13-4760, DAWN Series D-39.* Rockville, MD: Author

Substance Abuse and Mental Health Services Administration. (2014). Behavioral Health Trends in the United States: Results from the 2014 National Survey on Drug Use and Health.

Taffe, M. A., Huitron-Resendiz, S., Schroeder, R., Parsons, L. H., Henriksen, S. J., & Gold, L. H. (2003). MDMA exposure alters cognitive and electrophysiological sensitivity to rapid tryptophan depletion in Rhesus monkeys. *Pharmacology Biochemistry and Behavior, 76*(1), 141-152.

United Nations Office on Drugs and Crime. (2013). World drug report 2013. Retrieved June 21, 2016, from http://www.unodc.org/unodc/secured/wdr/wdr2013/World_Drug_Report_2013.pdf

U.S. Department of Justice. Controlled substances schedules. Retrieved June 21, 2016, from http://www.deadiversion.usdoj.gov/schedules/

Zuckerman, M. D., & Boyer, E. W. (2012). HIV and club drugs in emerging adulthood. *Current Opinion in Pediatrics, 24*(2), 219-224. doi:10.1097/MOP.0b013e32834faa9b

SUBSTANCE ABUSE: CLUB DRUGS—GHB

MAJOR CATEGORIES: Substance Abuse

DESCRIPTION

Club drugs are a group of psychotropic chemical substances also known as *recreational drugs* and used illicitly, often by teenagers and young adults and often at bars, nightclubs, concerts, and all-night dance parties called *raves*. Most club drugs distort perception, behavior, and mental function to some degree, ranging from impaired judgment to loss of memory, and the patterns of use of these drugs have expanded to include locations, circumstances, and users other than those implied by the name "club drugs." The U.S. Office of National Drug Control Policy identifies four specific club drugs: gamma-hydroxybutyrate (GHB), ketamine, 3,4-methylenedioxy-methamphetamine (MDMA, Ecstasy), and flunitrazepam (Rohypnol).

Gamma-hydroxybutyrate is a central nervous system (CNS) depressant initially synthesized for medical use, to treat conditions such as insomnia, clinical depression, the disorder known as narcolepsy, which is marked by an extreme tendency to fall asleep under relaxed circumstances, and the condition known as cataplexy, in which strong emotion or laughter causes sudden physical collapse without loss of consciousness (National Institute on Drug Abuse [NIDA], 2010). Gamma-hydroxybutyrate is approved by the U.S. Food and Drug Administration (FDA) for treating both narcolepsy and cataplexy, for which it is sold under the brand name of Xyrem and several other brand names, and it is used medically outside the United States to treat alcoholism.

As a club drug, GHB is used for its euphoric and sedative effects, and is used illegally by some athletes to aid in fat reduction and in muscle building because of its ability to increase the body's production of human growth hormone. It is known as a "date rape drug" because its sedative effects have led to its use to facilitate drug-related sexual assaults. Street names for GHB include "Scoop," "Easy Lay," "Chemical X," "Get-Her-to-Bed," "Liquid Dream," "Georgia Home Boy," "Grievous Bodily Harm," and "Liquid Ecstasy," although GHB is chemically unrelated to the club drug known as Ecstasy, for which MDMA is the abbreviated chemical name. Gamma-hydroxybutyrate is inexpensive and may be sold illicitly as a powder, often in the form of a gummy ball called a Booger, or as a colorless and odorless liquid that is virtually undetectable when diluted with other liquids. Overdosing of GHB is fairly common and can result in nausea, vomiting, muscle stiffness, confusion, seizures, the rapid heartbeat known as tachycardia, high blood pressure, and coma, with coma and death as particular risks when GHB is consumed together with alcohol or other drugs that depress the CNS.

The illegal use of club drugs in Western countries has increased over the past 20 years and is becoming an issue worldwide. With the use of chemicals found in household products, over-the-counter medications, and prescription drugs, the production of club drugs is inexpensive, making them easily accessible.

FACTS AND FIGURES

The U.S. Substance Abuse and Mental Health Services Administration (SAMHSA) reported 2,406 GHB-related visits to emergency rooms in 2011, with most of these visits made by White and male individuals (SAMHSA, 2013). However, overdoses of GHB and toxic incidents related to it are believed to be grossly underreported. The NIDA-funded 2014 Monitoring the Future survey, conducted by the Institute for Social Research at the University of Michigan, showed that in 2011, 0.6 percent of 8th-grade, 0.5 percent of 10th-grade, and 1.4 percent of

12th-grade students in the United States had used GHB. In 2014, the only data available were for 12th graders, among whom the rate of use of GHB had declined to 1.0 percent (Johnston et al., 2015). Between 1990 and 2015, 72 deaths resulting from GHB and 15,600 overdoses of it were reported in the United States (HealthResearchFunding.org, 2015).

RISK FACTORS

Research on risk factors for the use of club drugs, including GHB, has been limited. However, many behaviors associated with the use of GHB (e.g., attendance at clubs, raves, or concerts; use by peers) may be considered as risk factors for its use.

SIGNS AND SYMPTOMS

Psychological effects of GHB, as reported by users, include euphoria and an altered mental state. However, GHB can also cause hallucinations, insomnia, and amnesia, and

has been described as a sensual drug, inducing a feeling of pleasant disinhibition and numbness, which may account for reports of its ability to enhance sexual pleasure.

Behaviorally, GHB increases risk-taking and induces a loss of inhibition. Users commonly awaken from GHB-induced sleep without recall of events that occurred while they were under the influence of GHB. Physical effects of GHB begin from 15 to 30 minutes after its intake and last for approximately 4 hours. Low doses make users feel more sociable, less inhibited, and euphoric. Higher doses intensify these effects and can cause drowsiness and dizziness. Physically, GHB can cause tremors, sweating, slurred speech, and headache.

APPLICABLE LAWS AND REGULATIONS

During the 1980s, GHB was legally sold over the counter and used to enhance athletic performance, decrease body fat, and build muscle, but the FDA banned it in 1990 on the basis of its adverse effects (CampusHealthandSafety.org, n.d.).

TREATMENT

A complete biological, psychological, social, and spiritual assessment is helpful in understanding the extent and nature of a substance use disorder (SUD) such as that involving the use of GHB and the interaction of such a disorder with other aspects of the life of the user. This is essential for the accurate diagnosis, appropriate management, and successful treatment of an SUD. Individuals who meet the criteria for an SUD should be asked to provide a thorough history of their drug use, types of drugs used, and frequency of their use. In this content, it is important to know that GHB is rapidly excreted in urine and is not easily detected in the blood, and that routine toxicology screening tests may not be helpful in establishing its recent use.

Also requiring careful consideration in the diagnosis of SUDs is their frequent coexistence with personality disorders, anxiety and depression. To ensure that important information is obtained in an assessment, social workers and other providers of care for persons who may have an SUD should use standardized screening tools, assessment instruments, and interview protocols that have been established for the population to which these persons belong (e.g., adolescents, adults). A medical evaluation is important for persons with an SUD involving GHB because withdrawal from its use can produce physical effects that need to be addressed in a medical setting, such as an inpatient detoxification program. It is also important to explore barriers to treatment (e.g., housing, health insurance, transportation, financial) of individuals with SUDs and refer them services that can help overcome such barriers. Individuals at risk for drug-facilitated sexual assault should be advised about the need to closely monitor their food and drink in settings in which illicit drugs are used, such as at raves and clubs. They should be taught the signs and symptoms of GHB intoxication, and encouraged to adopt a "buddy system" in which friends and family members can assist in monitoring for the use and effects of illicit drugs.

Successful treatment of an SUD for GHB includes a medical evaluation, detoxification if necessary, psychotherapy and/or behavioral therapy for the SUD, medicinal treatment if needed, and support in a recovery group. A detoxification and drug treatment program provided by a multidisciplinary team to address the sleep difficulties, depression, and anxiety usually associated with use of GHB can be highly effective.

Cognitive behavioral therapy designed to help modify self-destructive thinking and behavior related to substance use, and to increase skills in coping with life stressors, is an important part of assistance toward a drug-free lifestyle. Also used in the treatment of an SUD, and contrasting with the more conventional treatment goal of abstinence, is the harm-reduction model, a motivational technique that attempts to minimize the hazards associated with the use of psychoactive drugs, rather than preventing their use.

Another technique for treating SUDs, which has been evaluated in more than 200 clinical trials and has been reported to have positive outcomes, is motivational interviewing (MI). This technique has three key elements, consisting of collaboration with the individual being treated (as opposed to confrontation), drawing out the individual's ideas about change (as opposed to imposing ideas on the treated individual), and emphasis on the treated individual's autonomy, and has been described as "a collaborative, person-centered form of guiding to elicit and strengthen motivation for change" (Miller et al., 2009). The MI model tends to involve fewer sessions than conventional psychotherapy, making it more cost effective.

Social workers assisting persons with an SUD, such as that involving GHB, should be aware of their own cultural values, beliefs, and biases, and develop specialized knowledge about the histories, traditions, and values of the individuals whom they seek to assist. They should adopt treatment methods that reflect their knowledge of the cultural diversity of these individuals and the societies in which they live.

SERVICES AND RESOURCES

The following resources can provide information about GHB and its effects:

- National Institute on Drug Abuse (NIDA), 1-877-643-2644, http://www.nida.nih.gov/DrugPages/Clubdrugs.html
- NIDA for Teens: the Science Behind Drug Abuse website, http://www.teens.drugabuse.gov
- Substance Abuse and Mental Health Services Administration (SAMHSA), http://store.samhsa.gov/home
- Harm Reduction Coalition, http://harmreduction.org/

Written by Laura McLuckey, MSW, LCSW, and Chris Bates, MA, MSW

Reviewed by Lynn B. Cooper, D. Crim, and Laura Gale, LCSW

REFERENCES

British Association of Social Workers. (2012). *The code of ethics for social work: Statement of principles.* Retrieved March 28, 2016, from http://cdn.basw.co.uk/upload/basw_112315-7.pdf

CampusHealthandSafety.org. (n.d.). Date rape and club drugs. Retrieved March 28, 2016, from http://campushealthandsafety.org/drugs/club-drugs/

Substance Abuse and Mental Health Services Administration. (2013). Drug Abuse Warning Network, 2011: National estimates of drug-related emergency department visits.

Engstrom, M., Mahoney, C. A., & Marsh, J. C. (2012). Substance use problems in health social work practice. In S. Gehlert & T. Arthur Browne (Eds.), *Handbook of health social work* (2nd ed., pp. 426-427). Hoboken, NJ: Wiley.

HealthResearchFunding.org. (2015, February 15). 17 remarkable GHB statistics. Retrieved March 28, 2016, from http://healthresearchfunding.org/17-remarkable-ghb-death-statistics/

International Federation of Social Workers. (2012, March 3). Statement of ethical principles. Retrieved March 28, 2016, from http://ifsw.org/policies/statement-of-ethical-principles/

Johnston, L. D., O'Malley, P. M., Miech, R. A., Bachman, J. G., & Schulenberg, J. E. (2014). Monitoring the future: National results on drug use 1975-2013: Overview key findings on adolescent drug use. Ann Arbor, MI: Institute for Social Research, The University of Michigan.

Johnston, L. D., O'Malley, D. M., Miech, R. A., Bachman, J. G., & Schulenberg, J. E. (2015). Monitoring the Future national survey results on drug use: 1975-2014 overview, key findings on adolescent drug use. Retrieved from http://www.monitoringthefuture.org/pubs/monographs/mtf-overview2014.pdf

Kamal, R. M., van Iwaarden, S., Dijkstra, B. A. G., & de Jong, C. A. J. (2014). Decision rules for GHB (gamma-hydroxybutyric acid) detoxification: A vignette study. *Drug and Alcohol Dependence, 135,* 146-151. doi:10.1016/j.drugalcdep.2013.12.003

McDowell, D. (2006). Club drugs and their treatment. *Psychiatric Times, 23*(1), 83-86.

McGinn, C. (2005). Close calls with club drugs. *New England Journal of Medicine, 352*(26), 2671-2672. doi:10.1056/NEJMp058107

Miller, E. R., & Rollnick, S. (2009). Ten things that Motivational Interviewing is not. *Behavioural and Cognitive Psychotherapy, 37*(2), 129-140. doi:10.1017/S1352465809005128

National Association of Social Workers. (2013). NASW standards for social work practice with clients with substance use disorders. Retrieved March 28, 2016, from http://www.socialworkers.org/practice/standards/NASWATODStatndards.pdf

National Institute on Drug Abuse. (2012). NIDA InfoFacts: Club drugs (GHB, ketamine, and Rohypnol). Retrieved March 28, 2016, from http://www.drugabuse.gov/drugs-abuse/club-drugs

Talbert, J. J. (2014). Club drugs: Coming to a patient near you. *The Nurse Practitioner, 39*(3), 20-26. doi:10.1097/01.NPR.0000443227.72357.72

Wheeler, D. (2015). NASW standards for cultural competence in social work practice. Retrieved March 28, 2016, from http://www.socialworkers.org/practice/standards/PRA-BRO-253150-CC-Standards.pd

SUBSTANCE ABUSE: CLUB DRUGS—ROHYPNOL

MAJOR CATEGORIES: Substance Abuse

DESCRIPTION

Club drugs are a group of recreational drugs used primarily by young adults, and often at all-night dance parties called *raves*, although the patterns of use of these drugs have evolved to include locations, circumstances, and users unrelated to those implied by the term "club drugs." The most commonly used club drugs are flunitrazepam (Rohypnol), ketamine, gamma-hydroxybutyrate (GHB), and 3,4-methylenedioxymethamphetamine (MDMA; "ecstasy").

Rohypnol is the trade name of the drug whose medicinal or pharmacological name is flunitrazepam. Flunitrazepam was developed for the short-term treatment of insomnia, as a premedication in surgical procedures, and for inducing anesthesia. It belongs to the family of psychoactive drugs known as benzodiazepines (of which Valium [diazepam] and Librium [chlordiazepoxide] are also members) and acts as a central nervous system (CNS) depressant, with sedative effects that are from 7 to 10 times stronger than those of Valium, and also has amnesic effects. Flunitrazepam is approved for medical use in more than 60 countries, and in Europe and South America is primarily used as a hypnotic or sedative drug, but is not legally available in the United States. into which it is smuggled primarily from Europe, South America, and Mexico, and where its illicit use began in the 1990s (Addiction Search, 2015). Under its trade name of Rohypnol, however, flunitrazepam is a popular club drug and has potent sedative and amnesic properties. Tablets of Rohypnol are often distributed on the street in bubble packaging, giving them an appearance of legitimacy and legality, and are usually sold for $2 to $4 each. The "street names" of Rohypnol include "circles," "roaches," "rib," "forget pills," "R2," "Mexican valium," and "roofies," with the last of these nicknames being perhaps the best known.

Rohypnol is usually taken orally, but can also be snorted into the nostrils, injected, or dissolved in beverages. It is odorless, tasteless, and virtually undetectable if diluted with liquid. The ability of Rohypnol to be undetected has led to its use in drug-facilitated sexual assaults. Because of this, the manufacturer added a blue dye to each tablet of Rohypnol that is released when the tablet is placed in liquid, allowing the drug to be detected.

Rohypnol has both physical and psychological effects, which may be intensified by the ingestion of alcohol and other drugs that depress the CNS when these drugs are used together with it, and can cause death when used in combination with such drugs. Rohypnol has been linked to a wide range of adverse physical and mental effects, including decreased blood pressure and body temperature, impaired cognitive and psychomotor function, dizziness, confusion, and gastrointestinal disturbance. Symptoms of withdrawal from Rohypnol include headaches, confusion, muscle pain, and hallucinations. Seizures may occur up to a week after users abstain from the drug. Additionally, and as noted earlier, Rohypnol has been used to facilitate drug-related sexual assaults because it causes profound sedation, and as noted above, can cause amnesia, leading to its having been given the name of a "date rape" drug.

As with other benzodiazepines, the prolonged use of Rohypnol can produce tolerance, in which increasing doses are required in order to experience its effects; dependence on it, in which the user becomes needful of it in order to continue to function; and addiction to it, in which the user becomes completely dependent on it. The Fifth Edition of the *Diagnostic and Statistical Manual of Mental Disorders* (*DSM-V*) includes flunitrazepam, the pharmacological name for Rohypnol, among the group of drugs with sedative, hypnotic, or anxiolytic activity. The *DSM-V* describes a disorder associated with the use of these drugs, including benzodiazepines, carbamates, and barbiturates, as a recurrent pattern of their use within a 12-month period that has an adverse effect on functioning or causes distress. The *DSM-5* divides the disorders related to the use of these drugs into the two categories named "substance use disorders" (SUD) and "substance-induced disorders" (e.g., intoxication, withdrawal), and further divides each of these two categories into mild, moderate, and severe subtypes.

Because withdrawal from benzodiazepines can be life-threatening, treatment for addiction to Rohypnol typically involves admission to a hospital and 3 to 5 days of detoxification with 24-hour intensive medical monitoring and management of withdrawal symptoms.

FACTS AND FIGURES

According to the 2014 Monitoring the Future survey, conducted by the Institute for Social Research at the University of Michigan, the annual prevalence of use of Rohypnol among 8th-, 10th-, and 12th-grade students in the United States declined slightly for all three groups from 2013 to 2014 (by –0.1 percent, –0.1 percent, and –0.2 percent, respectively), continuing a trend of stability of its use among 8th- and 10th-grade students and a trend of decline in its use among 12th graders (Johnston et al., 2015).

RISK FACTORS

Risk factors for using Rohypnol include attendance at raves or participation in a club setting in which illicit drugs are used, the consumption of alcohol or other drugs, and an inclination toward risk-taking behaviors.

SIGNS AND SYMPTOMS

Psychological effects of Rohypnol include euphoria, hallucinations, insomnia, and amnesia, with social effects including reduced anxiety and disinhibition. Behavioral effects of Rohypnol include impaired judgment, fearlessness, and aggressive behavior. The onset of effects of Rohypnol is rapid, occurring within 15 to 20 minutes of its ingestion, and its effects last for up to 12 hours. At low doses it produces muscle relaxation and sedation, and at higher doses causes visual disturbances, nausea, vomiting, problems of gait, memory loss, difficulty with motor function and speech, blackouts, coma, respiratory arrest, and death.

APPLICABLE LAWS AND REGULATIONS

Under the international Convention on Psychotropic Substances of 1971, which the United Nations drafted and adopted for the control of psychoactive substances, Rohypnol is classified as a Schedule III drug, within the category of barbiturates with medical uses and serious potential for abuse.

In 1984 Rohypnol was classified in the United States under the Controlled Substances Act as a Schedule IV drug, with a low potential for abuse and low risk of inducing dependence. However, according to the Drug Enforcement Administration (DEA), the possession, trafficking, and distribution of a gram or more of Rohypnol carries the same penalties as those for Schedule I drugs (i.e., drugs with high potential for abuse, no medical use, with possible severe dependence, and the highest levels of penalties).

In 1996 the United States Congress passed the Drug-Induced Rape Prevention and Punishment Act, which allows harsh penalties for persons who administer a controlled substance to another person without the latter person's knowledge or consent and with the intent of committing a criminal act. In the United States, any use, administration, or distribution of Rohypnol that causes death or serious injury can result in a lifelong prison term.

TREATMENT

The social worker of an individual with a known or suspected SUD involving Rohypnol should conduct a complete biological, psychological, social, and spiritual assessment of the individual. This should include a mental-health history, an evaluation for risk factors associated with the use of Rohypnol, and a thorough history of the individual's drug use, including the types of drugs used and frequency of their use, and the individual's risk for self harm or harm to others. This is essential for an accurate diagnosis of mental, physical, and drug-related disorders and for their appropriate management and successful treatment, particularly because SUDs often coexist with personality disorders, anxiety, and depression. Although Rohypnol is not included in standard urine drug screens, and is rapidly excreted in urine, laboratories that can test for its presence in urine can detect it for up to 72 hours after its ingestion.

To ensure the collection of important information from an individual with an SUD involving Rohypnol, the social worker should use standardized screening tools, assessment instruments, and interview protocols that have been established for the population to which the individual belongs (e.g., adolescents, adults). It is also important that the social worker explore possible barriers to such individuals' treatment (e.g., problems with housing, health insurance, transportation, expenses) and provide referrals for medical evaluation, drug treatment, and comprehensive multidisciplinary therapy.

Counseling of an individual with an SUD involving Rohypnol should include identifying triggers for his or her substance use, discussing alternatives to drug use, and helping the individual to improve his or her coping and problem-solving skills. Cognitive behavioral interventions designed to help modify behaviors, thinking, and expectancies related to drug use, and to increase skills in coping with life stressors, can help individuals with an SUD involving Rohypnol toward a drug-free lifestyle. Also used in treating the illicit use of Rohypnol and other drugs is the harm-reduction model. This contrasts with the traditional goal of abstinence from the use of illicit drugs, such as that in "zero tolerance" policies and 12-step-based practices, and instead uses a motivational approach to minimize rather than prevent the use of such drugs.

Social workers of individuals with SUDs involving Rohypnol and other illicit drugs should provide them with referrals to substance-abuse treatment programs, mental- health services, and recovery support groups as appropriate, to support their long-term drug-free recovery. These individuals may also need referrals for pregnancy testing and testing for HIV, hepatitis, and other sexually transmitted diseases. Social workers involved in this work should be aware of their own cultural values, beliefs, and biases, and develop specialized knowledge about the histories, traditions, and values of persons with SUDs. They should adopt treatment methods that reflect their knowledge of the cultural diversity of the communities in which these persons live.

SERVICES AND RESOURCES

The following resources can provide information about Rohypnol:

- National Institute on Drug Abuse, 1-877-643-2644, http://www.drugabuse.gov/drugs-abuse/club-drugs
- Teen Drug Abuse, http://www.teens.drugabuse.gov
- Substance Abuse and Mental Health Services Administration (SAMHSA), http://store.samhsa.gov/home
- Harm Reduction International, www.ihra.net/

Written by Laura McLuckey, MSW, LCSW

Reviewed by Lynn B. Cooper, D. Crim

REFERENCES

American Psychiatric Association. (2013). Diagnostic and statistical manual of mental disorders. In (5th ed., pp. 50-59). Arlington, VA: American Psychiatric Publishing.

Beynon, C. M., McVeigh, C., McVeigh, J., Leavey, C., & Bellis, M. A. (2008). The involvement of drugs and alcohol in drug-facilitated sexual assault: A systematic review of the evidence. *Trauma, Violence, and Abuse, 9*(3), 178-188.

British Association of Social Workers. (2012). The code of ethics for social work: Statement of principles. Retrieved March 29, 2016, from http://cdn.basw.co.uk/upload/basw_112315-7.pdf

Britt, G., & McCance-Katz, E. (2005). A brief overview of the clinical pharmacology of "club drugs". *Substance Use and Misuse, 40*(9-10), 1189-1201. doi:10.1081/JA-200066730

Gahlinger, M. P. (2004, June). Club drugs: MDMA, gamma-hydroxybutyrate (GHB), Rohypnol, and ketamine. *American Family Physician, 69*, 11. Retrieved March 24, 2014, from http://aafp.org/afp/2004/0601/p2619.html

International Federation of Social Workers. (2012). Statement of ethical principles. Retrieved March 29, 2016, from http://ifsw.org/policies/statement-of-ethical-principles/

Johnston, L. D., O'Malley, P. M., Miech, R. A., Bachman, J. G., & Schulenberg, J. E. (2015). Monitoring the Future national survey results on drug use: 1975-2014 overview, key findings on adolescent drug use. Ann Arbor, MI: Institute for Social Research, University of Michigan. Retrieved March 29, 2016, from http://www.monitoringthefuture.org/pubs/monographs/mtf-overview2014.pdf

McGinn, C. (2005). Close calls with club drugs. *New England Journal of Medicine, 352*(26), 2671-2672.

Mizrahi, T., & Mayden, R. W. (2001). NASW standards for cultural competence in social work practice. Retrieved March 29, 2016, from http://www.socialworkers.org/practice/standards/NASWCulturalStandards.pdf

National Institute on Drug Abuse. (2012, December). NIDA Info Facts: Club Drugs (GHB, Ketamine, and Rohypnol). Retrieved March 29, 2016, from https://www.drugabuse.gov/drugs-abuse/club-drugs

Ricaurte, G. A., & McCann, U. D. (2005). Recognition and management of complications of new recreational drug use. *Lancet, 365*(9477), 2137-2145.

Rohypnol addiction and abuse. (2015). *Addiction Search.* Retrieved from http://www.addiction-search.com/treatment_articles/article/rohypnol-addiction-and-abuse_26.html

Substance Abuse: Club Drugs & "Raves"

Major Categories: Substance Abuse

Description

Club drugs are a group of recreational drugs used primarily by teenagers and young adults, often at bars, nightclubs, concerts, and all-night dance parties called *raves*, although evolving patterns indicate that both the users of such drugs and the circumstances and locations of their use extend beyond those implied by the name *club drugs*. These drugs often are illegally diverted from laboratories, smuggled into the United States by mail or airline courier from other countries, and sold through the Internet. They are generally inexpensive to purchase, and are usually ingested orally, but can be snorted or inhaled into the nostrils, smoked, or injected.

The effects of club drugs are both physical and psychological, and may be intensified because their use is often accompanied by the ingestion of alcohol and other drugs. The prolonged use of club drugs can produce tolerance, dependence, and addiction.

The U.S. Office of National Drug Control Policy identifies four specific club drugs: 3-methylenedioxymethamphetamine (MDMA; Ecstasy), gamma-hydroxybutyrate (GHB), ketamine, and flunitrazepam (Rohypnol). Club drugs are often used to increase social interaction, libido, and energy; to enhance sensory perception; or because these drugs are thought to be safer and less addictive than "harder" drugs (e.g., cocaine, methamphetamine, heroin). Most club drugs cause some degree of temporary mental distortion, ranging from impaired judgment to memory loss. The effects of MDMA include sense of well-being, a sensation of empathy and emotional warmth for others, mental stimulation, and diminished anxiety. Through their ability to sedate and incapacitate unsuspecting victims, both GHB and Rohypnol have been used to commit the sexual assault also known as "date rape." Ketamine, known medically as a dissociative anesthetic, distorts perceptions of sight and sound and induces a sense of detachment from the environment and the self.

The Fifth Edition of the *Diagnostic and Statistical Manual of Mental Disorders* (*DSM-V*), published in 2013, removes the distinction between substance abuse and substance dependence that was used in the fourth edition of the manual (*DSM-IV*). It combines these two categories of disorder under the single heading of *substance use disorder* (SUD), which it defines as a recurrent pattern of use of a substance within a 12-month period that adversely affects functioning or causes distress (American Psychiatric Association, 2013). The *DSM-V* includes Rohypnol and GHB among sedative, hypnotic, or anxiolytic substances. Ketamine appears under the new classification of *phencyclidine use disorder* in the *DSM-V*, and

Ecstasy is included in the category of *other hallucinogen use disorder.*

Raves, which began in the 1980s in England, are among the most popular settings in which club drugs are distributed. They feature the fast, pounding electronic dance music known as techno music, choreographed laser-light shows, and manufactured fog, and often draw very large crowds of adolescents and young adults. Raves often take place in nightclubs, bars, open fields, or warehouses. Initially, raves were invitation-only dance parties, often held in gay clubs. Typically the location of the venue of a rave was kept secret until the night of the event, leading the rave culture to be described as an underground movement. Raves subsequently became increasingly popular, and in the late 1980s emerged in the United States. Rave parties now take place throughout the United States and in other countries around the world, and are characterized by the use of club drugs, overpriced bottled water, and "chill rooms" to help dancers cool down. Although they began in metropolitan areas, raves are now increasingly found in rural areas.

The rave culture is highly promoted, publicized, and commercialized. Its promoters maximize the profits gained from raves by using these gatherings to market clothes, toys, drugs, and music. Promoters of raves capitalize on the effects of club drugs, and often sell water, juice, and sports drinks at inflated prices to manage the dehydration and hypothermia that these drugs can cause. They may also sell lollipops and pacifiers to prevent the involuntary clenching of the teeth that is another effect of club drugs, and sell menthol nasal inhalers, medicated and scented salves to ease breathing, and other devices for enhancing the sensory effects of club drugs. Attendance at raves can range from 30 persons to tens of thousands, depending on the size of the venue in which a rave is held. Their attendees often pay a high entrance fee to dance in dark, often poorly ventilated rooms on overcrowded dance floors.

FACTS AND FIGURES

Under the United States Controlled Substances Act, which was enacted into law as Title II of the Comprehensive Drug Abuse Prevention and Control Act of 1970, club drugs are classified into one of five schedules according to their potential for abuse, risk of dependence, and medical utility. Thus, GHB and ketamine are classified as belonging under Schedule III, MDMA under Schedule I, and Rohypnol under Schedule IV.

According to the 2015 U.S. Monitoring the Future survey, conducted by the Institute for Social Research at the University of Michigan, use of ecstasy among 8th-, 10th-, and 12th-grade students in the United States stabilized or declined between 2010 and 2015. The prevalences of use of Rohypnol, GHB, and ketamine in 2015 were respectively 1 percent for 8th graders, 0.7 percent for 10th graders, and 1.4 percent for 12th graders (Johnston et al., 2016).

Group sex is associated with SUDs, and in a study of club-drug users in Miami, 46.3 percent of the male and 33.7 percent of the female study participants disclosed having had group-sex experiences after using such drugs (Buttram et al., 2015). Also found have been higher rates of sexually transmitted infection among club-drug users, and especially among HIV-infected men who have sex with other men, than among those who do not use such drugs (Rowlands et al., 2014; Sullivan, 2015).

RISK FACTORS

As is the case with all drugs, the use of club drugs carries various risks. Gamma-hydroxybutyrate reduces inhibition, can increase the libido, or sex drive, and can cause extreme euphoria, in addition to impairing memory and causing dizziness and drowsiness. Its ability to incapacitate those who ingest it is the reason for its having become known as a "date-rape" drug. This same property also applies to Rohypnol, which ios highly addictive even when used for a short period, and can interfere with memory, cause mood swings and loss of consciousness, interfere with motor skills and vision, and reduce the body's rates of heartbeat and breathing. Ketamine, which is used medically as an anesthetic agent, creates the mental state known as dissociation, in which perception of one's physical surroundings is distorted or severed. It can also cause amnesia and interfere with movement of the body. Other adverse effects of ketamine include muscle rigicidity, a rapid heart rate, increased blood pressure, respiratory depression, and vomiting. Adverse effects of MDMA include altered perception, an increased heart rate and blood pressure, which in some cases can be fatal, as well as muscle cramping, dangerous increases in body temperature, blurring of vision, nausea, sweating, and chills.

SIGNS AND SYMPTOMS

Psychological signs and symptoms of the use of MDMA, GHB, ketamine, and Rohypnol include euphoria, amnesia, impaired judgment, confusion, anxiety, depression, and paranoia. Social effects of these drugs include an increased sense of empathy, self-confidence, social/interpersonal connectedness, and friendliness. Behavioral effects of MDMA, GHB, ketamine, and Rohypnol include increased risk-taking behavior, including increased impulsivity and an increased frequency of unsafe sex, an increased risk of sexually transmitted diseases, anterograde amnesia (i.e., the inability to transfer current events into long-term memory), and the risk among these drugs' users of date rape. Physically, the drugs effects have a rapid onset, typically occurring within an hour after their consumption, with a varied duration of action.

APPLICABLE LAWS AND REGULATIONS

Both GHB and Rohypnol induce anterograde amnesia, or loss of the ability to retain memories after the occurrence of a particular event, such as an injury to the brain or the taking of a drug that acts on the brain, and it is this property that has led to the use of these drugs to facilitate sexual access to another person, as in the case of "date rape." The United States Drug-Induced Rape Prevention and Punishment Act of 1996 allows harsh penalties for giving a controlled substance such as GHB or Rohypnol without the knowledge or consent of the person to whom they are given and for the purpose of committing a criminal act. Local laws and professional requirements for reporting the abuse of these drugs should be known and observed.

TREATMENT

The social worker of an individual with a known or suspected SUD involving MDMA, GHB, ketamine, or Rohypnol should conduct a complete biological, psychological, social, and spiritual assessment of the individual. This should include a mental-health history, an evaluation for participation in the milieu of club drugs, risk factors associated with the use of these drugs, and a thorough history of the individual's drug use, including the types of drugs used and frequency of their use, an evaluation for persistent physical complaints such as fatigue and a persistent cough, and questioning about mood fluctuations, irritability, depression, feelings of worthlessness, and suicidal ideation. This is essential for the accurate identification

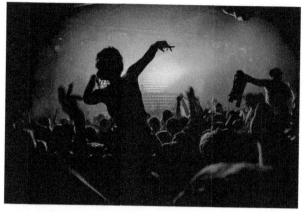

of club-drug use and its individual effects, and for diagnosis of the personality disorders, anxiety, depression, and other mental disorders that often coexist with SUDs. Because club drugs are often excreted rapidly in urine and are not easily detectable in blood, specialized tests may be needed for their detection.

It is important to concurrently treat both SUDs involving club drugs and the disorders of mental health that may accompany these SUDs, in order to avoid sending individuals with these two types of problem from having to attend both substance-abuse and mental-health treatment facilities. This can be accomplished through a program that works with a multidisciplinary team to provide comprehensive treatment of both an SUD and an accompanying psychiatric disorder. It also is important to explore possible barriers to treatment (e.g., housing, health insurance, transportation, finances) among individuals with these disorders and to provide referrals that can ease or eliminate such barriers.

Psychotherapy for an individual with an SUD involving club drugs is directed at identifying and changing troubling or self-destructive emotions, thoughts, and behavior,

and can be provided through one or more of several techniques, such as psychoanalysis, behavior therapy for the modification of behavior, cognitive therapy directed at changing an individual's thoughts and beliefs, humanistic therapy to improve an individual's reasoning and personal achiement, and cognitive behavioral therapy (CBT). Cognitive behavioral interventions for SUD are designed to help modify behaviors, thinking, and expectations related to an individual's drug use, and to increase skills important for coping with life stressors and supporting a drug-free lifestyle. Thus, the treatment of club-drug user who exhibits risk-taking behavior, poor judgment, and ignorance of the consequences of using club drugs might involve CBT addressing deficits in interpersonal and social skills, brief motivational interviewing addressing the consequences of substance use, and the suggestion and practice of alternative behaviors and habits.

Another approach to treating SUD uses the harm-reduction model. This motivational approach aims to increase the desire for better health and well-being and minimize the potential hazards associated with alcohol and drug use. The harm-reduction model contrasts with the more traditional treatment goal of abstinence, as in "zero tolerance" policies and 12-step-based practices; rather than requiring total abstinence, it instead promotes changes in behavior that will decrease harm to the individual who has chosen to engage in high-risk behavior.

Social workers assisting individuals with an SUD involving club drugs should be aware of their own cultural values, beliefs, and biases, and develop specialized knowledge about these individuals' histories, traditions, and values. They should adopt treatment methods that reflect their knowledge of the cultural diversity of the communities in which they practice.

SERVICES AND RESOURCES

The following resources can provide information about club drugs, their effects, and the treatment of these effects:

- National Institute on Drug Abuse (NIDA), 1-877-643-2644, https://www.drugabuse.gov/drugs-abuse/club-drugs
- NIDA for Teens, http://www.teens.drugabuse.gov
- Substance Abuse and Mental Health Services Administration (SAMHSA), http://www.samhsa.gov/
- Harm Reduction International, http://www.ihra.net/?no-splash=true

Written by Laura McLuckey, MSW, LCSW

Reviewed by Lynn B. Cooper, D. Crim, and Melissa Rosales Neff, MSW

REFERENCES

American Psychiatric Association. (2013). *Diagnostic and statistical manual of mental disorders: DSM-5* (5th ed.). Washington, DC: Author.

Bao, Y., Liu, Z., Li, J., Zhang, R., Hao, W., Zhao, M., ... Lu, L. (2015). Club drug use and associated high-risk sexual behavior in six provinces in China. *Addiction, 110*(1), 11-19. doi:10.1111/add.12770. pmid:25533860

British Association of Social Workers. (2012). *The code of ethics for social work: Statement of principles.* Retrieved April 12, 2016, from http://cdn.basw.co.uk/upload/basw_112315-7.pdf

Buttram, M., & Kurtz, S. (2015). Characteristics associated with group sex participation among men and women in the club drug scene. *Sexual Health, 12,* 560-562. doi:10.1071/SH15071

Conner, L. C., Wiener, J., Lewis, J. V., Phill, R., Peralta, L., Chandwani, S., & Koenig, L. J. (2013). Prevalence and predictors of drug use among adolescents with HIV infection acquired perinatally or later in life. *AIDS Behavior, 17*(3), 976-986. doi:10.1007/s10461-011-9950-x

Ding, Y., He, N., Shoptaw, S., Gao, M., & Detels, R. (2014). Severity of club drug dependence and perceived need for treatment among a sample of adult club drug users in Shanghai, China. *Social Psychiatry & Psychiatric Epidemiology, 49*(3), 395-404. doi:10.1007/s00127-013-0713-z

International Federation of Social Workers. (2012, March 3). Statement of ethical principles. Retrieved April 12, 2016, from http://ifsw.org/policies/statement-of-ethical-principles/

Johnston, L. D., O'Malley, P. M., Miech, R. A., Bachman, J. G., & Schulenberg, J. E. (2016). Monitoring the Future national survey results on drug use, 1975-2015: Overview, key findings on adolescent drug use. Ann Arbor, MI: Institute for Social Research, The University of Michigan.

Lea, T., Prestage, G., Mao, L., Zablotska, I., de Wit, J., & Holt, M. (2013). Trends in drug use among gay and bisexual men in Sydney, Melbourne and Queensland, Australia. *Drug and Alcohol Review, 32*(1), 39-46. doi:10.1111/j.1465-3362.2012.00494.x

National Association of Social Workers. (2008). Code of ethics. Retrieved April 4, 2016, from https://www.socialworkers.org/pubs/code/code.asp

Shimane, T., Hidaka, Y., Wada, K., & Funada, M. (2013). Ecstasy (3,4-methylenedioxymethamphetamine) use among Japanese rave population. *Psychiatry and Clinical Neurosciences, 67*(1), 12-19. doi:10.1111/j.1440-1819.2012.02402.x

Talbert, J. J. (2014). Club drugs: Coming to a patient near you. *The Nurse Practitioner, 39*(3), 20-26. doi:10.1097/01.NPR.0000443227.72357.72

Wheeler, D. (2015). NASW standards and indicators for cultural competence in social work practice. Retrieved March 2, 2016, from http://www.socialworkers.org/practice/standards/PRA-BRO-253150-CC-Standards.pdf

SUBSTANCE ABUSE: HARM REDUCTION

MAJOR CATEGORIES: Substance Abuse

DESCRIPTION

Harm reduction (HR) refers to any program, policy, or intervention that seeks to reduce or minimize adverse consequences of drug or alcohol use. It has been an established practice for decades, although only recently implemented in the United States. Strategies of HR are directed at individuals, families, and communities, with the goal of minimizing the negative effects of drugs and alcohol.

There are no universally defined strategies for HR, nor is there any established protocol for implementing them. Instead, HR is a philosophy built on a belief in and respect for the human rights of individuals who use drugs and alcohol, in addition to findings from evidence-based research that reducing the consumption of alcohol or drugs reduces the adverse effects of their use. The idea of meeting substance users "where they are," without requiring their abstinence from substance use, is a key component of HR and consistent with the belief in self-determination (National Association of Social Workers [NASW], 2013). The concept of HR recognizes that the use of alcohol and drugs (licit or illicit) is a reality, but is directed at minimizing its adverse consequences. Its goal is to promote changes in behavior that will decrease the harm done to the individual who continues to use substances, even when their use is excessive. This approach contrasts with the treatment goal of abstinence as reflected in "zero tolerance" policies and 12-step-based practices.

Harm reduction was first implemented in the late 1980s in Europe, Australia, and Canada. The movement for HR began in response to treatment systems that tended to be overwhelmingly punitive and judgmental toward drug users and heavy drinkers, and in 1996 the International Harm Reduction Association was created with the goal of advancing HR policies around the world.

The pragmatic approach of HR focuses on promoting health (e.g., supporting the prevention and treatment of infections such as that by human immunodeficiency virus [HIV]), and on social issues (e.g., countering social exclusion and stigma), on issues of justice (e.g., decriminalizing drug use), and economic issues (e.g., unemployment as a root cause of drug abuse, ineffective drug-containment policies). Examples of strategies for HR include hypodermic needle exchange and education for injection-drug users, to limit exposure to diseases transmitted via blood; methadone treatment programs for stabilizing the lives of individuals addicted to opiates, removing them from the danger and unpredictability of acquiring drugs illegally, and encouraging their education about and treatment for drug use; and the increased availability of naloxone, an opiate antagonist that rapidly counteracts the effects of opiates, and in the hands of persons trained in its safe and correct use, can be lifesaving in the event of opiate overdosage. Other strategies used in HR include voluntary counseling about and testing for HIV, education toward preventing drug use, the promotion of designated drivers as replacements for those who are intoxicated, sex education, and the distribution of condoms in schools.

Although popular in many European countries, the concept of HR for reducing or minimizing adverse consequences of drug or alcohol use has been less well received in the United States, where it remains controversial. Many individuals, particularly those with a conservative religious and/or political viewpoint, believe that efforts toward HR provide social approval for the abuse of drugs and alcohol and can have a negative effect on communities. As a result, they oppose large-scale efforts for HR, such as needle- exchange programs and condom distribution in schools. However, the societal stigma once associated with addiction to drugs and/or alcohol is being replaced with recognition that such addiction is a brain disease rather than a lack of individual self-control, and the frequent use of federal funding for drug treatment and other programs that seek to reduce harm has made HR an increasingly studied concept.

FACTS AND FIGURES

The overall cost of substance abuse in the United States, including losses in productivity and health- and crime-related costs, is estimated to exceed $600 billion annually (NIDA, 2012). During 2014 1.5 million persons in the United States were arrested on charges of non-violent drug-related behavior, and 47,055 persons died of drug overdoses (Drug Policy Alliance, n.d.). According to the U.S. Substance Abuse and Mental Health Services Administration, more than 7.9 million perons have both a disorder of mental health and a substance use disorder (SAMSHA, 2016).

Needle-exchange programs for the purpose of HR can significantly decrease the incidence of infection with hepatitis C virus, which is the most common chronic infectious disease among injection-drug users, and can have consequences that include cirrhosis, liver cancer, and liver failure (Smith-Spangler & Asch, 2012).

RISK FACTORS

Environmental, behavioral, mental, and genetic factors, as well as risk factors (e.g., drug availability, peer pressure, poverty) and protective factors (e.g., strong family and social attachments, academic competence, employability skills), influence the use of drugs and alcohol. Limiting the risks for it while enhancing the factors that countyeract it will help reduce substance abuse. Neurochemical changes in the brain induced by exposure to drugs and alcohol contribute to the development of drug- and/or alcohol-related problems. The earlier an individual begins using substances the greater the risk that he or she will develop substance-related problems. The abuse of drugs and alcohol is associated with many adverse consequences, from physical and psychological problems such as cirrhosis, mental aberratons, and accidents or injuries occurring during intoxication, to problems with interpersonal relationships, employment, and the criminal justice system. The

acquisition of drugs and alcohol often poses additional risks, through their users' exposure to potentially dangerous situations and environments.

SIGNS AND SYMPTOMS

Psychological effects of the use of drugs and alcohol include depression, elation, anxiety, and disorganized ideation. Its behavioral effects include irresponsibility, illegal and criminal dangerous behavior. Sexual effects of the use of drugs and alcohol can include high-risk sexual behavior, and the physical effects of their use can include changes in appetite or sleep patterns, weight loss or gain, changes in physical appearance, tremors, slurred speech, impaired coordination, increased drug and alcohol tolerance, and physical dependence or addiction. Social effects of drug and/or alcohol abuse include relational problems, loss of friends, isolation, neglect of responsibilities, abuse and neglect of children, and divorce.

APPLICABLE LAWS AND REGULATIONS

In December 2009, President Obama signed legislation that allowed federal funding of needle exchange programs both domestically and abroad with the goal of stopping the spread of HIV and other infections among drug users.

As of January 2017, 37 states and the District of Columbia had implemented 911 Good Samaritan Laws to encourage persons who thought they might have given themselves an overdose of a drug, or who sought treatment with naloxone for a drug overdose, to call their local emergency medical service at 911 for help without a penalty for their use of the drug in question, as long as the police obtain evidence for this only through the 911 call.

TREATMENT

The social worker engaged in an HR program should conduct a comprehensive biological, psychological, social, and spiritual assessment of individuals being considered for enrollment in it to include information on physical, mental, environmental, social, and financial factors in their lives. The social worker should ask these individuals about any history of physical/sexual/emotional abuse or neglect in their lives, exposure to violence or other trauma, family history, level of functioning; history of psychiatric symptoms, disorders. or issues that pose a risk to the individual or others (e.g., self-harm, thoughts about and/or attempts at suicide); family and community supports; and history of psychotropic medication. The social worker should evaluate the individual being assessed for risk factors associated with the use of drugs and alcohol (e.g., risk-taking behaviors, family history of drug or alcohol abuse, inadequate or unhealthy social or family attachment), and if family members are present, should obtain as much information from them as possible. Standardized tests (e.g., urine, breathalyzer, blood) can be administered to screen for drugs and alcohol in individuals being considered for enrollment in an HR program.

A complete psychological assessment is helpful for understanding the extent and nature of a substance use disorder (SUD) and its interaction with other aspects of the life of the affected individual. This is essential for the careful diagnosis, appropriate case management, and successful treatment of an SUD. Substance use disorders often coexist with disorders of mental health, and in such cases it is important to treat both disorders at the same time to prevent the affected individual from being sent back and forth between facilities for treating substance abuse and those that treat disorders of mental health. The possibility of this happening can be reduced by the use of standardized screening tools, assessment instruments, and interview protocols that have been established for the population being served (e.g., adolescents, adults). It is also important to explore barriers to treatment (e.g., housing, health insurance, transportation, cost) and to provide referrals to ameliorate potential obstacles.

The social worker assisting an individual with an SUD should provide referrals to programs for treating such disorders, mental-health services, and recovery support groups to support his or her long-term drug-free recovery. The social worker can refer such individuals as indicated for pregnancy testing and testing for HIV, hepatitis, and other sexually transmitted diseases. Individuals who exhibit risk-taking behavior, poor judgment, and disregard of the consequences of an SUD involving drugs or alcohol can be referred for cognitive behavioral therapy (CBT) to increase their knowledge of the disorder and its effects, increase their self-efficacy and self-esteem, and develop alternative coping skills. Those who meet the criteria for a moderate or severe substance use disorder can be referred for a medical evaluation and enrollment in a drug treatment program in which a multidisciplinary team provides comprehensive treatment.

Currently, the HR model is being used in limited settings in the United States for treating illicit drug and alcohol use, with the goal of increasing the users' desire for greater health and well-being. It often includes a comprehensive behavioral support plan that contains multiple strategies (e.g., motivational interviewing and cognitive-behavioral skills training) to address problem behaviors. Thus, for example, Harm reduction, Abstinence, and Moderation Support (HAMS) focuses on reducing alcohol consumption through peer-led support groups for individuals who recognize alcohol yet recognize that they have a problem with alcohol consumption and want to change.

Social workers assisting individuals who have an SUD should be aware of their own cultural values, beliefs, and biases, and develop specialized knowledge about the histories, traditions, and values of these individuals. They should adopt treatment methodologies that reflect their knowledge of the cultural diversity of the communities in which they these people live.

SERVICES AND RESOURCES
The following resources can provide information about HR programs and methods for substance abuse:

- Harm Reduction International, http://www.ihra.net/?no-splash=true
- Harm Reduction Coalition, http://harmreduction.org/
- Substance Abuse and Mental Health Services Administration (SAMHSA), http://store.samhsa.gov/home
- Burnet Institute, http://www.burnet.edu.au/health_themes/2_alcohol_drugs_and_harm_reduction
- Harm Reduction Journal, http://harmreductionjournal.biomedcentral.com/
- Harm reduction, Abstinence, and Moderation Support (HAMS), focuses on reducing alcohol consumption, www.hamsnetwork.org

Written by Laura McLuckey, MSW, LCSW

Reviewed by Lynn B. Cooper, D. Crim, and Chris Bates, MA, MSW

REFERENCES

Alcohol allowed here: Minn. center diverges from 12-Step model. (2013). *Alcoholism & Drug Abuse Weekly, 25*(13), 1-7.

Bartlett, R., Brown, L., Shattell, M., Wright, T., & Lewallen, L. (2013). Harm reduction: Compassionate care of persons with addictions. *MEDSURG Nursing, 22*(6), 349-358.

Beirness, D. J., Notarandrea, R., Jesseman, R., & Perron, M. (2008). Reducing the harm of "harm reduction.". *Clinical Pharmacology & Therapeutics, 83*(4), 523-525.

Bonar, E., & Rosenberg, H. (2014). Injection drug users' perceived barriers to using self-initiated harm reduction strategies. *Addiction Research & Theory, 22*(4), 271-278.

Davis, A. K., & Rosenberg, H. (2013). Acceptance of non-abstinence goals by addiction professionals in the United States. *Psychology of Addictive Behaviors, 27*(4), 1102-1109. doi:10.1037/a0030563

Drucker, E. (2013). Advocacy research in harm reduction drug policies. *Journal of Social Issues, 69*(4), 684-693. doi:10.1111/josi.12036

Drug Policy Alliance. (n.d.). Drug War Statistics. Retrieved April 6, 2016, from http://www.drugpolicy.org/drug-war-statistics

Eversman, M. (2015). "We want a living solution:" Views of harm reduction programs in black U.S. communities. *Journal of Ethnicity in Substance Abuse, 14*(2), 187-207. doi:10.1080/15332640.2014.976803

Henwood, B., Padgett, D., & Tiderington, E. (2014). Provider views of harm reduction versus abstinence policies within homeless services for dually diagnosed adults. *Journal of Behavioral Health Services & Research, 41*(1), 80-89. doi:10.1007/s11414-013-9318-2

International Federation of Social Workers. (2012). Statement of Ethical Principles. Retrieved April 6, 2016, from http://ifsw.org/policies/statement-of-ethical-principles/

Johnston, B. (2012). Harm reduction for unintentional poisoning. *Injury Prevention, 16*(4), 217-217.

Kreek, M. J., Levran, O., Reed, B., Schlussman, S.D., Zhou, Y., & Butelman, E. R. (2012). Opiate addiction and cocaine addiction: Underlying molecular neurobiology and genetics. *The Journal of Clinical Investigation, 122*(10), 3387-3393. doi:10.1172/JCI60390

McClean, K. (2013). Reducing risk, producing order: The surprisingly disciplinary world of needle exchange. *Contemporary Drug Problems, 40*(3), 415-445.

National Association of Social Workers. (2008). Code of ethics. Retrieved April 6, 2016, from https://www.socialworkers.org/pubs/code/code.asp

National Association of Social Workers. (2013). *NASW standards for social work practice with clients with substance use disorders.* Retrieved April 6, 2016, from https://www.socialworkers.org/practice/standards/Clients_with_Substance_Use_Disorders.asp

National Association of Social Workers. (2015). NASW standards and indicators for cultural competence in social work practice. Retrieved April 6, 2016, from http://www.socialworkers.org/practice/standards/PRA-BRO-253150-CC-Standards.pdf

National Institute on Drug Abuse (NIDA). (2012). Drug facts: Understanding drug abuse and addiction. Retrieved April 6, 2016, from https://www.drugabuse.gov/publications/drugfacts/understanding-drug-abuse-addiction

Pinkham, S., & Malinowska-Sempruch, K. (2008). Women, harm reduction, and HIV. *Reproductive Health Matters, 16*(31), 168-181.

The Policy, Ethics, and Human Rights Committee, British Association of Social Workers. (2012, January). The Code of Ethics for Social Work: Statement of principles. Retrieved April 6, 2016, from http://cdn.basw.co.uk/upload/basw_112315-7.pdf

Smith-Spangler, C. M., & Asch, S. M. (2012). Commentary on Vickerman et al. (2012): Reducing hepatitis C virus among injection drug users through harm reduction programs. *Addiction, 107*(11), 1196-1197. doi:10.1111/j.1360-0443.2012.04011.x

Substance Abuse and Mental Health Services Administration (SAMSHA). (n.d.). Common risk and protective factors for alcohol and drug use. Retrieved April 6, 2016, from http://www.samhsa.gov/capt/practicing-effective-prevention/prevention-behavioral-health/risk-protective-factors

Substance Abuse and Mental Health Services Administration (SAMHSA). (2016). Co-occurring disorders. Retrieved April 6, 2016, from http://www.samhsa.gov/co-occurring

WHO/UNAIDS/UNICEF. (2011). Global HIV/AIDS response: Epidemic update and health sector progress towards universal access. Progress report 2011. Retrieved May 2, 2016, from http://www.unaids.org/sites/default/files/media_asset/20111130_UA_Report_en_1.pdf

SUBSTANCE ABUSE: MARIJUANA

MAJOR CATEGORIES: Substance Abuse

DESCRIPTION

Marijuana is extracted from the upper leaves, flowering tops, and stems of the plant species *Cannabis sativa*, commonly known as cannabis and also known as Indian hemp. The plant contains cannabinoids, a group of more than 100 closely related chemical substances which, when ingested, act to obstruct the release of the substances known as neurotransmitters, which transmit signals between nerve cells in the body. The obstruction of these substances' release produces the psychoactive effects of marijuana and its products, which include drowsiness, euphoria, an increased appetite for food, giddiness, hallucinations, and anxiety.

The primary active ingredient in cannabis, tetrahydrocannabinol (THC), produces the mildly hallucinogenic effects of marijuana, which is one of the most commonly used drugs in the world, ranking fourth after caffeine, nicotine, and alcohol, and is the most commonly used illicit drug in the Western world. In the United States, marijuana, together with heroin, ecstasy, and other drugs, is classified under the Controlled Substances Act, passed by Congress in 1970, as a Schedule I drug (i.e., a drug without legitimate medical use and with a strong potential for abuse).

Of the cannabinoid compounds found in marijuana, two stand out: tetrahydrocannabinol (THC) and cannabidiol (CBD), with THC specifically known for its hallucinatory and other psychoactive properties.

Marijuana is typically is smoked in joints or pipes (including water pipes, also known as "bongs," or in "blunts," which are cigars filled with a mixture of marijuana and tobacco), because inhaling it is the fastest way for THC and its other ingredients to enter the bloodstream and pass from there to the brain and other parts of the nervous system, where it exerts its effects. Because it is fat soluble, marijuana can also be ingested by eating food to which it has been added or by drinking beverages to which an extract of it has been added. Users of marijuana may also combine it with other illicit substances (e.g., opium, cocaine, phencyclidine [PCP]) in a joint, pipe, or blunt). A trend gaining popularity among marijuana users is the use of synthetic marijuana (i.e., cannabinoids that have been artificially produced through chemistry), which is sprayed onto dry herbs and plant leaves (e.g., sage, mint) and sold under brand names such as Spice and K-2, which are among an increasing number of marketing-driven names being used to build customer bases for marijuana consumption.

Marijuana produces intoxication, euphoria, and a general sense of feeling "high" or "stoned." Symptoms of marijuana intoxication, such as euphoria, or feeling "high" or "stoned," can develop within minutes and last for 3 to 4 hours, depending on the method of consumption (e.g., smoking a marijuana cigarette or "joint," eating marijuana baked into food, applying to the skin a moisturizer that has been infused with cannabis oils). Chronic users of marijuana are less likely than chronic users of other illicit drugs to experience severe symptoms of its withdrawal, caused by the body's excretion of marijuana. Debate continues about the long-term consequences of using marijuana and whether it can result in a physical addiction. Research in the United States has been limited because of the classification of cannabis as a Schedule 1 drug.

The criteria for making a diagnosis of substance use disorder (SUD) are contained in the Fifth Edition of the *Diagnostic and Statistical Manual of Mental Disorders* (*DSM-5*), published by the American Psychiatric Association in 2013 and replacing DSM-IV-TR (where "TR" represents "Text Revision"). The chapter in *DSM-IV-TR* on substance-related disorders included substance dependence, substance abuse, substance intoxication, and substance withdrawal, and then discussed specific substances (e.g., alcohol, amphetamines). In *DSM-5* these disorders are divided into the two categories of substance use disorders and substance-induced disorders (intoxication, withdrawal, and other substance/medication-induced mental disorders). Thus, *DSM-5* removes the distinction between abuse and dependence and instead divides each type of disorder into mild, moderate, and severe subtypes, depending on the number of criteria met for each of these three categories within a particular disorder. Drug craving has been added as a criterion for substance use disorder (SUD), whereas "recurrent legal problems" has been removed as a criterion for SUD. The general criteria for SUD are the presence of significant problems in the user's life directly related to continued use of a particular substance. Cannabis use disorder would be the appropriate SUD diagnosis for the use of marijuana, hash, or synthetic marijuana that meets at least 2 of the 11 criteria for an SUD. The legal or medical status (i.e., prescribed or not prescribed) of a substance is not among the criteria for a diagnosis of SUD.

The severity of an SUD is related to several factors, including frequency of use of the substance in question, the method of entry of the substance into the body (e.g., inhalation, ingestion), and characteristics of the user. Treatment for cannabis use disorder is similar to the treatment for SUDs involving other drugs. Although hospitalization and detoxification are rarely required, persons engaged in marijuana use can benefit from a multifaceted approach consisting of drug counseling, individual and/or group therapy, motivation for behavioral change, random urine testing, and peer support.

The concentration of THC in marijuana has increased significantly over time. In 2012 the average concentration was almost 15 percent, whereas in the 1980s it averaged 4 percent. The increased concentration increases the risk of an adverse reaction to marijuana among new users and poses a greater risk for addiction to its use (NIDA, 2014).

FACTS AND FIGURES

According to the 2014 National Survey on Drug Use and Health, conducted by the Substance Abuse and Mental Health Services Administration (SAMHSA), marijuana is the most commonly used illicit drug in the United States. The survey found that approximately 22.2 million Americans, or 8.4 percent of the population aged 12 years or older, had used marijuana in the past month. The 2014 survey found that about 1.8 million, or 7.4 percent, of adolescents aged 12 to 17 had used marijuana in the past month, a rate similar to that for each year from 2003 to 2103. The survey also found that about 6.8 million, or 19.6 percent, of young adults aged 18 to 25 had used marijuana in the past month, a rate similar to that from 2010 to 2013 but higher than in 2003 to 2009; and that 13.5 million, or about 6.6 percent, of adults aged 26 and older had used marijuana in the past month, representing a slight

but steady increase in the annual rate that began in 2010 (SAMHSA, 2015).

Data from the 2015 Monitoring the Future Survey, which measures trends in attitudes and drug use among teenaged persons in the United States, reported that 11.8 percent of students in the eighth grade of school, 25.4 percent of those in the tenth grade, and 34.9 percent of those in the twelfth grade had used marijuana in the previous year, with corresponding figures of 3.1 percent, 4.3 percent, and 5.2 percent for the use of synthetic marijuana. A study conducted in 2014 found that adolescents who smoked marijuana chose to associate with peers who also smoked marijuana, making adolescence an age to consider as a time for intervention in stopping its use (Becker & Curry, 2014).

In 2013, the DSM-5 reported that 12-month rates for the diagnosis of cannabis SUD were higher among men than among women, with the highest rate being among 18- to 29-year-olds, followed by a steady decline with increasing age after age 29. The highest rates of cannabis SUD were among Native American and Alaska Natives (7.1 percent) aged 12 to 17, with the rates of the disorder not differing significantly among adult African Americans (1.8 percent), Whites (1.4 percent), and Hispanics (1.2 percent) (American Psychiatric Association, 2013).

RISK FACTORS

Use of marijuana is common among adults with a history of substance abuse, especially those who experimented with drug use as children. Children of single parents with limited supervision in the home and access to marijuana are at increased risk for cannabis SUD. Adults and adolescents with a mental illness are also at increased risk for the disorder, with the most common psychiatric conditions in this population being antisocial personality disorder, bipolar disorder, anxiety disorder, and schizophrenia. Marijuana users who have coexisting mental disorders are more likely to relapse than others. Men and adolescents are more likely than women and members of other age groups to become chronic users of cannabis and to have a diagnosis of cannabis SUD. Also, chronic users of marijuana are significantly more likely to engage in the use of multiple substances, comprising both legal (e.g., alcohol, nicotine) and illegal drugs (e.g., cocaine, lysergic acid diethylamide [LSD], methamphetamine).

SIGNS AND SYMPTOMS

The consumption of marijuana and its products has psychological, behavioral, physical, and social effects. Psychologically, it may be marked by sedation, lethargy, and difficulty in sleeping; distorted sensory perception; impaired cognition and motor skills; and a sensation of prolonged time. Behaviorally the consumption of marijuana is often experienced as a sense of euphoria, accompanied by inappropriate laughter and feelings of grandiosity; it may also be marked by a loss of motivation or of interest in typical activities; and by withdrawal accompanied by anger, aggressiveness, or irritability.

Physical effects of the use of marijuana may include tolerance, and interruptions in its use may create mild withdrawal symptoms (e.g., irritability, changes in appetite, sleep disturbances, insomnia, flu-like symptoms, diarrhea, constipation, aching, pain, abdominal cramps, weight loss, and restlessness). Other physical effects of marijuana can include disturbances in respiratory and immune system function; bloodshot eyes; an increased appetite; and dryness of the mouth.

Social effects of using marijuana may include withdrawal from social contact or a preference to spend time with other drug users, and impairment of the ability to work, attend school, or engage in social and familial activities.

APPLICABLE LAWS AND REGULATIONS

Marijuana was declared a drug under Schedule I of the Controlled Substances Act in 1972, and has remained under this classification to date. However, 23 states of the United States and the District of Columbia have legalized the medical use of marijuana for the treatment of certain conditions, including chronic pain, glaucoma, cancer, and neurodegenerative diseases, and for appetite stimulation. A memorandum on federal medical marijuana policy issued by the U.S. Department of Justice in 2009 instructed prosecutors and governing agencies not to target patients and their providers in states in which medical marijuana has been legalized. Colorado and Washington were the first two states to legalize, regulate, and tax small amounts of marijuana for recreational use by adults of age 21 and older (National Conference of State Legislatures, 2013; Governing, 2014), and since 2015, the recreational use of marijuana has also been legal in Alaska and Oregon (Governing, 2014). The legal status of marijuana is changing rapidly in the United States, with ballot initiatives for its legalization now being planned in many states.

TREATMENT

The social worker involved in assisting persons who may be using marijuana should conduct a preliminary assessment to determine whether a particular individual would benefit most from outpatient treatment or hospitalization. Those who meet the criteria for marijuana abuse or a cannabis SUD should have a biological, psychological, socials, and spiritual assessment to determine the means of treatment that will best address these problems. (e.g., cognitive behavioral therapy [CBT], psychodrama, psychotherapy for comorbid mental disorders, referral to a psychiatrist if pharmacological treatment is needed); help them to change maladaptive thoughts and behaviors and develop new coping mechanisms. The assessment should include an effort to determine the factors that precipitated the individual's marijuana abuse or cannabis SUD, such as a mental illness, a medical condition, or a traumatic experience, and an effort to determine whether the individual is also engaging in the use or abuse of more than one psychoactive or pharmacologically active substance. Also very important is to identify skills in a user that can help in overcoming the use of marijuana and other substances, if these are a problem, and to establish new patterns of functioning for the individual being treated. Other factors that should be included in the assessment are environmental, social, financial, and medical information relating to the affected individual. The individual's support system should be explored and used to identify private and professional persons who will be active in the recovery process. It is important to help develop a support network that includes family members, friends, and community members as part of the process of a marijuana user's recovery.

A urinalysis can detect the presence of marijuana-related cannabinoids for 1 to 5 days after the use of marijuana in non-chronic users and for up to 21 days or longer in chronic users. Blood samples taken within 8 days after the use of marijuana may also be used to detect and measure cannabinoids obtained from marijuana.

Medical detoxification is rarely is needed for users of marijuana, but may be necessary when it is being used together with other drugs. Upon referral for medical treatment, users who experience severe anxiety may be treated with benzodiazepines, although most symptoms of cannabis-related anxiety will resolve in a short time without the use of medications.

The behavioral/psychological approach to treating marijuana use resembles that for the use of other drugs. In general, it involves participating in a recovery program and individual and/or group therapy. Group therapy provides a safe environment in which persons with cannabis SUD can share experiences, offer support to others, and confront addictive behavior. Cognitive behavioral therapy (CBT) and psychodrama therapy can be used to address distorted thoughts and maladaptive behaviors while assisting the development of healthy coping mechanisms and effective behavior management. For clients who have sobriety as a goal, a relapse prevention program is vital in helping to maintain sobriety and minimizing the risk of relapse. An important goal for social workers and others involved in attempting to prevent relapse in persons with cannabis SUD is their achievement of coping skills for handling negative emotional states, situations involving social pressure, and situations involving interpersonal conflict (collectively referred to as triggers), all of which contribute to an increased likelihood of relapse.

Some persons with a cannabis SUD who cannot achieve complete sobriety may benefit from a harm-reduction approach, which focuses on reducing the adverse effects of using marijuana rather than on abstinence.

A new treatment modality is ecological momentary interventions (EMI), an intervention applied in real time in the user's own environment of daily functioning, rather than in a clinic or therapist's office, and often provided through smart phones or tablets. The intervention sends messages from 4 to 6 times a day to the user, with a reminder to self-assess both the desire for the use of marijuana and its actual use, as well as the user's feelings at both times. The program also prompts the user to report any triggers in a diary function included in the electronic intervention program. When the user reports a trigger, a desire to use marijuana, or the use of marijuana, a motivational message with coping strategies is sent via text or email (Shrier et al., 2014).

Social workers assisting persons engaged in assisting persons being treated for marijuana use should develop and aftercare plan that includes a referral to an outpatient treatment service, support groups, a recovery/sobriety coach, and a home for sober living. The social worker should educate the user's family members about signs of relapse, and encourage their attendance in support groups.

Social workers assisting persons who abuse marijuana should be aware of their own cultural values, beliefs, and biases, and develop specialized knowledge about these persons' histories, traditions, and values. They should adopt treatment methods that reflect their knowledge of the cultural diversity of the communities in which they practice.

SERVICES AND RESOURCES

The following sources can provide information for assisting persons engaged in marijuana use:

- The U.S. Drug Enforcement Administration (DEA) provides a list of controlled substances, http://www.deadiversion.usdoj.gov/schedules/index.html
- Drug Abuse Warning Network (DAWN) – database and information on trends that influence treatment and prevention, http://www.samhsa.gov/data/emergency-department-data-dawn
- Harm Reduction Coalition provides research, training, and policy advocacy for harm reduction approaches to treatment, http://www.harmreduction.org/
- Behavioral Health Treatment Services Locator, http://www.findtreatment.samhsa.gov

Written by Nikole Seals, MSW, ACSW, and Jessica Therivel, LMSW-IPR

Reviewed by Lynn B. Cooper, D. Crim, and Laura Gale, LCSW

REFERENCES

American Psychiatric Association. (2013). Panic Disorder. In *Diagnostic and statistical manual of mental disorders: DSM-5* (5th ed., pp. 481-589). Washington, DC: American Psychiatric Publishing.

Townsend, M. C. (2015). Substance-related and addictive disorders. In M. C. Townsend (Ed.),

Psychiatric mental health nursing: Concepts of care in evidence-based practice (8th ed., pp. 365-400). Philadelphia: F. A. Davis Company.

Becker, S. J., & Curry, J. F. (2014). Testing the effects of peer socialization versus selection on alcohol and marijuana use among treated adolescents. *Substance Use & Misuse, 49*(3), 234-242. doi:10.3109/10826084.2013.824479

Bender, K., Tripodi, S. J., Sarteschi, C., & Vaughn, M. G. (2011). A meta-analysis of interventions to reduce adolescent cannabis use. *Research on Social Work Practice, 21*(2), 153-164.

Blevins, C. E., Stephens, R. S., Walker, D. D., & Roffman, R. A. (2014). Situational determinants of use and treatment outcomes in marijuana dependent adults. *Addictive Behaviors, 39*(3), 546-552. doi:10.1016/j.addbeh.2013.10.031

British Association of Social Workers. (2012). The code of ethics for social work: Statement of principles. Retrieved March 7, 20196, from http://cdn.basw.co.uk/upload/basw_112315-7.pdf

Choo, E. K., Benz, M., Zaller, N., Warren, O., Rising, K. L., & McConnell, K. J. (2014). The impact of state medical marijuana legislation on adolescent marijuana use. *Journal of Adolescent Health, 55*(2), 160-166. doi:10.1016/j.jadohealth.2014.02.018

Copersino, M. L., Boyd, S. J., Tashkin, D. P., Huestis, M. A., Heishman, S. J., Dermand, J. C., & Gorelick, D. A. (2010). Sociodemographic characteristics of cannabis smokers and the experience of cannabis withdrawal. *American Journal of Drug and Alcohol Abuse, 36*(6), 311-319.

International Federation of Social Workers. (2012). Statement of Ethical Principles. Retrieved March 7, 2016, from http://ifsw.org/policies/statement-of-ethical-principles

Johnston, L. D., O'Malley, P. M., Miech, R. A., Bachman, J. G., & Shulenberg, J. E. (2015). Monitoring the Future national survey on drug use: 2015 overview key findings on adolescent drug use. *University of Michigan Institute for Social Research.* Retrieved March 7, 1970, from http://www.monitoringthefuture.org/pubs/monographs/mtf-overview2015.pdf

Lopez-Quintero, C., Hasin, D. S., los Cobos, J. P., Pines, A., Wang, S., Grant, B. F., & Blanco, C. (2010). Probability and predictors of remission from life-time nicotine, alcohol, cannabis or cocaine dependence: Results from the National Epidemiologic Survey on Alcohol and Related Conditions. *Addiction, 106*(3), 657-669.

National Institute on Drug Abuse (NIDA). (2014). Drug facts: Marijuana. Retrieved from http://www.drugabuse.gov/publications/drugfacts/marijuana

National Institute on Drug Abuse (NIDA). (2014). Marijuana: Research report series. Retrieved March 28, 2015, from http://www.drugabuse.gov/publications/finder/t/135-162/marijuana-research-reports

National Association of Social Workers. (2015). NASW Standards and Indicators for Cultural Competence in Social Work Practice. Retrieved March 7, 2016, from http://www.socialworkers.org/practice/standards/PRA-BRO-253150-CC-Standards.pdf

Peters, E. N., Hendricks, P. S., Clark, B., Vocci, F. J., & Cropsey, K. L. (2014). Association of race and age with treatment attendance and completion among adult marijuana users in community-based substance abuse treatment. *Journal of Addiction Medicine, 8*(2), 143-149. doi:10.1097/ADM.0000000000000030

Shrier, L. A., Rhoads, A. M., Fredette, M. E., & Burke, P. J. (2014). "Counselor in your pocket": Youth and provider perspectives on a mobile motivational Intervention for marijuana use. *Substance Use & Misuse, 49*(1/2), 134-144.

State marijuana laws map. (2014). *Governing.* Retrieved March 28, 2016, from http://www.governing.com/gov-data/state-marijuana-laws-map-medical-recreational.html

Substance Abuse and Mental Health Services Administration, U.S. (2015). Behavioral health trends in the United States: Results from the 2014 National Survey on Drug Use and Health. Retrieved March 7, 2016, from

http://www.samhsa.gov/data/sites/default/files/NSDUH-FRR1-2014/NSDUH-FRR1-2014.htm

SUBSTANCE ABUSE: OXYCONTIN

MAJOR CATEGORIES: Substance Abuse

DESCRIPTION

OxyContin is a prescription medication whose active ingredient is the opioid drug known as oxycodone. It is used for the management of moderate to severe pain (e.g., pain caused by cancer, trauma, or major surgery, and chronic back pain), and was first approved for use by the U.S. Food and Drug Administration (FDA) in 1995 for the treatment of chronic pain. The oxycodone that is the active ingredient in OxyContin acts in the brain, spinal cord, and the part of the nervous system known as the peripheral nervous system, in all three of which it blocks the transmission of nerve impulses that cause pain, thereby exerting a pain-blocking or analgesic effect. OxyContin is typically is prescribed in the form of 10-, 20-, 40-, or 80-mg tablets.

When taken orally, OxyContin provides pain relief for a 12-hour period. Its ability to gradually enter the blood from the stomach, over a long period after it is taken, was intended to extend its therapeutic, pain-blocking benefit as well as to deter its abuse.

OxyContin is abused more frequently than any other opioid drug prescribed for pain relief (e.g., codeine, hydrocodone) because its high concentration of oxycodone gives it a more potent pain-relieving effect. The abuse of OxyContin came about as the result of its ability to prompt a rapid, marked increase in the release, within the nervous system of the substance known as dopamine, which produces feelings of reward and pleasure when tablets of OxyContin are pulverized by chewing them, crushing and dissolving them in water, or crushing them and inserting them into the rectum. This led to rapid growth of the illicit use of OxyContin, bypassing its intended slow and controlled-release from its tablets as used medically to dampen or stop pain.

The consequence of the pleasurable effects of OxyContin by those who abuse it is a need to continue taking it, often in increasing quantities, in order to maintain these effects throughout the day and night and to prevent the abdominal cramping, nausea, vomiting, and other effects that occur when its illicit use is interrupted. This need to continue using OxyContin among its illicit users in turn creates a dependency on or addiction to it, which can be fatal because in excessive quantities it can block the contraction of the heart muscle that is needed to pump blood through the body, and can also block breathing, or respiration.

Many abusers of OxyContin obtain prescriptions for it by visiting local clinics with reports of chronic pain or by "doctor shopping," in which they visit various physicians to whom they complain of pain and obtain prescriptions that they have filled at different pharmacies. Other abusers of OxyContin may obtain the drug from friends or family members who have a prescription, or may buy the drug on the streets.

According to the Fourth Edition of the Diagnostic and Statistical Manual of *Mental Disorders* (*DSM-IV*), published by the American Psychiatric Association, "substance abuse" consists of a pattern of continued use of a substance (e.g., alcohol, cannabis, opioids, sedatives) that causes cognitive, physiological, and behavioral symptoms, resulting in problems in various areas of functioning. The substance being abused may be illegal (e.g., cannabis, cocaine, heroin), legal (e.g., alcohol), or a prescription medication (e.g., oxycodone)L used for purposes (i.e., recreational use) other than those for which the medication was intended. Additionally, abuse of a prescription drug such as OxyContin implies that the pattern in which it is used fails to correspond to the pattern of its legally prescribed use, and in order to meet the definition of substance abuse set forth in *DSM-IV*, this problematic pattern of use must continue for at least 12 months (APA, 2013).

A drug or other substance that is being abused may impair the self-control of the user, who may continue to abuse it even when this poses personal risks to health or life. Abuse of the substance may also create tolerance to it, in which its use may have to be continued or its dosage increased to maintain its effects, and stopping its use may cause symptoms of withdrawal. The Fifth Edition of the *Diagnostic and Statistical Manual of Mental Disorders* (*DSM-V*), published in 2013, and which replaced the *DSM-IV*, removes the distinction between substance abuse and substance dependence that existed in the *DSM-IV*, and adds drug craving as a criterion for substance use disorder (SUD).

FACTS AND FIGURES

The 2014 National Survey on Drug Use and Health estimated that the number of nonmedical users of OxyContin and other prescription pain-relieving drugs was 4.3 million people, of whom 1.9 million would meet the criteria for a prescription pain-reliever use disorder, and among whom 21.2 was the average age of the first use of such a drug (SAMHSA, 2015). In 2014, the Centers for Disease Control and Prevention (CDC) estimated that 46 people die every day from an overdose of a prescription drug and that in 2012, 259-million prescriptions were written for pain-relieving drugs in 2012 (CDC, 2014); according to the CDC, 10 of the states of the United States with the highest numbers of prescriptions were located in the South, and many states were having to cope with the proliferation of "pill mills," which are high-volume, profit-making pain clinics that prescribe a large number of pain-relieving drugs to persons who do not need them medically (CDC, 2014).

RISK FACTORS

Dependence on OxyContin was first recognized in rural communities that are sites of labor-intensive industries (e.g., logging, coal mining), in which the quest for medicinal treatment for work-related pain is a common and accepted practice. These industries also tend to be located in economically depressed areas in which persons see the selling of medications that are prescribed for them as a means of making money. Abuse of OxyContin, and the illegal practice of selling it for profit, have spread throughout the United States, with the highest rates of its abuse and largest number of prescriptions for it occurring in the state of Florida. Abuse of OxyContin is most common among White males living in small towns and rural areas (mean age = 34 years). Those with a history of substance abuse are at increased risk of developing an addiction to OxyContin. Also at increased risk for addiction to OxyContin are Native American adolescents and young adults living on or near Native American reservations.

When ease of access and cost grow too high for users of OxyContin, there is a risk that they will switch to heroin, which typically has a lower cost and is not hard to obtain (Mars, Bourgois, Karandinos, Montero, & Ciccarone, 2014).

SIGNS AND SYMPTOMS

Abuse of OxyContin typically produces any of a variety of psychological, behavioral, physical, and social effects. Its psychological effects include anxiety or moodiness, and a rationale for needing OxyContin such as control of pain (often referred to as "medication seeking"). Behaviorally its effects can include sedation, drowsiness, euphoria, lightheadedness, dry mouth, sweating, and constricted pupils, with interruption or cessation of its use causing irritability, sweating, tremors, nausea, and vomiting. Physically, effects of abusing OxyContin can include tolerance and/or withdrawal symptoms upon interruption or cessation of its use (e.g., profuse sweating, irritability, cravings, nausea, vomiting, digestive problems); and sleepiness, calmness, or a sedative effect. Social effects of OxyContin abuse may include withdrawal from social contact or a preference to spend time with other drug abusers; client may have involvement with criminal court due to drug-related charges; and impairment of the ability to work, attend school, manage familial responsibilities, and engage in social activities.

APPLICABLE LAWS AND REGULATIONS

Forty-nine states of the United States and the Territory of Guam currently have Prescription Drug Monitoring Programs (PDMPs) to combat drug abuse (Prescription Drug Monitoring Program Center for Excellence at Brandeis University, 2014). These programs collect, monitor, and analyze electronically transmitted drug-prescribing and drug-dispensing data submitted by pharmacies, dispensing practitioners, and law-enforcement authorities, and use these data for research, education, enforcement and abuse prevention.

In 2010 the U.S. Food and Drug Administration (FDA) approved a reformulated version of OxyContin with a new label that indicates that the new version of the drug has properties that interfere with its abuse via injection or nasal inhalation difficult. The FDA also stopped approving generic versions of OxyContin.

TREATMENT

The social worker assisting an individual engaged in the abuse of OxyContin should first determine whether the individual may require detoxification and whether this would best be done on an inpatient or outpatient basis. The presence of oxycodone can be determined through drug toxicology testing done on a urine sample. This should be followed by a biological, psychological, social, and spiritual assessment to include physical, mental, environmental, social, financial, and medical information relating to the individual's treatment, and should refer the individual for screening for coexisting psychiatric conditions. The assessment should include a determination of the factors that precipitated the individual's use of OxyContin, such as previous substance use, a medical condition, or any life trauma, and the factors that more immediately trigger its use; and should identify the individual's support system and the persons who will be active in his or her recovery process.

Approaches to treating OxyContin addiction resemble those for treating heroin addiction and typically consist of long-term residential treatment or long-term medication-assisted outpatient treatment. Both treatment methods take a dual approach of controlled withdrawal from the drug and behavioral counseling. Typically, medical detoxification, to eliminate addiction to and dependency on OxyContin, precedes other phases of treatment for its abuse. Detoxification is done under the supervision of a qualified medical professional and involves the use of medications such as methadone that block the effects of OxyContin and minimize the often severe effects of withdrawal from it. When detoxification is complete, stabilized, cognitive behavioral therapy (CBT) and psychodrama therapy can be used to address the underlying causes of addiction to OxyContin. A relapse-prevention program is developed and put in place prior to completion of therapy.

In working with an individual being treated for addiction to OxyContin, the social worker should develop a relapse prevention plan. This should include identifying skills and tools that the individual may use as an alternative to substance use/abuse; and referral to community-based programs for ongoing support.

Social workers assisting persons in the recovery from OxyContin abuse should be aware of their own cultural values, beliefs, and biases, and develop specialized knowledge about the histories, traditions, and values of the individuals they are assisting. They should adopt treatment methodologies that reflect their knowledge of the cultural diversity of the societies in which they practice

SERVICES AND RESOURCES

The following services provide information about OxyContin and its abuse:

- Information on OxyContin for healthcare providers, http://www.drugs.com/pro/oxycontin.html
- Substance Abuse Treatment Locator, http://www.findtreatment.samhsa.gov

Written by Nikole Seals, MSW, ACSW

Reviewed by Lynn B. Cooper, D. Crim, and Jessica Therivel, LMSW-IPR

REFERENCES

Aquina, C. T., Marques-Baptista, A., Bridgeman, P., & Merlin, M. A. (2009). OxyContin abuse and overdose. *Postgraduate Medicine, 121*(2), 163-167. doi:10.3810/pgm.2009.03.1988

British Association of Social Workers. (2012, January). The code of ethics for social work: Statement of principles. Retrieved January 25, 2015, from http://cdn.basw.co.uk/upload/basw_112315-7.pdf

Buer, L.-M., Havens, J. R., & Leukefeld, C. (n.d.). Does the new formulation of OxyContin deter misuse? A qualitative analysis. *Substance Use & Misuse, 49*(6), 770-774. doi:10.3109/10826084.2013.866963

Centers for Disease Control and Prevention (CDC). (n.d.). Opioid painkiller prescribing. *CDC Vital Signs.* Retrieved January 26, 2016, from http://www.cdc.gov/vitalsigns/opioid-prescribing/

Hansen, R. N., Oster, G., Edelsberg, J., Woody, G. E., & Sullivan, S. D. (2011). Economic costs of nonmedical use of prescription opioids. *Clinical Journal of Pain, 27*(3), 194-202.

Harris, S. C., Perrino, P. J., Smith, I., Shram, M. J., Colucci, S. V., Bartlett, C., & Sellers, E. M. (2014). Abuse potential, pharmacokinetics, pharmacodynamics, and safety of intranasally administered crushed oxycodone HCl abuse-deterrent controlled-release tablets in recreational opioid users. *Journal of Clinical Pharmacology, 54*(4), 468-477. doi:10.1002/jcph.235

Hays, L. R. (2004). A profile of OxyContin addiction. *Journal of Addictive Diseases, 23*(4), 1-9.

International Federation of Social Workers. (2012). Statement of Ethical Principles. Retrieved January 25, 2016, from http://ifsw.org/policies/statement-of-ethical-principles/

Levy, M. S. (2007). An exploratory study of Oxy-Contin use among individuals with substance use disorders. *Journal of Psychoactive Drugs, 39*(3), 271-276.

Mars, S. G., Bourgois, P., Karandinos, G., Montero, F., & Ciccarone, D. (2014). "Every 'Never' I ever said came true." Transitions from opioid pills to heroin injecting. *International Journal of Drug Policy, 25,* 257-266. doi:10.1016/j.drugpo.2013.10.004

Prescription Drug Monitoring Program Center of Excellence at Brandeis. (2014, September). Briefing on PDMP effectiveness. Retrieved January 25, 2016, from http://www.pdmpexcellence.org/sites/all/pdfs/Briefing percent20on percent-20PDMP percent20Effectiveness percent203rd percent20revision.pdf

Stanley, L. R., Harness, S. D., Swaim, R. C., & Beauvais, F. (2014). Rates of substance use of American Indian students in 8th, 10th, and 12th grades living on or near reservations: Update, 2009-2012. *Public Health Reports, 129*(2), 156-163.

Substance Abuse and Mental Health Services Administration, U.S. (2015). Behavioral health trends in the United States: Results from the 2014 National Survey on Drug Use and Health. Retrieved January 25, 2016, from http://www.samhsa.gov/data/sites/default/files/NSDUH-FRR1-2014/NSDUH-FRR1-2014.htm

U.S. and Mental Health Services Administration. (2008). OxyContin: Prescription drug abuse-2008 revision. *Substance Abuse Treatment Advisory: News for the Treatment Field, 7*(1), 1-8. Retrieved from

U.S. Drug Enforcement Administration. (2010). FDA approves a more tamper-resistant formulation of OxyContin. *Formulary, 45*(5), 166-167.

Wheeler, D. (2015). NASW Standards and Indicators for Cultural Competence in Social Work Practice. Retrieved January 25, 2016, from http://www.socialworkers.org/practice/standards/PRA-BRO-253150-CC-Standards.pdf

Zarbock, S. (2007). On the OxyContin scandal: Don't abandon patients in pain. *JAAPA: Official Journal of the American Academy of Physician Assistants, 20*(7), 12.

Substance Use & Conduct Disorder

Major Categories: Behavioral & Mental Health, Substance Abuse

What We Know
Substance use and conduct disorder (CD) frequently co-occur in children and adolescents. CD is one of the most common reasons for referrals to mental health services for children and adolescents.

Early-onset substance use can influence the development, continuation, and acceleration of the symptoms of CD.

In 2014, researchers found that 8th and 9th graders who reported alcohol and marijuana use had an increased risk of both parent-reported and adolescent-reported symptoms of CD.

Investigators for another study in 2014 found that 8th graders with higher levels of conduct problems had higher levels of marijuana and alcohol use than 8th graders with fewer conduct issues.

Ananalysis of data from a population-wide sample of 3,720 adults collected in Lausanne, Switzerland, in 2007 produced a sub-sample of 238 who had a diagnosis of attention-deficit/hyperactive disorder (ADHD), oppositional defiant disorder (ODD), and/or conduct disorder before age 15. Fifty-six percent of those with CD had an alcohol use disorder and 48 percent had a substance use disorder; 24 percent of those with ADHD had an alcohol use disorder and 7 percent had a substance use disorder.

The authors of a study of 9,154 adolescents who had been discharged from inpatient psychiatric services in the United States concluded that of all individuals with a mental health disorder, those with CD had the greatest probability of having a co-occurring substance use disorder.

For substance use disorder (SUD) to be diagnosed, an individual must experience impairment of performance at work or school, problems with functioning at home, or repeated negative consequences caused by ongoing substance use within a 12-month period. These criteria are used to diagnose substance use disorder in both youth and adults.

Substance abuse and substance dependence are now combined into one category, substance use disorder, in the *Diagnostic and Statistical Manual of Mental Disorders*, 5th edition (*DSM-5*), with each substance specified as a separate use disorder, such as alcohol use disorder and stimulant use disorder.

More than one symptom must be present for a diagnosis of substance use disorder in the *DSM-5*.

Drug craving has been added in the fifth edition of the *DSM* to the list of symptoms of substance use disorder; problems with law enforcement has been removed.

Typically CD is diagnosed prior to adulthood and is characterized by behavior that violates the rights of others or major societal norms, such as aggression toward people and animals, physical cruelty, property damage, theft, deceitfulness, and serious violations of rules. Symptoms must cause significant impairment in social, academic, or occupational functioning and three or more diagnostic criteria must have been met in the previous 12 months, with at least one criterion in the last 6 months. Symptoms may be present as early as preschool but more often they develop in middle childhood to middle adolescence.

The *DSM-5* adds a specifier to the diagnosis of conduct disorder that allows the clinician to identify a more serious pattern of behavior characterized as a callous and unemotional interpersonal style across multiple settings.

CD is strongly associated with poor educational performance, social isolation, substance misuse, and contact with the juvenile justice system. CD frequently follows young persons into adulthood, leading to poor educational and occupational outcomes.

After a year of outpatient treatment for SUD, adolescents who had co-occurring CD continued to report more psychiatric symptoms and increased utilization of further inpatient and outpatient treatment than adolescents with SUD alone.

Adolescents with CD typically have higher degrees of impulsivity than adolescents without CD.

Researchers in 2015 found that adolescents with CD had a more "black and white" thinking style, which diminished their ability to cope with stressful situations.

SUD and CD most commonly occur among adolescent boys who are chronically defiant and/or impulsive, who use drugs, and who partake in criminal activity.

CD is associated with child maltreatment, parents who abuse substances, family conflicts, poverty, and genetic factors which may predispose individuals to addiction.

Investigators in 2014 found that CD severity was increased among adolescents whose fathers had troubles with work due to substance use and among those whose mothers had legal problems related to substance use.

SUD is known to have lifelong adverse consequences for individuals and affects family systems through generations. In families in which parents have SUDs, children are more likely to be maltreated. Maltreated children, in turn, are susceptible to multiple psychosocial problems.

Investigators in a 2011 study found that adolescents with both ADHD and CD had significantly higher rates of SUDs in adulthood than those with ADHD alone.

Adolescents with mental health conditions often do not receive the care they need and are considered especially difficult to treat because of their resistance and noncompliance. Investigators in multiple studies suggest that this resistance is amplified, in part, by the increased level of vulnerability and sensitivity in this phase of development.

The persistence of coexisting psychosocial problems in adolescents has led to the creation of what is described as the matrix, or multi-systemic, approach to interventions. This approach incorporates relapse prevention; individual, group, and family therapies; self-help; and educational elements to help individuals better understand the effects and consequences of their behavior. Below are some recommended interventions and harm reduction approaches for CD and SUDs.

Outdoor behavioral healthcare is a residentially based therapeutic approach to CD and SUDs among adolescents. Researchers in 2013 found that this intervention significantly reduced symptoms. Further, reductions were maintained over a 12-month follow-up period.

The natural environment is used in these programs to help clients learn how to develop and expand a range of skills, including skills to promote social-cognitive growth, community involvement, and coping mechanisms; adolescents have to plan and set goals and depend upon each other in an environment in which they experience naturally occurring consequences of their behavior.

Group therapy enhances interpersonal learning and facilitates cognitive, affective, and behavioral changes. Groups of small to medium size are recommended for adolescents and should include didactic presentations covering the consequences of their behavior.

Cognitive behavioral therapy (CBT) addresses skills deficits and assists in the development and rehearsal of new skills. Therapists working in CBT examine with clients the situations that lead to substance use and suggest alternative ways of behaving. It can be used in one-on-one sessions or within groups.

WHAT CAN BE DONE

Develop an awareness of your own cultural values, beliefs, and biases and develop knowledge about the histories, traditions, and values of your clients. Adopt treatment methodologies that reflect the cultural needs of the client.

Practice with awareness of, and adherence to, the social work principles of respect for human rights and human dignity, social justice, and professional conduct as described in the International Federation of Social Workers (IFSW) Statement of Ethical Principles.

Become knowledgeable about substance use and conduct disorder so you can accurately assess your clients' unique characteristics and health/mental health education needs; share this information with your colleagues.

Learn about the link between substance use and conduct disorder and the psychosocial consequences of these conditions for youth.

Learn about the developmental characteristics of adolescents and how these can impact interventions.

Learn about the lifetime consequences of SUDs and CD, including how the co-occurrence of CD and ADHD has the potential to increase the risk of SUDs in adulthood.

Learn about the range of interventions used for SUDs and CD and make referrals as appropriate.

Written by Jan Wagstaff, MA, MSW, and Jessica Therivel, LMSW-IPR

Reviewed by Chris Bates, MA, MSW, and Melissa Rosales Neff, MSW

REFERENCES

American Psychiatric Association. (2013). Diagnostic and statistical manual of mental disorders. (5th ed.). Arlington, VA: American Psychiatric Publishing.

British Association of Social Workers. (2012). The code of ethics for social work: Statement of principles. Retrieved August 15, 2015, from http://cdn.basw.co.uk/upload/basw_112315-7.pdf

Conduct disorder. (2011). *MedlinePlus.* Retrieved June 23, 2016, from http://www.nlm.nih.gov/medlineplus/ency/article/000919.htm

Engstrom, M., Mahoney, C. A., & Marsh, J. C. (2012). Substance use problems in health social work practice. S. Gehlert & T. Browne (Eds.), *Handbook of health social work* (2nd ed.). Hoboken, NJ: John Wiley & Sons, Inc.

Harty, S. C., Ivanov, I., Newcorn, J. H., & Halperin, J. M. (2011). The impact of conduct disorder and stimulant medication on later substance use in an ethnically diverse sample of individuals with attention deficit/hyperactivity disorder in childhood. *Journal of Child & Adolescent Psychopharmacology, 21*(4), 331-339. doi:10.1089/cap.2010.0074

Hollen, V., & Ortiz, G. (2015). Mental health and substance use comorbidity among adolescents in psychiatric inpatient hospitals: Prevalence and covariates. *Journal of Child & Adolescent Substance Abuse, 24*(2), 102-112. doi:10.1080/1067828X.2013.768575

International Federation of Social Workers. (2012). Statement of Ethical Principles. Retrieved August 15, 2015, from http://ifsw.org/policies/statement-of-ethical-principles/

Lewis, S. F. (2013). Examining changes in substance use and conduct problems among treatment-seeking adolescents. *Child & Adolescent Mental Health, 18*(1), 33-38. doi:10.1111/j.1475-3588.2012.00657.x

Maslowsky, J., Schulenberg, J. E., & Zucker, R. A. (2014). Influence of conduct problems and depressive symptomatology on adolescent substance use: Developmentally proximal versus distal effects. *Developmental Psychology, 50*(4), 1179-1189. doi:10.1037/a0035085

National Association of Social Workers. (2015). Standards and indicators for cultural competence in social work practice. Retrieved June 23, 2016, from http://www.socialworkers.org/practice/standards/PRA-BRO-253150-CC-Standards.pdf

National Institute for Health and Care Excellence. (2013). Antisocial behavior and conduct disorders in children and young people: recognition, intervention and management. Retrieved from https://www.nice.org.uk/guidance/cg158

Reavy, R., Stein, L. A. R., Quina, K., & Paiva, A. L. (2014). Assessing conduct disorder: A new measurement approach. *Journal of Correctional Health Care, 20*(1), 4-17. doi:10.1177/1078345813505448

Rodgers, S., Muller, M., Rossler, W., Castelao, E., Preisig, M., & Ajdacid-Gross, V. (2015). Externalizing disorders and substance use: empirically derived subtypes in a population-based sample of adults. *Social Psychiatry & Psychiatric Epidemiology, 50*(1), 7-17. doi:10.1007/s00127-014-0898-9

Urben, S., Suter, M., Pihet, S., Straccia, C., & Stephan, P. (2015). Constructive thinking skills and impulsivity dimensions in conduct and substance use disorders: Differences and relationships in an adolescents' sample. *Psychiatric Quarterly, 86*(2), 207-218. doi:10.1007/s11126-014-9320-8

Watson, J. A., Greene, M. C., & Kelly, J. F. (2014). Outpatient alcohol and drug treatment for adolescents with co-occurring conduct disorder. *Alcoholism Treatment Quarterly, 32*(4), 393-415. doi:10.1080/07347324.2014.949119

Webb, N. B. (2011). Social work practice with children. New York, NY: The Guilford Press.

Wymbs, B. T., McCarty, C. A., Mason, W. A., King, K. M., Baer, J. S., Stoep, A. V., & McCauley, E. (2014). Early adolescent substance use as a risk factor for developing conduct disorder and depression symptoms. *Journal of Studies on Alcohol & Drugs, 75*(2), 279-289.

Substance Use Disorder & Adults: Treatment

Major Categories: Substance Abuse

What We Know

"Substance abuse" refers to a pattern of continued use of a substance (e.g., alcohol, cannabis, opioids, sedatives) that causes negative cognitive, physiological, and behavioral symptoms, resulting in problems in various areas of functioning. The pattern of use is pathological. The individual may experience impaired behavioral control, continued use despite risks, and social impairment. There also may be tolerance and withdrawal. This problematic pattern of use must persist for at least 12 months to be diagnosed as substance abuse.

The *Diagnostic and Statistical Manual of Mental Disorders,* fifth edition (*DSM-5*), was published in mid-2103 and replaced the fourth edition (*DSM-IV*). The *DSM-IV* chapter "Substance-Related Disorders" included substance dependence, substance abuse, substance intoxication, and substance withdrawal, and discussed specific substances (e.g., alcohol, amphetamines). The *DSM-5* divides these disorders into two categories: substance use disorders (SUD) and substance-induced disorders (intoxication, withdrawal, and other substance-/medication-induced mental disorders). The *DSM-5* removes the distinction between abuse and dependence that appeared in the *DSM-IV* and instead provides three specifiers, mild, moderate, or severe, depending on the number of

symptoms present. Drug craving has been added as a criterion for substance use disorder, whereas "recurrent legal problems" has been removed. In the *DSM-5*, substance abuse and dependence are referred to as "substance use disorder," whereas in the research literature and in treatment situations the terms "substance abuse" and "dependence" are still commonly used.

In 2014, the Substance Abuse and Mental Health Services Administration (SAMHSA) determined that 21.5 million persons in the United States over the age of 12 met criteria for a SUD within the past year.

- 7.1 million met criteria for an SUD for an illicit drug (e.g., marijuana [in some states], heroin, cocaine, nonmedical use of prescription medications)
- 17 million met criteria for alcohol use disorder
- 2.6 million met criteria for both alcohol and illicit use disorders
- In 2014, SAMHSA found that 4.1 million persons received treatment for a problem related to alcohol or illicit drug use.
- 2.6 million persons received their treatment in a facility
- 2.4 million persons received treatment for an alcohol use disorder

- 1 million persons received treatment for marijuana use disorder.

Smaller numbers of individuals received treatment for cocaine, heroin, and nonmedical use of prescription medications.

Screening for substance abuse within the client population requires maintaining awareness of risk factors and using validated tools.

Risk factors include family history of substance use, recent stressful events, a lack of social support, chronic pain, chronic illness, trauma, history of mental illness (e.g., depression, bipolar disorder), cognitive disabilities, physical disabilities, alcohol use before age 15, and presence of medical conditions associated with substance use (e.g., cirrhosis, respiratory disease, human immunodeficiency virus [HIV] infection).

Researchers found that, compared to the general population, adults entering a treatment program for co-occurring mental health disorders and substance use disorders had higher rates of hypertension, arthritis, asthma, and smoking. Substance use severity was higher as well.

The social worker needs to actively engage clients during initial screening to increase the likelihood of successful treatment.

The social worker must demonstrate empathy and be aware that the client may be embarrassed by his or her substance use.

The social worker needs to be able to distinguish between the client as a person and the client's substance-using behavior.

The social worker needs to complete an extensive biopsychosocial-spiritual assessment that includes obtaining information from a variety of sources (e.g., family, other clinicians, medical providers, friends).

Validated screening tools include the CAGE survey, Alcohol Use Disorders Identification Test (AUDIT), Substance Abuse Subtle Screening Inventory (SASSI), and Drug Abuse Screening Test (DAST).

The frequently used CAGE survey is a short, 4-question tool geared solely toward alcohol use.

The CAGE has been adapted to screen for abuse of other substances; this version is called the CAGE-AID (CAGE Adapted to Include Drugs).

The AUDIT is a 10-item tool that can be completed orally or in writing.

The SASSI-3 uses *DSM-5* criteria and language to identify probability of a SUD, level of defensiveness, desire to change, and acknowledgement of SUD as a problem.

The DAST is a 28-item self-report tool that measures use of drugs other than alcohol.

Particular populations may be more vulnerable to substance abuse than others and/or encounter more barriers to appropriate treatment.

Older adults are being admitted to treatment for substance abuse for the first time in growing proportions when compared to younger adults entering treatment for the first time; the most common referral source for older adults is self-referral.

Researchers found that older adults who were age 65 or older were less likely to have accessed treatment for SUDs or perceive a need for treatment than adults ages 35 to 49 were. Researchers also found that symptoms alone would not motivate older adults to seek treatment.

Some clinicians suggest not over-relying on the *DSM-5* criteria for identifying SUDs in older adults but instead suggest using a two-tier classification of either "at-risk use" or "problem use." "At-risk use" refers to the use of substances above recommended or prescribed levels but where the individual is not yet experiencing problems of use in the areas of physical, mental, emotional, or social functioning.

Adults with disabilities have decreased access and utilization rates for substance abuse treatment, with one study finding access and utilization for this population at rates about half those of the general population.

Investigators for the 2013 SAMHSA study, which was the most recent to examine race, found that American Indian/Alaskan Natives had the highest

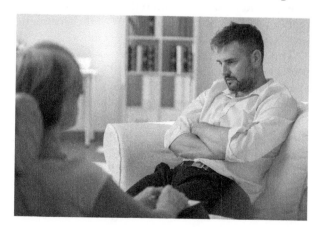

rates of SUDs, at 14.9 percent, followed by Native Hawaiians and Pacific Islanders at 11.3 percent and individuals reporting two or more races at 10.9 percent. Asian Americans had the lowest rate for SUDs, at 4.6 percent. black individuals, white individuals, and Hispanic individuals had comparable rates at 7.4 percent, 8.4 percent, and 8.6 percent respectively.

The criminal justice population has much higher rates of dependence than the general population, with 34 percent of adults over the age of 18 meeting criteria for dependence or abuse while on parole or supervised release from jail within the last year; among the general population, the rate was 8.6 percent.

Treatment interventions usually are developed based on a specific model of how and why substance abuse develops. Social workers need to be aware of the theories regarding the development of substance abuse upon which particular interventions are based to correctly apply interventions.

The most commonly researched and utilized models of substance abuse are the disease model, psychological models, motivation and change theories, transtheoretical/stages of change, and harm reduction (i.e., the public health model).

The *disease model* is most commonly associated with Alcoholics Anonymous (AA) and other 12-step programs, in which substance abuse is viewed as a disease. The theory that substance abuse is a medical condition recognizes the influence of biological, environmental, behavioral, and genetic factors.

The *psychological models* focus on the cognitive and behavioral perspectives on why an individual abuses substances and employ strategies for change that incorporate these perspectives. Addictive behaviors and traits are viewed as habits that can be studied and changed. Relapse is considered a likely occurrence that can be beneficially used as part of the treatment process and is not viewed as an abject failure.

The *motivation and change theory models* place emphasis on examining the individual's motivation for change and the nature and mechanics of change itself while working to establish a collaborative relationship between social worker and client. Motivational interviewing (MI) focuses on why people commit to making changes in behavior.

The central component of the *transtheoretical model* (also referred to as "the stages of change") outlines five stages of change for any behavior and has three key tenets. The five stages of change are precontemplation, contemplation, preparation, action, and maintenance. The three key tenets are that the change process can start no matter which stage the client is in, that relapse is a likely occurrence, and that interventions should match the client's stage (e.g., a client in precontemplation would not be ready for action-oriented interventions).

Harm reduction programs and policies aim to reduce harm to individuals who use or abuse alcohol or other substances. Examples range from designated driver programs and in-school sex education to needle-exchange and methadone programs and making naloxone widely available to counteract opiate overdoses. Harm reduction does not focus on abstinence but instead meets clients where they are in terms of their use of alcohol and substances.

Intervention strategies should be based on the model or theory to which the social worker or the agency subscribes. Disease model interventions focus on increasing abstinence, improving self-efficacy, and enhancing the client's socialization. There may be pharmacotherapy (e.g., disulfiram [Antabuse], acamprosate [Campral], topiramate [Topamax], methadone, or selective serotonin reuptake inhibitors [SSRIs]) included in a disease model of treatment. Psychological model interventions examine the client's negative behavior, the antecedents present in behavior or situations (e.g., interpersonal conflicts, negative emotions, social influences), and the client's expectations regarding the outcome of using the substance in question. Consequences of the behavior are also examined.

In MI interventions, which are based on the models of motivation and change theory, the social worker encourages the client to discover his or her personal perspectives, interests, and reasons for change. The client demonstrates that making changes in his or her pattern of substance use is a self-choice and not mandated by the social worker, family, or friends.

Transtheoretical model interventions focus on determining the client's stage of change and using treatment strategies that coordinate with the stage the client is in. Harm reduction engages the client in making changes to behaviors related to alcohol or substance use even if the client is not ready for total abstinence

Interventions are strengths-based, are empowering to clients, and look to help clients achieve goals that they set.

Public health reforms and projects can follow this model through public initiatives (e.g., clean needle programs, designated driver programs, affordable housing without abstinence requirements) and public policy (e.g., addressing sentencing disparities in the criminal justice system).

Complementary therapies may be a component of treatment programs. Researchers found that study subjects who were in alcohol treatment programs that included producing art through art therapy had improved mood and reduced anxiety.

Many individuals who would benefit from treatment for substance abuse do not receive treatment because of existing barriers.

Publicly supported treatment programs can be difficult to find, have long waiting lists, or be unavailable to clients who do not qualify.

A fear of being stigmatized or labeled an "addict" or "alcoholic" may prevent clients from seeking help.

Co-occurring disabilities and/or medical conditions can result in increased difficulty in accessing treatment.

A study using data from a U.S. national survey on substance use found that 46 percent of adults with a serious mental illness and a substance use disorder were not receiving any treatment and 65 percent of respondents with one or more mental health symptoms were not receiving substance abuse treatment.

WHAT CAN BE DONE

Learn about substance abuse treatment in adults so you can accurately assess your clients' personal characteristics and health education needs; share this information with your colleagues.

Develop an awareness of your own cultural values, beliefs, and biases and develop knowledge about the histories, traditions, and values of your clients. Adopt treatment methodologies that reflect the cultural needs of clients.

Understand risk factors and screen all clients for issues related to substance use.

Provide assistance as appropriate (e.g., financial and social supports, including housing, vocational rehabilitation programs, legal assistance).

Work to eliminate existing barriers to treatment for all clients who are in need of substance abuse treatment.

Provide interventions that follow the model and theory of practice in use at your practice, agency, or facility.

Maintain education and awareness of current best evidence-based practices.

Written by Jessica Therivel, LMSW-IPR

*Reviewed by Melissa Rosales Neff, MSW, and
Chris Bates, MA, MSW*

REFERENCES

American Psychiatric Association. (2013). Substance-related and addictive disorders. *Diagnostic and Statistical Manual of Mental Disorders* (5th ed.). Arlington, VA: American Psychiatric Publishing.

Anastas, J. W., & Clark, E. J. (2012). Alcohol, tobacco, and other drugs. In S. Lowman (Ed.), *Social Work Speaks: National Association of Social Workers Policy Statements* (9th ed., pp. 28-36). Washington, DC: NASW Press.

Arndt, S., Clayton, R., & Schultz, S. K. (2011). Trends in substance abuse treatment 1998-2008: Increasing older adult first-time admissions for illicit drugs. *American Journal of Geriatric Psychiatry, 19*(8), 704-711. doi:10.1097/JGP.0b013e31820d942b

British Association of Social Workers. (2012). *The code of ethics for social work: Statement of principles*. Retrieved February 1, 2015, from http://cdn.basw.co.uk/upload/basw_112315-7.pdf

Center for Behavioral Health Statistics and Quality. (2015). Behavioral health trends in the United States: Results from the 2014 National Survey on Drug Use and Health (HHS Publication No. SMA 15-4927, NSDUH Series H-50). Retrieved February 1, 2016, from http://www.samhsa.gov/data/sites/default/files/NSDUH-FRR1-2014/NSDUH-FRR1-2014.pdf

Chesher, N. J., Bousman, C. A., Gale, M., Norman, S. B., Twamley, E. W., Heaton, R. K.,... Judd, P. A. (2011). Chronic illness histories of adults entering treatment for co-occurring substance abuse and other mental health disorders. *The American Journal on Addictions, 21*(1), 1-4.

Choi, N. G., DiNitto, D. M., & Marti, C. N. (2014). Treatment use, perceived need, and barriers to seeking treatment for substance abuse and mental health problems among older adults compared to younger adults. *Drug and Alcohol Dependence, 145,* 113-120. doi:10.1016/j.drugalcdep.2014.10.004

Engstrom, M., Mahoney, C. A., & Marsh, J. C. (2012). Substance use problems in health social work practice. In S. Gehlert & T. Arthur Browne (Eds.), *Handbook of health social work* (2nd ed., pp. 426-427). Hoboken, NJ: Wiley.

Han, B., Hedden, S. L., Lipari, R., Copello, E. A. P., & Kroutil, L. A. (2015, September). Receipt of services for behavioral health problems: results from the 2014 National Survey on Drug Use and Health. Retrieved February 1, 2016, from http://www.samhsa.gov/data/sites/default/files/NSDUH-DR-FRR3-2014/NSDUH-DR-FRR3-2014/NSDUH-DR-FRR3-2014.htm

Harris, K. M., & Edlund, M. J. (2005). Use of mental health care and substance abuse treatment among adults with co-occurring disorders. *Psychiatric Services, 56*(8), 954-959.

International Federation of Social Workers. (2012). *Statement of ethical principles.* Retrieved February 1, 2015, from http://ifsw.org/policies/statements-of-ethical-principles

Krahn, G., Deck, D., Gabriel, R., & Farrell, N. (2007). A population-based study on substance abuse treatment for adults with disabilities: Access, utilization, and treatment outcomes. *The American Journal of Drug and Alcohol Abuse, 33*(6), 791-798.

Kuerbis, A., Sacco, P., Blazer, D. G., & Moore, A. A. (2014). Substance abuse among older adults. *Clinics in Geriatric Medicine, 30*(3), 629-654. doi:10.1016/j.cger.2014.04.008

Lauer, M., & van der Vennet, R. (2015). Effect of art production on negative mood and anxiety for adults in treatment for substance abuse. *Art Therapy: Journal of the American Art Therapy Association, 32*(4), 177-183. doi:10.1080/07421656.2015.1092731

Michigan Quality Improvement Consortium. (2009). Screening, diagnosis and referral for substance use disorders. Southfield, MI: Author.

Mizrahi, T., & Davis, L. E. (2011). Alcohol and drug problems. In T. Mizrahi & L. E. Davis (Eds.), *Encyclopedia of Social Work* (20th ed., pp. 121-130). Washington, D.C.: NASW Press.

Outlaw, F. H., Marquart, J. M., Roy, A., Luellen, J. K., Moran, M., Willis, A., & Doub, T. (2012). Treatment outcomes for older adults who abuse substances. *Journal of Applied Gerontology, 31*(1), 78-100. doi:10.1177/0733464810382906

Substance Abuse and Mental Health Services Administration. (2014). Results from the 2013 National Survey on Drug Use and Health: Summary of national findings, NSDUH Series H-48, HHS Publication No. (SMA) 14-4863. Retrieved February 1, 2016, from http://archive.samhsa.gov/data/NSDUH/2013SummNatFindDetTables/National-Findings/NSDUHresults2013.pdf

Wheeler, D. (2015). NASW standards and indicators for cultural competence in social work practice. Retrieved February 1, 2015, from http://www.socialworkers.org/practice/standards/PRA-BRO-253150-CC-Standards.pdf

SUBSTANCE USE DISORDERS: RISK-TAKING SEXUAL BEHAVIOR IN YOUNG PEOPLE—INTERVENTIONS TO PREVENT

MAJOR CATEGORIES: Substance Abuse

WHAT WE KNOW

Substance use disorders (SUDs) are patterns of substance use that cause, mental, or social impairment. SUDs constitute a widespread public health problem; they are associated with increased risk for unsafe behaviors, illness and injury, and mortality.

The *Diagnostic and Statistical Manual of Mental Disorders,* 5 edition (*DSM-5*), criteria for SUD include severity specifiers that are determined by the number of criteria met. For SUD to be diagnosed, distress or functional impairment must be present; severity is determined by how many of the additional 11 criteria occur within a 12-month period. At least two are needed for a diagnosis to be made.

SUDs can involve use of legal (e.g., alcohol, prescription medications) or illicit substances.

SUDs are common in individuals 16–25 years of age. A 2011 report by the National Center on Addiction and Substance Abuse (CASA) at Columbia University indicates that 1.6 million (roughly 1 in 8)

high school students in the United States have a diagnosable SUD.

Risk factors for SUDs in adolescence include a family history of SUD, low socioeconomic status, unemployment, family dysfunction or trauma, academic difficulties, criminal p involvement, depression, anxiety, antisocial personality disorder, bipolar disorder, and attention deficit disorder.

The Monitoring the Future project, which has surveyed 8, 10, and 12 grade students in the United States annually since 1975, found a slight decline during the 12 months prior to the 2015 survey in use of all illicit drugs among the 44,900 students who participated in the survey.

Lifetime prevalence for all survey respondents of use of any illicit drug including inhalants was 37.4 percent; for cannabis, 30.0 percent; alcohol, 45.2 percent; and 28.2 percent reported having been drunk.

The annual use for students in 12 grade of all illicit drugs including inhalants was 40.2 percent, which is about the midpoint between the high of 43.3 percent and the low of 37.0 percent since 1996; for cannabis alone, prevalence was 34.9 percent, which is about the midpoint between the high of 38.5 percent and the low of 31.5 percent since 1996; alcohol was 58.2 percent, which continues a trend of decline that started in the late 1990s from about 70 percent; and 37.7 percent reported having been drunk, which continues a trend of decline that started in the early 2000s from about 50 percent .

Young people with SUDs are more likely to engage in high-risk sexual behaviors than their peers without SUDs. SUDs are associated with increased risk for potentially devastating social and health consequences, including unintended pregnancy, sexual assault, sexually transmitted diseases (STDs), and the human immunodeficiency virus (HIV) infection.

One in five persons 13–24 years of age reports having unprotected sex after drinking alcohol or using other drugs.

Increased substance use/abuse correlates with decreased condom use.

Girls who began smoking before 16 years of age are more likely to engage in early sex leading to pregnancy when compared to those who never smoked or those who only experimented with smoking.

Use of alcohol at an early age is associated with an early age at first intercourse and pregnancy at a young age.

Adolescents who binge drink (commonly defined as consuming 5 or more alcoholic drinks on one occasion) are more likely to engage in high-risk sexual behaviors than non-drinkers. In a study involving over 15,000 teens, investigators found that those who binge drank were:

- 5.5 times more likely to engage in sexual activity,
- 10.3 times more likely to have used alcohol or other drugs before their last sexual intercourse,
- 4.7 times more likely to have become pregnant or made someone pregnant, and
- 3.7 times more likely to be raped.

High school students who have used heroin, methamphetamine, ecstasy, cocaine, or inhalants in their lifetime engage in high-risk sexual behaviors more than their non-using peers, with the degree of increased risk varying according to the specific drug used. Adolescents who use illicit drugs are:

- 3–10 times more likely than non-users to have had sex before age 13,
- 3–13 times more likely to report having multiple sex partners,
- 1.7–2.4 times more likely to have unprotected sex, and
- 3–16 times more likely to have become pregnant or make someone pregnant.

Healthcare providers often lack the training necessary to identify individuals with SUDs and to refer them to treatment. In adolescents, early intervention is particularly crucial because health-risk behaviors that are formed during this time often are continued into adulthood.

The Substance Abuse and Mental Health Services Administration (SAMHSA) is a public health service that provides resources for healthcare providers regarding SUD prevention, early detection, intervention, and treatment across the lifespan, including in adolescence.

Brief interventions can be utilized to educate and motivate behavioral changes to reduce or prevent use of nicotine, alcohol, and/or other substances; referral to specialty services is appropriate in individuals with SUDs who require more intensive treatment.

A brief (6-question) screen designed for adolescents is the CRAFFT, which has the advantages of being free, quick (about 2 to 3 minutes), and includes questions specific to both alcohol and drugs. If warranted the CRAFFT can be used as a starting point for a conversation using Motivational Interviewing techniques about substance use and risky sexual behavior.

Healthcare providers are more reluctant to address sexual risk behaviors than SUD with adolescents. Avoiding discussions of sexual health with young persons can convey a message that sexual risk behaviors are inconsequential or unimportant. Evaluation of sexual risk behaviors should be a standard part of assessment in young persons. It is important for these converstions to take place in a confidential environment in order to directly address their sexual risk behaviors offer opportunities for health promotion, intervention, screening, and treatment.

It may be helpful when working with adolescents to help facilitate conversation between them and their families and/or peers to opens a forum to explore values related to sex and to promote awareness of the serious consequences of risk-taking sexual behaviors.

More research is required to evaluate the effects on adolescent alcohol use and sexual behaviors of family variables (e.g., divorce), parent-child communication, attitudes about sex, peer relations, and knowledge and attitudes about HIV/acquired immunodeficiency syndrome (AIDS).

What Can Be Done

Develop an awareness of our own cultural values, beliefs, and biases and develop knowledge about the histories, traditions, and values of our clients. Adopt treatment methodologies that reflect the cultural needs of the client.

Learn about sexual risk behaviors in adolescents with SUDs and share this information with your colleagues.

Educate adolescent clients and their families, when appropriate, about screening, prevention, and treatment options for SUDs, STDs, unplanned pregnancy, and/or sexual assault. Refer to local resources for psychosocial support and addiction counseling, as appropriate.

Develop a therapeutic relationship with adolescent clients to better assess them and their health education needs, as well as to engage them in treatment.

Determine if family therapy sessions are appropriate.

Educate yourself on confidentiality rules regarding sexual risk behaviors and adolescents so your adolescent clients understand their confidentiality rights.

Educate yourself on your state's laws regarding STD screening of minors so you and your clients know what tests they may have without parental consent.

Collaborate with your facility's education department to provide ongoing interdisciplinary education about the prevalence of and relationship between SUDs and sexual risk-taking behaviors in young persons; advocate for the implementation of routine substance use/abuse screening and early intervention for young persons.

Written by Melissa Rosales Neff, MSW, and Chris Bates, MA, MSW

Reviewed by Jessica Therivel, LMSW-IPR

References

American Psychiatric Association. (2013). Diagnostic and statistical manual of mental disorders. (5th ed.). Arlington, VA: Author.

Clarke, S. L. (2015). Substance use disorders. In F. J. Domino (Ed.), *The 5-minute clinical consult standard 2016* (24th ed., pp. 1058-1059). Philadelphia, PA: Wolters Kluwer Health.

Connery, H. S., Albright, B. B., & Rodolico, J. M. (2014). Adolescent substance use and unplanned pregnancy: strategies for risk reduction. *Obstetrics & Gynecology Clinics of North America, 41*(2), 191-203. doi:10.1016/j.ogc.2014.02.011

Dembo, R., Briones-Robins, R., Winters, K. C., Belenko, S., Karas, L. M., Gulledge, L., & Wareham, J. (2014). Brief intervention for truant youth sexual risk behavior and marijuana use. *Journal of Child & Adolescent Substance Abuse, 23*(5), 318-333. doi:10.1080/1067828X.2014.928116

Fornili, K., & Haack, M. R. (2005). Policy watch. Promoting early intervention for substance use disorders through interdisciplinary education for health professionals. *Journal of Addictions Nursing, 16*(3), 153-160. doi:10.1080/10884600500231946

Hoff, T., Greene, L., & Davis, J. (2003). National survey of adolescents and young adults: Sexual health knowledge, attitudes and experiences. Retrieved February 13, 2014, from

http://kaiserfamilyfoundation.files.wordpress.
com/2013/01/national-survey-of-adolescents-and-
young-adults.pdf

Houck, C. (2010). Early adolescent sexual risk behavior: The clinician's role. *Brown University Child
and Adolescent Behavior Letter, 26*(7), 1, 5-6.

Joffe, A., & Morris, R. E. (2008). Adolescent substance use and abuse. In L. S. Neinstein (Ed.),
Adolescent health care: A practical guide (5th ed., pp.
863-877). Philadelphia: Wolters Kluwer Health/
Lippincott Williams & Wilkins.

Johnston, L. D., O'Malley, P. M., Miech, R. A., Bachman,
J. G., & Schulenberg, J. E. (2016). Monitoring the Fu-
ture - national survey results on drug use, 1975-2016:
Overview, key findings on adolescent use.

Miller, J. W., Naimi, T. S., Brewer, R. D., & Jones, S. E.
(2007). Binge drinking and associated health risk
behaviors among high school students. *Pediatrics,
119*(1), 76-85. doi:10.1542/peds.2006-1517

National Association of Social Workers. (2015). NASW
standards and indicators for cultural competence
in social work practice. Retrieved April 4, 2016,
from http://www.socialworkers.org/practice/stan-
dards/PRA-BRO-253150-CC-Standards.pdf

The National Center on Addiction and Substance
Abuse at Columbia University. (2011). Adolescent
substance use: America's #1 public health problem.
Retrieved February 13, 2014, from http://www.ca-
sacolumbia.org/upload/2011/20110629adolesce
ntsubstanceuse.pdf

Orgiles, M., Carratala, E., Carballo, J. L., Piqueras, J.
A., & Espada, J. P. (2013). Factors associated with
sex under the influence of alcohol among adolescents with divorced parents. *Journal of Child & Adolescent Substance Abuse, 22*(2), 150-162.

The Policy, Ethics, and Human Rights Committee,
British Association of Social Workers. (2012, January). *The Code of Ethics for Social Work: Statement
of Principles.* Retrieved February 13, 2014, from
http://cdn.basw.co.uk/upload/basw_112315-7.
pdf

Springer, A. E., Peters, R. J., Shegog, R., White, D. L.,
& Kelder, S. H. (2007). Methamphetamine use and
sexual risk behaviors in U.S. high school students:
Findings from a national risk behavior survey.
Prevention Science, 8(2), 103-113. doi:10.1007/
s11121-007-0065-6

Substance Abuse and Mental Health Services Administration. (2011). Strategic prevention framework.
Retrieved February 13, 2014, from http://www.
samhsa.gov/sbirt

Substance/Medication-Induced Psychotic Disorder

Major Categories: Behavioral & Mental Health, Substance Abuse

Description

A substance/medication-induced psychotic disorder is a psychosis induced by a drug or alcohol, and is included as a specific disorder in the Fifth Edition of the *Diagnostic and Statistical Manual of Mental Disorders* (*DSM-V*) (American Psychiatric Association, 2013). A substance/medication-induced psychotic disorder can have either or both of the two major symptoms of delusions and hallucinations, which indicate an individual's loss of contact with reality, and are usually associated with certain mental illnesses such as schizophrenia. However, although the symptoms of a substance-/medication-induced psychotic disorder, such as delusions or hallucinations, can resemble those of such an illness, the two are different conditions, with different causes and treatments. In the case of schizophrenia and other intrinsic mental illnesses these symptoms result from a disorder of the brain itself, whereas in the case of a substance-/medication-induced psychotic disorder they result from the effects on the brain of a chemical substance or a particular medication. Consequently, a diagnosis of substance-medication-induced psychotic disorder required evidence from an individual's medical history, physical examination, or findings in laboratory tests of the use of particular substance or of alcohol as the cause of the disorder (American Psychiatric Association, 2013). Apart from alcohol, substances that can cause a substance-/medication-induced psychotic disorder include amphetamines, cannabis (marijuana), cocaine, anxiolytic agents hallucinogens, hypnotic agents, opioids, phencyclidine (PCP) and related substances, and sedatives, such as barbiturates.

A defining characteristic of substance/medication-induced psychotic disorder is that when the substance or medication that causes the disorder is no longer used and the body has completely eliminated it, the psychotic symptoms of the disorder will cease or remit. However, care must be taken to recognize the distinction between hallucinations or delusions resulting directly from the use of a causative substance or medication and the occurrence of such symptoms as the result of cessation or withdrawal from the use of such a substance or medication. Further complicating the diagnosis of a substance/-medication-induced psychotic disorder is that it may exist concurrently with an intrinsic or endogenous psychosis whose symptoms resemble those of the disorder.

The symptoms of a substance-/medication-induced psychotic disorder will ordinarily cease or remit within 1 month after the cessation of its use, with the with the user returning to his or her same level of functioning as before the occurrence of the disorder. The frequently retroactive nature of a confirmed diagnosis and the wide variety of possible causes make research and evidence-based treatments difficult to develop. Depending on the severity and duration of the symptoms treatment might include hospitalization, medications, psychotherapy, and education of family and friends about the disorder.

FACTS AND FIGURES

Because of the possibility of its confusion with an intrinsic or endogenous psychotic disorder, few generally accepted facts and figures exists for the incidence or prevalence of substance-/medication-induced psychotic disorder. Moreover, most information about this comes from studies of substance use disorders (SUDs) that focus on a specific substance, and therefore does not apply to the many different possible causes of substance-/medication-induced psychotic disorder.

RISK FACTORS

Risk factors for a substance-/medication induced psychotic disorder include the recent use of a wide range of substance(s) or medication(s), both legal or illegal, prescribed or not prescribed, and consumed intentionally or unintentionally (e.g., organophosphate insecticides or volatile substances such as fuel or paint). Research has found that polydrug use is the strongest risk factor for substance-induced psychosis (Rognli et al., 2015).

SIGNS AND SYMPTOMS

Signs and symptoms of a substance-/medication induced psychotic disorder include prominent hallucinations or delusions in the absence of a long-term history of mental disorder and of other signs or symptoms that reflect or indicate an intrinsic or endogenous mental health disorder.

APPLICABLE LAWS AND REGULATIONS

The U.S. Government and individuals states of the United States have their own standards, procedures, and laws for the involuntary restraint and detention of persons who may be a danger to themselves or to others. Because individuals having delusions or hallucinations may be in danger of hurting themselves or others, it is important to become familiar with the local requirements for reporting potentially harmful behavior and for involuntary detention.

TREATMENT

The social worker assisting an individual with a substance-/medication-induced psychotic disorder should conduct a standard biological, psychological, social, and spiritual assessment of the individual, including an assessment of his or her risk for suicide and for inflicting harm on him- or herself and others. This should include an assessment of the individual's level of functioning and demeanor during the interview conducted for the assessment, with particular attention to the individual's affect and cognitive symptoms and to the collection of information on any prior or other mental-health disorders. The assessment should also include laboratory tests if and as needed to identify medical disorders and substance abuse, including the presence of potentially causative substances in the affected individual's urine and blood, and the collection of collateral information from the individual's family, friends, and co-workers. The evaluation of persons with a substance-/medication-induced psychotic disorder is especially important because of its possible coexistence with an intrinsic or endogenous mental disorder.

The treatments used to stop or decrease the use of a psychosis-inducing substance or medication will vary with the nature of such a substance or medication, but will typically include a monitored period of withdrawal and detoxification, with or without hospitalization; interactive therapy, such as psychotherapy, cognitive behavioral therapy (CBT), or participation in a 12-step support group; and intensive inpatient or outpatient rehabilitation.

The social worker should review the regimen of any medication prescribed as part of the treatment of an individual with a substance-/medication-induced psychotic disorder, follow-up to ensure adherence to the regimen of such medication, and make follow-up appointments for the affected individual with the agency or physician issuing the prescription for this medication. If appropriate, the affected individual should be referred to local support groups or treatment programs for SUDs. The social worker should also ascertain the stability of the affected individual's living situation and refer him or her, and family members if and as needed, to appropriate groups or organizations for support, including those for mental health disorders and substance use.

Social workers assisting individuals who have a substance-/medication-induced psychotic disorder should be aware of their own cultural values, beliefs, and biases, and develop specialized knowledge about these individuals' histories, traditions, and values. They should adopt treatment methods that reflect their knowledge of the cultural diversity of the communities to which these individuals belong.

SERVICES AND RESOURCES

The following resources can provide information about substance-/medication-induced psychotic disorder. The term "substance-induced psychosis" or "substance/medication-induced psychosis" should be entered in the online "search" box of a particular resource to access relevant information available at its website.

- U.S. National Institutes of Health (NIH), http://www.nih.gov/
- U.S. National Institute of Mental Health (NIMH), http://www.nimh.nih.gov/index.shtml
- National Association of Social Workers (NASW), http://www.socialworkers.org/

Written by Chris Bates, MA, MSW

Reviewed by Lynn B. Cooper, D. Crim, and Pedram Samghabadi

REFERENCES

American Psychiatric Association. (2013). Diagnostic and statistical manual of mental health disorders (DSM-5). (5th ed.). Arlington, VA: American Psychiatric Publishing.

British Association of Social Workers. (2012, January). The code of ethics for social work: Statement of principles. Retrieved February 26, 2016, from http://cdn.basw.co.uk/upload/basw_112315-7.pdf

Conner, K., Gamble, S., Bagge, C., He, H., Swogger, M., Watts, A., & Houston, R. (2014). Substance-induced depression and independent depression in proximal risk for suicidal behavior. *Journal of Studies on Alcohol & Drugs*, 75(4), 567-572.

International Federation of Social Workers. (2012, March 3). Statement of Ethical Principles. Retrieved February 26, 2016, from http://ifsw.org/policies/statement-of-ethical-principles/

Liang, H. J., Tang, O. K. L., Chan, O. F., Ungvari, O. G. S., & Tang, W. K. (2015). Ketamine users have high rates of psychosis and/or depression. *Journal of Addictions Nursing*, 26(1), 8-13. doi:10.1097/JAN.0000000000000060

National Association of Social Workers. (2015). NASW standards and indicators for cultural competence in social work practice. Retrieved February 26, 2016, from http://www.socialworkers.org/practice/standards/PRA-BRO-253150-CC-Standards.pdf

Rognli, E., Berge, J., Hakansson, A., & Bramess, J. (2015). Long-term risk factors for substance-induced and primary psychosis after release from prison. A longitudinal study of substance users. *Schizoprenia Research*, 168(1-2), 185-190. doi:10.1016/j.schres.2015.08.032

Schanzer, B. M., First, M. B., Dominguez, B., Hasin, D. S., & Caton, C. L. M. (2006). Diagnosing psychotic disorders in the emergency department in the context of substance use. *Psychiatric Services*, 57(10), 1468-1473.

Tyrer, P. (2011). People with psychosis should be asked about substance use. *Guidelines in Practice*, 14(10), 9-19.

SUDDEN TRAUMATIC LOSS & COMPLICATED GRIEF

MAJOR CATEGORIES: Behavioral & Mental Health

DESCRIPTION

Grief, defined as a reaction to major loss characterized by a period of sorrow, emotional numbness, and, in some cases, guilt and anger, is a healthy, normal response to losing a loved one that usually fades as the affected person accepts the loss. For some individuals, however, the grief state persists to the point of debilitation. In persons with complicated grief (also called *prolonged, traumatic,* and *pathological grief*), painful emotions, including nonacceptance of the loved one's death, are so long-lasting and severe that bereaved individuals are unable to resume their normal daily activities. Sudden traumatic loss, defined as a death resulting from an unexpected, destructive, or preventable event (e.g., car accident, suicide, homicide, natural disaster, war),is a risk factor for complicated grief.

The fifth edition of the *Diagnostic and Statistical Manual of Mental Disorders (DSM-5)* has codified the concept of complicated grief in the newly added condition "persistent complex bereavement disorder" in the chapter on conditions for further study. The proposed criteria are the death of someone close to one and the presence for at least 12 months (6 for children) of at least one of the following: longing for the deceased, intense emotional pain, preoccupation with the deceased, and preoccupation with the manner of the death. In addition, 6 of 12 other criteria dealing with distress related to the death and social or identity disruption must be present for the same amount of time (American Psychiatric Association, p. 789).

Complicated grief resulting from traumatic loss places a person at risk for comorbid mental health conditions, including major depression, posttraumatic stress disorder (PTSD), and substance use disorder. Please see the appropriate Quick Lesson for more information regarding these mental health disorders.

Treatment for complicated grief includes psychotherapy and pharmacotherapy. Grief-focused individual and group therapies have been associated with significant and lasting improvements in complicated grief. There are insufficient data regarding pharmacological interventions for complicated grief, although in cases of comorbid depression, medication may help clients sustain engagement in treatment.

FACTS AND FIGURES

An estimated 10 percent–20 percent of individuals who sustain a loss experience complicated grief (Jordan & Litz, 2014); studies from outside the United States often report lower numbers (3 percent–5 percent; Rosner, 2015).

Researchers in an Australian population-based study of bereavement found that among respondents who completed a risk assessment for prolonged grief disorder, 58.4 percent were at low risk for complicated grief, 35.2 percent were at moderate risk, and 6.4 percent were at high risk. Respondents who were at high risk often were grieving unexpected and untimely deaths (Aoun et al., 2015).

Significantly higher rates of complicated grief have been reported in studies of bereavement resulting from violence and natural disasters.

Investigators in a Norwegian study found that parents and siblings of youth who were victims of a mass shooting continued to experience high levels of distress and impaired work and school performance 1.5 years after the deaths. Complicated grief was identified in 82 percent of parents and 75 percent of siblings in the study (Dyregrov, & Kristensen, 2015).

Researchers in a study involving bereaved earthquake survivors in China reported that the prevalence of complicated grief was 71 percent a year after the disaster (Li, Chow, Shi, & Chan, 2015).

RISK FACTORS

Risk factors for complicated grief include the following:

- preexisting mental health and/or substance use problems;
- having poor coping skills, poor social support, multiple life stressors, or a lack of information about the details of the loved one's death;
- having an insecure attachment style;
- being a woman, child, adolescent, younger spouse who has lost a partner, or older adult who has lost a person with whom he/she had a long-standing relationship;
- having had conflict and/or a difficult relationship with the deceased loved one;
- having lost a person in traumatic or violent circumstances;

- having experienced a previous traumatic loss;
- potentially socially unrecognized or stigmatized losses (e.g., stillbirth, suicide); and
- childhood abuse or neglect.

SIGNS AND SYMPTOMS

Grief manifestations in persons with complicated grief persist longer than 6 months after the loss of a loved one.

Psychological: feelings of depression (episodic or pervasive), intense yearning, hopelessness, isolation, denial, anger, shame, guilt, fear, worthlessness, loss of pleasure in activities, stress, feelings of stigma, reliving of traumatic events, rumination, preoccupation with thoughts of deceased, hyperarousal, emotional numbness.

Behavioral: increase or decrease in sleep, nervousness, aggression, agitation, loss of interest in activities, isolation, nightmares.

Pharmacological: side effects of medications or combinations of medications may exacerbate existing symptoms.

Physical: somatic complaints (e.g., chronic muscle pain, back pain, headaches, fatigue, gastrointestinal disorders), sleep disturbances, changes in weight, neglect, frailty, debilitation.

ASSESSMENT

Complete a detailed patient history, including alcohol and tobacco use, unintentional weight loss, and sleep patterns; ask about any comorbid mental health conditions.

Assess your clients' responses to grief and screen for complicated grief and other bereavement complications.

Biopsychosocial-spiritual assessments should be used in conjunction with other assessment and screening tools to develop a better understanding of clients' physical and emotional support systems.

Evaluating social support relationships, presence of comorbidities, and physical health can help to determine any perceived or actual barriers to care and support and allow for the implementation of individualized interventions. In addition, individuals at risk should be assessed for suicidal ideation/plans, substance abuse, and risk to self.

ASSESSMENTS AND SCREENING TOOLS

Complicated grief can be measured utilizing the following tools: Inventory of Complicated Grief (ICG), Brief Grief Questionnaire (BGQ), Persistent Complex Bereavement Inventory (PCBI), Complicated Bereavement Risk Assessment (CBRA), and Extended Grief Inventory (EGI). Screening tools for posttraumatic stress disorder include the Clinician Administered PTSD Scale (CAPS) and the University of California–Los Angeles Post-Traumatic Stress Disorder Reaction Index. In addition, assessments for depression, anxiety, and substance abuse should be completed if indicated.

TREATMENT

Treatment for complicated grief includes a combination of psychotherapy and pharmacotherapy.

Some persons with complicated grief receive significant benefit from psychotherapy, particularly cognitive behavioral grief-specific therapies such as complicated grief treatment, cognitive behavioral therapy (CBT), and cognitive narrative intervention. Therapy may include psychoeducation about grief, exposure to painful aspects of loss, processing of loss, restoration of meaningful goals and social connections, and cognitive restructuring to deal with disruptive thoughts (e.g., self-blame). Additional interventions include a grief support group, stress management, progressive muscle relaxation, guided imagery, and meditation. Psychotherapy can help patients become more aware of their emotions, improve coping skills, and reduce feelings of self-blame and guilt.

Investigators who conducted a meta-analysis found that CBT and group therapy are effective in reducing signs and symptoms of complicated grief and have benefits that persist for 3–6 months (Wittouck, Van Autreve, De Jaegere, Portzky, & Van Heeringen, 2011).

Complicated grief treatment (CGT) is a time-limited, manualized model that focuses both on processing loss and restoring engagement.

In a randomized clinical trial, researchers found that although both CGT and grief-focused interpersonal psychotherapy were associated with a decrease in complicated grief symptoms, CGT was associated with greater symptom reduction (Shear et al., 2014).

Researchers in another randomized trial found that the CGT model adapted as a group therapy intervention was more effective than a standard grief support group (Supiano & Luptak, 2014).

In a small randomized controlled trial in Portugal, researchers found that a brief cognitive narrative intervention was linked with a significant decrease in complicated grief, depression, and trauma symptoms (Barbosa, Sá, & Rocha, 2014).

Although there is little research on prevention of complicated grief, participation in a brief psychotherapy program after the loss of a loved one may help prevent or reduce the severity of complicated grief, especially for individuals who have risk factors for complicated grief.

Social workers should be aware of their own cultural values, beliefs, and biases and develop specialized knowledge about the histories, traditions, and values of their clients. Social workers should adopt treatment methodologies that reflect their knowledge of the cultural diversity of the societies in which they practice

Problem	Goal	Intervention
Client has signs and symptoms of complicated grief	Reduce signs and symptoms of complicated grief	Use cognitive behavioral grief-targeted interventions to assist client to understand his or her grief, process loss, and learn to reengage in life and pleasurable activities. Provide or refer for other interventions as indicated. Interventions for comorbid disorders may need to be prioritized
Client is at risk for complicated grief	Reduce risk for complicated grief	See Treatment Summary above
Client has a lack of social support and/or poor coping skills	Improve social support and coping skills	Assist client in reengaging with support system; refer for grief-focused support groups

LAWS AND REGULATIONS
Social workers and other mental health and healthcare professionals are bound by the "duty to warn," which states that they must inform the proper authorities if a person is found to be a danger to him- or herself or others. Clinicians should be aware of the policies and procedures of their state's duty to warn law.

Each country has its own standards for cultural competence and diversity in social work practice. Social workers must be aware of the standards of practice set forth by their governing bodies (e.g., National Association of Social Workers in the United States, British Association of Social Workers in England) and practice accordingly.

SERVICES AND RESOURCES
- The National Social Worker Finder links individuals to mental health social workers, including those focused on grief and loss, www.helpstartshere.org

- The National Bereavement Resource Guide, a database of local bereavement services, http://www.moyerfoundation.org/nbrg/
- Local Veterans Affairs hospitals(http://www.va.gov/landing2_locations.htm), medical facilities, and community mental health organizations have resources to assist with grief and loss
- National Alliance for Grieving Children,http://childrengrieve.org/
- The Center for Complicated Grief http://complicatedgrief.org/

FOOD FOR THOUGHT
There is minimal research on the use of antidepressants in the treatment of complicated grief; selective serotonin reuptake inhibitors (SSRIs) may reduce manifestations of complicated grief in some patients.

Spiritual questioning and crises are more likely after a sudden or traumatic loss among spiritually inclined individuals and may place individuals at higher risk of developing complicated grief. Spiritually sensitive assessments, interventions, and referrals may assist in decreasing this risk.

Complicated grief has been linked with neurological findings (e.g., smaller brain volume, lower performance on cognitive tests). Although the direction of the relationship is not clear, it is notable that these differences are not seen in normal grief. Cognitive screening and support may be indicated for individuals with complicated grief.

RED FLAGS
Clients with complicated grief may develop comorbid mental health problems; monitor client for suicidal ideation.

Different groups of bereaved clients (e.g., parents who have lost a child, people who have lost a loved one to suicide) have distinct treatment needs; adapt interventions accordingly.

NEXT STEPS
Referrals for follow-up services for adults who have experienced sudden traumatic loss are an important step toward improving the mental health of those individuals and families. Biopsychosocial-spiritual, posttraumatic stress, and depression assessments should be conducted. Multiple resources are available for families experiencing sudden traumatic loss, including individual and group programs. Referrals should be based on assessments and client-specific needs (e.g., infant loss, loss of spouse, suicide).

Ensure that clients feel that their loss has been validated by the social worker.

Written by Amanda Becker, LCSW, and Jennifer Teska, MSW

Reviewed by Jessica Therivel, LMSW-IPR, and Chris Bates, MA, MSW

REFERENCES
Aoun, S. M., Breen, L. J., Howting, D. A., Rumbold, B., McNamara, B., & Hegney, D. (2015). Who needs bereavement support? A population based survey of bereavement risk and support need. *PLoS ONE, 10*(3), e0121101. doi:10.1371/journal.pone.0121101 American Psychiatric Association. (2013). Diagnostic and statistical manual of mental disorders. (5th ed.).

Arlington, VA: Author. Barbosa, V., Sá, M., & Rocha, J. C. (2014). Randomised controlled trial of a cognitive narrative intervention for complicated grief in widowhood. *Aging and Mental Health, 18*(3), 354-362. doi:10.1080/13607863.2013.833164

Boyer, J. L., Ginzburg, H. M., & Foote, A. (2008). A unique therapeutic approach to complicated grief. *Journal of the Oklahoma State Medical Association, 101*(12), 291-294.

British Association of Social Workers. (2012). The code of ethics for social work: Statement of principles. Retrieved December 29, 2015, from http://cdn.basw.co.uk/upload/basw_112315-7.pdf

Bui, E., Horonstein, A., Shah, R., Skritskaya, N. A., Mauro, C., Wang, Y., ... Simon, N. M. (2015). Grief-related panic symptoms in complicated grief. *Journal of Affective Disorders, 170*, 213-216. doi:10.1016/j.jad.2014.08.028

Burke, L. A., & Neimeyer, R. A. (2014). Complicated spiritual grief I: Relation to complicated grief symptomatology following violent death bereavement. *Death Studies, 38*(4), 259-267. doi:10.1080/07481187.2013.829372

Claxon, R., & Reynolds, C. F., III. (2012). Complicated grief #254. *Journal of Palliative Medicine, 15*(7), 829-830. doi:10.1089/jpm.2012.9577

Currier, J. M., Irish, J. E. F., Neimeryer, R. A., & Foster, J. D. (2015). Attachment, continuing bonds, and complicated grief following violent loss: Testing a moderated model. *Death Studies, 39*(4), 201-210. doi:10.1080/07481187.2014.975869

Dyregrov, K., Dyregrov, A., & Kristensen, P. (2015). Traumatic bereavement and terror: The psychosocial impact on parents and siblings 1.5 years after the July 2011 terror killings in Norway. *Journal of Loss and Trauma, 20*(6), 556-576. doi:10.1080/15325024.2014.957603

International Federation of Social Workers. (2012). Statement of Ethical Principles. Retrieved December 29, 2014, from http://ifsw.org/policies/statement-of-ethical-principles/

Jordan, A. H., & Litz, B. T. (2014). Prolonged grief disorder: Diagnostic, assessment, and treatment considerations. *Professional Psychology: Research and Practice, 45*(3), 180-187.

Lee, S. A. (2015). The persistent complex bereavement inventory: A measure based on the DSM-5. *Death Studies, 39*(7), 399-410. doi:10.1080/07481187.2015.1029144

Li, J., Chow, A. Y. M., Shi, Z., & Chan, C. L. W. (2015). Prevalence and risk factors of complicated grief among Sichuan earthquake survivors. *Journal of Effective Disorders*, *175*, 218-223. doi:10.1016/j.jad.2015.01.003

Lobb, E. A., Kristjanson, L. J., Aoun, S. M., Monterosso, L., Halkett, G. K., & Davies, A. (2010). Predictors of complicated grief: A systematic review of empirical studies. *Death Studies*, *34*(8), 673-698. doi:10.1080/07481187.2010.496686

Wheeler, D., & McClain, A. (2015). NASW standards for cultural competence in social work practice. Retrieved December 29, 2015, from http://www.socialworkers.org/practice/standards/PRA-BRO-253150-CC-Standards.pd

Robertson, T., & Scanlan, M. (2010). A discussion of the use of treatment approaches that can help individuals recover from complicated grief. *British Journal of Wellbeing*, *1*(8), 26-29.

Rosner, R. (2015). Prolonged grief: Setting the research agenda. *European Journal of Psychotraumatology*, *6*, 27303. doi:10.3402/ejpt.v6.27303

Saavedra Pérez, H. C., Ikram, M. A., Direk, N., Prigerson, H. G., Freak-Poli, R., ... Tiemeier, H. (2015). Cognition, structural brain changes and complicated grief. A population-based study. *Psychological Medicine*, *45*(7), 1389-1399. doi:10.1017/S0033291714002499

Shear, M. K. (2010). Complicated grief treatment: The theory, practice and outcomes. *Bereavement Care*, *29*(3), 10-14. doi:10.1080/02682621.2010.522373

Shear, M. K. (2015). Complicated grief. *New England Journal of Medicine*, *372*(2), 153-160. doi:10.1056/NEJMcp1315618

Shear, M. K., Wang, Y., Skritskaya, N., Duan, N., Mauro, C., & Ghesquiere, A. (2014). Treatment of complicated grief in elderly persons. *JAMA Psychiatry*, *71*(11), 1287-1295. doi:10.1001/jamapsychiatry.2014.1242

Sprang, G. (2001). The use of eye Movement desensitization and reprocessing (EMDR) in the treatment of traumatic stress and complicated mourning: Psychological and behavioral outcomes. *Research on Social Work Practice*, *11*(3), 300-320. doi:10.1177/104973150101100302

Supiano, K. P., & Luptak, M. (2014). Complicated grief in older adults: A randomized controlled trial of complicated grief group therapy. *Gerontologist*, *54*(5), 840-856. doi:geront/gnt076

Wagner, B., Keller, V., Knaevelsrud, C., & Maercker, A. (2012). Social acknowledgement as a predictor of post-traumatic stress and complicated grief after witnessing assisted suicide. *International Journal of Social Psychiatry*, *58*(4), 381-385. doi:10.1177/0020764011400791

Walijarvi, C. M., Weiss, A. H., & Weinman, M. L. (2012). A traumatic death support group program: Applying an integrated conceptual framework. *Death Studies*, *36*(2), 152-181. doi:10.1080/07481187.2011.553344

Wittouck, C., Van Autreve, S., De Jaegere, E., Portzky, G., & Van Heeringen, K. (2011). The prevention and treatment of complicated grief: A meta-analysis. *Clinical Psychiatry Review*, *31*(1), 69-78. doi:10.1016/j.cpr.2010.09.005

SUICIDE

MAJOR CATEGORIES: Behavioral & Mental Health

DESCRIPTION

The U.S. Centers for Disease Control and Prevention (CDC) defines suicide as "death caused by self-directed injurious behavior with an intent to die as a result of the behavior." The CDC defines a suicide attempt as "a non-fatal, self-directed, potentially injurious behavior with any intent to die that is a result of the behavior. A suicide attempt may or may not result in injury."

Suicidal ideation is thinking about or planning a suicide attempt. A combination of individual, familial, and community factors contribute to an individual's risk for suicide. A history of mental illness, particularly depression, and a history of physical or sexual abuse or alcohol or substance abuse increase the risk for suicide. A previous unsuccessful suicide attempt is a strong predictor of future death by suicide. Persons who have been imprisoned or otherwise legally institutionalized are at a higher risk for suicide after their release, possibly because of mental illness and the stress of their reintegration into the community. Familial factors that contribute to suicide include a family history of suicide or suicide attempts. Local epidemics of suicide among young persons (sometimes called *copycat suicides*) may also heighten the risk for suicide.

Despite these risk factors, many suicides are preventable with early intervention by mental-health professionals because persons who commit suicide often give warnings of their intent to do so. Common warning signs of suicide include giving away personal items, verbalizing suicidal thoughts, and withdrawing from friends and family; a further warning is that most persons who take their own lives have made previous suicide attempts.

FACTS AND FIGURES

Worldwide, suicide is the second leading cause of death among persons 15 to 44 years of age. In 2013, there were 41,149 suicides in the United States, a rate of 12.6 suicides per 100,000 people (CDC, 2015a), and in 2015, the CDC estimated that suicide in the United States cost $44.6 billion in medical expenses and lost work annually (CDC, 2015b).

In the United States, men are four times more likely to commit suicide than are women, and chiefly use firearms for this purpose, whereas women most often use poison. Among persons in the United States in the age group of 15 to 34, years, Native Americans have the highest rate of suicide. On average, Black men who commit suicide do so earlier in life than do White men who commit suicide. Lesbian and gay Americans have higher rates of suicide than heterosexual Americans. Individuals with chronic depression are 20 times more likely to commit suicide than those without any mental disorder. Black women have the lowest rate of suicide in the United States, and are 9 times less likely than White women to commit suicide.

RISK FACTORS FOR SUICIDE

Groups considered at high risk for suicide are veterans and military personnel, adolescents, and older adults. More United States military personnel died of suicide from 2009 to 2013 than died in active duty. A combination of factors can increase the risk of an individual's suicide attempts and completions. Persons who have already attempted suicide or who have a family history of suicide are at heightened risk for it, especially when they experience a physical illness and/or depression. One study found that that 80 percent of those who completed suicide had made a previous attempt at it (Coletsoset al., 2016). A major psychiatric disorder is a feature in the lives of most victims of suicide, and depressed individuals are among those at risk for attempting and completing it. Adolescents with mood, anxiety, or disruptive behavior disorders are at an increased risk for suicide, as are those who have been victims of bullying or who have been incarcerated.

Substance abuse is a common factor among those who complete suicide, and is therefore a risk factor for it. Bisexuality or homosexuality increases the risk of suicide, particularly among young persons. Other factors that increase the risk of suicide are recent loss, such as through divorce or separation, the death of a loved one, or job loss. Having experienced childhood sexual or physical abuse can also increase the risk. Others at risk for suicide are persons who as children were the subjects of intervention by child welfare agencies. Also at risk are individuals who have access to lethal items such as firearms and prescription drugs. In terms of occupation, physicians have been considered at the greatest risk of committing suicide.

The most overt sign of a risk of suicide is a verbal statement about wanting to die or taking one's own life. Suicidal individuals may appear depressed, with feelings of loneliness, despair, and hopelessness. They may have experienced a recent loss or know that they have a serious physical illness. Other signs of risk include substance abuse, with alcohol abuse especially common among older male victims of suicide. As noted earlier, a previous attempt at suicide or a history of such an attempt increases its risk, and mood, anxiety, or disruptive disorders or confusion about their sexuality are risk factors for suicide among adolescents. Rapid significant weight loss can also be a sign of depression and suicidal thinking. Serious warning signs are suicidal ideation, a plan for how to accomplish suicide, and a means for carrying out the plan.

EVALUATION OF RISK FOR SUICIDE

Social workers and other healthcare professionals should conduct an assessment of persons who may be at risk of suicide to establish whether they have any suicidal thinking and its severity. A psychiatric consultation with persons who appear to be at risk for suicide is usually necessary. It is especially important to monitor persons in whom treatment with antidepressant drugs has just begun or after it ends. Treating any underlying mental illness or substance abuse is essential in persons at risk for suicide. Research has indicated that cognitive behavioral therapy (CBT) has halved the rate of re-attempts at suicide in persons who have previously attempted it (Coletsoset al., 2016).

Questioning depressed clients about suicidal thinking is considered an essential measure in suicide prevention (e.g., "Have you ever felt that life is not worth living?" "Do you ever wish you could go to sleep and not wake up?" "Are you having thoughts about killing yourself"). However, some people will deny that they are at risk for suicide even if they are questioned about it. Someone who discloses suicidal ideation, should immediately be evaluated for having any risk factors for suicide, their mental status, and their thinking. They should also be asked whether there is any history of suicide in their family.

Persons who have a plan to accomplish their suicide are at especially high risk for doing so. Social workers can question individuals about any previous attempts at suicide, recent personal losses, or history of substance abuse, and about their physical and mental health. Persons who exhibit suicidal thinking should be asked about their relationships with family members and social support systems, who may be able to assist in maintaining their safety. It is critical to ask whether someone who expresses suicidal thinking has access to firearms and prescription and/or nonprescription drugs and, if so, to encourage that person to remove them from the home.

It is also important that the social worker educate family members about warning signs of suicide. In adults these can include hopelessness, isolation, and significant losses (e.g., spouse, job). For youths, warning signs can include family stress, bullying at school or electronically (via text or social media), changes in eating or sleeping patterns, and a friend's having committed suicide.

Persons at risk for suicide, and their family members, should be provided with with resources for its prevention that are available on a 24-hour-a-day/7-day-per-week basis. Support groups appear to be very beneficial for the survivors of someone who has committed suicide, who typically experience a great feelings of guilt.

Social workers engaged in working with potentially suicidal individuals should be aware of their own cultural values, beliefs, and biases, and develop specialized knowledge about the histories, traditions, and values of these individuals. They should also use treatment methods that reflect their knowledge of the cultures of these individuals and their communities.

APPLICABLE LAWS AND REGULATIONS

In many jurisdictions, suicidal ideation is considered an exception to the confidentiality that typically exists between a patient and a social worker, psychiatrist, or other therapist.

SERVICES AND RESOURCES

The following resources are available for helping to prevent suicide:

- National Suicide Prevention Lifeline, http://www.suicidepreventionlifeline.org [(800) 273-8255]
- http://www.suicide.org/, a nonprofit organization working for suicide prevention, awareness, and support [(800) 784-2433]
- The Trevor Project, a national organization providing crisis intervention for lesbian, gay, bisexual, transgender, and questioning youth, http://www.thetrevorproject.org [(866) 488-7386]
- Indian Health Service (HIS), the American Indian and Alaska Native Suicide Prevention Program, https://www.ihs.gov/suicideprevention/ [(800) 273-8255]
- Veterans Crisis Line, http://www.veteranscrisisline.net [(800) 273-8255, press 1]
- Suicide Prevention Resource Center, http://www.sprc.org
- Training Institute for Suicide Assessment and Clinical Interviewing (TISA), http://www.suicideassessment.com

Written by Jan Wagstaff, MA, MSW, and Laura Gale, LCSW

Reviewed by Lynn B. Cooper, D. Crim, and Melissa Rosales Neff, MSW

REFERENCES

Anestis, M., Khazem, L., Law, K., Houtsma, C., LeTard, R., Moberg, R., & Martin, R. (2015). The association between state laws regulating handgun ownership and statewide suicide rates. *American Journal of Public Health, 105*(10), 2059-2067. doi: 10.2105/AJPH.2014.302465

British Association of Social Workers. (2012). The code of ethics for social work: Statement of principles. Retrieved March 10, 2015, from http: //cdn.basw.co.uk/upload/basw_112315-7.pdf

Centers for Disease Control and Prevention. (2015). Suicide: facts at a glance. Retrieved March 10, 2016, from http: //www.cdc.gov/violenceprevention/pdf/suicide-datasheet-a.pdf

Centers for Disease Control and Prevention. (2015). Understanding suicide. Retrieved March 10, 2016, from http: //www.cdc.gov/violenceprevention/pdf/suicide_factsheet-a.pdf

Coletsos, I. C., & Bursztajn, H. J. (2016). Suicide. In F. J. Domino (Ed.), *The 5-minute clinical consult 2016* (24th ed., pp. 1062-1063). Philadelphia, PA: Wolters Kluwer Health/Lippincott Williams & Wilkins.

Definitions: Self-directed violence. (2015, August 28). *Centers for Disease Control and Prevention.* Retrieved March 10, 2016, from http: //www.cdc.gov/violenceprevention/suicide/definitions.html

International Federation of Social Workers. (2012). Statement of Ethical Principles. Retrieved March 10, 2016, from http: //ifsw.org/policies/statement-of-ethical-principles/

Jones, D., & Maynard, A. (2013). Suicide in recently released prisoners: A systematic review. *Mental Health Practice, 17*(3), 20-27.

Mallett, C. (2014). Youthful offending and delinquency: The comorbid impact of maltreatment, mental health problems, and learning disabilities. *Child and Adolescent Social Work Journal, 31*(4), 369-392. doi: 10.1007/s10560-013-0323-3

Montross, T., Palinkas, L., Meier, E., Iglewicz, A., Kirkland, T., & Zisook, S. (2014). Yearning to be heard: What veterans teach us about suicide risk and effective interventions. *Crisis, 35*(3), 161-167. doi: 10.1027/0227-5910/a000247

Mueller, A., Welsey, J., Abrutyn, S., & Levin, M. (2015). Suicide ideation and bullying among adolescents: Examining the intersections of sexual orientation, gender, and race/ethnicity. *American Journal of Public Health, 105*(5), 980-985. doi: 10.2105/AJPH.2014.302391

Osteen, P. J., Jacobson, J. M., & Sharpe, T. L. (2014). Suicide prevention in social work education: How prepared are social work students? *Journal of Social Work Education, 50*(2), 349-364. doi: 10.1080/10437797.2014.885272

(2015). Psychiatric emergencies: 29.1 suicide. In B. J. Sadock, V. A. Sadock, & P. Ruiz (Eds.), *Kaplan & Sadock's comprehensive textbook of psychiatry* (11th ed., Vol. 2, pp. 763-774). Philadelphia, PA: Wolters Kluwer Health/Lippincott Williams & Wilkins.

Wheeler, D. (2015). NASW standards and indicators for cultural competence in social work practice. Retrieved February 23, 2016, from http: //www.socialworkers.org/practice/standards/PRA-BRO-253150-CC-Standards.pdf

World Health Organization (WHO). (2014). Preventing suicide: A global imperative. Geneva: World Health Organization. Retrieved March 10, 1970, from http: //www.who.int/mental_health/suicide-prevention/exe_summary_english.pdf?ua=1

SUICIDE & MAJOR DEPRESSIVE DISORDER

MAJOR CATEGORIES: Behavioral & Mental Health

DESCRIPTION

The U.S. Centers for Disease Control and Prevention (CDC) defines suicide as death caused by self-directed injurious behavior with any intent to die as a result of the behavior. In 2013 in the United States, suicide was the second leading cause of death in persons between the ages of 15 and 34 (CDC, 2015). For those suffering from major depressive disorder (MDD) or major depressive episodes (MDE), the risk for suicide increases dramatically. Studies have shown that the majority of individuals who completed suicide were depressed at the time of their death, making depression one of the greatest risk factors for suicidal behavior. The *Diagnostic and Statistical Manual of Mental Disorders* (*DSM-5*) criteria for MDD are at least five of the following symptoms for more than 2 weeks, creating a change in functional ability: depressed mood, significant loss of interest or pleasure in all or most things, weight loss or gain, insomnia or hypersomnia, psychomotor agitation or retardation, feelings of worthlessness or excessive guilt, diminished ability to think or concentrate, and recurrent thoughts of death (APA, 2013). The *DSM-5* excludes bereavement from the definition of MDD because the symptoms of bereavement may mirror MDD initially but tend to decrease over time.

FACTS AND FIGURES

In 2013, 41,149 persons in the United States committed suicide and nearly 500,000 were treated for self-inflicted injuries, resulting in $44.6 billion in medical expenses and lost productivity costs(CDC, 2015).Current facts and figures about suicide in the United States are available at http://www.cdc.gov/violenceprevention/suicide/statistics.

RISK FACTORS

Undiagnosed or untreated major depressive disorder is thought to be the leading risk factor for attempted suicide. Other risk factors are previous attempts at suicide; comorbid personality disorders, especially borderline personality disorder; alcohol dependence or use; and chronic disease. Lack of social supports and longer depressive episodes also are risk factors for suicide among persons experiencing depression. Stress, history of abuse or neglect, impulsive behavior, loss, physical illness, family history of depression or suicide, and feelings of stigma may also be risk factors for suicide. American Indians, Native Alaskans, persons who live in rural communities, and active or retired military personnel are at higher risk for suicide than others (CDC, 2015).Transgender persons are also at high risk for suicidal ideation because of the social exclusion and discrimination that these individuals face (Bauer et al., 2015).

SIGNS AND SYMPTOMS

Psychological: feelings may be episodic or pervasive and may include, hopelessness, sadness, emptiness, isolation, shame, guilt, worthlessness, loss of pleasure in activities, sudden elation after extended depressive state, bereavement, stress, dementia, feeling stigmatized, recurrent thoughts of death, inability to concentrate, indecisiveness.

Behavioral: increase or decrease in sleep, nervousness, aggression, agitation, loss of interest in activities including activities of daily living, isolation, giving

away of treasured personal belongings, history of violence or abuse (physical, emotional, or sexual).

Physical: chronic disease, somatic complaints (e.g., chronic muscle and back pain, headaches, fatigue, gastrointestinal disorders), sleep disturbances, weight loss or gain, pain without physical explanation.

ASSESSMENT

Biopsychosocial-spiritual assessments should be used in conjunction with other assessment and screening tools to develop a better understanding of the clients' physical, emotional, social, and spiritual support systems. Evaluating social relationships, cognitive functioning, and physical health can help identify any perceived or actual barriers to care and support and allow for the implementation of an intervention that will be effective for each individual. In addition, individuals at risk should be assessed for suicide ideation, suicidal planning, and risk to self. Specific care should be taken to assess for past or familial suicidal ideation and substance use.

ASSESSMENTS AND SCREENING TOOLS

Several suicide and depression assessment tools are available to determine the level of intervention need for clients, including the Beck Depression Inventory (BDI), Schedule for Affective Disorders and Schizophrenia (SADS), Beck Anxiety Inventory (BAI), Beck Scale for Suicide Ideation (BSSI), and Hospital Anxiety and Depression Scale (HADS). In addition, assessments for cognitive impairments, such as the Mini Mental State Examination (MMSE), and for substance abuse should be completed if indicated. All assessments and screening tools must be done in conjunction with a physical examination and medication review.

TREATMENT

Treatment planning for someone who is suicidal should never be done in isolation. Clinical consultation with supervisors and colleagues should be utilized as routine practice because of the complex nature of the clients' clinical presentation (i.e., a combination of factors affect clients' symptomology simultaneously) and potential for morbidity. All suicidal ideation should be taken seriously; if it is present, ensuring the safety of the client should be the first treatment priority. Once the safety of the client has been established, interventions may be provided to address both the issues leading to the depressive disorder and the manifestation of the disorder itself. Cognitive behavioral therapy can be useful in helping clients identify the connections between thoughts, feelings, and behaviors and challenging inaccurate thoughts that might be contributing to feelings of depression. Psychodynamic interventions can be useful in assisting clients in

addressing underlying issues that might be contributing to the depression.

Social workers should be aware of their own cultural values, beliefs, and biases and develop specialized knowledge about the histories, traditions, and values of their clients. Social workers should adopt treatment methodologies that reflect their knowledge of the cultural diversity of the communities in which they practice.

Problem	Goal	Intervention
Client is experiencing suicidal ideation	Client will not harm him- or herself, suicidal ideation will be reduced or eliminated	Safety planning: Assess to determine whether the client has a plan for how to commit suicide and a means to carry out the plan. If client is in immediate danger of harming him- or herself, take the necessary steps to initiate an evaluation for psychiatric hospitalization per agency/facility protocol; if client's suicidal ideation is nonspecific and/or client does not have a plan or a means to carry out the plan, provide psychotherapy if qualified or refer client to a qualified mental health professional. Refer client for pharmacological assessment and intervention. Continue to assess client on a regular basis for changes in suicidal status
Client is showing signs and symptoms of major depression but is not expressing or demonstrating suicidal ideation	Client will have reduced symptoms of depression and improved functioning	Provide psychotherapy if qualified, or refer to a qualified mental health professional. If qualified, utilize cognitive behavioral or psychodynamic interventions to address immediate symptoms and underlying issues. Continue to assess regularly for suicidal ideation, and create safety plan as necessary

LAWS AND REGULATIONS

Social workers and healthcare professionals are bound by the "duty to warn," which requires that they inform the proper authorities if a person is found to be a danger to him- or herself or others. Clinicians should be aware of the policies and procedures laid out in their state's duty-to-warn law.

Each country has its own standards for cultural competence and diversity in social work practice. Social workers must be aware of the standards of practice set forth by their governing body (e.g., National Association of Social Workers in the United States,

British Association of Social Workers in England) and practice accordingly.

SERVICES AND RESOURCES

Many individuals are treated for depression by their primary care physicians. Mental health social workers, psychiatrists, counselors, and other mental health providers should care for individuals with MDD as part of their treatment team. Utilization of community mental health resources, support groups, and psychoeducation can assist in preventing suicide for those individuals with MDD.

- National Suicide Prevention Lifeline, 1-800-273-TALK (8255)
- The American Foundation for Suicide Prevention (www.afsp.org) and www.helpguide.org are national resources that can be used to locate resources within each community
- Suicide Prevention Resource Center, http://www.sprc.org/
- National Alliance on Mental Illness, http://www.nami.org/
- Yellow Ribbon Suicide Prevention Program, http://yellowribbon.org/

FOOD FOR THOUGHT

The American Foundation for Suicide Prevention estimates that 3 out of 4 suicidal individuals show warning signs to close family or friends before they attempt suicide (American Foundation for Suicide Prevention, 2010).

One study showed that 15.8 percent of teens in high school reported having seriously considered suicide in the last 12 months and 7.8 percent reported having attempted suicide, 2.4 percent of whom needed medical attention (CDC, 2012).

RED FLAGS

According to the U.S. Food and Drug Administration, certain antidepressants such as selective serotonin reuptake inhibitors have been found to increase risk of suicidal thoughts and actions.

Many individuals who completed suicide either received a diagnosis of depressive disorder or were seen at their physician's office within 6 months of their deaths.

NEXT STEPS

Client should not be discharged from services if suicidal ideation is present unless they have been connected to a higher or more appropriate level of care such as admission to an inpatient psychiatric hospital.

Ensure that clients are aware of confidentiality restrictions related to harm to self or others.

Provide local and multimedia resources to assist with depression and suicide ideation, including referrals to appropriate agencies and services.

Written by Amanda Becker, LCSW

Reviewed by Jessica Therivel, LMSW-IPR

REFERENCES

American Association of Suicidology. (n.d.). Know the Warning Signs of Suicide. Retrieved December 9, 2015, from http://www.suicidology.org/resources/warning-signs

American Foundation for Suicide Prevention. (n.d.). Understanding suicide. Retrieved December 9, 2015, from http://www.afsp.org/understanding-suicide

American Psychiatric Association. (2013). Major depressive disorder. *Diagnostic and statistical manual of mental disorders: DSM-V-TR.* Arlington, VA: American Psychiatric Publishing.

Bauer, G. R., Scheim, A. I., Pyne, J., Travers, R., & Hammond, R. (2015). Intervenable factors associated with suicide risk in transgender persons: A respondent driven sampling study in Ontario, Canada. *BMC Public Health, 15,* 525. doi:10.1186/s12889-015-1867-2

British Association of Social Workers. (2012). The code of ethics for social work: Statement of principles. Retrieved December 9, 2015, from http://cdn.basw.co.uk/upload/basw_112315-7.pdf

Butt, T. (2005). Constructive social work and personal construct theory: The case of psychological trauma. *British Journal of Social Work, 35*(6), 793-806. doi:10.1093/bjsw/bch210

Centers for Disease Control and Prevention. (2015). Understanding suicide. Retrieved December 9, 2015, from http://www.cdc.gov/violenceprevention/pdf/suicide_factsheet-a.pdf

Gehlert, S., & Browne, T. A. (2006). *Handbook of health social work.* Hoboken, NJ: Wiley.

Holma, K. M., Melartin, T. K., Haukka, J., Holma, I. A., Sokero, T. P., & Isometsä, E. T. (2010). Incidence and predictors of suicide attempts in DSM-IV major depressive disorder: A five-year prospective study. *American Journal of Psychiatry, 167*(7), 801-808. doi:10.1176/appi.ajp.2010.09050627

Hyler, S. E. (2002). APA Online CME practice guideline for the treatment of patients with major depressive disorder. *Journal of Psychiatric Practice, 8*(5), 315-319. doi:10.1097/00131746-200209000-00008

International Federation of Social Workers. (2012). Statement of ethical principles. Retrieved December 9, 2015, from http://ifsw.org/policies/statement-of-ethical-principles/

McGirr, A., Renaud, J., Seguin, M., Alda, M., & Turecki, G. (2008). Course of major depressive disorder and suicide outcome: A psychological autopsy study. *Journal of Clinical Psychiatry, 69*(6), 966-970. doi:10.4088/JCP.v69n0612

O'Hare, T., & Sherrer, M. (2009). Impact of the most frequently reported traumatic events on community mental health clients. *Journal of Human Behavior in the Social Environment, 19*(2), 186-195. doi:10.1080/10911350802687158

Wheeler, D. (2015). NASW standards and indicators for cultural competence in social work practice. Retrieved December 9, 2015, from http://www.socialworkers.org/practice/standards/PRA-BRO-253150-CC-Standards.pdf

T

Terrorism, Victims: Psychosocial Effects & Social Work Interventions

Major Categories: Terrorism

What We Know

Terrorism has been defined by the United Nations Security Council as "any action that is intended to cause death or serious bodily harm to civilians or noncombatants, when the purpose of such an act, by its nature or context, is to intimidate a population, or to compel a government or an international organization to do or to abstain from doing any act." In addition to being physically harmed, victims of terrorism may experience serious short-term and long-term psychological effects as a result of traumatic stress, although there has not been extensive research on trauma caused by terrorism. It is estimated that 28 percent of individuals who have experienced a terrorist attack develop post-traumatic stress disorder (PTSD).

Researchers in Israel who studied victims of terrorist attacks found that PTSD symptoms typically are less severe among affected individuals who have a tendency to forgive and if they utilize problem-focused coping versus avoidance coping.

PTSD may be experienced by persons directly affected by a terrorist event and by those who are indirectly affected.

Direct exposure means that the individual was injured or in close physical contact with someone who was killed or injured during an attack. Indirect exposure results from living under the threat of an attack or having other secondary exposure to an attack (e.g., watching news reports of an attack, repeatedly discussing an attack with others, identifying oneself as being similar to a victim).

Psychological stress may be experienced when resources (e.g., empowerment, sense of belonging to the community) are lost or threatened as a result of a terrorist attack.

Anticipatory fear often lingers after a terrorist attack. Long after the event has passed, affected individuals may fear another attack, which may influence life choices such as where to live, travel plans, etc..

Researchers also found that public trust in government frequently goes up after a terrorist attack and this can help buffer anticipatory fear.

Children and adolescents are at high risk for having their mental health affected by an act of terrorism.

Direct exposure has been found to magnify this risk. Physical proximity to a terrorist attack increases the likelihood that one will experience intrusive thoughts and avoidance symptoms of PTSD; psychological proximity (i.e., being close emotionally or personally to the terrorist act, such as having a parent who worked at the site of an attack even if the parent was unharmed) increases intrusive thoughts.

Children and adolescents who experience a traumatic loss as a result of a terrorist event (e.g., those who lost a parent in the 9/11 terrorist attack in the United States) may continue to experience behavioral and psychological reactions that extend past what is typical for a loss. The combination of the loss and the environmental and external circumstances surrounding a terrorist attack (e.g., search for remains, constant public and private memorials, anniversary memorials, public nature of victims' grief) greatly increases the risk of a complicated grief reaction.

For children and adolescents who live under continual threat of terrorism (e.g., Israelis, Iraqis, Afghans) studies have indicated two different typical reactions to the stress.

Continual exposure to terrorist trauma may result in cumulative stress: chronic PTSD, attachment issues, distorted thoughts regarding the future, and problems in cognitive and emotional development.

Some children and adolescents are able to adjust and cope even in the face of constant stress. Resilience is enhanced by protective factors such as strong family relationships and support from peers.

Social workers may fill a number of roles after a terrorist event, including providing information, support, and counseling.

In the support role, the social worker can assist victims by:

reducing feelings of isolation in order to decrease anxiety and depression;

working with parents who are purposefully isolating their children out of fear (e.g., keeping children home from school after an attack elsewhere in the country on a school) on discontinuing that isolation and rejoining society;

discussing with the client the trauma itself and the client's perception of the trauma;

allowing for and encouraging any expressions of grief;

monitoring the client for physical, psychological, and emotional symptoms resulting from the trauma;

if seeing the client long-term, maintaining awareness of anniversary issues related to the trauma and/or the client's sense of loss;

recognizing any resilience and positive coping and encouraging this with the client.

In the counseling role, the social worker can utilize the counseling intervention that is the most appropriate for the client. Interventions may include elements of psychoeducation, psychopharmacology, and psychotherapy (individual or group), and may use the following techniques.

- Cognitive behavioral therapy
- Psychological debriefing
- Prolonged exposure techniques
- Relaxation exercises
- Optimism training
- Imagery rehearsal
- Present-centered group therapy (The current situation of each group member is what is focused on; recall of the traumatic event is discouraged.)
- Trauma-focused group therapy (Recall of the traumatic event is emphasized using cognitive restructuring and prolonged exposure.)

WHAT CAN BE DONE

Learn about terrorism, the difficulties victims encounter, and interventions that may assist victims so you can accurately assess your client's personal characteristics and education needs; share this information with your colleagues.

Enhance resources for clients, especially through community interventions and community involvement.

Maintain awareness and understanding of the impact of a terrorist act upon members of the same ethnic group as the terrorists (e.g., American Muslims after 9/11).

Provide counseling interventions or referrals to appropriate counseling interventions for victims of a terrorist event.

Provide education and support to school systems and community groups as requested.

Develop an awareness of your own cultural values, beliefs, and biases and develop knowledge about the histories, traditions, and values of your clients. Adopt treatment methodologies that reflect the cultural needs of the client.

Written by Jessica Therivel, LMSW-IPR

Reviewed by Lynn B. Cooper, D. Crim

REFERENCES

Ai, A. L., Evans-Campbell, T., Santangelo, L. K., & Cascio, T. (2006). The traumatic impact of the September 11, 2001, terrorist attacks and the potential protection of optimism. *Journal of Interpersonal Violence, 21*(5), 689-700.

Antonius, D., Sinclair, S. J., & contributing writers. (2013). The impact of terrorism fears. *Security: Solutions for Enterprise Security Leaders, 50*(11), 128-132.

British Association of Social Workers. (2012, January). The code of ethics for social work: Statement of principles. Retrieved January 25, 2015, from http://cdn.basw.co.uk/upload/basw_112315-7.pdf

Carter, B. G. (2010). The strengths of Muslim American couples in the face of religious discrimination following September 11 and the Iraq War. *Smith College Studies in Social Work (Haworth), 80*(2-3), 323-343. doi:10.1080/00377317.2010.481462

Christ, G. (2010). Social work contribution to a comprehensive model of mourning: The experience of bereaved families of fire-fighters killed on 9/11/01. *Progress in Palliative Care, 18*(4), 228-236. doi:10.1179/096992610X12624290277060

Cohen, M., & Eid, J. (2007). The effect of constant threat of terror on Israeli Jewish and Arab adolescents. *Anxiety, Stress, and Coping, 20*(1), 47-60.

Duffy, M., Gillespie, K., & Clark, D. M. (2007). Post-traumatic stress disorder in the context of terrorism and other civil conflict in Northern Ireland: Randomized controlled trial. *British*

Medical Journal (Clinical Research Ed.), 334(7604), 1147-1150.

Fischer, P., & Ai, A. L. (2008). International terrorism and mental health: Recent research and future directions. *Journal of Interpersonal Violence, 23*(3), 339-361. doi:10.1177/0886260507312292

International Federation of Social Workers. (2012). Statement of ethical principles. Retrieved November 22, 2015, from http://ifsw.org/policies/statement-of-ethical-principles/

Itzhaky, H., & Dekel, R. (2008). Community intervention with Jewish Israeli mothers in times of terror. *British Journal of Social Work, 38*(3), 462-475.

Monahan, K., & Lurie, A. (2007). Reactions of senior citizens to 9/11: Exploration and practice guidelines for social workers. *Social Work in Health Care, 45*(1), 33-47.

Precin, P. (2011). Return to work after 9/11. *Work, 38*(1), 3-11. doi:10.3233/WOR-2011-1099

Ron, P., & Shamai, M. (2011). Assessing the impact of ongoing national terror: Social workers in Israel. *Social Work Research, 35*(1), 36-45.

Schiff, M., Benbenishty, R., McKay, M., Devoe, E., Liu, X., & Hasin, D. (2006). Exposure to terrorism and Israeli youths' psychological distress and alcohol use: An exploratory study. *The American Journal on Addictions/American Academy of Psychiatrists in Alcoholism and Addictions, 15*(3), 220-226.

Sever, I., Somer, E., Ruvio, A., & Soref, E. (2008). Gender, distress, and coping in response to terrorism. *Affilia: Journal of Women & Social Work, 23*(2), 156-166.

Sweifach, J., Heft LaPorte, H. L., & Linzer, N. (2010). Social work responses to terrorism: Balancing ethics and responsibility. *International Social Work, 53*(6), 822-835. doi:10.1177/0020872809360036

Weinberg, M., Gil, S., & Gilbar, O. (2014). Forgiveness, coping, and terrorism: Do tendency to forgive and coping strategies associate with the level of posttraumatic symptoms of injured victims of terror attacks?. *Journal of Clinical Psychology, 70*(7), 693-703. doi:10.1002/jclp.22056

Wheeler, D. (2015). NASW Standards and Indicators for Cultural Competence in Social Work Practice. Retrieved November 15, 2015, from http://www.socialworkers.org/practice/standards/PRA-BRO-253150-CC-Standards.pdf

THERAPEUTIC FOSTER CARE: AN OVERVIEW

MAJOR CATEGORIES: Adoption/Foster Care

DESCRIPTION

Therapeutic foster care, also sometimes called treatment foster care, (TFC), is a family-based treatment model for children with severe emotional and/or behavioral issues who require out-of-home placement due to child abuse or neglect, mental health needs, and/or delinquency. TFC represents the least restrictive out-of-home treatment setting available and serves as an alternative to group or residential care. Placement in TFC has the benefit of allowing children to remain in a family and community setting whileavoiding the introduction of negative peer influences that may be found in a group home or residential treatment facility.

Children may be referred to a TFC program by a child welfare services social worker, mental health clinician,and/or juvenile court judge. Although some children are placed voluntarily by their parents, the majority are in the legal custody of a child welfare agency because of abuse, neglect, or dependency or are wards of the juvenile court because of delinquency. The implementation of TFC varies considerably among agencies in terms of administration, therapeutic approach, and whether the agency is primarily oriented toward child welfare, mental health, or juvenile corrections perspectives. Some common standards for programs in North America have been established by the Foster Family-Based Treatment Association, which has grown to over 400 member agencies. Despite individual variations, TFC programs generally share the following core components:

Foster parents receive specialized training, are licensed to care for only one or two children at a time, and receive a higher rate of compensation than parents in nontherapeutic foster homes.

Foster parents are regarded as full members of the child's treatment team and are expected to implement treatment goals in accordance with the child's individualized service plan and to provide more structure and supervision than parents in non-therapeutic foster homes.

Agency workers carry a small caseload of families and are expected to provide a high level of guidance, support, crisis intervention, and respite to families.

Agency workers may provide consultation and service coordination for school staff, mental health clinicians, medical providers, and other team members.

Programs include a family component to engage birth parents in education, visits, and/or family therapy and an aftercare plan to support transition to birth family or other permanent placement.

One evidence-based TFC model, multidimensional treatment foster care (MTFC), has demonstrated positive effects including reduced violence and delinquency, enhanced resilience, and increased probability of successful placement in permanent homes. Certified MTFC programs have been established in the United States, England, Norway, Denmark, Sweden, the Netherlands, and New Zealand. The majority of MTFC homes serve youth ages 12–17, although there are also programs for preschoolers ages 3–6 and children ages 7–11. The MTFC model is time-limited, typically involving 6 to 9 months of treatment and 3 months of aftercare. Critical elements that distinguish this model include grounding in social learning theory, vigilant attention and response to children's behaviors in home and community settings, consistent limits, predictable rewards and consequences for behavior, skills training for children, daily contact between staff and foster parents, implementation of behavior management strategies by foster parents, and supportive therapy for the child and involved adults.

FACTS AND FIGURES

Current facts and figures specific to TFC are limited. As of September 30, 2014, there were 415,129 individuals 20 years old or younger in any kind of foster care in the United States; 52 percent were male and 48 percent female; 2 percent were American Indian/Alaskan Native, 1 percent Asian, 24 percent black, 0 percent Native Hawaiian/other Pacific Islander, 22 percent Hispanic of any race, 42 percent white, 3 percent of unknown ethnicity, and 7 percent two or more races (Children's Bureau, 2105).

A large multisite sample of youths in TFC in the United States found that the TFC population includes children from 3 to 20 years of age, with a mean age of 13.59 and a higher proportion of males (64.7 percent) than of females (Baker et al., 2007). As many as 90 percent are prescribed psychotropic medication, 38.3 percent have experienced previous psychiatric hospitalization, 33 percent have a history of criminal offenses, 18.5 percent have substance abuse issues, and 6.9 percent have a history of sexual offenses. A high percentage are in the clinical range on one or more scales on the Child Behavior Checklist (CBCL), including externalizing (e.g., lying, stealing; 47.9 percent), internalizing (e.g. depressed, anxious, withdrawn; 35.9 percent), delinquency (24.5 percent), attention problems (21.8 percent), and aggression (20.6 percent).

RISK FACTORS

The majority of youths in TFC have displayed behaviors that have presented significant challenges in home, school, and other settings, jeopardizing their ability to remain in the community. Risk factors for disruptive or antisocial behavior in childhood include inconsistent or harsh discipline; chaotic, multiproblem families; and child abuse or neglect. As maladaptive behaviors become entrenched, children become increasingly at risk for academic difficulties, negative peer relationships, and other social difficulties. Children who display disruptive behaviors in foster-home settings are also more likely to experience multiple placements, which in turn increases the probability of poor long-term outcomes.

SIGNS AND SYMPTOMS

The majority of children served in TFC exhibit disruptive, defiant, aggressive, antisocial behaviors that have created significant difficulties in home and school settings. They may have a history of substance abuse, truancy, school suspensions and failures, chronic delinquency, sexual assault psychiatric hospitalizations, multiple living arrangements, and runaway episodes.

ASSESSMENT

Client history includes a complete comprehensive bio-psychosocial-spiritual assessment with particular attention to trauma and placement history, substance abuse, psychiatric symptoms, issues that pose a risk to self and others (e.g., suicidal ideation, runaway behaviors, fire setting, aggression, sexual offenses), involvement in other systems (e.g., school, child welfare, corrections), family and community supports.

ASSESSMENTS AND SCREENING TOOLS

- Child and Adolescent Functional Assessment Scale (CAFAS) for children 6–17 or Preschool and Early Childhood Functional Assessment Scale (PECFAS) for children 3–7; Child Behavioral Checklist (CBCL) for ages 1.5–18.
- Child and Adolescent Needs and Strengths, Mental Health (CANS-MH).

TREATMENT

A system of care framework is recommended to manage the complex needs of youths in TFC, who typically are involved with one or more public agencies (e.g., mental health, juvenile delinquency, child welfare) and multiple service providers. Although TFC is itself a psychosocial intervention, many children also need specialized treatment (e.g., trauma-focused therapy, medication management, substance abuse services), individual and/or group skills training, special education, and/or vocational training.

TFC is rooted in recognition that the home is a natural learning environment for children, with foster parents serving as powerful change agents in children's treatment. Preparation and support of both foster parents and the caregivers whom children will reside with upon discharge is critical. A good alliance between therapeutic parents and children is associated with more positive outcomes, as is the foster parents' identifying themselves more as parents than as professionals.

The social worker will utilize an ecological approach to ensure that the child's individual needs are addressed; that both foster parents have adequate training and support; that ongoing and aftercare services include the child's biological, foster, or adoptive family that will care for the child upon discharge; and that involved agencies and systems work in coordination, addressing any barriers that arise.

Social workers should be aware of their own cultural values, beliefs, and biases and develop specialized knowledge about the histories, traditions, and values of their clients. Social workers should adopt treatment methodologies that reflect their knowledge of the cultural diversity of the communities in which they practice.

Problem	Goal	Intervention
Child is exhibiting maladaptive and/or disruptive behaviors, lack of prosocial skills and behaviors	Reduce problem behaviors, teach and reinforce prosocial skills and behaviors	Individualized behavioral strategies focused on reinforcing positive behaviors, close supervision, limiting negative peer associations, and strengthening adult–child relationship; individual and group skills coaching for parents and children; mentoring
Child has underlying mental health condition, trauma	Support resolution of mental health symptoms and/or trauma, enhance adaptive coping	Refer for specialized mental health therapy (e.g., trauma-focused cognitive behavioral therapy, anger coping, substance abuse treatment, psychotropic medication)
Parent lacks skills to establish limits, rewards, and consequences to promote and reinforce prosocial behavior; parenting approach may be inconsistent or coercive	Increased parental understanding and capacity to respond to and shape child's behaviors	Parent–child interaction therapy, parent-management training
Frequency or severity of child's negative behaviors is causing high degree of parental stress	Parent will have realistic expectations of child, sense of competence in responding to child's behaviors, enhanced coping skills, and reduction in stress	Provide education regarding child's emotional/behavioral issues and strategies for reducing stress, assist parent in identifying supports and coping strategies, offer respite services, refer to parent support groups

LAWS AND REGULATIONS

The licensure and operation of TFC homes are governed by laws and regulations on the national and local levels.

Each country has its own standards for cultural competency and diversity in social work practice. Social workers must be aware of the standards of practice set forth by their governing body (e.g., National Association of Social Workers in the United States, British Association of Social Workers in England) and practice accordingly.

SERVICES AND RESOURCES

- Foster Family-Based Treatment Association, http://www.ffta.org
- Multidimensional Treatment Foster Care, http://mtfc.com

FOOD FOR THOUGHT

Girls in TFC are more likely to have been sexually abused, are at higher risk for suicide attempts and runaway behavior, and show less long-term improvement than boys in TFC do.

Hundreds of programs identify themselves as TFC and share common elements, but there are also significant differences between programs in their implementation of an evidence-based model or best practices and standards.

RED FLAGS

A significant number of youths in TFC are on psychotropic medication, but foster parents and staff often do not receive adequate training in administering and monitoring medications and side effects. Additional training is needed in this area.

Many youths in TFC have a history of suicidal ideation and previous psychiatric hospitalization. TFC and program staff should be adequately trained to recognize warning signs and have a plan for responding to psychiatric crises.

Youths with a history of sexual assault should immediately be assessed and provided with intensive treatment. Therapeutic foster parents must be adequately trained to recognize problematic behaviors related to sexual history.

NEXT STEPS

Ensure that transitions occur in a planned and coordinated manner with input from all providers, parents, and youths.

Provide linkage to community services (e.g., support groups, mentors, recreational programs) as appropriate to provide additional supports.

Provide written information regarding the child's mental health condition or needs as applicable (e.g., parent handouts available through MedLinePlus, http://www.nlm.nih.gov/medlineplus/childmentalhealth.html).

Written by Jennifer Teska, MSW

Reviewed by Laura McLuckey, MSW, LCSW

REFERENCES

Baker, A. J., Kurland, D., Curtis, P., Alexander, G., & Papa-Lentini, C. (2007). Mental health and behavioral problems of youth in the child welfare system: Residential treatment centers compared to therapeutic foster care in the Odyssey Project population. *Child Welfare, 86*(3), 97-123.

Breland-Noble, A. M., Farmer, E. M. Z., Dubs, M. S., Potter, E., & Burns, B. J. (2005). Mental health and other service use by youth in therapeutic foster care and group homes. *Journal of Child & Family Studies, 14*(2), 167-180. doi:10.1007/s10826-005-5045-5

British Association of Social Workers. (2012). The code of ethics for social work: Statement of principles. Retrieved November 27, 2015, from http://cdn.basw.co.uk/upload/basw_112315-7.pdf

Chamberlain, P. (2002). Treatment foster care. In B. J. Burns & K. Hoagwood (Eds.), *Community treatment for youth* (pp. 117-138). New York, NY: Oxford University Press.

Children's Bureau. (2015). The AFCARS report: Preliminary FY 2014 estimates as of July 2015. Retrieved November 27, 2015, from https://www.acf.hhs.gov/sites/default/files/cb/afcarsreport22.pdf

Dore, M. M., & Mullin, D. (2006). Treatment family foster care: Its history and current role in the foster care continuum. *Families in Society: The Journal of Contemporary Social Services, 87*(4), 475-482. doi:10.1606/1044-3894.3562

Farmer, E. M. Z., Burns, B. J., Wagner, H. R., Murray, M., & Southerland, D. G. (2010). Enhancing "usual practice" treatment foster care: Findings from a randomized trial on improving youths' outcomes. *Psychiatric Services, 61*(6), 555-561. doi:10.1176/appi.ps.61.6.555

Fisher, P. A., Kim, H. K., & Pears, K. C. (2009). Effects of multidimensional treatment foster care for preschoolers (MTFC-P) on reducing permanent placement failures among children with placement instability. *Children and Youth Services Review, 31*(5), 541-546. doi:10.1016/j.childyouth.2008.10.012

International Federation of Social Workers. (2012, March 3). Statement of ethical principles. Retrieved November 27, 2015, from http://ifsw.org/policies/statement-of-ethical-principles/

Jonkman, C. S., Bolle, E. A., Lindeboom, R., Schuengel, C., Oosterman, M., Boer, F., & Lindauer, R. J. L. (2012). Multidimensional treatment foster care for preschoolers: Early findings of an implementation in the Netherlands. *Child & Adolescent Psychiatry & Mental Health, 6*(38), 1-5. doi:10.1186/1753-2000-6-38

Leve, L. D., Fisher, P. A., & Chamberlain, P. (2009). Multidimensional treatment foster care as a preventative intervention to promote resiliency among youth in the child welfare system. *Journal of Personality, 77*(6), 1869-1902. doi:10.1111/j.1467-6494.2009.00603.x

Pavkov, T. W., Hug, R. W., Lourie, I. S., & Negash, S. (2010). Service process and quality in therapeutic foster care: An exploratory study of one county system. *Journal of Social Service Research, 36*(3), 174-187. doi:10.1080/01488371003697897

Southerland, D., Mustillo, S., Farmer, E., Stambaugh, L., & Murray, M. (2009). What's the relationship got to do with it? Understanding the therapeutic relationship in therapeutic foster care. *Child & Adolescent Social Work Journal, 26*(1), 49-63. doi:10.1007/s10560-008-0159-4

Wheeler, D. (2015). NASW standards and indicators for cultural competence in social work practice. Retrieved November 27, 2015, from http://www.socialworkers.org/practice/standards/PRA-BRO-253150-CC-Standards.pdf

THERAPEUTIC FOSTER CARE: CHILD WELFARE

MAJOR CATEGORIES: Adoption/Foster Care

DESCRIPTION

Therapeutic foster care (TFC) is a family-based treatment model for children with severe emotional and/or behavioral issues. Although children may be referred to TFC by mental health or juvenile justice agencies, the majority are referred by child welfare services (CWS) agencies subsequent to being placed in foster care as a result of child maltreatment (CM) or dependency. For children in the custody of CWS because of abuse, neglect, or dependency, foster care placement is necessary in order to provide a safe, stable living situation while CWS makes efforts to reunify them with their birth parents or establish permanency through legal custody or guardianship with relatives or adoption. Children's initial placements usually are with relatives, extended family members, or traditional foster homes, but those children with significant emotional and/or behavioral issues may experience multiple disruptions and escalating difficulties. Placement in TFC is often the least restrictive setting available for a child with challenging behaviors and has the benefit of allowing children to remain in a family and community setting as well as avoiding the introduction of negative peer influences such as may be found in a group home or residential care facility. Referral to TFC may be initiated by the child welfare social worker, but authorization for payment purposes also requires a clinical assessment indicating that the child needs a higher level of care than can be provided in a traditional family foster-care setting.

The implementation of TFC varies considerably among agencies in terms of administration and therapeutic approach, although some common standards for programs in North America have been established by the Foster Family-Based Treatment Association. Despite individual variations, TFC programs generally share the following core components:

Foster parents receive specialized training, are licensed to care for only one or two children at a time, and receive a higher rate of compensation than parents in nontherapeutic foster homes;

Foster parents are regarded as full members of the child's treatment team and are expected to implement treatment goals in accordance with the child's individualized service plan and to provide more structure and supervision than parents in nontherapeutic foster homes;

Agency workers carry a small caseload of families and are expected to provide a high level of guidance, support, crisis intervention, and respite to families; and

Agency workers may provide consultation and/or service coordination for school staff, mental health clinicians, medical providers, and other team members.

Programs include a family component to engage birth parents in education, visits, and/or family therapy and an aftercare plan to support transition to birth family or other permanent placement.

One evidence-based TFC model, multidimensional treatment foster care (MTFC), has demonstrated positive effects including reducing violence and delinquency, enhancing resilience, and increasing the probability of successful placement in permanent homes. Certified MTFC programs have been established in the United States, England, Norway, Denmark, Sweden, and New Zealand. The majority of MTFC homes serve youth ages 12–17, although there also are programs for preschoolers 3–6 years old and children ages 7–11. The MTFC model is time-limited, typically involving 6 to 9 months of treatment and 3 months of aftercare. Critical elements that distinguish this model include grounding in social learning theory, vigilant attention and response to children's behaviors in home and community settings, consistent limits, predictable rewards and consequences for behavior, skills training for children, daily contact between staff and foster parents, implementation of behavior management strategies by foster parents, and supportive therapy for the child and involved adults. Early intervention foster care (EIFC/MTFC-P), for preschool children, also incorporates a therapeutic playgroup, in-home behavioral services, and parent training for parents who are expected to reunify with their children.

Research shows that therapeutic mentoring for foster children can reduce trauma symptoms significantly. Therapeutic mentoring involves mentors who are in helping professions and are extensively trained and supervised to mentor foster youth. The trainings received by the therapeutic mentors include information about working with children with emotional and behavioral disorders, therapeutic crisis interventions, and boundaries. Each mentor–mentee relationship is closely monitored by a master's-level clinician.

The mentors see their mentees on a weekly basis for 3–5 hours and engage in activities with them such as playing outdoors, attending cultural events, or going to sporting events. Investigators in 2013 found that foster youth who participated in a therapeutic mentoring program for 18 months experienced a significant decrease in their trauma symptoms compared to foster youth who did not participate in the therapeutic mentoring (Johnson & Pryce, 2013).

Researchers for another study reported that adolescents in long-term therapeutic foster care emphasized positive aspects of their placement such as being treated like adults, being listened to, and being made to feel safe. The researchers noted positive changes in the adolescents' attachment security over time (Dallos et al., 2015).

Outcomes for children in foster care are influenced by a number of factors. Most children in foster care have experienced significant trauma and disruption, which in turn is associated with high rates of mental health problems and attachment issues. Children with severe emotional and behavioral issues are more likely to have families with multiple adversities, experience changes in placement, and stay longer in foster care. Trauma-informed practices, service coordination, and engagement of birth parents, relatives, or others who are committed to providing a permanent home for the child support more favorable outcomes.

FACTS AND FIGURES

In 2014, approximately 415,000 children in the United States were in foster care. Of these children, 39 percent were 5 years of age and under and 46 percent were placed in foster care with a nonrelative; the average time in care was 20.8 months (U.S. Department of Health & Human Services, 2015). Children in foster care have significantly higher prevalence rates for mental health disorders than the general population, and most have also experienced significant trauma. Researchers studying children in foster care who were referred to a National Child Traumatic Stress Network site for services found that 50 percent of the children had suffered neglect, traumatic loss or separation, caregiver impairment, intimate partner violence, and/or emotional abuse; 48 percent had experienced physical abuse, and 32 percent had experienced sexual abuse (Greeson et al., 2011).

RISK FACTORS

Children in foster care are at significant risk for medical, developmental, educational, behavioral, and mental health problems. Most have experienced an array of adversities prior to placement, including parental substance abuse and/or mental health issues, the incarceration of one or both parents, exposure to intimate partner violence, poverty, unstable living situations, prenatal exposure to drugs and alcohol, lack of adequate stimulation and care during early childhood, developmental delays, and maltreatment (physical, sexual, and emotional abuse and/or neglect). Foster care introduces additional stressors, including the trauma of removal from the child's family and resulting losses and having to adjust to new environments. These children may have difficulty with attachment, self-regulation, and prosocial behaviors. As maladaptive behaviors become entrenched, children become increasingly at risk for academic difficulties, negative peer relationships, and other social difficulties. Children with severe emotional and/or behavioral issues are more likely to experience multiple placements,which in turn is strongly associated with escalating behavioral issues and poor long-term outcomes. Serious mental health issues are also the greatest predictor for children having extended lengths of stay in foster care.

SIGNS AND SYMPTOMS

The majority of children in TFC demonstrate disruptive, defiant, aggressive, antisocial behaviors that have created significant difficulty in home and school settings. They may have a history of substance abuse, truancy, school suspensions and failures, chronic delinquency, stealing,sexual abuse perpetration, psychiatric hospitalizations, multiple living situations, and episodes of running away. Diagnoses may include attention deficit hyperactivity disorder, oppositional defiant disorder, conduct disorder, posttraumatic stress disorder, and mood disorders. Children entering TFC from CW tend to be younger than children referred by mental health or juvenile justice. They are likely to have had several disrupted foster care placements prior to placement in TFC.

ASSESSMENT

Complete a comprehensive biopsychosocial-spiritual assessment to include information on physical, mental, environmental, social, and financial factors as they relate to the child and his/her family.

Ask about history of physical/sexual/emotional abuse or neglect, exposure to violence or other trauma, family history, placement history, level of functioning, history of psychiatric symptoms or issues that pose risk to self or others (e.g., suicide ideation/ attempts, self-harm, substance abuse, aggression, fire setting, running away, sexual abuse perpetration), history of mental health treatment and psychotropic medication, child's involvement with other systems (e.g. school, corrections), family and community supports.

ASSESSMENTS AND SCREENING TOOLS

- Child and Adolescent Functional Assessment Scale (CAFAS) for children 6–17 or Preschool and Early Childhood Functional Assessment Scale (PECFAS) for children 3–7
- Child Behavioral Checklist (CBCL) for ages 6–18
- Child and Adolescent Needs and Strengths, Mental Health (CANS-MH)
- Strengths and Difficulties Questionnaire (SDQ)
- UCLA Posttraumatic Stress Disorder Reaction Index (PTSD-R)

There may be a need for a toxicology screen for drug and/or alcohol use.

TREATMENT

A system-of-care framework is recommended for managing the complex needs of youth in TFC, who typically are involved with one or more public agencies in addition to child welfare services (e.g., mental health, juvenile delinquency) and multiple service providers. Although TFC is itself a psychosocial intervention, many children also need specialized treatment, individual and/or group skills training, special education, and/or vocational training.

TFC recognizes that the home is a natural learning environment for children, with foster parents serving as powerful change agents in the child's treatment. Preparation and support of both foster parents and the caregivers with whom the child will reside upon discharge are critical. A good alliance between therapeutic parents and children is associated with more positive outcomes, as is the foster parents' identifying themselves more as parents than as professionals.

The social worker should utilize an ecological approach to ensure that the child's individual needs are addressed; that foster parents have adequate training and support; that ongoing and aftercare services include the biological, foster, or adoptive family that will care for the child upon discharge; and that involved agencies and systems work in coordination, addressing any barriers that arise.

Social workers should be aware of their own cultural values, beliefs, and biases and develop specialized knowledge about the histories, traditions, and values of their clients. Social workers should adopt treatment methodologies that reflect their knowledge of the cultural diversity of the communities in which they practice.

Problem	Goal	Intervention
Child in TFC is exhibiting maladaptive and/or disruptive behaviors, lacks prosocial skills and behaviors	Reduce problem behaviors, teach and reinforce prosocial skills and behaviors	Individualized behavioral strategies focused on reinforcing positive behaviors, close supervision, limiting negative peer associations, and strengthening adult-child relationships; individual and group skills coaching for parents and children; mentoring
Child in TFC has underlying mental health condition	Support resolution of mental health symptoms, enhance adaptive coping	Refer for specialized mental health therapy (e.g., anger coping, substance abuse treatment, psychotropic medication)
Child in TFC experiences symptoms resulting from history of trauma	Support resolution of symptoms related to exposure to trauma	Screen all youth in TFC for trauma history, refer for trauma-focused cognitive behavioral therapy (TF-CBT), abuse-focused cognitive behavioral therapy (AF-CBT); ensure that foster parent is adequately informed regarding history of trauma so he or she can recognize symptoms and provide support
Foster parent lacks skills to establish limits, rewards, and consequences to promote and reinforce prosocial behavior; parenting approach may be inconsistent or coercive	Parent will gain increased understanding and capacity to respond to and shape child's behaviors	Provide information and coaching regarding effective discipline, strengthen parent–child relationship, refer to parent–child interaction therapy (PCIT), parent management training
Frequency or severity of behaviors causes high degree of parental stress	Parent will have realistic expectations of child, sense of competence in responding to child's behaviors, enhanced coping skills, and reduction in stress	Provide education regarding child's emotional/behavioral issues and strategies for reducing stress, assist parent to identify supports and coping strategies, offer respite services, refer to parent support groups

LAWS AND REGULATIONS
The licensure and operation of TFC homes generally are governed by laws and regulations on the national and local levels.

In the United States, professionals are mandated by state statutes to report suspected or known child maltreatment to child protective services and/or law enforcement.

The 1980 United States Adoption Assistance and Child Welfare Act requires that states provide out-of-home placement for children in CW agency custody in the least restrictive, most family-like setting appropriate for their needs and facilitate reunification or placement in a permanent home in a timely manner.

The 2011 Child and Family Services Improvement and Innovation Act requires that states specifically address trauma, psychotropic medications, and developmental needs of children in foster care as part of their healthcare plan.

Each country has its own standards for cultural competence and diversity in social work practice. Social workers must be aware of the standards of practice set forth by their governing body (e.g., National Association of Social Workers in the United States, British Association of Social Workers in the UK) and practice accordingly.

Services and Resources

- Child Welfare Information Gateway, https://www.childwelfare.gov/
- Foster Family-Based Treatment Association, http://www.ffta.org
- Treatment Foster Care Oregon, formerly known as Multidimensional Treatment Foster Care, http://www.tfcoregon.com/
- National Child Traumatic Stress Network (NCTSN), www.nctsn.org

Food for Thought

Hundreds of programs identify themselves as TFC and share common elements, but there are also significant differences between programs in terms of their implementation of an evidence-based model or best practices and standards. These differences may lead to significant differences in outcomes and should be considered during the referral process.

Regulations commonly restrict TFC to one or two children, which works against placing siblings together.

Red Flags

Child welfare social workers often approach readiness for reunification primarily in terms of parental progress toward resolving safety concerns that led to the child's removal and are less attuned to the impact of the child's mental health issues on reunification or to the parents' ambivalence or lack of readiness to manage the child's behaviors.

A significant number of youth in TFC are on psychotropic medication, but caregivers and staff often do not receive adequate training in administering and monitoring medications and side effects. Additional training is needed in this area.

The educational needs of children in TFC often are overlooked. Greater attention is needed to ensuring that children are referred for early intervention or special education if indicated, as well as encouraging foster parents to participate in school meetings.

Many youth in TFC have a history of suicidal ideation and previous psychiatric hospitalization. TFC and program staff should be adequately trained to recognize warning signs and have a plan for responding to psychiatric crises.

Youth with a history of sexual perpetration should immediately be assessed and provided with intensive treatment. Therapeutic foster parents must be adequately trained to recognize problematic behaviors.

Youth from undocumented families can be at a higher risk for placement with a nonrelative rather than in kinship care when these youth come into the child welfare system. Researchers in Texas found that the undocumented youth were placed with a nonrelative 84.16 percent of the time, compared to legal citizen youth, who were placed with a nonrelative 69.83 percent of the time. This difference may be due to issues related to socioeconomics, immigration status, or language barriers that impede relatives from coming forward to provide kinship care (Scott et al., 2014)

Next Steps

Ensure that parents/caregivers are adequately prepared for reunification, understand the child's diagnoses and needs, are educated about psychotropic medications if applicable, have realistic expectations for the child's behaviors, and are prepared to manage challenges.

Ensure that transitions occur in a planned and coordinated manner, with input from all providers, parents, and child.

Provide linkage to community services (e.g., support groups, mentors, recreational programs) as appropriate to provide additional supports.

Provide written information regarding the child's mental health condition or needs as applicable (e.g., parent handouts available through MedLinePlus, http://www.nlm.nih.gov/medlineplus/childmentalhealth.html).

Written by Jennifer Teska, MSW

Reviewed by Laura McLuckey, MSW, LCSW, and Melissa Rosales Neff, MSW

REFERENCES

Akin, B. A., Bryson, S. A., McDonald, T., & Walker, S. (2012). Defining a target population at high risk of long-term foster care: Barriers to permanency for families of children with serious emotional disturbances. *Child Welfare, 91*(6), 79-101.

Baker, A. J., Kurland, D., Curtis, P., Alexander, G., & Papa-Lentini, C. (2007). Mental health and behavioral problems of youth in the child welfare system: Residential treatment centers compared to therapeutic foster care in the Odyssey Project population. *Child Welfare, 86*(3), 97-123.

Boyd, L., Brylske, P., & Wall, E. (2013). Beyond safety and permanency: Promoting social and emotional well-being for youth in treatment foster care. *Foster Family Based Treatment Association.*

Breland-Noble, A. M., Farmer, E. M. Z., Dubs, M. S., Potter, E., & Burns, B. J. (2005). Mental health and other service use by youth in therapeutic foster care and group homes. *Journal of Child & Family Studies, 14*(2), 167-180. doi:10.1007/s10826-005-5045-5

British Association of Social Workers. (2012). The code of ethics for social work: Statement of principles. Retrieved February 1, 2016, from http://cdn.basw.co.uk/upload/basw_112315-7.pdf

Child Welfare Information Gateway. (2013). Mandatory reporters of child abuse and neglect. Washington, DC: U. S. Department of Health and Human Services, Children's Bureau. Retrieved February 1, 2016, from https://www.childwelfare.gov/pubPDFs/manda.pdf

Child Welfare Information Gateway. (2015). Major federal legislation concerned with child protection, child welfare, and adoption. Retrieved February 1, 2016, from https://www.childwelfare.gov/pubpdfs/majorfedlegis.pdf

Dallos, M., Morgan-West, K., & Denam, K. (2015). Changes in attachment representations for young people in long-term therapeutic foster care.

Clinical Child Psychology and Psychiatry, 20(4), 657-676. doi:10.1177/1359104514543956

Dore, M. M., & Mullin, D. (2006). Treatment family foster care: Its history and current role in the foster care continuum. *Families in Society: The Journal of Contemporary Social Services, 87*(4), 475-482. doi:10.1606/1044-3894.3562

Dorsey, S., Burns, B. J., Southerland, D. G., Cox, J. R., Wagner, H. R., & Farmer, E. M. Z. (2012). Prior trauma exposure for youth in treatment foster care. *Journal of Child and Family Studies, 21*(5), 816-824.

Fisher, P. A., Kim, H. K., & Pears, K. C. (2009). Effects of multidimensional treatment foster care for preschoolers (MTFC-P) on reducing permanent placement failures among children with placement instability. *Children and Youth Services Review, 31*(5), 541-546. doi:10.1016/j.childyouth.2008.10.012

Greeson, J. K. P., Briggs, E. C., Kisiel, C. L., Layne, C. M., Ake, G. S., Ko, S. J., ... Fairbanks, J. A. (2011). Complex trauma and mental health in children and adolescents placed in foster care: Findings from the National Child Traumatic Stress Network, *90*(6), 91-108.

Hussey, D. L., & Guo, S. (2005). Characteristics and trajectories of treatment foster care youth. *Child Welfare, 84*(4), 485-506. International Federation of Social Workers. (2012). Statement of ethical principles. Retrieved February 1, 2016, from http://ifsw.org/policies/statement-of-ethical-principles/

Jamora, M. S., Brylske, P. D., Martens, P., Braxton, D., Colantuoni, E., & Belcher, H. M. E. (2009). Children in foster care: Adverse childhood experiences and psychiatric diagnoses. *Journal of Child & Adolescent Trauma, 2*, 198-208. doi:10.1080/19361520903120491

Johnson, S., & Pryce, J. (2013). Therapeutic mentoring: Reducing the impact of trauma for foster youth. *Child Welfare, 92*(3), 9-25.

Jonkman, C. S., Bolle, E. A., Lindeboom, R., Schuengel, C., Oosterman, M., Boer, F., & Lindauer, R. J. L. (2012). Multidimensional treatment foster care for preschoolers: Early findings of an implementation in the Netherlands. *Child & Adolescent Psychiatry & Mental Health, 6*(38), 1-5. doi:10.1186/1753-2000-6-38

Leve, L. D., Fisher, P. A., & Chamberlain, P. (2009). Multidimensional treatment foster care as a preventative intervention to promote resiliency among youth in the child welfare system. *Journal of Personality, 77*(6), 1869-1902. doi:10.1111/j.1467-6494.2009.00603.x

Madden, E. E., Maher, E. J., McRoy, R. G., Ward, K. J., Peveto, L., & Stanley, A. (2012). Family reunification of youth in foster care with complex mental health needs: Barriers and recommendations. *Child & Adolescent Social Work Journal, 29*(3), 221-240. doi:10.1007/s10560-012-0257-1

McAuley, C., & Davis, T. (2009). Emotional well-being and mental health of looked after children in England. *Child and Family Social Work, 14*, 147-155. doi:10.1111/j.1365.2206.2009.00619.x

Neely-Barnes, S., & Whitted, K. (2011). Examining the social, emotional and behavioral needs of youth involved in the child welfare and juvenile justice systems. *Journal of Health & Human Services Administration*, 206-238.

Pavkov, T. W., Hug, R. W., Lourie, I. S., & Negash, S. (2010). Service process and quality in therapeutic foster care: An exploratory study of one county system. *Journal of Social Service Research, 36*(3), 174-187. doi:10.1080/01488371003697897

Shipman, K., & Taussig, H. (2009). Mental health treatment of child abuse and neglect: The promise of evidence-based practice. *Pediatric Clinics of North America, 56*(2), 417-428. doi:10.1016/j.pcl.2009.02.002

Scott, J., Faulkner, M., Cardoso, J. B., & Burstain, J. (2014). Kinship care and undocumented Latino children in the Texas foster care system: Navigating child welfare – immigration crossroads. *Child Welfare, 93*(4), 53-69.

Southerland, D., Mustillo, S., Farmer, E., Stambaugh, L., & Murray, M. (2009). What's the relationship got to do with it? Understanding the therapeutic relationship in therapeutic foster care. *Child & Adolescent Social Work Journal, 26*(1), 49-63. doi:10.1007/s10560-008-0159-4

U.S. Department of Health and Human Services, Administration for Children and Families, Administration on Children, Youth and Families, & Children's Bureau. (2015). The AFCARS report no. 22: Preliminary FY 2014 estimates as of July 2015. Retrieved February 1, 2016, from http://www.acf.hhs.gov/sites/default/files/cb/afcarsreport22.pdf

Westermark, P. K., Hansson, K., & Olsson, M. (2010). Multidimensional treatment foster care (MTFC): Results from an independent replication. *Journal of Family Therapy, 33*, 20-41. doi:10.1111/j.1467-6427.2010.00515.x

Wheeler, D. (2015). NASW standards and indicators for cultural competence in social work practice. Retrieved February 1, 2016, from http://www.socialworkers.org/practice/standards/PRA-BRO-253150-CC-Standards.pdf

THERAPEUTIC FOSTER CARE: CHILDREN WITH MENTAL HEALTH ISSUES

MAJOR CATEGORIES: Adoption/Foster Care, Behavioral & Mental Health

DESCRIPTION

Therapeutic foster care (TFC) is a family-based treatment model for children with serious mental health issues that is utilized when it is determined that out-of-home care is necessary because of the severity of the child's behaviors. In the mental health continuum of care, TFC represents the least restrictive out-of-home treatment setting available and may be utilized as either an alternative to or a step down from group or residential care for youth who can safely reside in a community setting but need a supportive, therapeutic environment to attain treatment goals or maintain gains already made

in treatment. Children may be referred to a TFC agency by a parent, mental health provider, social worker, or other professional working with the child. Acceptance into TFC generally is based on the child meeting clinical criteria established by the child's insurer or payment entity.

The implementation of TFC varies considerably among agencies in terms of administration and therapeutic approach, although the Foster Family-based Treatment Association has established some common standards for programs in North America. Despite individual variations, TFC programs generally share the following core components:

Foster parents receive specialized training, are licensed to care for only one or two children at a time, and receive a higher rate of compensation than parents in non-therapeutic foster homes.

Foster parents are regarded as full members of the child's treatment team and are expected to implement treatment goals in accordance with the child's individualized service plan and provide more structure and supervision than parents in non-therapeutic foster homes.

Agency workers carry a small caseload of families and are expected to provide a high level of guidance, support, crisis intervention, and respite to families.

Agency workers may provide consultation and/or service coordination for school staff, mental health clinicians, medical providers, and other team members.

Programs include a family component to engage the child's parents in education, visits, and/or family therapy and an aftercare plan to support transition to birth family or other permanent placement.

One evidence-based TFC model, Treatment Foster Care Oregon (TFCO) (formerly known as Multidimensional Treatment Foster Care [MTFC]), has demonstrated positive effects including reducing violence and delinquency, reducing behavior problems, and enhancing resilience. Certified MTFC programs have been established in the United States, England, Norway, Denmark, Sweden, and New Zealand. The majority of MTFC homes serve youth ages 12–17 years, although there are also programs for preschoolers ages 3–6 years and children ages 7–11 years. The MTFC model is time-limited, typically involving 6 to 9 months of treatment and 3 months of aftercare. Critical elements that distinguish this model include grounding in social learning theory, vigilant attention and response to children's behaviors in home and community settings, consistent limits, predictable rewards and consequences for behavior, skills training for children, daily contact between staff and foster parents, implementation of behavior management strategies by foster parents, and supportive therapy for the child and involved adults.

FACTS AND FIGURES

The prevalence rate for mental health disorders among children and adolescents is estimated to be approximately 1 in 5, with studies in various countries reporting findings in a similar range. In one such study in the United States, researchers found that 17.1 percent of youth ages 11 to 17 years had a mental health disorder, 5.3 percent of whom evidenced significant impairment. The most prevalent disorders were anxiety (6.9 percent), disruptive (oppositional or conduct) disorders (6.5 percent), and substance use disorders (5.3 percent) (Roberts et al., 2007). In Chile, 22.5 percent of youth ages 4 to 11 years had a disorder causing moderate impairment in at least one area. Disruptive disorders (14.6 percent) were most common, followed by anxiety (8.3 percent) and affective disorders (5.1 percent). Substance use disorders were identified for 1.2 percent (Vicente et al., 2012).

Children and adolescents in foster care have disproportionately high rates of emotional and behavioral problems. They are significantly more likely to receive at least one psychiatric *DSM* diagnosis in their lifetime; many will receive more than three diagnoses in their lifetime. These diagnoses include oppositional defiant disorder, conduct disorder, major depressive disorder, post-traumatic stress disorder (PTSD), and attention deficit hyperactivity disorder (ADHD) (Pecora et al., 2009).

A large multi-site sample of youth in TFC in the United States found that the TFC population includes children from 3 to 20 years of age, with a mean age of 13.59 and a higher proportion of males (64.7 percent) than females. As many as 90 percent are prescribed psychotropic medication, 38.3 percent have previous psychiatric hospitalization, 33 percent have a history of criminal offenses, 18.5 percent have substance abuse issues, and 6.9 percent have a history of sexual offenses. A high percentage are in the clinical range on one or more scales on the Child Behavior Checklist (CBCL), including externalizing (e.g., lying, stealing) (47.9 percent), internalizing (e.g., is depressed, anxious, withdrawn) (35.9 percent), delinquency (24.5 percent), attention problems (21.8 percent), and aggression (20.6 percent) (Baker et al., 2007).

In a 2014 study of 334 adolescents (ages 15–18 years) in foster care in the United States, 25 percent reported dealing with anxiety or depression and 28 percent reported delinquent or aggressive behavior. Furthermore, 39 percent reported alcohol use and 35 percent reported marijuana use. The researchers reported that the foster youth who had used marijuana in the past 6 months also engaged in the most human immunodeficiency virus (HIV)-related sexual risk behaviors (e.g., vaginal or anal intercourse without a condom, IV drug use) (Auslander et al., 2014).

Trauma increasingly is recognized as a significant contributor to children's emotional and behavioral difficulties. In one study of youth from 5 to 18 years of age, 93 percent had experienced at least one traumatic event, with the highest rates being for emotional abuse (85 percent), exposure to domestic violence (65.4 percent), sexual abuse (52.7 percent), neglect (51.5 percent), physical abuse (49.5 percent), and the loss of a parent to incarceration or death (46.8 percent). Most children experienced more than one type of trauma, and 48.5 percent experienced at least four types (Dorsey et al., 2012).

RISK FACTORS

The majority of youth in TFC have displayed behaviors that have presented significant challenges in home, school, and other settings, jeopardizing their ability to remain in the community. Risk factors for disruptive or conduct issues in childhood include low family income;inconsistent or harsh discipline; chaotic, multi-problem families;parent-child conflict;child abuse and neglect;lack of positive parental involvement and/ or absent parent;low IQ;poor school achievement; and impulsiveness. As maladaptive behaviors become entrenched, children become increasingly at risk for academic difficulties, negative peer relationships, involvement with the juvenile justice system, and other social difficulties. They are at significantly high risk for PTSD, depression, and drug dependency.

SIGNS AND SYMPTOMS

The majority of children in TFC have disruptive, defiant, aggressive, antisocial behaviors that have created significant difficulty in home and school settings. Diagnoses may include ADHD, oppositional defiant disorder, conduct disorder, PTSD, and mood disorders. Children may have a history of substance abuse, truancy, school suspensions and failures, chronic delinquency, sexual perpetration, psychiatric hospitalizations, multiple living situations, and episodes of running away.

ASSESSMENT

Complete a comprehensive biopsychosocialspiritual assessment to include information on physical, mental, environmental, social, and financial factors as they relate to the child and his/her family.

Ask about history of physical/sexual/emotional abuse or neglect, exposure to violence or other trauma, family history, placement history, level of functioning, history of psychiatric symptoms or issues that pose risk to self or others (e.g., suicide ideation/attempts,

self-harm, substance abuse, aggression, fire setting, running away, sexual perpetration), history of mental health treatment and psychotropic medication, child's involvement with other systems (e.g., school, corrections), and family and community supports.

ASSESSMENTS AND SCREENING TOOLS

- Child and Adolescent Functional Assessment Scale (CAFAS) for children ages 6–17 years or Preschool and Early Childhood Functional Assessment Scale (PECFAS) for children ages 3–7 years
- CBCL for ages 1.5-18 years
- Child and Adolescent Needs and Strengths, Mental Health (CANS-MH)
- Strengths and Difficulties Questionnaire (SDQ)
- UCLA PTSD Reaction Index (PTSD-RI)

There may be a need for a toxicology screen for drug and/or alcohol use.

TREATMENT

A system of care framework is recommended to manage the complex needs of youth in TFC, who typically are involved with one or more public agencies in addition to mental health services (e.g.,child welfare, juvenile delinquency) and multiple service providers. Although TFC is itself a psychosocial intervention, many children also need specialized treatment, individual and/or group skills training, special education, and/or vocational training. In some programs, TFC may be supplemented by day treatment or partial hospitalization.

TFC recognizes that the home is a natural learning environment for children, with foster parents serving as powerful change agents in the child's treatment. Preparation and support of both foster parents and the caregivers whom the child will reside with upon discharge is critical. A good alliance between therapeutic parents and children is associated with more positive outcomes, as is the foster parents' identifying themselves more as parents than as professionals.

The social worker will utilize an ecological approach to ensure that the child's individual needs are addressed; that foster parents have adequate training and support; that ongoing and aftercare services include the child's biological, foster, or adoptive family that will care for the child upon discharge; and that involved agencies and systems work in collaboration, addressing any barriers that arise.

Social workers should be aware of their own cultural values, beliefs, and biases and develop specialized knowledge about the histories, traditions, and values of their clients. Social workers should adopt treatment methodologies that reflect their knowledge of the cultural diversity of the societies in which they practice.

Problem	Goal	Intervention
Child is exhibiting maladaptive and/or disruptive behaviors and lack of prosocial skills and behaviors	Reduce problem behaviors, teach and reinforce prosocial skills and behaviors	Individualized behavioral strategies focused on reinforcing positive behaviors, close supervision, limiting negative peer associations, and strengthening adult-child relationships; individual and group skills coaching for parents and children
Child has underlying mental health condition	Support resolution of mental health symptoms, enhance adaptive coping	Refer for specialized mental health therapy, e.g., anger coping, substance abuse treatment, psychotropic medication
Child experiences symptoms resulting from history of trauma	Support resolution of symptoms related to exposure to trauma	Screen all youth in TFC for trauma history, refer for trauma-focused cognitive behavioral therapy (TF-CBT) and abuse-focused cognitive behavioral therapy (AF-CBT), ensure that foster parent is adequately informed of history of trauma so he or she can recognize symptoms and provide support
Parent lacks skills to establish limits, rewards, and consequences to promote and reinforce prosocial behavior; parenting approach may be inconsistent or coercive	Parent will gain increased understanding and capacity to respond to and shape child's behaviors	Provide information and coaching regarding effective discipline, strengthen parent-child relationship, refer to parent-child interaction therapy (PCIT) and parent management training
Frequency or severity of behaviors is causing high degree of parental stress	Parent will have realistic expectations of child, sense of competence in responding to child's behaviors, enhanced coping skills, and reduction in stress	Provide education regarding child's emotional/behavioral issues and strategies for reducing stress, assist parent to identify supports and coping strategies, offer respite services, refer to parent support groups

LAWS AND REGULATIONS
The licensure and operation of TFC homes are governed by laws and regulations on the national and local levels.

Each country has its own standards for cultural competency and diversity in social work practice. Social workers must be aware of the standards of practice set forth by their governing body (National Association of Social Workers, British Association of Social Workers, etc.) and practice accordingly.

SERVICES AND RESOURCES
- Foster Family-based Treatment Association, http://www.ffta.org
- Treatment Foster Care Oregon (TFCO), http://www.tfcoregon.com/
- The National Child Traumatic Stress Network (NCTSN), www.nctsn.org
- National Institute of Mental Health (NIMH), http://www.nimh.nih.gov/health/topics/child-and-adolescent-mental-health/index.shtml

FOOD FOR THOUGHT
Hundreds of programs identify themselves as TFC and share common elements, but there are also significant differences between programs in terms of their implementation of an evidence-based model or best practices and standards.

Subgroups of children in TFC may have distinct needs; for instance, children with serious mental illness, attachment disorders, and those with histories of significant trauma often require that the TFC program be able to incorporate an array of specialized mental health treatment and supportive services.

Investigators in a study in the United Kingdom reported that adolescents in long-term TFC emphasized positive aspects of their placement such as being treated as adults, being listened to, and being made to feel safe. The study noted positive changes in the adolescents' attachment security over time (Dallos et al., 2015).

RED FLAGS.

A significant number of youth in TFC are on psychotropic medication, but foster parents and staff often do not receive adequate training in administering and monitoring medications and side effects. Additional training is needed in this area.

Many youth in TFC have a history of suicidal ideation and previous psychiatric hospitalization. Therapeutic foster parents and program staff should be adequately trained to recognize warning signs and have a plan for responding to psychiatric crises.

Youth with a history of sexual perpetration should immediately be assessed and provided with intensive treatment. Therapeutic foster parents must be adequately trained to recognize problematic behaviors.

NEXT STEPS

Ensure that transitions occur in a planned and coordinated manner, with input from all providers, parents, and youth.

Provide linkage to community services (e.g., support groups, mentors, recreational programs), as appropriate, to provide additional supports.

Provide written information regarding the child's mental health condition or needs, as applicable (e.g., parent handouts available through MedLinePlus, http://www.nlm.nih.gov/medlineplus/childmentalhealth.html)

Written by Jennifer Teska, MSW

Reviewed by Laura McLuckey, MSW, LCSW, and Melissa Rosales Neff, MSW

REFERENCES

Auslander, W., Thompson, R., & Gerke, D. (2014). The moderating effect of marijuana use on the relationship between delinquent behavior and HIV risk among adolescents in foster care. *Journal of HIV/AIDS & Social Services, 13*(2), 179-197. doi:10.1080/15381501.2013.859112

Baker, A. J., Kurland, D., Curits, P., Alexander, G., & Papa-Lentini, C. (2007). Mental health and behavioral problems of youth in the child welfare system: Residential treatment centers compared to therapeutic foster care in the Odyssey Project population. *Child Welfare, 86*(3), 97-123.

Bertram, J. E., Narendorf, S. C., & McMillen, J. C. (2013). Pioneering the psychiatric nurse role in foster care. *Archives of Psychiatric Nursing, 27*(6), 285-292. doi:10.1016/j.apnu.2013.09.003

Breland-Noble, A. M., Farmer, E. M. Z., Dubs, M. S., Potter, E., & Burns, B. J. (2005). Mental health and other service use by youth in therapeutic foster care and group homes. *Journal of Child & Family Studies, 14*(2), 167-180. doi:10.1007/s10826-005-5045-5

Chamberlain, P. (2002). Treatment foster care. In B. J. Burns & K. Hoagwood (Eds.), *Community treatment for youth: Evidence-based interventions for severe emotional and behavioral disorders* (pp. 117-138). New York, NY: Oxford University Press.

Dallos, M., Morgan-West, K., & Denam, K. (2015). Changes in attachment representations for young people in long-term therapeutic foster care. *Clinical Child Psychology and Psychiatry, 20*(4), 657-676. doi:10.1177/1359104514543956

Dore, M. M., & Mullin, D. (2006). Treatment family foster care: Its history and current role in the foster care continuum. *Families in Society: The Journal of Contemporary Social Services, 87*(4), 475-482. doi:10.1606/1044-3894.3562

Dorsey, S., Burns, B. J., Southerland, D. G., Cox, J. R., Wagner, H. R., & Farmer, E. M. Z. (2012). Prior trauma exposure for youth in treatment foster care. *Journal of Child and Family Studies, 21*(5), 816-824.

Fisher, P. A., Kim, H. K., & Pears, K. C. (2009). Effects of multidimensional treatment foster care for preschoolers (MTFC-P) on reducing permanent placement failures among children with placement instability. *Children and Youth Services Review, 31*(5), 541-546. doi:10.1016/j.childyouth.2008.10.012

Hornor, G. (2014). Children in foster care: What forensic nurses need to know. *Journal of Forensic Nursing, 10*(3), 160-167. doi:10.1097/JFN.0000000000000038

Hussey, D. L., & Guo, S. (2005). Characteristics and trajectories of treatment foster care youth. *Child Welfare, 84*(4), 485-506.

Leve, L. D., Fisher, P. A., & Chamberlain, P. (2009). Multidimensional treatment foster care as a preventive intervention to promote resiliency among youth in the child welfare system. *Journal of Personality, 77*(6), 1869-1902. doi:10.1111/j.1467-6494.2009.00603.x

Minnis, H., Everett, K., Pelosi, A. J., Dunn, J., & Knapp, M. (2006). Children in foster care: Mental health, service use and costs. *European Child & Adolescent Psychiatry, 15*(2), 63-70. doi:10.1007/s00787-006-0452-8

Oswald, S. H., Heil, K., & Goldbeck, L. (2010). History of maltreatment and mental health problems in foster children: A review of the literature. *Journal of Pediatric Psychology, 35*(5), 462-472. doi:10.1093/jpepsy/jsp114

Pavkov, T. W., Hug, R. W., Lourie, I. S., & Negash, S. (2010). Service process and quality in therapeutic foster care: An exploratory study of one county system. *Journal of Social Service Research, 36*(3), 174-187. doi:10.1080/01488371003697897

Pecora, P. J., Jensen, P. S., Romanelli, L. H., Jackson, L. J., & Ortiz, A. (2009). Mental health services for children placed in foster care: An overview of current challenges. *Child Welfare, 88*(1), 5-26.

Pinto, R. J., & Maia, A. C. (2013). Psychopathology, physical complaints and health risk behaviors among youths who were victims of childhood maltreatment: A comparison between home and institutional interventions. *Children & Youth Services Review, 35*(4), 603-610. doi:10.1016/j.childyouth.2013.01.008

The Policy, Ethics and Human Rights Committee, British Association of Social Workers. (2012, January). The code of ethics for social work: Statement of principles. Retrieved January 18, 2016, from http://cdn.basw.co.uk/upload/basw_112315-7.pdf

Roberts, R. E., Roberts, C. R., & Xing, Y. (2007). Rates of DSM-IV psychiatric disorders among adolescents in a large metropolitan area. *Journal of Psychiatric Research, 41*(11), 959-967.

Shipman, K., & Taussig, H. (2009). Mental health treatment of child abuse and neglect: The promise of evidence-based practice. *Pediatric Clinics of North America, 56*(2), 417-428. doi:10.1016/j.pcl.2009.02.002

Southerland, D. G., Mustillo, S. A., Farmer, E. M. Z., Stambaugh, L. F., & Murray, M. (2009). What's the relationship got to do with it? Understanding the therapeutic relationship in therapeutic foster care. *Child & Adolescent Social Work Journal, 26*(1), 49-63. doi:10.1007/s10560-008-0159-4

Statement of ethical principles. (2012, March 3). *International Federation of Social Workers.* Retrieved from http://ifsw.org/policies/statement-of-ethical-principles/

Vicente, B., Saldivia, S., de la Barra, F., Kohn, R., Pihan, R., Valdivia, M., ... Melipillan, R. (2012). Prevalence of child and adolescent mental disorders in Chile: A community epidemiological study. *The Journal of Child Psychology and Psychiatry, 53*(10), 1026-1035. doi:10.1111/j.1469-7610.2012.02566.x

Westermark, P. K., Hansson, K., & Olsson, M. (2010). Multidimensional treatment foster care (MTFC): Results from an independent replication. *Journal of Family Therapy, 33*, 20-41. doi:10.1111/j.1467-6427.2010.00515.x

Wheeler, D. (2015). NASW Standards and Indicators for Cultural Competence in Social Work Practice. Retrieved January 18, 2016, from http://www.socialworkers.org/practice/standards/PRA-BRO-253150-CC-Standards.pdf

THERAPEUTIC FOSTER CARE: JUVENILE COURT SYSTEM

MAJOR CATEGORIES: Adoption/Foster Care

DESCRIPTION

Therapeutic foster care (TFC) is a family-based treatment model for youth with severe emotional and/or behavioral issues. Youth who have been mandated to out-of-home care through delinquency proceedings may be referred to TFC by the juvenile justice system. TFC represents the least restrictive out-of-home treatment setting available and serves as an alternative to group or residential care or a step down from incarceration for youth who need a supportive, therapeutic environment to successfully transition back into the community.

The implementation of TFC varies considerably among agencies in terms of administration and therapeutic approach, although some common standards for programs in North America have been established by the Foster Family-Based Treatment Association. Despite individual variations, TFC programs generally share the following core components:

Foster parents receive specialized training, are licensed to care for only one or two children at a time, and receive a higher rate of compensation than parents in nontherapeutic foster homes;

Foster parents are regarded as full members of the youth's treatment team and are expected to implement treatment goals in accordance with the youth's individualized service plan and to provide more structure and supervision than parents in nontherapeutic foster homes;

Agency workers carry a small caseload of families and are expected to provide a high level of guidance, support, crisis intervention, and respite to families;

Agency workers may provide consultation and/or service coordination for school staff, mental health clinicians, medical providers, and other team members.

Programs include a family component to engage birth parents in education, visits, and/or family therapy and an aftercare plan to support transition to birth family or other permanent placement.

One evidence-based TFC model, multidimensional treatment foster care (MTFC), which was originally developed for adjudicated delinquents (i.e., youths who have violated criminal laws), has demonstrated positive effects including reducing violence and other problematic behaviors as well as decreasing the risk of reoffending. Certified MTFC programs have been established in the United States, England, Norway, Denmark, Sweden, and New Zealand. The majority of MTFC homes serve youth ages 12–17, although there also are adaptations for younger children. The MTFC model is time-limited, typically involving 6 to 9 months of treatment and 3 months of aftercare. Critical elements that distinguish this model include grounding in social learning theory, vigilant attention and response to the youth's behaviors in home and community settings, consistent limits, predictable rewards and consequences for behavior, skills training for youth, daily contact between staff and foster parents, implementation

of behavior management strategies by foster parents, and supportive therapy for the youth and involved adults. Discharge occurs when the youth has completed treatment goals and the parent has gained the skills to manage future behavior issues at home.

Research shows that therapeutic mentoring for foster children can reduce trauma symptoms significantly. Therapeutic mentoring involves mentors who are in helping professions and are extensively trained and supervised to mentor foster youth. The trainings received by the therapeutic mentors include information about working with children with emotional and behavioral disorders, therapeutic crisis interventions, and boundaries. Each mentor–mentee relationship is closely monitored by a master's-level clinician. The mentors see their mentees on a weekly basis for 3–5 hours and engage in activities with them such as playing outdoors, attending cultural events, or going to sporting events. Researchers in 2013 found that foster youth who participated in a therapeutic mentoring program for 18 months experienced a significant decrease in their trauma symptoms compared to the foster youth who did not participate in the therapeutic mentoring (Johnson & Pryce, 2013).

Other investigators reported that adolescents in long-term therapeutic foster care emphasized positive aspects of their placement such as being treated like adults, being listened to, and being made to feel safe. The investigators noted positive changes in the adolescents' attachment security over time (Dallos et al., 2014).

Although not the primary concern of the juvenile justice system, the mental health needs and trauma histories of involved youth have begun to receive increased recognition. Long-term outcomes for youth involved with the juvenile justice system are improved by incorporating trauma-informed services that treat underlying mental health issues.

FACTS AND FIGURES

In a study of youth involved with juvenile justice, 70.4 percent were found to have at least one mental health diagnosis. Of those youth with any diagnosis, 60 percent had three or more diagnosable conditions. Disruptive disorders were present in 46.5 percent of youth, substance use disorders in 46.2 percent, anxiety disorders in 34.4 percent, and mood disorders in 18.3 percent (Shufelt & Cocozza, 2006).

A large multisite sample in the United States found that the TFC population includes children from 3 to

20 years of age, with a mean age of 13.59 and a higher proportion of males (64.7 percent) than of females. As many as 90 percent are prescribed psychotropic medication, 38.3 percent have experienced previous psychiatric hospitalization, 33 percent have a history of criminal offenses, 18.5 percent have substance abuse issues, and 6.9 percent have a history of sexual offenses. A high percentage are in the clinical range on one or more scales on the Child Behavior Checklist (CBCL), including externalizing (e.g., lying, stealing) (47.9 percent), internalizing (e.g., being depressed, anxious, withdrawn) (35.9 percent), delinquency (24.5 percent), attention problems (21.8 percent), and aggression (20.6 percent) (Baker et al., 2007), 2007).

Trauma is increasingly recognized as a significant contributor to children's emotional and behavioral difficulties. In one study of youth from 5 to 18 years of age, 93 percent had experienced at least one traumatic event, with the highest rates being for emotional abuse (85 percent), exposure to domestic violence (65.4 percent), sexual abuse (52.7 percent), neglect (51.5 percent), physical abuse (49.5 percent), and the loss of a parent to incarceration or death (46.8 percent). Most children experienced more than one type of trauma, and 48.5 percent experienced at least four types (Dorsey et al., 2012).

RISK FACTORS

Youth involved with the juvenile justice system often come from impoverished, multiproblem families; have a history of abuse and neglect; and lack positive relationships with adults in their lives. Inadequate parental involvement, supervision, and discipline contribute to the risk for antisocial behavior, as does having a delinquent peer group. Mental health issues such as conduct disorders and substance abuse increase the likelihood of juvenile justice system involvement. Chronic maltreatment also is a significant risk factor for delinquency, with one group of investigators finding that the likelihood of temporary detention and/or commitment to a juvenile facility increased with each report of maltreatment (Yampolskaya et al., 2011). Among Yampolskaya et al.'s sample of youth between ages 7 and 17 who were reported to have been maltreated, being older, male, victims of sexual abuse, and/or African American also were associated with increased juvenile justice involvement. Similar to other youth in TFC, youth involved with the juvenile

justice system have displayed behaviors that have presented significant challenges in home, school, and other settings. Their behaviors may have alienated and endangered family members as well as violated laws and community safety, leaving them at high risk for out-of-home placement and/or incarceration.

SIGNS AND SYMPTOMS

The majority of youth in TFC have disruptive, defiant, aggressive, antisocial behaviors that have created significant difficulty in home and school settings. They may have a history of substance abuse, truancy, school suspensions and failures, chronic delinquency, stealing, sexual abuse perpetration, psychiatric hospitalizations, multiple living situations, and episodes of running away. Diagnoses may include attention deficit hyperactivity disorder, oppositional defiant disorder, conduct disorder, substance use disorder, posttraumatic stress disorder, and mood disorders.

ASSESSMENT

Complete a comprehensive biopsychosocial-spiritual assessment to include information on physical, mental, environmental, social, and financial factors as they relate to the youth and his/her family.

Ask about history of physical/sexual/emotional abuse or neglect, exposure to violence or other trauma, family history, placement history, level of functioning, history of psychiatric symptoms or issues that pose risk to self or others (e.g., suicide ideation/attempts, self-harm, substance abuse, aggression, fire setting, running away, sexual abuse perpetration), history of mental health treatment and psychotropic medication, youth's involvement with other systems (e.g., school, corrections), family and community supports.

ASSESSMENTS AND SCREENING TOOLS

- Child and Adolescent Functional Assessment Scale (CAFAS) for children 6–17
- Child Behavioral Checklist (CBCL) for ages 6–18
- Child and Adolescent Needs and Strengths, Mental Health (CANS-MH)
- Strengths and Difficulties Questionnaire (SDQ)
- UCLA Posttraumatic Stress Disorder Reaction Index (PTSD-R)
- Global Appraisal of Individual Needs Short Screener (GAIN-SS)

There may be a need for a toxicology screen for drug and/or alcohol use.

TREATMENT

A system-of-care framework is recommended for managing the complex needs of youth in TFC, who typically are involved with one or more public agencies in addition to juvenile justice (e.g., mental health, child welfare) and multiple service providers. Although TFC is itself a psychosocial intervention, many youth also need specialized treatment, individual and/or group skills training, substance abuse treatment, special education, and/or vocational training.

TFC recognizes that the home is a natural learning environment for children, with foster parents serving as powerful change agents in the youth's treatment. Preparation and support of both foster parents and the caregivers with whom the youth will reside upon discharge is critical. A good alliance between therapeutic parents and youth is associated with more positive outcomes, as is the foster parents' identifying themselves more as parents than as professionals.

The social worker will utilize an ecological approach to ensure that the youth's individual needs are addressed; that foster parents have adequate training and support; that ongoing and aftercare services include the youth's biological, foster, or adoptive family that will care for the youth upon discharge; and that involved agencies and systems work in coordination, addressing any barriers that arise.

Social workers should be aware of their own cultural values, beliefs, and biases and develop specialized knowledge about the histories, traditions, and values of their clients. Social workers should adopt treatment methodologies that reflect their knowledge of the cultural diversity of the communities in which they practice.

Problem	Goal	Intervention
Youth is exhibiting maladaptive and/or disruptive behaviors, lack of prosocial skills and behaviors	Reduce problem behaviors, teach and reinforce prosocial skills and behaviors	Individualized behavioral strategies focused on reinforcing positive behaviors, close supervision, limiting negative peer associations, and strengthening adult–youth relationships; individual and group skills coaching for parents and youth; mentoring
Youth has underlying mental health condition	Support resolution of mental health symptoms, enhance adaptive coping	Refer for specialized mental health therapy (e.g., anger coping, substance abuse treatment, psychotropic medication)
Youth experiences symptoms resulting from history of trauma	Support resolution of symptoms related to exposure to trauma	Screen all youth in TFC for trauma history, refer for trauma-focused cognitive behavioral therapy (TF-CBT), abuse-focused cognitive behavioral therapy (AF-CBT); ensure that foster parent is adequately informed regarding history of trauma so he or she can recognize symptoms and provide support
Parent lacks skills to establish limits, rewards, and consequences to promote and reinforce prosocial behavior; parenting approach may be inconsistent or coercive	Parent will gain increased understanding and capacity to respond to and shape youth's behaviors	Provide information and coaching regarding effective discipline, strengthen parent–youth relationship, provide parent management training
Frequency or severity of behaviors is causing high degree of parental stress	Parent will have realistic expectations of youth, sense of competence in responding to youth's behaviors, enhanced coping skills, and reduction in stress	Provide education regarding youth's emotional/behavioral issues and strategies for reducing stress, assist parent to identify supports and coping strategies, offer respite services, refer parent to support groups

LAWS AND REGULATIONS

The licensure and operation of TFC homes are governed by laws and regulations on the national and local levels.

The Juvenile Justice and Delinquency Prevention Act of 1974 sets standards for juvenile justice systems throughout the United States.

Each country has its own standards for cultural competency and diversity in social work practice. Social workers must be aware of the standards of practice set forth by their governing body (e.g., National Association of Social Workers in the United States, British Association of Social Workers in the UK) and practice accordingly.

SERVICES AND RESOURCES

- Foster Family-Based Treatment Association, http://www.ffta.org
- Treatment Foster Care Oregon, http://www.tfcoregon.com
- National Center for Mental Health and Juvenile Justice, http://www.ncmhjj.com/
- National Child Traumatic Stress Network (NCTSN), www.nctsn.org
- Office of Juvenile Justice and Delinquency Prevention, http://www.ojjdp.gov/

FOOD FOR THOUGHT

Hundreds of programs identify themselves as TFC and share common elements, but there are also significant differences between programs in terms of their implementation of an evidence-based model or best practices and standards.

Delinquent girls tend to have higher levels of individual and family risk factors than boys do, but they also appear to be at the lowest risk for recidivism after completing MFTC.

RED FLAGS

A significant number of youth in TFC are prescribed psychotropic medication, but foster parents and staff often do not receive adequate training in administering and monitoring medications and side effects. Additional training is needed in this area.

Many youth in TFC have a history of suicidal ideation and previous psychiatric hospitalization. TFC and program staff should be adequately trained to recognize warning signs and have a plan for responding to psychiatric crises.

Youth with a history of sexual perpetration should immediately be assessed and provided with intensive treatment. Therapeutic foster parents must be adequately trained to recognize problematic behaviors.

NEXT STEPS

Ensure that transitions occur in a planned and coordinated manner, with input from all providers, parents, and youth.

Provide linkage to community services (e.g., support groups, mentors, recreational programs) as appropriate to provide additional supports.

Provide written information regarding the youth's mental health condition or needs as applicable (e.g., parent handouts available through MedlinePlus, http://www.nlm.nih.gov/medlineplus/childmentalhealth.html).

Written by Jennifer Teska, MSW

Reviewed by Laura McLuckey, MSW, LCSW, and Melissa Rosales Neff, MSW

REFERENCES

Baker, A. J., Kurland, D., Curtis, P., Alexander, G., & Papa-Lentini, C. (2007). Mental health and behavioral problems of youth in the child welfare system: Residential treatment centers compared to therapeutic foster care in the Odyssey Project population. *Child Welfare, 86*(3), 97-123.

Breland-Noble, A. M., Farmer, E. M. Z., Dubs, M. S., Potter, E., & Burns, B. J. (2005). Mental health and other service use by youth in therapeutic foster care and group homes. *Journal of Child & Family Studies, 14*(2), 167-180. doi:10.1007/s10826-005-5045-5

Chamberlain, P. (2002). Treatment foster care. In B. J. Burns & K. Hoagwood (Eds.), *Community treatment for youth: Evidence-based interventions for severe emotional and behavioral disorders* (pp. 117-138). New York, NY: Oxford University Press.

Dallos, M., Morgan-West, K., & Denam, K. (2015). Changes in attachment representations for young people in long-term therapeutic foster care. *Clinical Child Psychology and Psychiatry, 20*(4), 657-676. doi:10.1177/1359104514543956

Dore, M. M., & Mullin, D. (2006). Treatment family foster care: Its history and current role in the foster care continuum. *Families in Society: The*

Journal of Contemporary Social Services, 87(4), 475-482. doi:10.1606/1044-3894.3562

Dorsey, S., Burns, B. J., Southerland, D. G., Cox, J. R., Wagner, H. R., & Farmer, E. M. Z. (2012). Prior trauma exposure for youth in treatment foster care. *Journal of Child and Family Studies, 21*(5), 816-824.

Fisher, P. A., Kim, H. K., & Pears, K. C. (2009). Effects of multidimensional treatment foster care for preschoolers (MTFC-P) on reducing permanent placement failures among children with placement instability. *Children and Youth Services Review, 31*(5), 541-546. doi:10.1016/j.childyouth.2008.10.012

Hahn, R. A., Bilukha, O., Lowy, J., Crosby, A., Fullilove, M. T., Liberman, A., ... Schofield, A. (2005). The effectiveness of therapeutic foster care for the prevention of violence: A systematic review. *American Journal of Preventive Medicine, 28*(2SI), 72-90. doi:10.1016/j.ampre.2004.10.007

International Federation of Social Workers. (2012, March 3). Statement of ethical principles. Retrieved February 1, 2016, from http://ifsw.org/policies/statement-of-ethical-principles/

Johnson, S., & Pryce, J. (2013). Therapeutic mentoring: Reducing the impact of trauma for foster youth. *Child Welfare, 92*(3), 9-25.

Leve, L. D., Fisher, P. A., & Chamberlain, P. (2009). Multidimensional treatment foster care as a preventative intervention to promote resiliency among youth in the child welfare system. *Journal of Personality, 77*(6), 1869-1902. doi:10.1111/j.1467-6494.2009.00603.x

Minnis, H., Everett, K., Pelosi, A. J., Dunn, J., & Knapp, M. (2006). Children in foster care: Mental health, service use and costs. *European Child & Adolescent Psychiatry, 15*(2), 63-70. doi:10.1007/s00787-006-0452-8

Wheeler, D. (2015). NASW standards and indicators for cultural competence in social work practice. Retrieved February 1, 2016, from http://www.socialworkers.org/practice/standards/PRA-BRO-253150-CC-Standards.pdf

Oswald, S. H., Heil, K., & Goldbeck, L. (2010). History of maltreatment and mental health problems in foster children: A review of the literature. *Journal of Pediatric Psychology, 35*(5), 462-472. doi:10.1093/jpepsy/jsp114

Pavkov, T. W., Hug, R. W., Lourie, I. S., & Negash, S. (2010). Service process and quality in therapeutic foster care: An exploratory study of one county

system. *Journal of Social Service Research, 36*(3), 174-187. doi:10.1080/01488371003697897

Pinto, R. J., & Maia, A. C. (2013). Psychopathology, physical complaints and health risk behaviors among youths who were victims of childhood maltreatment: A comparison between home and institutional interventions. *Children & Youth Services Review, 35*(4), 603-610. doi:10.1016/j.childyouth.2013.01.008

Pullman, M. D. (2010). Predictors of criminal charges for youth in public mental health during the transition to adulthood. *Journal of Child Family Studies, 19*(4), 438-491. doi:10.1007/s10826-009-9320-8

Shipman, K., & Taussig, H. (2009). Mental health treatment of child abuse and neglect: The promise of evidence-based practice. *Pediatric Clinics of North America, 56*(2), 417-428. doi:10.1016/j.pcl.2009.02.002

Shufelt, J. L., & Cocozza, J. J. (2006). Youth with mental disorders in the juvenile justice system: Results from a multi-state prevalence study. Delmar, NY: National Center for Mental Health and Juvenile Justice.

Smith, D. K. (2004). Risk, reinforcement, retention in treatment, and reoffending for boys and girls in multidimensional treatment foster care. *Journal of Emotional and Behavioral Disorders, 12*(1), 38-48. doi:10.1177/10634266040120010501

Southerland, D., Mustillo, S., Farmer, E., Stambaugh, L., & Murray, M. (2009). What's the relationship got to do with it? Understanding the therapeutic relationship in therapeutic foster care. *Child & Adolescent Social Work Journal, 26*(1), 49-63. doi:10.1007/s10560-008-0159-4

British Association of Social Workers. (2012). The code of ethics for social work: Statement of principles. Retrieved February 1, 2016, from http://cdn.basw.co.uk/upload/basw_112315-7.pdf

Westermark, P. K., Hansson, K., & Olsson, M. (2010). Multidimensional treatment foster care (MTFC): Results from an independent replication. *Journal of Family Therapy, 33*, 20-41. doi:10.1111/j.1467-6427.2010.00515.x

Yampolskaya, S., Armstrong, M. I., & McNeish, R. (2011). Children placed in out-of-home care: Risk factors for involvement with the juvenile justice system. *Violence & Victims, 26*(2), 231-245. doi:10.1891/0886-6708.26.2.231

TRANSGENDER ADULTS: PSYCHOSOCIAL ISSUES

MAJOR CATEGORIES: Behavioral & Mental Health, Gender/Identity

WHAT WE KNOW

Transgender is an umbrella term used to describe individuals whose gender identity and behaviors fall outside gender norms and do not conform to their biological sex.

Transgender individuals may be transsexuals (who identify opposite to their assigned biological sex), bi-gendered persons (who exhibit both genders), intersex persons (whose chromosomal structure or sex organs are not distinctly male or female), or transvestites (i.e., men who dress as women or women who dress as men).

Gender-nonconforming and *gender-variant* are also terms used to describe individuals whose gender identity does not conform to the binary of female or male.

Transgender individuals may identify, and frequently are referred to in the literature, as either male-to-female (MTF) or female-to-male (FTM) transgender.

Experiences of being transgender vary with the age of the individual and should be placed in historical context of changing societal attitudes.

The internal experience of masculinity and femininity for each individual increasingly is understood as an idiosyncratic experience that exists on a spectrum of gender identification, rather than being a fixed, binary characteristic.

Many transgender individuals are aware of their gender variance in childhood and describe feeling a "mind-body dissonance." One study showed that MTF transgender individuals were aware of their gender dissonance earlier in childhood than FTMs were.

Coming out as transgender can be a process that requires the individual to reestablish all of his or her relationships; because of this, it is an experience that is different from revealing oneself as gay, lesbian, or bisexual.

Researchers who carried out a study of transgender individuals living in rural versus urban environments noted significant differences in access to mental healthcare, along with similar levels of alcohol and marijuana use.

Sexual identity and gender are related, but often are conflated and should not be confused: Being transgender does not imply a particular sexual orientation.

A study of the impact of testosterone treatment found that some participants changed their self-defined sexual orientation after starting treatments.

Scholars, advocates, and transgender individuals have been critical of state and medical requirements that insist on sex reassignment surgery and hormone replacement treatment before establishing the preferred gender of the transgender individual.

In 2011 the United Nations High Commission for Human Rights adopted a resolution explicitly supporting the human rights of transgender individuals(as well as lesbian, gay, and bisexual individuals).

The report expresses grave concern about the global abuse of and discrimination toward these populations.

Verbal and physical abuse of transgender individuals occurs frequently and may come from family, peers, and religious and other authority figures.

Transgender identity is persistently over-sexualized by society, and transgender individuals are extremely vulnerable to sexual abuse.

Researchers of one study found widespread negative attitudes among heterosexual adults in the United States toward transgender individuals. More frequent negativity toward transgender individuals was reported by heterosexual men than by heterosexual women. Less frequent negativity was reported by heterosexuals who had contact with sexual minorities.

Discrimination in the housing market is reported by transgender individuals buying and renting homes: 1 in 5 have been homeless at some point since identifying as transgender.

Results from a review of 33 studies indicated that between 35 percent and 72 percent of transgender individuals had been arrested at some point. Transgender individuals are targeted by law enforcement with illegal police stops, abuse, and harassment; the abuse includes condoning violence toward transgender prison inmates by other inmates. Transgender individuals may not seek assistance when they are victims of crime because of fear of secondary victimization by law enforcement.

Two thirds of transgender adults report experiencing discrimination in the workplace.

In California, transgender individuals are twice as likely to have a bachelor's degree than Californians overall, but they earn 40 percent less than other graduates.

As a result of discrimination in California, transgender individuals are twice as likely to live below the poverty threshold as the general population is.

Transgender individuals have an elevated risk of poor mental health. Rates of depression and suicidal ideation among transgender persons are described as high; they are highest among younger transgender individuals. These rates may lessen with age due to improved coping mechanisms.

Statistics from Europe, the United States and Canada reveal that 22 percent–43 percent of transgender individuals report a history of suicide attempts, 9 percent–10 percent having attempted suicide in the past year.

A strong social support system, protection from transphobia, and undergoing a full medical transition (with hormone use and/or surgical procedures) are significant protective factors from suicide risk among transgender individuals.

Results from one study indicated that FTM transgender individuals were at a higher risk of attempting suicide in their lifetime compared to MTF transgender individuals.

Non-suicidal self-injury (NSSI) (when individuals intentionally harm themselves without lethal intent) is prevalent among transgender individuals. Examples of NSSI are cutting, burning, severe scratching, and hitting.

Results from a study of transgender adults in the United States indicated that 41.9 percent of participants reported a history of NSSI. The mean age of NSSI initiation was 13 years of age, and the behaviors continued well into adulthood.

Results from a study of older transgender adults indicated that they had significantly poorer health (i.e., physical health, disabilities, symptoms of depression, and perceived stress) than nontransgender lesbian, gay, and bisexual older adults.

Transgender adults who experience more daily discrimination are more likely to participate in health-harming behaviors such as drug and alcohol abuse, smoking, and suicide attempts.

A lower overall quality of life was found among Dutch FTMs than in the overall Dutch male population; Dutch MTFs showed no significant difference in quality of life compared to the overall female population, however.

In a U.S. study, quality of life was significantly lower among FTM transgender persons compared to the overall male and female population.

Younger transgender individuals are at risk of being institutionalized and subjected to gender-conforming interventions.

Gender dysphoria, as outlined in the *Diagnostic and Statistical Manual of Mental Disorders 5* (*DSM-5*),may be diagnosed in some transgender individuals. In the *DSM-5*, the disorder is now separate from other sexual dysfunctions and paraphilic disorders. Diagnosis in *DSM-5* requires that there be a marked difference between an individual's expressed or experienced gender and the gender that others wish to assign him or her, which must cause clinically significant distress or impairment in social, occupational, or other areas of functioning for at least6 months. To ensure access to treatment, the*DSM-5* includes a post-transition specifier for individuals living full-time as their desired gender.

Substance abuse and HIV reportedly are high among transgender individuals. HIV is highest among transgender women, specifically black MTF transgender persons. A significant connection has been shown between substance abuse and sexual risk-taking. Transgender sex workers are especially at risk for substance abuse and HIV infection.

Some scholars emphasize the tendency to misdiagnose mental health problems in transgender individuals. One study showed no difference in physical and mental health between stably housed transgender adults and the overall U.S. population. Another study found that 9 of the 10 individual case studies researchers examined at a gender identity clinic demonstrated at least one significant pathology. Transgender individuals have difficulties accessing social and health services because of discrimination.

Researchers found that 42 percent of FTM transgender adults reported verbal harassment, physical assault or lack of access to equal treatment in a medical office setting or hospital.

Research indicates that communities and social workers lack knowledge and information about transgender individuals and therefore require educational interventions to prevent discrimination and victimization.

Transgender parents and their children report experiencing a tremendous amount of stress: Parents feel stress from being rejected by their family and from job discrimination. Their children report feeling stressed from bullying, having to change their perception of their parents, and feeling like they are caught in the middle of family relationships and strife. Both transgender parents and their children report viewing therapy as a beneficial resource.

WHAT CAN BE DONE

Learn about the psychosocial issues of transgender individuals and help create trans-positive environments by providing education and sensitivity trainings to colleagues.

Clinical practice and research should recognize the unique experience of transgender individuals and be alert to the convenience and oversimplification of consolidating all LGBT individuals together.

Learn about the discrimination and prejudice that transgender individuals experience, and advocate for legislation that prohibits it.

Work closely with transgender individuals on developing healthy coping strategies to decrease stress associated with being transgender. Educate clients on self-soothing techniques to replace any present maladaptive coping mechanisms.

Advocate for more specific training for clinicians on transgender issues and therapeutic approaches and interventions.

Connect clients and their families to local support groups.

Develop an awareness of your own cultural values, beliefs, and biases and develop knowledge about the histories, traditions, and values of your clients. Adopt treatment methodologies that reflect the cultural needs of the client.

Written by Jan Wagstaff, MA, MSW

Reviewed by Jessica Therivel, LMSW-IPR, and Chris Bates, MA, MSW

REFERENCES

American Psychiatric Association. (2013). Gender dysphoria. Retrieved November 22, 2014, from http://www.dsm5.org/Documents/Gender percent20Dysphoria percent20Fact percent20Sheet.pdf

Bauer, G., Scheim, A., Pyne, J., Travers, R., & Hammond, R. (2015). Intervenable factors associated with suicide risk in transgender persons: A respondent-driven sampling study in Ontario, Canada. *BMC Public Health, 15*, 525. doi:10.1186/s12889-015-1867-2

Bess, J. A., & Stabb, S. D. (2009). The experiences of transgendered persons in psychotherapy: Voices and recommendations. *Journal of Mental Health Counseling, 31*(3), 264-282.

Biblarz, T. J., & Savci, E. (2010). Lesbian, gay, bisexual, and transgender families. *Journal of Marriage & Family, 72*(3), 480-497. doi:10.1111/j.1741-3737.2010.00714.x

Brill, S., & Pepper, R. (2008). The transgender child: A handbook for families and professionals. San Francisco, CA: Cleis.

British Association of Social Workers. (2012, January). The Code of Ethics for Social Workers: Statement of Principles. Retrieved November 22, 2015, from ttp://cdn.basw.co.uk/upload/basw_112315-7.pdf

Centers for Disease Control and Prevention. (2015). HIV among transgender people. Retrieved November 22, 2015, from http://www.cdc.gov/hiv/group/gender/transgender/

Childs, J. M. (2009). Transsexualism: Some theological and ethical perspectives. *Dialog: A Journal of Theology, 48*(1), 30-41. doi:10.1111/j.1540-6385.2009.00428.x

Collazo, A., Austin, A., & Craig, S. L. (2013). Facilitating transition among transgender clients: Components of effective clinical practice. *Clinical Social Work Journal, 41*(3), 228-237. doi:10.1007/s10615-013-0436-3

Conron, K. J., Scott, G., Stowell, G. S., & Landers, S. J. (2012). Transgender health in Massachusetts: Results from a household probability sample of adults. *American Journal of Public Health, 102*(1), 118-122. doi:10.2105/AJPH.2011.300315

Davis, M., & Wertz, K. (2012). When laws are not enough: A study of the economic health of transgender people and the need for a multidisciplinary approach to economic justice. *Seattle Journal for Social Justice, 8*(2), 3.

Davis, S. A., & Colton, M. S. (2014). Effects of testosterone treatment and chest reconstruction surgery on mental health and sexuality in female-to-male transgender people. *International Journal of*

Sexual Health, 26(2), 113-128. doi:10.1080/19317 611.2013.833152

Dickey, L., Resiner, S., & Juntunen, C. (2015). Non-suicidal self-injury in a large online sample of transgender adults. *Professional Psychology: Research and Practice, 46*(1), 3-11.

Factor, R. J., & Rothblum, E. (2008). Exploring gender identity and community among three groups of transgender individuals in the United States: MTFs, FTMs, and genderqueers. *Health Sociology Review, 17*(3), 235-253. doi:10.5172/hesr.451.17.3.235

Fredriksen-Goldsen, K., Cook-Daniels, L., Kim, H., Erosheva, E., Emlet, C., Hoy-Ellis, C., & Muraco, A. (2013). Physical and mental health of transgender older adults: An at-risk and underserved population. *The Gerontologist, 54*(3), 488-500.

Hines, S. (2009). A pathway to diversity? Human rights, citizenship and the politics of trans-gender. *Contemporary Politics, 15*(1), 87-102. doi:10.1080/13569770802674238

Horvath, K. J., Iantaffi, A., Swinburne-Romine, R., & Bockting, W. (2014). A comparison of mental health, substance use, and sexual risk behaviors between rural and non-rural transgender persons. *Journal of Homosexuality, 61*(8), 1117-1130. doi:10.1 080/00918369.2014.872502

International Federation of Social Workers. (2012). Statement of ethical principles. Retrieved November 22, 2015, from http://ifsw.org/policies/statement-of-ethical-principles/

International Federation of Social Workers. (2012, March 3). Statement of Ethical Principles. Retrieved November 22, 2015, from http://ifsw.org/policies/statement-of-ethical-principles/

Keuroghlian, A., Reisner, S., Weiss, J., & Roger, D. (2015). Substance use and treatment of substance use disorders in a community sample of transgender adults. *Drug and Alcohol Dependence, 152,* 139-146. doi:10.1016/j.drugalcdep.2015.04.008

Koken, J. A., Bimbi, D. S., & Parsons, J. T. (2009). Experiences of familial acceptance-rejection among transwomen of color. *Journal of Family Psychology, 23*(6), 853-860. doi:10.1037/a0017198

Levine, S. B., & Solomon, A. (2009). Meanings and political implications of "psychopathology" in a gender identity clinic: A report of 10 cases. *Journal of Sex & Marital Therapy, 35,* 40-57. doi:10.1080/00926230802525646

Male-to-female transgender youth: Gender expression milestones, gender atypicality, victimization, and parents' responses. (2006). *Journal of GLBT Family Studies, 2*(1), 71-92. doi:10.1300/J461v02n01_04R

Miller, L., & Grollman, E. (2015). The social costs of gender noncomformity for transgender adults: Implications for discrimination and health. *Sociological Forum, 30*(3), 809-831. doi:10.1111/socf.12193

Morgan, S. W., & Stevens, P. E. (2008). Transgender identity development as represented by a group of female-to-male transgendered adults. *Issues in Mental Health Nursing, 29*(6), 585-599. doi:10.1080/01612840802048782

Motmans, J., Meier, P., Ponnet, K., & T'Sjoen, G. (2012). Female and male transgender quality of life: Socioeconomic and medical differences. *Journal of Sexual Medicine, 9*(3), 743-750. doi:10.1111/j.1743-6109.2011.02569.x

National Center for Transgender Equality. (2011). Peer violence and bullying against transgender and gender nonconforming youth: Submission to the United States Commission on Civil Rights. Retrieved November 22, 2015, from http://www.eusccr.com/10. percent20national percent20center percent20for percent20transgender percent20equality.pdf

Newfield, E., Hart, S., Dibble, S., & Kohler, L. (2006). Female-to-male transgender quality of life. *Quality of Life Research, 15*(9), 1447-1457. doi:10.1007/s11136-006-0002-3

Norton, A. T., & Herek, G. M. (2013). Heterosexuals' attitudes toward transgender people: Findings from a national probability sample of U.S. adults. *Sex Roles, 68*(11/12), 738-753. doi:10.1007/s11199-011-0110-6

Nuttbrook, L., Hwahng, S., Bockting, W., Rosenblum, A., Mason, M., Macri, M., & Becker, J. (2010). Psychiatric impact of gender-related abuse across the life course of male-to-female transgender persons. *Journal of Sex Research, 47*(1), 12-23. doi:10.1080/00224490903062258

O'Neil, M. E., McWhirter, E. H., & Cerezo, A. (2008). Transgender identities and gender variance in vocational psychology: Recommendations for practice, social advocacy and research. *Journal of Career Development, 34*(3), 286-308. doi:10.1177/0894845307311251

Perez-Brumer, A., Hatzenbueler, M., Oldenburg, C., & Bockting, W. (0205). Individual and structural level risk factors for suicide attempts among transgender adults. *Behavioral Medicine, 41*(3), 164-171. doi:10.1080/08964289.2015.1028322

Rands, K. E. (2009). Considering transgender people in education: A gender-complex approach. *Journal of Teacher Education, 60*(4), 419-431.

Riley, E. A., Sitharthan, G., Clemson, L., & Diamond, M. (2011). The needs of gender-variant children and their parents: A parent survey. *International Journal of Sexual Health, 23*(3), 181-195.

Shaw, S. Y., Lorway, R. R., Deering, K. N., Avery, L., Mohan, H. L., Bhattacharjee, P.,... Blanchard, J. F. (2012). Factors associated with sexual violence against men who have sex with men and transgendered individuals in Karnataka, India. *PLOS One, 7*(3), e31705. doi:10.1371/journal.pone.0031705

Shires, D., & Jaffee, K. (2015). Factors associated with health care discrimination experiences among a national sample of female-to-male transgender individuals. *Health and Social Work, 40*(2), 134-141. doi:10.1093/hsw/hlv025

Siverskog, A. (2014). "They just don't have a clue": Transgender aging and implications for social work. *Journal of Gerontological Social Work, 57*(2-4), 386-406. doi:10.1080/01634372.2014.895472

Stotzer, R. L. (2014). Law enforcement and criminal justice personnel interactions with transgender people in the United States: A literature review. *Aggression & Violent Behavior, 19*(3), 263-277. doi:10.1016/j.avb.2014.04.012

Transgender Law Center. (2008). The state of transgender California report. Retrieved November 22, 2015, from http://www.scribd.com/fullscreen/95219573?access_key=key-m5tdtfnmqfypcyumpe9

Veldorale-Griffin, A. (2014). Transgender parents and their adult children's experiences of disclosure and transition. *Journal of GLBT Family Studies, 10*(5), 475-501. doi:10.1080/1550 428X.2013.866063

Wheeler, D. (2015). NASW standards and indicators for cultural competence in social work practice. Retrieved from http://www.socialworkers.org/practice/standards/PRA-BRO-253150-CC-Standards.pdf

TRAUMATIC BRAIN INJURY IN MILITARY PERSONNEL & VETERANS: CONCUSSION

MAJOR CATEGORIES: Medical & Health, Military & Veterans

WHAT WE KNOW

A concussion, also known as a mild traumatic brain injury (mTBI), is a structural injury to the brain caused by blunt trauma, acceleration or deceleration forces acting on the brain, penetration by a foreign body, or exposure to a blast. The primary causes of mTBI in a military setting are blasts, fragments, bullets, falls, and motor vehicle accidents. It is now the most common injury suffered by military service members who have served in Iraq or Afghanistan.

A concussion results in one or more of the following:

Temporary confusion, disorientation, or a change in consciousness.

Memory dysfunction immediately after the injury.

Loss of consciousness for less than 30 minutes.

Any observed signs or symptoms of neurological or neuropsychological problems (e.g., headache, dizziness, fatigue, trouble concentrating, irritability).

Concussions are a common injury among military personnel and can have lasting effects for veterans. The U.S. Department of Defense (DOD) reports that in 2014 there were 25,111 concussions sustained by military personnel. A high proportion of military personnel experience repeated concussions.

Researchers in a DOD study found that 20 percent of service members studied had a repeat concussion within 2 weeks of the first concussion and 87 percent had a repeat concussion within 3 months of the first concussion. In comparison, among professional football players who were studied only 4 percent experienced a repeated concussion within 2 weeks and 20 percent had another concussion within 3 months.

Common symptoms of concussions include headache, nausea, balance problems, dizziness, vision problems, light and noise sensitivity, feeling sluggish or fatigued, trouble concentrating, memory problems, changes in sleep patterns, and insomnia.

Research indicates that concussions may cause not only structural changes in the brain as a result of the impact but also metabolic changes. Individuals who experience metabolic imbalance as a result of a concussion may be at risk for second-impact syndrome, in which a subsequent concussion, even if the subsequent concussion presents as a minor injury, may result in death.

Trauma that occurs to the pituitary gland as a result of an mTBI can create ongoing, persistent symptoms that mimic the immediate aftereffects of a TBI.

Some individuals experience post-concussion syndrome (PCS), TBI symptoms that continue for weeks or months instead of resolving in a few days as is typical. PCS may be found in returning military personnel and veterans; frequently it co-occurs with posttraumatic stress disorder (PTSD).

According to one model, PCS is more likely to develop after mTBI among individuals with predisposing factors (e.g., anxiety, depression, negative life experiences, negative attitude) who have limited social support and who have a negative cognitive, behavioral, or emotional state that perpetuates the predisposing factors. When the perpetuating factors interact with pre-existing conditions and a poor social environment, there is a higher risk for PCS.

Individuals who have experienced a concussion are at increased risk for mental health disorders. Social workers working with military or veteran populations should screen clients for mTBIs since they are a contributing factor in mental health problems.

Early identification of concussions in active-duty military personnel is crucial in order to provide appropriate medical care and prevent personnel from returning to duty prematurely. The brain has an increased vulnerability to a second concussion within 10 days of the primary concussion.

There are three opportunities for screening for concussions: during deployment after the injury event, upon return from deployment, or when a veteran enters the VA healthcare system after leaving active-duty status.

The DOD requiers all military personnel involved in a "potentially concussive event" to be medically evaluated if they answer yes to their commander on any of the items on the Injury/Evaluation/Distance (I.E.D.) Checklist. The affected service member is also supposed to complete the Military Acute Concussion Evaluation (MACE).

The MACE is not intended to diagnose a concussion but is a screening tool that can trigger a more thorough evaluation to determine diagnosis.

Service members who have experienced a first concussion are supposed to rest for at least 24 hours and not return to duty during that time. Those who receive a second concussion within 12 months are supposed to wait 7 days after symptoms resolve before returning to duty. If three or more concussions happen within 12 months, the service member is supposed to remain off duty until a recurrent concussion evaluation is completed.

The recurrent concussion evaluation consists of a comprehensive neurological evaluation, neuroimaging, a neurophysical assessment, a functional assessment, and a duty-status determination.

Active-duty personnel who are returning from deployment are supposed to be screened with either a variation of the Brief Traumatic Brain Injury Screen (BTBIS) or the Automated Neuropsychological Assessment Metrics (ANAM). Both of these instruments have been shown to have questionable validity and reliability when used at any time other than shortly after the event however.

The ANAM has been shown to be a successful diagnostic tool for concussions if utilized within 72 hours of an injury.

Veterans who are entering the VA system and who began service after September 11, 2001, are supposed to be screened for TBI with a four-question screening tool; if the result is positive the veteran is referred for a more comprehensive evaluation.

Occupational therapist have recently started to promote a performance-based assessment of concussion-related deficits called the Assessment of Military Multitasking Performance (AMMP)and are gathering data to determine if tht AMMP is a valid and reliable tool. This assessment consists of six individual tasks designed to assess concussion-related deficits.

Participants are given thorough instructions and a written list of the tasks to be performed. They are also required to visit four areas (e.g., a bulletin board, supply closet) to complete certain tasks (e.g., assemble a footstool out of PVC pipe, report the number of empty rooms in service members' living quarters, locate a service member's room using a map).

The goal of this type of assessment is to aid occupational therapists in screening for and characterizing concussion-related deficits in order to construct individualized treatment plans for their military clients.

Underreporting of mTBIs by military personnel is common. The reasons for this may have roots in the military culture.

Service members may minimize symptoms to avoid longer evaluations, to stay with their units, and to facilitate a quicker return to duty or return home.

The emphasis in the military on perseverance, self-sacrifice, and stoicism, and the fact that concussion is an "invisible" injury, may lessen the acceptance of reporting mTBI.

There is no curative course of treatment for concussions,only symptom management. Early detection, evaluation, and management of a concussion and its symptoms are paramount to protect the individual while he or she is vulnerable to further injury or experiencing the negative effects of a concussion. Social workers need to understand the effects of concussion and assess their impact on clients' mental health and quality of life.

Treatment for concussions consists of symptom management, supervised rest, and adequate recovery time. The social worker should educate the client on the need to follow the treatment plan in the acute post-concussion phase. Preventing further injury should be emphasized; a premature return to duty may worsen existing symptoms.

Individuals with persistent symptoms may benefit from pharmacological treatment (e.g., sleep medications, preventive headache medications, medications for dizziness).

WHAT CAN BE DONE

Develop an awareness of your own cultural values, beliefs, and biases and develop knowledge about the histories, traditions, and values of your clients. Adopt treatment methodologies that reflect the cultural needs of the client.

Learn about concussions in military personnel so you can accurately assess your client's personal characteristics and health/mental health education needs; share this information with your colleagues.

Create a safe, therapeutic environment to encourage military personnel and veterans you are working with to disclose any mTBIs in order to receive the proper assistance and reduce risk for further concussions.

Screen for mTBI in any veteran who is receiving substance use or mental health services from you or your agency.

Screen any military service member or veteran with an mTBI for the common co-existing conditions of anxiety, depression, substance use, and sleep disorders.

Utilize the biopsychosocialspiritual assessment to fully analyze and address the symptoms and negative life impact the mTBI potentially is having on the client. Utilize this assessment information to develop a comprehensive treatment plan.

Social workers should prioritize treating the identified problem and symptoms over trying to determine conclusively if the issues stem from a concussion.

Advocate for continued education for providers and military personnel on the risks of early return to duty when an mTBI has occurred.

Advocate for continued research on concussions in the military.

Written by Jessica Therivel, LMSW-IPR

Reviewed by Laura Gale, LCSW

REFERENCES

Buck, P. W. (2011). Mild traumatic brain injury: A silent epidemic in our practices. *Health and Social Work, 36*(4), 299-302. doi:10.1093/hsw/36.4.299

Coldren, R. L., Kelly, M. P., Parish, R. V., Dretsch, M., & Russell, M. L. (2010). Evaluation of the Military Acute Concussion Evaluation for use in combat operations more than 12 hours after injury. *Military Medicine, 175*(7), 477-481.

Coldren, R. L., Russell, M. L., Parish, R. V., Dretsch, M., & Kelly, M. P. (2012). The ANAM lacks utility as a diagnostic or screening tool for concussion more than 10 days following injury. *Military Medicine, 177*(2), 179-183. doi:10.7205/MILMED-D-11-00278

DOD numbers for traumatic brain injury: Worldwide totals. (2014). *Defense and Veterans Brain Injury Center.* Retrieved October 19, 2015, from http://dvbic.dcoe.mil/sites/default/files/Worldwide-Totals-2014.pdf

D. of D. (2012). DOD policy guidance for management of mild traumatic brain injury/concussion in the deployed setting. Report no. 6490.11. Washington, DC: Author.

Department of Veterans Affairs, Department of Defense. (2009). VA/DOD clinical practice guideline for management of concussion/mild traumatic brain injury (mTBI). Washington, DC: Author.

Hou, R., Moss-Morris, R., Peveler, R., Mogg, K., Bradley, B. P., & Belli, A. (2012). When a minor head injury results in enduring symptoms: A prospective investigation of risk for post-concussional syndrome after mild traumatic brain injury. *Journal of Neurology, Neurosurgery, and Psychiatry, 83*(2), 217-223. doi:10.1136/jnnp-2011-300767

International Federation of Social Workers. (2012, March 3). Statement of Ethical Principles. Retrieved December 2, 2013, from http://ifsw.org/policies/statement-of-ethical-principles/

Kelly, M. P., Coldren, R. L., Parish, R. V., Dretsch, M. N., & Russell, M. L. (2012). Assessment of acute concussion in the combat environment. *Archives of Clinical Neuropsychology, 27*(4), 375-388. doi:10.1093/arclin/acs036

Lovell, M., Collins, M., Pardini, J. E., Parodi, A., & Yates, A. (2005). Management of cerebral concussion in military personnel: lessons learned from sports medicine. *Operative Techniques in Sports Medicine, 13*(4), 212-221.

MacGregor, A. J., Dougherty, A. L., Morrison, R. H., Quinn, K. H., & Galarneau, M. R. (2011). Repeated concussion among U.S. military personnel during Operation Iraqi Freedom. *Journal of Rehabilitation Research and Development, 48*(10), 1269-1277. doi:10.1682/JRRD.2011.01.0013

Marshall, K. R., Holland, S. L., Meyer, K. S., Martin, E. M., Wilmore, M., & Grimes, J. B. (2012). Mild traumatic brain injury screening: Diagnosis and treatment. *Military Medicine, 177*(8 Suppl), 67-75.

Mizrahi, T., & Mayden, R. W. (2001). NASW Standards for Cultural Competency in Social Work Practice. Retrieved December 2, 2013, from http://www.socialworkers.org/practice/standards/NASWCulturalStandards.pdf

Moore, M. (2013). Mild traumatic brain injury: Implications for social work research and practice with civilian and military populations. *Social Work in Health Care, 52*(5), 498-518. doi:10.1080/00981389.2012.714447

Pogoda, T., Iverson, K., Meterko, M., Baker, E., Hendricks, A., Stolzmann, K.,... Lew, H. (2014). Concordance of clinician judgement of mild traumatic brain injury history with a diagnostic standard. *Journal of Rehabilitation Research & Development, 51*(3), 363-375. doi:10.1682/JRRD.2013.05.0115

Sayer, N. A., Nelson, D., & Nugent, S. (2011). Evaluation of the Veterans Health Administration traumatic brain injury screening program in the upper Midwest. *Journal of Head Trauma Rehabilitation, 26*(6), 454-467. doi:10.1097/HTR.0b013e3181ff393c

Smith, L., Radomski, M., Davidson, L., Finkelstein, M., Weightman, M., McCulloch, K., & Scherer, M. (2014). Development and preliminary reliability of a multitasking assessment for executive functioning after concussion. *American Journal of Occupational Therapy, 68*(4), 439-443.

Terrio, H. P., Nelson, L. A., Betthauser, L. M., Harwood, J. E., & Brenner, L. A. (2011). Post deployment traumatic brain injury screening questions: Sensitivity, specificity, and predictive values in returning soldiers. *Rehabilitation Psychology, 56*(1), 26-31. doi:10.1037/a0022685

The Policy, Ethics, and Human Rights Committee, British Association of Social Workers. (2012, January). The Code of Ethics for Social Work: Statement of Principles. Retrieved December 2, 2013, from http://cdn.basw.co.uk/upload/basw_112315-7.pdf

Tsai, J., Whealin, J. M., Scott, J. C., Harpaz-Rotem, I., & Piertzak, R. H. (2012). Examining the relation between combat-related concussion, a novel 5-factor model of posttraumatic stress symptoms, and health-related quality of life in Iraq and Afghanistan veterans. *The Journal of Clinical Psychiatry, 73*(8), 1110-1118. doi:10.4088/JCP.11m07587

Walker, R. L., Clark, M. E., & Sanders, S. H. (2010). The "post deployment multi-symptom disorder": An emerging syndrome in need of a new treatment paradigm. *Psychological Services, 7*(3), 136-147.

Williams, K. (2013). After concussion: treatment considerations in the U.S. service member, *4*(1), 14-18.

TUBERCULOSIS: HIGH-RISK GROUPS IN THE UNITED STATES

MAJOR CATEGORIES: Medical & Health

WHAT WE KNOW

Tuberculosis (TB) is a disease caused by a particular bacterium that most commonly attacks the lungs. It is the leading cause of death from an infectious disease. Worldwide, in 2014 an estimated 9.6 million persons developed TB and 1.5 million died from it. Approximately one-third of the world's population has TB. Of the 9.6 million new cases of TB in 2014, 58 percent were in the Southeast Asia and Western Pacific regions. TB is caused most often by the bacterium *Mycobacterium tuberculosis*, although it can be caused by other *Mycobacterium* species of bacteria. TB usually is acquired through close contact with or prolonged exposure to a person with active TB.

Smoking increases the risk of developing TB. Globally, approximately 20 percent of TB cases can be attributed to smoking. Once acquired, TB may become active, remain dormant, or reactivate. TB in a dormant state is called latent TB infection (LTBI). HIV infection is the strongest risk factor for the reactivation of TB from LTBI state. Individuals infected with HIV are 20 to 30 times more likely to develop TB. Treatment of LTBI can prevent the disease from reactivating and is recommended for those who are at risk of contracting TB or for persons who have LTBI (e.g., individuals in refugee camps, those who live with someone who has active TB).

In the United States, TB disproportionately affects immigrants, non-whites, homeless individuals, residents of correctional facilities, healthcare workers, individuals infected with HIV, and individuals who inject illegal drugs. The risk for TB among these groups is increased by poverty, unsanitary living conditions, malnutrition, lack of access to healthcare, mental health disorders, substance abuse, diabetes mellitus, overcrowded living conditions, and the greater numbers of inmates with HIV in correctional facilities.

TB is classified as an occupational disease in the United States, meaning that it is considered a risk for individuals who work in the healthcare field. In 2014 there were 9,421 new cases of TB reported in the United States, a rate of 2.96 cases per 100,000 persons. This is a 2.2 percent decrease of cases from 2013, when the rate was 3.02 cases of TB per 100,000 persons.

In 2014, the incidence of TB among foreign-born individuals living in the United States was 13.4 times higher than that among U. S.-born persons, even though the number and rate of cases among foreign-born persons have decreased annually since a resurgence in 1992. The number of TB cases among persons born in the United States also has decreased annually since 1992.

The majority of foreign-born individuals who come to the United States as immigrants, refugees, and on student visas currently are not screened for TB, increasing the risk of the disease progressing to symptomatic, active TB and increasing the likelihood of transmission of the disease while in the United States. In 2014 the Centers for Disease Control and Prevention reported the TB rates per 100,000 for different races and ethnicities in the United States as 4.3 for American Indians, Alaska Natives, Native Hawaiians, and Pacific Islanders; 17.9 for Asians; 5.1 for blacks; 5.0 for Hispanics; and 0.6 for whites.

The countries of origin most associated with foreign-born carriers of TB in the United States are Mexico, the Philippines, Vietnam, India, and China. Cases of active TB among foreign-born persons are most often due to reactivation of LTBI. It is unclear whether this is due to an increased risk for TB to progress from LTBI to active disease in foreign-born persons or if the reactivation of LTBI is due to an increased prevalence of LTBI among foreign-born persons. Current U.S. guidelines recommend tuberculin testing for and treatment of LTBI for foreign-born individuals who entered the United States within the previous 5 years.

Adherence to treatment of TB often is poor and not completed. The lack of adherence to necessary treatment and prescribed medication regimen may be related to several factors including poverty, mental health disorders, substance abuse, difficulty accessing healthcare, and cultural beliefs. Even with adherence, in 2014 approximately 1.0 percent of reported cases of TB exhibited signs of multidrug resistance. This percentage has remained essentially stable for the last 10 years.

The failure to complete the treatment regimen fosters the development of drug-resistant TB. Drug resistance is passed along the entire strain of bacteria which causes TB. Drug-resistant TB can be spread from person to person and requires treatment with second-line TB agents. Second-line drugs often are less effective than first-line drugs and are more likely to have adverse side effects. Mortality from drug-resistant TB is a serious risk in the United States.

Directly observed therapy (DOT; i.e., clinical supervision to ensure that the client follows the prescribed medication regimen) is a strategy proven to improve an individual's adherence to treatment. DOT increases the rate of completion of the treatment regimen and decreases disease transmission and drug resistance.

WHAT CAN BE DONE

Social workers, mental health professionals, and medical professionals can learn about TB in high-risk groups and assess high risk clients' personal, social, and medical needs including support, treatment, and resources. Assessments should include the identification of individual risk factors and screenings for at-risk individuals. If necessary, professionals should use an interpreter to ensure effective communication of needs. Social workers can advocate for required routine screening for TB for immigrants, refugees, and temporary visa holders (e.g., students). Social workers and helping professionals can become familiar with the community they work and serve in to recognize specific cultural needs and risk factors for TB.

All professionals working with clients who may have TB should follow facility protocols for infection control/airborne precautions and mandatory reporting of infectious disease so the public health department can initiate a contact investigation and screen other contacts of the client.

Culturally sensitive written material should be provided to clients and their family members, if available, that includes information on prevention, signs/symptoms, treatment, and when to seek medical attention.

Social workers and healthcare professionals should be sensitive to the literacy levels of clients and their families and adapt education materials and verbal information to best meet individualized client ability. The healthcare professional and social worker should encourage and stress importance of strict adherence to the prescribed medication regimen and maintaining scheduled follow-up care. The social worker or healthcare professional may encourage and recommend DOT as part of the adherence plan.

The social worker should help identify the client's barriers to adherence to the treatment regimen. The social worker may collaborate with community representatives to increase availability of clinics and treatment resources for high-risk clients to improve adherence to the treatment regimen. Social workers may assist clients in obtaining their medications for their treatment regimens if they will otherwise be noncompliant because of access issues or cost issues.

Social workers can collaborate with community members and healthcare providers in the development of community outreach screening programs that focus on TB screening in homeless shelters, correctional facilities, and substance abuse treatment programs. As appropriate, social workers may request referrals for at-risk persons, including referrals to subsidized mental health/counseling agencies, food banks, homeless shelters, 12-step programs, and financial assistance programs.

More information on tuberculosis may be obtained from the following resources:

- Daily Strength, http://www.dailystrength.org/c/Tuberculosis-TB/support-group
- Tuberculosis Patients Support, http://tbpatientssupportgroup.blogspot.com/
- The American Lung Association, http://www.lung.org/

Written by Suzanne Pinto, MSW, and
Jennifer Kornusky, RN, MS

Reviewed by Jessica Therivel, LMSW-IPR

REFERENCES

British Association of Social Workers. (2012). The code of ethics for social work: Statement of principles. Retrieved June 9, 2016, from http://cdn.basw.co.uk/upload/basw_112315-7.pdf

Cain, K. P., Haley, C. A., Armstrong, L. R., Garman, K. N., Wells, C. D., Iademarco, M. F., & Laserson, K. F. (2007). Tuberculosis among foreign-born persons in the United States: Achieving tuberculosis elimination. *American Journal of Respiratory and Critical Care Medicine, 175*(1), 75-79. doi:10.1164/rccm.200608-11780C

Centers for Disease Control and Prevention. (2016). Leveling of tuberculosis incidence – United States, 2013-2015. *Morbidity and Mortality Weekly Report, 65*(11), 273-278.

Centers for Disease Control and Prevention (CDC). (2014). Executive commentary highlights of 2014 report. Retrieved September 9, 2016, from https://www.cdc.gov/tb/statistics/reports/2014/pdfs/2014-surveillance-report_summary.pdf

Centers for Disease Control and Prevention (CDC). (2015). Morbidity and Mortality Weekly Report: Tuberculosis trends- United States, 2014. Retrieved June 9, 2016, from http://www.cdc.gov/mmwr/preview/mmwrhtml/mm6410a2.htm#Tab

Chai, S. J., Mattingly, D. C., & Varma, J. K. (2013). Protecting health care workers from tuberculosis in China: A review of policy and practice in China and the United States. *Health Policy and Planning, 28*(1), 100-109. doi:10.1093/heapol/czs029

Collins, J. M., Reves, R. R., & Belknap, R. W.`. (2016). High rates of tuberculosis and opportunities for prevention among international students in the United States. *Annals of the American Thoracic Society, 13*(4), 522-528. doi:10.1513/AnnalsATS.201508-547OC

International Federation of Social Workers. (2012, March 3). Statement of Ethical Principles. Retrieved June 23, 2016, from http://ifsw.org/policies/statement-of-ethical-principles

Kim, S., & Crittenden, K. (2007). Treatment completion among TB patients returned to the community from a large urban jail. *Journal of Community Health, 32*(2), 135-147. doi:10.1007/s10900-006-9036-2

Lashley, M. (2007). A targeted testing program for tuberculosis control and prevention among Baltimore City's homeless population. *Public Health Nursing, 24*(1), 34-39. doi:10.1111/j.1525-1446.2006.00605.x

National Association of Social Workers. (2008). Code of ethics. Retrieved June 9, 2016, from https://www.socialworkers.org/pubs/code/code.asp

National Association of Social Workers. (2015). Standards and indicators for cultural competence in social work practice. Retrieved June 9, 2016, from http://www.socialworkers.org/practice/standards/PRA-BRO-253150-CC-Standards.pdf

Patel, S., Parsyan, A. E., Gunn, J., Barry, M. A., Reed, C., Sharnprapai, S., & Horsburgh, C. R. (2007). Risk of progression to active tuberculosis among foreign-born persons with latent tuberculosis. *Chest, 131*(6), 1811-1816.

Price, P. (2015). Public health control measures in response to global pandemics and drug resistance. *Journal of Law, Medicine, & Ethics, 43*(S2), 49-56. doi:10.1111/jlme.12266

Restrepo, B. I., Fisher-Hoch, S. P., Crespo, J. G., Whitney, E., Perez, A., Smith, B., & McCormick, J. B. (2007). Type 2 diabetes and tuberculosis in a dynamic bi-national border population. *Epidemiology and Infection, 135*(3), 483-491. doi:10.1017/S0950268806006935

World Health Organization. (2016). Tuberculosis: Fact sheet 104. Retrieved June 9, 2016, from http://www.who.int/mediacentre/factsheets/fs104/en/

Yew, W. W., & Leung, C. C. (2008). Update in tuberculosis 2007. *American Journal of Respiratory and Critical Care Medicine, 177*(5), 479-485. doi:10.1164/rccm.200710-1561UP

U

ULCERATIVE COLITIS: HEALTHCARE COSTS

MAJOR CATEGORIES: Medical & Health

WHAT WE KNOW

Ulcerative colitis (UC) is a long lasting, inflammatory bowel disease.

UC is responsible for major healthcare costs in North America. Healthcare costs for UC can be high as a result of high death rates and decreased quality of life. Annual direct costs that can be credited to UC are approximately $2.7 billion.

In 2008, the average annual total costs for individuals with UC were $7,948. Hospitalization accounted for 37.6 percent of the costs, outpatient services for 34.9 percent, and pharmaceutical costs for 27.5 percent

Costs are higher for pediatrics (i.e. infant, children and adolescents).

Researchers from a 2014 study found that total yearly medical costs per individual ranged from $9,663 to $12,679 depending on the therapies that were provided.

Surgery is required in up to 35 percent of individual cases of UC. Individuals who have laparoscopic surgery typically have lower rates of postsurgical death and shorter recovery times, which result in lower costs. Restorative proctocolectomy (RP) surgery is common and places individuals at high risk for postoperative readmission and increased medical costs.

Treatment goals for UC are individualized according to disease location, activity, and severity. Medical treatment of UC commonly includes aminosalicylates (i.e., anti-inflammatory medications for the gut), glucocorticoids (i.e., specific steroid hormones), tumor necrosis factor (TNF) inhibitors, immunomodulators, antibiotics, and antidiarrheal drugs.

First-line treatment often includes a 5-aminosalicylic acid (5-ASA) preparation, given rectally or orally. Costs for an 8-week supply of 5-ASA vary by formulation, as follows:

- Balsalazide (Colazal), 2.25 g given 3 times daily: $504
- Mesalamine (Asacol), 800–1,600 mg given 3 times daily: $273–$545

- Mesalamine (Pentasa), 1 g given 4 times daily: $445
- Mesalamine is also called mesalazine
- Olsalazine (Dipentum), 500 mg given 4 times daily: $436
- Olsalazine has not been approved for use by the U.S. Food and Drug Administration (FDA)
- Sulfasalazine (generic, generic delayed release, Azulfidine, Azulfidine Entabs), 500 mg pills given as 1 g twice daily: $28, $43, $65, $78, respectively

TNF inhibitors (e.g., infliximab, adalimumab) may be used in individuals with moderate to severe UC that is unresponsive to regular therapies.

Annual drug costs for TNF inhibitors in Canada range from CA$23,000 to CA$38,000.

Compared with individuals whose UC symptoms are managed with treatment, those with uncontrolled UC are more likely to require hospitalization and surgery and to have higher healthcare costs.

During 2001–2005, the total annual healthcare costs for individuals in the United States with severe UC were $26,875, whereas total annual healthcare costs for individuals with mild or moderate UC were $12,154.

Researches in the UK found that relapse frequency is related to the direct medical cost of individuals with UC. Persons with 2 or more relapses had higher annual UC-related medical costs: £6,660 compared to £1,168 for clients without a relapse.

Treatment failure of medications for UC increases the risk of hospitalization and surgery and results in higher healthcare costs. The estimated cost of treatment failure of 5-ASA over a period of 150 days is $36,173 per person, with an additional cost of $18,231 experienced for a colectomy (i.e., resection of the large intestine). Treatment failure is more likely in individuals who do not follow their prescribed medication regimen of 5-ASA.

Total healthcare costs are 12.5 percent higher for individuals who do not follow prescribed treatment plans compared to individual who do follow them. Lower medical costs are linked with individuals who are compliant with their medication despite the increased cost for the medication.

Treatment failure rates can be reduced by improving individual obedience and by clinician selection of the most effective drug.

Treatment with balsalazide (a prodrug that is cleaved in the colon to produce 5-ASA) capsules results in a 16 percent reduction in total healthcare costs compared to treatment with oral mesalamine (a formulation of 5-ASA).

WHAT YOU CAN DO

Learn about the healthcare costs connected with UC so that you can expand your resources.

If working with a social worker they will educate you about UC as a disease, its management, and connected costs.

They will also encourage you to follow the prescribed treatment program recommended by your primary care physician.

If appropriate, they will encourage you to discuss and identify reasons for not following through with the treatment plan, which may include forgetfulness, not feeling that you need treatment, lack of information or emotional support, and not being able to afford medications.

If you are lacking emotional support, your social worker can provide counseling and support to assist you in following through with your treatment plan.

If you are unable to pay for medications, your social can assist to enroll you (if eligible) in a prescription assistance program such as Partnership for Prescription Assistance:https://www.pparx.org/en

Lastly, the can provide written guides or information sheets regarding your condition, including online supports—http://www.ccfa.org/living-with-crohns-colitis/find-a-support-group/, http://www.crohnsforum.com/, http://www.crohnsandcolitis.org.uk/—and the GI Buddy app,an interactive disease management tool for iPhone and Android devices that allows a client to track all aspects of his or her disease (i.e., symptoms, treatment, and diet).

Written by Sharon Richman, MSPT, and Tanja Schub, BS

Reviewed by Jessica Therivel, LMSW-IPR

REFERENCES

Brereton, N., Bodger, K., Kamm, M. A., Hodgkins, P., Yan, S., & Akehurst, R. (2010). A cost-effectiveness analysis of MMX mesalazine compared with mesalazine in the treatment of mild-to-moderate ulcerative colitis from a UK perspective. *Journal of Medical Economics, 13*(1), 148-161. doi:10.3111/13696990903562861

British Association of Social Workers. (2012, January). The code of ethics for social work: Statement of principles. Retrieved March 15, 2016, from http://cdn.basw.co.uk/upload/basw_112315-7.pdf

Buskens, C. J., Sahami, S., Tanis, P. J., & Bemelman, W. A. (2014). The potential benefits and disadvantages of laparoscopic surgery for ulcerative colitis: A review of current evidence. *Best Practice & Research in Clinical Gastroenterology, 28*(1), 19-27. doi:10.1016/j.bpg.2013.11.007

Gibson, T. B., Ng, E., Ozminkowski, R. J., Wang, S., Burton, W. N., Goetzel, R. Z., & McClean, R. (2008). The direct and indirect cost burden of Crohn's disease and ulcerative colitis. *Journal of Occupational and Environmental Medicine, 50*(11), 1261-1272. doi:10.1097/JOM.0b013e318181b8ca

Higgins, P. D., Rubin, D. T., Kaulback, K., Schoenfield, P. S., & Kane, S. V. (2009). Systematic review: Impact of non-adherence to 5-aminosalicylic acid products on the frequency and cost of ulcerative colitis flares. *Alimentary Pharmacology and Therapeutics, 29*(3), 247-257. doi:10.1111/j.1365-2036.2008.03865.x

Hillson, E., Dybicz, S., Waters, H. C., Stuart, B., Schaneman, J., Dabbous, O., ... Broussard, D. (2008). Health care expenditures in ulcerative colitis: The perspective of a self-insured employer. *Journal of Occupational and Environmental Medicine, 50*(8), 969-977. doi:10.1097/JOM.0b013e31816fd663.

International Federation of Social Workers. (2012). Statement of ethical principles. Retrieved March 15, 2016, from http://ifsw.org/policies/statement-of-ethical-principles/

Kane, S. V. (2006). Systematic review: Adherence issues in the treatment of ulcerative colitis. *Alimentary Pharmacology and Therapeutics, 23*(5), 577-585. doi:10.1111/j.1365-2036.2006.02809.x

Kappelman, M. D., Rifas-Shiman, S. L., Porter, C., Ollendorf, D., Sandler, R. S., Galanko, J. A., & Finkelstein, J. A. (2008). Direct health care costs of Crohn's disease and ulcerative colitis in US children and adults. *Gastroenterology, 135*(6), 1907-1913. doi:10.1053/j.gastro.2008.09.012

Mackowiak, J. I. (2006). A two-stage decision analysis to assess the cost of 5-aminosalicylic acid failure and the economics of balsalazide versus mesalamine in the treatment of ulcerative colitis. *Managed Care Interface, 19*(10), 39-46, 56.

Mitra, D. (2012). Nonadherence to 5-ASAs for ulcerative colitis occurred often, raised health care costs. *BMC Gastroenterology, 12,* 132. doi:10.1186/1471-230X-12-132

Wheeler, D. (2015). NASW Standards and Indicators for Cultural Competence in Social Work Practice. Retrieved March 15, 2016, from http://www.socialworkers.org/practice/standards/PRA-BRO-253150-CC-Standards.pdf

Rubin, D. T., Mody, R., David, K. L., & Wang, C. C. (2014). Real-world assessment of therapy changes, suboptimal treatment and associated costs in patients with ulcerative colitis or Crohn's disease. *Alimentary Pharmacology & Therapeutics, 39*(10), 1143-1155. doi:10.1111/apt.12727

Tindall, W. N., Boltri, J. M., & Wilhelm, S. M. (2007). Mild-to-moderate ulcerative colitis: Your role in patient compliance and health care costs. *Journal of Managed Care Pharmacy, 13*(7 Suppl. A), S2-S12.

Xie, F., Blackhouse, G., Assasi, N., Gaebel, K., Robertson, D., & Goeree, R. (2009). Cost-utility analysis of infliximab and adalimumab for refractory ulcerative colitis. *Cost Effectiveness and Resource Allocation, 7,* 20. doi:10.1186/1478-7547-7-20

Hanzlik, T. P., Tevis, S. E., Suwanabol, P. A., Carchman, E. H., Harms, B. A., Heise, C. P., & Kennedy, G. D. (2015). Characterizing readmission in ulcerative colitis patients undergoing restorative proctocolectomy. *Journal of Gastrointestinal Surgery, 19*(3), 564-569. doi:10.1007/s11605-014-2734-7

Gray, L. (2015). Implications and benefits of the NICE appraisal for ulcerative colitis. *British Journal of Healthcare Management, 21*(8), 356-357. doi:10.12968/bjhc.2015.21.8.356

Kidhu, P. S., Karwa, R., Kenneth, V., Oxley, D., & Agrawal, A. (2014). Which 5-ASA? Understanding the choices in ulcerative colitis therapy. *Gastrointestinal Nursing, 12*(5), 17-26. doi:10.12968/gasn.2014.12.5.17

Bodger, K., Yen, L., Szende, A., Sharma, G., Chen, Y. J., McDermott, J., & Hodgkins, P. (2014). Medical resource utilization and costs in patients with ulcerative colitis in the UK: A chart review analysis. *European Journal of Gastroenterology & Hepatology, 26*(2), 213-221.

UNEMPLOYMENT & ECONOMIC HARDSHIP: PSYCHOSOCIAL ISSUES

MAJOR CATEGORIES: Community, Behavioral & Mental Health

WHAT WE KNOW

Although the economy has recovered to some extent, unemployment remains a major problem in the United States. In the years 2007–2009, 10 million jobs disappeared from the U.S. economy and the gross domestic product (GDP) fell by more than 5 percent, the largest decline since World War II.

In November 2015 the U.S. Labor Department reported the unemployment rate to be 5.0 percent (BLS CPS).

Long-term unemployment is defined as unemployment for 27 weeks or more.

Discouraged workers are individuals who have stopped looking for work because they feel that there are no jobs available for them.

Individuals who have greater financial, social, and personal resources experience less of a negative effect from job loss compared to individuals with fewer financial resources, less social support, and/or preexisting mental health challenges.

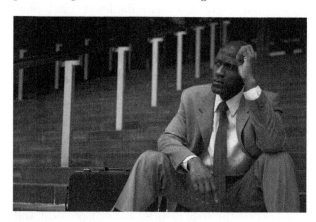

Among adult men in the United States, 5.2 percent are unemployed, whereas 4.9 percent of adult women are.

For the major worker groups, in November 2015 the highest rate of unemployment was found to be 15.7 percent for teenagers, 9.4 percent for Blacks, and 6.4 percent for Hispanics.

In 2010, researchers found that young workers (ages 16–24) were more likely than prime-age workers (ages 25–54) to be unemployed.

In November 2015, men who were ages 24 and younger had unemployment rates that were in double digits, with 19 percent of 16- to 17-year-olds unemployed and 11.3 percent of 20- to 24-year-olds. Among women, adolescents also had high rates of unemployment, ranging from 7.9 percent to 15.1 percent depending on the age breakdown for women ages 24 or younger.

Poverty and lower socioeconomic status are risk factors for unemployment. There are fewer job opportunities in poorer areas of the country, and poor individuals are more likely to work in fields that are the most vulnerable to recession (e.g., wholesale and retail trade, hospitality). Urban areas are not necessarily the most impoverished: Rural communities often have higher rates of unemployment and joblessness.

Persons of lower socioeconomic status have fewer employment opportunities and face more competition for jobs. Lower-wage workers who lose their jobs are at a higher risk of having their utilities shut off or losing their homes than higher-wage employees. The fragile financial equilibrium of many low-wage workers can easily be upset by a job loss.

Education is a protective factor against unemployment. College graduates have the lowest unemployment rate whereas individuals without high school diplomas have the highest.

The Bureau of Labor Statistics published 2014 unemployment data based on education attainment. Individuals who were 25 years old or older without a high school diplomas had an unemployment rate of 9 percent; high school graduates who were age 25 or older saw their unemployment rate decrease to 6 percent, and the unemployment rate for college graduates who were 25 or older decreased even further, to 3.5 percent

Unemployment may result in acute negative consequences in the areas of social, familial, physical, and psychological functioning. Work is a source of social support and interaction for many people. With job loss this support can disappear, leaving individuals socially isolated. Strong social supports can serve as a protective factor against the negative consequences of job loss.

Economic pressure has been shown to produce emotional distress, which in turn has an effect on marital and familial quality, with marital problems frequently resulting. Family stress as a result of economic pressure can trickle down to children. Relationship problems can create disruptions in parenting and normal family routines. As a result the children in a family affected by unemployment can experience decreases in competent functioning (e.g., school achievement, social skills), internalize symptoms (e.g., anxiety, reduced "meaning of life, " depression), and externalize behaviors (e.g., aggression, social isolation, antisocial behaviors, acting-out behaviors).

Parents who are experiencing stress may inadvertently change their parenting style and become more punitive or arbitrary in their punishments.

Physical functioning can be negatively affected by unemployment for two main reasons.

Unemployment often results in loss of health insurance. Because they lack access to preventive care, unemployed individuals may ignore health problems until they experience a crisis. They may be unable to afford medications that are taken to control chronic conditions.

Job loss and financial strain have been shown to be primary causes of stress. This stress may exacerbate any existing health problems. Poor health then may make it more difficult for the unemployed individual to find work.

The burden of a home mortgage can cause additional financial stress and a decline in health status.

Poor psychological functioning as a result of unemployment is very common. This may include symptoms of depression, anxiety, hopelessness, helplessness, and sleep disturbances. The loss of daily structure can result in decreased feelings of competence.

Researchers have found that unemployment has a more marked effect on the mental health of men than on that of women. It is proposed that this is due to traditional expectations that men are more responsible for the family's financial well-being, as a result of which their self-esteem is derived primarily from work.

Unemployment is a risk factor for suicide because of the increase in mental health symptoms that often result from job loss.

Unemployment benefits (i.e., money and medical insurance) may help mitigate the negative mental health effects of a job loss and reduce the incidence of suicide.

Internal resilience is a protective factor that can mitigate the negative psychological effects of job loss.

There are five primary models utilized in studying the effect of unemployment on the individual and in structuring counseling interventions for clients who are unemployed:

Economic deprivation models follow a classic sociology principle that when people have less money, they will have poorer quality food, housing, clothing, etc., and in turn poorer physical and mental health.

Control models employ the assumption that an individual who feels more in control of his or her environment will have a less negative response to unemployment, will approach the job search with a more positive attitude, and will be less likely to blame external forces for the unemployment.

Stress models are conceptualized around coping mechanisms as a means to mitigate negative physical and psychological consequences of stress.

Social support models are closely related to stress models and have two main subsets:

The direct effect version looks at the disappearance of a social network as having immediate consequences for physical and mental health.

The buffer version looks to social support as a defense against stress.

Latent functions models theorize that work provides latent functions (e.g., a time structure for the day, opportunities for social contact, status and identity). Losing these latent functions because of job loss adversely affects physical and mental health.

Kübler-Ross's stages of grieving have been adapted by a researcher, Gary Blau, to stage the experience of job loss. The stages are not always experienced in a linear fashion but are more of an overall framework. The stages are:

- *denial* following the shock of the job loss (e.g., still getting up and taking the train into the city, not telling anyone what has happened);

- *anger* resulting from feeling betrayed by the employer (This is also called *psychological contract violation*: the individual who loses his or her job, especially in a layoff, feels as if the employer has reneged on or violated an agreement. The higher the degree of contract violation the individual feels, the more difficult it may be for him or her to move through the stages.);
- *bargaining* with the employer to try to reverse the termination;
- *depression*, including sadness and withdrawal;
- *exploration*, as a willingness to begin to explore options; and
- *acceptance* or being at peace with what has happened.

Individuals who have lost their jobs may employ positive or negative coping strategies.

Positive coping mechanisms have a problem-solving focus. They include:
- trying to find work or start a business;
- pursuing further education or training to expand available options;
- networking with other unemployed individuals;
- scheduling or arranging daily life so it has structure and feels like a workday;
- reaching out to people who might be able to help in locating a new job; and
- maintaining a positive core self-evaluation (CSE).

CSE is a stable personality trait that consists of self-esteem, self-efficacy, neuroticism, and locus of control. Core self-evaluations (CSE) represent a stable personality trait which encompasses an individual's subconscious, fundamental evaluations about themselves, their own abilities and their own control. People who have high core self-evaluations will think positively of themselves and be confident in their own abilities. Conversely, people with low core self-evaluations will have a negative appraisal of themselves and will lack confidence.

Positive self-efficacy can result in more intrinsic motivation, higher self-esteem, and better performance and results. Promoting this follows the social work tradition of employing a strengths perspective.

A negative coping mechanism focus is called *avoidant coping*. This includes the following:
- avoiding thinking about possible work options;
- avoiding being seen by neighbors or friends to hide unemployment status;

- keeping worries to oneself, not sharing with loved ones;
- blaming oneself; and
- having a poor CSE.

Interventions with unemployed clients may take place at the individual level or in a group setting. These interventions should include a focus on empowerment: helping clients recognize power dynamics in their lives, develop skills that allow them to regain a feeling of control, and utilize that control without interfering with the rights of others. To accomplish this, scaffolding (i.e., using multiple levels of intervention such as counseling, group work, case management, social support, and advocacy) is usually recommended.

Cognitive behavioral therapy(CBT) is the most common treatment type when working with unemployed clients. Clients who have lost their jobs frequently experience negative cognitions and anger, which results in negative behaviors. CBT focuses on eliminating ruminating on the negative, accepting what can be changed and what cannot be changed, and finding acceptable behaviors that can come from changing cognitions.

Group work can provide a source of social support and opportunities to observe other participants or group leaders modeling job search skills. Participants in groups are able to explore the emotional effects of job loss while building skills.

Encouraging mindfulness is an intervention strategy that can be used with individuals or groups to reduce stress and anxiety. Mindfulness is intentional consciousness or awareness: being attentive and present in the moment rather than focusing on the future or the past. This includes meditation along with mindfulness exercises. Social workers can teach mindfulness techniques to clients who are stuck in anxious thought patterns related to their unemployment.

Awareness has three components: stopping, observing, and returning:

Stopping is teaching clients to interrupt automatic thoughts and also to slow down.

Observing refers to focusing on sensations, feelings, thoughts, and sensory experiences.

Returning refers to returning intentional consciousness to the activity in the present moment.

WHAT CAN BE DONE

Become knowledgeable about the effects of unemployment and economic hardship and strategies to counter these negative effects so you can accurately assess your clients' personal characteristics and physical and mental health education needs; share this information with your colleagues.

Develop an awareness of your own cultural values, beliefs, and biases and develop knowledge about the histories, traditions, and values of your clients. Adopt treatment methodologies that reflect the cultural needs of your clients.

Educate yourself on job search resources to share with your clients and colleagues.

Assist when comfortable with résumé advising and/or refer clients to career websites or community resources for résumé assistance.

Provide appropriate interventions to reduce stress, anxiety, and/or any physical symptoms the client is experiencing as a result of unemployment or financial stress.

Provide linkage to community services, such as referrals for medical, financial, childcare, housing, counseling, and educational services as appropriate.

Provide clients with a list of online resources. Examples include the following:
- Simply Hired aggregates job listings from all over the Web, http://www.simplyhired.com/.
- Intuit Quicken Online assists in creating a budget, http://quicken.intuit.com/personal-finance-software/mint-online-money-management.jsp.
- Desperate Dollars is filled with ideas for making money (e.g., volunteering for paid clinical tests, donating blood), http://desperatedollars.com/
- Meetup provides a platform for like-minded individuals to meet and exchange information about job opportunities that are not posted, job fairs, and other events, http://www.meetup.com/
- Wise Bread provide blogs about personal finance, careers, ways to reduce daily expenditures, daily Web deals, green living, and frugal buying, http://www.wisebread.com/

Advocate for state and federal funding of job training and reemployment programs that will address the psychological needs of clients.

REFERENCES

Association for Behavioral and Cognitive Therapies. (2010). Coping with unemployment: Some tips from cognitive-behavioral therapy. *Association for Behavioral and Cognitive Therapies Fact Sheet*, 1-3.

American Psychological Association. (n.d.). Psychological effects of unemployment and underemployment. *APA Government Relations Socioeconomic Issues*. Retrieved January 3, 2016, from http://www.utexas.edu/law/journals/tlr/sources/Volume percent2092/Issue percent206/Rogers/DSB/Rogers.fn210.1.SB.pdf

Artacoz, L., Benach, J., Borrell, C., & Cortes, I. (2004). Unemployment and mental health: Understanding the interactions among gender, family roles, and social class. *American Journal of Public Health*, *94*(1), 82-88.

Belle, D., & Bullock, H. E. (n.d.). The psychological consequences of unemployment. *Society for the Psychological Study of Social Issues Policy Statement*. Retrieved January 3, 2013, from http://www.spssi.org/index.cfm?fuseaction=page.viewpage&pageid=1457

Bernhardt, A., & Rubin, K. (2003). Recession and 9/11: Economic hardship and the failure of the safety net for unemployed workers in New York City. *Brennan Center for Justice at NYU School of Law*. Retrieved January 3, 1970, from http://www.brennancenter.org/sites/default/files/legacy/d/Recession_9_11_Report.pdf

Bhat, C. S. (2010). Assisting unemployed adults find suitable work: A group intervention embedded in community and grounded in social action. *Journal for Specialists in Group Work*, *35*(3), 246-254. doi:10.1080/01933922.2010.492898

Blau, G. (2008). Exploring antecedents of individual grieving stages during an anticipated worksite closure. *Journal of Occupational and Organizational Psychology*, *81*(3), 529-550. doi:10.1348/096317907X241560

Bruckner, T. A. (2014). Invited commentary: Are there unrealized benefits of unemployment insurance among the employed?. *American Journal of Epidemiology*, *180*(1), 53-55. doi:10.1093/aje/kwu104

Burke, C., Johnson, E. E., Bourgault, C., Borgia, M., & O'Toole, T. P. (2013). Losing work: Regional unemployment and its effect on homeless demographic characteristics, needs, and health care.

Journal of Health Care for the Poor and Underserved, *24*(3), 1391-1402. doi:10.1353/hpu.2013.0150

Chan, W. S., Yip, P. S., Wong, P. W., & Chen, E. Y. (2007). Suicide and unemployment: What are the missing links? *Archives of Suicide Research*, *11*(4), 327-335.

Christensen, U., Schmidt, L., Kriegbaum, M., Hougaard, C. O., & Holsten, B. (2006). Coping with unemployment: Does educational attainment make any difference? *Scandinavian Journal of Public Health*, *34*(4), 363-370.

Conger, R. D., Conger, K. J., & Martin, M. J. (2010). Socioeconomic status, family processes, and individual development. *Journal of Marriage and Family*, *72*(3), 685-704. doi:10.1111/j.1741-3737.2010.00725.x

Cook, J. F., Alford, K. A., & Conway, P. (2012). Introduction to rural families and reshaping human services. *Journal of Family Social Work*, *15*(5), 351-358. doi:10.1080/10522158.2012.721122

Cylus, J., Glymour, M. M., & Avendano, M. (2014). Do generous unemployment benefit programs reduce suicide results? A state fixed-effect analysis covering 1968-2008. *American Journal of Epidemiology*, *180*(1), 45-52. doi:10.1093/aje/kwu106

Gagin, R., & Shinan-Altman, S. (2012). Is work beneficial to good health? *Social Work in Health Care*, *51*(4), 296-311. doi:10.1080/00981389.2011.638420

Goldman-Mellor, S. J., Saxton, K. B., & Catalano, R. C. (2010). Economic contraction and mental health: A review of the evidence, 1990-2009. *International Journal of Mental Health*, *39*(2), 6-31. doi:10.2753/IMH0020-7411390201

Goldsmith, A., & Diette, T. (2012). Exploring the link between unemployment and mental health outcomes. *The Socioeconomic Indicator*. Retrieved January 3, 2013, from http://www.apa.org/pi/ses/resources/indicator/2012/04/unemployment.aspx

International Federation of Social Workers. (2012, March 3). Statement of ethical principles. Retrieved January 6, 2015, from http://ifsw.org/policies/statement-of-ethical-principles/

Jacobs, S. J., & Blustein, D. L. (2008). Mindfulness as a coping mechanism for employment uncertainty. *Career Development Quarterly*, *57*(2), 1-7. doi:10.1002/j.2161-0045.2008.tb00045.x

Janlert, U., & Hammarstrom, A. (2009). Which theory is best? Explanatory models of the relationship between unemployment and health. *BMC Public Health, 9,* 235-244. doi:10.1186/1471-2458-9-235

Lau, C., & Leung, L. A. (2014). Mortgage debt as a moderator in the association between unemployment and health. *Public Health, 128*(3), 239-245. doi:10.1016/j.puhe.2013.12.012

Leahy, R. L. (2009). Unemployment anxiety. *The Behavior Therapist, 32*(3), 1-2.

U. S. Congress Joint Economic Committee. (2010). Understanding the economy: Unemployment among young workers. Washingtion, D. C.: Author.

McDonald, C., & Marston, G. (2008). Motivating the unemployed? Attitudes at the front line. *Australian Social Work, 61*(4), 315-326.

McKee-Ryan, F., Song, Z., Wanberg, C. R., & Kinicki, A. J. (2005). Psychological and physical well-being during unemployment: A meta-analytic study. *The Journal of Applied Psychology, 90*(1), 53-76.

Pelzer, B., Schaffrath, S., & Vernaleken, I. (2014). Coping with unemployment: The impact of unemployment on mental health, personality, and social interaction skills. *Work, 48*(2), 289-295. doi:10.3233/WOR-131626

The Policy, Ethics, and Human Rights Committee, British Association of Social Workers. (2012). The Code of Ethics for Social Work: Statement of Principles. Retrieved January 3, 2016, from http://cdn.basw.co.uk/upload/basw_112315-7.pdf

U.S. Bureau of Labor Statistics. (2013). Economic news release: Employment situation summary. (Report (Report No. USDL-15-0001). Retrieved January 3, 2016, from http://www.bls.gov/news.release/pdf/empsit.pdf

U. S. Bureau of Labor Statistics. (2015, December 4). Labor force statistics from the current population surve. Retrieved January 3, 2016, from http://www.bls.gov/web/empsit/cpseea10.htm

U. S. Bureau of Labor Statistics. (2015, December 4). Earning and unemployment rates by educational attainment. Retrieved January 3, 2016, from http://www.bls.gov/emp/ep_chart_001.htm

Wheeler, D. (2015). NASW Standards and Indicators for Cultural Competence in Social Work Practice. Retrieved January 3, 2015, from http://www.socialworkers.org/practice/standards/PRA-BRO-253150-CC-Standards.pdf

V

VETERANS & SUBSTANCE USE DISORDER

MAJOR CATEGORIES: Military & Veterans, Substance Abuse

WHAT WE KNOW

Substance use disorders are a significant problem among military veterans and active-duty service members. The *Diagnostic and Statistical Manual of Mental Disorders* (*DSM-5*) was published in 2013, replacing the *DSM-IV*. The *DSM-IV* chapter on "Substance-Related Disorders" included substance dependence, substance abuse, substance intoxication, and substance withdrawal and then discussed specific substances (e.g., alcohol, amphetamines). The *DSM-5* instead separates these disorders into two categories: substance use disorders and substance-induced disorders (intoxication, withdrawal, and other substance-/medication-induced mental disorders). Thus, it removes the distinction between abuse and dependence and instead divides each disorder into mild, moderate, and severe subtypes. Drug craving was added as a criterion for substance use disorder, whereas "recurrent legal problems" was removed. Substance use disorders refer to a pattern of continued use of a substance (e.g., alcohol, cannabis, opioids, sedatives) that causes cognitive, physiological, and behavioral symptoms, resulting in problems in various areas of functioning. The substance may be illegal (e.g., cannabis, cocaine, heroin), legal (e.g., alcohol), or a prescription medication used for purposes (i.e., recreational use) other than for which it was prescribed. The pattern of use is pathological. The individual may experience impaired self-control and may continue to use even when risks are present. There also may be tolerance and withdrawal.

Prevalence rates for substance use disorders among veterans vary between studies depending on a number of variables, including whether data are collected for veterans of all ages or for a subpopulation (e.g., those returning from recent conflicts in Iraq and Afghanistan).

Investigators found that of a sample of over 4 million United States veterans seen for primary care, an estimated 8.3 percent were diagnosed with a substance use disorder.

Analysis of data from the National Survey on Drug Use and Health (NSDUH) in the United States showed that 18 percent of veterans ages 21 to 34 years old met criteria for a substance use disorder.

Researchers found higher rates among a sample of veterans returning to impoverished areas in New York City, reporting that 32 percent had a substance use disorder.

In a longitudinal study of veterans returning from deployment, young veterans (i.e., under 26 years of age) were more likely than older veterans to experience worsening of excessive alcohol use and PTSD symptoms at 6 month follow-up.

The current demands of military service may increase the risk of substance use disorders. Multiple tours of duty, improvements in body armor, and medical advances may result in additional exposure to trauma as well as increase the likelihood of surviving injuries that once would have been fatal. Service members injured in combat return home with life-altering injuries: amputated limbs, brain and spinal injuries, vision and hearing loss, disfigurements, and psychological problems, resulting in significant medical and financial challenges that increase the risk of substance use disorders.

Substance use disorders often co-occur with another mental health condition such as depression, posttraumatic stress disorder (PTSD), anxiety disorder, or serious mental illness.

Veterans and service members may use alcohol and drugs as a means of coping with exposure to traumatic events. PTSD has been linked with more severe alcohol use and higher rates of illicit drug use in veterans, and moderate to severe depression is seen more frequently in veterans with PTSD who also have more severe alcohol use.

Coping style moderates the association between PTSD and alcohol outcomes. Veterans who reported using fewer action-oriented coping strategies (reframing, planning, instrumental and emotional support, acceptance, religion, humor, and distraction) and more avoidant strategies (disengagement, self-blame, denial, and venting) were more likely to have an alcohol use disorder than veterans who utilized more action-oriented coping.

Physical injuries and associated pain are prevalent among veterans;as a result, legally prescribed narcotics are abused by injured veterans at an increasing rate.

Prescription drug use quadrupled among U.S. military personnel from 2001 to 2009. Twenty-four percent of active-duty service members reported past-year use of prescription drugs, predominantly pain relievers.

The prevalence of opioid use disorder is 7 times higher among recipients of VA services than among members of commercial insurance plans. Opiate use among veterans who have recently served is on the rise. Because Afghanistan is one of the world's leading producers of opium, soldiers who served in Afghanistan and Iraq are more likely to have been exposed to opiates. Opiates may be used to cope with injury and chronic pain, which may lead to the development of opioid use disorder.

Alcohol use disorder is the most common substance use problem among veterans. Alcohol use has been a tradition in military culture and is more socially acceptable and involves fewer negative repercussions in the workplace than illicit drug use.

In a 2011 survey of active-duty service members, 33 percent reported recent binge drinking and 11.3 percent could be classified as problem drinkers; 1.5 percent reported they were in treatment or likely to seek treatment for their alcohol use.

Although many soldiers return from deployment meeting the criteria for alcohol use disorder, few are referred to alcohol treatment. In a study of veterans returning from deployment with a substance use disorder, the rate of past-year treatment was only 10 percent, and treatment rates were lower among blacks and Hispanics than among whites.

Alcohol use disorders predispose military veterans and service members to health problems and greater health-related expenditures as well as alcohol-related crimes (e.g., driving under the influence, use of illicit drugs).

More women are serving in the U.S. military than at any other point in history. The percentage of women in the military increased from 2 percent in 1973 to 15 percent in 2002. Women make up approximately 5 percent of veterans with access to healthcare services in the Veterans Health Administration system (VA).

In 2008, the VA provided treatment to women for substance use disorders in 139 facilities. In a study of over 15,000 women veterans with substance use disorders, researchers found that 41 percent had an alcohol use disorder, 32 percent had a drug use disorder, and 27 percent had a combination of drug and alcohol use disorders.Approximately one-third of female veterans, compared with 30 percent of male veterans, participated in a program that offered specialty treatment services for substance use disorders.

Women who received services at facilities that offered gender-specific treatment (e.g., education, counseling, peer support) attended more outpatient sessions overall than those served at facilities that did not offer gender-specific services.

Military values of self-sufficiency, adherence to codes of conduct, and emotional restraint can inhibit service men and women from seeking treatment for mental health and substance use disorders. Instead, many attempt to cope with the effects of trauma without seeking treatment.

There are multiple barriers to care for veterans and active-duty service members.

Underdiagnosis and undertreatment of substance use disorders in the VA is a serious problem.

Military personnel often have difficulty admitting that they need treatment, do not trust mental health professionals, fear their superiors may treat them differently, or are concerned that their units will lose confidence in them, posing additional barriers to treatment. Increasingly veterans are accessing treatment services for substance use disorders outside the military.

Service providers who are not employed within the VA may not be equipped to deal with men and women who have served in combat. Additionally, civilian mental health providers may not understand the military culture, which can pose additional barriers to treatment.

Improved screening and access to care is recommended for all veterans and active-duty service members with substance use disorders.

Screening tools include the Alcohol Use Disorders Identification Test (AUDIT-C), thee Drug Abuse Screening Test (DAST-10), and the Alcohol, Smoking, and Substance Involvement Screening Test (ASSIST).

Brief interventions can be enhanced by motivational interviewing techniques and providing personalized feedback that can be delivered verbally in one session as well as provided in printed form.

Cognitive behavioral therapy (CBT), motivational enhancement therapy, behavioral couples therapy, and pharmacological treatment have been shown to be effective interventions for substance use disorders.

Internet-based intervention offering online treatment services is an effective means to increase access to drug treatment.

Integrated treatments address both the substance abuse and PTSD to decrease risk of relapse and improve management of symptoms.

WHAT CAN BE DONE

Learn about the challenges faced by military veterans and active-duty service members with substance use disorders in order to better evaluate their needs and provide support; share this information with your colleagues.

Clinicians working with this population should utilize an ecological perspective that takes into account the multiple systems that may affect the client's treatment and help-seeking behavior, including the client's worldview, military culture, ethnicity, family, community, impact of trauma, co-occurring disorders, and culture.

To more competently serve service members, veterans, and their families, civilian social workers should

- become knowledgeable about military culture, military and governmental systems of care, issues affecting military and veteran populations, and appropriate policy and practice interventions;
- develop an awareness their own cultural values, beliefs, and biases and develop knowledge about the histories, traditions, and values of their clients. Adopt treatment methodologies that reflect the cultural needs of the client;
- develop a comprehensive directory of resources and programs available to service members, veterans, and their families;
- collaborate with military systems to provide continuity of care; and

- review and understand assessments and treatment(s) used by the VA (e.g., VA/DoD Clinical Practice Guidelines for Management of Substance Use Disorder, available at http://www.healthquality.va.gov/guidelines/MH/sud).

Provide support to veterans and active-duty service members by recognizing and acknowledging the emotional, physical, and financial stress of serving in the armed forces, and by

- evaluating the range and quality of available social support;
- taking sufficient time to assess the individual needs of the veteran by actively listening and answering questions;
- educating and assisting veterans to access military benefits; and
- based on the needs of the veteran, providing referrals to community-based services (e.g., non-profit agencies, veteran service organizations, treatment programs for substance use disorders, support groups, mental health services, vocational training).

Provide military veterans and active-duty service members with a list of online resources such as:

- United States Department of Veteran Affairs, http://www.vetcenter.va.gov/.
- Substance Abuse and Mental Health Services Administration (SAMHSA), http://www.samhsa.gov/.
- National Institute on Drug Abuse, http://www.drugabuse.gov/.
- Veterans Crisis Line, (800) 273-8255, http://www.veteranscrisisline.net.

*Written by Laura McLuckey, MSW, LCSW, and
Jennifer Teska, MSW*

*Reviewed by Laura Gale, LCSW, and
Chris Bates, MA, MSW*

REFERENCES

American Psychiatric Association. (2013). Diagnostic and statistical manual of mental disorders. (5th ed.). Arlington, VA: American Psychiatric Publishing.

Baser, O., Xie, L., Mardekian, J., Schaaf, D., Wang, L., & Joshi, A. V. (2014). Prevalence of diagnosed opioid abuse and its economic burden in the veterans health administration. *Pain Practice, 14*(5), 437-445. doi:10.1111/papr.12097

Benda, B. B. (2005). A study of substance abuse, traumata, and social support systems among homeless veterans. *Journal of Human Behavior in the Social Environment, 12*(1), 59-82. doi:10.1300/J137v12n01

British Association of Social Workers. (2012). The code of ethics for social work: Statement of principles. Retrieved December 21, 2015, from http://cdn.basw.co.uk/upload/basw_112315-7.pdf

Claiborne, N., Videka, L., Postiglione, P., Finkelstein, A., McDonnell, P., & Krause, R. D. (2010). Alcohol screening, evaluation, and referral for veterans. *Journal of Social Work Practice in the Addictions, 10*(3), 308-326. doi:10.1080/1533 256X.2010.500963

Cucciare, M. A., Weingardt, K. R., Valencia-Garcia, D., & Ghaus, S. (2015). Post-traumatic stress disorder and illicit drug use in veterans presenting to primary care with alcohol misuse. *Addiction Research and Theory, 23*(4), 287-293. doi:10.3109/160 66359.2014.984700

Department of Defense. (2013). 2011 health related behavior survey of active duty military personnel. Retrieved December 21, 2015, from http://www.murray.senate.gov/public/_cache/files/889efd07-2475-40ee-b3b0-508947957a0f/final-2011-hrb-active-duty-survey-report.pdf

Enggasser, J. L., Hermos, J. A., Rubin, J. A., Lachowicz, M., Rybin, D., Brief, D. J.,... Keane, T. M. (2015). Drinking goal choice and outcomes in a Web-based alcohol intervention: Results from VetChange. *Addictive Behaviors, 42*, 63-68.

Franklin, E. (2009). The emerging needs of veterans: A call to action for the social work profession. *Health & Social Work, 34*(3), 163-167. doi:10.1093/hsw/34.3.163

Golub, A., Vazan, P., Bennett, A. S., & Liberty, H. J. (2013). Unmet need for treatment of substance use disorders and serious psychological distress among veterans: A nationwide analysis using the NSDUH. *Military Medicine, 178*, 107-114. doi:10.7205/MILMED-D-12-00131

Grosso, J. A., Kimbrel, N. A., Dolan, S., Meyer, E. C., Kruse, M. I., Gulliver, S. B., & Morissette, S. B. (2014). A test of whether coping styles moderate the effect of PTSD symptoms on alcohol outcomes, *27*(4), 478-482. Retrieved from Journal of Traumatic Stress, doi:10.1002/jts.21943

International Federation of Social Workers. (2012, March 3). Statement of ethical principles. Retrieved December 21, 2015, from http://ifsw.org/policies/statement-of-ethical-principles/

McDevitt-Murphy, M. E., Williams, J. L., Murphy, J. G., Monahan, C. J., & Bracken-Minor, K. L. (2015). Brief intervention to reduce hazardous drinking and enhance coping among OEF/OIF/OND veterans. *Professional Psychology: Research and Practice, 46*(2), 83-89. doi:10.1037/a0036771

National Institute on Drug Abuse. (2013). Substance abuse in the military. Retrieved December 21, 2015, from http://www.drugabuse.gov/publications/drugfacts/substance-abuse-in-military

Oliva, E. M., Gregor, A., Rogers, J., Dalton, A., Harris, A., & Trafton, J. A. (2012). Correlates of specialty substance use disorder treatment among female patients in the veterans' health administration. *Journal of Social Work Practice in the Addictions, 12*(3), 282-301. doi:10.1080/1533256X.2012.702620

Savitsky, L., Illingworth, M., & DuLaney, M. (2009). Civilian social work: Serving the military and veteran populations. *Social Work, 54*(4), 327-339. doi:10.1093/sw/54.4.327

Schultz, M., Glickman, M. E., & Eisen, S. V. (2014). Predictors of decline in overall mental health, PTSD and alcohol use in OEF/OIF veterans. *Comprehensive Psychiatry, 55*(7), 1654-1664. doi:10.1016/j.comppsych.2014.06.003

Skidmoore, W. C., & Roy, M. (2011). Practical considerations for addressing substance use disorders in veterans and service members. *Social Work in Health Care, 50*(1), 85-107. doi:10.1080/00981389.2010.522913

Trivedi, R. B., Post, E. P., Sun, H., Pomerantz, A., Saxon, A. J., Piette, J. D.,... Nelson, K. (2015). Prevalence, comorbidity, and prognosis of mental health among US veterans. *American Journal of Public Health, 105*(12), 2564-2569. doi:10.2105/AJPH.2015.302836

Vazan, P., Golub, A., & Bennett, A. S. (2013). Substance use and other mental health disorders among veterans returning to the inner city: Prevalence, correlates, and rates of unmet treatment need. *Substance Use & Misuse, 48*(10), 880-893. doi:10.3109/10826084.2013.796989

Weiss, E. L., Coll, J. E., Mayeda, S., Mascarenas, J., Lawlor, K., & Debraber, T. (2012). An ecosystemic perspective in the treatment of posttraumatic stress and substance use disorders in veterans. *Journal of Social Worker Practice in the Addictions, 12*(2), 143-162. doi:10.1080/1533256X.2012.676471

Wheeler, D. (2015). NASW standards and indicators for cultural competence in social work practice. Retrieved December 21, 2015, from http://www.socialworkers.org/practice/standards/PRA-BRO-253150-CC-Standards.pdf

VETERANS: NUTRITION-RELATED HEALTH PROBLEMS

MAJOR CATEGORIES: Community, Medical & Health, Military & Veterans

WHAT WE KNOW

United States veterans are a highly vulnerable population with significant mental, physical, and economic challenges. These challenges place individuals at greater risk for nutrition-related illnesses (e.g., diabetes, obesity, vitamin deficiencies). Veterans experience many of these illnesses simultaneously. Therefore, they are in greater need of health- and nutrition-related resources than the general population.

A major nutrition-related health problem for veterans is obesity. Many health conditions have been found to be related to or worsened by obesity (e.g., heart disease, diabetes, mental illness, prostate cancer).

Veterans have been found to engage in more sedentary leisure activities than the general population and to spend less time engaging in physical activity generally. Sedentary behavior and obesity in veterans can be related to mental and physical disabilities caused by military service. For example, the loss of limb(s) can lead to difficulty engaging in physical activity. Veterans with posttraumatic stress disorder (PTSD) may be treated with medications that cause lethargy and obesity.

Age, marital status, tobacco use, mental health, and socioeconomic status all affect an individual's likelihood of developing obesity and ability to adhere to nutritional interventions.

Poor food choices increase the risk of obesity and nutrient deficiencies, which are correlated with significant health problems in veterans (e.g., diabetes, prostate cancer, tooth decay, cardiovascular disease, mental illness).

Calcium and vitamin D deficiencies are prevalent among veterans, placing them at greater risk for prostate cancer.

Improving nutrition is strongly correlated with improving depression among veterans with dementia.

Increasing fruit and vegetable intake is essential for addressing vitamin deficiencies and related health problems. This can be particularly challenging for poor and homeless veterans.

Veterans have high rates of mental illness, PTSD, poverty, and homelessness compared to the general population. Homelessness among veterans is estimated to be double the rate of homelessness in the general population. Poverty and homelessness decrease access to resources and prevent individuals from obtaining adequate nutrition.

The federal government's Supplemental Nutritional Assistance Program (SNAP) provides benefits to 7 percent of veterans. Veterans comprise 6 percent of all SNAP recipients. Between 2008 and 2012, the percentage of veterans receiving SNAP benefits increased in 47 states.

There is a high percentage of veterans with mental illness. Mental illness increases the risk for poor nutrition and obesity in the veteran population.

The population of female veterans is increasing. Female veterans have specific health and nutrition needs that differ from those of male veterans, including treatment for eating disorders and military sexual trauma (MST).

Eating disorders affect a greater percentage of women than of men. Eating disorders may result in vitamin deficiencies and organ failure. In addition, eating disorders in veterans have been found to be correlated with PTSD, depression, and other mood disorders.

MST affects more female veterans than it does male veterans. MST contributes to a higher prevalence of PTSD in female veterans.

Studies have found that veterans are a highly motivated population. With proper intervention, changes in lifestyle and dietary habits are possible. There are existing programs and resources that have demonstrated positive results for veterans.

The Veterans Health Administration (VA), one of the major resources available to veterans, provides many programs and services that address veteran health and nutrition needs. These programs include Healthcare for Homeless Veterans (HCHV); psychological services and counseling; MOVE!, an obesity management program; temporary housing for homeless veterans; benefits education; hospitals; and general health services.

The VA needs to adapt and improve services for female veterans; this growing population requires more in-depth screening and treatment for women's health issues, MST, and eating disorders.

The MOVE! program has demonstrated positive results in creating lasting dietary and lifestyle changes in veterans who are overweight or obese.

Wellness coaching and individual case managers have been demonstrated to be effective tools for assisting veterans in maintaining lasting weight loss. Unpaid interns are needed to provide this service in a cost-effective way.

WHAT CAN BE DONE

Become knowledgeable about the nutritional deficiencies and health problems that veterans experience so you can accurately assess and provide interventions for the veterans you treat.

Share your knowledge with your colleagues.

Learn about the programs that exist for veterans in order to properly provide referrals to them for veterans.

Develop an awareness of your own cultural values, beliefs, and biases and develop knowledge about the histories, traditions, and values of your clients. Adopt treatment methodologies that reflect the cultural needs of the client.

Written by Emma Tiffany-Malm, MSW

Reviewed by Melissa Rosales Neff, MA, MSW

REFERENCES

Balshem, H., Christensen, V., Tuepker, A., & Kansagara, D. (2011). A critical review of the literature regarding homelessness among veterans. VA-ESP Project #05-225. Washington, DC: Department of Veterans Affairs.

Batuman, E., Bean-Mayberry, B., Goldzweig, C. L., Huang, C., Miake-Lye, I. M., Washington, D. L.,... Shekelle, P. G. (2011). Health effects of military service on women veterans. Washington, DC: Department of Veterans Affairs.

Brown, E., Roberts, R., Bearden, R., & O'Donohue, J. (2012). 7 stepping stones—Using spirituality to enhance nutrition and wellness programs for Jesse Brown Veterans Administration (VA) Medical Center veterans. *Journal of the Academy of Nutrition & Dietetics, 112*(9), A84. doi:http://dx.doi.org/10.1016/j.jand.2012.06.300

Ceresa, C. L., Foley, S., Shahnazari, M., Fong, A., Zidaru, E., & Moddy, S. Y. (2012). Wellness coaching promotes healthy eating behavior in veterans. *Journal of the Academy of Nutrition & Dietetics, 112*(9), A15. doi:http://dx.doi.org/10.1016/j.jand.2012.06.038

Der, T., Bailey, B. A., Youssef, D., Manning, T., Grant, W. B., & Peiris, A. N. (2014). Vitamin D and prostate cancer survival in veterans. *Military Medicine, 179*(1), 81-84. doi:10.7205/MILMED-D-12-00540

Goldberg, R. W., Reeves, G., Tapscott, S., Medoff, D., Dickerson, F., Goldberg, A. P.,... Dixon, L. B. (2013). "MOVE!": Outcomes of a weight loss program modified for veterans with serious mental illness. *Psychiatric Services, 64*(8), 737-744. doi:10.1176/appi.ps.201200314

Haskell, S. G., Gordon, K. S., Mattocks, K., Duggal, M., Erdos, J., Justice, A., & Brandt, C. A. (2010). Gender differences in rates of depression, PTDS, pain, obesity, and military sexual trauma among Connecticut war veterans of Iraq and Afghanistan. *Journal of Women's Health, 19*(2), 267-271. doi:10.1089/jwh.2008.1262

Ko, L. K., Allicok, M., Campbell, M. K., Valle, C. G., Armstrong-Brown, J., Carr, C.,... Anthony, T. (2011). An examination of sociodemographic, health, psychological factors, and fruit and vegetable consumption among overweight and obese U.S. veterans. *Military Medicine, 176*(11), 1281-1286.

Koepsell, T. D., Littman, A. J., & Forsberg, C. W. (2012). Obesity, overweight, and their life course trajectories in veterans and non-veterans. *Obesity, 20*(2), 434-439. doi:10.1038/oby.2011.2

Littman, A. J., Forsberg, C. W., & Boyko, E. J. (2013). Associations between compulsory physical activity during military service and activity in later adulthood among male veterans compared to nonveterans. *Journal of Physical Activity & Health, 10*(6), 784-791.

Mizrahi, T., & Mayden, R. W. (2001). NASW standards for cultural competency in social work practice. Retrieved October 11, 2015, from http://www.socialworkers.org/practice/standards/NASWCulturalStandards.pdf

Osborne, V. A., Gage, L. A., & Rolbiecki, A. J. (2012). Psychosocial effects of trauma on military women serving in the National Guard and Reserves. *Advances in Social Work, 13*(1), 166-184. Retrieved from https://journals.iupui.edu/index.php/advancesinsocialwork/article/view/1878/1961

Romanova, M., Liang, L. J., Deng, M. L., Li, Z., & Herber, D. (2013). Effectiveness of the MOVE! Multidisciplinary weight loss program for veterans in Los Angeles. *Preventing Chronic Disease, 10,* E112. doi:10.5888/pcd10.120325

Schwartz, N., Kaye, E. K., Nunn, M. E., Spiro, A., & Garcia, R. I. (2012). High-fiber foods reduce periodontal disease progression in men aged 65 and older: The Veterans Affairs Normative Aging Study/Dental Longitudinal Study. *Journal of the American Geriatrics Society, 60*(4), 676-683. doi:10.1111/j.1532-5415.2011.03866.x

Shahnazari, M., Ceresa, C., Foley, S., Fong, A., Zidaru, E., & Moody, S. (2013). Nutrition-focused wellness coaching promotes a reduction in body weight in overweight US veterans. *Journal of the Academy of Nutrition and Dietetics, 113*(7), 928-935. doi:10.1016/j.jand.2013.04.001

Soroka, O., Tseng, C. L., Rajan, M., Maney, M., & Pogach, L. (2012). A clinical action measure to assess glycemic management in the 65-74 year old veteran population. *Journal of the American Geriatrics Society, 60*(8), 1442-1447. doi:10.1111/j.1532-5415.2012.04079.x

Williams, C. D., Whitley, B. M., Hoyo, C., Grant, D. J., Schwartz, G. G., Presti, J. C., Jr,... Freedland, S. J. (2012). Dietary calcium and risk for prostate cancer: A case-control study among US veterans. *Preventing Chronic Disease, 9,* E39. doi:10.5888/pcd9.110125

Wu, H. S., & Lin, L. C. (2013). The moderating effect of nutritional status on depressive symptoms in veteran elders with dementia: A spaced retrieval combined with Montessori-based activities. *Journal of Advanced Nursing, 69*(10), 2229-2241. doi:10.1111/jan.12097

VIDEO GAME ADDICTION

MAJOR CATEGORIES: Behavioral & Mental Health

DESCRIPTION

Video game addiction (VGA) is a relatively new area of research and clinical study and practice. There is debate within the mental health community over whether VGA is a disorder deserving inclusion in the *Diagnostic and Statistical Manual of Mental Disorders,* which is a manual used to diagnose mental health disorders. In the *Diagnostic and Statistical Manual of Mental Disorders,* fifth edition *(DSM-5),* gambling disorder is the only non-substance-related disorder included in the Substance-Related and Addictive Disorders section. However, many researchers have argued that video game addiction should be considered a disorder. The *DSM-5* includes Internet gaming disorder (IGD) in its section on conditions for further study, which includes proposed criteria for conditions for which further research is advised. IGD is defined as the persistent and recurrent use of the Internet to engage in games, often with other players, leading to clinically significant impairment or distress as indicated by at least five of the following proposed criteria: preoccupation with Internet games, withdrawal symptoms when access to Internet gaming is lost (e.g., irritability, anxiety, sadness, tolerance (i.e., the need to spend increasing amounts of time engaged in Internet games), unsuccessful attempts to control participation in Internet games, loss of interest in previous hobbies because of Internet games, continued excessive use of Internet games despite knowledge of the possible psychosocial problems that result, deception of family members and friends with regard to the amount of Internet gaming, use of Internet games to escape or relieve a negative mood, and loss of a significant relationship or job because of participation in Internet games.

Video games may be grouped into the following categories: first-person shooter games, real-time strategy games, multi-user dungeons/domains, and massively multiplayer online role-playing games (MMORPG). MMORPG are complex and realistic virtual worlds in which a player interacts with other players through fantasy roles. Although other types of games have an end point, MMORPG are endless, which increases the potential for problematic use. Furthermore, because MMORPG are played online by participants from around the world, the distinction between real-time day and night disappears. Players in other time zones may gain an advantage in the game while a player sleeps or goes to work, thereby increasing one's urge to play continuously. Another difference between stand-alone video games (games not played through the Internet) and MMORPG is that the latter requires social interaction within the game and frequently involves team play within the game, both of which require different levels of motivation and involvement than stand-alone video games.

There is debate over how to think about and address VGA and IGD, including how, or if, they differ from one another and whether either or both conditions should be included in the DSM-5. Many argue that since video games can be played both online and offline, the term Internet gaming disorder is inaccurate and the condition should instead be called video gaming disorder. Other researchers assert that it is important to make a clear distinction between an addiction to an activity (e.g., video gaming) and use of a delivery system (e.g., the Internet). Others argue that MMORPG have distinct qualities that make them a separate category of games, use of which should be assessed and treated uniquely. Another conceptualization of video games equates the points and rewards accumulated in games to forms of currency, and concludes that video games and gambling share enough traits to be measured and treated using the same tools and interventions. As noted above, Internet gaming disorder is being considered for inclusion in future editions of the DSM. As the debate continues, the definition of the proposed disorder and its criteria may change. Video game addiction includes both online and offline video gaming, unless otherwise noted, for the purpose of this article.

VGA does not have the clearly defined and established symptom clusters that typically characterize addiction. Research has been inconsistent in regard to how problematic gaming is for individuals. There is evidence of individuals being unable to quit their video gaming habits and playing to the point of neglecting their psychological and physical health, which is similar to what occurs in other addictions. No universal theory for video game addiction exists,

but intense internal conflict is a hallmark. Excessive video game play may be a coping mechanism, an escape from reality, or a mood modifier. The act of playing may provide the user with a sense of euphoria; repetitive activation of the brain's reward circuit can create actual neurological changes in brain anatomy. VGA commonly has substance use, anxiety, and depression as co-occurring conditions. Attention problems and impulsivity are also commonly present in individuals with VGA but it is not clear if the causality is bidirectional where attention problems and impulsivity cause VGA and VGA causes attention problems and impulsivity.

Determining at what point an individual's video gaming behavior has moved from healthy engagement in the activity to excessive or addictive behavior is not simple since there is no scientific consensus to rely on. Common criteria to determine an addiction to video games for most individuals include cravings of playing the game, feeling a loss of control, experiencing withdrawal symptoms, preoccupation with gaming, and relapse. Traditionally, addiction refers to behavior that is out of control; the diagnostic criteria for substance dependence, salience, and relapse often are used with VGA. Salience can be behavioral or cognitive. With behavioral salience, the user might be missing meals, sleep, work, or school in order to play video games. Cognitive salience refers to thinking about video gaming taking up much of the user's time. The individual may require more and more time with the video game to achieve the same levels of euphoria. A side effect of VGA is the effect on the social development or experiences of the user. Excessive time spent playing video games in isolation takes away from opportunities to engage with the outside world in positive experiences.

FACTS AND FIGURES

The prevalence of VGA is difficult to determine since VGA is not universally accepted as a diagnosis and there is no consensus on how to measure it. Researchers have found that VGA is a clinically significant problem, with internationally between 4.9 percent and 9 percent of video gamers showing addiction. Other investigators have found significantly higher rates of VGA in men than women. A 2008 study in which researchers examined MRIs of potentially addicted video gamers who played World of Warcraft, an MMORPG, found that the area of the brain that was activated during play was the same area that has been associated with cravings in individuals with substance use disorders. A 2013 study conducted in Hong Kong of secondary school students used the five-factor personality model (i.e., openness to experience, conscientiousness, extraversion, agreeableness, and neuroticism) to measure the association of personality traits with addictive online gaming and social networking. Study participants who were addicted to online gaming measured low in conscientiousness and openness, while those addicted to social networking were high in neuroticism and extraversion.

The *DSM-5* includes some information about the prevalence of IGD, first noting the difficulties of measurement and then stating that prevalence seems to be highest among 12- to 20-year-old males, with more studies conducted in China and South Korea than elsewhere.

RISK FACTORS

Males seem to be at a higher risk for VGA, which may be due to video gaming being a male-dominated activity. Males or females with depression, anxiety, social isolation, low self-esteem, and introverted personalities are at risk for VGA. Having access to a computer with an Internet connection can be an environmental risk factor.

SIGNS AND SYMPTOMS

The signs and symptoms of video game use becoming problematic include a preoccupation with playing video games, needing to spend more and more time engaged in games while disengaging from family and friends, numerous attempts to reduce use, experiencing symptoms of withdrawal when video game use is reduced, conflict with family, work, or friends as a result of video game use, changes in mood, and dishonesty with family or friends regarding how much time is spent playing video games.

ASSESSMENT

The social worker should complete a thorough biological, psychological, social, and spiritual assessment to determine the extent of the client's addiction, including the client's daily functioning, the type of video game(s) used, the influence of video game use on the client's mood, behaviors, and relationships, what supports are available, how to frame any interventions, and the client's desire for change. The social worker should assess for any co-occurring conditions that may need attention such as symptoms of depression.

ASSESSMENTS AND SCREENING TOOLS

The social worker may utilize standardized assessment and screening tools as part of their assessment process to identify the client's emotional and social intervention needs. The Video Game Addiction Test (VAT) is a 14-item scaled test that measures loss of control, conflict, preoccupation, coping/mood symptoms, and withdrawal. The Game Addiction Scale for Adolescents developed by Lemmens and Valkenburg is a 21-item scale that uses criteria similar to those for pathological gambling, with three questions for each of seven criteria: salience, tolerance, mood modification, relapse, withdrawal, conflict, and problems. In Germany researchers developed the Video Game Dependency Scale, KFN-CSAS-II, which is similar in design to the Game Addiction Scale for Adolescents. The Problem Video Game Playing Scale is a survey with 9 yes or no questions to assess addiction to playing video games.

TREATMENT

Because of the difficulty measuring VGA and its relative newness as a concern, there is limited evidence-based information about treatment. The *DSM-5* reports that the Chinese government has set up a treatment system, but does not include details. Research that has been published about treatment is mostly conducted in China and South Korea.

INTERVENTION

If it is determined that the client is experiencing problematic use of video games, the social worker should provide interventions to help reduce the client's negative emotions regarding their video game use. The social worker may recommend that the client decrease video game use and increase social interactions to improve relationships that were negatively affected by gaming. The social worker should support the client when asking about video game use. The social worker may assist the client in finding alternative activities and work with the client on determining alternative or replacement activities. The social worker should help the client determine if an abstinence or harm reduction model is appropriate to assist with their video game addiction. The social worker may provide or refer the client for cognitive-behavioral treatment if appropriate. The social worker and treating clinician should utilize the client's preferred therapy techniques to reduce negative emotions and improve the client's self-esteem.

APPLICABLE LAWS AND REGULATIONS

There are currently no laws in the United States that restrict video game use. In South Korea a law was passed requiring video game manufacturers of a certain size and revenue to include a mechanism in their games that enables parents to lock the game after a specified amount of time. Some U.S. manufacturers have put warnings or reminders on the loading screens of games advising video gamers to use the games in moderation.

SERVICES AND RESOURCES

- The Center for Internet Addiction is a source of information and resources for professionals and families, http://www.netaddiction.com/
- On-Line Gamers Anonymous operates as a resource for support, education, discussion, and referrals for individuals struggling with computer, video, console, or online gaming addictions, http://www.olganon.org/
- The Restart Internet Addiction Recovery Center provides treatment for VGA along with resources and information, http://www.netaddictionrecovery.com/

FOOD FOR THOUGHT

VGA has a frequent co-occurrence with diagnosis of depression, anxiety, social isolation, impulsivity, attention-deficit/hyperactivity disorder, and poor school performance. Excessive video gaming negatively influences proactive cognitive control. Proactive cognitive control is keeping a goal actively in the brain (e.g., to control a plan to stop at the grocery store, the individual keeps in mind the goal of going to the store before getting to the turnoff to the store).

RED FLAGS

There is a difference between users who are introverted or antisocial versus users who are showing signs of VGA. Introverted users of multiplayer online games may not be forgoing external sources of social activity (e.g., bars, clubs, parties) to play, which is a sign of addiction, but instead are using time they would have spent alone anyway to play.

The social worker needs to be aware of personal cultural biases he or she may hold against video games, such as viewing playing as a sign of laziness or social awkwardness. Many games require skill and intelligence to play, as well as interaction with team members. Stereotypes about "video gamers" can lead to internalization by clients if these biases are present in practice and can therefore interfere with the effectiveness of interventions provided and interfere with the client and social worker relationship.

NEXT STEPS

The social worker may provide a referral for long-term therapy if necessary. The social worker may make referrals for the client's family members for continued education and support. Individuals experiencing video game addiction may need ongoing counseling and support.

Written by Jessica Therivel, LMSW IPR

Reviewed by Lynn B. Cooper, D. Crim, and Melissa Rosales Neff, MSW

REFERENCES

American Psychiatric Association. (2013). Diagnostic and statistical manual of mental disorders. (5th ed.). Arlington, VA: American Psychiatric Publishing.

Bleckmann, P., Eckert, J., & Jukschat, N. (2012). Futile search for a better life? Two biographical case studies on women with depression and video game dependency. *Advances in Dual Diagnosis, 5*(3), 137-146. doi:10.1108/17570971211253711

British Association of Social Work. (2012, January). The code of ethics for social work: Statement of principles. Retrieved October 31, 2015, from http://cdn.basw.co.uk/upload/basw_112315-7.pdf

Gentile, D. A., Swing, E. L., Lim, C. G., & Khoo, A. (2012). Video game playing, attention problems, and impulsiveness: Evidence of bidirectional causality. *Psychology of Popular Media Culture, 1*(1), 62-70. doi:10.1037/a0026969

Griffiths, M. (2010). The role of context in online gaming excess and addiction: Some case study evidence. *International Journal of Mental Health and Addiction, 8*, 119-125. doi:10.1007/s11469-009-9229-x

Hellman, M., Schoenmakers, T. M., Nordstrom, B. R., & van Holst, R. J. (2013). Is there such a thing as online video game addiction? A cross-disciplinary review. *Addiction Research & Theory, 21*(2), 102-112. doi:10.3109/16066359.2012.693222

Hussain, Z., Griffiths, M. D., & Baguley, T. (2011). Online gaming addiction: Classification, prediction and associated risk factors. *Addiction Research and Theory, 20*(5), 359-371. doi:10.3109/16066359.2011.640442

International Federation of Social Workers. (2012, March 3). Statement of Ethical Principles. Retrieved from http://ifsw.org/policies/statement-of-ethical-principles

King, D. L., & Delfabbro, P. H. (2012). Issues for DSM-5: video-gaming disorder? *Australian & New Zealand Journal of Psychiatry, 47*(1), 20-22. doi:10.1177/0004867412464065

Kuhn, S., Romanowski, A., Schilling, C., Lorenz, R., Morsen, C., Seiferth, N., ... Gallinat, J. (2011). The neural basis of video gaming. *Translational Psychiatry, 1*, e53. doi:10.1038/tp.2011.53

Kuss, D. J., & Griffiths, M. D. (2012). Online gaming addiction in children and adolescents: A literature review of empirical research. *Journal of Behavioural Addiction, 1*, 3-22.

Petry, N. M. (2010). Commentary on Van Rooij et al. (2011) : 'Gaming addiction' - a psychiatric disorder or not?. *Addiction, 106*(1), 213-214.

Ream, G. L., Elliott, L. C., & Dunlap, E. (2011). Patterns of and motivation for concurrent use of video games and substances. *International Journal of Environmental Research and Public Health, 8*(10), 3999-4012. doi:10.3390/ijerph8103999

Starcevic, V. (2013). Video-gaming disorder and behavioural addictions. *Australian & New Zealand Journal of Psychiatry, 47*(3), 285-286. doi:10.1177/0004867413476145

van Holst, R. J., Lemmens, J. S., Valkenburg, P. M., Peter, J., Veltman, D. J., & Goudriaan, A.

E. (2012). Attentional bias and disinhibition toward gaming cues are related to problem gaming in male adolescents. *Journal of Adolescent Health, 50*(6), 541-546. doi:10.1016/j.jadohealth.2011.07.006

Van Rooij, A. J., Kuss, D. J., Griffiths, M. D., Shorter, G. W., Schoenmakeres, M. T., & Van de Mheen, D. (2014). The (co-) occurrence of problematic video gaming, substance use, and psychosocial problems in adolescents. *Journal of Behavioral Addictions, 3*(3), 157-165. doi:10.1556/JBA.3.2014.013

van Rooij, A. J., Meerkerk, G. J., Schoenmakers, T. M., Griffiths, M., & Van de Mheen, D. (2010). Video game addiction and social responsibility. *Addiction Research & Theory, 18*(5), 489-493. doi:10.3109/16066350903168579

Wang, C. W., Ho, R. T. H., Chan, C. E. W., & Tse, S. (2015). Exploring personality characteristics of Chinese adolescents with internet-related addictive behaviors: Trait differences for gaming addiction and social networking addiction. *Addictive Behaviors, 42*, 32-35. doi:10.1016/j.addbeh.2014.10.039

Wheeler, D. (2015). NASW standards and indicators for cultural competence in social work practice. Retrieved April 11, 2016, from http://www.socialworkers.org/practice/standards/PRA-BRO-253150-CC-Standards.pdf

20 Wong, U., & Hodgins, D. C. (2014). Development of the Game Addiction Inventory for Adults (GAIA). *Addiction Research & Theory, 22*(3), 195-209. doi:10.3109/16066359.2013.824565

Violence against Lesbian, Gay, Bisexual & Transgender Persons

Major Categories: Gender/Identity, Violence

Description

The victimization and persecution of sexual minorities around the world is described as a human rights issue and an urgent public health problem. *Sexual minority* is an umbrella term used to describe individuals who do not conform to normative heterosexual identity, forms of behavior, relationships, or community structure. Their sexual orientation may be heterosexual, homosexual, or bisexual. Most visibly, the sexual minority population consists of gay men and lesbians. Bisexual, intersex, transsexual, trans-identified, and transgender individuals, along with those identifying as queer or questioning, are also included as sexual minorities, with the term *intersex* referring to persons with atypical genitalia. *Transsexual* refers to a person who identifies as belonging to a gender other than that culturally assigned to him or her; *transgender* is a broader term that describes persons who vary from conventional gender roles. Several acronyms collectively identify these groups of people: LGBT (lesbian, gay, bisexual, and transgender), LGBTQ (lesbian, gay, bisexual, transgender, and queer or questioning), LGBTQQ (lesbian, gay, bisexual, transgender, and queer or questioning), and LGBTIQ (lesbian, gay, bisexual, transgender, intersex, queer or questioning). The acronyms are used collectively because persons in these groups encounter similar as well as unique forms of discrimination and oppression. Members of these communities may also experience a variety of biopsychosocial problems.

For many members of sexual minority groups, violence is a pervasive aspect of living. The global victimization of gender-variant individuals has been described as a "pandemic of focused prejudice" (Kidd & Witten, 2007). In the extreme, an individual identifying as a member of a sexual minority, or an individual who is perceived as one, may be punished by incarceration or execution in countries in which gender variance and nonconforming sexualities are criminalized. In more legally and socially tolerant countries, the prevalence of homophobia and transphobia leads to frequent verbal and physical attacks against members of sexual minority groups. *Homophobia* is a term used to describe hatred of gay men and lesbians, while *transphobia* defines hatred of those who do not conform to traditional gender identities.

Media coverage of hate crimes against sexual minorities, and especially of youths belonging to sexual minorities, has drawn attention to the need for policies and interventions that promote tolerance and respect for members of these populations. Youths belonging to sexual minorities, gay men, and older LGBTQ adults living in long-term care facilities are especially vulnerable to violence stemming from hatred. Youthful members of sexual minorities report extremely high levels of abuse from family members and others familiar to them, as well as from strangers. Because youthful members of sexual minorities have fewer protective factors, such as family support or school connectedness, they have high levels of depression, suicidal ideation, and attempted suicide. To avoid victimization, some individuals of LGBTQ identity may actively pass as "straight," but the self-monitoring required to achieve this can impose enormous strains on such individuals.

Preventing violence against sexual minorities requires challenging the attitudes and behaviors that foster it. Schools can do this by organizing alliances between gay and other LGBTQ groups and the rest of the student population, which can promote understanding and harmony by supporting sexual minorities and helping them to feel fully included as members of school populations. Professionals working with younger persons should avoid assuming that all adolescents are heterosexual. Organizations that provide care, services, and information to the LGBTQ community should ensure that their workers are trained in cultural competence so that they can effectively accomplish these objectives.

FACTS AND FIGURES

High-school students who identify as gay, lesbian, or bisexual experience more violence and bullying at school than students who identify as heterosexual. A study done in 2014 found that 43.1 percent of boys who identified as gay and 35.2 percent who identified as bisexual reported being bullied on school property, as compared to 18.3 percent of boys who identified as heterosexual (O'Malley Olsen et al., 2014). According to the 2013 National School Climate Survey 55.5 percent of LGBT students felt unsafe at school because of their sexual orientation; 74.1 percent of LGBT students were verbally harassed (e.g., called names), 36.2 were physically harassed (e.g., pushed), and 16.5 percent were physically assaulted (e.g., punched, kicked) because of their sexual orientation (Kosciw et. al., 2014). Transgender women of color are especially at risk for violence; in 2013, 72 percent of LGBT victims of homicide were transgender women and 67 percent of those victims were women of color (National Coalition of Anti-Violence Programs, 2013). Lesbian, gay, and bisexual youths are twice as likely as heterosexual youths to be victims of physical violence when dating (Luo et al., 2014). Sexual minorities are also more likely than heterosexuals to be victims of both child abuse and intimate partner violence (IPV) (Koeppel& Bouffard, 2014).

RISK FACTORS

Lesbian, gay, bisexual, transgender, and questioning individuals have a significantly greater than average risk for post-traumatic stress disorder (PTSD). Research has found that higher proportions of LGBTQ adults than heterosexual adults were abused sexually and physically as children and adolescents. Lesbian, gay, bisexual, transgender, and questioning adolescents have a greater risk of violent victimization than do other adolescents or adult members of sexual minority groups. Alcohol use by both the victim and the perpetrator is the best predictor of sexual assault for lesbians, whereas childhood sexual assault is the best predictor of sexual assault for adult gay men (Han et al., 2013). Data also suggest that gay men have a higher risk of being victims of property crime and physical violence than do lesbian or bisexual individuals. Being a member of a stigmatized group targeted for violence creates chronic stress, putting members of such a group at risk for problems of mental-health and stress-related illness.

SIGNS AND SYMPTOMS
High proportions of LGBTQ adults have been victims of violence and child maltreatment and may have symptoms of PTSD that affect their daily functioning. Members of sexual minority groups who are victims of hate crimes are at higher risk for depression, PTSD, anxiety, and anger than do victims of hate crimes who are not members of sexual minority groups. Young LGBTQ persons may feel alienated from or be pushed out of their families, be increasingly absent from school, and lack a connection with school and peers, and are especially likely to have suicidal ideation and to attempt suicide.

APPLICABLE LAWS AND REGULATIONS
In 2011 the United Nations High Commission for Human Rights adopted Resolution 17/19, which explicitly supports the human rights of lesbian, gay, transgender, and bisexual persons. The report presented to the High Commission in support of the resolution expressed grave concern about the global abuse and discrimination confronting this population.

The Hate Crime Statistics Act of 1990 became the first federal law in the United States to recognize and name gay, lesbian, and bisexual people as such. It requires the Attorney General of the United States to collect data on crimes committed because of the victim's race, religion, disability, sexual orientation, or ethnicity, and since 1992, the Department of Justice and the Federal Bureau of Investigation have jointly published an annual report on hate crime statistics. More than 30 states now have laws for preventing

hate crimes based on sexual orientation or gender identity. On October 28, 2009 President Barack Obama signed the Matthew Shepard and James Byrd, Jr. Hate Crimes Prevention Act, which expanded existing United States federal hate crime law to apply to crimes motivated by a victim's actual or perceived gender, sexual orientation, gender identity, or disability, and which eliminated the requirement that the victim be engaging in a federally protected activity.

Schools can be held liable for failing to protect LGBTQ youth from violence and harassment.

TREATMENT
The social worker assisting an LGBTQ individual should conduct a biological, psychological, social, and spiritual assessment that provides information about physical, mental, environmental, social, financial, spiritual, and medical factors as they relate to the individual and his or her family.

ASSESSMENTS AND SCREENING TOOLS
The mental status exam (MSE) can be used in conjunction with other questioning to establish risk.

The Scale for Suicidal Ideation (SSI) measures the intensity, pervasiveness, and characteristics of suicidal ideation.

The Center for Epidemiological Studies Depression Scale (CES-D) is an online questionnaire useful for detecting depression in adolescents.

The Beck Depression Inventory (BDI) for adults has 12 multiple-choice questions and is widely used.

The Trauma Screening Questionnaire (TSQ) has 10 items and can be used with survivors of all types of traumatic stress.

The Short Screening Test for PTSD is for survivors of all types of trauma and has seven items.

TREATMENT
Cognitive behavioral therapy (CBT) can assist individuals with histories of trauma to develop and practice new skills, and has been effective in dealing with PTSD (National Institute of Mental Health, 2016). The social worker can assist an LGBTQ individual in reducing recollections of trauma, reactions that involve avoidance and numbing of memories, and sleep problems, and in stabilizing his or her emotions. This can be facilitated by the individual's recording of intrusive thoughts or feelings, and \writing about any

traumatic experiences and exploring alternative responses to them. The social worker can also help by introducing the affected individual to a peer support group, which can help LGBTQ individuals to feel supported and less isolated, and to share information and resources (Browne et al., 2011). If no such group is available, the social workers can help to establish one. Schools can create gay–straight alliance groups to help inform and empower sexual minority adolescents (Grossman et al., 2009).

In the case of LGBTQ individuals who have lost interest or pleasure in activities, the social worker can explore the perceived causes of this and these individuals' internal dialogue about their feelings. Cognitive behavioral techniques can be used to help these individuals to identify negative cognitions and replace them with healthier ways of thinking The social worker can also refer these individuals for psychiatric medication and support if appropriate, and can help them to become part of a peer support group or network, and locate community LGBT centers.

Additionally, school-based programs and peer mediation groups have proven successful in promoting respectful relationships between LGBTQ and non-LGBTQ students, and social workers can help prevent violence toward and bullying of sexual minorities in schools by promoting and working with school administrators and community representatives to develop alliances of LGBTQ with non-LGBTQ students that enhance their communication and mutual understanding.

Social workers assisting LGBTQ individuals should be aware of their own cultural values, beliefs, and biases, and develop specialized knowledge about these individuals' histories, traditions, and values. They should adopt treatment methods that reflect their knowledge of this and of the means for promoting intergroup understanding in the communities in which they work.

APPLICABLE LAWS AND REGULATIONS

In 2009 the United States passed comprehensive hate-crime legislation that extended the 1969 federal hate-crime law to include gender, sexual orientation, gender identity, and disability.

Hate crime is also known as "bias-motivated violence."

Schools can be held liable for failing to protect LGBTQ youth from violence and harassment.

"Gay panic" is a controversial concept suggesting a negative psychosocial response by a heterosexual man to a gay man; it has been successfully used in the United States and Europe to defend men who have murdered gay men.

In some countries homosexuality is illegal and punishable with death.

Each country has its own standards for cultural competency and diversity in social work practice. Social workers must be aware of the standards of practice set forth by their governing body (National Association of Social Workers, British Association of Social Workers, etc.) and practice accordingly.

In 2011 the United Nations High Commission for Human Rights adopted Resolution 17/19, which explicitly supports the human rights of lesbian, gay, transgender, and bisexual persons. The report presented to the High Commission in support of the resolution expressed grave concern about the global abuse and discrimination this population faces.

SERVICES AND RESOURCES

The following resources can provide information about the rights of and legal protections for LGBTQ individuals:

- LAMBDA Legal, provides legal information and professional allies to the LGBTQ community, http://www.lambdalegal.org/
- The Anti-Violence Project, a New York–based nonprofit organization working toward ending hate crime against members of the LGBTQ community, http://www.avp.org
- PFLAG, http://community.pflag.org/page.aspx?pid=194
- Gay–Straight Alliance Network, fights homophobia and transphobia in schools, http://gsanetwork.org
- OutRight Action International, has information with a global perspective, https://www.outrightinternational.org/

FOOD FOR THOUGHT

Homosexuality was eliminated as a mental disorder in the *Diagnostic and Statistical Manual of Mental Disorders* (DSM) in 1973.

The World Health Organization removed homosexuality from its international classification of diseases in 1990.

Heterosexism is defined as "an ideological system that denies, denigrates, and stigmatizes any non-heterosexual form of behavior, identity, relationship, or community" (Goldberg & Smith, 2009).

Sexuality often is conflated with gender: sexuality refers to sexual attraction whereas gender refers to identity.

RED FLAGS

Being a member of a stigmatized group can cause chronic stress and put individuals at risk for mental health problems.

PTSD is extremely common among members of the LGBTQ community.

Although intimate partner violence occurs in LGBT subgroups at rates similar to those among heterosexual couples, gay men are less likely than heterosexual women to seek help and/or report the abuse (Oliffe et al., 2014).

NEXT STEPS

Ensure your client has contact details for a local LGBTQ center, where specialized information and services can be sought.

Provide referrals when indicated and linkage to support and advocacy groups and legal support if indicated.

Written by Jan Wagstaff, MA, MSW

Reviewed by Lynn B. Cooper, D. Crim, and Laura Gale, LCSW

REFERENCES

Adams, R. (1997). Preventing verbal harassment and violence toward gay and lesbian students. *Journal of School Nursing, 13*(3), 24-28.

Bakker, L. S., & Cavender, A. (2003). Promoting culturally competent care for gay youth. *Journal of School Nursing, 19*(2), 65-72.

British Association of Social Workers. (2012, January). *The Code of Ethics for Social Work: Statement of principles.* Retrieved March 23, 2016, from http://cdn.basw.co.uk/upload/basw_112315-7.pdf

Browne, K., Bakshi, L., & Lim, J. (2011). "It's something you just have to ignore": Understanding and addressing contemporary lesbian, gay, bisexual and trans safety beyond hate crime paradigms. *Journal of Social Policy, 40*(4), 739-736.

Cahill, S., & Cianciotto, J. (2004). U.S. policy interventions that can make schools safer. *Journal of Gay and Lesbian Issues in Education, 2*(1), 3-17.

Cook-Daniels, L. (2011). Institutional abuse of LGBT long-term care facility residents. *Victimization of the Elderly & Disabled, 14*(3), 37-47.

Dank, M., Lachman, P., Zweig, J., & Yahner, J. (2014). Dating violence experiences of lesbian, gay, bisexual, and transgender youth. *Journal of Youth & Adolescence, 43*(5), 846-857. doi:10.1007/s10964-013-9975-8

Estrada, R., & Marksamer, J. (2006). The legal rights of LGBT youth in state custody: What child welfare juvenile justice professionals need to know. *Child Welfare, 85*(2), 171-194.

Friedman, M. S., Marshal, M. P., Guadamuz, T. E., Wei, C., Wong, C. F., Saewyc, E. M., & Stall, R. (2011). A meta-analysis of disparities in childhood sexual abuse, parental physical abuse, and peer victimization among sexual minority and sexual nonminority individuals. *American Journal of Public Health, 101*(8), 1481-1493.

Fuller, C. B., Chang, D. F., & Rubin, L. R. (2009). Sliding under the radar: Passing and power among sexual minorities. *Journal of LGBT Issues in Counseling, 3*(2), 128-151.

Goldberg, A. E., & Smith, J. Z. (2009). Perceived parenting skill across the transition to adoptive parenthood among lesbian, gay, and heterosexual couples. *Journal of Family Psychology, 23*(6), 861-870. doi:10.1037/a0017009

Grossman, A. H., Haney, A. P., Edwards, P., Alessi, E. J., Ardon, M., & Jarrett Howell, T. (2009). Lesbian, gay, bisexual and transgender youth talk about experiencing and coping with school violence: A qualitative study. *Journal of LGBT Youth, 6*(1), 24-46.

Guarnero, P. A. (2007). Family and community influences on the social and sexual lives of Latino gay men. *Journal of Transcultural Nursing, 18*(1), 12-18.

Han, S. C., Gallagher, M. W., Franz, M. R., Chen, M. S., Cabral, F. M., & Marx, B. P. (2013). Childhood sexual abuse, alcohol use, and PTSD symptoms as predictors of adult sexual assault among lesbians and gay men. *Journal of Interpersonal Violence, 28*(12), 2505-2520. doi:10.1177/0886260513479030

Herek, G. M. (2009). Hate crimes and stigma-related experiences among sexual minority adults in the United States: Prevalence estimates from a national probability sample. *Journal of Interpersonal Violence, 24*(1), 54-74.

Hightow Weidman, L. B., Phillips, G., Jones, K. C., Outlaw, A. Y., Fields, F. D., & Smith, J. C. (2011). Racial and sexual identity-related maltreatment among minority YMSM: Prevalence, perceptions, and the association with emotional distress. *AIDS Patient Care & STDs, 25*(1), 39-45.

Home Office of the United Kingdom. (2015). Hate crime action plan: Challenge it, report it, stop it. Retrieved March 23, 2016, from https://www.gov.uk/government/publications/hate-crime-action-plan-challenge-it-report-it-stop-it

Huebner, D. M., Rebchook, G. M., & Kegeles, S. M. (2004). Experiences of harassment, discrimination, and physical violence among young gay and bisexual men. *American Journal of Public Health, 94*(7), 1200-1203.

Hyman, B. (2008). Violence in the lives of lesbian women: Implications for mental health. *Social Work in Mental Health, 7*(1-3), 204-225.

International Federation of Social Workers. (2012, March 3). Statement of Ethical Principles. Retrieved March 24, 2016, from http://ifsw.org/policies/statement-of-ethical-principles/

Kidd, J. D., & Witten, T. M. (2008). Transgender and transsexual identities: The next strange fruit-hate crimes, violence and genocide against the global trans community. *Journal of Hate Crimes, 6*(31), 31-63.

Koeppel, M. D. H., & Bouffard, L. (2014). Sexual orientation, child abuse, and intimate partner violence victimization. *Violence and Victims, 29*(3), 436-450.

Kosciw, J. G., Greytak, E. A., Palmer, N. A., & Boesen, M. J. (2014). The 2013 National School Climate Survey. Retrieved March 23, 2016, from http://www.glsen.org/sites/default/files/2013 percent-20National percent20School percent20Climate percent20Survey percent20Full percent20Report_0.pdf

Kuhar, R., & Svab, A. (2008). Homophobia and violence against gays and lesbians in Slovenia. *Revija za Sociologiju, 39*(4), 267-281.

Luo, F., Stone, D. M., & Tharp, A. T. (2014). Physical dating violence victimization among sexual minority youth. *American Journal of Public Health, 104*(10), e66-73. doi:10.2105/AJPH.2014.302051

Meyer, D. (2008). Interpreting and experiencing anti-queer violence: Race, class, and gender differences among LGBT hate crime victims. *Race, Gender & Class, 15*(3-4), 262-282.

National Association of Social Workers. (2015). Standards and Indicators for Cultural Competence in Social Work Practice. Retrieved January 22, 2016, from http://www.socialworkers.org/practice/standards/PRA-BRO-253150-CC-Standards.pdf

National Coalition of Anti-Violence Programs. (2013). Lesbian, gay, bisexual, transgender, queer, and HIV-affected hate violence in 2013. Retrieved March 23, 2016, from http://avp.org/storage/documents/2013_ncavp_hvreport_final.pdf

National Institute of Mental Health. (2016). Posttraumatic stress disorder. Retrieved April 19, 2016, from http://www.nimh.nih.gov/health/topics/post-traumatic-stress-disorder-ptsd/index.shtml

Oliffe, J. L., Han, C., Maria, E. S., Lohan, M., Howard, T., Stewart, D. E., & MacMillan, H. (2014). Gay men and intimate partner violence: A gender analysis. *Sociology of Health & Illness, 36*(4), 564-579. doi:10.1111/1467-9566.12099

O'Malley Olsen, E., Kann, L., Vivolo-Kantor, A., Kinchen, S., & McManus, T. (2014). School violence and bullying among sexual minority high school students, 2009-2011. *Journal of Adolescent Health, 55*(3), 432-480. doi:10.1016/j.jadohealth.2014.03.002

Quick Hits: Sex in the News. Lawyers debate 'gay panic' defense in murder cases. (2006). *Contemporary Sexuality, 40*(9), 8.

Roberts, A. L., Austin, B., Corliss, H. L., Vandermorris, A. K., & Koenen, K. C. (2010). Pervasive trauma exposure among US sexual orientation minority adults and risk of posttraumatic stress disorder. *American Journal of Public Health, 100*(12), 2433-2441.

Ryan, C., & Rivers, I. (2003). Lesbian, gay, bisexual and transgender youth: Victimization and its correlates in the USA and UK. *Culture, Health & Sexuality, 5*(2), 103-119.

Savage, T. A., & Harley, D. A. (2009). A place at the blackboard: Including lesbian, gay, bisexual, transgender, intersex, and queer/questioning issues in the education process. *Multicultural Education, 16*(4), 2-9.

U. S. Department of Veteran Affairs. (2015). Treatment of PTSD. Retrieved April 21, 2016, from

http://www.ptsd.va.gov/public/treatment/ther-
apy-med/treatment-ptsd.asp

Vincent, W., Parrott, D. J., & Peterson, J. L. (2011).
Combined effects of masculine gender-role stress
and sexual prejudice on anger and aggression toward gay men. *Journal of Applied Social Psychology*,
41(5), 1237-1257.

Walls, N. E., Freedenthal, S., & Wisneski, H. (2008).
Suicide ideation and attempts among sexual minority youths receiving social services. *Social Work*,
53(1), 21-29.

Wells, K. (2009). Research exploring the health, wellness, and safety concerns of sexual minority youth.
Canadian Journal of Human Sexuality, *43*(1-2), 221-229.

VIOLENCE IN ADOLESCENCE & SUBSTANCE ABUSE

MAJOR CATEGORIES: Adolescents, Substance Abuse, Violence

DESCRIPTION

Adolescent violence occurs within families, in inti-mate relationships, between friends and acquain-tances, and within communities. It includes sexual and other physical violence, emotional violence, stalking, gang violence, and bullying. Suicide and non-fatal suicidal behavior may also be considered forms of youth violence.

All forms of violence affect biological, physical, psychological, and social well-being, whether of indi-viduals, families, or entire communities. Adolescent violence is often an apparent consequence of sub-stance abuse, whereas early exposure to violence and other maltreatment by parents, which leads to feelings of worthlessness and hopelessness, and gang violence, may conversely lead to substance abuse.

Studies have found that adolescents' use of al-cohol, cigarettes, marijuana, and hard drugs, such as cocaine and heroin, increases their exposure to violence both as victims and perpetrators of it. Risk-taking behavior increases with substance use, and as substance use increases, so does violent behavior and the risk of injury. The adverse psychosocial effect in adolescence of growing up in an abusive environ-ment is well documented.

Because successful intervention in adolescent sub-stance abuse will reduce violent behavior, addressing such substance abuse should be a priority of any in-tervention plan. Intervention plans that extend be-yond individual therapy and programs are recom-mended, such as group work and family therapy. Studies stress that programs for reducing adolescent violence and substance abuse should be of sufficient duration to succeed, with brief therapies reported to have yielded mixed results.

The early identification and treatment of sub-stance abuse improves the outcomes of its treatment. Adolescents with acute levels of maltreatment tend to fare better in residential than in outpatient pro-grams. Treatment techniques underpinned by social learning theory, in which cognitive approaches are used to help the individuals being treated to develop and practice new skills, have successfully reduced substance abuse and violence. Rapport within groups and between therapists and the individuals they treat is critical for this. Motivational interviewing (MI) is effective with adolescents and has reduced violence and alcohol misuse. Family involvement is often dif-ficult to sustain but if appropriate should be pursued as a means of reducing substance abuse and violent behavior because a close emotional relationship with a parent acts as a buffer against both of these problems.

Because material deprivation, violence, and child maltreatment are strongly linked with one another at both the family and community levels, it is es-sential that social workers become knowledgeable about their effective management. For example, on a neighborhood level, the collective efficacy theory holds that neighborhood involvement by adults and communal responsibility for monitoring and, when needed, correcting the behavior of adolescents, builds trust and cohesion among all members of a community and in turn reduces both interpersonal and public violence in the community.

FACTS AND FIGURES

The 2015 Monitoring the Future national survey, an annual survey of 8th-, 10th-, and 12th-grade students in the United States, revealed that during the 30 days prior to the survey, the prevalence of the use of any illicit substance in all three grades combined was 15.9 percent; the prevalence of use of any illicit drug including inhalants was 16.8 percent; that of alcohol was 21.8 percent; and that of having been drunk was 11.0 percent. The same survey found a lifetime prevalence of use among 12th-grade students of any illicit drug of 48.9 percent; of any illicit drug including inhalants of 51.4 percent; of alcohol of 64 percent; and of having been drunk of 45.7 percent (Johnston et al., 2016).

The Youth Risk Behavior Surveillance—United States, 2013 survey revealed that nationwide, 17.9 percent of 9th- to 12th-grade students had carried a weapon (e.g., knife, gun, club) on at least one day during the prior 30 days. The same survey found that during the previous 12 months, 6.9 percent of students had been threatened with a weapon or injured on school property one or more times; 24.7 percent had been in a physical fight one or more times; 3.1 percent had sustained injury in a physical fight one or more times that required treatment by a medical professional; 14.8 percent had been bullied via electronic communications (e.g., e-mail, texting, social media); 7.3 percent had been physically forced to have sexual intercourse; and of the 73.9 percent of students who dated, 10.3 percent had been physically assaulted (e.g., hit) by the person they were dating (Kann et al., 2014). Child protective services (CPS) agencies in the United States report receiving an estimated 3.3 million reports of child abuse annually, involving the maltreatment of 6 million children, 25 percent of whom are adolescents (Temple et al., 2013). Only 10 percent of youth of 12 to 17 years of age who need treatment for substance abuse receive it (Vassalo et al., 2014).

RISK FACTORS

Exposure to substance abuse in the home, intimate partner violence (IPV), material deprivation, and childhood maltreatment can lead to depression and increase an adolescent's risk of involvement in violence and substance abuse later in life. Aggressive behavior can also lead to substance abuse and violence, and frequent consumption of alcohol during adolescence is associated with an increased risk of violence in early adulthood. Adolescents whose peers use drugs or alcohol are more likely to themselves start using them, which may lead to their persistent use. Correlations have also been found between opioid use and violent thoughts and behaviors in adolescents. Adolescents belonging to the lesbian, gay, bisexual, transgender, and questioning (LGBTQ) population, as well as adolescents growing up in the foster care system, have been found to have higher rates of substance use than others not belonging to these groups. Electronic sites used in social networking can reflect high-risk behavior among adolescents relating to sexual activity, substance abuse, and violence.

SIGNS AND SYMPTOMS

Physical signs of substance abuse include fatigue, problems with sleep, repeated health complaints, and lapses of memory. Low self-esteem, poor judgment, depression, suicidal ideation, a general lack of interest in activities, and disagreements with family members may be other signs of such abuse, as may changes in personality, sudden changes in mood, violent outbursts, irritability, lying, and irresponsible behavior. The affected adolescent may make new friendships and develop a negative attitude toward school, with falling grades, tardiness, truancy, and disciplinary problems. An adolescent's sudden loss or gain of large amounts of money can also indicate involvement in substance use.

APPLICABLE LAWS AND REGULATIONS

In the United States, the minimum legal age for the consumption of alcohol is 21 years.

The production, sale, and use of psychoactive substances, such as cannabis, amphetamines, cocaine, and opioids, and the nonprescribed use of psychoactive prescription medications, has legal consequences that depend on the jurisdiction in which such sale and use occurs.

ASSESSMENT

The social worker assisting an adolescent who exhibits substance abuse and violent behavior should conduct a biological, psychological, social, and spiritual assessment of the youngster and seek to identify any psychological or physical trauma he or she may experience as a result of maltreatment. This should include questions about mood fluctuations, irritability, depression, feelings of worthlessness, and suicidal ideation; attitudes toward school; academic performance; disciplinary problems; and legal problems. The social worker should also explore the use of drugs and alcohol by members of the adolescent's immediate and extended family, his or her familial relationships and personal friendships, and the activities that the adolescent shares with his or her family.

Ask about mood fluctuations, irritability, depression, feelings of worthlessness, and suicidal ideation.

Explore attitudes toward school; ask about academic performance, discipline problems, and legal problems.

ASSESSMENTS AND SCREENING TOOLS

The Drug Use Screening Inventory (DUSI-R) has 159 questions covering 10 psychosocial domains and includes a validated violence proneness scale for adolescents.

The CRAFFT assessment tool, designed for adolescents, has six questions about alcohol and other drugs. CRAFFT is an acronym of key words in the six screening questions.

The Simple Screening Instrument for Alcohol and Other Drugs (SSI-AOD) has 16 questions that require a yes or no response.

The Adolescent Alcohol Involvement Scale (AAIS) is a 14-item, self-report questionnaire that examines the type and frequency of alcohol use as well as several behavioral and perceptual aspects of drinking.

The Adolescent Drinking Index has 24 items that examine adolescent drinking by measuring psychological symptoms, physical symptoms, social symptoms, and loss of control.

The Rutgers Alcohol Problem Index (RAPI) uses a 23-item measure of consequences of adolescent alcohol use pertaining to family life, social relations, psychological functioning, delinquency, physical problems, and neuropsychological functioning.

The Adolescent Obsessive–Compulsive Drinking Scale (A–OCDS) has 14 items that assess for problem drinking. This instrument contains one scale that measures obsessive thoughts about drinking and a second scale that measures compulsive drinking behaviors.

The Conflict Tactics Scales (CTS) measure the presence (although not the motivation or context) of violence between partners (CTS2) or parents and children (CTSPC). They are used primarily in research but can be used in clinical settings.

Appropriate medical and/or laboratory tests can be ordered for injuries from violence experienced by the adolescent and for substances that he or she may be using.

Tests (e.g., urine, blood, breathalyzer) may be done to check for the presence of substances.

TREATMENT

MI can teach risk-benefit analysis and help increase consequential awareness. CBT can help address skill deficits and teach alternative responses.

Adolescent is experiencing poor family relations and community dysfunction.

Multidimensional family therapy with individual and family sessions, visitations with extended family members if indicated.

Group therapy for adolescents can enhance their interpersonal learning and facilitate cognitive, affective, and behavioral changes in them (Dartnell, 2013). Groups of small to medium size are recommended, and can help adolescents who have feelings of worthlessness, mistrust, or anger. Individual and group therapy can increase adolescents' self-esteem; and anger-management techniques can help adolescents with regulation of their emotions. Group therapies for adolescents should include didactic presentations covering the consequences of their behavior.

Cognitive behavioral therapy (CBT) can help address deficits in skills, and assists in the development and rehearsal of new skills (Becker, 2013). It can be used in one-to-one sessions or within groups, and can help adolescents to stop engaging in violence, substance abuse, and risk-taking behavior. Therapists using CBT, together with the adolescents they are assisting to cease violence and substance abuse, examine the situations that lead to these problems and suggest alternative ways of behaving.

Motivational interviewing (MI) has been shown to work well with adolescents. In MI the social worker creates a positive, empathic atmosphere that avoids argumentation, facilitates mutual trust, and encourages self-efficacy as the individual being treated engages in risk-benefit analysis of the use of drugs (McKenna et al., 2013).

Multidimensional family therapy (MDFT) is an intensive intervention that focuses on roles, interactions, and other problem areas at the individual, family, and community level (Schaub et al., 2014). With MDFT the therapist meets with individuals, organizes family-group sessions, meets with the extended family, and makes information-gathering visits to schools and neighborhoods. This technique can be helpful to adolescents experiencing poor family relations and community dysfunction.

Another technique, which has been found to be effective in helping young persons in foster-care settings, is Multidimensional Treatment Foster Care (MTFC). In this technique, the foster parents of a young person go through detailed training regimens in behavioral management and participate in weekly support meetings for families. The program also has individual therapy sessions for the young person involved in it (Rhoades et al., 2013). The support of parents/caregivers and other family members is found to be a universal protective factor for adolescents against violence and substance abuse.

Social workers should be aware of their own cultural values, beliefs, and biases, and develop specialized knowledge about the histories, traditions, and values of the young persons they assist in managing violence and substance abuse. They should adopt treatment methods that reflect their knowledge of the cultural diversity of the communities in which these youngsters live.

APPLICABLE LAWS AND REGULATIONS
In the United States, the minimum legal age for the consumption of alcohol is 21 years.

Alcohol use by adolescents is a leading cause of global morbidity and mortality; the vast majority of countries set a legal age at which individuals can buy and consume alcohol. The most common age is 18 years, in some countries it is 16, and in a small number of countries, including the United States, the age requirement is 21. In a small number of countries drinking is forbidden; dozens of others have no laws limiting alcohol consumption or purchase by age.

Each country has its own standards for cultural competency and diversity in social work practice. Social workers must be aware of the standards of practice set forth by their governing body (e.g., in the United States the National Association of Social Workers, in England the British Association of Social Workers) and practice accordingly.

SERVICES AND RESOURCES
The following resources can provide information about adolescent substance abuse and violence:
- YourHealthCheck has various online screening and treatment tools for substance abuse and mental health, http://www.yourhealthcheck.org
- National Institute on Drug Abuse (NIDA); information and a rapid screening tool for alcohol and other substance abuse, http://www.drugabuse.gov
- NIDA for Teens; educational material, blogs, games, and videos for youth, parents, and teachers

on the science behind drug abuse, http://www.teens.drugabuse.gov
- Substance Abuse and Mental Health Services Administration (SAMHSA); information about substance abuse, prevention, and treatment, http://www.samhsa.gov/
- KidsHealth; provides information and advice on health for parents, kids, and teens, http://kidshealth.org
- U.S. Centers for Disease Control & Prevention, Division of Violence Prevention; provides resources for parents and youth, http://www.cdc.gov/ViolencePrevention/youthviolence/index.html
- The Center for the Study and Prevention of Violence at the University of Colorado Boulder; information and resources available for school-based prevention of violence, http://www.colorado.edu/cspv

FOOD FOR THOUGHT
High-risk behavior by adolescents, such as sexual activity, substance abuse, and violence, frequently is displayed on social networking sites.

Some studies have shown that because adolescents learn from their experiences, exposure to risk can help youth build resiliency and avoid victimization. At which point this exposure becomes detrimental is highly individualized.

Girls are more likely to internalize their stress responses and have higher rates of depression and anxiety in response to violence whereas boys tend to externalize their responses with antisocial behavior and risk-taking.

Having a strong connection to parents/caregivers and parents'/caregivers' physical presence in the home have been associated with lower levels of substance use among adolescents.

RED FLAGS
Adolescents involved in violence and substance abuse are highly likely to have histories of maltreatment.

Adolescents in the United States are more likely to be victims of violent crime than adults.

NEXT STEPS
Adolescents and their families may need extensive support with frequent follow-ups and reinforcements.

Assist client in identifying triggers for substance use. Discuss alternatives to substance use and identify strategies to improve coping and problem-solving skills.

Provide referrals to substance abuse treatment programs, mental health services, and recovery support group to support long-term substance-free recovery.

Written by Jan Wagstaff, MA, MSW, and Michael James White, MSW, PPSC

Reviewed by Laura McLuckey, MSW, LCSW

REFERENCES

Becker, S. J. (2013). Adolescent substance abuse: National trends, consequences, and promising treatments. *Brown University Child & Adolescent Behavior Letter, 29*(5), 1-7.

Brunelle, N., Tremblay, J., Blanchette-Martin, N., Gendron, A., & Tessier, M. (2014). Relationships between drugs and delinquency in adolescence: Influence of gender and victimization experiences. *Journal of Child & Adolescent Substance Abuse, 23*(1), 19-28. doi:10.1080/1067828X.2012.735488

Butler Center for Research. (2011). Research update: Youth violence and alcohol/drug abuse. Retrieved April 16, 2015, from http://www.hazelden.org/web/public/researchupdates.page

Casanueva, C., Stambaugh, L., Urato, M., Fraser, J. G., & Williams, J. (2014). Illicit drug use from adolescence to young adulthood among child-welfare involved youths. *Journal of Child and Adolescent Substance Abuse, 23*(1), 29-48. doi:10.1080/1067828X.2012.735514

Dartnell, D. (2013, July). Group therapy for bereaved adolescents: If you are old enough to love you are old enough to grieve. In *The Group Psychologist* (pp. 7-10).

Doherty, E., Robertson, J. A., Green, K. M., Fothergill, K. E., & Ensminger, M. E. (2012). A longitudinal study of substance use and violent victimization in adulthood among a cohort of urban African Americans. *Addiction, 107*(2), 339-348. doi:10.1111/j.1360-0443.2011.03665.x

Draucker, C. B., & Mazurczyk, J. (2013). Relationships between childhood sexual abuse and substance use and sexual risk behaviors during adolescence: An integrative review. *Nursing Outlook, 61*(5), 291-310. doi:10.1016/j.outlook.2012.12.003

Espelage, D. L., Low, S., Rao, M, Hong, J. S., & Little, T. D. (2014). Family violence, bullying, fighting, and substance use among adolescents: A longitudinal mediational model. *Journal of Research on Adolescence, 24*(2), 337-349. doi:10.1111/jora.12060

Fagan, A. A., Wright, E. M., & Pinchevsky, G. M. (2014). The protective effects on neighborhood collective efficacy on adolescent substance use and violence following exposure to violence. *Journal of Youth & Adolescence, 43*(9), 1498-1512.

Green, K. M., Doherty, E. E., Zebrak, K. A., & Ensminger, M. E. (2011). Association between adolescent drinking and adult violence: Evidence from a longitudinal study of urban African Americans. *Journal of Studies on Alcohol & Drugs, 72*(5), 701-710.

Haggerty, K. P., McGlynn-Wright, A., & Klima, T. (2013). Promising parenting programs for reducing adolescent problem behaviors. *Journal of Children's Services, 8*(4), 229-243. doi:10.1108/JCS-04-2013-0016

International Federation of Social Workers. (2012, March 3). Statement of Ethical Principles. Retrieved April 16, 2015, from http://ifsw.org/policies/statement-of-ethical-principles/

Johnston, L. D., O'Malley, P. M., Miech, R. A., Bachman, J. G., & Schulenberg, J. E. (2016). Monitoring the future national survey result on drug use, 197502015: Overview, key findings on adolescent drug use.

Jolly, K., Archibald, C., & Liehr, P. (2013). Risk taking in first and second generation Afro-Caribbean adolescents: An emerging challenge for school nurses. *Journal of Nursing, 29*(5), 353-360. doi:10.1177/1059840513475819

Kann, L., Kinchen, S., Shanklin, S. L., Flint, K. H., Hawkins, J., Harris, W. A., ... Zaza, S. (2014). Youth Risk Behavior Surveillance – United States, 2013. *MMWR, 63*(4). Retrieved from http://www.cdc.gov/mmwr/pdf/ss/ss6304.pdf

Lamont, A., Woodlief, D., & Malone, P. (2014). Predicting high-risk versus higher-risk substance use during late adolescence from early adolescent risk factors using latent class analysis. *Addiction Research and Theory, 22*(1), 78-89. doi:10.3109/16066359.2013.772587

Mckenna, C., Gines, B., Hatfield, C., Helman, S., Meyer, L., Rennick, C., ... Zaremski, J. (2013). Implementation of a screening, brief intervention, and referral to treatment program using the electronic medical record in a pediatric trauma center. *Journal of Trauma Nursing, 20*(1), 16-23. doi:10.1097/JTN.0b013e3182866221

Mills, R., Alati, R., Strathearn, L., & Najman, J. (2014). Alcohol and tobacco use among maltreated and non-maltreated adolescents in a birth cohort. *Addiction, 109*(4), 672-680. doi:10.1111/add.1244

Murphy, S. M., McPHerson, S., & Robinson, K. (2014). Non-medical prescription opioid use and violent behavior among adolescents. *Journal of Child & Adolescent Mental Health, 26*(1), 35-47.

National Institute on Drug Abuse. (2014). Drug facts: Nationwide Trends. Retrieved April 16, 2015, from http://www.drugabuse.gov/publications/drugfacts/nationwide-trends

\http://cdn.basw.co.uk/upload/basw_112315-7.pdf

Principles of adolescent substance use disorder treatment: A research-based guide. (2014). *National Institute on drug abuse.* Retrieved April 16, 2015, from http://www.drugabuse.gov/sites/default/files/podata_1_17_14.pdf

Rhoades, K. A., Chamberlain, P., Roberts, R., & Leve, L. D. (2013). MFTC for high-risk adolescent girls: A comparison of outcomes in England and the United States. *Journal of Child & Adolescent Substance Abuse, 22*(5), 435-449.

Saldana, L., Smith, D., & Weber, E. (2013). Adolescent onset of maternal substance abuse: Descriptive findings from a feasibility trail. *Journal of Child & Adolescent Substance Abuse, 22*(5), 407-420.

Sartor, C. E., Waldron, M., Duncan, A. E., Grant, J. D., McCutcheon, V. V., Nelson, E. C., ... Heath, A. C. (2013). Childhood sexual abuse and early substance use in adolescent girls: The role of familial influences. *Addiction (Abington, England), 108*(5), 993-1000. doi:10.1111/add.12115

Schaub, M. P., Henderson, C. E., Pelc, I., Tossmann, P., Phan, O., Hendriks, V., ... Rigter, H. (2014). Multidimensional family therapy decreases the rate of externalising behavioural disorder symptoms in cannabis abusing adolescents: Outcomes of the INCANT trial. *BMC Psychiatry, 14*(1), 1-16. doi:10.1186/1471-244X-14-26

Schiff, M., Plotnikova, M., Dingle, K., Williams, G. M., Najman, J., & Clavarino, A. (2014). Does adolescent's exposure to parental intimate partner conflict and violence predict psychological distress and substance use in young adulthood? A longitudinal study. *Child Abuse & Neglect, 38*(12), 1945-1954.

Smith, D. K., & Saldana, L. (2013). Trauma, delinquency, and substance use: co-occurring problems for adoelscent girls in the juvenile justice system. *Journal of Child & Adolescent Substance Abuse, 22*(5), 450-465.

Temple, J., Shorey, R., Fite, P., Stuart, G., & Le, V. (2013). Substance use as a longitudinal predictor of the perpetration of teen dating violence. *Journal of Youth & Adolescence, 42*(4), 596-606. doi:10.1007/s10964-012-9877-1

Vassallo, S., Edwards, B., Renda, J., & Olsson, C. C. (2014). Bullying in adolescents and antisocial behavior and depression six years later: What are protective factors? *Journal of School Violence, 13*(1), 100-124. doi:10.1080/15388220.2013.840643

Wheeler, D. (2015). NASW standards and indicators for cultural competence in social work practice. Retrieved April 4, 2016, from http://www.socialworkers.org/practice/standards/PRA-BRO-253150-CC-Standards.pdf

Whiteside, L. K., Walton, M. A., Bohnert, A., Blow, F. C., Bonar, E., Ehrlich, P., & Cunningham, R. (2013). Nonmedical prescription opioid and sedative use among adolescents in the emergency department. *Pediatrics, 132*(5), 825-832. doi:10.1542/peds.2013-0721

VIOLENCE IN ADOLESCENCE: BULLYING

MAJOR CATEGORIES: Adolescents, Violence

DESCRIPTION/ETIOLOGY
Bullying among adolescents is intentional and repeated aggressive behavior on the part of one individual toward another that causes injury or discomfort. It most often takes the form of attacks or intimidation of a less powerful person with the intention to cause fear, harm, or distress(American Psychological Association, n.d.).Bullying may consist of verbal, physical, or social aggression (e.g., gossip, demeaning gestures, social exclusion). Bullying is a crime and criminal investigations and charges can result. Among adolescents, peer harassment peaks between the ages of 11 and 15 and then declines among older adolescents. Adolescents may be perpetrators of bullying, victims, or both.

Bullying frequently occurs when adolescents are unsupervised; for instance, on playgrounds, in lunchrooms and bathrooms, and on school buses. Boys bully more often than girls and are more likely to use physical forms of aggression, which is considered a direct form of harassment. Females who bully are more likely to use indirect harassment, such as slandering and social exclusion. A growing number of adolescents experience sexual harassment at school. Cyberbullying, a growing phenomenon, is an indirect form of aggression that occurs via personal computers and cell phones. Adolescents who are cyberbullied often are bullied in person as well.

Adolescent bullying occurs predominantly within the school context because school is a peer-intensive social environment. Victims typically are younger than the perpetrator, and boys are bullied more often than girls. Victims often are different in physical appearance from the bully. Adolescents can be bullied because of disability, race, sexual orientation, or gender nonconformity. They may be bullied because they have same-sex parents. It is important to understand that bullying extends beyond the bully/victim dyad: an entire peer group may be involved in bullying, in which individuals fulfill different roles in the social context of the harassment, most frequently as passive bystanders.

Being victimized can adversely impact academic achievement and participation in extracurricular school activities. Bullying can cause poor physical and mental health and increase the risk of substance abuse and suicide. Victims feel lonely and isolated. Adolescents with the lowest self-esteem are more likely to be victimized. There is disagreement as to whether perpetrators also have low self-esteem: some

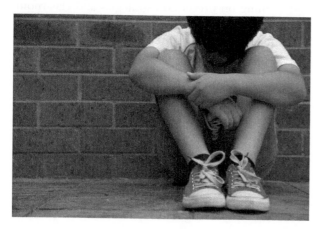

bullies are well connected with their peers and like to dominate, whereas others are more isolated and appear depressed or anxious. In most cases, both bullies and their victims have lower school attachment and often are uninvolved with their peers. Some adolescents oscillate between being a victim and being a bully; such children have high levels of social avoidance and conduct problems. Adolescent bullying victims are especially vulnerable to psychiatric disorders.

Victimized adolescents are unlikely to seek help from teachers or other adults. It is recommended that school staff consider possible bullying when students report with somatic symptoms such as headaches, stomachaches, and/or trouble eating or sleeping. Researchers have found that parental support and a good parent and child relationship help prevent adolescents from becoming bullies and protect them from being bullied. Friendship can also help protect children from becoming targets of bullies. Peer mediation, conflict-resolution classes, anger-management training, diversity and tolerance education, and increased adult supervision all help to lessen, prevent, and stop bullying in schools. Preventive efforts need to be community-wide.

FACTS AND FIGURES

It is estimated that nearly 30 percent of all school-aged children in the United States are involved in bullying, either as perpetrators, victims, or bystanders (National Center for Educational Statistics, 2013)

In the United States 56 percent of students have witnessed some type of bullying at school (MBNBD, n.d.)

Students with physical and mental disabilities as well as those who identify as gay, lesbian, bisexual, transgender, or queer/questioning (LGBTQ) are at a higher risk of being victims of bullying

Most bullying is unreported. Many students decide not to report instances of bullying because of social pressure, fear, guilt, or embarrassment. More than 25 percent of bullied youth do not tell anyone and nearly 20 percent do not talk about it with their parents (Anti-Bullying Alliance, n.d.)

Fifty percent of all bullying is seen to cease when someone intervenes, whether a peer, parent, or teacher

In the United States 15 percent of school absenteeism is directly related to fears of being bullied at school (MBNBD, n.d.)

RISK FACTORS

There is an increased risk of depression, self-harm, violent ideation, suicidal ideation, and suicide among perpetrators and victims of bullying. Victimization also causes emotional distress, anger, and embarrassment; increases risk for drug and/or alcohol use; and is linked with a drop in school performance and attendance. Studies of perpetrators indicate that adolescents who bully also have an elevated risk for these problems (Centers for Disease Control and Prevention, 2012). Adolescents who are perceived to be physically different from their peers have an elevated risk of being bullied. LGBTQ adolescents are much more likely to be bullied than heterosexual adolescents. Adolescents perceived as weak or unable to defend themselves, those who are depressed or anxious, those with physical or mental disabilities, those with low self-esteem, and those who are less popular or who do not get along well with others are at risk of being bullied. Having witnessed intimate partner violence at home also increases the risk of being bullied. Bullies are at risk for continuing patterns of antisocial behavior in later adolescence.

SIGNS AND SYMPTOMS

Victims of bullying often exhibit sleeplessness, nightmares, depression, and somatic symptoms such as headaches and stomachaches. Changes in eating habits, such as binge eating or skipping meals, may occur. As bullying continues, the adolescent may increasingly be absent from school and may avoid certain activities. A change in academic performance or loss of interest in schoolwork may be a sign of victimization. There may be unexplained injuries. Victims may exhibit self-destructive behaviors such as running away, using drugs and/or alcohol, and threatening or attempting suicide. They may fantasize about violence and/or express a desire to carry a weapon.

ASSESSMENT

Complete a biopsychosocialspiritual assessment to include information on physical, mental, environmental, social, and spiritual factors as they relate to the adolescent and his or her family.

The social worker should include parents, siblings, and teachers in the assessment process because they are a valuable source of information about the adolescent.

Ensure adolescents have ample opportunity to talk about their past and present experiences.

Gather the adolescent's history and ask him or her to describe any victimizing events he or she has experienced.

Interview the family and assess for poor communication and intimate partner violence.

ASSESSMENTS AND SCREENING TOOLS

The Scale for Suicidal Ideation (SSI) measures the intensity, pervasiveness, and characteristics of suicidal ideation and can be used with adolescents.

The Center for Epidemiological Studies—Depression Scale (CES-D) is an online questionnaire useful for detecting depression in adolescents.

The Children's Depression Inventory has 28 items and can be used to screen children ages 7 to 17.

Tools used to assess family/systems relationships include genograms and ecomaps.

TREATMENT

When an adolescent is suspected of bullying, the parent should talk with the adolescent and his or her teacher, principal, school counselor, pediatrician and/or family physician; a plan of action to stop the bullying should be established (ACAP, 2011). If he or she does not stop bullying then the adolescent should be evaluated by a mental health professional (ACAP, 2011). Victims of bullying should be given opportunities to talk about their experiences and should be reassured that the bullying is not their fault (ACAP, 2011). Peer mediation, conflict resolution classes, anger management training, and increased adult supervision in schools can help lessen, stop, and prevent bullying (ACAP, 2011). Clinical programs involving intensive staff training on prevention strategies and classroom education programs have been found to be effective as well. Supportive and preventive counseling for students both ameliorates past instances of bullying and discourages future ones (Tsiantis et al., 2013). Programs increasing the ability and willingness of school staff to notice and interfere with instances of bullying, as well as encouraging students to do the same, yield positive results (Banas, 2014). Another strategy is for schools to include diversity and tolerance education in their curricula (NCPC, n.d.). Poster campaigns addressing bullying were shown in several schools to reduce bullying (Wesley Perkins et al., 2011). Programs focusing on building and maintaining a positive school community and increasing connectedness of staff members have been found effective in reducing instances of bullying as well as preventing escalation of any bullying that does take place (O'Brennan et al., 2014). The Olweus Bullying Prevention Program has had success in reducing bullying in schools (Violence Prevention Works, n.d.).

Social workers should be aware of their own cultural values, beliefs, and biases and develop specialized knowledge about the histories, traditions, and values of their clients. Social workers should adopt treatment methodologies that reflect their knowledge of the cultural diversity of the communities in which they practice.

Problem	Goal	Intervention
Adolescent is bullying another	Stop bullying	Talk to the child and his/her parent/s about what is happening. If bullying does not stop, suggest an evaluation from a mental health professional. These are important steps to follow for victims and perpetrators alike
Adolescent is a victim of bullying	Stop the bullying	Gather adolescent's history of victimization. Provide opportunity for the adolescent to explain what is happening. Have the adolescent practice what he or she will say to the bully. Help the adolescent practice being assertive. Pursue peer mediation. Encourage the adolescent to travel back and forth to school with friends. Contact the police if there are any threats of harm
Bullying is occurring in a school	Prevent bullying	Diversity and tolerance education, conflict resolution classes, anger management training, and/or increased adult supervision in school

APPLICABLE LAWS AND REGULATIONS

Every U.S. state has enacted laws and/or policies that address bullying (FindLaw, n.d.). State laws and policies address bullying in different ways.

School bullying can result in criminal charges of assault, battery, and harassment. Parents can also bring civil lawsuits on behalf of their victimized children.

Laws, ordinances, and policies in the United Kingdom that address acts committed by bullies include the Protection from Harassment Act of 1997, the Malicious Communication Act of 1998, the Communication Act of 2003, the Crime Disorder Act of 1998, and the Computer Misuse Act of 1999 (NoBullying.com, 2014).

Each country has its own standards for cultural competency and diversity in social work practice.

Social workers must be aware of the standards of practice set forth by their governing body (National Association of Social Workers, British Association of Social Workers, etc.) and practice accordingly.

SERVICES AND RESOURCES

- BullyVille, http://www.bullyville.com
- Violence Prevention Works!, http://www.violencepreventionworks.org
- StopBullying.gov, http://www.stopbullying.gov
- Bullying. No Way! http://www.bullyingnoway.gov.au
- Anti-Bullying Alliance, http://www.anti-bullyingalliance.org.uk/
- Teaching Tolerance, http://www.tolerance.org
- National Crime Prevention Council, http://www.ncpc.org

FOOD FOR THOUGHT

Adolescents frequently do not seek adult assistance with their conflicts and often must deal with bullying by themselves.

Adolescents may seek emotional support without identifying a specific bullying problem.

Countries with greater wealth inequality have higher rates of adolescent bullying (Elgar et al., 2009).

Bullying can lead to emotional disturbances in adulthood for victims and perpetrators.

The strongest motivation for perpetrators of school shootings is revenge for bullying (MBNBD, n.d.).

RED FLAGS

Unlike other types of victimization among adolescents, racial victimization has been shown not to diminish as perpetrators age.

Adolescents who are bullied may suddenly for undisclosed reasons not want to attend school or spend time with peers who had been their friends.

Adolescents exposed to parental conflict and physical punishment may be more prone to bully. Likewise, adolescents who experience more parental warmth and guidance are less likely to be perpetrators and show more resilience if they are victims of bullying.

Adolescents who bully are more likely to perpetrate intimate partner violence and their relationships are more likely to be characterized by negative qualities such as lack of communication skills and use of coercion or threats (Ellis & Wolfe, 2014).

NEXT STEPS

Provide referrals when indicated and link families to services that support the entire family system.

Maintain contact and follow up with adolescents whenever possible.

Provide additional information about bullying, including:

- Bullying: What Parents Can Do About It, http://extension.psu.edu/publications/ui368/view
- Creating a Safe and Caring Home, http://www.schoolclimate.org/parents/safeHome.php

Written by Jan Wagstaff, MA, MSW, and Laura McLuckey, MSW, LCSW

Reviewed by Lynn B. Cooper, D. Crim, and Jennifer Teska, MSW

REFERENCES

Academy of Child & Adolescent Psychiatry (ACAP). (2011). Facts for families: Bullying. Retrieved April 10, 2015, from http://aacap.org/page.ww?name=Bullying&section=Facts+for+Families

Albdour, K. (2014). Bullying and victimization among African American adolescents: a literature review. *Journal of Child and Adolescent Psychiatric Nursing, 27*(2), 68.

Ami, A., & Chandra-Mouli, V. (2014). Empowering adolescent girls: Developing egalitarian gender norms and relations to end violence. *Reproductive Health, 11*(1), 75-77. doi:10.1186/1742-4755-11-75

Anti Bullying Alliance. (n.d.). The problem of bullying in the U.K. Retrieved April 9, 2015, from http://www.antibullyingalliance.org.uk/

Banas, J. R. (2014). Impact of authentic learning exercises on preservice teachers' self-efficacy to perform bullying prevention tasks. *American Journal of Health Education, 45*(4), 239-248. doi:10.1080/19325037.2014.916634

Blood, G. (2014). BULLYING BE GONE. *ASHA Leader, 19*(5), 36-43.

British Association of Social Workers. (2012). The Code of Ethics for Social Work: Statement of Principles. Retrieved April 8, 2015, from http://cdn.basw.co.uk/upload/basw_112315-7.pdf

Chan, H. C. O., & Chui, W. H. (2013). Social bonds and school bullying: A study of Macanese male adolescents on bullying perpetration and peer victimization. *Child & Youth Care Forum, 42*(6), 599-616. doi:10.1007/s10566-013-9221-2

Chui, W. H., & Chan, H. C. (2013). Association between self-control and school bullying among Macanese adolescents. *Child Abuse & Neglect, 37*(4), 237-242. doi:10.1016/j.chiabu.2012.12.003

Debnam, K. J., Johnson, S. L., & Bradshaw, C. P. (2014). Examining the association between bullying and adolescent concerns about dating violence. *The Journal of School Health, 84*(7), 421-428. doi:10.1111/josh.12170

Elgar, R. J., Craig, W., Boyce, W., Morgan, A., & Vella-Zarb, R. (2009). Income inequality and school bullying: Multilevel study of adolescents in 37 countries. *Journal of Adolescent Health, 45*(4), 351-359. doi:10.1016/j.jadohealth.2009.04.004

Ellis, W. E., & Wolfe, D. A. (2014). Bullying predicts reported dating violence and observed qualities in adolescent dating relationships. *Journal of*

Interpersonal Violence. Advance online publication. doi:10.1177/0886260514554428 1-22

Espelage, D. L., Low, S., Rao, M, Hong, J. S., & Little, T. D. (2014). Family violence, bullying, fighting, and substance use among adolescents: A longitudinal mediational model. *Journal of Research on Adolescence, 24*(2), 337-349. doi:10.1111/jora.12060

Garandeau, C. F., Lee, I. A., & Salmivalli, C. (2014). Inequality matters: Classroom status hierarchy and adolescents' bullying. *Journal of Youth and Adolescence, 43*(7), 1123-1133. doi:10.1007/s10964-013-0040-4

Hellstrom, L., Beckman, L., & Hagquist, C. (2013). Self-reported peer victimization: Concordance and discordance between measures of bullying and peer aggression among Swedish adolescents. *Journal of School Violence, 12*(4), 395-413. doi:10.1080/15388220.2013.825626

Hilliard, L. J., Bowers, E. P., Greenman, K. N., Hershberg, R. M., Geldof, G. J., Glickman, S. A., ... Lerner, R. M. (2014). Beyond the deficit model: Bullying and trajectories of character virtues in adolescents. *Journal of Youth and Adolescence, 43*(6), 991-1003. doi:10.1007/s10964-014-0094-y

International Federation of Social Workers. (2012). Statement of Ethical Principles. Retrieved April 8, 2015, from http://ifsw.org/policies/statement-of-ethical-principles/

Kira, I. A., Lewandowski, L., Ashby, J. S., Somers, C., Chiodo, L., & Odenat, L. (2014). Does bullying victimization suppress IQ? The effects of bullying on IQ in Iraqi and African American adolescents: A traumatology perspective. *Journal of Aggression, Maltreatment & Trauma, 23*(5), 431-453. doi:10.1080/10926771.2014.904463

Kodzopeljic, J., Smederevac, S., Miltrovic, D., Dinic, B., & Colovic, P. (2014). School bullying in adolescence and personality traits: A person-centered approach. *Journal of Interpersonal Violence, 29*(4), 536-757. doi:10.1177/0886260513505216

Melander, L. A., Sittner Harshorn, K. J., & Whitbeck, L. B. (2013). Correlates of bullying behaviors among a sample of North American indigenous adolescents. *Journal of Adolescents, 36*(4), 675-684. doi:10.1016/j.adolescence.2013.05.003

Mizrahi, T., & Mayden, R. W. (2001). NASW Standards for Cultural Competence in Social Work Practice. Retrieved April 8, 2015, from http://www.socialworkers.org/practice/standards/NASWCulturalStandards.pdf

National Crime Prevention Center (NCPC). Strategies. Retrieved April 10, 2015, from http://www.ncpc.org/topics/bullying/strategies

O'Brennan, L. M., Waasdorp, T. E., & Bradshaw, C. P. (2014). Strengthening bullying prevention through school staff connectedness. *Journal of Educational Psychology, 106*(3), 870-880. doi:10.1037/a0035957

Tsiantis, A. J., Beratis, I. N., Syngelaki, E. M., Stefanakou, A., Asimopoulos, C., Sideridis, G. D., & Tsiantis, J. (2013). The effects of a clinical prevention program on bullying, victimization, and attitudes toward school of elementary school students. *Behavioral Disorders, 38*(4), 243-257.

Vassallo, S., Edwards, B., Renda, J., & Olsson, C. C. (2014). Bullying in adolescents and antisocial behavior and depression six years later: What are protective factors? *Journal of School Violence, 13*(1), 100-124. doi:10.1080/15388220.2013.840643

Violence Prevention Works. Olweus Bullying Prevention Program (BPP). Retrieved April 10, 2015, from http://www.violencepreventionworks.org

Wesley Perkins, H., Craig, D. W., & Perkins, J. M. (2011). Using social norms to reduce bullying: A research intervention among adolescents in five middle schools. *Group Processes & Intergroup Relations, 14*(5), 703-702.

Yen, C. F., Yang, P., Wang, P. W., Lin, H. C., Liu, T. L., Wu, Y. Y., & Tang, T. C. (2014). Association between school bullying levels/types and mental health problems among Taiwanese adolescents. *Comprehensive Psychiatry, 55*(3), 405-413. doi:10.1016/j.comppsych.2013.06.001

Ziv, Y., Leibovich, I., & Shechtman, Z. (2013). Bullying and victimization in early adolescence: Relations to social processing patterns. *Aggressive Behavior, 39*(6), 482-492. doi:10.1002/ab.21494

Zottis, G., Salum, G. A., Isolan, L. R., Manfro, G. G., & Heidi, E. (2014). Associations between child disciplinary practices and bullying behavior in adolescents. *Jornal De Pediatria, 93*(4), 408. doi:10.1016/j.jped.2013.12.009

U.S. Department of Education, National Center for Educational Statistics. (2013). Student reports of bullying and cyber-bullying: Results from the 2011 School Crime Supplement to the National Crime Victimization Survey. Retrieved

April 11, 2015, from http://nces.ed.gov/pubs2013/2013329.pdf

U.S. Department of Education, National Center for Educational Statistics. (2013). *Student reports of bullying and cyber-bullying: Results from the 2011 School Crime Supplement to the National Crime Victimization Survey.* Retrieved April 11, 2015, from http://nces.ed.gov/pubs2013/2013329.pdf

Centers for Disease Control, National Center for Injury Prevention and Control. (2012). Understanding bullying. Retrieved April 11, 2015, from http://www.cdc.gov/violenceprevention/pdf/bullyingfactsheet2012-a.pdf

American Psychological Association. (n.d.). Bullying. Retrieved April 11, 2015, from http://www.apa.org/topics/bullying/

Bullying and the law in the U.K. (2014). *NoBullying.com.* Retrieved April 11, 2015, from http://nobullying.com/bullying-and-the-laws-in-the-uk/

Facts & statistics: The numbers continue to rise every month. (n.d.). *MBNBD.* Retrieved April 30, 2015, from http://www.makebeatsnotbeatdowns.org/facts_new.html

Specific state laws against bullying. (n.d.). *FindLaw.* Retrieved June 26, 2015, from http://education.findlaw.com/student-conduct-and-discipline/specific-state-laws-against-bullying.html

VIOLENCE IN ADOLESCENCE: GENDER DIFFERENCES IN PERPETRATORS

MAJOR CATEGORIES: Adolescents, Violence

WHAT WE KNOW

Adolescent violence perpetration is a complex global public health problem, interconnected with gender, ethnicity, race, family, community, peers, delinquency, poverty, and disadvantage.

Adolescent violence may include bullying; sexual or physical assault, including intimate partner violence (IPV or dating violence) and community violence (i.e., violence that takes place in public places, such as gang violence or school shootings); and homicide.

The majority of adolescent homicide perpetrators and victims worldwide are males.

Homicide is the fourth leading cause of death among youth 10–29 years of age worldwide; it is the leading cause of death for black males 12–19 years of age in the United States.

In the United States, juvenile offenders accounted for 17 percent of all serious violent crime arrests in 2013. The rate of serious violent crimes among youth ages 12–17 is 9 crimes per 1, 000 youth.

In a 2013 United States sample of youth in grades 9–12, 28 percent of males and almost 8 percent of females reported that they had carried a weapon (e.g., knife, gun) during the past 30 days; 8 percent of males and 3 percent of females reported that they had carried a weapon to school.

Males were significantly more likely than females to carry a gun (9.4 percent versus 1.6 percent).

One in four respondents (30 percent of males, 19 percent of females) reported being in a physical fight during the past year. Cross-national research also shows that adolescent males are more likely than adolescent females to carry weapons and engage in physical fights. Over 5 percent of adolescents 13–15 years old in the Czech Republic, Russia, and United States report carrying a weapon to school.

In a study comparing weapon-carrying among adolescents 11–15 years old in Belgium, Canada, Israel, Macedonia, and the United States, weapon-carrying by boys ranged from approximately 11 percent in Belgium to 22 percent in the United States; and for girls, from almost 2 percent in Belgium to 7 percent in the United States.

Engagement in frequent physical fighting among adolescent boys ranges from approximately 13 percent in the United States to 26 percent in Belgium. Among adolescent girls, physical fighting ranges from 3 percent in Israel to almost 13 percent in Belgium.

In a study of middle school youth in California, 11.3 percent of male students and 7.9 percent of female students reported being members of a gang. Researchers found that gang membership did not on its own predict school violence; additional risk factors such as truancy, substance use, and negative peer influences in youth who self-identified as gang members were associated with increased school violence.

In another United States study, the ratio of violent to nonviolent offenses increased by 10 percent after youth joined a gang and was 21 percent higher among youth who were gang members compared to non-gang youth.

IPV among adolescents is a precursor to IPV in adult intimate relationships. Researchers have found that nearly 30 percent of girls ages 15–19 worldwide have experienced IPV. In a United States study, 10 percent of male respondents reported perpetrating IPV in the 8–9 grade, and 22 percent reported past-year IPV in the 9–10 grade. Male adolescents indicate that IPV can be a way of maintaining power and control in their intimate relationships.

Researchers found that the combination of traditional beliefs about gender roles and acceptance of dating violence is associated with increased risk of IPV perpetration by male adolescents.

School violence (i.e., violence that occurs on school property, on the way to or from school, during school-sponsored events, or on the way to or from school-sponsored events) can include aggravated assault (i.e., an assault which causes serious bodily harm), bullying, cyberbullying (i.e., electronic aggression), rape, sexual assault, and homicide.

Researchers in transnational studies have found that among youth ages 11–15, close to 1 in 3 reports occasional bullying and 1 in 8 reports chronic bullying; the prevalence of youth who report bullying others ranges from 0.73 percent in Finland to 11.02 percent in Lithuania.

Boys are more likely to engage in physical aggression at school whereas girls are more likely to engage in verbal aggression (also called relational aggression; such as ostracism, manipulation, and rumors).

School shootings, although relatively rare, have increased dramatically in the past 30 years. In a study of attempted and completed mass shootings and/or killings at schools worldwide, researchers found that 96 percent of perpetrators were male.

In contrast to adolescent perpetrators of other forms of community violence, perpetrators of school shootings are more likely to be middle-class and white, and typically do not have a history of significant academic or discipline issues, violent behaviors, or substance abuse.

Risk factors for the perpetration of violent acts by adolescents include:

- Neighborhood and community disadvantage and poverty (Although female adolescents are consistently involved in less violent crime than males, as community disadvantage and poverty increase this gender gap in violent offending decreases.);
- Alcohol and substance abuse (Researchers found that among adolescent males in the Czech Republic, Russia, and the United States, and adolescent girls in the United States, substance use was linked with a higher likelihood of weapon-carrying. Perpetrators and victims of bullying are 3–5 times more likely to use alcohol and 5–6 times more likely to use drugs than adolescents who are not involved in bullying.)
- Child maltreatment, exposure to violence, and intimate partner violence (Children become highly sensitized to conflict and threats and perceive violence as a legitimate response. More than 3,500 studies have confirmed that witnessing violence increases the acceptance of aggressive attitudes and behavior.);
- Inconsistent discipline, poor monitoring and supervision;
- Peer victimization (Victims of bullying are more likely to carry weapons to school as a means of self-defense, particularly if they perceive their school as unsafe. In a longitudinal study, researchers reported that youth who were frequently victimized initially reported higher levels of aggression than youth who were not victimized or reported occasional victimization; initial levels of aggression declined over the course of the study, particularly for those youth who perceived strong family support. Researchers in one study reported that bullying has been linked with an estimated 19 percent of attempted or completed mass shootings and/or killings at schools.);
- Neurobiological risk factors, personality traits, mental illness. (Impulsive aggression occurs more often in male than female adolescents.);
- In males, the assumption of a "jock" identity (although not involvement in athletics per se);
- Poor academic achievement;
- Exposure to violent media and/or video games. (Researchers have found significant correlations between time spent by youths playing violent video games and youth aggression, delinquency, and violence.);
- Access to firearms.

Protective factors that have been found to reduce violence in adolescence include:

- Low-conflict families can impart resiliency against community and neighborhood violence for teenage males;
- Family connectedness and support can buffer the effects of peer victimization and have been associated with more rapid decline in aggression among youth who are bullied;
- Female friendships and relational intimacy can moderate and may reduce peer violence among teenage girls;
- Early exposure to maltreatment and violence is not deterministic; with opportunities and corrective experiences, early negative experiences can be offset.

Adolescents learn from their experiences: some studies have shown that exposure to psychosocial risk (e.g., dangerous people, places, and activities) can help youth build resiliency and avoid violent encounters. At what point exposure to risk becomes detrimental rather than protective is highly individualized. Having positive expectations for their future also serves as a protective factor for adolescents.

WHAT CAN BE DONE

Develop an awareness of your own cultural values, beliefs, and biases and develop knowledge about the histories, traditions, and values of your clients. Adopt treatment methodologies that reflect the cultural needs of the client.

Practice with awareness of, and adherence to, the social work principles of respect for human rights and human dignity, social justice, and professional conduct as described in the International Federation of Social Workers (IFSW) Statement of Ethical Principles. Become knowledgeable of the IFSW ethical standards as they apply to social work with adolescents and practice accordingly.

Learn about working with adolescent perpetrators of violence so you can accurately assess your clients' personal characteristics and health education needs; share this information with your colleagues.

Promote prevention and intervention programs that improve parenting, reduce child maltreatment, enhance family bonds, and promote positive monitoring and discipline (e.g., Triple P Positive Parenting, Multisystemic Therapy, Strengthening Families).

Become knowledgeable about childrearing and socialization patterns that typically are promoted in males and promote warm interpersonal relations and nonaggressive communication.

Work with schools to identify forms of school violence, educate staff and students on school violence, and work to implement evidence-based prevention and intervention programs.

Build skills in social competence, self-regulation, conflict resolution, problem-solving, communication, and anger management (e.g., life-skills training).

Become knowledgeable about adolescent IPV/dating violence and help promote healthy, respectful relationships between young persons; share knowledge with colleagues.

Work with schools to implement school-based dating violence interventions.

Encourage implementation of community-based programs that address attitudes and behaviors underlying physical and sexual violence toward women and promote more equitable gender norms.

Interventions that are longer, involve familiar adults (e.g., parents, teachers), and take place in multiple settings (e.g., school, community) have been associated with reductions in IPV.

Become knowledgeable about local child advocacy centers so you can link families to resources that focus on violence among youth.

Utilize assessment scales (such as the Aggression Scale and the Bullying Behavior Scale) with students who have bullied to better understand the dynamics and reasons for their bullying.

Provide additional information about violence and bullying, including:

- Bullying: What Parents Can Do About It, http://extension.psu.edu/publications/ui368/view
- Creating a Safe and Caring Home, http://www.schoolclimate.org/parents/safeHome.php
- Veto Violence, http://www.cdc.gov/features/veto-violence/index.html
- StopBullying.gov, http://www.stopbullying.gov/

Written by Melissa Rosales Neff, MSW, and Jennifer Teska, MSW

Reviewed by Lynn B. Cooper, D. Crim

REFERENCES

Agnich, L. E. (2015). A comparative analysis of attempted and completed school-based mass murder attacks. *American Journal of Criminal Justice, 40*(1), 1-22. doi:10.1007/s12103-014-9239-5

Bushman, B. J., Newman, K., Calvert, S. L., Downey, G., Dredze, M., Gottfredson, M., ... Webster, D. W. (2016). Youth violence: What We Know and what we need to know. *American Psychologist, 71*(1), 17-39. doi:10.1037/a0039687

Champion, H., & Sege, R. (2008). Youth violence. In L. S. Neinstein (Ed.), *Adolescent health care: A practical guide* (pp. 984-990). Philadelphia, PA: Lippincott Williams & Wilkins.

Chester, K. L., Callaghan, M., Cosma, A., Donnelly, P., Craig, W., Walsh, S., & Molcho, M. (2015). Cross-national time trends in bullying victimization in 33 countries among children aged 11, 13 and 15 from 2002 to 2010. *European Journal of Public Health, 25*(Supplement 2), 61-64. doi:10.1093/eurpub/ckv029

David-Ferdon, C., & Simon, T. R. (2014). Preventing youth violence: Opportunities for Action. *National Center for Injury Prevention and Control, Centers for Disease Control and Prevention.* Atlanta, GA.

De Koker, P., Mathews, C., Zuch, M., Bastien, S., & Mason-Jones, A. J. (2014). A systematic review of interventions for preventing adolescent intimate partner violence. *Journal of Adolescent Health, 54*(1), 3-13. doi:10.1016/j.jadohealth.2013.08.008

DeLisi, M., Vaughn, M. G., Gentile, D. A., Anderson, C. A., & Shook, J. (2012). Violent video games, delinquency, and youth violence: New evidence. *Youth Violence and Juvenile Justice, 11*(2), 132-142.

Duggins, S., Kuperminc, G. P., Henrich, C. C., Smalls-Glover, C., & Perilla, J. L. (2016). Aggression among adolescent victims of school bullying: Protective roles of family and school connectedness. *Psychology of Violence, 6*(2), 205-212. doi:10.1037/s0039439

Duke, N. N., Pettingell, S. L., McMorris, B. J., & Borowsky, I. W. (2010). Adolescent violence perpetration: Associations with multiple types of adverse childhood experiences. *Pediatrics, 125*(4), 778-786.

Elgar, F. J., Pickett, K. E., Pickett, W., Craig, W., Molcho, M., Hurrelmann, K., & Lenzi, M. (2013). School bullying, homicide and income inequality: A cross-national pooled time series analysis.

International Journal of Public Health, 58(2), 237-245. doi:10.1007/s00038-012-0380-y

Espelage, D. L., Low, S., Rao, M, Hong, J. S., & Little, T. D. (2014). Family violence, bullying, fighting, and substance use among adolescents: A longitudinal mediational model. *Journal of Research on Adolescence, 24*(2), 337-349. doi:10.1111/jora.12060

Esselmont, C. (2014). Carrying a weapon to school: The roles of bullying victimization and perceived safety. *Deviant Behavior, 35*(3), 215-232.

Estrada, J. N., Gilreath, T. D., Astor, R. A., & Benbenishty, R. (2013). Gang membership of California middle school students: Behaviors and attitudes as mediators of school violence. *Health Education Research, 28*(4), 626-639. doi:10.1093/her/cyt037

Federal Interagency Forum on Child and Family Statistics. (2015). America's Children: Key National Indicators of Well-Being, 2015. Washington, DC: U.S. Government Printing Office. Retrieved April 10, 2016, from http://www.childstats.gov/pubs/

Garaigordobil, M., Maganto, C., Pérez, J. I., & Sansinenea, E. (2009). Gender differences in socioemotional factors during adolescence and effects of a violence prevention program. *Journal of Adolescent Health, 44*(5), 468-477.

Hamburger, M. E., Basile, K. C., & Vivolo, A. M. (2011). Measuring bullying victimization, perpetration, and bystander experiences: A compendium of assessment tools. Retrieved from http://stacks.cdc.gov/view/cdc/5994

International Federation of Social Workers. (2012, March 3). *Statement of ethical principles.* Retrieved April 9, 2016, from http://ifsw.org/policies/statement-of-ethical-principles/

Kann, L., Kinchen, S., Shanklin, S. L., Flint, K. H., Hawkins, J., Harris, W. A., ... Zaza, S. (2014). Youth risk behavior surveillance—United States, 2013. *Morbidity and Mortality Weekly Report, 63*(4), 1-168.

Lundgren, R., & Amin, A. (2015). Addressing intimate partner violence and sexual violence among adolescents: Emerging evidence of effectiveness. *Journal of Adolescent Health, 56*(5), S42-S50. doi:10.1016/j.jadohealth.2014.08.012

Marsh, S. C., Evans, P. W., & Weigel, D. J. (2009). Exploring models of resiliency by gender in relation to adolescent victimization. *Victims & Offenders, 4*(3), 230-248.

McKelvey, L. M., Whiteside-Mansell, L., Bradley, R. H., Casey, P. H., Conners-Burrow, N. A., & Barrett,

K. W. (2011). Growing up in violent communities: Do family conflict and gender moderate impacts on adolescents' psychosocial development? *Journal of Abnormal Child Psychology, 39*(1), 95-107.

Melde, C., & esbensen, F.-A. (2013). Gangs and violence: Disentangling the impact of gang membership on the level and nature of offending. *Journal of Quantitative Criminology, 29*(2), 143-166. doi:10.1007/s10940-012-9164-z

Miller, K. E., Melnick, M. J., Farrell, M. P., Sabo, D. F., & Barnes, G. M. (2006). Jocks, gender, binge drinking, and adolescent violence. *Journal of Interpersonal Violence, 21*(1), 105-120.

Miller, S., Gorman-Smith, D., Sullivan, T., Orpinas, P., & Simon, T. R. (2009). Parent and peer predictors of physical dating violence perpetration in early adolescence: Tests of moderation and gender differences. *Journal of Clinical Child & Adolescent Psychology, 38*(4), 538-550.

Miniño, A. M. (2010). Mortality among teenagers aged 12-19 years: United States, 1999-2006. NCHS Data Brief, 37. Retrieved April 9, 2016, from http://www.cdc.gov/nchs/data/databriefs/db37.htm

Mizrahi, T., & Davis, L. (2008). Violence. In *Encyclopedia of social work* (20th ed., Vol. 4, pp. 259-264). Washington, DC: National Association of Social Workers.

National Association of Social Workers. (2015). NASW standards and indicators for cultural competence in social work practice. Retrieved April 9, 2016, from http://www.socialworkers.org/practice/standards/PRA-BRO-253150-CC-Standards.pdf

Nasr, I., Sivarajasingam, V., Jones, S., & Shepherd, J. (2009). Gender inequality in the risk of violence: Material deprivation is linked to higher risk for adolescent girls. *Emergency Medicine Journal, 27*(11), 811-814.

The Policy, Ethics and Human Rights Committee, British Association of Social Workers. (2012, January). *The Code of Ethics for Social Work: Statement of principles.* Retrieved April 9, 2016, from http://cdn.basw.co.uk/upload/basw_112315-7.pdf

Próspero, M. (2007). Young adolescent boys and dating violence: The beginning of patriarchal terrorism? *Journal of Women & Social Work, 22*(3), 271-280.

Reyes, H. L. M., Foshee, V. A., Niolon, P. H., Reidy, D. E., & Hall, J. E. (2016). Gender role attitudes and male adolescent dating violence perpetration: Normative beliefs as moderators. *Journal of Youth & Adolescence, 45*(2), 350-360. doi:10.1007/s10964-015-0278-0

Rice, T. (2014). Violence among young men: The importance of a gender-specific developmental approach to adolescent male suicide and homicide. *International Journal of Adolescent Medicine and Health, 27*(2), 177-181. doi:10.1515/ijamh-2015-5008

Stickley, A., Koyanagi, A., Koposov, R., Blatny, M., Hrdlicka, M., Schwab-Stone, M., & Ruchkin, V. (2015). Correlates of weapon carrying in school among adolescents in three countries. *American Journal of Health Behavior, 39*(1), 99-108. doi:10.5993/AJHB.39.1.11

Walsh, S. D., Molcho, M., Craig, W., Harel-Fisch, Y., Huynh, Q., Kukaswadia, A., ... Pickett, W. (2013). Physical and emotional health problems experienced by youth engaged in physical fighting and weapon carrying. *PLOS ONE, 8*(2), e56403. doi:10.1371/journal.pone.0056403

Webb, N.B. (2011). The interpersonal violence of bullying. In *Social work practice with children* (3rd ed., pp. 355-366). New York, NY: The Guilford Press.

Wolfe, D. A., Crooks, C., Chiodo, D., & Jaffe, P. (2009). Child maltreatment, bullying, gender-based harassment, and adolescent dating violence: Making the connections. *Psychology of Women Quarterly, 33*(1), 21-24.

World Health Organization. (2013). Global and regional estimates of violence against women: Prevalence and health effects of intimate partner violence and non-partner sexual violence. Retrieved April 9, 2016, from http://apps.who.int/iris/bitstream/10665/85239/1/9789241564625_eng.pdf?ua=1

World Health Organization. (2015, October). Youth violence. Fact sheet no. 356. Retrieved April 9, 2016, from http://www.who.int/mediacentre/factsheets/fs356/en/

Zimmerman, G. M., & Messner, S. F. (2010). Neighborhood context and the gender gap in adolescent violent crime. *American Sociological Review, 75*(6), 958-980.

VIOLENCE IN ADOLESCENCE: GENDER DIFFERENCES IN VICTIMS

MAJOR CATEGORIES: Adolescents, Violence

WHAT WE KNOW

The World Health Organization defines violence as "the intentional use of physical force or power, threatened or actual, against oneself, another person, or against a group or community, which either results in or has a high likelihood of resulting in injury, death, psychological harm, maldevelopment, or deprivation."

Violence in adolescence may include bullying; sexual or physical assault, including intimate partner violence (IPV, also called dating violence); community violence (violence that takes place in public places, such as gang violence or school shootings),and homicide.

Simple assault is the most common violent crime experienced by adolescents in the United States, constituting 77 percent of all instances of victimization among those ages 12–14 years and 63 percent of victimization among those ages 15–17.

In the United States adolescents are more likely than adults to be victims of violent crime.

The United States has the highest teenage homicide rate in the advanced industrialized world. Homicide (at 13 percent) is the second leading cause of death for adolescents after accidents (48 percent), and the leading cause of death of black teenagers.

Adolescent males and females are at risk for different types of violent victimization. Adolescent males are more likely than adolescent females to be victims of all crimes except sexual assault and IPV. Among young adolescents (12–14 years old) the overall rate of victimization is 52 per 1,000, with more males experiencing violence (66 per 1,000) than females (39 per 1,000).

Female adolescents have the highest risk of any group of sexual assault. In a multi-country study of violence victimization, researchers found that among female adolescents who had a history of having a romantic or sexual partner, 8.8 percent to 30.9 percent reported experiencing physical violence victimization during the previous year and 1.8 percent to 18.3 percent reported experiencing sexual violence victimization during the previous year.

Males are more likely to be involved in gangs and community violence (e.g., gang shootings) than females. Males account for 83 percent of youth homicide victims worldwide. In the United States male adolescents are 6 times more likely to be victims of homicide than females.

Rates of bullying are similar for boys and girls. Data from the Global School-based Student Health Survey (GSHS) revealed that 42 percent of male adolescents and 37 percent of female adolescents reported bullying during the previous 30 days. In a study of adolescents in Portugal, researchers found that boys were more often victims of bullying that includes physical aggression than were girls.

Male and female adolescents cope with violence and the risk of victimization differently. Female adolescents are much more likely than male adolescents to internalize their stress responses to community and family violence and they have higher rates of depression and anxiety. Female adolescents typically develop an awareness of their sexual vulnerability during adolescence and may express fears of being raped. Male adolescents are more likely than female adolescents to express a fear of gangs.

Females who have experienced community violence engage in more binge drinking than males who have experienced community violence.

To protect themselves, males report trying to be non-provocative in the face of danger, whereas females report acting confidently as a way to avoid being perceived as weak or vulnerable.

For male adolescents, residing in a family in which violence is not present is a protective factor against community violence. Having a low-conflict family does not protect female adolescents from the effects of community violence, however.

Both boys and girls who are involved in dating violence, either as victims or perpetrators, report lower levels of social support. However, boys who are victims reported lower levels of social support from their families compared to their non-victim counterparts, whereas girls who are victims report lower levels of support from their peers.

In a survey of Latino youth, male and female adolescents who perceived high levels of caring from and communication with their parents were less likely to report physical violence in dating relationships. The girls were also less likely to report sexual victimization in their dating relationships.

WHAT CAN BE DONE

Become knowledgeable about violence in adolescence and gender differences in victims; share knowledge with colleagues.

Develop an awareness of our own cultural values, beliefs, and biases and develop knowledge about the histories, traditions, and values of our clients. Adopt treatment methodologies that reflect the cultural needs of the client.

Work with school leadership to implement evidence-based school violence prevention programs and school-based dating violence interventions.

Encourage the implementation of community-based programs that address attitudes and behaviors underlying physical and sexual violence toward females and promote more equitable gender norms.

Encourage the development of social support for adolescents, both within families and among peers.

Teach non-violent parenting and communication skills to parents of adolescents, particularly those with a history of high conflict and/or aggression.

Become knowledgeable about interventions that enhance resilience in individuals, families, and communities to provide support and education.

Become knowledgeable about local child advocacy centers and mental health clinics in order to link families and adolescents to resources.

Written by Jan Wagstaff, MA, MSW

Reviewed by Lynn B. Cooper, D. Crim

REFERENCES

British Association of Social Workers. (2012). *The code of ethics for social work: Statement of principles.* Retrieved January 11, 2016, http://cdn.basw.co.uk/upload/basw_112315-7.pdf

Champion, H., & Sege, R. (2008). Youth violence. In L. S. Neinstein (Ed.), *Adolescent health care: A practical guide* (pp. 984-990). Philadelphia, PA: Lippincott Williams & Wilkins.

Child Trends. (2015). Violent crime victimization: Indicators on children and youth. Retrieved from http://www.childtrends.org/?indicators=violent-crime-victimization

Decker, M. R., Peitzmeier, S., Olumide, A., Acharya, R., Ojengbede, O., Covarrubias, L., ... Brahmbhatt, H. (2014). Prevalence and health impact of intimate partner violence and non-partner sexual violence among female adolescents aged 15—19 years in vulnerable urban environments: A multi-country study. *Journal of Adolescent Health, 55*(6 Suppl), S58-S67. doi:10.1016/j.jadohealth.2014.08.022

Hallman, K. K., Kenworthy, N. J., Diers, J., Swan, N., & Devnarain, B. (2015). The shrinking world of girls at puberty: Violence and gender-divergent access to the public sphere among adolescents in South Africa. *Global Public Health, 10*(3), 279-295. doi:10.1080/17441692.2014.964746

Henson, B., Wilcox, P., Reyns, B. W., & Cullen, F. T. (2010). Gender, adolescent lifestyles, and violent victimization: Implications for routine activity theory. *Victims & Offenders, 5*(4), 303-328.

International Federation of Social Workers. (2012, March 3). Statement of ethical principles. Retrieved January 11, 2016, from http://ifsw.org/policies/statement-of-ethical-principles/

Johansson, K., Laflamme, L., & Eliasson, M. (2012). Adolescents' perceived safety and security in public space-a Swedish focus group study with a gender perspective. *Young, 20*(1), 68-88.

Kast, N. R., Eisenberg, M. E., & Sieving, R. E. (2015). The role of parent communication and connectedness in dating violence victimization among Latino adolescents. *Journal of Interpersonal Violence.* doi:10.1177/0886260515570750

Lundgren, R., & Amin, A. (2015). Addressing intimate partner violence and sexual violence among adolescents: Emerging evidence of effectiveness. *Journal of Adolescent Health, 56*(1 Suppl), S42-S50. doi:10.1016/j.jadohealth.2014.08.012

Marsh, S. C., Evans, P. W., & Weigel, D. J. (2009). Exploring models of resiliency by gender in relation to adolescent victimization. *Victims & Offenders, 4,* 230-248.

McKelvey, L. M., Whiteside-Mansell, L., Bradley, R. H., Casey, P. H., Conners-Burrow, N. A., & Barrett, K. W. (2011). Growing up in violent communities: Do family conflict and gender moderate impacts on adolescents' psychosocial development? *Journal of Abnormal Child Psychology, 39*(1), 95-107.

Miniño, A. M. (2010). Mortality among teenagers aged 12-19 years: United States, 1999-2006. NCHS

Data Brief, 37. Retrieved January 11, 2016, from http://www.cdc.gov/nchs/data/databriefs/db37.htm

Wheeler, D. (2015). NASW standards and indicators for cultural competence in social work practice. Retrieved January 11, 2016, from http://www.socialworkers.org/practice/standards/PRA-BRO-253150-CC-Standards.pdf

Pinchevsky, G. M., Wright, E. M., & Fagan, A. A. (2013). Gender differences in the effects of exposure to violence on adolescent substance use. *Violence and Victims, 28*(1), 122-44.

Richards, T. N., & Branch, K. A. (2012). The relationship between social support and adolescent dating violence: A comparison across genders. *Journal of Interpersonal Violence, 27*(8), 1540-1561. doi:10.1177/0886260511425796

Silva, M. A. I., Pereira, B., Mendonca, D., Nunes, B., & de Oliveira, W. A. (2013). The Involvement of girls and boys with bullying: An analysis of gender differences. *International Journal of Environmental Research and Public Health, 10*(12), 6820-6831. doi:10.3390/ijerph10126820

Voisin, D. R., & Neilands, T. B. (2010). Community violence and health risk factors among adolescents on Chicago's southside: Does gender matter? *Journal of Adolescent Health, 46*(6), 600-602.

Webb, N. B. (2011). Social work practice with children. New York, NY: The Guilford Press.

Wilson, C. W., Rosenthal, B. S., & Battle, W. S. (2007). Effects of gender, ethnicity and educational status on exposure to community violence and psychological distress in adolescents. *Journal of Aggression, Maltreatment & Trauma, 15*(1), 93-111.

World Health Organization. (n.d.). Health topics: Violence. Retrieved January 11, 2016, from http://www.who.int/topics/violence/en/

World Health Organization. (2011, August). Youth violence. Fact sheet no. 356. Retrieved January 11, 2016, http://www.who.int/mediacentre/factsheets/fs356/en/

World Health Organization. (2015). Preventing youth violence: An overview of the evidence. Retrieved January 11, 2016, from http://www.who.int/violence_injury_prevention/violence/youth/youth_violence/en/

VIOLENCE IN SCHOOLS: AN OVERVIEW

MAJOR CATEGORIES: Violence

DESCRIPTION

Throughout the world, large numbers of children are threatened with or experience violence while at school. In addition to physical violence, violence at school includes bullying and electronic aggression, or so-called *cyberbullying*. Bullying is intentional and repeated aggression that is most often verbal, with cyberbullied youngsters often also being bullied in person. It is also important to understand that physical and emotional violence in schools often extends beyond the bully/victim dyad: An entire peer group may be involved, with individuals fulfilling different roles in the social context of the bullying incident. Moreover, school-aged young persons may oscillate between being victims and being perpetrators of violence, with its perpetrators likely to have of social avoidance and conduct problems.

In industrialized nations, violence at school manifests in its most extreme form as mass shootings. Although students constitute the vast majority of victims of violence in schools, teachers and other school staff members are sometimes also its victims. Although school shootings are extremely rare, they have expanded to become a global phenomenon since the 1999 Columbine High School shooting in the United States, in which 12 students and 1 teacher died and 21 further people were injured. These tragic events, which draw intensive media attention, reinforce a climate of fear in communities, promoting anxiety about schools as dangerous places. School violence is portrayed in the media as unpredictable and increasing, suggesting schools as places for potential tragedy. Contrary to this portrayal, however, statistics show that schools are generally safe places for children.

Data indicate that youth violence within and outside of schools is a highly gender-weighted experience, with larger proportions of boys than of girls being perpetrators of violence. One fifth of high-school students in the United States, chiefly boys, report carrying a weapon to school. More school-aged boys than girls report threats and injury; and more boys die from violence, whereas higher proportions of girls than of boys are sexually assaulted. Also, although data on intimate partner violence (IPV) in adolescence (frequently referred to as *teen dating violence* [TDV]) suggests that boys and girls are equally likely to be victims of it, girls are much more likely than boys to be severely injured in IPV.

Discussions of school violence often omit sexual assault and IPV, with an emphasis instead on highly visible physical violence, such as gang violence. However, it is worth noting that 43 percent of incidents of IPV between adolescents reportedly occur on school premises at times when young couples are alone.

High-risk environments and behaviors that can lead to school violence exist in both urban and rural settings, with incidents of violence occurring more often in settings with limited resources. In the United States, such violence tends to have disadvantaged inner cities as its nuclei, with violent encounters being the leading cause of death for young black males, who are far more likely than average to be inhabitants of inner cities.

Being the victim of or even witnessing a violent act can have serious effects on school-age students' psychological development, and may result in poor social functioning, substandard academic achievement, and a greater-than-average propensity for violence and related criminal activity later in life. Early exposure to violence in the media, IPV in the home, and physical punishment are common in the lives of individuals involved in school violence. Delinquent behavior, risk-taking, and impulsivity increase the exposure to violence, with peer attitudes being highly influential in the consequences of this. For such reasons, fostering respectful, quality relationships between young people and their peers and teachers is a significant strategy for preventing school violence. Attention to emotional, social, and behavioral issues at schools should be as important as attention to academic performance. Young persons at high-risk for being perpetrators and/or victims of violence should be identified for intervention, preferably with an approach that is multidimensional and culturally sensitive, and which includes interventional measures at the individual, family, and community levels.

FACTS AND FIGURES

In 2014, 94 percent of public middle- and high-school administrators in the United States reported one or more incidents of violent crime among their students. Likewise, 1 in 10 school-aged children report having been being threatened or injured by a weapon while on school grounds. It is estimated that 75 percent of students in the United States witness verbally aggressive behavior and physical violence while at school. Members of sexual minorities (e.g., lesbians and homosexual males) are at higher risk than are heterosexual students for victimization while at school, and for not going to school because of fear of victimization (O'Malley Olsen, Kann, Vivolo-Kantor, Kinchen, & McManus, 2014). The 2013 Youth Risk Behavior Survey found that among teens who were dating, approximately 21 percent of females and 10 percent of males experienced some form of violence in dating (Vagi, O'Malley Olsen, Basile, & Vivolo-Kantor, 2015).

RISK FACTORS

Students are most at risk for physical injuries from peer violence when going to or from school. Older adolescents are at greater risk for being victims and perpetrators of violence at school than are younger children. Using alcohol and drugs, having access to firearms, carrying weapons, and being involved in gangs increase the risk of violence in schools. Exposure to violence, such as witnessing IPV, being physically punished, and witnessing the maltreatment of another child, increases the risk of involvement in violence in adolescence and adulthood. Violent television shows and video games increase the acceptance of violence and aggression as means for solving conflicts.

SIGNS AND SYMPTOMS

As noted earlier, victims of violence can also be perpetrators of it, and this overlap means that its victims and its perpetrators may exhibit similar signs and symptoms. Females frequently internalize their responses to violence and abuse, and experience depression and low self-esteem as a consequence, whereas males tend to externalize their responses to violence, in the form of substance abuse and aggression. Apart from the more obvious signs of violence, it may cause unexplained injuries. Somatic symptoms such as headaches, stomachaches, and sleeplessness can all be signs of violence, as can depression. Students who are victims of violence may have increasingly absenteeism from school, avoid certain activities, show changes in their academic performance, or show decreasing connectedness with their schools. They may also be especially vulnerable to suicidal ideation, or may attempt suicide; fantasize about violence; or express a desire to carry a weapon. Gang affiliation has been found to have a high correlation with students' involvement as both perpetrators and victims of violence. Schools with a higher reported gang presence have more reports of violence.

APPLICABLE LAWS AND REGULATIONS

Social workers in the United States are mandated to report child maltreatment, which is understood as being any condition that could reasonably result in harm to a child, and the failure to report this is punishable by law. Local police departments can investigate criminal charges against juvenile perpetrators of violence, IPV, and bullying, which can result in charges against them of assault, battery, and harassment. Additionally, the parents of a child who has been victimized by violence while at school can bring civil lawsuits against the school officials and school district.

TREATMENT

The social worker assisting a youngster involved in violence at school should first determine whether he or she has been a victim or perpetrator of it, its nature, and its duration. The social worker should also identify the perpetrator or victim of the violence, as the case may be, and the circumstances in which the violence occurred. This should be followed by a complete biological, psychological, social, and spiritual assessment of the youngster who is being assisted, with a specific focus on his or her personal and family history with regard to childhood trauma, family structure, history of alcohol/substance abuse, community climate, academic performance, social functioning, medical and mental health, and suicidal ideation. The social worker should also assess the youngster's stress-management skills and coping mechanisms, and obtain permission to ask any available family members for additional relevant information about the youngster's personal history and family background. The social worker should also speak with school officials to obtain further information about the violence involving the youngster.

If the youngster is known to have been involved or is suspected of involvement in physical violence, a medical examination may be helpful. Tests of the youngster's blood and urine for alcohol and/or substance use, tests of girls for pregnancy, and tests for sexually transmitted diseases (STDs) may be indicated and useful in planning treatment interventions.

ASSESSMENTS AND SCREENING TOOLS

The Drug Use Screening Inventory (DUSI-R) has 159 questions covering 10 psychosocial domains and includes a validated violence proneness scale (VPS) that is suitable for use with adolescents.

The Scale for Suicidal Ideation (SSI) measures the intensity, pervasiveness, and characteristics of suicidal ideation and can be used with adolescents.

The Center for Epidemiological Studies—Depression Scale (CES-D) is an online questionnaire useful for detecting depression in adolescents.

The Aggression Scale is a self-reporting tool that is used to assess aggressive behavior in middle school students.

The California Healthy Kids Survey measures victimization in students and is administered in 7th, 9thand 11th grades.

The Forms of Bullying Scale (FBS) is used to measure levels of both perpetration (FBS-P) and victimization (FBS-V) of bullying in adolescents aged 12 to 15 years old.

If physical violence is suspected but not visible, a medical examination may be helpful.

TREATMENT

Multidimensional and culturally sensitive interventions at the individual and group levels are recommended for treating young persons involved as victims or perpetrators of school violence (Ellis, Chung-Hall, & Dumas, 2013; Vagi, Rothman, Latzman, Tharp, Hall, & Breiding, 2013). Motivational interviewing (MI) has proven successful in work with adolescents, in creating between the social worker and a youngster involved in violence a positive, empathic atmosphere that avoids argumentation, facilitates mutual trust, and encourages self-efficacy as the youngster engages in risk–benefit analyses of his or her behaviors (Cunningham et al., 2013). Educating youngsters about respectful relationships and anger management is also critical (Burt, Patel, Butler, & Gonzalez, 2013). As elements in a school curriculum, anger-management programs can help young persons to navigate conflict, and peer-mediation programs can help reduce conflict. Education about individual beliefs and attitudes, behavior, and peer relationships, included in a school's health curriculum, has proven successful for promoting positive and respectful relationships (Vagi et al., 2013), and it is suggested that school curricula focus on peer relationships because many instances of violence have been found to have roots in peer-group dynamics (Ellis et al., 2013).

Programs designed to build social awareness and develop character have also reduced risk-taking and violent behaviors among adolescents. One such program is Coaching Boys into Men, in which athletic coaches educate their players on topics such as respect and responsibility throughout the sport season in an effort to reduce the likelihood that they will commit acts of violence (University of Pittsburgh Schools of the Health Sciences, 2013). The *Shifting Boundaries program, supported by the U.S. National Institute of Justice,* and which includes both classroom and schoolwide elements, is an evidence-based, multi-level program for preventing sexual harassment and factors leading to dating violence among middle-school students.

School climate committees can help assess school violence and the potential for it, and teachers and school counselors can implement curriculum tools to foster more positive school communities and help children deal with conflicts that arise both at home and at school (O'Brennan, Waasdorp, & Bradshaw, 2014).

Social workers should be aware of their own cultural values, beliefs, and biases, and develop specialized knowledge about the histories, traditions, and values of the youngsters with whom they work in reducing victimization by violence and its perpetration. They should adopt treatment methods that reflect the cultural diversity of the young people with whom they work, and these young peoples' peer groups and schools.

APPLICABLE LAWS AND REGULATIONS

Social workers in the United States are mandated to report child maltreatment, which is understood as any condition that could reasonably result in harm; failure to do so is punishable by law. This is not the case in other countries such as the United Kingdom and Australia, although professionals are expected to cooperate fully with law enforcement. The police can investigate criminal charges against juvenile perpetrators of violence, IPV, and bullying, and this may result in charges of assault, battery, and harassment. Parents can also bring civil lawsuits against school officials and districts on behalf of their children if a child has been victimized.

Each country has its own standards for cultural competence and diversity in social work practice. Social workers must be aware of the standards of practice set forth by their governing body (e.g., the British Association of Social Workers in England, the National Association of Social Workers in the United States) and practice accordingly.

SERVICES AND RESOURCES

The following resources can provide information about violence in schools:

- The National School Climate Center has information, resources, and tools for setting up climate committees, http://www.schoolclimate.org
- Kelso's Choice is a widely used conflict management tool for children; curriculum information is available at http://kelsoschoice.com
- VetoViolence: Violence Education Tools Online explains all types of violence within the social ecological model and offers online courses and information for professionals, http://www.vetoviolence.org
- Futures Without Violence is an organization that works to end all types of violence, http://www.futureswithoutviolence.org
- The Center for the Study and Prevention of Violence at the University of Colorado Boulder has information and resources available for school-based prevention, http://www.colorado.edu/cspv
- The Childhood Violent Trauma Center provides information and resources to professionals, http://www.nccev.org
- The Office of Juvenile Justice and Delinquency Prevention (OJJDP) has news, research, and information on youth violence, http://www.ojjdp.gov

FOOD FOR THOUGHT

Students attending schools with metal detectors reported less fear of violence than students at schools without them, even though levels of violence were equivalent.

It is recommended that all schools be routinely assessed for levels of violence and safety using a social ecological model.

It has been argued that policies promoting zero tolerance and police presence in schools increase negative interactions between students and law enforcement, sometimes unnecessarily, and this contributes to the passage from school to prison for some youth.

When students have quality relationships with teachers, they are more willing to seek help in dealing with school violence.

RED FLAGS

Students often fail to report threats by peers of their intention to bring guns to school.

Violence most frequently emerges from interpersonal disputes and reputational concerns.

NEXT STEPS

Refer to appropriate services (e.g., medical treatment, mental health assessment, academic tutoring) to address problem stemming from school violence.

If possible, check in regularly with student to assess and amend interventions.

Written by Jan Wagstaff, MA, MSW and Michael James White, MSW, PPSC

Reviewed by Lynn B. Cooper, D. Crim, and Chris Bates, MA, MSW

REFERENCES

Agnich, L. E., & Miyazaki, Y. (2013). A multilevel cross-national analysis of direct and indirect forms of school violence. *Journal of School Violence, 12*(4), 319-339. doi:10.1080/15388220.2013.807737

Banas, J. R. (2014). Impact of authentic learning exercises on preservice teachers' self-efficacy to perform bullying prevention tasks. *American Journal of Health Education, 45*(4), 239-248. doi:10.1080/193 25037.2014.916634

Bondii, R., Cornell, D. G., & Scheithauer, H. (2011). Student homicidal violence in schools: An international problem. *New Directions for Youth Development, 129,* 13-30.

British Association of Social Workers. (2012, January). *The Code of Ethics for Social Workers: Statement of Principles.* Retrieved December 7, 2015, from http://cdn.basw.co.uk/upload/basw_112315-7.pdf

Burt, I., Patel, S. H., Butler, S. K., & Gonzalez, T. (2013). Integrating leadership skills into anger management groups to reduce aggressive behaviors: The LIT Model. *Journal of Mental Health Counseling, 35*(2), 124-141.

Cawood, N. D. (2013). Addressing interpersonal violence in the school context: Awareness and use of evidence-supported programs. *Children & Schools, 35*(1), 41-52. doi:10.1093/cs/cds013

Charles, G., & DeGagne, M. (2013). Student-to-student abuse in the Indian residential schools in Canada: Setting the stage for further understanding. *Child & Youth Services, 34*(4), 343-359. doi:10.1080/0145935X.2013.859903

Centers for Disease Control & Prevention (CDC). (2012). About school violence. Retrieved December 7, 2015, from http://www.cdc.gov/ViolencePrevention/youthviolence/schoolviolence

Cunningham, R., Whiteside, L., Chermack, S., Zimmerman, M., Shope, J., Bingham, C., ... Walton, M. (2013). Dating violence: Outcomes following a brief motivational interviewing intervention among at-risk adolescents in an urban emergency department. *Academic Emergency Medicine, 20*(6), 562-569. doi:10.1111/acem.12151

Ellis, W., Chung-Hall, J., & Dumas, T. (2013). The role of peer group aggression in predicting adolescent dating violence and relationship quality. *Journal of Youth & Adolescence, 42*(4), 487-499. doi:10.1007/s10964-012-9797-0

Estrada, J. N., Gilreath, T. D., Astor, R. A., & Benbenishty, R. (2013). Gang membership of California middle school students: Behaviors and attitudes as mediators of school violence. *Health Education Research, 28*(4), 626-639. doi:10.1093/her/cyt037

Estrada, J. N., Gilreath, T. D., Astor, R. A., & Benbenishty, R. (2014). Gang membership, school violence, and the mediating effects of risk and protective behaviors in California high schools. *Journal of School Violence, 13*(2), 228-251. doi:10.1080/15388220.2013.846860

Foster, H., & Brooks-Gunn, J. (2013). Neighborhood, family, and individual influences on school physical victimization. *Journal of Youth & Adolescence, 42*(10), 1596-1610. doi:10.1007/s10964-012-9890-4

Green, J. G., Furlong, M. J., Astor, R. A., Benbenishty, R., & Espinoza, E. (2011). Assessing school victimization in the United States, Guatemala, and Israel: Cross-cultural psychometric analysis of the school victimization scale. *Victims & Offenders, 6*(3), 290-305.

Hemphill, S. A., Tollit, M., & Herrenkohl, T. I. (2014). Protective factors against the impact of school bullying perpetration and victimization on young adult externalizing and internalizing problems. *Journal of School Violence, 13*(1), 125-145. doi: 10.1080/15388220.2013.844072

Hildenbrand, A. K., Daly, B. P., Nicholls, E., Brooks-Holliday, S., & Kloss, J. D. (2013). Increased risk for school violence-related behaviors among adolescents with insufficient sleep. *Journal of School Health, 83*(6), 408-414. doi:10.1111/josh.12044

Hoglund, W. L. G., & Hosan, N. E. (2013). The context of ethnicity: Peer victimization and adjustment problems in early adolescence. *Journal of Early Adolescence, 33*(5), 585-609. doi:10.1177/0272431612451925

International Federation of Social Workers. (2012, March 3). Statement of Ethical Principles. Retrieved December 7, 2015, from http://ifsw.org/policies/statement-of-ethical-principles/

Mendard, S., & Grotpeter, J. K. (2014). Evaluation of bully-proofing your school as an elementary school antibullying intervention. *Journal of School Violence, 13*(2), 188-209. doi:10.1080/15388220.2013.840641

O'Brennan, L. M., Waasdorp, T. E., & Bradshaw, C. P. (2014). Strengthening bullying prevention through school staff connectedness. *Journal of Educational Psychology, 106*(3), 870-880. doi:10.1037/a0035957

O'Malley Olsen, E., Kann, L., Vivolo-Kantor, A., Kinchen, S., & McManus, T. (2014). School violence and bullying among sexual minority high school students, 2009-2011. *Journal of Adolescent Health, 55*(3), 432-438. doi:10.1016/j.jadohealth.2014.03.002

Schultes, M., Stefanek, E., de Schoot, R., Strohmeier, D., & Spiel, C. (2014). Measuring implementation of a school-based violence prevention program. *Zeitschrift fur Psychologie, 222*(1), 49-57. doi:10.1027/2151-2604/a000165

Shaw, T., Dooley, J. J., Cross, D., Zubrick, S. R., & Waters, S. (2013). The Forms of Bullying Scale (FBS): Validity and reliability estimates for a measure of bullying victimization and perpetration in adolescence. *Psychological Assessment, 25*(4), 1045-1057. doi:10.1037/a0032955

Skubak Tillyer, M., Fisher, B. S., & Wilcox, P. (2011). The effects of school crime prevention on students' violent victimization, risk perception, and fear of crime: A multilevel opportunity perspective. *Justice Quarterly, 28*(2), 249-277. doi:10.1080/07418825.2010.493526

Sumiala, J., & Tikka, M. (2011). Reality on circulation – School shootings, ritualised communication, and the dark side of the sacred. *Journal of Communication Studies, 4*(2), 145-159.

Taylor, B. G., Mumford, E. A., & Stein, N. D. (2015). Effectiveness of "Shifting Boundaries" teen dating violence prevention program for subgroups of middle school students. *Journal of Adolescent Health, 56*(2 Suppl 2), S20-S26.

Teasley, M. L. (2013). School violence reduction and related services personnel. *Children & Schools, 35*(4), 195-198.

Temple, J., Shorey, R., Fite, P., Stuart, G., & Le, V. (2013). Substance use as a longitudinal predictor of the perpetration of teen dating violence. *Journal of Youth & Adolescence, 42*(4), 596-606. doi:10.1007/s10964-012-9877-1

Thompkins, A. C., Chauveron, L. M., Harel, O., & Perkins, D. F. (2014). Optimizing violence prevention programs: An examination of program effectiveness among urban high school students. *Journal of School Health, 84*(7), 435-443. doi:10.1111/josh.12171

United Nations Children's Fund (UNICEF). (2011). Swaziland convenes first national dialogue on violence against children in schools. Retrieved December 7, 2014, from http://www.unicef.org/protection/swaziland_60286.html

University of Pittsburgh Schools of the Health Sciences. (2013, April 30). Coaching Boys Into Men program proves effective in preventing teen dating violence, follow-up study finds. doi:10.1037/e566782013-001 Retrieved December 7, 2015, from http://www.upmc.com/media/NewsReleases/2013/Pages/coaching-boys-into-men-program-teen-dating-violence.aspx

Vagi, K., O'Malley Olsen, E., Basile, K., & Vivolo-Kantor, A. M. (2015). Teen dating violence (physical and sexual) among U.S. high school students: Findings from the 2013 National Youth Risk Survey. *JAMA Pediatrics, 169*(5), 474-782. doi:10.1001/jamapediatrics.2014.3577

Vagi, K., Rothman, E., Latzman, N., Tharp, A., Hall, D., & Breiding, M. (2013). Beyond correlates: A review of risk and protective factors for adolescent dating violence perpetration. *Journal of Youth & Adolescence, 42*(4), 633-649. doi:10.1007/s10964-013-9907-7

Wheeler, D. (2015). NASW Standards and Indicators for Cultural Competence in Social Work Practice. Retrieved December 7, 2015, from http://www.socialworkers.org/practice/standards/PRA-BRO-253150-CC-Standards.pdf

Zweig, J., Dank, M., Yahner, J., & Lachman, P. (2013). The rate of cyber dating abuse among teens and how it relates to other forms of teen dating violence. *Journal of Youth & Adolescence, 42*(7), 1063-1077. doi:10.1007/s10964-013-9922-8

VIOLENCE IN SCHOOLS: ELECTRONIC AGGRESSION

MAJOR CATEGORIES: Violence

DESCRIPTION

The increasing use of cell phones and computers by children has given rise to the growing phenomenon of so-called cyberbullying, digital bullying, or electronic aggression, in which children use technology to hurt others. Electronic aggression may take the form of teasing, telling lies, making crude, sexually explicit, rude, or mean comments, spreading rumors, and making threats. Electronic aggression takes place through instant messaging, text, email, chat rooms, blogs, and social networking websites and applications such as Facebook, Instagram, and Snapchat. Young people may send or post videos or photographs as a form of harassment.

Electronic aggression is an emerging field of research; few studies to date have focused on it. Some studies have included cyberbullying in broader examinations of bullying. All forms of bullying are defined as the intentional, repeated aggression on the part of one individual toward another, less powerful individual. Most often, electronic aggression takes place between known peers; however, perpetrators of the electronic aggression may be anonymous or may be individuals pretending to be others, including adults posing as children.

Among children, physical bullying declines with age, whereas verbal bullying and cyberbullying peak between the ages of 11 and 15 before decreasing with maturity. Even though girls send texts more frequently than boys, research suggests that boys are more likely than girls to be perpetrators of cyberbullying. Cyberbullying, which is considered an indirect form of aggression, has been defined as "an aggressive, intentional act carried out by a group or individual, using electronic forms of contact, repeatedly and over time against a victim who cannot easily defend him or herself". Those who are cyberbullied often are bullied in person as well.

The most frequent forms of cyberbullying are spreading lies online; violations of trust, in which private messages are forwarded without permission; and digital disrespect, which is spreading negative or embarrassing information about another person. Sending sexually explicit photos or videos via cell phone is called sexting. Only a small proportion of children send sexts, and those who do engage in sexting tend to be older adolescents. Some sexting occurs when girls send images to their male romantic partners. Many girls who send images to their romantic partners indicate that they do so under pressure from their partner. Problems occur when these explicit images are shared with others. Criminal prosecutions of teenagers involved in sexting have included charges of sexual exploitation of children.

Victims of electronic aggression may feel lonely and isolated. They may experience physical and mental health problems; diminished academic achievement and diminished participation in extracurricular school activities. Victims of electronic aggression may be at an increased risk for substance abuse and suicidal ideation or suicide completion. The media has drawn public attention to extreme cases of electronic aggression in which adolescents have committed suicide as a result of cyberbullying. Victims often are reluctant to seek help from teachers or other adults. A third of those who do seek help indicate that nothing changes after they seek help, and for some the bullying increases. Parental support and friendships act as protective factors for children. Peer mediation, conflict-resolution classes, anger-management training, diversity and tolerance education, and increased adult supervision all help to lessen, prevent, and stop bullying.

FACTS AND FIGURES

Results of the 2013 Youth Risk Behavior Surveillance System survey of U.S. students in 9 through 12 grades indicated that 14.8 percent had been electronically bullied in the 12 months before the survey. Broken down by gender, 21.0 percent females had been bulled and 8.5 percent of males had been bullied. The prevalence of victimization declined as females grew older, starting at 22.8 percent in 9th grade, 21.9 percent in 10th grade, 20.6 percent in 11th grade, and 18.3 percent in 12th grade, whereas the rates for males were 9.4 percent in 9th grade, 7.2 percent in 10th grade, 8.9 percent in 11th grade, and 8.6 percent in 12th grade. The highest rates of cyberbullying are found to occur at the middle school level (ages 12 to 14). Youth ages 8 to 18 are found to spend an average of 7.5 hours a day utilizing various forms of electronic entertainment, much of it social networking media. Researchers have found that 93 percent of youth regularly use the Internet and 47 percent of parents screened feel that their children know more about the Internet than they do. Similarly, 70 percent of health professionals working with youth state that they have not received training focusing on online risk assessment. More than 25 percent of bullied youth do not tell anyone about the bullying and nearly 20 percent do not talk about it with their parents.

RISK FACTORS

Girls are more at a higher risk for cyberbullying than are boys. Some groups, such as youth with disabilities, lesbian, gay, bisexual, and transgender youth, socially isolated children, new students, children from low-income families, and students who are perceived as weak, antisocial, or unpopular, also are at risk for cyberbullying. Victims of bullying are found to suffer academically in terms both of declining grades and poor school attendance. Victimization causes emotional distress, anger, and embarrassment and increases the risk of depression, self-harm, violent ideation, suicidal ideation, and suicide. Studies of perpetrators of bullying indicate they also have an elevated risk for these problems. Children who bully often are concerned with popularity, have friends who bully, like to be in charge of others, have family problems or have uninvolved parents, and view violence positively. Children who bully are also at risk for continuing patterns of antisocial behavior into adulthood.

SIGNS AND SYMPTOMS

When a child unexpectedly stops using his or her computer or cell phone, this can indicate cyberbullying. Children may also act nervous when an instant message or email appears or may quickly switch screens or close programs when a parent or other adult nears. Somatic symptoms which present through physical manifestations such as headaches and stomachaches; sleeplessness and nightmares; and depression may be symptoms of victimization, as may be changes in eating habits, such as binge eating or skipping meals. Absenteeism from school, loss of interest in schoolwork, and a change in academic performance may be signs that the child is experiencing bullying. Victims of bullying may exhibit self-destructive behaviors such as running away, using drugs and/or alcohol, and threatening or attempting suicide.

ASSESSMENT

Social workers assisting children who may be perpetrators or victims of bullying should complete a thorough biological, psychological, social, and spiritual assessment to include information on the physical, mental, environmental, social, and spiritual factors as they relate to the child. Information gathered from the assessment can help in the design of interventions. The social worker should include parents, siblings, and teachers in the assessment process because they are a valuable source of information about the child. The social worker should ensure that the child has ample opportunity to talk about past and present life experiences.

ASSESSMENTS AND SCREENING TOOLS

The social worker may utilize standardized assessment and screening tools to determine the child's level of need. Assessment and screening tools that may be used include The Scale for Suicidal Ideation (SSI) which measures the intensity, pervasiveness, and characteristics of suicidal ideation and can be used with adolescents; The Center for Epidemiological Studies Depression Scale (CES-D) which is an online questionnaire useful for detecting depression in adolescents; The Reynolds Child Depression Scale which has short and long versions that screen children from grades 2 to 6; The Children's Depression Inventory has 28 items and can be used to screen children ages 7 to 17; The Bullying Prevalence Questionnaire (BPQ) which is a 20-item scale that includes questions that measure for being a bully, being a victim, and the presence of pro-social activities; and The Peer Relations Assessment Questionnaire – Revised (PRAQ –R) which is designed to give schools an overall assessment of bullying, and includes separate questionnaires for younger students, older students, teachers, and parents. Tools that may be used to assess the relationships within the child's family and systems, such as the school, include genograms and ecomaps.

TREATMENT

Some adolescents oscillate between being a victim and being a bully. Young persons involved in cyberbullying should be given opportunities to talk about their experiences and victims should be reassured that the bullying is not their fault. Schools need to encourage students to report acts of electronic aggression. Peer mediation, conflict-resolution classes, anger-management training, and increased adult supervision in schools can help lessen, stop, and prevent bullying. Another strategy is for schools to include diversity and tolerance education. Poster campaigns addressing bullying were shown to reduce bullying in several schools. Schools are advised to attend to the emotional well-being of students by providing counseling support as a form of early intervention. Programs designed to educate both students and their families about the nature and repercussions of cyberbullying have also been found to decrease prevalence of cyberbullying. School-climate committees can assess schools for bullying, make recommendations, and disseminate information to students, staff, and parents.

INTERVENTION

If it is determined that a child is cyberbullying, the social worker should provide interventions to prevent further cyberbullying. Possible interventions may include talking to the child and his/her parent/s about what is happening. Children who bully often are victims of bullying as well as perpetrators and this should be explored. If bullying does not stop, the social worker may suggest an evaluation form a mental health professional such as a psychiatrist.

It it is determined that the child is being victimized by means of electronic aggression, the social worker provide interventions to prevent further cyberbullying from occurring. The social worker can gather history of the victimization and provide

an opportunity for the child to explain what is happening. The social worker should assess the child for suicide ideation and depression. The social worker may have the child practice what he or she will say or text to the bully and let the child practice being assertive. The social worker should recommend peer mediation. The social worker may talk to the perpetrator's parent/s about what is happening and if it does not stop, suggest that the perpetrator have an evaluation from a mental health professional such as a psychiatrist. The social worker and school personnel should contact the police if there are any threats of harm made to any student.

If the child who is a victim of electronic aggression experiences somatic symptoms such as headaches, stomachaches, or sleeplessness, the social worker should provide interventions to help reduce the experienced symptoms including improved sleep and an overall sense of well-being. Possible interventions may include speaking to the student, teachers, school administrators, and family members of the victim. The social worker should assess the child for symptoms of depression and risk for suicidal ideation. The child may be referred to the school nurse or a physician, if needed. The social worker may also provide a referral for individual, group, and family therapy as necessary for additional support.

If it is determined that the victim of electronic aggression is experiencing symptoms of depression, the social worker may provide interventions to help reduce the depressive symptoms. The social worker should complete a thorough biological, psychological, and social assessment to determine the child's needs. The social worker should include information gathered from teachers, school administrators, and family members of the child. The social worker should assess the child for suicidal ideation and risk. If needed, the child may be referred for individual, group, and family therapy. The social worker should build a relationship with the student and check in regularly with him/her for continued support.

If it is determined that the child is a victim of electronic aggression and has repeated absences from school, the social worker should establish what the problem is regarding the inability to come to school and provide interventions to increase school attendance. The social worker may talk with the student, his or her family, and teachers to identify the problem and make appropriate referrals for support.

Possible referrals may include counseling and continued check-ins with the student and family.

If known instances of cyberbullying are taking place among student at a school, the social worker should provide interventions to prevent and reduce the bullying. Possible interventions may include setting up a climate committee at school and evaluating the school for bullying. Education regarding diversity, conflict-resolution classes, anger-management training and peer mediation may be helpful to reduce bullying in schools. Social workers may provide educational tutorials to help the children understand the effects of cyberbullying and ways to manage it.

APPLICABLE LAWS AND REGULATIONS

Prosecuting individuals for electronic aggression has been difficult because of a lack of laws directly addressing the issue. Teenagers in the United States involved in sexting have been prosecuted for disorderly conduct, illegal use of a minor in nudity-oriented material, sexual abuse of children, criminal use of a communications facility, and open lewdness. Laws and policies increasingly are being adapted and new laws put in place to specifically criminalize acts of electronic aggression. Police can investigate criminal charges against juveniles who bully. School bullying can result in charges of assault, battery, and harassment. Parents can bring civil lawsuits on behalf of their children if a child has been victimized.

SERVICES AND RESOURCES

- Cyberbullying Research Center is a help site with a range of information and resources, http://www.cyberbullying.us
- MTV's A Thin Line, designed for young people, provides information about and resources for what to do about digital bullying, http://www.athinline.org
- StopBullying.gov is a government help site with a range of information and resources, http://www.stopbullying.gov
- Bullying. No Way! has resources and information for parents, professionals, and students, http://www.bullyingnoway.gov.au
- Anti-Bullying Alliance is a help site with a range of information and resources, http://www.anti-bullyingalliance.org.uk/
- KidsHealth has a section on bullying, http://kidshealth.org

- Teaching Tolerance has resources for teachers and other professionals who work with children, http://www.tolerance.org
- The National School Climate Center has information, resources, and tools for setting up climate committees, http://www.schoolclimate.org
- VetoViolence: Violence Education Tools Online explains all types of violence within the social ecological model and offers online courses and information for professionals, http://www.vetoviolence.org
- The Center for Civic Mediation has a section on youth and provides information and resources, http://centerforcivicmediation.org

FOOD FOR THOUGHT

It is not always clear who the perpetrator is in some forms of electronic aggression: students are known to have set up accounts using false identities on social media platforms in order to pursue and victimize others. Students may use electronic aggression to improve their popularity and position in their peer hierarchy. Students are found to be more adept at navigating social media platforms than parents and health professionals, making it difficult for adults to effectively monitor their activities.

RED FLAGS

Children frequently do not seek adult assistance with their conflicts and often are left to deal with bullying by themselves. Children may seek emotional support without identifying a specific bullying problem. Without disclosing a reason children may suddenly not want to attend school or spend time with children who had been their friends.

NEXT STEPS

Social workers can provide referrals for victims and perpetrators of bullying when indicated and help link families to services that support the entire family system in coping with the bullying. The social worker should maintain contact and follow up with students whenever possible for continued support.

Written by Michael James White, MSW, PPSC, and Laura McLuckey, MSW, LCSW

Reviewed by Lynn B. Cooper, D. Crim

REFERENCES

Academy of Child & Adolescent Psychiatry (ACAP). (2011). Facts for families: Bullying. Retrieved April 10, 2015, from http://www.aacap.org/AACAP/Families_and_Youth/Facts_for_Families/FFF-Guide/Bullying-080.aspx

Anti Bullying Alliance. (n.d.). The problem of bullying in the U.K. Retrieved April 9, 2015, from http://www.antibullyingalliance.org.uk/

Badaly, D., Kelly, B. M., Schwartz, D., & Dabney-Lieras, K. (2013). Longitudinal associations of electronic aggression and victimization with social standing during adolescence. *Journal Of Youth And Adolescence, 42*(6), 891-904. doi:10.1007/s10964-012-9787-2

British Association of Social Workers. (2012). The code of ethics for social work: Statement of principles. Retrieved November 2, 2015, from http://cdn.basw.co.uk/upload/basw_112315-7.pdf

Children's MH forum addresses innovative approaches to avert crisis. (2014). *Mental Health Weekly, 24*(23), 1-3.

Donegan, R. (2012). Bullying & cyberbullying: History, statistics, law, prevention and analysis. *The Elon Journal of Undergraduate Research in Communications, 3*(1), 33-42.

Estrada, J. N., Gilreath, T. D., Astor, R. A., & Benbenishty, R. (2014). Gang membership, school violence, and the mediating effects of risk and protective behaviors in California high schools. *Journal of School Violence, 13*(2), 228-251. doi:10.1080/15388220.2013.846860

Forward, C. (2014). Information and resources on internet safety for children. *British Journal of School Nursing, 9*(3), 147-150.

Gibson-Young, L., Martinasek, M., Clutter, M., & Forest, J. (2014). Are students with asthma at increased risk for being a victim of bullying in school or cyberspace? *Journal of School Health, 84*(7), 429-434. doi:10.1111/josh.12167

Greif Green, J., Dunn, E. C., Johnson, R. M., & Molnar, B. E. (2011). A multilevel investigation of the association between school context and adolescent nonphysical bullying. *Journal of School Violence, 10*, 133-149.

Hinduja, S., & Patchin, J. W. (2011). Cyberbullying fact sheet: Electronic dating violence. Cyberbullying Research Center. Retrieved April 3, 2015, from http://www.cyberbullying.us/electronic_dating_violence_fact_sheet.pdf

Hinduja, S., & Patchin, J. W. (2013). Cyberbullying Research Summary: The Influence of Parent, Educators, and Peers. Retrieved April 3, 2015, from http://www.cyberbullying.us/Social_Influences_on_Cyberbullying.pdf

International Federation of Social Workers. (2012). Statement of Ethical Principles. Retrieved April 8, 2015, from http://ifsw.org/policies/statement-of-ethical-principles/

Kann, L., Kinchen, S., Shanklin, S. L., Flint, K. H., Hawkins, J., ... Harris, W. A. (2014, June 13). Youth Risk Behavior Surveillance – United States, 2013. *Centers for Disease Control and Prevention, MMWR, Surveillance Summaries, 63*(4).

Kowalski, R. M., & Limber, S. P. (2013). Psychological, physical, and academic correlates of cyberbullying and traditional bullying. *Journal of Adolescent Health, 53*(1), S13-S20. doi:10.1016/j.jadohealth.2012.09.018

Messias, E., Kindrick, K., & Castro, J. (2014). School bullying, cyberbullying, or both: Correlates of teen suicidality in the 2011 CDC youth risk behavior survey. *Comprehensive Psychiatry, 55*(5), 1063-1068. doi:10.1016/j.comppsych.2014.02.005

National Crime Prevention Center (NCPC). (n.d.). Strategies. Retrieved April 28, 2016, from http://www.ncpc.org/topics/bullying/strategies

Padilla-Walker, L. M., Coyne, S. M., & Fraser, A. M. (2012). Getting a high-speed family connection: Associations between family media use and family connection. *Family Relations, 61*(3), 426-440. doi:10.1111/j.1741-3729.2012.00710.x

Patchin, J. W., & Hinduja, S. (2013). Cyberbullying among adolescents: Implications for empirical research. *Journal of Adolescent Health, 53*(4), 431-432. doi:10.1016/j.jadohealth.2013.07.030

Renda, J., Vassallo, S., & Edwards, B. (2011). Bullying in early adolescence and its association with antisocial behavior, criminality, and violence 6 to 10 years later. *Criminal Behavior and Mental Health, 21*, 117-127.

Rideout, V. J., Goehr, U., & Roberts, D. F. (2010). Generation M2 media in the lives of 8- to 18-year-olds. Retrieved from http://files.eric.ed.gov/fulltext/ED527859.pdf

Roberto, A., Eden, J., Savage, M., Ramos-Salazar, L., & Deiss, D. (2014). Outcome evaluation results of school-based cybersafety promotions and cyberbullying prevention intervention for middle school students. *Health Communication, 29*(10), 1029-1042. doi:10.1080/10410236.2013.831684

Thompkins, A. C., Chauveron, L. M., Harel, O., & Perkins, D. F. (2014). Optimizing violence prevention programs: An examination of program effectiveness among urban high school students. *Journal of School Health, 84*(7), 435-443. doi:10.1111/josh.12171

U.S. Department of Health and Human Services. (n.d.). Age trends in the prevalence of bullying. Retrieved April 8, 2015, from http://www.prevnet.ca/sites/prevnet.ca/files/fact-sheet/PREVNet-SAMHSA-Fact-sheet-Age-Trends-in-the-Prevalence-of-Bullying.pdf

Violence Prevention Works! Olweus Bullying Prevention Program (BPP). Retrieved April 3, 2015, from http://www.violencepreventionworks.org

Wesley Perkins, H., Craig, D. W., & Perkins, J. M. (2011). Using social norms to reduce bullying: A research intervention among adolescents in five middle schools. *Group Practices & Intergroup Relations, 14*(5), 703-702.

Wheeler, L. (2015). NASW standards and indicators for cultural competence in social work practice. Retrieved April 9, 2016, from http://www.socialworkers.org/practice/standards/PRA-BRO-253150-CC-Standards.pdf

VISUAL IMPAIRMENT IN CHILDREN: AN OVERVIEW

MAJOR CATEGORIES: Medical & Health

DESCRIPTION

Visual impairment is vision loss that cannot be corrected to a "normal" level and interferes with daily activities. The World Health Organization divides visual function into four levels: normal vision, moderate visual impairment, severe visual impairment, and blindness. Moderate and severe visual impairment are also referred to as "low vision"; blindness ranges from visual acuity of 20/400 or less to no light perception. 'Legal blindness' refers to having a level of vision loss that meets eligibility criteria for publically funded benefits and services. In the United States, criteria for legal blindness include having a central visual acuity of 20/200 or less in the better eye with the best possible correction, and/or having a visual field of 20 degrees or less. Many people who are legally blind still have some usable vision. An individual with 20/200 vision, for example, can discern at 20 feet the same size letter (or number or image) that someone with normal visual acuity (20/20) can see at 200 feet.

The World Health Organization classifies blindness and low vision of children in two ways. The first is a descriptive category that refers to the anatomical site most affected. The categories are:

whole globe (e.g., anophthalmos [when an infant is born with orbital tissue missing from one or both eyes]);

microphthalmos (infant is born with smaller than average mass of orbital tissue);

cornea (e.g., corneal scarring);

lens (e.g., cataract [clouding of the lens that causes blurry vision]);

uvea (the pigmented layer of the eye);

retina (the layer at the back of the eyeball that contains cells that are sensitive to light and trigger nerve impulses that pass via the optic nerve to the brain);

optic nerve (e.g., atrophy [loss of some or all of the fibers of the optic nerve]);

glaucoma and conditions in which the eye appears normal (e.g., refractive errors [eye disorder in which the eye cannot clearly focus images]);

cortical (loss of vision due to damage to the brain's occipital cortex).

The second type of classification categorizes conditions that lead to blindness and low vision based on underlying cause and time of onset:

hereditary (at conception [e.g., genetic diseases, chromosomal abnormalities]).

intrauterine (during pregnancy [e.g., caused by rubella or thalidomide]).

perinatal (e.g., retinopathy of prematurity [potentially blinding eye disorder in some infants born before 31 weeks' gestational age]).

birth injury (e.g., cerebral palsy).

neonatal conjunctivitis (inflammation or infection of the tissue lining the eyelids of a newborn).

childhood (e.g., vitamin A deficiency disorder, trauma, measles).

unknown/cannot be determined (e.g., congenital abnormalities).

Causes of childhood blindness vary greatly among world regions, with an especially large divide between developing and developed countries. In wealthier countries, for example, lesions of the optic nerve (which often are related to prematurity) and hereditary eye diseases are the most common causes of childhood blindness. In contrast, the majority of causes of childhood blindness in poorer countries are preventable conditions such as vitamin A deficiency, corneal scarring caused by measles, and newborn conjunctivitis.

Eliminating preventable childhood visual impairment and blindness is a priority for the World Health Organization, which has initiated a global campaign called VISION 2020—The Right to Sight. The campaign is made up of several international, nongovernmental, and private organizations that share the goal of eradicating avoidable blindness as a public health problem by 2020. They plan to accomplish this goal through disease prevention and control (spreading access to immunization against measles, vitamin A supplementation), training of personnel in the eye care system, strengthening the existing eye care infrastructure, use of appropriate and affordable technology, and mobilization of resources in poor and developing countries.

In developed countries, in which childhood visual impairment largely is not preventable, it is vital for visually impaired children and their families to have access to resources that will help alleviate the burdens and obstacles they may face. For example, school-aged children who are visually impaired sometimes require the assistance of a paraeducator, a school employee who is trained to work with and alongside educators in the classroom to support children with special needs physically, socially, and instructionally. Paraeducators who work with visually impaired children use the Expanded Core Curriculum (ECC). The ECC is a specific curriculum of skills and knowledge for visually impaired students based on their unique needs:

communication mode (e.g., children using Braille, large print, sign language, or recorded materials to communicate);

social interaction (e.g., children learning how to greet adults and other children and learning how close to be when in conversation with another person);

assistive technology (e.g., screen magnification software on a computer so that a visually impaired child can read on the computer more easily);

career education (e.g., children having the opportunity to explore firsthand their strengths and interests in a vocational or career setting in a well-planned manner, such as visiting banks to learn what a bank teller does or visiting a nursery to learn what a gardener does);

orientation and mobility (e.g., children learning about body image and how to move as independently as possible);

independent living skills (e.g., children learning daily living tasks such as personal hygiene, money management, food preparation);

*sensory efficiency skill*s (e.g., children learning to optimize the use of their senses other than vision to find their personal belongings);

recreational and leisure activities (e.g., children actively participating in recreational activities and learning to follow rules in a game);

self-determination (e.g., children building skills to advocate for themselves such as asking a teacher for more time to complete assignments).

Studies have found that visually impaired children are much more successful in school settings with the aid of a paraeducator. There are also rehabilitation workers who work closely with visually impaired children on mobility training. Mobility training is focused on teaching skills that visually impaired children need to travel safely and independently to school, use public transportation, and participate in sports and social activities. Workers also address independence skill training, which focuses on areas such as eating, hygiene, home care, and relationships.

FACTS AND FIGURES

The World Health Organization (WHO) estimates that approximately 285 million people worldwide are visually impaired. Of this number, 39 million are blind and 246 million have low vision. Ninety percent live in developing countries; 19 million are children. Of these children, 12 million are visually impaired because of refractive errors that could be easily corrected and 1.4 million are irreversibly blind. The prevalence of visual impairment or blindness ranges from 0.3/1,000 in developed countries to 1.5/1,000 in developing countries.

In the United Kingdom it is estimated that severe visual impairment or blindness will be diagnosed in 4 of 10,000 children by their first birthday and in 6 of 10,000 by their 16th birthday. Approximately 1 percent of children in New Zealand are blind or visually impaired. An estimated 1.1 percent of junior high students in Ghana have moderate visual impairment and 7.3 percent have mild visual impairment; just over 20 percent have had an eye examination. In the United States, it is estimated that 468,000 3- to 5-year-olds have vision problems (1 in 3) and 12.1 million school-aged children have eye disorders (1 in 4).

Children who are blind or otherwise visually impaired have a higher mortality rate than children who are not visually impaired. Moreover, 60 percent of blind children in the developing world die within 1 year of becoming blind. This high mortality is attributed to the fact that children who are born blind often have associated conditions such as measles, rubella, prematurity, head injuries, or genetic diseases.

RISK FACTORS
Risk factors for loss of vision include age, gender, poverty, and limited access to healthcare. Females are 1.5 to 2 times more likely than males to have vision loss. For children, the greatest risk factor is living in a developing country that has an increased prevalence of measles and ineffective treatments for treating neonatal conjunctivitis at birth. For children in developed countries, the greatest risk factors are retinal conditions, which are mainly hereditary, and optic nerve disorders resulting from premature birth.

SIGNS AND SYMPTOMS
The cost of pediatric visual impairment is high for both societies and affected children and their families. There are associated educational and healthcare costs as well as social and emotional costs for children and their families. Vision plays an important role in children's development in their first 3 years as they use their sight to establish motor functions, bond with their parent(s) or caregiver, and develop their balance. Therefore, a child without full vision will have to overcome obstacles that their counterparts with normal vision may not encounter. Children who are visually impaired have a much higher prevalence of emotional and behavioral issues than children with normal vision. Some commonly noted

problems as children get older are poor educational outcomes resulting from lack of access to resources needed to teach children who are visually impaired, reduced recreational activities, and difficult social experiences. A child may not have access to assistive technology in his or her classroom, for example; may not be given the opportunity to participate fully in physical education classes; or may be embarrassed to go to school because he or she feels less capable than his or her peers. Visually impaired children tend to have fewer friends, fewer chances to socialize, and fewer opportunities to develop interpersonal skills. They may feel rejected, have low self-esteem, struggle with depression, and be withdrawn. They also tend to spend the majority of their time indoors doing individual activities as opposed to being outside with full-sighted peers. Blind or visually impaired children are twice as likely as their full-sighted peers to be bullied because of their disability.

ASSESSMENT
An assessement may require a biopsychosocial-spiritual assessment.

Obtain medical records from the child's ophthalmologist or vision specialist to determine severity of visual impairment, causes, and medical interventions.

A parent/caregiver interview should be used to gather information regarding the prenatal, perinatal, and developmental history of the child, including age of onset and progression of visual impairment or blindness.

Assess for any emotional or behavioral issues that may be associated with the visual impairment, especially for school-aged children.

Assess for the presence and effectiveness of current or past interventions related to blindness or visual impairment.

Visual acuity tests can be used to determine child's diagnosis.

TREATMENT
Social workers working with visually impaired children and their families may assist families to receive an accurate diagnosis for their visually impaired child; help the family and the child come to terms with the diagnosis and possible long-term limitations; provide case management to ensure that the child is receiving needed services; and/or provide psychosocial support to the child experiencing depression,

anxiety, or social isolation. Therefore, it is vital for all social workers to become familiar with blindness and visual impairment, its consequences, and effective interventions.

Social workers should be aware of their own cultural values, beliefs, and biases and develop specialized knowledge about the histories, traditions, and values of their clients. Social workers should adopt treatment methodologies that reflect their knowledge of the cultural diversity of the communities in which they practice. It is important that social workers not assume that those who are visually impaired are unable to work, have families, or participate in activities such as sports or travel. Social workers also should not assume that the visual impairment is the presenting problem in the initial assessment. Social workers should advocate for and assist with access to services for visually impaired individuals and fight the discrimination and exclusion often faced by these individuals. They can also assist in facilitating learning of skills and adaptations so that visually impaired

children can enjoy and participate fully in the activities they want to take part in.

What is most important in a therapeutic relationship with a child with vision issues is to incorporate a strengths-based perspective. A visually impaired child receives many messages about what he or she cannot do. As an advocate, a social worker can help the child identify all the things that he or she can do. In a case management role, a social worker can work closely with medical staff and school staff to ensure that the child has access to needed resources. Specifically, it is important that the social worker be present when the family has an individualized education plan (IEP) meeting for the child at the school with other school personnel. An IEP is an individualized plan containing specific educational goals and objectives for a child with a disability. The IEP identifies the child's current performance, any special assistance or resources needed, special accommodations, and measurements of progress.

Problem	Goal	Intervention
Visual impairment is diagnosed in child and family is fearful, distressed, confused in response	Acceptance of diagnosis	Provide family with accurate information about services and resources available to their child and to them. Validate their feelings. Work on coping skills. Support the grief process that accompanies acceptance of a chronic diagnosis of any kind
Child is experiencing depression and/or anxiety related to visual impairment	Reduce negative mood symptoms and improve emotional support	Teach child relaxation techniques that may help with anxiety. Provide psychosocial support through active listening and supportive counseling to address fears or worries resulting from coping with a visual impairment. Help child develop coping strategies to minimize negative peer interactions related to visual impairment and reduce feelings of embarrassment. Assess for any thoughts of harm to self or others
Visually impaired child is having a difficult time at school academically	Improve academic situation	Collaborate with teachers to create an individualized education plan (IEP) to address areas of need. Share information on technological devices and alternative methods that allow vision-impaired children to participate in music, art, sports, and academic activities in school

LAWS AND REGULATIONS

The Individuals with Disabilities Education Act (IDEA) is a law that ensures services to children with disabilities throughout the United States. It governs how states and public agencies provide early intervention, special education, and related services to more than 6.5 million eligible infants, toddlers, children, and youth with disabilities.

The U.S. Social Security Administration defines legal blindness as having a central visual acuity of 20/200 or less in one's better eye with correction. If a child is legally blind, he or she may be eligible for Supplemental Security Income.

Each country has its own standards for cultural competence and diversity in social work practice. Social workers must be aware of the standards of practice set forth by their governing body (e.g., National Association of Social Workers in the United States, British Association of Social Workers in the UK), and practice accordingly.

SERVICES AND RESOURCES

- Blind Children UK, www.blindchildrenuk.org
- Family Connect, http://www.familyconnect.org/parentsitehome.aspx
- Helen Keller National Center for Deaf-Blind Youths and Adults, http://www.hknc.org/
- National Federation of the Blind, https://nfb.org/
- National Foundation for Blind Children, http://www.foundationforblindchildren.org/
- National Library Service for the Blind and Physically Handicapped, http://www.loc.gov/nls/: a free library program of braille and audio materials circulated to borrowers in the United States by postage-free mail
- National Organization of Parents of Blind Children, http://nopbc.org/

FOOD FOR THOUGHT

WHO's VISION 2020—The Right to Sight Program, is a global initiative to eliminate avoidable visual impairment and blindness by 2020.

Children who are visually impaired often are overlooked in physical education classes in schools because teachers assume that they cannot participate. Therefore, visually impaired children are more sedentary than their sighted peers. There is a need for physical educators to receive more training on how to adapt their classes to include activities for children who have vision issues.

Different resources work for different visually impaired children. They may use braille, canes or guide dogs, recorded materials, live readers, or adapted computers. Working collaboratively with the child's school and medical team can help determine the best resources for each child.

RED FLAGS

Early detection and intervention are crucial if there is any possibility of improving vision outcomes for a child with visual impairment. Visual experience is essential during the critical period (beginning in infancy and gradually declining until around age 8 in most children) in order for the brain's visual system to develop properly. Amblyopia is decreased vision resulting from abnormal vision development during early childhood and results in permanent impairment.

The majority of parents with a visually impaired child report high levels of stress resulting from worry over their ability to meet their child's needs and the uncertainty of the future.

NEXT STEPS

Ensure that children and families have information on appropriate resources available to them.

Encourage parents to utilize early intervention and other services to maximize children's vision and functional abilities.

Written by Melissa Rosales Neff, MSW

Reviewed by Laura Gale, LCSW, and Jennifer Teska, MSW

REFERENCES

Abu, E. K., Yeboah, A. A., Ocansey, S., Kyei, S., & Abokyi, S. (2015). Epidemiology of ocular disorders and visual impairment among school pupils in the Cape Coast Metropolis, Ghana. *British Journal of Visual Impairment, 33*(1), 45-53.

Alimovic, S. (2013). Emotional and behavioural problems in children with visual impairment, intellectual and multiple disabilities. *Journal of Intellectual Disability Research, 57*(2), 153-160. doi:10.1111/j.1365-2788.2012.01562.x

American Foundation for the Blind. (2008). Key definitions of statistical terms. Retrieved December 11, 2015, from http://www.afb.org/info/living-with-vision-loss/blindness-statistics/key-definitions-of-statistical-terms/125

Heijthuijsen, A., Beunders, A., Jiawan, D., Mesquita-Voigt, A., Pawiroredjo, J., Mourits, M., ... Saeed, P. (n.d.). Causes of severe visual impairment and blindness in children in the Republic of Suriname. *The British Journal of Ophthalmology, 97*(7), 812-815. doi:10.1136/bjophthalmol-2011-301000

Begeer, S., Dik, M., voor de Wind, M., Asbrock, D., Brambring, M., & Kef, S. (2014). A new look at the Theory of Mind with ocular and ocular-plus congenital blindness. *Journal of Visual Impairment & Blindness, 108*(1), 17-27.

Bello, S., Meremikwu, M. M., Ejemot-Nwadiaro, R. I., & Oduwole, O. (2014). Routine vitamin A supplementation for the prevention of blindness due to measles infection in children. *The Cochrane Database of Systematic Reviews,* 1. Art. No.: CD007719. doi:10.1002/14651858.CD007719.pub3

British Association of Social Workers. (2012, January). The Code of Ethics for Social Workers: Statement of principles. Retrieved December 13, 2015, from http://cdn.basw.co.uk/upload/basw_112315-7.pdf

Chong, C., & Dai, S. (2013). Cross-sectional study on prevalence, causes and avoidable causes of visual impairment in Maori children. *The New Zealand Medical Journal, 126*(1379), 31-38.

Ganesh, S., Sethi, S., Srivastav, S., Chaudhary, A., & Arora, P. (2013). Impact of low vision rehabilitation on functional vision performance of children with visual impairment. *Journal of Ophthalmology, 6*(3), 170-174. doi:10.4103/0974-620X.122271

Gray, C. (2008). Support for children with a visual impairment in Northern Ireland: The role of the rehabilitation worker. *British Journal of Visual Impairment, 26*(3), 239-254. doi:10.1177/0264619608093642

Gogate, P., & Gilbert, C. (2007). Blindness in children: A worldwide perspective. *Community Eye Health, 20*(62), 32-33. Junior Blind of America. (2014). FAQS about Blindness. Retrieved April 29, 2014, from http://www.juniorblind.org/site/faqs-about-blindness

Khadka, J., Ryan, B., Margrain, H., Woodhouse, T., & Margaret, J. (2012). Listening to voices of children with a visual impairment: A focus group study. *British Journal of Visual Impairment, 30*(3), 182-196.

Lieberman, L. J., & Conroy, P. (2013). Training of paraeducators for physical education for children with visual impairments. *Journal of Visual Impairment & Blindness, 107*(1), 17-28.

Mitry, D., Bunce, C., Wormald, R., & Bowman, R. (2013). Childhood visual impairment in England: A rising trend. *Archives of Disease in Childhood, 98*(5), 378-380. doi:10.1136/archdischild-2012-301970

Mizrahi, T., & Davis, L. E. (2008). Blindness and visual impairment. In *Encyclopedia of social work* (20th ed., Vol. 1, pp. 206-214). Washington, DC: National Association of Social Workers.

Perkins, K., Columna, L., Liberman, L., & Bailey, J. (2013). Parents' perceptions of physical activity for their children with visual impairments. *Journal of Visual Impairment & Blindness, 107*(2), 131-142.

Philip, S. S., & Dutton, G. N. (2014). Identifying and characterising cerebral visual impairment in children: A review. *Clinical and Experimental Optometry: Journal of the Australian Optometrical Association, 97*(3), 196-208. doi:10.1111/cxo.12155

Premsenthil, M., Menju, R., Askokumaran, T., Rahman, S., & Aik Kah, T. (2013). The screening of visual impairment among preschool children in an urban population in Malaysia. *Biomed Central Ophthalmology, 13*(1), 16-21. doi:10.1186/1471-2415-13-16

Ravenscroft, J., Blaikie, A., Macewen, C., O'Hare, A., Creswell, L., & Dutton, G. N. (2008). A novel method of notification to profile childhood visual impairment in Scotland to meet the needs of children with visual impairment. *British Journal of Visual Impairment, 26*(2), 170-189.

Roe, J. (2008). Social inclusion: Meeting the socio-emotional needs of children with vision needs. *British Journal of Visual Impairment, 26*(2), 147-158.

Rolebo, A. L., & Rahi, J. (2014). Epidemiology, aetiology and management of visual impairment in children. *Archives of Disease in Childhood, 99*(4), 375-379. doi:10.1136/archdischild-2012-303002

Wheeler, D., & McClain, A. (2015). NASW standards and indicators for cultural competence in social work practice. Retrieved December 13, 2015, from http://www.socialworkers.org/practice/standards/PRA-BRO-253150-CC-Standards.pdf

World Health Organization. (2012). Visual Impairment and Blindness Fact Sheet. Retrieved

December 13, 2015, from http://www.who.int/
blindness/GLOBALDATAFINALforweb.pdf?ua=1
World Health Organization. (2012). Global Data
on Visual Impairments. Retrieved April 29, 2014,
from http://www.who.int/blindness/GLOBAL-
DATAFINALforweb.pdf?ua=1

World Health Organization. (2001). *International
Classification of Functioning, Disability and Health
(ICF)*. Geneva, Switzerland: World Health Organization. World Health Organization. (2007). *Global
initiative for the elimination of avoidable blindness*. Geneva, Switzerland: WHO.

War: Child Soldiers

MAJOR CATEGORIES: Military & Veterans

WHAT WE KNOW

UNICEF defines a child soldier as any child, boy or girl, under age 18 who has been made part of any kind of armed force or group, whether regular (i.e., government sanctioned) or irregular (i.e., guerilla groups). This definition refers to children used in any capacity, including but not limited to cooks, porters, and messengers. This definition also includes any child who is brought into the armed force or armed group for sexual reasons, including forced marriage.

This is a broad definition that encompasses roles beyond carrying weapons or engaging in combat.

Sexual abuse of child soldiers includes not only children as victims of abuse but children forced to witness or perpetrate forcible sexual acts as part of combat.

Six dimensions interact to facilitate the institutionalization of the military use of children. Politics, policies or the absence of policies, and the cultural and religious beliefs of the region are the three macrolevel dimensions that contribute to the use of child soldiers. Although the majority of African states have a voluntary recruitment age of 18, this is often violated by government militias and opposing forces that recruit child soldiers to further their political agendas. Families may also encourage their children to join, as the military training offered is considered by some as an opportunity for upward social mobility. At the micro level, family, community, and individual psychosocial factors interact with the macro dimensions to foster an environment that allows for children to be abducted and forced to join armies as well as to be non-forcibly recruited and utilized.

There are approximately 300,000 children under age 18 serving in some capacity as child soldiers in 30 conflicts worldwide, including conflicts in Afghanistan, Angola, Burundi, Colombia, the Democratic Republic of the Congo, Guinea-Bissau, Liberia, Mozambique, Rwanda, Sierra Leone, Somalia, Sri Lanka, Sudan, and Uganda.

Researchers studying former child soldiers in Uganda found the average age at which children entered the armed forces to be 10.8 years old; these children served for an average of 19.8 months. Except for one respondent who was born into captivity, all were abducted from their families.

An additional study by the same researchers found that tasks for child soldiers were divided into three categories: front-line tasks (e.g., fighting, looting, abductions), logistics (e.g., carrying cargo, spying, escorting commanders), and domestic tasks (e.g., cooking, child care, cleaning).

An additional study on Ugandan former child soldiers found equal numbers of boys and girls utilized as soldiers. The mean abducted age for this group of respondents was 11.9 years and service was a mean of 24 months.

Former child soldiers from Sierra Leone had a comparable average age of abduction, approximately 10 years old. Of these former child soldiers, girls experienced similar levels of exposure to violence and participation in front-line combat. These girls were not being utilized for domestic tasks only, which has been found in studies of child soldiers in other areas.

Child soldiers are exposed to trauma while involved with armed forces or groups, with the most common being the abduction that led to their involvement with the armed force. Additional traumas include witnessing or perpetrating war-related violence (e.g., massacres or village raids, abductions, assaults, sexual violence, murders), being beaten by members of the armed group, being the victim or forced perpetrator of sexual violence and rape, seeing dead bodies, food and sleep deprivation, electric shocks, mutilation, being used as human shields to protect other soldiers, being ordered to sweep mine fields before military advance, and being threatened on a regular basis with violence.

Researchers found that half of the child soldiers studied had killed someone and one quarter had been raped. This study listed 19 possible traumatic events for child soldiers; on average the former child soldiers had experienced 15 of the 19.

Children were also forced to commit criminal or violent acts, with investigators finding that 65.2 percent had looted houses and 59.1 percent had abducted other children.

Investigators found that 90.6 percent of the children reported having been beaten, 87.9 percent witnessed murder, 86.4 percent were threatened with their own death, and 25.8 percent were raped. Rape was reported almost equally by boys and girls: it was experienced by 22.4 percent of boys and 29.4 percent of girls.

Researchers found that girls and boys experienced equal rates overall for abuse and were equally likely to have been involved in violent acts including physical assaults and murder.

In addition to the trauma suffered during service and combat, there are also traumas that occur post-conflict during what is referred to for child soldiers as the time of disarmament, demobilization, and reintegration. The aftereffects of having served as soldiers create hostile post-conflict realities for children.

Physical injuries and the emotional wounds that accompany injury and disability can have a lasting impact on former child soldiers. Some children are even physically branded by the armed forces they are forced to join.

Loss of family occurs for many of these children, either because they become geographically separated from their families or family members died during the conflict while they were gone.

Long-term traumatic memories can cause nightmares and additional signs and symptoms that lead to post-traumatic stress disorder (PTSD).

In a study of child soldiers 72.4 percent of respondents were found by the investigators to be showing significant symptoms consistent with mental health issues, with 33 percent meeting criteria for PTSD and 36.4 percent meeting criteria for depression.

Grief, guilt, and shame commonly are experienced by former child soldiers and can contribute to anxiety, depression, and PTSD.

Suicidal ideation was found by researchers in 30 percent of the children that were studied.

Traumatic experiences as a perpetrator can lead to feelings of guilt for child soldiers. Researchers found that guilt is associated with externalizing behaviors and the development of PTSD.

Anxiety and depression were found at higher rates among respondents who had been raped, held for longer periods of time, or experienced stigma.

Investigators found that female child soldiers had higher scores for depression and anxiety when compared to males.

Stigma and community rejection can occur when child soldiers try to return to their family or community but as former combatants are rejected, discriminated against, or otherwise stigmatized.

Girls frequently are rejected because assumptions are made that they experienced sexual violence, which culturally can lead to rejection, including inability to find a suitor.

Girls are vulnerable to sexual violence during war and are at increased risk of unwanted pregnancy, chronic pelvic pain, sexually transmitted infections (e.g., HIV), infertility, and incontinence.

Community acceptance has been shown to be a crucial protective factor for more positive outcomes post-conflict by reducing negative symptoms such as depression and anxiety while increasing prosocial attitudes.

The youth studied who experienced stigma post-conflict were found to have higher rates of externalizing issues.

Educational and economic marginalization is a risk since former child soldiers often missed educational opportunities and missed chances to learn marketable skills. This lack of education or career training makes escaping an impoverished situation even more unlikely.

Children who were able to return to a school setting and had higher levels of community acceptance operated at a higher baseline of functioning.

Researchers have found that as child soldiers become parents themselves, they can transmit symptoms such as emotional numbness, anxiety, aggression, and emotional distress to their own children, creating a pattern of intergenerational trauma.

Drugs and alcohol often are given to child soldiers to prepare them for battle. Drug and/or alcohol addiction can impede rehabilitation.

Disarmament, demobilization, and reintegration is a time during which social workers and humanitarian aid workers have an opportunity to help these youth process the trauma they have experienced.

Narrative exposure therapy, which is a short-term therapy often used with multiple traumas, was found by investigators to significantly reduce PTSD symptoms among the Ugandan former child soldiers who participated in the study.

Traditional healing or cleansing rituals or ceremonies can help children reintegrate with families and the community and may reduce the negative effects of trauma.

Community sensitization campaigns may increase community acceptance of returning child soldiers.

Formalized peer support can reduce the feelings of isolation and shame that affect former child soldiers.

A holistic approach that addresses both mental health issues (e.g., anxiety, depression, PTSD) and postwar stressors (e.g., lack of education, poverty, unemployment, inadequate housing, stigma, lack of social support) is important to mitigate the psychological and psychosocial problems faced by child soldiers.

WHAT CAN BE DONE

Learn about the needs of child soldiers so you can accurately assess your client's personal characteristics and education needs; share this information with your colleagues.

Develop an awareness of your own cultural values, beliefs, and biases and develop knowledge about the histories, traditions, and values of your clients. Adopt treatment methodologies that reflect the cultural needs of the client.

Advocate for the ratification of the United Nations Optional Protocol to the Convention on the Rights of the Child on the involvement of children in armed conflict by nations that have not yet made legal strides to protect children during times of armed conflict.

Promote demobilization of child soldiers worldwide while supporting reintegration.

Recognize child soldiers as being the victims of institutionalized child abuse.

Work to develop psychological intervention efforts that can be used within communities in which returned child soldiers live or in refugee camps.

If working as a social worker in a community with former child soldiers, work with the community on a sensitization program to increase awareness and acceptance of former child soldiers and potentially develop a ceremony or healing ritual for them.

If working as a social worker in a Western nation, become knowledgeable about child soldiers to be prepared for potential former child soldiers being part of a caseload after those children have relocated.

Utilize culturally sensitive and appropriate trauma counseling techniques when working with any former child soldiers.

Written by Jessica Therivel, LMSW-IPR

Reviewed by Lynn B. Cooper, D. Crim, and Laura McLuckey, MSW, LCSW

REFERENCES

Amone-P'Olak, K., Stochl, J., Ovuga, E., Abbott, R., Meiser-Stedman, R., Croudace, T. J., & Jones, P. B. (2014). Postwar environment and long-term mental health problems in former child soldiers in Northern Uganda: The WAYS study. *Journal of Epidemiology & Community Health, 68*(5), 425-430. doi:10.1136/jech-2013-203042

Awodola, B. (2012). An examination of methods to reintegrate former child soldiers in Liberia. *Intervention, 10*(1), 30-42.

Betancourt, T. S., Agnew-Blais, J., Gilman, S. E., Williams, D. R., & Ellis, B. H. (2010). Past horrors, present struggles: The role of stigma in the association between war experiences and psychosocial adjustment among former child soldiers in Sierra Leone. *Social Science & Medicine, 70*(1), 17-26. doi:10.1016/j.socscimed.2009.09.038

Betancourt, T. S., Borisova, I. I., de la Soudiere, M., & Williamson, J. (2011). Sierra Leone's child soldiers: War exposures and mental health problems by gender. *The Journal of Adolescent Health: Official Publication of the Society for Adolescent Medicine, 49*(1), 21-28. doi:10.1016/j.jadohealth.2010.09.021

Betancourt, T. S., Borisova, I. I., Williams, T. P., Brennan, R. T., Whitfield, T. H., de la Soudiere, M.,.... Gilman, S. E. (2010). Sierra Leone's former child soldiers: A follow-up study of psychosocial adjustment and community reintegration. *Child Development, 81*(4), 1077-1095. doi:10.1111/j.1467-8624.2010.01455.x

Betancourt, T. S., Brennan, R. T., Rubin-Smith, J., Fitzmaurice, G. M., & Gilman, S. E. (2010). Sierra Leone's former child soldiers: A longitudinal study of risk, protective factors, and mental health. *Journal of the American Academy of Child and Adolescent Psychiatry, 49*(6), 606-615. doi:10.1016/j.jaac.2010.03.008

British Association of Social Workers. (2012, January). The code of ethics for social work: Statement of principles. Retrieved from http://cdn.basw.co.uk/upload/basw_112315-7.pdf

Denov, M. (2010). Coping with the trauma of war: Former child soldiers in post-conflict Sierra Leone. *International Social Work, 53*(6), 791-806. doi:10.1177/0020872809358400

Derluyn, I. (2011). Toward a new agenda for rehabilitation and reintegration processes for child soldiers. *The Journal of Adolescent Health: Official Publication of the Society for Adolescent Medicine, 49*(1), 3-4. doi:10.1016/j.jadohealth.2011.05.006

Ertl, V., Pfeiffer, A., Schauer, E., Elbert, T., & Neuner, F. (2011). Community-implemented trauma therapy for former child soldiers in Northern Uganda: A randomized controlled trial. *JAMA: The Journal of the American Medical Association, 306*(5), 503-512. doi:10.1001/jama.2011.1060

International Federation of Social Workers. (n.d.). Statement of ethical principles. Retrieved December 10, 2015, from http://ifsw.org/policies/statement-of-ethical-principles/

Johannessen, S., & Holdersen, H. (2014). Former child soldiers' problems and needs: Congolese experiences. *Qualitative Health Research, 24*(1), 55-66. doi:10.1177/1049732313513655

Kerig, P. K., & Wainryb, C. (2013). Introduction to the special issue, part I: New research on trauma, psychopathology, and resilience among child soldiers around the world. *Journal of Aggression, Maltreatment & Trauma, 22*(7), 685-697. doi:10.1080/10926771.2013.817816

Kerig, P. K., & Wainryb, C. (2013). Introduction to the special issue, part II: Interventions to promote reintegration of traumatized youth conscripted as child soldiers. *Journal of Aggression, Maltreatment & Traum, 22*(8), 797-802. doi:10.1080/10926771.2013.823591

Kimmel, C. E., & Roby, J. L. (2007). Institutionalized child abuse: The use of child soldiers. *International Social Work, 50*(6), 740-754.

Klasen, F., Oettingen, G., Daniels, J., & Adam, H. (2010). Multiple trauma and mental health in former Ugandan child soldiers. *Journal of Traumatic Stress, 23*(5), 573-581. doi:10.1002/jts.20557

Klasen, F., Oettingen, G., Daniels, J., Post, M., Hoyer, C., & Adam, H. (2010). Posttraumatic resilience in former Ugandan child soldiers. *Child Development, 81*(4), 1096-1113. doi:10.1111/j.1467-8624.2010.01456.x

Klasen, F., Reissmann, S., Voss, C., & Okello, J. (2015). The guiltless guilty: Trauma-related guilt and psychopathology in former Ugandan child soldiers. *Child Psychiatry and Human Development, 46*(2), 180-193. doi:10.1007/s10578-014-0470-6

Moscardino, U., Scrimin, S., Cadei, F., & Altoe, G. (2012). Mental health among former child soldiers and never-abducted children in northern Uganda. *The Scientific World Journal*, 1-7.

Song, S. J., Tol, W., & de Jong, J. (2014). Indero: Intergenerational trauma and resilience between Burundian former child soldiers and their children. *Family Process, 53*(2), 239-251. doi:10.1111/famp.12071

Stevens, A. J. (2014). The invisible soldiers: Understanding how the life experiences of girl child soldiers impacts upon their health and rehabilitation needs. *Archives of Disease in Childhood, 99*(5), 458-462. doi:10.1136/archdischild-2013-305240

United Nations Children's Fund (UNICEF), &. (2002). Adult wars, child soldiers: Voices of children involved in armed conflict in the East Asia and Pacific region. *UNICEF East Asia and Pacific Region Regional Office*. Retrieved December 10, 2015, from http://www.unicef.org/sowc06/pdfs/pub_adultwars_en.pdf

United Nations Children's Fund (UNICEF). (2007, February). The Paris principles: Principles and guidelines on children associated with armed forces or armed groups. *UNICEF*. Retrieved December 10, 2015, from http://www.unicef.org/emerg/files/ParisPrinciples310107English.pdf

Wheeler, D. (2015). NASW standards for cultural competency in social work practice. Retrieved December 10, 2015, from http://www.socialworkers.org/practice/standards/PRA-BRO-253150-CC-Standards.pdf

WAR: EFFECTS ON CHILDREN

MAJOR CATEGORIES: Child & Family

WHAT WE KNOW

An estimated 230 million children worldwide live in areas involved in armed conflict.

In the 21 century children n are considered more vulnerable in war than previously: often there are no clearly defined battlefields, warring parties are complex and multiple, previously safe sites such as schools and hospitals come under deliberate attack, and children frequently are targeted as victims or forced participants.

The impacts of war on children vary, but may include the following:

- Direct victimization (e.g., death and maiming, abduction, imprisonment, torture, sexual abuse, recruitment as soldiers or forced participation in violent acts).
- Witnessing maiming and killing.
- Victimization of close friend and relatives.
- Separation from family; displacement from home and/or country (At the end of 2014, 59.5 million persons worldwide were forcibly displaced, of which 38.2 million were displaced within their countries of origin, 19.5 million were refugees, and 1.8 million were asylum seekers (i.e., persons whose claim of refugee status has not yet been confirmed). Just over half of all refugees in 2014 were children.
- Removal from families by force or coercion and placement for adoption, often under the guise of "rescue."
- Restricted access to medical care, education, and humanitarian assistance.
- Exposure to war-related experiences is associated in children with high rates of post-traumatic stress disorder (PTSD), depression,and anxiety.

Children exposed to severe trauma during war often experience lifelong intrusive memories, the inability to verbalize emotions, and poor psychological development as a result of the impact of severe stress.

Researchers in a study of students between 18 and 25 years old who were exposed to war in the Balkans as children found that 15 years after the conflict, approximately two-thirds of respondents reported clinically significant symptoms of anxiety and one third reported clinically significant symptoms of depression.

Children who utilize primarily emotion-focused coping strategies (e.g., avoidance, self-control) have a higher likelihood of having emotional and behavioral issues than children who utilize problem-focused coping strategies (e.g., problem-solving, seeking support).

A child's risk of developing PTSD after exposure to war increases if the child had a psychological disorder or experienced trauma prior to war (e.g., family violence, neglect, abuse).

Secure attachment to a parental figure acts as a protective factor for children exposed to war, reducing their risk for developing a psychological disorder.

Children imprisoned during wartime are at risk for multiple physical and mental health conditions.

Depression, irritability, aggression, withdrawal, and PTSD symptoms such as insomnia, nightmares, and paranoia are frequent. Respiratory infections, kidney malfunction, and visual disorders also are common. Boys tortured with electric shocks to their genitals frequently become sexually impotent and unable to marry.

Children are sometimes detained in prison with adults during war and are vulnerable to abuse. Researchers in a longitudinal study of youth who were abducted and held captive by rebels in Northern Uganda found that rhe majority (70 percent) reported mental health difficulties, including anxiety, irritability, and nightmares; 10 percent of males and 65 percent of females reported being sexually abused by their captors.

Many youth continued to experience long-term effects associated with war experiences, including increased risk of psychotic symptoms in youth who were involved in combat, experienced sexual abuse in captivity, or witnessed violence and/or deaths. Post-war stressors were also found to contribute to individual differences in long-term mental health issues for these youth.

The majority of youth were receptive to mental health services and those who had received mental health services in the past reported better functioning than those who did not; stigma, fear of family break-up, and lack of available services were barriers to youth receiving needed mental health services.

Some scholars draw attention to the resourcefulness of children living in conditions of war. Children often show self-efficacy and resilience, overcome hardships, and seek psychosocial safety and security under dire circumstances.

War often deprives children of an adequate education, reducing their potential for economic independence and increasing the risk that they will live in extreme economic hardship as adults.

When war is over, postwar conditions, including displacement, poverty, poor living conditions, social exclusion, and inadequate support systems (e.g. healthcare and employment training) are reported to hinder the reintegration of children into the community.

It is recommended that education, training, and physical and mental healthcare needs be prioritized once war is over.

In some countries child protection workers are inadequately trained to deal with the problems facing children who have experienced war; in addition, there often is limited government support for initiatives to assist them.

In addition to children who live in areas experiencing conflict, the children of soldiers who are deployed to combat are also affected by war.

Children of soldiers who return from war with physical and mental health conditions are at risk of developing high levels of distress and anxiety, which is understood as secondary trauma or secondary traumatic stress: anxiety-related behaviors, depressed mood, withdrawal, and somatic symptoms are common.

Children of parents deployed to war are especially vulnerable to adverse consequences if their families have histories of mental health problems, poverty, and intimate partner violence.

Military families have low participation rates in interventions: additional help removing the barriers to treatment, such as transportation and stigma, may need to be addressed.

WHAT CAN BE DONE

Learn about the effects of war upon children and how these effects may impact their childhood, adolescence, and adulthood so you can accurately assess your client's personal characteristics and effectively

advocate for his or her rights; share this information with your colleagues.

Develop an awareness of your own cultural values, beliefs, and biases and develop knowledge about the histories, traditions, and values of your clients. Adopt treatment methodologies that reflect the cultural needs of the client.

Social workers working with children affected by war are advised to use the definitions of health and illness that are used by the child's culture when making assessments. Using an ethnically sensitive ecological framework is critical.

Learn about the child's strengths and resilience during and after war.

Early detection of PTSD and psychological distress after children are exposed to war is critical to reduce the likelihood of long-term psychological impairment.

A comprehensive description of screening and assessment tools can be found online,http://www.cpcnetwork.org/wp-content/uploads/2014/06/Measuring-Child-MHPSS-in-Emergencies_CU_Compendium_March-2014-.pdf.

Learn about interventions for children who are at risk for or who are experiencing mental health difficulties as a result of war-related experiences

In a review of research regarding interventions for children exposed to war-related events, investigators noted that there are not sufficient data regarding effective strategies to prevent mental health issues or to reduce the chance of recurrence of symptoms in children affected by war. There is a stronger knowledge base for interventions effective for treating mental health symptoms associated with war experiences.

Trauma-focused cognitive-behavioral therapy (TF-CBT) and eye-movement desensitization and reprocessing (EMDR) have been recognized as effective treatments for PTSD.

Researchers in a randomized controlled study found that TF-CBT group therapy was associated with significant reductions in PTSD symptoms in boys affected by war.

Narrative exposure therapy, and an adaptation for youth aged 12-17 (KidNET),has also been associated with reduction in PTSD symptoms.

School-based interventions are often referenced in the literature, but research findings vary and some investigators assert that classroom-based interventions that use universal treatment approaches to target large groups of children are less effective than individual assessment and treatment modalities for children experiencing PTSD, anxiety, and/or depression as a result of war exposure.

School-based interventions can be beneficial for strengthening coping and resilience.

Social support networks can alleviate the psychological effects of war experienced by children. Social workers should incorporate a child's social support network into treatment.

Learn about the range of injuries parents serving in the military may experience in order to understand what their children are having to adjust to (e.g., amputations, traumatic brain injuries, PTSD).

Learn about parenting programs that may support positive functioning in families affected by deployment.

Written by Jan Wagstaff, MA, MSW, and Jennifer Teska, MSW

Reviewed by Jessica Therivel, LMSW-IPR, and Emma Tiffany-Malm, MSW

REFERENCES

Amone-P'Olak, K., Jones, P., Meiser-Stedman, R., Abbott, R., Ayella-Ataro, P. S., Amone, J., & Ovuga, E. (2014). War experiences, general functioning and barriers to care among former child soldiers in Northern Uganda: The WAYS Study. *Journal of Public Health, 36*(4), 568-576. doi:10.1093/pubmed/fdt126

Amone-P'Olak, K., Otim, B. N., Opio, G., Ovuga, E., & Meiser-Stedman, R. (2015). War experiences and psychotic symptoms among former child soldiers in Northern Uganda: The mediating role of post-war hardships – the WAYS Study. *South African Journal of Psychology, 45*(2), 155-167.

Amone-P'Olak, K., Stochl, J., Ovuga, E., Abbott, R., Meiser-Stedman, R., Croudace, T. J., & Jones, P. B. (2014). Postwar environment and long-term mental health problems in former child soldiers in Northern Uganda: The WAYS study. *Journal of Epidemiology & Community Health, 68*(5), 425-430. doi:10.1136/jech-2013-203042

Betancourt, T. S., Meyers-Ohki, S. E., Charrow, A. P., & Tol, W. A. (2013). Interventions for children affected by war: An ecological perspective on psychosocial support and mental health care. *Harvard*

Review of Psychiatry, 21(2), 70-91. doi:10.1097/HRP.0b013e31828bf8f

British Association of Social Workers. (2012, January). The Code of Ethics for Social Work: Statement of Principles. Retrieved from http://cdn.basw.co.uk/upload/basw_112315-7.pdf

Denov, M. (2010). Coping with the trauma of war: Former child soldiers in post-conflict Sierra Leone. *International Social Work, 53*(6), 791-806. doi:10.1177/0020872809358400

Ertl, V., & Neuner, F. (2014). Are school-based mental health interventions for war-affected children effective and harmless?. *BMC Medicine, 12*(1), 84. doi:10.1186/1741-7015-12-84

Ertl, V., Pfeiffer, A., Schauer, E., Elbert, T., & Neuner, F. (2011). Community-implemented trauma therapy for former child soldiers in Northern Uganda: A randomized controlled trial. *Journal of the American Medical Association, 306*(5), 503-512. doi:10.1001/jama.2011.1060

Feldman, R., Vengrober, A., & Ebstein, R. P. (2014). Affiliation buffers stress: cumulative genetic risk in oxytocin-vasopressin genes combines with early caregiving to predict PTSD in war-exposed young children. *Translational Psychiatry, 4*, e370. doi:10.1038/tp.2014.6

Fletcher, K. L. (2013). Helping children with the psychosocial effects of a parent's deployment: Integrating today's needs with lessons learned from the Vietnam War. *Smith College Studies in Social Work, 83*(1), 78-96. doi:10.1080/00377317.2013.746924

Gewirtz, A. H., & Zamir, O. (2014). The impact of parental deployment to war on children: The crucial role of parenting. *Advances in Child Development and Behavior, 46*, 89-112. doi:10.1016/B978-0-12-8002855-8-00004-2

Herzog, J., Everson, R., & Whitworth, J. (2011). Do secondary trauma symptoms in spouses of combat-exposed National Guard soldiers mediate impacts of soldiers' trauma exposure on their children? *Child & Adolescent Social Work Journal, 28*(6), 459-473. doi:10.1007/s10560-011-0243-z

International Federation of Social Workers. (2012). Statement of ethical principles. Retrieved January 10, 2016, from http://ifsw.org/policies/statement-of-ethical-principles/

Kamya, H. (2009). The impact of war on children: How children perceive their experiences. *Journal of Immigrant & Refugee Studies, 7*(2), 211-216. doi:10.1080/15562940902936587

Karam, E. G., Fayyad, J., Karam, A. N., Melham, N., Mneimneh, Z., Dimassi, H., & Tabet, C. C. (2014). Outcome of depression and anxiety after war: a prospective epidemiologic study of children and adolescents. *Journal of Traumatic Stress, 27*(2), 192-199. doi:10.1002/jts.21895

Khamis, V. (2015). Coping with war trauma and psychological distress among school-age Palestinian children. *American Journal of Orthopsychiatry, 85*(1), 72-79. doi:10.1037/ort0000039

Lincoln, A. J., & Sweeten, K. (2011). Considerations for the effects of military deployment on children and families. *Social Work in Health Care, 50*(1), 73-84. doi:10.1080/00981389.2010.513921

Llabre, M. M., Hadi, F., La Greca, A. M., & Lai, B. S. (2013). Psychological distress in young adults exposed to war-related trauma in childhood. *Journal of Clinical Child and Adolescent Psychology, 44*(1), 169-80. doi:10.1080/15374416.2013.828295

McMullen, J., O'Callaghan, P., Shannon, C., Black, A., & Eakin, J. (2013). Group trauma-focused cognitive-behavioural therapy with former child soldiers and other war-affected boys in the DR Congo: A randomised controlled trial. *Journal of Child Psychology and Psychiatry, 54*(11), 1231-1241. doi:10.1111/jcpp.12094

Mooren, T. T., & Kleber, R. J. (2013). The significance of experiences of war and migration in older age: long-term consequences in child survivors from the Dutch East Indies. *International Psychogeriatrics/ IPA, 25*(11), 1783-1794. doi:10.1017/S1041610213

Ochen, E. A., Jones, A. D., & McAuley, J. W. (2012). Formerly abducted child mothers in Northern Uganda: A critique of modern structures for child protection and reintegration. *Journal of Community Practice, 20*(1/2), 89-111. doi:10.1080/10705422.2012.644228

Rashid, J. (2012). An analysis of self-accounts of children-in-conflict-with-law in Kashmir concerning the impact of torture and detention on their lives. *International Social Work, 55*(5), 629-644. doi:10.1177/0020872812447640

Snyder, C. S., May, J. D., Zulcic, N. N., & Gabbard, W. J. (2005). Social work with Bosnian Muslim refugee children and families: A review of the literature. *Child Welfare, 84*(5), 607-630.

Tol, W. A., Komproe, I. H., Jordans, M. J. D., Ndayisaba, A., Ntamutumba, P., Sipsma, H., & de Jong, J. T. V. M.,. (2014). School-based mental health intervention for children in war-affected Burundi: A cluster randomized trial. *BMC Medicine, 12*(1), 56. doi:10.1186/1741-7015-12-56

Wheeler, D. (2015). NASW Standards and Indicators for Cultural Competence in Social Work Practice. Retrieved January 10, 2016, from http://www.socialworkers.org/practice/standards/PRA-BRO-253150-CC-Standards.pdf

Robinson, S., Metzler, J., & Ager, A. (2014). *A compendium of tools for the assessment of the mental health and psychosocial wellbeing of children in the context of humanitarian emergencies.* New York: Columbia University, Columbia Group for Children in Adversity and Child Protection in Crisis (CPC) Network. Retrieved January 16, 2016, from http://www.cpcnetwork.org/wp-content/uploads/2014/06/Measuring-Child-MHPSS-in-Emergencies_CU_Compendium_March-2014-.pdf

Rotabi, K. S. (2014). Child adoption and war: 'Living disappeared' children and the social worker's post-conflict role in El Salvador and Argentina. *International Social Work, 57*(2), 169180. doi:10.1177/0020872812454314

UNICEF. (2014). Children and emergencies in 2014: Facts & Figures. Retrieved January 16, 2016, from http://www.unicef.org/media/files/UNICEF_Children_and_Emergencies_2014_fact_sheet.pdf

United Nations Children's Fund. (2009). Machel Study 10-year strategic review: Children and conflict in a changing world. Retrieved January 16, 1970, from https://childrenandarmedconflict.un.org/publications/MachelStudy-10YearStrategicReview_en.pdf

United Nations High Commissioner for Refugees. (2014). Global trends: Forced displacement in 2014. Retrieved December 6, 2015, from http://www.unhcr.org/556725e69.html

Zikic, O., Krstic, M., Randjelovic, D., Nikolic, G., Dimitrijevic, B., & Jaredic, B. (2015). Anxiety and depressiveness in students with childhood war-related experiences. *Journal of Loss and Trauma, 20*(2), 95-108. doi:10.1080/15325024.2013.828560

WORKPLACE VIOLENCE: AN OVERVIEW

MAJOR CATEGORIES: Physical Abuse, Violence

DESCRIPTION

Workplace violence is any act or threat of physical violence, verbal abuse, sexual harassment, intimidation, or property damage occurring at a place of work. It affects employees, clients, customers, and visitors in work environments, and in extreme cases can include homicide, which in the United States is a leading cause of fatal occupational injury. Besides causing death or injury, workplace violence may have significant acute and long-term psychosocial consequences for the victim, and may result in lost productivity and financial losses for organizations.

Although workplace violence is a serious public health concern affecting many different industries, it especially affects employees in the healthcare and social service professions. Asserting that corporate and other organizations have a duty to protect their employees from all forms of workplace violence, many studies have issued a call to action for preventing such violence.

A major source of workplace conflict is employee frustration, which is often the result of role conflicts, poor managerial responses to workers' expressed needs, and lack of adequate staffing. Work environments can foster bullying that extends beyond the dyad of a perpetrator and a victim. Organizations in which supervisors aggressively assert their authority, make decisions without consultation, and yell at employees experience increased levels of conflict between workers, as well as more accidents and absenteeism. Less workplace violence occurs in organizations whose managers are respectful and understanding, who problem solve with workers, and who compromise. Sexual harassment, a form of violence that constitutes an abuse of power, is reportedly increasing among both men and women in the workplace.

In addition to violence between employees and within organizations, workplace violence may also take the form of violent acts perpetrated by individuals from outside the workplace. Occupations in which workers have high levels of contact with the public, such as law enforcement, nursing, and the social service professions, are more vulnerable to this type of workplace violence. Work-related violence perpetrated by individuals outside an organization also occurs in the form of robbery, mugging, and intimate partner violence (IPV), or results from road rage. The location of a workplace is also a factor in workplace violence: Studies have found increased rates of violence in healthcare workplaces in urban communities with high levels of poverty.

For all of the foregoing reasons, conflict resolution within organizations is critically important. A high level of collaboration between employees has been shown to result in fewer conflicts. Employee advocacy programs can help workers to report, discuss, and resolve conflicts. In high-risk work environments, coworker support, high-quality supervision, respect for diversity, and consensual decision making have been identified as factors protecting employees from violence.

Employee assistance programs (EAPs) can provide counseling, support, and conflict resolution services to workers, and should be created or strengthened in organizations at high risk for workplace violence. Plans for preventing and managing violent events should be implemented, and occupations in which there is a high risk of violence against employees should provide them with training to recognize the warning signs of violence and to respond, defuse, and document potentially violent events. Among recommendations for this are lobbying for stricter gun control legislation by health and social service professionals.

FACTS AND FIGURES

In the United States, nearly 2 million workers a year report having been a victim of workplace violence. However, the actual number is probably greater than this because many incidents of violence go unreported. Healthcare and social service workers are four times more likely to be victims of violence than are employees in the private sector. In a study done in 2008, 18.3 of 10,000 social service workers reported experiencing some form of workplace-related violence, making them the group at highest risk for such violence, with the corresponding figure for all other occupational groups collectively being 2.7 of every 10,000 workers. In 2012, homicide was the fourth leading cause of fatal occupational injury in the United States, accounting for 11 percent of all workplace fatalities.

RISK FACTORS

Younger workers have a greater risk than older ones of being victims of workplace-related violence. Beyond this, an increased risk of work-related violence can occur in settings in which staffing levels are low; in which staff members work alone or handle money; and in which customers, clients, or patients must endure long waits for services or in which services are unavailable. As noted earlier, employment in which there is a high level of contact with the public, such as police and security work, nursing, and social work, also carry an increased risk for workplace violence, as do occupations that require working late at night or during early morning hours, working with unstable or volatile persons, working in high-crime areas, guarding valuable property or possessions, or working in community-based settings. Organizations that permit guns on their premises may create an increased risk of homicide for workers.

The assessment of an individual's risk of perpetrating violence must include factors such as a personal history of violence, gender, gender attitudes, and behavior. Behavior that is deemed unacceptable should be described in an organization's violence-prevention policy, and all employees of the organization should be informed of the criteria considered to constitute appropriate behavior.

SIGNS AND SYMPTOMS

Victims and witnesses of workplace violence can experience shock, disbelief, guilt, anger, depression, and overwhelming fear. Other signs of such violence are physical injury; increased stress; physical disorders (migraine, vomiting); loss of self-esteem and of belief in professional competence; paralyzing self-blame; feelings of powerlessness and of being exploited; sexual disturbances; avoidance behavior that may negatively affect performance; impairment of interpersonal relationships; loss of job satisfaction; absenteeism; and loss of morale and efficiency. Organizations in which workplace violence has occurred may experience increased staff turnover.

TREATMENT

Employees who report having been victims of violence, and those who appear to be stressed and isolated,

should be given a medical, psychological, social, and spiritual assessment that includes information about their physical, mental, environmental, social, financial, and medical characteristics as part of helping in development of the most suitable treatment for them, and their well-being should be monitored. These individuals and the organizations for which they work should be questioned about workplace conflict, and such individuals should be helped with means for resolving such conflict and referred to the appropriate services, such as an Employee Assistance Program (EAP). Pictograms can be helpful if an assessment indicates that an individual has a low level of literacy.

Persons who have experienced or witnessed a traumatic violent event may need ongoing support and counseling, and those who exhibit depression should be examined for its perceived causes and for their individual internal dialogue about their feelings. Cognitive behavioral interventions can help in identifying negative cognitions and replacing them with healthier ways of thinking. Membership in a peer support group and social support network can help in this regard. Individuals who have experienced trauma through a violent incident should initially be offered reassurance and support. They should be helped to desensitize themselves to the trauma they experienced and asked to record and explore any intrusive thoughts or feelings. The social worker should provide referrals and linkage to support and advocacy groups and legal support if indicated.

Employees should be advised against trying to handle dangerous workplace situations alone, but to call for security. They should be advised not to ignore an agitated person, and should be counseled to neither threaten nor demand obedience of another employee or other individual, or to argue, become defensive, laugh, move suddenly, or make threatening gestures against such an individual, and to avoid invading a potential perpetrator's personal space.

Social workers should be aware of their own cultural values, beliefs, and biases and develop specialized knowledge about the histories, traditions, and values of the individuals they serve, and should adopt methodologies that reflect a knowledge of the cultural diversity of the societies in which they practice. They should provide educational information in a culturally sensitive manner, using language that can be easily understood by the persons they seek to assist. Social workers should utilize evidence-based practices, ensure the privacy and confidentiality of their work with an individual client, and keep accurate records of the services they provide to the client.

Applicable Laws and Regulations

The California Division of Occupational Safety and Health Administration (Cal/OSHA) has defined the following four types of workplace violence, and these definitions are accepted internationally:

Type I: The aggressor has no legitimate relationship, on the basis of employment, to the worker or the workplace, and the main object of violence is usually to obtain cash or valuable property or to demonstrate power. Examples of this type of violence are robbery, mugging, and road rage.

Type II: The aggressor is someone who is the recipient of a service provided by the affected workplace or by the worker who is the victim of violence. Examples of such violence are assaults or verbal threats to healthcare workers by patients, caregivers, or relatives of hospitalized patients.

Type III: The aggressor is another employee, a supervisor, or a manager. Examples of such violence are bullying and harassment.

Type IV: The aggressor has no workplace relationship to the employee who is a victim of violence other than being a current or former intimate partner, relative, or friend of the employee.

In developed countries, employers have a duty of care towards workers that is outlined in organizational policies and regulated through domestic laws. In the United States, the Occupational Safety and Health Administration (OSHA) has created a directive designed to prevent workplace violence and ensure prompt, informed intervention by all employers to prevent or stop such violence through precautionary measures such as implementing a zero-tolerance policy for violence and implementing a written protocol and preventive and interruptive procedures against violence.

Services and Resources

- The United States Department of Labor, http://www.osha.gov/SLTC/workplaceviolence

Written by Jan Wagstaff, MA, MSW

Reviewed by Lynn B. Cooper, D Crim, and Jennifer Mary Dorrell, ASW

References

Abu A lRub, R. F., & Al Khaldeh, A. T. (2013). Workplace physical violence among hospital nurses and physicians in underserved areas in Jordan. *Journal of Clinical Nursing, 23*(13-14), 1937-1947. doi: 10.1111/jocn.124736

American Academy of Experts in Traumatic Stress (AAETS). (2012). Workplace violence. Retrieved April 21, 2016, from http://www.aaets.org/article179.htm

Bentley, T. A., Catley, B., Forsyth, D., & Tappin, D. (2014). Understanding workplace violence: The value of a systems perspective. *Applied Ergonomics, 45*(4), 839-848. doi: 10.1016/j.apergo.2013.10.016

Booth, B., Vecchi, G. M., Finney, E. J., Van Hasselt, V. B., & Romano, S.J. (2009). Captive-taking incidents in the context of workplace violence: Descriptive analysis and case examples. *Victims & Offenders, 4*(1), 76-92. doi: 10.1080/15564880802675935

British Association of Social Workers. (2012). *The code of ethics for social work: Statement of principles.* Retrieved April 22, 2016, from http://cdn.basw.co.uk/upload/basw_112315-7.pdf

Bureau of Labor and Statistics. (2012). National consensus of fatal occupation injuries in 2012. Retrieved April 21, 2016, from http://www.bls.gov/iif/oshwc/cfoi/cfch0011.pdf

Centers for Disease Control and Prevention. (2014). Occupational violence. Retrieved April 21, 2016, from http://www.cdc.gov/niosh/topics/violencend

DePuy, J., Romain-Glassey, N., Gut, M., Pascal, W., Mangin, P., & Danuser, B. (2014). Clinically assessed consequences of workplace physical violence. *International Archives of Occupational and Environmental Health, 88*(2), 213-224. doi: 10.1007/s00420-014-0950-9

Fute, M., Mengesha, Z. B., Wakgari, N., & Tessema, G. A. (2015). High prevalence of workplace violence among nurses working at public health facilities in Southern Ethiopia. *BMC Nursing, 14*(1), 1-5. doi: 10.1186/s12912-015-0062-1

Gillespie, G. L., Gates, D. M., & Fisher, B. S. (2014). Individual, relationship, workplace, and societal recommendations for addressing healthcare workplace violence. *Work, 51*(1), 67-71. Advance online publication. doi: 10.3233/WOR-141890

Harrell, E. (2011). Workplace violence, 1993-2009: National crime victimization survey and the census of fatal occupational injuries. Retrieved

April 21, 2016, from http://bjs.ojp.usdoj.gov/index.cfm?ty=pbdetail&iid=2377

International Federation of Social Workers. (2012). Statement of ethical principles. Retrieved April 21, 2016, from http://ifsw.org/policies/statement-of-ethical-principles/

Loomis, D., Marshall, S. W., & Ta, M. L. (2005). Employer policies toward guns and the risk of homicide in the workplace. *American Journal of Public Health, 95*(5), 830-832. doi: 10.2105/AJPH.2003.033535

Malik, S., & Farooqi, Y. N. (2014). General and Sexual Harassment as Predictors of Posttraumatic Stress Symptoms among Female Health Professionals. *World Journal of Medical Sciences, 10*(1), 43-49. doi: 10.5829/idosi.wjms.2014.10.1.81128

Morken, T., Johansen, H. J., & Alsaker, K. (2015). Dealing with workplace violence in emergency primary health care: A focus group. *BMC Family Practice, 16*(1), 1-7. doi: 10.1186/s12875-015-0276-z

Notelaers, G., De Witte, H., & Einarsen, S. (2010). A job characteristics approach to explain workplace bullying. *European Journal of Work and Organizational Psychology, 19*(4), 487-504. doi: 10.1080/13594320903007620

Office for National Statistics. (2015). Crime in England and Wales: Year ending March 2015. Retrieved April 21, 2016, from http://www.ons.gov.uk/peoplepopulationandcommunity/crimeandjustice/bulletins/crimeinenglandandwales/2015-07-16

Park, M., Sung-Hyun, C., & Hong, H. (2015). Prevalence and perpetrators of workplace violence by nursing unit and the relationship between violence and the perceived work environment. *Journal of Nursing Scholarship, 47*(1), 87-95.

Paterson, B., McKenna, K., & Bowie, V. (2014). A charter for trainers in the prevention and management of workplace violence in mental health settings. *Journal of Mental Health Training, Education & Practice, 9*(2), 101-108. doi: 10.1108/JMHTEP-08-2013-0028

Pollack, K. M., Austin, W., & Grisso, J. A. (2010). Employee assistance programs: A workplace resource to address intimate partner violence. *Journal of Women's Health, 19*(4), 729-733. doi: 10.1089/jwh.2009.1495

Powell, M. (2010). Ageism and abuse in the workplace: A new frontier. *Journal of Gerontological Social Work, 53*(7), 654-658. doi: 10.1080/01634372.2010.508510

Respass, G., & Payne, B. K. (2008). Social services workers and workplace violence. *Journal of Aggression, Maltreatment & Trauma, 16*(2), 131-143. doi: 10.1080/10926770801921287

Ridenour, M., Lanza, M., Hendricks, S., Hartley, D., Rierdan, J., Zeiss, R., & Amandus, H. (2013). Incidence and risk factors of workplace violence on psychiatric staff. *Work.* doi: 10.3233/WOR-141894

Ringstad, R. (2005). Conflict in the workplace: Social workers as victims and perpetrators. *Social Work, 50*(4), 305-313. doi: 10.1093/sw/50.4.305

Slattery, S. M., & Goodman, L. A. (2009). Secondary traumatic stress among domestic violence advocates: Workplace risk and protective factors. *Violence Against Women, 15*(11), 1358-1379. doi: 10.1177/1077801209347469

State of California Department of Industrial Relations. (1995). Cal/OSHA guidelines for workplace security. Retrieved from http://www.dir.ca.gov/dosh/dosh_publications/worksecurity.html

Ta, M. L., Marshall, S. W., Kaufman, J. S., Loomis, D., Casteel, C., & Land, K. C. (2009). Area-based socioeconomic characteristics of industries at high risk for violence in the workplace. *American Journal of Community Psychology, 44*(3-4), 249-260. doi: 10.1007/s10464-009-9263-7

United States Department of Labor. (2015). OSHA updates guidance for protecting healthcare and social service workers from workplace violence. Retrieved April 21, 2016, from https://www.osha.gov/newsrelease/nat-20150403.html

United States Department of Labor and Statistics. (n.d.). Workplace violence. Retrieved April 21, 2016, from https://www.osha.gov/SLTC/workplaceviolence/

Versola-Russo, J. M., & Russo, F. (2009). When domestic violence turns into workplace violence: Organizational impact and response. *Journal of Police Crisis Negotiations, 9*, 141-148. doi: 10.1080/15332580902865193

Wheeler, D. (2015). NASW standards and indicators for cultural competence in social work practice. Retrieved April 21, 2016, from http://www.socialworkers.org/practice/standards/PRA-BRO-253150-CC-Standards.pdf

Winstanley, S., & Hales, L. (2008). Prevalence of aggression towards residential social workers: Do qualifications and experience make a difference?

Child and Youth Care Forum, 37(2), 103-110. doi: 10.1007/s10566-008-9051-9

Zelnick, J. R., Slayter, E., Flanzbaum, B., Butler, N. G., Domingo, B., Perlstein, J., & Trust, C. (2013). Part of the job? Workplace violence in Massachusetts social service agencies. *Health & Social Work, 38*(2), 75-85. doi: 10.1093/hsw/hlt007

WORKPLACE VIOLENCE: SEXUAL HARASSMENT

MAJOR CATEGORIES: Violence

DESCRIPTION

Sexual harassment (SH) is defined as any behavior, comment, gesture, or contact of a sexual nature in the workplace that may cause offense, humiliation, or intimidation. SH may be physical or nonphysical. It includes offensive remarks made about an individual's sex, such as derogatory comments made about women in general. Perpetrators most often are men and victims most often are women, although women may sexually harass men and SH may take place between persons of the same sex. The victim does not need to be the individual being directly harassed for SH charges to be filed; they can be filed by a third party exposed to SH. SH may be a one-time incident or be committed repeatedly. Women are most likely to experience extended patterns of SH. It is often the case that individuals in more powerful positions in the workplace, such as supervisors and managers, sexually harass subordinates (employees that work under them). However, studies show that women in senior roles may be subjected to SH from male subordinates, which is perceived by the committer to act as a power equalizer. Fundamentally, SH is the assertion of power by one individual over another. Any level of SH can have significant psychosocial outcomes for victims.

SH is committed in the workplace by colleagues, clients, and customers. A study conducted in a Taiwanese hospital reported that the most common form of SH experienced by women was the telling of sexual jokes not only by colleagues but also by patients and their family members. Men in this study were more likely to be exposed to pornography while at work, which they experienced as a form of SH. A Japanese study found that SH in the workplace extended beyond SH, constituting criminal offenses such as rape, assault and battery, obscenity, and false imprisonment. Perpetrators may devalue their target by criticizing his or her work; frequently they reinterpret their actions to minimize them or they blame others for their behavior. Perpetrators often cover up their acts of SH by ensuring that there are no witnesses. Scholarly opinion is that SH regularly goes underreported and that victims rarely use formal complaint procedures to tackle it. Organizations with poor workplace relations and weak coworker social ties report high levels of SH.

The *Diagnostic and Statistical Manual of Mental Disorders,* Fifth Edition *(DSM-5),* expanded the single entry related to SH to four different identifiable variations of SH. They appear in the chapter "Other Conditions That May Be a Focus of Clinical Attention" and are included not as mental health disorders but as conditions that may come up during assessment and that may provide insight into an individual's condition as well as inform the selection of intervention(s).

Scholars suggest that SH takes place on a continuum of intimate violence that extends beyond the workplace and is best understood within a broader social framework. Like other forms of sexual violence, workplace SH has significant consequences to a person's biological, social, and psychological health. Most frequently it reduces job satisfaction and

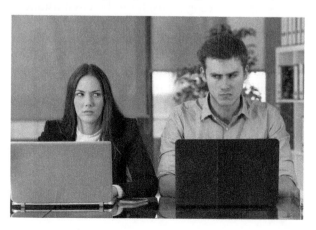

commitment and leads to resignations. It may also cause decreased productivity in the workplace, poor time management, and low-quality relationships between management and employees. Members of the armed services are less likely to reenlist when they have experienced SH. SH can cause irritation, anger, and stress and lead to mental health conditions such as depression and anxiety. Posttraumatic stress disorder (PTSD) can develop or be triggered when individuals are sexually harassed at work.

To eliminate SH, zero tolerance policies and interventions at small, moderate, and large levels are recommended. Law, policy, and training restrict SH in the workplace; however, some research reports a backlash in response to these efforts. Men are less likely to mentor women because of SH laws. Trainees in sessions promoting equality struggle with trainers over rights, responsibilities, and obligations in the workplace, which may displace the importance of the social justice aspect of removing SH. However, the benefits of organizational policy and procedure outweigh any opposing outcomes. Organizations need to be proactive in tackling SH, with clear procedures in place so victims know how to make complaints, understand objectives, and understand how to get help as well as support. When complaints are made, it is important that victims are not seen as being oversensitive or complaining about innocuous events. Each state in the United States has its own commission or agency that oversees matters related to SH (for example, New Hampshire Commission for Human Rights, Nevada Equal Rights Commission). At the federal level, the U.S. Equal Employment Opportunity Commission (EEOC) investigates allegations of SH in workplaces. In its investigations, both the circumstances of the alleged harassment (the nature of the sexual conduct) and the context in which the alleged incidents occurred are examined. In 2011, the EEOC received 11,364 complaints of SH in the workplace. Males filed 16.3 percent of the complaints; females filed 83.7 percent.

FACTS AND FIGURES

Estimations of SH vary greatly due to a lack of standardized definitions, but studies report extremely high levels within the workplace worldwide. A study of nurses and midwives in a hospital setting in Australia reported that 34.4 percent of the nurses and midwives had been sexually harassed in their workplace, a hospital that has zero tolerance policies towards aggression. In a study of 265 female hospital personnel in Italy, 54 percent stated that they had been sexually harassed at work in the previous 12 months. In the United States, between 40 and 75 percent of women are victimized each year compared to between 13 and 31 percent of men. However, the number of SH charges filed in the United States under Title VII of the Civil Rights Act has been falling since 1997. Between 17 and 81 percent of women across Europe report victimization. In the United States, 90 percent of large organizations have anti-SH policies.

RISK FACTORS

Being female puts an individual at risk of experiencing SH in the workplace. Both women in subordinate positions and women in supervisory roles are vulnerable to SH. A history of intimate violence and sexual abuse can also increase the risk of being targeted for SH. One study found that men with previous anxiety and depression are at risk for victimization.

SIGNS AND SYMPTOMS

Stress, anxiety, depression, and PTSD may be signs of victimization.

ASSESSMENT

Social workers should complete an assessment to get more detailed information and history regarding the individual's biological (physical), social, psychological and spiritual health in order to help in the development of individual interventions.

ASSESSMENT AND SCREENING TOOLS

The following are some surveys the social worker may ask the individual and/or his or her coworkers to complete when SH may be an issue.

The Rahim Organizational Conflict Inventory has 21 items that evaluate interpersonal, intragroup, and intergroup conflict in work environments.

The Beck Depression Inventory (BDI) for adults has 12 multiple-choice questions and is widely used to determine whether an individual is experiencing depression.

The Trauma Screening Questionnaire (TSQ) has 10 items and can be used with survivors of all types of traumatic stress.

The Hopkins Symptom Checklist has 25 questions and is commonly used to measure anxiety and depression.

TREATMENT

Social workers should work together with workplace or company personnel to ensure that SH policies are in place and are widely spread, and they should help with any SH training. If in a clinical setting working with an offender, the social worker should use appropriate therapeutic techniques to address accountability for the person's behavior, improve appropriate social skills, correct impulse control, and develop relapse prevention (psychoeducation, role play, cognitive behavioral therapy). If in a clinical setting working with a victim, the social worker should use appropriate therapeutic techniques (cognitive behavioral therapy, solution-focused therapy, psychotherapy) to address anxiety, depression, sleep disturbances, and PTSD symptoms.

Social workers can also provide SH prevention training for workplaces. In one study, administrators in three workplaces were interested in conducting evidence-based SH training for their staff, yet could not devote much time to the training. Therefore, a 1-hour workshop followed by best practice recommendations was given to the staff. The staff's knowledge regarding SH prevention increased significantly from its level prior to the workshop, demonstrating that even a short workshop can be extremely helpful.

APPLICABLE LAWS AND REGULATIONS

In many countries around the world, SH in the workplace is illegal. Employers have a duty of care to protect workers from SH. In the United States, individuals who are victims of SH in the workplace may sue under Title VII of the Civil Rights Act of 1964.

There are two types of unlawful SH: quid quo pro, in which sexual cooperation is required in return for employment, promotion, and so forth, and the existence of workplace environments in which the atmosphere is intimidating, hostile, or offensive.

Defense lawyers may use an individual's personal history of sexual and physical abuse to minimize any effects attributed to workplace SH in order to limit compensation.

SH is a continuing and expensive problem for organizations; in the 1990s, for example, Mitsubishi paid $34 million to plaintiffs as a result of rampant SH at its manufacturing plant in Chicago.

SERVICES AND RESOURCES

- The U.S. Equal Employment Opportunity Commission has resources and information available for victims and professionals, http://www.eeoc.gov
- Equal Rights Advocates provides information and advice to victims of SH in the workplace, http://www.equalrights.org/
- Workplace Fairness offers information and resources to victims of SH, http://www.workplace-fairness.org
- The Legal Aid Society Employment Law Center has information and resources on SH and work discrimination and holds workplace clinics, http://www.las-elc.org/
- The United States Department of Labor has a range of information about workplace harassment and how to file complaints, http://www.dol.gov

FOOD FOR THOUGHT

Studies show that a work environment with a social climate that is lenient of SH is the strongest predictor of harassment occurring. To eradicate SH, organizations need to actively promote equality and respect.

Organizations that implement policies to eradicate SH often find those policies met with resistance at all levels of staffing.

Workplace bonds between colleagues can be a protective factor for women working in intimidating environments.

One study found that psychological distress (measured on the Hopkins Symptom Checklist) predicted victimization among men but not among women.

Individuals frequently minimize behaviors that signify SH.

SH frequently is underreported.

A 2013 study of youth residential care reported that 81 percent of the group workers (often social workers) stated that they had experienced verbal threats, physical violence, and SH from the youths living in residential care.

RED FLAGS

Lack of support for victims deters workers from reporting incidents.

Previous abuse such as childhood sexual assault can increase the risk for victimization.

All levels of SH can have significant consequences on an individual's psychological and social health outcomes.

Verbal SH is just as damaging to individuals as physical SH.

Adolescents aged 16 to 18 reported violence and SH in their workplaces (retail stores, food service) from coworkers, supervisors, and customers. Schools can educate adolescents on how to handle workplace aggression.

Written by Jan Wagstaff, MA, MSW

Reviewed by Melissa Rosales Neff, MSW, and Chris Bates, MA, MSW

REFERENCES

Alink, L., Euser, S., Bakermans-Kranenburg, M., & Ijzendoorn, M. (2014). A challenging job: Physical and sexual violence towards group workers in youth residential care. *Child Youth & Care Forum, 43*(2), 243-250. doi:10.1007/s10566-013-9236-8

American Psychiatric Association. (2013). Diagnostic and statistical manual of mental health disorders (DSM-5). (5th ed.). Arlington, VA: American Psychiatric Publishing.

Bell, M. P., Campbell Quick, J., & Cycyota, C. S. (2012). Assessment and prevention of sexual harassment of employees: An applied guide to creating healthy organizations. *International Journal of Selection & Assessment, 10*(1/2), 160-167. doi:10.1111/1468-2389.00203

British Association of Social Workers. (2012). The code of ethics for social work: Statement of principles. Retrieved November 14, 2015, from http://cdn.basw.co.uk/upload/basw_112315-7.pdf

Campbell, C., Kramer, A., Woolman, K., Staecker, E., Visker, E., & Cox, C. (2013). Effects of a brief pilot sexual harassment prevention workshop on employees' knowledge. *Workplace Health & Safety, 61*(10), 425-428. doi:10.3928/21650799-20130925-26

Demir, D., & Rodwell, J. (2012). Psychological antecedents and consequences of workplace aggression for hospital nurses. *Journal of Nursing Scholarship, 44*(4), 376-384. doi:10.1111/j.15475069.2012.01472.x

Dionisi, A. M., Barling, J., & Dupré, K. E. (2012). Revisiting the comparative outcomes of workplace aggression and sexual harassment. *Journal of Occupational Health Psychology, 17*(4), 398-408. doi:http://psycnet.apa.org/doi/10.1037/a0029883

Firestone, J. M., Hackett, J. D., & Harris, R. J. (2012). Testing relationships between sex of respondent, sexual harassment and intentions to reenlist in the U. S. military. *Public Administration Research, 1*(1), 1-13. doi:10.5539/par.v1n1p1

Harrison, J. (2012). Women in law enforcement: Subverting sexual harassment with social bonds. *Women & Criminal Justice, 22*, 228-236. doi:10.1080/08974454.2012.687964

McDonald, P. (2012). Workplace sexual harassment 30 years on: A review of the literature. *International Journal of Management Reviews, 14*(1), 1-17. doi:10.1111/j.1468-2370.2011.00300.x

McLaughlin, H., Uggen, C., & Blackstone, A. (2012). Sexual harassment, workplace authority, and the paradox of power. *American Sociological Review, 77*(4), 625-647. doi:10.1177/0003122412451728

Menendez, C., Snyder, J., Scherer, H., & Fisher, B. (2012). Social organization and social ties: Their effects on sexual harassment victimization in the workplace. *Work, 42*(1), 137-150. doi:10.3233/WOR-2012-1325

Munkres, S. A. (2008). Claiming "victim" to harassment law: Legal consciousness of the privileged. *Law & Social Inquiry, 33*(2), 447-472. doi:10.1111/j.1747-4469.2008.00109.x

Nielsen, M. B., & Einarsen, S. (2012). Prospective relationships between workplace sexual harassment and psychological distress. *Occupational Medicine, 62*(3), 226-228. doi:10.1093/occmed/kqs010

Perry, E. L., Kulik, C. T., & Bustamante, J. (2012). Factors impacting the knowing-doing gap in sexual harassment training. *Human Resource Development International, 15*(5), 589-608. doi:10.1080/13678868.2012.726540

Romito, P., Ballard, T., & Maton, N. (2004). Sexual harassment among female personnel in an Italian hospital: Frequency and correlates. *Violence Against Women, 10*(4), 386-417. doi:10.1177/1077801204263505

Smith, C. R., Fisher, B. S., Gillespie, G. L., Beery, T. A., & Gates, D. M. (2013). Adolescents' experience with workplace aggression: School health implications. *The Journal of School Nursing, 29*(6), 464-474. doi:10.1177/1059840513479036

Snyder, J. A., Scherer, H. L., & Fisher, B. S. (2012). Social organization and social ties: Their effects on sexual harassment victimization in the workplace. *Work, 42*(1), 137-150. doi:10.3233/WOR-2012-1325

Stockdale, M. S., & Nadler, J. T. (2012). Situating sexual harassment in the broader context of interpersonal violence: Research, theory, and policy implications. *Social Issues and Policy Review, 6*(1), 148-176. doi:10.1111/j.1751-2409.2011.01038.x

Tinkler, J. E. (2012). Resisting the enforcement of sexual harassment law. *Law & Social Inquiry, 37*(1), 1-24. doi:10.1111/j.1747-4469.2011.01279.x

U.S. Equal Opportunity Employment Commission. (2012). Sexual harassment charges: EEOC & FEPAs combined: FY 1997-FY 2011. Retrieved November 14, 2015, from http://www.eeoc.gov/eeoc/statistics/enforcement/sexual_harassment.cfm

Wang, L., Chen, C., Sheng, Y., Lu, P., Chen, Y., Chen, H., & Lin, J. (2012). Workplace sexual harassment in two general hospitals in Taiwan: The incidence, perception, and gender differences. *Journal of Occupational Health, 54*(1), 56-63. doi:10.1539/joh.11-0063-FS

Wheeler, D. (2015). NASW standards and indicators for cultural competency in social work practice. Retrieved November 14, 2015, from http://www.socialworkers.org/practice/standards/PRA-BRO-253150-CC-Standards.pdf

Zhang, X., & Zhang, Z. (2012). Investigation and analysis of sexual harassment in corporate workplace of China. *Sociology Mind, 2*(3), 289-292. doi:10.4236/sm.2012.23038

Facts about sexual harassment. (2002). *U.S. Equal Opportunity Employment Commission.* Retrieved November 14, 2015, from http://www.eeoc.gov/facts/fs-sex.html

International Federation of Social Workers. (2012, March 3). Statement of ethical principles. Retrieved November 14, 2015, from http://ifsw.org/policies/statement-of-ethical-principles/

GLOSSARY OF TERMS

Access: The extent to which an individual who needs care and services is able to receive them. Access is more than having insurance coverage or the ability to pay for services. It is also determined by the availability of services, acceptability of services, cultural appropriateness, location, hours of operation, transportation needs, and cost.

Accessible services: Services that are affordable, located nearby, and open during evenings and weekends. Staff is sensitive to and incorporates individual and cultural values. Staff is also sensitive to barriers that may keep a person from getting help. For example, an adolescent may be more willing to attend a support group meeting in a church or club near home than to travel to a mental health center. An accessible service can handle consumer demand without placing people on a long waiting list.: Accreditation: An official decision made by a recognized organization that a health care plan, network, or other delivery system complies with applicable standards.

Activity therapy: Includes art, dance, music, recreational and occupational therapies, and psychodrama.

Alternative therapy: An alternative approach to mental health care is one that emphasizes the interrelationship between mind, body, and spirit. Although some alternative approaches have a long history, many remain controversial.

Alzheimer's disease (AD): A slowly progressive form of dementia, which is a progressive, acquired impairment of intellectual functions. Memory impairment is a necessary feature for the diagnosis. Change in one of the following areas must also be present for any form of dementia to be diagnosed: language, decision-making ability, judgment, attention, and other related areas of cognitive function and personality. The rate of progression is different for each person. If AD develops rapidly, it is likely to continue to progress rapidly. If it has been slow to progress, it will likely continue on a slow course. The cause of Alzheimer's disease (AD) is not known, but it is not a part of normal aging. Prior theories regarding the accumulation of aluminum, lead, mercury, and other substances in the brain have been disproved. A diagnosis of AD is made based on characteristic symptoms and by excluding other causes of dementia. It can be confirmed by microscopic examination of a sample of brain tissue after death. By causing both structural and chemical problems in the brain, AD appears to disconnect areas of the brain that normally work together. There are two types of AD — early onset and late onset. In early onset AD, symptoms first appear before age 60. Some early onset disease runs in families and involves autosomal dominant, inherited mutations that may be the cause of the disease. So far, three early onset genes have been identified. Early onset AD is less common, resulting in about 5–10 percent of cases. Late onset AD, the most common form of the disease, develops in people 60 and older and is thought to be less likely to occur in families. Late onset AD may run in some families, but the role of genes is less direct and definitive. These genes may not cause the problem itself, but simply increase the likelihood of formation of plaques and tangles or other AD-related pathologies in the brain. In the early stages, the symptoms may be very subtle. Symptoms may often include: repeating statements frequently, frequently misplacing items, trouble finding names for familiar objects, getting lost on familiar routes, personality changes, becoming passive and losing interest in things previously enjoyed. AD cannot be cured and the impaired functions cannot be restored. Currently, the progression can be slowed but not stopped. Treatment focuses on attempting to slow the progression; managing the behavior problems, confusion, and agitation; modifying the home environment; and most importantly, supporting the family. As the disease progresses, it may take a greater toll on the family than the patient.

American Indian or Alaska Native: A person having origins in any of the original peoples of North and South America (including Central America), and who maintains tribal affiliations or community attachment.

Anorexia: An eating disorder characterized by refusal to maintain a minimally accepted body weight, intense fear of weight gain, and distorted body image.

Inadequate calorie intake or excessive energy expenditure results in severe weight loss. The exact cause of this disorder is not known, but social attitudes towards body appearance and family factors are believed to play a role in its development. The condition usually occurs in adolescence or young adulthood. It is more common in women, affecting 1–2 percent of the female population and only 0.1–0.2 percent of males. Anorexia is seen mainly in Caucasian women who are high academic achievers and have a goal-oriented family or personality. However, this eating disorder is not more common in higher socioeconomic groups. Some experts have suggested that conflicts within a family may also contribute to anorexia. It is thoughts that anorexia is a way for a child to draw attention away from marital problems, for example, and bring the family back together. Other psychologists have suggested that anorexia may be an attempt by young women to gain control and separate from their mothers. The causes, however, are still not well understood. The purpose of treatment is first to restore normal body weight and eating habits, and then attempt to resolve psychological issues. Hospitalization may be indicated in some cases (usually when body weight falls below 30 percent of expected weight). Supportive care by health care providers, structured behavioral therapy, psychotherapy, and anti-depressant drug therapy are some of the methods that are used for treatment. Severe and life-threatening malnutrition may require intravenous feeding.

Anxiety: Anxiety is an emotion that can signal just the right response to a situation. It can spur you on, for example, to add the finishing touches that transform an essay, painting, or important work document from good to excellent. However, if you have an anxiety disorder, exaggerated anxiety can stop you cold and disrupt your life. Like many other illnesses, anxiety disorders often have an underlying biological cause and frequently run in families. Anxiety disorders range from feelings of uneasiness to immobilizing bouts of terror. Symptoms range from chronic, exaggerated worry, tension, and irritability and appear to have no cause or are more intense than the situation warrants. Physical signs, such as restlessness, trouble falling or staying asleep, headaches, trembling, twitching, muscle tension, or sweating, often accompany these psychological symptoms. Anxiety is among the most common,

most treatable mental disorders. Effective treatments include cognitive behavioral therapy, relaxation techniques, and biofeedback to control muscle tension. Medication, most commonly anti-anxiety drugs, such as benzodiazepine and its derivatives, also may be required in some cases. Some commonly prescribed anti-anxiety medications are diazepam, alprazolam, and lorazepam. The non-benzodiazepine anti-anxiety medication buspirone can be helpful for some individuals.

Anxiety disorders: Anxiety disorders range from feelings of uneasiness to immobilizing bouts of terror. Most people experience anxiety at some point in their lives and some nervousness in anticipation of a real situation. However if a person cannot shake unwarranted worries, or if the feelings are jarring to the point of avoiding everyday activities, he or she most likely has an anxiety disorder.

Appropriate services: Designed to meet the specific needs of each individual child and family. For example, one family may need day treatment, while another may need home-based services. Appropriate services for one child and family may not be appropriate for another. Appropriate services usually are provided in the child's community.

Appropriateness: The extent to which a particular procedure, treatment, test, or service is clearly indicated, not excessive, adequate in quantity, and provided in the setting best suited to a patient's or member's needs. (See also, medically necessary)

Asian: A person having origins in any of the original peoples of the Far East, Southeast Asia, or the Indian subcontinent including, for example, Cambodia, China, India, Japan, Korea, Malaysia, Pakistan, the Philippine Islands, Thailand, and Vietnam.

Assessment: A professional review of child and family needs that is done when services are first sought from a caregiver. The assessment of the child includes a review of physical and mental health, intelligence, school performance, family situation, and behavior in the community. The assessment identifies the strengths of the child and family. Together, the caregiver and family decide what kind of treatment and supports, if any, are needed.

Attention Deficit Hyperactivity Disorder (ADD-ADHD): Attention Deficit Hyperactivity Disorder (ADD-ADHD) is a neurobiological condition characterized by developmentally inappropriate level of attention, concentration, activity, distractability, and impulsivity. The symptoms typically begin by 3 years of age-Attention deficit: does not pay close attention to details; may make careless mistakes at work, school, or other activities; failure to complete tasks; has difficulty maintaining attention in tasks or play activities; does not listen when spoken to directly; has difficulty organizing tasks; is easily distracted; unable to follow more than one instruction at a time. Many different methods of treatment have been used for ADD including psychotropic medications, psychosocial interventions, dietary management, herbal and homeopathic remedies, biofeedback, meditation, and perception stimulation/training. Of these treatment strategies, the most research has been done on stimulant medications and psychosocial interventions. Overall, these studies suggest stimulants to be superior relative to psychosocial interventions. However, there is no long term information comparing the two. The primary medications used to treat attention deficit disorder include: Dexedrine (dextroamphetamine), Ritalin (methylphenidate), Cylert (magnesium pemoline), tranquilizers (such as thioridazine), alpha-adrenergic agonist (clonidine), and others. Psychosocial therapeutic techniques include: contingency management (e.g., point reward systems, time out...), cognitive-behavioral treatment (self monitoring, verbal self instruction, problem solving strategies, self reinforcement), parent counseling, individual psychotherapy.

Autism: Autism, also called autistic disorder, is a complex developmental disability that appears in early childhood, usually before age 3. Autism prevents children and adolescents from interacting normally with other people and affects almost every aspect of their social and psychological development.

Auto-enrollment: The automatic assignment of a person to a health insurance plan (typically done under Medicaid plans).

Average length of stay: This represents the average time a client receives a specified service during a specified time period. This is generally computed by counting all the days that clients received the service during the time period and dividing by the number of clients that received the service during the same period. (Days a person was on furlough or not receiving are not counted.)

Behavioral therapy: As the name implies, behavioral therapy focuses on behavior-changing unwanted behaviors through rewards, reinforcements, and desensitization. Desensitization, or Exposure Therapy, is a process of confronting something that arouses anxiety, discomfort, or fear and overcoming the unwanted responses. Behavioral therapy often involves the cooperation of others, especially family and close friends, to reinforce a desired behavior.

Beneficiary: A person certified as eligible for health care services. A beneficiary may be a dependent or a subscriber.

Binge eating: Binge Eating is an eating disorder characterized by eating more than needed to satisfy hunger. It is a feature of bulimia, a disorder that also includes abnormal perception of body image, constant craving for food and binge eating, followed by self-induced vomiting or laxative use.

Biofeedback: Biofeedback is learning to control muscle tension and "involuntary" body functioning, such as heart rate and skin temperature; it can be a path to mastering one's fears. It is used in combination with, or as an alternative to, medication to treat disorders such as anxiety, panic, and phobias.

Biomedical treatment: Medication alone, or in combination with psychotherapy, has proven to be an effective treatment for a number of emotional, behavioral, and mental disorders. Any treatment involving medicine is a biomedical treatment. The kind of medication a psychiatrist prescribes varies with the disorder and the individual being treated.

Bipolar disorder: A chronic disease affecting over 2 million Americans at some point in their lives. The American Psychiatric Association's "Diagnostic and Statistical Manual of Mental Disorders" describes two types of bipolar disorder, type I and type II. In type I (formerly known as manic depressive disorder), there has been at least one full manic episode.

However, people with this type may also experience episodes of major depression. In type II disorder, periods of "hypomania" involve more attenuate (less severe) manic symptoms that alternate with at least one major depressive episode. When the patients have an acute exacerbation, they may be in a manic state, depressed state, or mixed state. People who suffer from bipolar disorder, however, have pathological mood swings from mania to depression, with a pattern of exacerbation and remission that are sometimes cyclic. The manic phase is characterized by elevated mood, hyperactivity, over-involvement in activities, inflated self-esteem, a tendency to be easily distracted, and little need for sleep. The manic episodes may last from several days to months. In the depressive phase, there is loss of self-esteem, withdrawal, sadness, and a risk of suicide. While in either phase, patients may abuse alcohol or other substances which worsen the symptoms. The disorder appears between the ages of 15 and 25, and it affects men and women equally. The exact cause is unknown, but it is a disturbance of areas of the brain which regulate mood. There is a strong genetic component. The incidence is higher in relatives of people with bipolar disorder. Hospitalization may be required during an acute phase to control the symptoms and to ensure safety of individuals. Medications to alleviate acute symptoms may include: neuroleptics (antipsychotics), antianxiety agents (such as benzodiazepines), and antidepressant agents. Mood stabilizers, such as lithium carbonate, and anticonvulsants (including carbamazepine and valproic acid) are started as maintenance therapy to relieve symptoms and to prevent relapse.

Black or African American: A person having origins in any of the black racial groups of Africa. Terms such as "Haitian" or "Negro" can be used in addition to "black or African American."

Borderline personality disorder: Symptoms of borderline personality disorder, a serious mental illness, include pervasive instability in moods, interpersonal relationships, self-image, and behavior. The instability can affect family and work life, long-term planning, and the individual's sense of self-identity.

Bulimia: An illness characterized by uncontrolled episodes of overeating usually followed by self-induced vomiting or other purging. In bulimia, eating binges may occur as often as several times a day. Induced vomiting known as purging allows the eating to continue without the weight gain; it may continue until interrupted by sleep, abdominal pain, or the presence of another person. The person is usually aware that their eating pattern is abnormal and may experience fear or guilt associated with the binge-purge episodes. The behavior is usually secretive, although clues to this disorder include overactivity, peculiar eating habits, eating rituals, and frequent weighing. Body weight is usually normal or low, although the person may perceive themselves as overweight. The exact cause of bulimia is unknown, but factors thought to contribute to its development are family problems, maladaptive behavior, self-identity conflict, and cultural overemphasis on physical appearance. Bulimia may be associated with depression. The disorder is usually not associated with any underlying physical problem although the behavior may be associated with neurological or endocrine diseases. The disorder occurs most often in females of adolescent or young adult age. The incidence is estimated to be 3 percent in the general population; but 20 percent of college women suffers from it. Treatment focuses on breaking the binge-purge cycles of behavior since the person is usually aware that the behavior is abnormal. Outpatient treatment may include behavior modification techniques and individual, group, or family counseling. Antidepressant drugs may be indicated for some whether or not they have coincident depression.

Caregiver: A person who has special training to help people with mental health problems. Examples include social workers, teachers, psychologists, psychiatrists, and mentors.

Case manager: An individual who organizes and coordinates services and supports for children with mental health problems and their families. (Alternate terms: service coordinator, advocate, and facilitator.)

Child protective services: Designed to safeguard the child when abuse, neglect, or abandonment is suspected, or when there is no family to take care of the child. Examples of help delivered in the home include financial assistance, vocational training, homemaker services, and daycare. If in-home supports are insufficient, the child may be removed from the home on a temporary or permanent basis. Ideally, the goal is to keep the child with the family whenever possible.

Children and adolescents at risk for mental health problems: Children are at greater risk for developing mental health problems when certain factors occur in their lives or environments. Factors include physical abuse, emotional abuse or neglect, harmful stress, discrimination, poverty, loss of a loved one, frequent relocation, alcohol and other drug use, trauma, and exposure to violence.

Claim: A request by an individual (or his or her provider) to that individual's insurance company to pay for services obtained from a health care professional.

Clinical psychologist: A clinical psychologist is a professional with a doctoral degree in psychology who specializes in therapy.

Clinical social worker (CSW): Clinical social workers are health professionals trained in client-centered advocacy that assist clients with information, referral, and direct help in dealing with local, State, or Federal government agencies. As a result, they often serve as case managers to help people "navigate the system." Clinical social workers cannot write prescriptions.

Cognitive/behavioral therapy: A combination of cognitive and behavioral therapies, this approach helps people change negative thought patterns, beliefs, and behaviors so they can manage symptoms and enjoy more productive, less stressful lives.

Cognitive therapy: Cognitive therapy aims to identify and correct distorted thinking patterns that can lead to feelings and behaviors that may be troublesome, self-defeating, or even self- destructive. The goal is to replace such thinking with a more balanced view that, in turn, leads to more fulfilling and productive behavior.

Community services: Services that are provided in a community setting. Community services refer to all services not provided in an inpatient setting.

Conduct disorders: Children with conduct disorder repeatedly violate the personal or property rights of others and the basic expectations of society. A diagnosis of conduct disorder is likely when these symptoms continue for 6 months or longer. Conduct disorder is known as a "disruptive behavior disorder" because of its impact on children and their families, neighbors, and schools.

Continuum of care: A term that implies a progression of services that a child moves through, usually one service at a time. More recently, it has come to mean comprehensive services. Also see system of care and wraparound services.

Coordinated services: Child-serving organizations talk with the family and agree upon a plan of care that meets the child's needs. These organizations can include mental health, education, juvenile justice, and child welfare. Case management is necessary to coordinate services. Also see family-centered services and wraparound services.

Couples counseling and family therapy: These two similar approaches to therapy involve discussions and problem-solving sessions facilitated by a therapist- sometimes with the couple or entire family group, sometimes with individuals. Such therapy can help couples and family members improve their understanding of, and the way they respond to, one another. This type of therapy can resolve patterns of behavior that might lead to more severe mental illness. Family therapy can help educate the individuals about the nature of mental disorders and teach them skills to cope better with the effects of having a family member with a mental illness- such as how to deal with feelings of anger or guilt.

Cultural competence: Help that is sensitive and responsive to cultural differences. Caregivers are aware of the impact of culture and possess skills to help provide services that respond appropriately to a person's unique cultural differences, including race and ethnicity, national origin, religion, age, gender, sexual orientation, or physical disability. They also adapt their skills to fit a family's values and customs.

Day treatment: Day treatment includes special education, counseling, parent training, vocational training, skill building, crisis intervention, and recreational therapy. It lasts at least 4 hours a day. Day treatment programs work in conjunction with mental health, recreation, and education organizations and may even be provided by them.

Deductible: The amount an individual must pay for health care expenses before insurance (or a self-insured company) begins to pay its contract share. Often insurance plans are based on yearly deductible amounts.

Delusions: Delusions are bizarre thoughts that have no basis in reality.

Dementia: Refers to a group of symptoms involving progressive impairment of all aspects of brain function. Disorders that cause dementia include conditions that impair the vascular (blood vessels) or neurologic (nerve) structures of the brain. A minority of causes of dementia are treatable. These include normal pressure hydrocephalus, brain tumors, and dementia due to metabolic causes and infections. Unfortunately, most of the disorders associated with dementia are progressive, irreversible, degenerative conditions. The two major degenerative causes of dementia are Alzheimer's disease, which is a progressive loss of nerve cells without a known cause or cure and vascular dementia, which is loss of brain function due to a series of small strokes. Dementia may be diagnosed when there is impairment of two or more brain functions, including language, memory, visual-spatial perception, emotional behavior or personality, and cognitive skills (such as calculation, abstract thinking, or judgment). Dementia usually appears first as forgetfulness. Other symptoms may be apparent only on neurologic examination or cognitive testing. Loss of functioning progresses slowly from decreased problem solving and language skills to difficulty with ordinary daily activities to severe memory loss and complete disorientation with withdrawal from social interaction.

Depression: A term that people commonly use to refer to states involving sadness, dejection, lack of self-esteem, and lack of energy. Feelings of depression are synonymous with feeling sad, blue, down in the dumps, unhappy, and miserable. Most feelings of depression are a reaction to an unhappy event. It is natural to have some feelings of sadness after a loss such as the death of a relative, or after a major disappointment at home or at work. Depression is more prevalent in women than men and is especially common among adolescents. Mild depression comes and goes and is characterized by downheartedness, sadness, and dejection. Short-term episodes of depression or other mood changes can occur with hormone changes, including those that accompany pregnancy or premenstrual syndrome (PMS), and those occurring shortly after the birth of a baby (postpartum "blues"). Sleep disruption and lack of sunlight during the winter months are other biological factors that can precipitate depressive symptoms. Distorted thought patterns, characterized by feelings of worthlessness, helplessness, and hopelessness are part of the "cognitive triad of depression," and can be a risk factor for depression. It appears that a tendency toward depression is often genetic, but that stressful life circumstances usually play a major role in bringing on depressive episodes. Problems with depression usually begin in adolescence, and are about twice as common in women as in men. Noticeably disturbed thought processes, poor communication and socialization, and sensory dysfunction indicate moderate depression. People with severe depression are withdrawn, indifferent toward their surroundings, and may show signs of delusional thinking and limited physical activity.

Diagnostic evaluation: The aims of a general psychiatric evaluation are 1) to establish a psychiatric diagnosis, 2) to collect data sufficient to permit a case formulation, and 3) to develop an initial treatment plan, with particular consideration of any immediate interventions that may be needed to ensure the patient's safety, or, if the evaluation is a reassessment of a patient in long-term treatment, to revise the plan of treatment in accord with new perspectives gained from the evaluation.

Discharge: A discharge is the formal termination of service, generally when treatment has been completed or through administrative authority.

Drop-in center: A social club offering peer support and flexible schedule of activities: may operate on evenings and/ weekends.

DSM-V (Diagnostic and Statistical Manual of Mental Disorders, Fifth Edition): An official manual of mental health problems developed by the American Psychiatric Association. Psychiatrists, psychologists, social workers, and other health and mental health care providers use this reference book to understand and diagnose mental health problems. Insurance companies and health care providers also use the terms and explanations in this book when discussing mental health problems.

Dyslexia: A reading disability resulting from a defect in the ability to process graphic symbols. There are about 2 to 8 percent of elementary-age children that have some degree of reading disability. Developmental reading disorder (DRD) or dyslexia is not attributable to eye problems but instead is a defect of higher cortical (brain) processing of symbols. Children with DRD may have trouble rhyming and separating the sounds in spoken words. These abilities appear critical in the process of learning to read. Initial reading skills are based on word recognition. More developed reading skills require the linking of words into a coherent sentence (thought). DRD children may be unable to form images from the meanings of the words or to process the words into an idea which is understandable. At this level, reading may fail at its primary function, which is to convey information. Dyslexia or developmental reading disorder may appear in combination with developmental writing disorder and developmental arithmetic disorder. All of these processes involve the manipulation of symbols and the conveyance of information by their manipulation. These conditions may appear singly or in any combination. Other causes of learning disability and, in particular, reading disability, must be ruled out before a diagnosis of DRD can be made. Cultural and educational shortfalls, emotional problems, mental retardation, and diseases of the brain (for example AIDS) can all cause learning disabilities. Remedial instruction has remained the best approach to this type of reading disorder.

Electroconvulsive therapy: Also known as ECT, this highly controversial technique uses low voltage electrical stimulation of the brain to treat some forms of major depression, acute mania, and some forms of schizophrenia. This potentially life-saving technique is considered only when other therapies have failed, when a person is seriously medically ill and/or unable to take medication, or when a person is very likely to commit suicide. Substantial improvements in the equipment, dosing guidelines, and anesthesia have significantly reduced the possibility of side effects.

Emergency: A planned program to provide psychiatric care in emergency situations with staff specifically assigned for this purpose. Includes crisis intervention, which enables the individual, family members and friends to cope with the emergency while maintaining the individual's status as a functioning community member to the greatest extent possible.

Emergency and crisis services: A group of services that is available 24 hours a day, 7 days a week, to help during a mental health emergency. Examples include telephone crisis hotlines, suicide hotlines, crisis counseling, crisis residential treatment services, crisis outreach teams, and crisis respite care.

Emergency Medical Treatment and Labor Act (EMTALA): EMTALA, also referred to as the Federal Anti- patient Dumping Law link An act pertaining to emergency medical situations. EMTALA requires hospitals to provide emergency treatment to individuals, regardless of insurance status and ability to pay (EMTALA, 2002).

Employed: This is a broad category of employment that includes competitive, supported, and sheltered employment.

Employment/vocational rehabilitation services: A broad range of services designed to address skills necessary for participation in job- related activities.

Enrollee: A person eligible for services from a managed care plan.

Family-centered services: Help designed to meet the specific needs of each individual child and family. Children and families should not be expected to fit into services that do not meet their needs. Also see appropriate services, coordinated services, wraparound services, and cultural competence.

Family-like arrangements: A broad range of living arrangements that simulate a family situation. This includes foster care and small group homes.

Family support services: Help designed to keep the family together, while coping with mental health problems that affect them. These services may include consumer information workshops, in-home supports, family therapy, parenting training, crisis services, and respite care.

Foster care: Provision of a living arrangement in a household other than that of the client's/patient's family.

Gatekeeper: Primary care physician or local agency responsible for coordinating and managing the health care needs of members. Generally, in order for specialty services such as mental health and hospital care to be covered, the gatekeeper must first approve the referral.

General hospital: A hospital that provides mental health services in at least one separate psychiatric unit with specially allocated staff and space for the treatment of persons with mental illness.

General support: Includes transportation, childcare, homemaker services, day care, and other general services for clients/patients.

Group therapy: This form of therapy involves groups of usually 4 to 12 people who have similar problems and who meet regularly with a therapist. The therapist uses the emotional interactions of the group's members to help them get relief from distress and possibly modify their behavior.

Hallucinations: Hallucinations are experiences of sensations that have no source. Some examples of hallucinations include hearing nonexistent voices, seeing nonexistent things, and experiencing burning or pain sensations with no physical cause.

Health Insurance Portability and Accountability Act (HIPAA): This 1996 act provides protections for consumers in group health insurance plans. HIPAA prevents health plans from excluding health coverage of pre-existing conditions and discriminating on the basis of health status.

Hispanic or Latino: A person of Cuban, Mexican, Puerto Rican, South or Central American, or other Spanish culture or origin, regardless of race. The term, "Spanish origin," can be used in addition to "Hispanic or Latino."

Home-based services: Help provided in a family's home either for a defined period of time or for as long as it takes to deal with a mental health problem. Examples include parent training, counseling, and working with family members to identify, find, or provide other necessary help. The goal is to prevent the child from being placed outside of the home. (Alternate term: in-home supports.)

Homeless: A person who lives on the street or in a shelter for the homeless.

Horizontal consolidation: When local health plans (or local hospitals) merge. This practice was popular in the late 1990s and was used to expand regional business presence.

Housing services: Assistance to clients/patients in finding and maintaining appropriate housing arrangements.

In-home family services: Mental health treatment and support services offered to children and adolescents with mental illness and to their family members in their own homes or apartments.

Independent living services: Support for a young person living on his or her own. These services include therapeutic group homes, supervised apartment living, and job placement. Services teach youth how to handle financial, medical, housing, transportation, and other daily living needs, as well as how to get along with others.

Individual therapy: Therapy tailored for a patient/client that is administered one-on-one.

Individualized services: Services designed to meet the unique needs of each child and family. Services are individualized when the caregivers pay attention to the needs and strengths, ages, and stages of development of the child and individual family members. Also see appropriate services and family-centered services.

Information and referral services: Information services are those designed to impart information on the availability of clinical resources and how to access them. Referral services are those that direct, guide, or a client/patient with appropriate services provided outside of your organization.

Inpatient hospitalization: Mental health treatment provided in a hospital setting 24 hours a day. Inpatient hospitalization provides: (1) short-term treatment in cases where a child is in crisis and possibly a danger to his/herself or others, and (2) diagnosis and treatment when the patient cannot be evaluated or treated appropriately in an outpatient setting.

Intake/screening: Services designed to briefly assess the type and degree of a client's/patient's mental health condition to determine whether services are needed and to link him/her to the most appropriate and available service. Services may include interviews, psychological testing, physical examinations including speech/hearing, and laboratory studies.

Intensive case management: Intensive community services for individuals with severe and persistent mental illness that are designed to improve planning for their service needs. Services include outreach, evaluation, and support.

Intensive residential services: Intensively staffed housing arrangements for clients/patients. May include medical, psychosocial, vocational, recreational or other support services.

Interpersonal psychotherapy: Through one-on-one conversations, this approach focuses on the patient's current life and relationships within the family, social, and work environments. The goal is to identify and resolve problems with insight, as well as build on strengths.

Legal Advocacy: Legal services provided to ensure the protection and maintenance of a client's/patient's rights.

Living independently: A client who lives in a private residence and requires no assistance in activities of daily living.

Local mental health authority: Local organizational entity (usually with some statutory authority) that centrally maintains administrative, clinical, and fiscal authority for a geographically specific and organized system of health care.

Medicaid: Medicaid is a health insurance assistance program funded by Federal, State, and local monies. It is run by State guidelines and assists low-income persons by paying for most medical expenses.

Medicaid client: Mental health clients to whom some services were reimbursable through Medicaid.

Medical group practice: A number of physicians working in a systematic association with the joint use of equipment and technical personnel and with centralized administration and financial organization.

Medical review criteria: Screening criteria used by third-party payers and review organizations as the underlying basis for reviewing the quality and appropriateness of care provided to selected cases.

Medically necessary: Health insurers often specify that, in order to be covered, a treatment or drug must be medically necessary for the consumer. Anything that falls outside of the realm of medical necessity is usually not covered. The plan will use prior authorization and utilization management procedures to determine whether or not the term "medically necessary" is applicable.

Medicare: Medicare is a Federal insurance program serving the disabled and persons over the age of 65. Most costs are paid via trust funds that beneficiaries have paid into throughout the courses of their lives; small deductibles and some co-payments are required.

Medication therapy: Prescription, administration, assessment of drug effectiveness, and monitoring of potential side effects of psycho-tropic medications.

Mental disorders: Another term used for mental health problems.

Mental health: How a person thinks, feels, and acts when faced with life's situations. Mental health is how people look at themselves, their lives, and the other people in their lives; evaluate their challenges and problems; and explore choices. This includes handling stress, relating to other people, and making decisions.

Mental Health Parity (Act): Mental health parity refers to providing the same insurance coverage for mental health treatment as that offered for medical and surgical treatments. The Mental Health Parity Act was passed in 1996 and established parity in lifetime benefit limits and annual limits.

Mental health problems: Mental health problems are real. They affect one's thoughts, body, feelings, and behavior. Mental health problems are not just a passing phase. They can be severe, seriously interfere with a person's life, and even cause a person to become disabled. Mental health problems include depression, bipolar disorder (manic-depressive illness), attention-deficit/ hyperactivity disorder, anxiety disorders, eating disorders, schizophrenia, and conduct disorder.

Mental illnesses: This term is usually used to refer to severe mental health problems in adults.

MHA Administration: Activities related to the planning, organization, management, funding, and oversight of direct services.

MI and MR/DD services: Services designed to address the needs of people with both psychiatric illness and mental retardation or developmental disabilities.

Mobile treatment team: Provides assertive outreach, crisis intervention, and independent-living assistance with linkage to necessary support services in the client's/patient's own environment. This includes PACT, CTTP, or other continuous treatment team programs.

Native Hawaiian or Other Pacific Islander: A person having origins in any of the original peoples of Hawaii, Guam, Samoa, or other Pacific Islands.

Network: The system of participating providers and institutions in a managed care plan.

Network adequacy: Many States have laws defining network adequacy, the number and distribution of health care providers required to operate a health plan. Also known as provider adequacy of a network.

New generation medications: Anti-psychotic medications which are new and atypical.

Non-institutional services: A facility that provides mental health services, but not on a residential basis, other than an inpatient facility or nursing home.

Non-Medicaid services: Services other than those funded by Medicaid.

Nurse practitioner (NP): A nurse practitioner is a registered nurse who works in an expanded role and manages patients' medical conditions.

Nursing home: An establishment that provides living quarters and care for the elderly and the chronically ill. This includes assisted living outside a nursing home.

Obsessive-compulsive disorder (OCD): One of the anxiety disorders, OCD is a potentially disabling condition that can persist throughout a person's life. The individual who suffers from OCD becomes trapped in a pattern of repetitive thoughts and behaviors that are senseless and distressing but extremely difficult to overcome. OCD occurs in a spectrum from mild to severe, but if severe and left untreated, can destroy a person's capacity to function at work, at school, or even in the home. Obsessions are unwanted ideas or impulses that repeatedly well up in the mind of the person with OCD. Persistent fears that harm may come to self or a loved one, an unreasonable concern with becoming contaminated, or an excessive need to do things correctly or perfectly, are common. Again and again, the individual experiences a disturbing thought, such as, "My hands may be contaminated– I must wash them"; "I may have left the gas on"; or "I am going to injure my child." These thoughts are intrusive, unpleasant, and produce a high degree of anxiety. Sometimes the obsessions are of a violent or a sexual nature, or concern illness. In response to their obsessions, most people with OCD resort to repetitive behaviors called compulsions. The most common of these are washing and checking. Other compulsive behaviors include counting (often while performing another compulsive action such as hand washing), repeating, hoarding, and endlessly rearranging objects in an effort to keep them in precise alignment with each other. Mental problems, such as mentally repeating phrases, listmaking, or checking are also common. These behaviors generally are intended to ward off harm to the person with OCD or others. Some people with OCD have regimented rituals while others have rituals that are complex and changing. Performing rituals may give the person with OCD some relief from anxiety, but it is only temporary. People with OCD show a range of insight into the senselessness of their obsessions. Often, especially when they are not actually having an obsession, they can recognize that their obsessions and compulsions are unrealistic. At other times they may be unsure about their fears or even believe strongly in their validity. OCD is sometimes accompanied by depression, eating disorders, substance abuse disorder, a personality disorder, attention deficit disorder, or another of the anxiety disorders. Co-existing disorders can make OCD more difficult both to diagnose and to treat.

Outcomes: The results of a specific health care service or benefit package.

Outcomes research: Studies that measure the effects of care or services.

Panic disorder: Panic Disorder is when people experience white-knuckled, heart-pounding terror that strikes suddenly and without warning. Since they cannot predict when a panic attack will seize them, many people live in persistent worry that another one could overcome them at any moment. Most panic attacks last only a few minutes, but they occasionally go on for ten minutes, and, in rare cases, have been known to last for as long as an hour. They can occur at any time, even during sleep. The good news is that proper treatment helps 70 to 90 percent of people with panic disorder, usually within six to eight weeks. Symptoms include pounding heart, chest pains, lightheadedness or dizziness, nausea, shortness of breath, shaking or trembling, choking, fear of dying, sweating, feelings of unreality, numbness or tingling, hot flashes or chills, and a feeling of going out of control or going crazy. Cognitive behavioral therapy and medications such as high-potency anti-anxiety drugs

like alprazolam can be used to treat panic disorders. Several classes of antidepressants (such as paroxetine, one of the newer selective serotonin reuptake inhibitors) and the older tricyclics and monoamine oxidase inhibitors (MAO inhibitors) are considered "gold standards" for treating panic disorder. Sometimes a combination of therapy and medication is the most effective approach to helping people manage their symptoms.

Pastoral counseling: Pastoral counselors are counselors working within traditional faith communities to incorporate psychotherapy, and/or medication, with prayer and spirituality to effectively help some people with mental disorders. Some people prefer to seek help for mental health problems from their pastor, rabbi, or priest, rather than from therapists who are not affiliated with a religious community.

Phobias: Irrational fears that lead people to altogether avoid specific things or situations that trigger intense anxiety. Phobias occur in several forms. Specific phobia is an unfounded fear of a particular object or situation-such as being afraid of dogs, yet loving to ride horses, or avoiding highway driving, yet being able to drive on city and country roads. Virtually an unlimited number of objects or situations- such as being afraid of flying, heights, or spiders-can be the target of a specific phobia. Agoraphobia is the fear of being in any situation that might trigger a panic attack and from which escape might be difficult. Many people who have agoraphobia become housebound. Others avoid open spaces, standing in line, or being in a crowd. Many of the physical symptoms that accompany panic attacks – such as sweating, racing heart, and trembling – also occur with phobias. Social phobia is a fear of being extremely embarrassed in front of other people. The most common social phobia is fear of public speaking. Cognitive behavioral therapy has the best track record for helping people overcome most phobic disorders. The goals of this therapy are to desensitize a person to feared situations or to teach a person how to recognize, relax, and cope with anxious thoughts and feelings. Medications, such as anti-anxiety agents or antidepressants, can also help relieve symptoms. Sometimes therapy and medication are combined to treat phobias.

Physician assistant: A physician assistant is a trained professional who provides health care services under the supervision of a licensed physician.

Plan of care: A treatment plan especially designed for each child and family, based on individual strengths and needs. The caregiver(s) develop(s) the plan with input from the family. The plan establishes goals and details appropriate treatment and services to meet the special needs of the child and family.

Play therapy: Geared toward young children, play therapy uses a variety of activities-such as painting, puppets, and dioramas-to establish communication with the therapist and resolve problems. Play allows the child to express emotions and problems that would be too difficult to discuss with another person.

Posttraumatic stress disorder (PTSD): Posttraumatic stress disorder (PTSD) affects people of all ages if they have experienced, witnessed, or participated in a traumatic occurrence-especially if the event was life threatening. PTSD can result from terrifying experiences such as rape, kidnapping, natural disasters, or war or serious accidents such as airplane crashes. The psychological damage such incidents cause can interfere with a person's ability to hold a job or to develop intimate relationships with others. The symptoms of PTSD can range from constantly reliving the event to a general emotional numbing. Persistent anxiety, exaggerated startle reactions, difficulty concentrating, nightmares, and insomnia are common. In addition, people with PTSD typically avoid situations that remind them of the traumatic event, because they provoke intense distress or even panic attacks. A rape victim with PTSD, for example, might avoid all contact with men and refuse to go out alone at night. Many people with PTSD also develop depression and may, at times, abuse alcohol or other drugs as "self-medication" to dull their emotional pain and to forget about the trauma. Psychotherapy can help people who have PTSD regain a sense of control over their lives. Many people who have this disorder need to confront what has happened to them and, by repeating this confrontation, learn to accept the trauma as part of their past. They also may need cognitive behavior therapy to change painful and intrusive patterns of behavior and thought and

to learn relaxation techniques. Another focus of psychotherapy is to help people who have PTSD resolve any conflicts that may have occurred as a result of the difference between their personal values and how behaviors and experiences during the traumatic event violated them. Support from family and friends can help speed recovery and healing. Medications, such as antidepressants and anti- anxiety agents to reduce anxiety, can ease the symptoms of depression and sleep problems. Treatment for PTSD often includes both psychotherapy and medication.

Prader-Willi syndrome: A congenital (present from birth) disease characterized by obesity, decreased muscle tone, decreased mental capacity, and hypogonadism. Prader-Willi is caused by the deletion of a gene on chromosome 15. For unkown reasons, only the copy of this gene on chromosome 15 that is received from the father is active. The maternal copy of this gene is turned off in all people. When there is a deletion of this gene on the copy received from the father, the disease occurs. This is because the patient is left with only the maternal copy — which is inactive in all people. Signs of Prader-Willi may be seen at birth. New infants with the condition are often small and very floppy (hypotonic). Male infants may have undescended testicles. The growing child exhibits slow mental and delayed motor development, increasing obesity, and characteristically small hands and feet. Rapid weight gain may occur during the first few years because the patient develops uncontrollable hunger which leads to morbid obesity. Mental development is slow, and the IQ seldom exceeds 80. However, children with Prader-Willi generally are very happy, smile frequently, and are pleasant to be around. Affected children have an intense craving for food and will do almost anything to get it. This results in uncontrollable weight gain. Morbid obesity (the degree of obesity that seriously affects health) may lead to respiratory failure with hypoxia (low blood oxygen levels), cor pulmonale (right-sided heart failure), and death.

Pre-existing condition: A medical condition that is excluded from coverage by an insurance company because the condition was believed to exist prior to the individual obtaining a policy from the insurance company. Many insurance companies now impose waiting periods for coverage of pre-existing conditions. Insurers will cover the condition after the waiting period (of no more than 12 months) has expired. (See also, HIPAA)

Prior authorization: The approval a provider must obtain from an insurer or other entity before furnishing certain health services, particularly inpatient hospital care, in order for the service to be covered under the plan.

Psychiatric emergency walk- in: A planned program to provide psychiatric care in emergency situations with staff specifically assigned for this purpose. Includes crisis intervention, which enables the individual, family members and friends to cope with the emergency while maintaining the individual's status as a functioning community member to the greatest extent possible and is open for a patient to walk-in.

Psychiatrist: A psychiatrist is a professional who completed both medical school and training in psychiatry and is a specialist in diagnosing and treating mental illness.

Psychoanalysis: Psychoanalysis focuses on past conflicts as the underpinnings to current emotional and behavioral problems. In this long-term and intensive therapy, an individual meets with a psychoanalyst three to five times a week, using "free association" to explore unconscious motivations and earlier, unproductive patterns of resolving issues.

Psychodynamic psychotherapy: Based on the principles of psychoanalysis, this therapy is less intense, tends to occur once or twice a week, and spans a shorter time. It is based on the premise that human behavior is determined by one's past experiences, genetic factors, and current situation. This approach recognizes the significant influence that emotions and unconscious motivation can have on human behavior.

Psychosocial rehabilitation: Therapeutic activities or interventions provided individually or in groups that may include development and maintenance of daily and community-living skills, self-care, skills training includes grooming, bodily care, feeding, social skills training, and development of basic language skills.

Registered Nurse (RN): A registered nurse is a trained professional with a nursing degree who provides patient care and administers medicine.

Report card: An accounting of the quality of services, compared among providers over time. The report card grades providers on predetermined, measurable quality and outcome indicators. Generally, consumers use report cards to choose a health plan or provider, while policy makers may use report card results to determine overall program effectiveness, efficiency, and financial stability.

Residential services: Services provided over a 24-hour period or any portion of the day which a patient resided, on an on-going basis, in a State facility or other facility and received treatment.

Residential treatment centers: Facilities that provide treatment 24 hours a day and can usually serve more than 12 young people at a time. Children with serious emotional disturbances receive constant supervision and care. Treatment may include individual, group, and family therapy; behavior therapy; special education; recreation therapy; and medical services. Residential treatment is usually more long- term than inpatient hospitalization. Centers are also known as therapeutic group homes.

Respite care: A service that provides a break for parents who have a child with a serious emotional disturbance. Trained parents or counselors take care of the child for a brief period of time to give families relief from the strain of caring for the child. This type of care can be provided in the home or in another location. Some parents may need this help every week.

Respite residential services: Provision of periodic relief to the usual family members and friends who care for the clients/patients.

Retired: Clients who are of legal age, stopped working and have withdrawn from one's occupation.

Risk: Possibility that revenues of the insurer will not be sufficient to cover expenditures incurred in the delivery of contractual services. A managed care provider is at risk if actual expenses exceed the payment amount.

Risk adjustment: The adjustment of premiums to compensate health plans for the risks associated with individuals who are more likely to require costly treatment. Risk adjustment takes into account the health status and risk profile of patients.

Schizophrenia: A serious brain disorder. It is a disease that makes it difficult for a person to tell the difference between real and unreal experiences, to think logically, to have normal emotional responses to others, and to behave normally in social situations. Schizophrenia is a complex and puzzling illness. Even the experts in the field are not exactly sure what causes it. Some doctors think that the brain may not be able to process information correctly. Genetic factors appear to play a role, as people who have family members with schizophrenia may be more likely to get the disease themselves. Some researchers believe that events in a person's environment may trigger schizophrenia. For example, problems during intrauterine development (infection) and birth may increase the risk for developing schizophrenia later in life. Psychological and social factors may also play some role in its development. However, the level of social and familial support appears to influence the course of illness and may be protective against relapse. There are five recognized types of schizophrenia: catatonic, paranoid, disorganized, undifferentiated, and residual. Features of schizophrenia include its typical onset before the age of 45, continuous presence of symptoms for six months or more, and deterioration from a prior level of social and occupational functioning. People with schizophrenia can have a variety of symptoms. Usually the illness develops slowly over months or even years. At first, the symptoms may not be noticed. For example, people may feel tense, may have trouble sleeping, or have trouble concentrating. They become isolated and withdrawn, and they do not make or keep friends. No single characteristic is present in all types of schizophrenia. The risk factors include a family history of schizophrenia. Schizophrenia is thought to affect about 1 percent of the population worldwide. Schizophrenia appears to occur in equal rates among men and women, but women have a later onset. For this reason, males tend to account for more than half of clients in services with high proportions of young adults. Although the onset of schizophrenia is typically in young adulthood, cases of the disorder with a late onset (over 45 years) are known. Childhood-onset schizophrenia begins after five years of age and, in most cases, after relatively normal development. Childhood schizophrenia is rare and can be difficult to differentiate from other pervasive developmental disorders of childhood, such as autism.

School attendance: Physical presence of a child in a school setting during scheduled class hours. "Regular" school attendance is attendance at least 75 percent of scheduled hours.

School-based services: School-based treatment and support interventions designed to identify emotional disturbances and/or assist parents, teachers, and counselors in developing comprehensive strategies for addressing these disturbances. School-based services also include counseling or other school-based programs for emotionally disturbed children, adolescents, and their families within the school, home and community environment.

Seasonal affective disorder (SAD): Seasonal affective disorder (SAD) is a form of depression that appears related to fluctuations in the exposure to natural light. It usually strikes during autumn and often continues through the winter when natural light is reduced. Researchers have found that people who have SAD can be helped with the symptoms of their illness if they spend blocks of time bathed in light from a special full-spectrum light source, called a "light box."

Self-help: Self-help generally refers to groups or meetings that: involve people who have similar needs; are facilitated by a consumer, survivor, or other layperson; assist people to deal with a "life-disrupting" event, such as a death, abuse, serious accident, addiction, or diagnosis of a physical, emotional, or mental disability, for oneself or a relative; are operated on an informal, free-of-charge, and nonprofit basis; provide support and education; and are voluntary, anonymous, and confidential. Many people with mental illnesses find that self-help groups are an invaluable resource for recovery and for empowerment.

Serious emotional disturbances: Diagnosable disorders in children and adolescents that severely disrupt their daily functioning in the home, school, or community. Serious emotional disturbances affect one in 10 young people. These disorders include depression, attention- deficit/hyperactivity, anxiety disorders, conduct disorder, and eating disorders. Pursuant to section 1912(c) of the Public Health Service Act "children with a serious emotional disturbance" are persons: (1) from birth up to age 18 and (2) who currently have, or at any time during the last year, had a diagnosable mental, behavioral, or emotional disorder of sufficient duration to meet diagnostic criteria specified within DSM- III-R. Federal Register Volume 58 No. 96 published Thursday May 20, 1993 pages 29422 through 29425.

Serious mental illness: Pursuant to section 1912(c) of the Public Health Service Act, adults with serious mental illness SMI are persons: (1) age 18 and over and (2) who currently have, or at any time during the past year had a diagnosable mental behavioral or emotional disorder of sufficient duration to meet diagnostic criteria specified within DSM-IV or their ICD-9-CM equivalent (and subsequent revisions) with the exception of DSM-IV "V" codes, substance use disorders, and developmental disorders, which are excluded, unless they co-occur with another diagnosable serious mental illness. (3) That has resulted in functional impairment, which substantially interferes with or limits one or more major life activities. Federal Register Volume 58 No. 96 published Thursday May 20, 1993 pages 29422 through 29425.

Service: A type of support or clinical intervention designed to address the specific mental health needs of a child and his or her family. A service could be provided only one time or repeated over a course of time, as determined by the child, family, and service provider.

Single-stream funding: The consolidation of multiple sources of funding into a single stream. This is a key approach used in progressive mental health systems to ensure that "funds follow consumers."

State Children's Health Insurance Plan (SCHIP): Under Title XXI of the Balanced Budget Act of 1997, the availability of health insurance for children with no insurance or for children from low-income families was expanded by the creation of SCHIP. SCHIPs

operate as part of a State's Medicaid program (Centers for Medicare and Medicaid Services, 2002).

State coverage: The total unduplicated count of mental health patients/clients served through State programs, exclusive of Medicaid and Other Coverage.

State hospital: A publicly funded inpatient facility for persons with mental illness.

State mental health authority or agency: State government agency charged with administering and funding its State's public mental health services.

Stress: Defined as a feeling of tension that can be both emotional and physical. Emotional stress usually occurs when situations are considered difficult or unmanageable. Therefore, different people consider different situations as stressful. Physical stress refers to a physiological reaction of the body to various triggers. The pain experienced after surgery is an example of physical stress. Physical stress often leads to emotional stress, and emotional stress is frequently experienced as physical discomfort (e.g., stomach cramps). Stress management refers to various efforts used to control and reduce the tension that occurs in these situations. The attitude of an individual can influence whether a situation or emotion is stressful or not. Negative attitude can be a predictor of stress, because this type of person will often report more stress than a person with a more positive attitude. Stress is not a disease and is a normal part of everyone's life. Stress in small quantities is good: it makes us more productive. For example, the fear of a bad grade can make the a student study more attentively. However, too much stress is unhealthy and counterproductive. The same student, if he was recently mugged and or is getting over the sudden death of a friend will not be able to study as well. Persistent and unrelenting stress is called anxiety.

Suicide: A successful or unsuccessful attempt to intentionally kill oneself. Suicidal behaviors indicate that a person wishes to, intends to, or actually attempts to commit suicide. Suicidal behaviors can accompany many emotional disturbances, including depression, schizophrenia, and other psychotic illnesses. In fact, more than 90 percent of all suicides are related to an emotional or psychiatric illness.

Suicidal behaviors occur as a response to a situation that the person views as overwhelming, such as social isolation, death of a loved one, emotional trauma, serious physical illness, growing old, unemployment or financial problems, guilt feelings, drug abuse, and alcohol abuse. In the U.S., suicide accounts for about 1 percent of all deaths each year. The highest rate is among the elderly, but there has been a steady increase in the rate among young people (particularly adolescents). Suicide is now the third leading cause of death for those 15 to 19 years old (after accidents and homicide). The incidence of reported suicides varies widely from country to country in the world; however, this may be in part related to reporting (especially in cultures where suicide is considered sinful or shameful). Suicide attempts (where the person tries to harm him- or herself but the attempt does not result in death) far outnumber actual suicides. The method of suicide attempt varies from relatively nonviolent methods (such as poisoning, overdose, or inhaling car exhaust) to violent methods (such as shooting or cutting oneself). Males are more likely to choose violent methods, which probably accounts for the fact that suicide attempts by males are more likely to be successful. Many unsuccessful suicide attempts are carried out in a manner or setting that makes rescue possible. They must be viewed as a cry for help.

Supported employment: Supportive services that include assisting individuals in finding work; assessing individuals' skills, attitudes, behaviors, and interest relevant to work; providing vocational rehabilitation and/or other training; and providing work opportunities. Includes transitional and supported employment services.

Supported housing: Services to assist individuals in finding and maintaining appropriate housing arrangements.

Supportive residential services: Moderately staffed housing arrangements for clients/patients. Includes supervised apartments, satellite facilities, group homes, halfway houses, mental health shelter- care facilities, and other facilities.

System of care: A system of care is a method of addressing children's mental health needs. It is developed on the premise that the mental health needs of children, adolescents, and their families can be met within their home, school, and community environments. These systems are also developed around the principles of being child-centered, family- driven, strength-based, and culturally competent and involving interagency collaboration.

Telephone hotline: A dedicated telephone line that is advertised and may be operated as a crisis hotline for emergency counseling, or as a referral resource for callers with mental health problems.

Therapeutic foster care: A service which provides treatment for troubled children within private homes of trained families. The approach combines the normalizing influence of family-based care with specialized treatment interventions, thereby creating a therapeutic environment in the context of a nurturant family home.

Third-party payer: A public or private organization that is responsible for the health care expenses of another entity.

Unable to Work: This on-line forum was created especially for the nation's jobless and underemployed workers. This resource is available to help the unemployed learn more about the unemployment system, to share their experiences and concerns, and to participate in the national debate over aid to the jobless.

Unmet needs: Identified treatment needs of the people that are not being met as well as those receiving treatment that is inappropriate or not optimal.

Vocational rehabilitation services: Services that include job finding/development, assessment and enhancement of work-related skills, attitudes, and behaviors as well as provision of job experience to clients/patients. Includes transitional employment.

White: A person having origins in any of the original peoples of Europe, the Middle East, or North Africa.

CATEGORIZED LIST OF CONTENTS

Abandonment
Abandoned Children
Children of Incarcerated Parents: An Overview
Children of Incarcerated Parents: Psychosocial Issues

Adolescents
Anxiety Disorders: Adolescents
Asperger's Syndrome in Children & Adolescents
Asthma in Children & Adolescents: An Overview
Asthma in Children & Adolescents: Family Support
Asthma in Children & Adolescents: Influence of Emotional Factors
Child Welfare: Children with Developmental Disabilities
Depression in Adolescence: An Overview
Depression in Adolescence: Black Adolescents
Depression in Adolescence: Korean American Adolescents
Depression in Adolescence: Smoking
Fathers' Contributions to Children's Development
Homeless Adolescents
Intimate Partner Violence: In Adolescence
Juvenile Delinquency & Substance Abuse
Juvenile Delinquency in the United States
Juvenile Delinquency: Prevention
Lesbian, Gay, Bisexual, Transgender, and Questioning Youth: Psychosocial Issues
Mental Health Screening of Adolescents
Mental Health Screening of Adolescents: Racial Disparities
Mental Health Treatment for Adolescents: Racial Disparities
Obesity in Children & Adolescents: Healthcare Costs
Pregnancy in Adolescence: Abortion Trends—Global Perspective
Pregnancy in Adolescence: Prevention—Beyond Abstinence
Pregnancy in Adolescence: Prevention—Emergency Contraception
Pregnancy in Adolescence: Prevention—Female Use of Contraception
Pregnancy in Adolescence: Prevention—Male Use of Contraception
Pregnancy in Adolescence: Prevention—Nonhormonal Contraception
Pregnancy in Adolescence: Prevention—Progestin-Only Contraception
Pregnancy in Adolescence: Risk Factors
Problematic Internet Use in Adolescents
Restorative Justice Programs: Juvenile Offenders
Sexual harassment: Peer Harassment in Middle & High School
Sexual Harassment: Peer Harassment in School—Supporting Victims
Sexual Harassment: Peer Harassment in School—Working with Perpetrators
Sexually Transmitted Diseases in Adolescents: Risk Factors for Gonorrhea & Chlamydia
Smoking Cessation in Adolescence
Social Media: Psychosocial Implications for Adolescents
Substance Abuse & Adolescents: Treatment
Substance Abuse in Adolescence: Risk & Protective Factors
Violence in Adolescence & Substance Abuse
Violence in Adolescence: Bullying
Violence in Adolescence: Gender Differences in Perpetrators
Violence in Adolescence: Gender Differences in Victims

Adoption/Foster Care
Adoption Disruption: Legal Issues in the United States
Adoption Disruption: Psychosocial Effects on Children
Adoption: Access to Birth Records
Adoption: An Overview
Bipolar Disorder in Children & Adolescents
Child Maltreatment & Foster Care: Military Families
Children with Developmental Disabilities: Foster Care & Adoption
Foster Care: Adolescents
Foster Care: An Overview
Foster Care: Children–Psychosocial Issues
Foster Care: Infants
Foster Care: Mental Health of Children
Foster Care: Racial Disparities of Children
Gay & Lesbian Adoption
Gay & Lesbian Transracial Adoption
Grandparents as Kinship Guardians: Legal Aspects

SUBJECT INDEX

H

I